DISEASE IS AN EXPIATION OF THE SINS

Dr Mira Bajirova

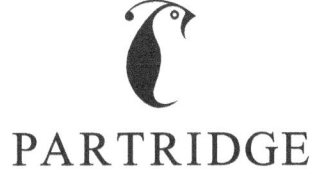

PARTRIDGE

Copyright © 2019 by Dr Mira Bajirova.

ISBN:	Hardcover	978-1-5437-5250-2
	Softcover	978-1-5437-5248-9
	eBook	978-1-5437-5249-6

All rights reserved. No part of this book may be used or reproduced by any means, graphic, electronic, or mechanical, including photocopying, recording, taping or by any information storage retrieval system without the written permission of the author except in the case of brief quotations embodied in critical articles and reviews.

Because of the dynamic nature of the Internet, any web addresses or links contained in this book may have changed since publication and may no longer be valid. The views expressed in this work are solely those of the author and do not necessarily reflect the views of the publisher, and the publisher hereby disclaims any responsibility for them.

Print information available on the last page.

To order additional copies of this book, contact
Toll Free +65 3165 7531 (Singapore)
Toll Free +60 3 3099 4412 (Malaysia)
orders.singapore@partridgepublishing.com

www.partridgepublishing.com/singapore

CONTENTS

Preface xxv
Acknowledgement xxix
Introduction xxxi
    Diseases happen by Allah's Decree xxxii
The Origin and Purpose of Human Creation xxxiii
Medicine of Calamities and Trials xxxix
Allah Send Down the Diseases for Three Reasons xlvii
    I. Disease Is A Test xlvii
        1.1. Story of the Prophet Ayub xlvii
        1.2. Story of the Sheikh Abd al Aziz ibn Abdullah Ibn Baaz ... xlviii
        1.3. Story of Three Men from the Children of Israel: a Leper, a
            Bald-headed and a Blind xlviii
        1.4. Testing According to one's Faith xlix
        1.5. Martyr will be in Paradise lii
    II. Disease is an Expiation of Sins liii
        Universal Law of "Cause and Effect" and "Action and Reaction" ... liv
        Epidemics are the Jinn Possession because of Humanity's Sins ... liv
        Disease is a Wake-Up Call lv
        Disease is a Blessing for the Disbelievers if they Repent lv
        This Temporary Life is Imperfect and the Enjoyment of Delusion ... lvii
    III. Disease is a Punishment lvii
Diseases are Caused by Positive Ions lix
    1. Diseases caused by Decreased Oxygen Utilization lix
        Positive Ions lix
        Hadith of Black Woman of Paradise lix
    2. Diseases caused by Evil Jinn (Demons) lx
        From the Qur'an: lx
        From Ahadith: lx
        Hippocrates and Jinn (Demonic) Possession lxvii
    Prophet Jesus and Jinn (Demonic) Possession lxvii
    Prophet Muhammad and Jinn (Demonic) Possession lxviii
        Hadith: Epilepsy by Jinn Possession lxviii
        Hadith: Aphasia by Jinn Possession lxviii
        Hadith: Epidemics are Jinn Possession because of Sins lxix
    Jinn Possession Reasons lxix
Why Do Sinless Children Suffer? lxxi
    Among the reasons why children suffer are the following: lxxii
    The measures for protecting children from the accursed Satan ... lxxvii
        Before Conception lxxvii

'Aqeeqah on the 7th day after the birth as a protection from Satan lxxvii
Righteous Parents – Protected Children lxxvii
Supplication (Du'a) is a means of protecting children lxxviii
Ruqyah is a means of protecting children lxxviii
Children should be prevented from going out after sunset lxxviii
Early teaching of the Qur'an and Sunnah for Protection from the Jinn lxxviii
Children are accountable for their deeds from the puberty lxxviii
Types of Sins lxxix
Major and Minor Sins lxxxi
When Minor Sin Becomes Major Sin and Shirk lxxxiii

715 SINS

1. Religion Other than Islam 1
    1.1. Islam is a Deen, Not to be Confused with Religion 1
        1.1.1. Deen is a Debt 2
        1.1.2. Submission to the Divine Will and Decree of Allah 3
        1.1.3. Deen Means Day of Judgment, Yawm al-Qiyamah or Yawm ad-Deen 5
        1.1.4. Deen Means Disciplining Yourself 6
        1.1.5. Islam is the Complete Code of Life for Humanity 6
        1.1.6. Deen Means Rain 7
        1.1.7. Angel Jibreel Said: "O Muhammad, Tell me About Islam" 8
        1.1.8. Islam is a Justice 8
    1.2. Why is this Religion Called Islam? 9
2. Ascribing Associates to Allah (Shirk) 11
    Major Shirk 12
    Minor Shirk 13
    Some of Idol Worship Forms 16
    Why Are The Most of People Disbelievers 26
    Final Destination of Muslims and Non-Muslims 31
3. Bowing to Someone is Shirk 32
4. Insulting Others' False Gods 32
5. Making Idols 32
6. Atheism 34
7. Darwinism 35
8. Speaking about Allah Without Knowledge 36
9. Disbelieving in Allah 36
10. Thinking Negative about Allah 37
11. Neglecting any Obligatory Act Ordered by our Creator 38
12. Questioning Allah for What He Does 39
13. Not Remembering Allah 39
14. Feeling Secure from the Plot of Allah 42
15. Despair of the Mercy of Allah 43
16. Seeking Help of Other than Allah is Shirk 45
17. Abomination of Saying "Forgive me if You Wish, O Allah!" 47
18. To Have No Fear of Allah 48
19. Saying "Don't Judge me!" or "Only God Can Judge me!" 49

20.	Lying about Allah and the Prophet	54
21.	Exchanging the Signs of Allah for a Small Price	55
22.	Prohibiting the Invocation of Allah in Mosques	56
23.	Believing that Allah is Everywhere	56
24.	Believing that Allah is Without Image and is Formless and Disbelieving in His Attributes	57
25.	Reciting the Names of Allah in Certain Combinations	62
26.	Calling Allah by the names which are not in the Qur'an or Ahadith	62
27.	Repeating the Name of Allah on its Own or the Pronoun Huwa (He) is a Sufi Bid'ah	63
28.	Writing the Name of Allah on the Cars	66
29.	Comparing the Creator to His creation	66
30.	Belief in Pantheism	67
31.	Rejection or Denial of what Allah Has Revealed to Prophet	68
32.	Claiming that the Story of the Isra' and Mi'raj is a Myth	70
33.	Celebrating the Night of Ascension the Isra' and Mi'raj	71
34.	Forgetting Sending Salat to the Prophet Muhammad	72
35.	Visiting Places and Mosques in which the Prophet Prayed (apart from Quba', Uhud, al-Baqee)	73
36.	Denying the Rights of the Ahl Al-Bayt	74
37.	Cursing the Companions of the Prophet	77
38.	Claiming that Ali Was Given Specific knowledge of Khilafah (Caliphate), which Was Not Given to Anybody else	77
39.	Disrespect of the Noble Qur'an	78
40.	Reciting Verses of the Qur'an a Specific Number of Times and with Specific Intention	79
41.	Distributing and Selling the Verses of the Qur'an for the Protection	80
42.	Hanging Verses of the Qur'an and/or Allah's Name on Walls	80
43.	Swearing or Taking an Oath by Placing Hand on the Mushaf	81
44.	Leaving the Broadcast of the Holy Qur'an Playing at the Places of Business and at Home	82
45.	Arguing About the Qur'an	82
46.	Rejection of the Qur'an as the Word of God	82
47.	Reciting the Qur'an During the Funeral, at the Grave and During the Days of Condolence on the Death Anniversary of the Person	83
48.	Prohibition of Carrying the Qur'an into the Land of Enemy	84
49.	Saying "Sadaqa Allaah al-'Azeem" (Allah has spoken the Truth)	85
50.	Disrespect of Ka'bah	85
51.	Reciting Specific Supplications in Each Circuit of Tawaf or Lap of Sa'i during Hajj and 'Umrah	86
52.	Doing Mischief in the Masjid Al-Haram in Makkah	87
53.	Disbelieving in Destiny (Qadar)	88
54.	Saying: "If Only I Had Done Such-and-Such"	93
55.	Using Allah's Decree (Qadar) as an Excuse for Your Sin	94
56.	Talking About Future Without "In Shaa Allah"	94
57.	Abomination of Saying- "What Allah Wills and so-and-so Wills"	95

58.	Ruling on one who Rejects a Saheeh Hadith	95
59.	Not Making Room in the Assemblies	96
60.	Excessive Questioning and Disagreement (in Disputed Religious Matters)	96
61.	Not Performing the Prayers	97
62.	Praying Without Intention, Ablution, Mentioning the Name of Allah and Seeking the Refuge with Allah from the Accursed Satan	110
63.	Actions by Intentions	110
64.	Washing Mouth and Nose Separately During Wudu	113
65.	Prayer Without Recitation of the Surah Al-Fatihah	113
66.	Closing the Eyes while Praying	113
67.	Ruling on Tahiyyat Al-Masjid - Greeting the Mosque	114
68.	Omitting Prayer Intentionally	114
69.	The Severity of Punishment for Missing the Asr Prayer	114
70.	Disapproval of Delaying the Prayer from its Prescribed Time	115
71.	Excellence of Congregational Prayers and Warning for Missing it	115
72.	Du'a After Iqamah	117
73.	Obligation to Straighten the Rows	118
74.	Undesirability of Observing Nafl Prayer when the Mu'adhdhin Begins Iqamah	119
75.	Regular Recitation of the Qunut During the Fajr Prayer	120
76.	Missing the Friday Prayer Without Valid Excuse	120
77.	Prayers Before and After Jumu'ah	132
78.	Using Anything to Count Adhkar Other than the Fingers	133
79.	Prohibition on Stepping over People when Coming to Jumu'ah Prayer	134
80.	Undesirability of Sitting with Legs Drawn Up to Belly During Friday Sermon	134
81.	Deal or Sale During Friday's Prayers	135
82.	Congratulating "Jumu'ah Mubarak"	135
83.	A Man Should Not Make his Brother Get up to Sit in his Place	135
84.	Rushing when Reciting Qur'an and Praying	136
85.	Not Separating the Obligatory and Voluntary Prayers	137
86.	Putting Two Prayers Together Without any Excuse	137
87.	Ruling on Joining and Shortening Prayers for Travelers	138
88.	Preventing Women from Praying in the Mosque	138
89.	Women Praying Differently from Men	140
90.	Breaking the Ruling in the Mosque	142
91.	Prohibition of Raising one's Head Before the Imam	142
92.	Prohibition of Raising one's Eyes Towards the Sky During Prayer	143
93.	Undesirability of Glancing in One Direction of the Other During Prayer	143
94.	Prohibition of Placing the Hands on the Sides During Prayer	144
95.	Prohibition of Praying with one's Hands on one's Waist	144
96.	Prohibition of Sitting with Left Hand Behind the Back and Leaning on the Fleshy Part of it	144
97.	Ruling on Raising the Hands in the Prayer	144
98.	Prohibition of Passing in Front of a Worshipper While he is Praying	146
99.	Prohibition to Recite Qur'an when Bowing and Prostrating	147
100.	Not Settling his Spine when Bowing and Prostrating	147
101.	Ruling on Forgetting a Prostration of Forgetfulness	147

102.	Prostrating for the Sake of Du'a is an Innovation	148
103.	Prohibition of Putting the Forearms on the Ground (in the Prostration) Like a Dog	148
104.	Saying "Taqabbal Allah (May Allah accept it)" after Prayer	149
105.	Praying Witr with Three Rak'ahs Like Maghrib	149
106.	Prohibition of Spitting in the Mosque	150
107.	Using the Mosque for Urinating or Easing Oneself	150
108.	Undesirability of Quarrelling or Raising Voices in the Mosque	151
109.	Undesirability of Entering the Mosque After Eating Raw Onion or Garlic	153
110.	Forbiddance to Go out of the Mosque After the Adhan Has Been Announced	154
111.	Building Lofty Mosques	154
112.	Praying at Forbidden Times	154
113.	Praying in the Bathroom	156
114.	Prayer in a House Taken Illegally	156
115.	Preventing from Praying	156
116.	Prohibition to Pray Istikhara on Behalf of Someone Else	157
117.	Abomination of Holding Conversation After Isha (Night) Prayer	157
118.	Ruling on Making up of Missed Prayer and Fast	158
119.	Disrespect of the Ruling of Ramadan	161
120.	Breaking One's Fast During Ramadan Without Valid Excuse	163
121.	Singling out the first third of Ramadan to pray for mercy, the second third to pray for forgiveness and the last third to pray for ransom from Hell is an innovation	164
122.	There is No Specific Du'a for Each Day and Night of Ramadan	164
123.	Ruling on I'tikaaf	165
124.	Ruling of Zakat Al-Fitr	167
125.	Ruling on One Who Does Not Pay Zakah on Wealth	169
126.	Not Paying Khums	172
127.	Not Performing the Hajj When Able to	172
128.	Disrespect of Ihram Clothes	174
129.	Prohibition of Having a Hair Cut or Paring one's Nail During the First Ten Days of Dhul-Hijjah for one Who Intends to Sacrifice an Animal	174
130.	Disrespect of Rulings of Udhiyah (Sacrifice)	174
131.	Congratulating the Pilgrim after he Returns and Decorating the House for him	177
132.	Violation of the Ruling of Four Sacred Months	178
133.	Rajab Month Innovations	179
134.	Shaban Month Innovations	181
135.	Muharram Month Innovations	183
136.	Salat al-Hajah is Innovation Worship Allah the Prophet's way	184
137.	Prohibition of Heresies in Religion	186
138.	Religious Excessiveness	187
139.	Prohibition of Monasticism	189
140.	Avoiding Jihad	189
141.	Islamic Rules of War	193
142.	Prohibition of Killing Women and Children in War	195
143.	Treatment of Prisoners of War in Islam	195

144.	Misappropriation of Spoils of War, Muslim Funds or Zakah	196
145.	Impatience	197
146.	Fighting when Enemy Asked for a Peace	198
147.	Fighting Among the Believers Without Making Reconciliation	199
148.	Frowning, Turning Away or Neglecting Those who Come to you Seeking Knowledge	199
149.	Learning Sacred Knowledge for the Sake of this World or Concealing It	199
150.	Killing Muslim	200
151.	Supplying Weapons to Disbelievers which Shall be Used Against Muslims	200
152.	Prohibition of Reviling a Muslim Without any Cause	201
153.	Prohibition of Spying on Muslims and to be Inquisitive About Others	201
154.	Prohibition of Despising Muslims	203
155.	Harming and Insulting Muslims	203
156.	Rights and Obligations of Muslim Over Another Muslim	205
157.	Shaking Hands with Both Hands	209
158.	Forsaking his Muslim Brother for More than Three Days	210
159.	Causing Trouble Between Muslims	210
160.	Prohibition of Calling a Muslim a Disbeliever	211
161.	Muslims Taking Non-Muslims as Auliya (friends, protectors, helpers, etc.)	211
162.	Greeting the Non-Muslims and Prohibition of Taking an Initiative	213
163.	Greeting with a Gesture	214
164.	Standing up for Someone to Venerate him	215
165.	Saluting the Flag, Standing up for it and Singing the National Anthem	216
166.	Undesirability of Praising a Person in his Presence	216
167.	Committing Evil After Embracing Islam	217
168.	Breach of Faith, Apostasy from Islam	217
169.	Calling People to Misguidance	219
170.	Condemnation of Double-Faced People – Hypocrisy	220
171.	Condemnation and Prohibition of Falsehood	221
172.	Prohibition of Lying and Listening to Lies	224
173.	Defamation	228
174.	Speaking Without Knowledge	229
175.	Following his Own Desire	230
176.	Preoccupation with this Life	231
177.	Bad Character and Manners	232
178.	Warning Against Persecution of the Pious, the Weak and the Indigent	237
179.	Prohibition of Disobeying Parents and Severance of Relations	238
180.	Responsibilities and Obligations of the Parents Forward their Children	241
181.	Ruling for Naming Children	243
182.	Not Commanding Your Children to Pray when they are Seven Years Old	246
183.	Stern Warning Against Disowning One's Child	246
184.	Prohibition of Giving Preference to Children Over one Another in Giving Gifts, etc.	248
185.	Child Abuse	249
186.	Killing Your Children	249
187.	Killing Your Daughters	250

188.	Prohibition of Legal Adoption	251
189.	Ruling of Sponsoring Orphan	252
190.	Adoption Fraud	254
191.	Elder Abuse	254
192.	Prohibition of Breaking Ties and Relationships	256
193.	Insult Families	258
194.	Prohibition of Deriding one's Lineage	258
195.	Prohibition of Attributing Wrong Fatherhood	259
196.	Changing his Father's/Family Name	260
197.	Looking Inside the House Without Permission	261
198.	Rights of Neighbours	261
199.	Inheritance Judgment by Any law Other than the Laws of Allah	263
200.	Bringing Loss to the Bequest (Wasiyya)	264
201.	Inheritance: Who Has the Right to Claim the Deceased's Estate?	265
202.	Inheritance Division Among the Heirs of a Deceased Muslim	268
203.	No Inheritance Between Muslim and non-Muslim	271
204.	No Inheritance for Illegitimate Child	271
205.	No Inheritance for Adopted Child	272
206.	No Inheritance for Murderer	272
207.	Prohibition of Celibacy	272
208.	Ruling on Choosing Your Wife/Husband	274
209.	Refusing Marriage Proposal	277
210.	Prohibited Marriage Proposals	277
211.	Prohibition of Marriage Proposal or Arranging the Marriage of	278
212.	Prohibition of Marriage Proposal to Woman Already Engaged	278
213.	Prohibition on a Woman Proposing to a Man who Has Proposed to Another Woman	279
214.	Prohibited Marriages	279
215.	Prohibition of Marriage Without Woman's Guardian Arrangement	281
216.	Prohibition of Marriage Without Two Legally Acceptable Witnesses	282
217.	Forced/Unconsented Marriage	282
218.	Prohibition of Marriage Without Obligatory Mahr Paid	283
219.	Prohibition of Dowry	284
220.	Dowry Abuse	284
221.	Dishonoring Woman	285
222.	Prohibition of Marriage Between Muslim Man and Non-Muslim Woman	289
223.	Prohibition of Marriage Between Muslim Woman and Non-Muslim Man	291
224.	Prohibition of Marriage to al-Maharim, the Relatives to whom	291
225.	Prohibition of Marriage to Two Sisters at the Same Time	292
226.	Prohibition of Marriage to a Woman whom Your Father Married	293
227.	Prohibition of Marriage to a Woman if he is Married to her Paternal or Maternal Aunt at the Same Time	293
228.	Prohibition of Marriage to a Woman Having a Foster Suckling Relationship	293
229.	Prohibition of Secret Marriage	294
230.	Prohibition of Shighar Marriage	295
231.	Prohibition of Al-Mut'ah Marriage	295

232. Prohibition of Marriage to a Woman Already Married 295
233. Prohibition of Marriage to his Illegitimate Daughter 295
234. Prohibition of the Marriage to the Orphan Girl under the Guardianship of her Guardian who Likes her Beauty and Wealth and Wishes to (Marry her and) Curtails her Mahr 296
235. Prohibition of Marriage to a Divorced or Widowed Woman During her Iddah (the Waiting Period During which she is Not Allowed to Marry Again) 297
236. Prohibition of Marriage to a Woman who is Ungrateful and Displeased with Allah's Decree 299
237. Prohibition of Plural Marriage if he Cannot Treat Wives Equally 300
238. Prohibition of Same-Sex Marriage 303
239. Prohibition of "Paper" Marriage 304
240. Prohibition of Marriage between Human and Jinn 305
241. Prohibition of Islamic Concubinage 307
242. Wearing Engagement and Wedding Ring..308
243. Refusing Wedding Invitation Without Valid Excuse 309
244. Extravagance in Wedding Party and Honeymoon... 309
245. Husband's Rights Concerning his Wife..310
246. Non-Fulfillment of Husband's Obligations 314
247. Wife's Rights Concerning his Husband 319
248. Non-Fulfillment of Wife's Obligations 321
249. Disobedience to Husband..324
250. Prohibition of Refusal by a Woman when her Husband Calls her to his Bed 325
251. Ingratitude to Husband 325
252. Forcing Your Wife..326
253. Prohibition of Observing Silence from Dawn till Night 327
254. Disclosing Bedroom Secrets..327
255. Prohibition of Observing an Optional Saum (Fast) by a Woman Without the Permission of her Husband 328
256. Prohibition of Describing the Charms of a Woman to a Man Without Valid Reason 328
257. Stoning of a Married Adulterer 329
258. Divorce is Mischief 329
259. Giving an Option to Divorce to Wife 331
260. Divorce Not Following Allah's Law 331
261. Condemnation of Divorce Without Compelling Reason.....................................336
262. Divorce Before Consumption of the Marriage...336
263. Annulment of Marriage by Husband's Vow to Refrain from Intercourse (Ila).......336
264. Atonement is Essential for the One who Made his Wife Unlawful for Himself Without the Intention to Divorce 337
265. Ruling on Divorce at a Moment of Anger...338
266. Divorce by One Strong Pronouncement of Divorce...338
267. Pronouncements of Three Divorces 339
268. Divorce Women at their Iddah (Prescribed Periods) 341
269. Prohibition of Divorcing Woman During Menstruation 342
270. Concealing What is in the Wombs 342

271. Taking Back Mahr ... 343
272. Khula' Divorce Initiated by the Wife ... 343
273. Marriage Dissolution Not following the Law of Li'an in Husband's Accusation Against his Spouse or Denying Paternity ... 344
274. Divorce of Breastfeeding Woman ... 347
275. Rights of Revocably and Irrevocably Divorced Women ... 348
276. Revocably Divorced Woman Should Stay in her Husband's House Until her Iddah is Over ... 349
277. The Iddah of Divorced Woman by Talaq ... 349
278. Prohibition to Marry a Woman Divorced by Three Pronouncements Until she is Married to Another Man and he has a Sexual Intercourse with her and then he Abandons her and she Completes her Iddah ... 350
279. Prohibition of Tahleel Marriage ... 351
280. When Husband Disappears and the Wife Doesn't Know Where he is ... 352
281. Alimony ... 352
282. Woman Stipulating the Divorce of the Wife of the would-be-Husband ... 355
283. Prohibition of Inciting a Woman Against her Husband or a Slave Against his Master ... 355
284. Unlawful Sexual Intercourse - Zina ... 355
285. Zina of the Eyes, Ears, Tongue, Hands, Feet and Heart ... 357
286. Prohibition of Incest ... 359
287. Prescribed Punishment for Adultery and Fornication ... 359
288. Prohibition of Sodomy ... 362
289. Lesbianism and Homosexuality ... 363
290. Rape ... 365
291. Prostitution ... 365
292. Bestiality ... 366
293. The Pimp and the One Who Permits His Wife to Fornicate ... 366
294. Masturbation ... 367
295. Prohibition of Gazing at Women and Beardless Handsome Boys Except in Exigency ... 367
296. Looking at Non-Mahram ... 368
297. Looking at the Sexual Organs of the Same or the Opposite Sex ... 369
298. Prohibition of Meeting a Non-Mahram Woman in Seclusion ... 373
299. Prohibition of Shaking Hands with Non-Mahram Women ... 374
300. Meeting and Mixing of Men and Women ... 374
301. Correspondence Between the Sexes ... 375
302. Dating and Romance Scam ... 376
303. Revealing one's Nudity ... 377
304. Touching the Body of a Stranger ... 378
305. Accusation of Immorality Without Proof ... 378
306. Accusation of Pedophilia Against Prophet Muhammad ... 380
307. Prohibition of Sexual Intercourse During Menstruation and Post-Natal Bleeding ... 381
308. Not Performing Ghusl after Menstruation and Post-Natal Bleeding ... 382
309. Praying and Fasting while Menstruating ... 382
310. Not Performing Ghusl After Sexual Intercourse or Seminal Emission ... 383

311.	Not Performing Ghusl for a Woman After Experiencing Orgasm in Dream	384
312.	Pornography	384
313.	Distributing Massage Parlour Cards	386
314.	Public Massage and Bathhouse	386
315.	Night, Strip, Sex Clubs	388
316.	Begging	388
317.	About Begging in the Name of Allah	393
318.	Greediness	393
319.	Not Spending of Good for Parents, Kindred, Orphans, Poor and Wayfarers	394
320.	Not Giving in Charity	396
321.	Taking Advantages of Other People for their Own Benefit	398
322.	Undesirability of Giving a Gift and then Ask Back for it	399
323.	Looking Down Upon the Gift	400
324.	Not Rewarding People for the Gift or Favor	400
325.	Prohibition of Miserliness	400
326.	Prohibition of Consumption of Unlawful Food and Income	401
327.	Slaughtering for Other than Allah	408
328.	Non-Islamic Slaughtering of Animal	409
329.	Do Not Mentioning the Name of Allah Before Eating and Drinking	410
330.	Prohibition of Using Utensils Made of Gold and Silver	411
331.	Throwing Leftover Food	411
332.	Gluttony	412
333.	Prohibition of Criticizing Food	413
334.	Prohibition of Eating Two Date-Fruits Simultaneously	414
335.	Prohibition of Selling and Buying Unripe Fruit	414
336.	Alcohol and Intoxicants	414
337.	Prescribed Punishment for Drinking Alcohol	416
338.	Blowing and Breathing into the Vessel	417
339.	Prohibited Drinking Directly from the Mouth of a Waterskin	418
340.	Undesirability of Drinking While Standing	418
341.	Declining the Invitation to a Meal Without Valid Reason	418
342.	Dishonoring the Guest	420
343.	Remaining in the Invited Home Unnecessarily After a Meal	421
344.	Uninvited Guests	422
345.	Abomination of Selecting Friday, Single Day, for Fasting	422
346.	Fasting on Saturday, Single Day	423
347.	Prohibition of Extending Fast Beyond One Day	423
348.	Fasting on Eid Al-Fitr, Eid Al-Adha and Three Days of Tashreeq	424
349.	Relieving Oneself Facing Qiblah or Turning Back Towards	424
350.	Prohibition of Relieving Nature on the Paths	425
351.	Not Concealing One's' Private Part while Bathing or Relieving Oneself	425
352.	Greeting, Speaking and Eating in the Toilet	426
353.	Prohibition of Using the Right Hand for Cleaning After Toilet Without Valid Reason	426
354.	Not Cleaning Oneself from All Traces of Urine	427
355.	Urinating in a Hole	428

356.	Prohibition of Urinating into Stagnant Water	428
357.	Uncleanliness	428
358.	Prohibition of Magic – Sorcery - Witchcraft	429
359.	Prohibition of Consultation with Soothsayers	435
360.	Forbiddance of Believing in Ill Omens	437
361.	Believing in Horoscope and Astrology	438
362.	Prohibition of Attributing Rain to the Stars	439
363.	Prohibition of Wearing String and Thread	440
364.	Prohibition of Wearing the Evil Eye Jewelry	441
365.	Belief in Superstitions	441
366.	Seeking Decision Through Divining Arrows	442
367.	Playing Games of Chance Without Betting	442
368.	Prohibition of Envy	443
369.	Amulets to Ward off the Evil Eye and Hasad (Envy)	445
370.	Saying "Ma Shaa Allah" to Prevent the Evil Eye is a Bid'ah	448
371.	Belief in Reincarnation	449
372.	Prohibition of Suspicion	451
373.	Prohibition of Spying on Muslims and to be Inquisitive about Others	451
374.	Spying in Order to Catch the Faults of Others	453
375.	Spying on Phones	453
376.	Prohibition of Obscenity	454
377.	Abomination of Self-Condemnation	455
378.	Prohibition of Maligning	455
379.	Prohibition of Nursing Rancor and Enmity	456
380.	Prohibition of Two Holding Secret Counsel to the Exclusion of the Third in a Gathering of Three People	457
381.	Prohibition of Rejoicing Over Another's Trouble	458
382.	Prohibition of Cruelty	458
383.	Throwing Stones	460
384.	Killing a Human Being	460
385.	Answering to Evil by the Greater Evil	461
386.	Spreading and Exposing his Own Sins	463
387.	Spreading and Exposing Someone's Sins	463
388.	Throwing a Fault or a Sin on to Someone Innocent	464
389.	Committing Evil Deeds Openly and Blatantly	464
390.	Not Denouncing or Advising the Sinner Committing Evil Deeds	465
391.	Accusing Innocent Person	465
392.	Condemning Instead of Advising	466
393.	Claiming Yourselves to be Pure	468
394.	Prohibition of Taking Ar-Riba (The Usury)	468
395.	Mortgage	470
396.	Credit Card as Riba	471
397.	Stock Market	471
398.	Money Exchange	472
399.	Bitcoin and Cryptocurrency	473
400.	Prohibition of Devouring the Property of an Orphan	474

401.	Taking People's Property Unjustly	475
402.	Illegally Using Someone's Property	476
403.	Consuming One Another's Wealth	477
404.	Carelessness in Guarding the Trust	477
405.	Taking More than Your Allotment	479
406.	Prohibition of Seeking out a Position of Authority	480
407.	The Leader Who Misleads his Followers, the Tyrant and the Oppressor	481
408.	The Unjust Ruler	481
409.	Obligation of Obedience to the Ruler in what is Lawful and	482
410.	Fighting the Ruler, Rebelling Against Him Even if He Oppresses	484
411.	Strike	487
412.	Betraying the Leader	487
413.	Betrayal of Trust and Cheating Others	488
414.	Acceptance of Gifts on the Part of State Officer is Forbidden	488
415.	Legislation Not Following Allah's Laws	489
416.	Usurping the Rights of Others or Non-Fulfillment of Rights	489
417.	Not Enjoining Good and Forbidding Evil	492
418.	Chastisement for One who Enjoins Good and Forbids Evil but Acts Otherwise	495
419.	Extortion	495
420.	Prohibition of Following the Manners of Satan and Disbelievers	496
421.	Condemnation of Pride and Self-Conceit	496
422.	Prohibition of Arrogance, Vanity and Haughtiness	498
423.	Prohibition of Oppression	500
424.	Unlawfulness of Oppression and Restoring Others Rights	504
425.	Terrorism, Extremism	507
426.	Humble before a Disbeliever, Transgressor, Arrogant People	508
427.	Prohibition of Conferring a Title of Honor upon a Sinner, a Hypocrite and the Like	509
428.	Saying "You are our Master"	509
429.	To Honor a Wealthy and Powerful Person for his Wealth and Power	509
430.	To Point a Sharp Object at Someone	510
431.	Prohibition of Pointing with a Weapon at Another Brother in Faith	510
432.	Prohibition of Chastisement with Fire	510
433.	Prohibition of Leaving the Fire Burning	511
434.	Prohibition of Putting Oneself to Undue Hardship	512
435.	Democracy, Telling "Rules of People"	512
436.	Electoral Fraud	513
437.	Discrimination	514
438.	Freedom	516
439.	Freedom of Expression	522
440.	Prohibition of Making Fun and Mockery	525
441.	Prohibition of Excessive Laughing	526
442.	Skepticism	527
443.	Abusive Language	528
444.	Calling Others with Bad Names	528
445.	Listening to the People's Private Conversations	529

446.	Disclosing Secret	529
447.	Reading the Other's Letter	529
448.	Prohibition of Calumny	530
449.	Prohibition of Carrying Tales of the Officers	531
450.	Arguing, Picking Apart Another's Words and Quarreling	531
451.	Prohibition of Backbiting and Slander	532
452.	Prohibition of Listening to Backbiting and Slander	533
453.	Ascertainment of What One Hears and Narrates	536
454.	Useless Talk or Talk too Much About Others	537
455.	Anger	538
456.	Harming and Insulting Others	540
457.	Prohibition of Cursing one Particular Man or Animal	541
458.	Prohibition of Invoking the Curse or Wrath of Allah	542
459.	Ignorance	544
460.	Seeing Oneself as Superior to Others in Any Way	546
461.	Disputes and the Virtue of Reconciling Between Two Disputing Parties	547
462.	Debt	548
463.	Prohibition of Procrastinating by a Rich Person to Fulfill his Obligation	552
464.	Borrowing the Item with No Intention of Return or Without Taking Care	553
465.	Public Nuisance	554
466.	Prohibition of Giving False Testimony	555
467.	Concealing Evidence	556
468.	Prohibition of Swearing in the Name of Anyone or Anything Besides Allah	557
469.	Illegality of Swearing Falsely	557
470.	Cheating on Exams No Matter what the Motives	558
471.	Smoking	559
472.	Gambling	560
473.	Theft	560
474.	Prohibition of Recession Regarding Prescribed Punishment for the Theft and Other (Crimes) in Case of Important Persons	561
475.	Highwaymen Who Menace the Road	562
476.	Stopping Others in the Street and Taking their Money	562
477.	Prohibition of the Treachery and Breaking One's Covenant	562
478.	Abomination of Swearing in Transaction	565
479.	Collecting Taxes	565
480.	Injustice	567
481.	Dishonest Judge	568
482.	Ruling on Financial Penalties	570
483.	Prohibition to Judge while Judge Being in a State of Anger	571
484.	Doubtful Matters	571
485.	Bribery	572
486.	Make People Pay in Order to Pass Through, though it is Not a Rule from the Authority	574
487.	Prohibition of Show-Off	575
488.	Prohibition of Recounting of Favors	577
489.	Not Returning a Favor (Kindness) to the One Who Did you a Favor	578

490.	Stinging to "Jazak Allah"	578
491.	Answering to "Jazak Allah Khayran" by "Wa ʾantum fa-jazākumu-llahu khayran"	579
492.	Ingratitude	579
493.	Preoccupation with What Does Not Concern Him	583
494.	Prohibition of Vowing	583
495.	Breaking Promise	584
496.	Prohibition of Drawing Portraits	584
497.	Photography	587
498.	Prohibition of Bewailing the Deceased or When Afflicted with Adversity	587
499.	Praying at the Grave, in the Graveyard	589
500.	Prohibition of Facing the Graves During Prayer	590
501.	Congregational Du'a after Funeral Prayer	591
502.	Prohibition of Mourning Beyond Three Days (for Women)	591
503.	Prohibition of Sitting on the Graves	592
504.	Prohibition of Plastering and Building over the Graves	592
505.	Touching Graves and Looking for Help from the Occupants	593
506.	Prohibition of Abusing the Deceased Without a Valid Legal Reason	596
507.	Prohibition of Disclosing the Physical Defects of the Deceased	596
508.	Not Performing Funeral Prayer for the Muslim Believer	597
509.	Burying the Dead at Three Forbidden Times	598
510.	Mourning on the 3rd, 10th, 40th and on the Yearly Death Anniversary of the Deceased	598
511.	Women Wearing Black Clothes at Times of Calamity and Death	599
512.	Prohibition of Funeral Prayer for the Disbeliever	600
513.	Abomination of Longing for Death	600
514.	Suicide	602
515.	Asking Forgiveness for the Disbelievers Alive and Dead	603
516.	Overburdening Against Others	603
517.	Prohibition for a Slave to Run Away from his Master	605
518.	Employer Keeping the Passports of Their Employees	605
519.	Salary Not Paid or Delayed Without Legal Reason	606
520.	Benefit Fraud	606
521.	Withholding Excess Water from Others	608
522.	Prohibition of the Sale of Excess Water in the Barren Lands and Preventing	609
523.	Prohibition of Malpractices in Commerce	609
524.	Selling the Commodity Before Taking the Possession of it	613
525.	Short Weighing or Cheating in Business	614
526.	Mixing Bad Articles with Good Ones and Selling at the Higher Price	615
527.	Falsifying the Origin, Quality or Expiration Date of Goods	615
528.	Lying and Concealing the Defects of Goods	616
529.	Misleading Others About Real Price	616
530.	Ba'i al-Najsh, a type of Impermissible Sale	617
531.	Selling a Product at Different Prices to Different Customers	617
532.	Hoarding, Black Marketing, Adulteration and Profiteering	618
533.	Trade and Traffic in Haram (Unlawful) and Doubtful Things	620

534.	Selling Something that Will Be Used for Sinful Purposes	621
535.	Prohibition of Deceiving Others	621
536.	Taking Things that Do Not Belong to You	622
537.	Internet Fraud	624
538.	Website Redirects	624
539.	Phishing	624
540.	Email Fraud	624
541.	Charitable Organization Fraud	625
542.	Pyramid Scheme	625
543.	Lottery Scam	626
544.	Bank Fraud	626
545.	Credit Card Fraud	627
546.	Check Fraud	627
547.	Job Offer Fraud	627
548.	University Admission Fraud	627
549.	Work from Home Scam	628
550.	Online Shopping Fraud	628
551.	Identity Fraud and Identity Theft	628
552.	Passport Fraud	628
553.	False Advertising	629
554.	Advertising Interrupting Allah's Words, the Qur'an Recitation	629
555.	Telecommunication Fraud	629
556.	Prize and Winning Fraud	630
557.	Scientific Article Publication Fraud	630
558.	Congress Fraud	630
559.	Visa Fraud	631
560.	Immigration Fraud	631
561.	Online Travel Agency Fraud	631
562.	Airline Baggage Lost Coverage Insurance Fraud	631
563.	Property Management Fraud	632
564.	Car Repair Fraud	632
565.	Prohibition of Squandering Wealth	632
566.	Buying Distinct Mobile Phone Numbers and Car Fancy Plate Numbers	633
567.	Saying "Wealth of People"	635
568.	568. Rulings on Dress for Men	635
569.	Rulings on Dress for Women	637
570.	Prohibition of Wearing Saffron-Colored Dress for Men	640
571.	Prohibition of Wearing Plain Red Colored Garments for Men	640
572.	Woman Not Covering Whole Body	640
573.	Hijab Ban	642
574.	Women Praying with Uncovered Feet	644
575.	Displaying the Beauty and Ornaments	644
576.	Women Doing Da'wah on Television	645
577.	Shoes Making Noise and High Heels	647
578.	Undesirability of Wearing one Shoe or Sock	647
579.	Prohibition of Using the Skin of the Leopard	647

580.	Man Wearing the Garment Below the Ankles (Isbaal)	648
581.	Man who Drags his Clothes Out of Pride	648
582.	Men Wearing Silk or Brocade and Gold	648
583.	Prohibition for Men and Women Apeing One Another	649
584.	Men Wearing the Earring, Necklace, Bracelet, Piercing	650
585.	Men with Whips Like the Tails of Cattle, Women with the Humps of Camels on their Heads	650
586.	Hair Extension	651
587.	Prohibition of Wearing False Hair, Tattooing and Filling of Teeth	651
588.	Prohibition to Dye Hair Black	653
589.	Prohibition of Shaving a Part of Head	654
590.	Prohibition of Plucking Grey Hairs	655
591.	Trimming or Plucking Eyebrows	655
592.	Wearing Fake Eyelashes	655
593.	Removing Excess Facial Hair	655
594.	Not Removing Pubic and Armpit Hair	656
595.	Mustache Hair Touching the Upper Lip	656
596.	Shaving the Beard	657
597.	Growing Fingernails and Using Nail Polish	657
598.	Using any Kind of Perfume Going Out for Women	657
599.	Wearing Colored Contact Lenses	658
600.	Makeup, Henna, Jewelry are Forbidden in front of Non-Mahram Men	658
601.	Sleeping and Lying on the Abdomen	659
602.	Christmas Celebration	660
603.	New Year Celebration	663
604.	Birthday Celebration	664
605.	Ruling on Celebrating Valentine's Day	665
606.	Conditions for the Acceptance of Good Deeds by Allah	666
607.	Unlawful Innovations (Bid'ah)	683
608.	Sitting with the Innovators in Religion or Listening to them	697
609.	Prohibition of the Music, Singing and Dancing	697
610.	Parties and Gathering Without Remembering Allah	698
611.	Settling in Non-Muslim Country if he is Unable to Practice his Religion Openly	699
612.	Driving or Accompanying People to the Place of Sins	700
613.	Renting or Offering the Place for the Gathering with Sins	700
614.	Television, Internet	701
615.	Reading Books about Unlawful Things	702
616.	Preserving Books that Lead to Deviation in Religion	702
617.	Branding Animals on the Face	702
618.	Killing, Torturing Animals, Birds, Not Feeding Them	702
619.	Prohibition of Keeping a Dog Except as a Watchdog or Hunting Dog	704
620.	Undesirability of Hanging Bells Round the Necks of Animals	706
621.	Buying and Selling Dogs and Cats	706
622.	Cursing the Beasts	707
623.	Disturbance to the Natural Environment	707
624.	Not Preserving the Blessings of Allah on Earth	708

625.	Prohibition of Reviling the Wind	710
626.	Football and Other Sport Games	711
627.	Yoga	711
628.	Persistence in Minor Sins	712
629.	Being Pleased with a Sinful Act	714
630.	Staying in an Assembly of Sin	714
631.	Prohibiting Woman from Traveling Alone	715
632.	Prohibition Traveling Alone at Night	716
633.	Trip to Mars	716
634.	Commercial Insurance Fraud	717
635.	Ruling on Medico-Surgical Treatment	719
636.	Health Care Fraud and Abuse	722
637.	Misdiagnosis of Jinn Diseases	723
638.	Medico-Surgical Treatment in Jinn Diseases	726
639.	Undesirability of Departing from or Coming to a Place Stricken by an Epidemic	736
640.	Undesirability of Reviling Fever	737
641.	Pharma Fraud	738
642.	Vaccination Fraud	739
643.	Children Vaccination	741
644.	Coronavirus Vaccination	741
645.	Post-Vaccination Diseases	743
646.	Death Following Vaccination	743
647.	Making Vaccination Obligatory	745
648.	Fine for Vaccination Refusal	746
649.	Penalties for Anti-Vaccination Claims	746
650.	Repeated Vaccination	747
651.	Multivalent Vaccines	747
652.	Telling that if you Don't Take this Medicine or Vaccine	747
653.	Buying and Selling Expensive Drugs	748
654.	Gene Therapy	749
655.	Cancer Treatment	750
656.	Chemotherapy and Nanotherapy	750
657.	Radiotherapy	751
658.	Immunotherapy	751
659.	Proton-Pump Inhibitors (PPIs) in Cancer Treatment	751
660.	Melatonin in Cancer Treatment	752
661.	Prophylactic Mastectomy	752
662.	Heart Diseases Treatment	752
663.	Obesity Treatment	754
664.	Diabetes Treatment	756
665.	Autoimmune Diseases Treatment	757
666.	Psychiatric Diseases Treatment	757
667.	Anti-HIV/AIDS Therapy	759
668.	Epilepsy Treatment	760
669.	Paralysis Treatment	761
670.	Treatment of Pain	763

671.	Autism Treatment	767
672.	Dementia and Alzheimer's Disease Treatment	767
673.	Infertility Treatment	768
674.	Anti-Allergy Treatment	768
675.	Ruling on Using Relaxants and Sleeping Pills to Treat Anxiety and Insomnia	769
676.	Ruling on Stem Cells Therapy	770
677.	Stem Cells from Induced Abortion	770
678.	Ruling on Medicines that are Mixed with Alcohol and Intoxicants	772
679.	Ruling on Medicine that Contain Pork	772
680.	Homeopathy	773
681.	Ruling on Treating Patients with Music	774
682.	Ruling on Dealing in so-called "Healing Crystals"	774
683.	Ruling on Believing in Auras and Energy Healing	776
684.	Ruling on Using a "Biodisc" and the Ruling on Wearing "Chi Pendants" for Healing	777
685.	Believing that Doctors or Drugs Cure	778
686.	Ordering Unnecessary Medical Tests, Medications	779
687.	Surgical Operations Without Medico-Legal Indication	779
688.	Euthanasia, Taking a Patient off a Respirator and the Ruling on Mercy Killing	780
689.	Telling that these Food or Drugs Increase Longevity	780
690.	Do Not Applying Ruqyah, Negative Ions and Prophetic Medicine	782
691.	Non-Islamic Exorcism	798
692.	Jinn Catching	811
693.	Not Performing Circumcision	817
694.	Ruling on Surgery that Causes Sterility	817
695.	Abortion	817
696.	Foeticide	820
697.	Prohibition on Selling Blood	820
698.	Cosmetic Surgical Procedures	821
699.	Ruling on Face-Lift, Botox, Skin Exfoliating	822
700.	Sex-Change Operation from Male to Female or Vice Versa	823
701.	Fertility Fraud	825
702.	Ruling on Sperm Donation	825
703.	Ruling on Egg Donation	826
704.	Prohibition of Mitochondrial Donation IVF	826
705.	Human Embryo Model Made from Stem Cells	826
706.	Prohibition of Infertility Treatment for the Single, Lesbian and Gay Couples	827
707.	Prohibition of Surrogacy	827
708.	Prohibition of Cloning of Human Beings	829
709.	Prohibition of Hypnotherapy	830
710.	Ruling on Organ Transplants	830
711.	Prohibition of Doing that which Allah and His Messenger Have Prohibited	831
712.	Undesirability of Intercession in Hudud	832
713.	Disbelief on Judgment Day	833
714.	Disbelief in Paradise	837
715.	Disbelief in Hellfire	840

Bibliography 877

I dedicate this book to my family, descendant of the Prophet Muhammad (peace and blessings of Allah be upon him).

Allah, the Exalted, says:

"And We have enjoined on man (to be dutiful and good) to his parents. His mother bore him in weakness and hardship upon weakness and hardship, and his weaning is in two years give thanks to Me and to your parents, unto Me is the final destination." (Qur'an, Luqman 31:14)

"We have enjoined upon man to be good to his parents. His mother carried him with hardship and gave birth to him with hardship, and his gestation and weaning is thirty months. He grows until, when he matures and reaches the age of forty years, he says: My Lord, enable me to be grateful for Your favor You have bestowed upon me and upon my parents, and to work righteousness of pleasing to You, and to make my offspring righteous for me. Verily, I have repented to You, and I am of the Muslims who surrender to You." (Qur'an, Al-Ahqaf 46:15)

Hadith on Parents: Honoring your mother, then your father

Abu Huraira reported: A man asked the Messenger of Allah, peace and blessings be upon him, "Who is most deserving of my good company?" The Prophet said, "**Your mother**." The man asked, "Then who?" The Prophet said "**Your mother**." The man asked again, "Then who?" The Prophet said, "**Your mother**." The man asked again, "Then who?" The Prophet said, "**Your father**." (Bukhari and Muslim) (https://www.abuaminaelias.com/dailyhadithonline/2010/09/12/honor-mother-then-father)

Anas ibn Malik (May Allah be pleased with him) reported: "I heard the Messenger of Allah (May Allah's peace and blessings be upon him) say: "Whoever loves to have his sustenance expanded and his term of life prolonged should maintain ties of kinship." (Bukhari and Muslim)

Explanation
This Hadith urges us to uphold our kinship ties and highlights some of the benefits of doing so, in addition to winning the pleasure of Allah, the Almighty. Maintaining ties of kinship is a cause for immediate rewards in worldly life, by the occurrence of pleasant things, like the expansion of sustenance and prolongation of lifespan. Some people may see the Hadith, in its literal meaning, as contradicting with the Verse that says: "But never will Allah delay a soul when its time has come." [Surah Al-Munafiqun 63:11] Answering this, we say that someone's lifespan is dependent on certain causes. Let us say, for example, that someone's life is set to be 60 years, if he were to maintain the ties of kinship, and 40, if he were to cut them off. So, Allah will extend his life, if he maintains ties of kinship, beyond the period fixed in case he does not uphold them.

PREFACE

Allah, the Exalted, says:

"Evil (sins and disobedience of Allah, etc.) has appeared on land and sea because of what the hands of men have earned (by oppression and evil deeds, etc.), that Allah may make them taste a part of that which they have done, in order that they may return (by repenting to Allah, and begging His Pardon)." (Qur'an, Ar-Rum 30:41)

"...whosoever works evil, will have the recompense thereof, and he will not find any protector or helper besides Allah." (Qur'an, An-Nisa 4:79)

"And whoever among you does wrong, We shall make him taste a great torment." (Qur'an, Al-Furqan 25:19)

Sins (disobedience to God) cause diseases, calamities, disasters, hardships, difficulties...

It is a Universal Law of **"cause and effect"** or **"action and reaction."**

Narrated 'Umar bin Khattab: "I heard the Messenger of Allah (peace and blessings be upon him) say:
'Whoever hoards food (and keeps it from) the Muslims, Allah will afflict him with leprosy and bankruptcy.'" (Ibn Majah)

Tubba, King of Yemen, Abu Karab As'ad intended in his heart to destroy Ka'bah and kill its people who did not welcome him without informing anybody about his plan. Suddenly, he was hit with a painful headache, and stinky fluid burst from his eyes, ears, nose and mouth. Everybody resisted away from him as a result of his bad odour. His minister then gathered the doctors, but they could not come near him to treat him due to his bad smell. At night one of the scholars came to the minister and informed him that he may know the cause of Tuba's sickness and that he knows its cure. The minister was delighted at hearing the news and he took him to see the King. The scholar said to the King: "Tell me the truth, did you intend to do something bad to this House (meaning the Ka'bah)." To that the King said: "Yes, I intended to destroy it and to kill its people." The scholar then said: "Know that your pain and affliction is the result of your bad intentions." He then said to him: "The Lord (Owner) of this House has the complete Power and nothing happens in His dominion except what He willed, He knows about the secrets and about the hidden things." That scholar, who was a follower of Prophet Ibrahim (Abraham), then taught the King about the Religion of Islam. The King embraced Islam immediately and was cured from his sickness." (1, 2)

Ibn Abi Khalid told us, from Abu Bakr bin Abi Zuhair: "I think he said: 'Abu Bakr said: 'O Messenger of Allah, how could we be in a good state after this reverse?' He said: `May Allah have mercy on you, O Abu Bakr. Do you not fall sick? Do you not feel sad? Don't calamities befall you? Do you not...?' He said: 'Of course.' He said: `That is for that. It was narrated that Abu Bakr ath-Thaqafi said: 'Abu Bakr said: 'O Messenger of Allah, how could we be in a good state after this Verse: `*whosoever works evil, will have the recompense thereof.*`" *(An-Nisa 4:123)* and he narrated the same Hadith." (Ahmad)

95% of diseases are caused by the Evil Jinn because of sins. Almighty Allah, the Only One True God, gave me the knowledge and confirmed me this statement by answering to my Istikhara prayer and Du'a.

"Shall I inform you (O people!) upon whom the Shayateen (Devils) descend? They descend on every lying (one who tells lies), sinful person." (Qur'an, Ash-Shu'ara 26:221-222)

"O Children of Adam! Let not Shaitan (Satan) deceive you, as he got your parents [Adam and Hawwa (Eve)] out of Paradise, stripping them of their raiments, to show them their private parts. Verily, he and Qabiluhu (his soldiers from the Jinns or his tribe) see you from where you cannot see them. Verily, We made the Shayateen (Devils) Auliya' (protectors and helpers) for those who believe not." (Qur'an, Al-A'raf 7:27)

The book describes 715 sins with their effects and consequences, and the conditions of repentance.

Medicine gone astray as didn't follow Hippocrates oath and warning that drugs cannot help in Jinn Possession disease; didn't follow Jesus' and Muhammad's teachings (May Allah have mercy on them) that sins cause diseases. There is nothing in medical education about the Qur'an and Negative Ions healing and Prophetic Medicine. How to expect cure when disbelieving people forgot Allah, the Only One Healer?

Allah, the Exalted, says:

"O Prophet (Muhammad SAW)! Keep your duty to Allah, and obey not the disbelievers and the hypocrites (i.e. do not follow their advices). Verily! Allah is Ever All-Knower, All-Wise." (Qur'an, Al-Ahzab 33:1)

It is our Creator Who send the diseases when people disobey Him and His Messenger and the cure relies in giving up sins, repentance and following Divine Guidance (the Qur'an and Sunnah). Medicine has gone from focusing on the wholeness to focusing on the part. While the soul of the human beings is the first which is affected by diseases (hypocrisy, showing off, vanity, jealousy, lying, backbiting, mockery, malice, pride, arrogance, love of praise, love of status, love of world, love of fame, following desires and whims, ingratitude, stinginess, hostility against truth, treachery, breach of trust, cruelty, committing sins openly, forgetfulness of death and the Judgment Day, not remembering and fearing Allah, etc.)

Abu Barzah reported: The Prophet (peace and blessings be upon him) said, "Verily, among what I fear most for you are seductive temptations in your stomachs and passions, and the misguidance of whims." (Aḥmad)

Medicine has become de-humanized, commercial and contributes to disease progression as excites the Evil Jinn as the majority people are Jinn Possessed. Toxicity of drugs is another serious issue causing new diseases and death.

ACKNOWLEDGEMENT

I am grateful to the One Who created the heavens and earth and everything between and beneath the soil, seen and unseen.

"Who created me, and He (it is Who) guides me.

And it is He Who feeds me and gives me drink.

And when I am ill, it is He Who cures me.

And Who will cause me to die and then bring me to life.

And Who I aspire that He will forgive me my sin on the Day of Recompense." (Qur'an, Ash-Shu'ara 26:78-81)

It is He, Allah, Who takes and returns back my soul every night.
It is by His Mercy, I breathe, I speak, I see, I hear, I understand, I walk, I work, I sleep, I eat and drink…
It is He Who has chosen the noble profession for me, being doctor, and blessed me with a special knowledge: the Qur'an Healing and Prophetic Medicine.
It is He, the Creator of all people, Who has chosen for me my family.
It is He Who forgives, guides, cures, supports, protects, provides, elevates.
He is the Only One Who gives the inner peace, tranquility, happiness and success.
He is the Best Planner and Disposer of all affairs.

Miraculous effects of Negative Ions (which are in the Noble Qur'an) on me and my patients, have changed completely my medical practice.

One of the country Rulers came to see me for repeated miscarriage and in every miscarriage the chromosomal studies showed male embryo; they wanted to have a boy after having two girls. I have explained the Negative Ions and Ruqyah treatment. Miscarriage is caused by the Evil Jinn. They followed my recommendations and she became pregnant naturally and delivered twin, two boys, Allah's Miracle!

Allah is the Source of all Goodness.

"And (remember) when your Lord proclaimed: 'If you give thanks (by accepting faith and worshipping none but Allah), I will give you more (of My blessings)…" (Qur'an, Ibrahim 14:7)

INTRODUCTION

Allah, the Exalted, says:

"Whatever of good reaches you, is from Allah, but whatever of evil befalls you, is from yourself. And We have sent you (O Muhammad SAW) as a Messenger to mankind, and Allah is Sufficient as a Witness." (Qur'an, Taha 20:120)

Adam disobeyed His Creator following the incitement of Satan. That was the first sin of the first man.

Allah, the Exalted, says:

"And O Adam! Dwell you and your wife in Paradise, and eat thereof as you both wish, but approach not this tree otherwise you both will be of the Zalimun (unjust and wrong-doers)." (Qur'an, Al-A'raf 7:19)

"Then Shaitan (Satan) whispered to him, saying: "O Adam! Shall I lead you to the Tree of Eternity and to a kingdom that will never waste away?" (Qur'an, Taha 20:120)

"Then they both ate of the tree, and so their private parts appeared to them, and they began to stick on themselves the leaves from Paradise for their covering. Thus, did Adam disobey his Lord, so he went astray." (Qur'an, Taha 20:121)

Adam and his wife realized their wrongdoing and turned in repentance with regret and sincerety, and Allah, the Creator, accepted their repentance and gave a guidance.

"(Allah) said: "Get you down (from the Paradise to the earth), both of you, together, some of you are an enemy to some others. Then if there comes to you guidance from Me, then whoever follows My Guidance shall neither go astray, nor fall into distress and misery." (Qur'an, Taha 20:123)

Allah, the Exalted, sent many Messengers with His Books to many nations. The last Book, the Qur'an, was sent to His last Messenger to guide all mankind and Jinn, by which will be judged on Judgment Day.

Allah, the Exalted, says

"O mankind! There has come to you a good advice from your Lord (i.e. the Qu'ran, ordering all that is good and forbidding all that is evil) and a Healing for that (disease of ignorance, doubt, hypocrisy and differences, etc.) in your breasts, - a Guidance and a Mercy (explaining lawful and unlawful things, etc.) for the believers." (Qur'an, Yunus 10:57)

Allah created this short temporary life only to test people; to distinguish truth from falsehood, belief in Allah from disbelief, morality from immorality, gratitude from ingratitude, patience from impatience and then to reward (Paradise) or punish (Hellfire) accordingly.
Allah, the Exalted, says

"Who has created death and life that He may test you which of you is best in deed. And He is the All-Mighty, the Oft-Forgiving." (Qur'an, Al-Mulk 67:2)

Sins (Disobedience to Allah) cause diseases, calamities, disasters, hardships, difficulties.

It is a Universal Law of "cause and effect" or "action and reaction".

Those who disobey Allah, authomatically guided by Satan, the temporary god for the disbelievers. Satan's role to misguide and bring maximum people to the Hellfire.

Diseases happen by Allah's Decree

Allah, the Exalted, says:

"No calamity befalls on the earth or in yourselves but it is inscribed in the Book of Decrees (Al-Lawh Al-Mahfuz) before We bring it into existence. Verily, that is easy for Allah. In order that you may not grieve at the things over that you fail to get, nor rejoice over that which has been given to you. And Allah likes not prideful boasters." (Qur'an, Al-Hadid 57:22-23)

"Say: "Nothing shall ever happen to us except what Allah has ordained for us. He is our Maula (Lord, Helper and Protector)." And in Allah let the believers put their trust." (Qur'an, At-Tawbah 9:51)

What Allah wills, happens and what He does not will, does not happen; there is nothing that can block the Will of Allah from being executed. The believer, who affirms the Oneness of Allah, knows that there is no room for regret or grief in this life, because everything happens by Allah's Will and Decree.

THE ORIGIN AND PURPOSE OF HUMAN CREATION

Allah, the Exalted, says:

"And (remember) when your Lord said to the angels: 'I am going to create a human (Adam) from sounding clay of altered black smooth mud. So, when I have fashioned him and breathed into him (his) soul created by Me, then you fall down prostrate to him." (Qur'an, Sad 38:71-72)

"It is He Who created you from dust, then from a sperm-drop, then from a clinging clot; then He brings you out as a child; then (He develops you) that you reach your (time of) maturity, then (further) that you become elders. And among you is he who is taken in death before (that), so that you reach a specified term; and perhaps you will use reason." (Qur'an, Ghafir 40:67)

When Adam's soul joined with his body, he sneezed, then said, "Al-Hamdulillah" which means "All praises and thanks to Allah". Adam was created Muslim.

Narrated Abu Hurairah: The Prophet (peace and blessings be upon him) said, "Allah created Adam, making him 60 cubits tall. When He created him, He said to him, 'Go and greet that group of angels and listen to their reply, for it will be your greeting (salutation) and the greeting (salutations of your offspring.' So, Adam said (to the angels), 'As-Salamu Alaikum (i.e. peace be upon you).' The angels said, 'As-salamu Alaika wa Rahmatullahi' (i.e. peace and Allah's Mercy be upon you). Thus, the angels added to Adam's salutation the expression, 'Wa Rahmatullahi,' Any person who will enter Paradise will resemble Adam (in appearance and figure). People have been decreasing in stature since Adam's creation." (Bukhari)

'Imran ibn al-Husayn (May Allah be pleased with him) reported: "A man came to the Prophet (May Allah's peace and blessings be upon him) and said: "Assalamu 'alaykum (peace be upon you)." The Prophet responded to his greeting and the man sat down. The Prophet (May Allah's peace and blessings be upon him) said: 'Ten.' Then another man came and said: "Assalamu 'alaykum wa rahmatullah (May the peace and mercy of Allah be upon you)." The Prophet replied to his greeting and the man sat down. Then another man came and said: "Assalamu 'alaykum wa rahmatullāh wa barakatuh (May the peace, mercy and blessings of Allah be upon you)." The Prophet replied to his greeting and the man sat down. The Prophet (May Allah's peace and blessings be upon him) said: 'Thirty.'" (Tirmidhi) (https://hadeethenc.com/en/browse/hadith/3587)

Allah, the Exalted, says:

"Their greeting on the Day they shall meet Him will be "Salam: Peace (i.e. the angels will say to them: Salamu 'Alaikum)!" And He has prepared for them a generous reward (i.e. Paradise)." (Qur'an, Al-Ahzab 33:44)

Other Verse: *Ar-Ra'd 13:24, Yasin 36:58, Az-Zumar 39:73.*

On the Day of Arafat (day 9th of Dhul-Hijjah (the month of Hajj), Allah, the Exalted, has extracted the souls of all people from Adam's loin which He created all Muslims and made them testify that Allah is their Lord. On that Day (Friday), Allah has chosen Islam as the Deen (code of life) for all humanity. (3)

Allah, the Exalted, says:

"This day, I have perfected your religion for you, completed My Favor upon you, and have chosen for you Islam as your religion." (Qur'an, Al-Ma'idah 5:3)

"And (remember) when your Lord brought forth from the Children of Adam, from their loins, their seed (or from Adam's loin his offspring) and made them testify as to themselves (saying): "Am I not your Lord?" They said: "Yes! We testify," lest you should say on the Day of Resurrection: "Verily, we have been unaware of this. Or lest you should say: "It was only our fathers aforetime who took others as partners in worship along with Allah, and we were (merely their) descendants after them; will You then destroy us because of the deeds of men who practiced Al-Batil (i.e. polytheism and committing crimes and sins, invoking and worshipping others besides Allah)?" (Tafsir At-Tabari). (Qur'an, Al-A'raf 7:172-173)

The covenant which the soul of every human being made to Allah during pre-creation was that he would recognize Allah as his Lord and not direct any form of worship to others besides Him. Because man has declared that Allah is his Lord, he must consider righteous deeds to be only those defined by His Creator and His Prophet.

Man's Fitrah is the basis of Islam, so when he practices Islam, his outer actions and deeds come into harmony with the very nature in which Allah created man's inner being. When this takes place, man unites his inner being with his outer being which is a key aspect of Tawheed. The result of this aspect of Tawheed is the creation of the truly pious man in the mould of, Adam, to whom Allah made the angels bow and whom Allah chose to rule the earth. Because, only man who lives Tawheed can judge and rule the earth with true justice. (4)

Everyone is responsible for belief in Allah and on Judgment Day, the excuses will not be accepted. Every human being has the belief in Allah imprinted on his soul (Fitrah). Allah shows every idolater sign that his idol is not a God. Allah created life and death for the purpose of testing.

Allah, the Exalted, says:

"And be not like her who undoes the thread which she has spun after it has become strong, by taking your oaths a means of deception among yourselves, lest a nation may be more numerous than another nation. Allah only tests you by this [i.e who obeys Allah and fulfills Allah's Covenant and who disobeys Allah and breaks Allah's Covenant]. And on the Day of Resurrection, He will certainly make clear to you that wherein you used to differ [i.e. a believer confesses and believes in the Oneness of Allah and in the Prophethood of Prophet Muhammad SAW which the disbeliever denies it and that was their difference amongst them in the life of this world]." (Qur'an, An-Nahl 16:92)

"Did you think that We had created you in play (without any purpose), and that you would not be brought back to Us?" So, Exalted be Allah, the True King: Laa ilaaha illa Huwa (none has the right to be worshipped but He), the Lord of the Supreme Throne!" (Qur'an, Al-Mu'minun 23:115-116)

"And We created not the heavens and the earth and all that is between them, for mere play. We created them not except with Truth (i.e. to examine and test those who are obedient and those who are disobedient and then reward the obedient ones and punish the disobedient ones), but most of them know not." (Qur'an, Ad-Dukhan 44:38-39)

Allah sent Guidance for all people to follow (the Qur'an) and warned those who turn away from Him.

"The revelation of the Book (this Qur'an) is from Allah, the All-Mighty, the All-Wise. We created not the heavens and the earth and all that is between them except with Truth, and for an appointed term. But those who disbelieve, turn away from that whereof they are warned." (Qur'an, Al-Ahqaf 46:2-3)

Allah is a Protector of those who follow His Laws and will save them from the Hellfire.

"Shall We treat those who believe (in the Oneness of Allah Islamic Monotheism) and do righteous good deeds as Mufsidoon (those who associate partners in worship with Allah and commit crimes) on earth? Or shall We treat the Muttaqoon (the pious) as the Fujjaar (criminals, disbelievers, the wicked)?" (Qur'an, Sad 38:28)

Allah has not created man just to eat, drink, enjoy and multiply, in which case he would be like the animals. Allah has honored man and favored him far above all creatures He has created, but many people insist on disbelief, so they are ignorant or deny the true wisdom behind their creation, and all they care about is enjoying the pleasures of this world. The life of such people is like that of animals, and indeed, they are even more astray; the animals prostrate to Allah.

Human beings will consistently misuse their God-given intelligence when they lack knowledge of their purpose of existence. The degraded human mind uses its abilities to create drugs and bombs and becomes engrossed in fornication, pornography, homosexuality, fortunetelling, corruption, etc.

Without knowledge of the purpose of life, human existence loses all meaning and is consequently wasted, and the reward of an eternal life of happiness in the Hereafter is completely destroyed. Therefore, it is of the utmost importance that human beings correctly answer the question "Why are we here?" It was necessary that God reveal the purpose of life to man through His Prophets, because human beings are incapable of arriving at the correct answers by themselves. All of the Prophets of God taught their followers the answers to the question "Why did God create man?" (5)
Allah has created mankind to know and worship Him.

"And I (Allah) created not the jinn and mankind except that they should worship Me (Alone)." *(Qur'an, Adh-Dhariyat 51:56)*

When a child is born, it has with it a natural belief in Allah. This natural belief is called in Arabic the "Fitrah". If the child were left alone, it would grow up aware of Allah in His unity, but all children are affected by their parents and the pressures of their environment whether directly or indirectly.

Abu Hurairah reported Allah's Messenger (peace and blessings be upon him) as saying: "The mother of every person gives him birth according to his true nature. It is subsequently his parents who make him a Jew or a Christian, or a Magian. Had his parents been Muslim he would have also remained a Muslim. Every person to whom his mother gives birth (has two aspects of his life); when his mother gives birth, Satan strikes him but it was not the case with Mary and her son (Jesus Christ)." (Muslim)

Adam disobeyed Allah and ate from the forbidden tree following Satan's deceptive prodding, and most of mankind ignored their responsibility to believe in Allah and worship Him Alone, and followed the footsteps of Satan, denying the Creator and worshipping Allah's creation instead of the Creator.

If someone sincerely believes in Allah and tries to do good, Allah will give him many opportunities to improve his belief and increase his good deeds. Allah will never cause sincere belief to be wasted even if the believer falls off the Path, He will help him back on it. Allah may punish him in this life when he goes off the right track to remind him of his errors and wake him up to make amends. In fact, Allah will be so Merciful as to take the life of the sincere believer while doing a good deed, thereby insuring that the believer will be among the fortunate dwellers of Paradise.

If someone, on the other hand, disbelieves in Allah and rejects righteousness, Allah then makes evil deeds easy for him. Allah gives him success when he does bad and that encourages him to do more evil until he dies in such a sinful state and is flung into the everlasting Fire. Humans are created to worship the Creator, but Satan leads them astray.

People should be aware of Satan's whispers (waswasa) and do not act upon the evil inclinations. Man must struggle between their Fitrah and desires. If he chooses his Fitrah, Allah will help him overcome his desires.

The ultimate goal of every human is to pass multiples tests in this temporary and short life and to attain his permanent residence made of gold and bliss in Paradise in Hereafter.

MEDICINE OF CALAMITIES AND TRIALS

Allah, the Exalted, says:

"Whatever of good reaches you, is from Allah, but whatever of evil befalls you, is from yourself. And We have sent you (O Muhammad SAW) as a Messenger to mankind, and Allah is Sufficient as a Witness." (Qur'an, An-Nisa 4:79)

"And certainly, We shall test you with something of fear, hunger, loss of wealth, lives and fruits, but give glad tidings to As-Sabirin (the patient ones, etc.)." (Qur'an, Al-Baqarah 2:155)

"Do people think that they will be left alone because they say: "We believe," and will not be tested. And We indeed tested those who were before them. And Allah will certainly make (it) known (the truth of) those who are true, and will certainly make (it) known (the falsehood of) those who are liars, (although Allah knows all that before putting them to test)." (Qur'an, Al-'Ankabut 29:1-3)

Umm Salamah reported: The Messenger of Allah (peace and blessings be upon him) said, "No Muslim is afflicted with a calamity but that he should say what Allah has commanded him: *"Indeed, to Allah we belong and to Allah we will return." (2:156)* O Allah, reward me in my affliction and replace it with something better than it. If he does so, Allah will replace it with something better." (Muslim)

Wisdom behind calamities, including the following:

1 - To Attain True Submission and Servitude to the Lord of the Worlds

Many people are slaves to their whims and desires and are not true slaves of Allah.

Allah, the Exalted, says:

"And among mankind is he who worships Allah as it were upon the edge (i.e. in doubt): if good befalls him, he is content therewith; but if a trial befalls him, he turns back on his face (i.e. reverts to disbelief after embracing Islam). He loses both this world and the Hereafter. That is the evident loss." (Qur'an, Al-Hajj 22:11)

2 - Trials Prepare the Believers to Prevail on Earth

It was said to Imam al-Shaafa'i (May Allah have mercy on him): "Which is better, patience or tests, or prevailing?" He said: "Prevailing is the level attained by the Prophets, and there can be no prevailing except after trials. If a person is tried, he will become patient, and if he remains patient, he will prevail." (6)

3 - Expiation of Sins

Abu Hurairah (May Allah be pleased with him) reported: The Messenger of Allah (peace and blessings be upon him) said, "The believing men and women continue to be under trial in their lives, their children and their wealth, until they meet Allah without any sin." (Tirmidhi)

4 - Attainment of Reward and a Rise in Status

Abu Sa'id and Abu Hurairah (May Allah be pleased with them) reported that the Prophet (May Allah's peace and blessings be upon him) said: "No fatigue, disease, sorrow, sadness, harm or distress befalls a Muslim, even if it were a prick of a thorn, but Allah will expiate some of his sins thereby." (Bukhari and Muslim) (https://hadeethenc.com/en/browse/hadith/3701)

5 - Calamities Provide an Opportunity to Think about one's Faults and Shortcomings and Past Mistakes

Because if it is a punishment, what was the sin?

6 - Calamity is a Lesson in Tawheed, Faith and Trust in Allah

Ibn al-Qayyim (May Allah have mercy on him) said:

"Were it not that Allah treats His slaves with the remedy of trials and calamities, they would transgress and overstep the mark. When Allah wills good for His slaves, He gives him the medicine of calamities and trials according to his situation, so as to cure him from all fatal illnesses and diseases, until He purifies and cleanses him, and then makes him qualified for the most honorable position in this world, which is that of being a true slave of Allah ('uboodiyyah), and for the greatest reward in the Hereafter, which is that of seeing Him and being close to Him." (End quote, Zad Al-Ma'ad) (7)

7 - Calamities Drive out Self-Admiration from the Hearts and Bring them Closer to Allah

Allah, the Exalted, says:

"And that Allah may purify the believers (through trials) and destroy the disbelievers."
(Qur'an, Ali 'Imran 3:141)

8 - Calamities Demonstrate the True Nature of People, for there are People whose Virtue is Unknown until Calamity Strikes

al-Fudayl Ibn 'Iyaad said,

"As long as people are doing fine, their true nature is concealed, but when calamity strikes, their true natures are revealed, so the believer resorts to his faith and the hypocrite resorts to his hypocrisy."

9 - Calamities Strengthen People's Resolve

Allah chose for His Prophet (peace and blessings of Allah be upon him) a hard life filled with all kinds of hardship from a young age, in order to prepare him for the great mission, which none could bear but the strongest of men, who are tested with calamities and bear them with patience.

Allah reminded the Prophet (peace and blessings of Allah be upon him):

"Did He not find you (O Muhammad) an orphan and give you a refuge?" (Qur'an, Ad-Duha 93:6)

10 - Another Reason behind Calamities and Hardship is that a Person Becomes Able to Distinguish between True Friends and Friends who only Have their Own Interests at Heart

11 - Calamities Remind you of your Sins so that you can Repent from them

Allah, the Exalted, says:

"Whatever of good reaches you, is from Allah, but whatever of evil befalls you, is from yourself." (Qur'an, An-Nisa 4:79)

"And verily, We will make them taste of the near torment (i.e. the torment in the life of this world, i.e. disasters, calamities) prior to the supreme torment (in the Hereafter), in order that they may (repent and) return (i.e. accept Islam)." (Qur'an, As-Sajdah 32:21)

The "near torment" is hardship in this world and bad things that happen to a person. If life continues to be easy, a person may become conceited and arrogant, and think that he has no need of Allah, so by His Mercy, He tests people, so that they may return to Him.

12 - Calamities Show you the True Nature of this World and its Transience, and that it is Temporary Conveniences, and Shows us that True Life is that which is Beyond this World, in a Life in which there is No Sickness or Exhaustion

Allah, the Exalted, says:

"Verily, the home of the Hereafter that is the life indeed (i.e. the eternal life that will never end), if they but knew." (Qur'an, Al-'Ankabut 29:64)

13 - Calamities Remind you of the Great Blessings of Good Health and Ease

The calamity shows you in the clearest way the meaning of health and ease that you enjoyed for many years, but did not taste their sweetness or appreciate them fully. Calamities remind you of Allah's blessings and cause you to thank and praise Allah for His Infinite Mercy.

14 - Longing for Paradise

You will never long for Paradise until you taste the bitterness of this world. How can you long for Paradise when you are content with this world? This is a wisdom behind calamities and the interests attained by them. Sometimes, natural disasters are very intense and crush even the innocent people living in the affected area. These innocent people will get reward of Allah on Judgment Day for the affliction they faced.

Allah, the Exalted, says:

"And fear the Fitnah (affliction and trial, etc.) which affects not in particular (only) those of you who do wrong (but it may afflict all the good and the bad people), and know that Allah is Severe in punishment." (Qur'an, Al-Anfal 8:25)

Allah Almighty narrated the incidents of different tribes and people who were hit by natural disasters. People should remember the past stories and lessons to avoid sins.

Prophet Noah

Prophet Nooh (Noah) (May Allah have mercy on him) warned his people, who were plunged in depravity and sins (idolatry, etc.) calling them for repentance and Allah's Mercy and Forgiveness, promising them the glad tidings if they stop sins. The people who denied the message of Nooh were drowned.

"So, We opened the gates of heaven with water pouring forth. And We caused the earth to gush forth with springs. So, the waters (of the heaven and the earth) met for a matter predestined. And We carried him on a (ship) made of planks and nails, floating under Our eyes, a reward for him who had been rejected! And indeed, We have left this as a sign, then is there any that will remember (or receive admonition)? Then how (terrible) was My torment and My warnings?" (Qur'an, Al-Qamar 54:9-16)

Prophet Hud

The people of Ad practiced polytheism and rejected the teachings of a monotheism by Prophet Hud (May Allah have mercy on him). They denied Allah and oppressed people. Allah sent a three years famine, but they took no warning. A terrible blast of violent storm destroyed them and their land.

"As for 'Ad, they were arrogant in the land without right, and they said: "Who is mightier than us in strength?" See they not that Allah, Who created them was mightier in strength than them. And they used to deny Our Ayat (proofs, evidences, verses, lessons, revelations, etc.)!" (Qur'an, Fussilat 41:15)

Prophet Lot

Prophet Lot (May Allah have mercy on him) was sent to the cities Sodom and Gomorrah, invited people to the Right Path, to preach monotheism and to stop their sinful lustful and violent acts (gang-rape).

The entire nation was destroyed by God due to their obscene behavior, homosexuality and rape, with a rain of stone. (https://sunnahonline.com/library/stories-of-the-prophets/297-story-of-prophet-lut)

Pharaoh

Pharaoh was disobedient to Allah and denied the clear signs brought to him by Prophet Musa (May Allah have mercy on him). Allah showed His signs to Pharaoh in the form of calamities, so that he may repent.

"And indeed, We punished the people of Fir'aun (Pharaoh) with years of drought and shortness of fruits (crops, etc.) that they might remember (take heed)." (Qur'an, Al-A'raf 7:130)

Because of his persistent disobedience, he was finally drowned. His repentance was not accepted.

Qaroon

Qaroon was a wealthy person unwilling to admit that his wealth was given to him by Allah, the Creator. He thought it was the result of his efforts and denied the blessings and right of Allah, the Owner of all things, on his wealth. Allah, the Most High, caused the earth to swallow him and his dwelling place.

"So, We caused the earth to swallow him and his dwelling place. Then he had no group or party to help him against Allah, nor was he one of those who could save themselves." (Qur'an, Al-Qasas 28:81)

Prophet Muhammad

Polytheists of Makkah brought a big army against Prophet Muhammad (peace and blessings of Allah be upon him) and his companions. Allah, the Most High, helped Muslims in a hidden way by sending a windstorm that pushed the enemy army back.

Allah, the Exalted, says:

"We sent against them a wind and forces that you saw not (angels during the battle of Al-Ahzab) (the Confederates)]. And Allah is Ever All-Seer of what you do." (Qur'an, Al-Ahzab 33:9)

Committing sin, disobeying Allah is one of the causes of Allah's Wrath and of loss of blessings and withholding of rain and being overtaken by the enemy, disease. Allah sends hardship to get you in the right track. And if it doesn't break you, it makes you stronger and better person.

Allah, the Exalted, says:

"And it may be that you dislike a thing which is good for you and that you like a thing which is bad for you. Allah knows but you do not know." (Qur'an, Al-Baqarah 2:216)

Through the trials and tribulations, we learn more, we become stronger and careful and if we seek the help of our Creator, being patient, then, the trials and tribulations will bring only benefits.
It is Allah's Wisdom, his servant endures the temporary trials of this world instead of eternal punishment in the Hereafter with the accumulated sins.

"And Allah will save those who feared Him by their attainment; no evil will touch them, nor will they grieve." (Qur'an, Az-Zumar 39:61)

Such remedy is created to protect one's faith and devotion, to expel through purgation the negative effects of a corrupt mind and spirit, and to bring forth the original intended purity. **The bitter taste of this life will bring the sweet taste of the Hereafter if the person follows the Qur'an and Sunnah, and patient.** For the Muslim, every pain is an expiation of sins and any test is a blessing in disguise!

Jabir narrated: The Prophet (peace and blessings of Allah be upon him) said: "On the Day of Judgment, when the people who were tried (in this world) are given their rewards, the people who were pardoned (in life), will wish that their skins had been cut off with scissors while they were in the world." (Tirmidhi)

And the opposite is true too; the sweet taste of this life projects a bitter end in the Hereafter.

Anas bin Malik narrated that the Messenger of Allah (peace and blessings of Allah be upon him) said: "Whoever makes the Hereafter his goal, Allah makes his heart rich, and organizes his affairs, and the world comes to him whether it wants to or not. And whoever makes the world his goal, Allah puts his poverty right before his eyes, and disorganizes his affairs, and the world does not come to him, except what has been decreed for him." (Tirmidhi)

ALLAH SEND DOWN THE DISEASES FOR THREE REASONS

I. Disease is a Test
II. Disease is an Expiation of Sins
III. Disease is a Punishment

Calamity can be a test and expiation of sins at the same time.

I. Disease Is A Test

Allah, the Exalted, says:

"Do people think that they will be left alone because they say: 'We believe,' and will not be tested. And We indeed tested those who were before them. And Allah will certainly make (it) known (the truth of) those who are true, and will certainly make (it) known (the falsehood of) those who are liars, (although Allah knows all that before putting them to test)." (Qur'an, Al-'Ankabut 29:2-3)

"We shall certainly test you, until We ascertain those of you who (sincerely) strive and those who are steadfast (in Allah's Religion); and We shall test your affairs (to distinguish the liars from the truthful)." (Qur'an, Muhammad 47:31)

1.1. Story of the Prophet Ayub

The Prophet Ayub (May Allah have mercy on him) was a humble man of great piety, constantly glorifying and devoutly thanking his Lord. Allah, the Exalted, tested his faith, gratitude and patience by sending the Devil to remove his health, wealth and children. But Ayub remained firm and continued to glorify his Lord, patient and grateful. Then, after many years, in his suffering, the Prophet Ayub cried to Allah.

"And remember Our slave Ayub (Job), when he invoked his Lord (saying): "Verily! Shaitan (Satan) has touched me with distress (by losing my health) and torment (by losing my wealth)!" (Qur'an, Sad 38:41)

"And (remember) Ayub (Job), when he cried to his Lord: "Verily, distress has seized me, and You are the Most Merciful of all those who show mercy." (Qur'an, Al-Anbya 21:83)

Allah, the Exalted, answered his Du'a and removed the Devil by the Negative Ions (spring water):

"So, We answered his call, and We removed the distress that was on him, and We restored his family to him (that he had lost), and the like thereof along with them, as a mercy from Ourselves and a Reminder for all who worship Us." (Qur'an, Al-Anbya 21:84)

"(Allah said to him): "Strike the ground with your foot: This is a spring of water to wash in, cool and a (refreshing) drink." (Qur'an, Sad 38:42)

1.2. Story of the Sheikh Abd al Aziz ibn Abdullah Ibn Baaz

His father died when he was only three. By the time he was thirteen, he had begun working. When he was sixteen, he started losing his eyesight. By the time he was twenty, he had totally lost his sight and had become blind. Ibn Baaz wrote more than sixty works. He was a Judge, Grand Mufti of Saudi Arabia, President of the Constituent Assembly of the Muslim World League.

Narrated Anas bin Malik (May Allah have mercy on him): "I heard Allah's Apostle (peace and blessings be upon him) saying, "Allah said, 'If I deprive my slave of his two beloved things (i.e. his eyes) and he remains patient, I will let him enter Paradise in compensation for them.'" (Bukhari)

Abu Qatadah (May Allah have mercy on him) reported: The Prophet (peace and blessings be upon him) said, "Verily, you will never leave anything for the sake of Allah Almighty but that Allah will replace it with something better for you." (Ahmad)

1.3. Story of Three Men from the Children of Israel: a Leper, a Bald-headed and a Blind

Allah, the Exalted, says:

"and We shall make a trial of you with evil and with good. And to Us you will be returned." (Qur'an, Al-Anbya 21:35)

Abu Hurairah (May Allah be pleased with him) reported that he heard the Prophet (May Allah's peace and blessings be upon him) say: ''There were three (men) from the Children of Israel: a leper, a bald-headed and a blind. Allah wanted to test them, so He sent to them an angel. The angel went to the leper and said: 'Which thing do you like most?' He said: 'A good color, fine skin, and to get rid of what makes me disgusting in the eyes of people.' He wiped over his body, so his illness went away and he was given a good color and fine skin. He (the angel) said: 'Which wealth do you like most?' He said: 'Camels, or cows (the sub-narrator Is'hāq was in doubt).' So, he was given a she-camel in an advanced stage of pregnancy, and he (the angel) said: 'May Allah bless it for you.' Then he went to the bald-headed man and said: 'Which thing do you like most?' He said: 'Good hair, and to get rid of what makes me disgusting in the eyes of people.' He wiped over his head, so his condition went away and he was given good hair. Then the angel said: 'Which wealth do you like most?' He said: 'Cows or camels.' So, he was given a pregnant cow and the angel said: 'May Allah bless it for you.' Then he went to the blind man and said: 'Which thing do you like most?' He said: 'That Allah restores to me my eyesight so that I can see people.' He wiped over his eyes, so Allah restored to him his eyesight. Then the angel said: 'Which wealth do you like most?' He said: 'Sheep.' So, he was given a pregnant ewe. The three then had offspring from the ones given to them: one had a valley of camels, the second a valley of cows, and the third a valley of sheep. Later, the angel went to the leper in his (past) appearance and said: 'I am a poor person, and I am running out of provision in my journey, so I cannot reach my destination except with the help of Allah and then your favor. I ask you by the One Who gave you good color, fine skin and wealth to give me one camel to carry me in my journey.' He said: 'I have many rights to fulfill.' Thereupon, he (the angel) said: 'It seems to me that I know you. Were you not a leper whom people found disgusting, and a poor man then Allah gave you wealth?' He said: 'I have inherited this wealth from my forefathers.' Thereupon, the angel said: 'If you are lying, may Allah change you to your past condition.' He then went in his (past) appearance to the bald-headed man and said to him the same as what he had said to the leper, and he replied to him in the same way the leper did. So, the angel said: 'If you are lying, may Allah change you to your past condition.' Then he went in his (past) appearance to the blind man and said: 'I am a poor man and a wayfarer. My provisions have run short in my journey, and today there is no way to reach my destination except with the help of Allah and then with your help. So, I ask you by the One Who restored to you your eyesight to give me one sheep by which I should be able to make provisions for the journey.' The man said: 'I was blind and Allah restored to me my eyesight. You may take whatever you like and leave whatever you like. By Allah, I shall not stand in your way today for what you take in the Name of Allah.' Thereupon, the angel said: 'Keep your property. The fact is that the three of you were put to test. Now, Allah is pleased with you and is displeased with your two companions.'" (Bukhari and Muslim) (https://hadeethenc.com/en/browse/hadith/5926)

1.4. Testing According to one's Faith

Abu Hurairah (May Allah be pleased with him) reported that the Prophet (May Allah's peace and blessings be upon him) said: "If Allah wills good for someone, He makes him suffer affliction."
(Bukhari) (https://hadeethenc.com/en/browse/hadith/4204)

Anas (May Allah be pleased with him) reported: The Messenger of Allah (May Allah's peace and blessings be upon him) said: ''If Allah willed to do good to His slave, He expedites his punishment in the life of this world, and if He willed to do ill to His slave, He withholds the punishment for his sins until He comes with all his sins on the Day of Resurrection."
(Tirmidhi) (https://hadeethenc.com/en/browse/hadith/3332)

Narrated Anas bin Malik: The Messenger of Allah (peace and blessings be upon him) said: "The greatest reward comes with the greatest trial. When Allah loves a people, He tests them. Whoever accepts, that wins His Pleasure but whoever is discontent with that, earns His Wrath." (Ibn Majah)

Narrated Musab bin Saad that his father, Saad bin Abu Waqqas, said: "I said: 'O Messenger of Allah, which people are most severely tested?' He said: 'The Prophets, then the next best and the next best. A person is tested according to his religious commitment. If he is steadfast in his religious commitment, he will be tested more severely, and if he is frail in his religious commitment, his test will be according to his commitment. Trials will continue to afflict a person until they leave him walking on the earth with no sin on him.'" (Ibn Majah)

Narrated Aisha (May Allah be pleased with her): "I never saw anybody suffering so much from sickness as Allah's Messenger (peace and blessings be upon him)." (Bukhari)

Suhaib reported: The Messenger of Allah (peace and blessings be upon him) said: "Strange are the ways of a believer for there is good in every affair of his and this is not the case with anyone else except in the case of a believer for if he has an occasion to feel delight, he thanks (God), thus there is a good for him in it, and if he gets into trouble and shows resignation (and endures it patiently), there is a good for him in it." (Muslim)

Ibn al-Qayyim (May Allah have mercy on him) gave the following precious advice in his valuable book Zad Al-Ma'ad:

1) If a person looks at what has befallen him, he will find that what his Lord has left for him is similar to it or better than it, and if he is patient and accepts it, He has stored up for him something that is many times greater than what he has lost through this calamity, and if He willed, He could have made the calamity even greater.

2) The fire of calamity can be extinguished by thinking of those who have been hit even harder. If you laugh a little, you will weep a lot, and if you are happy for a day, you will be miserable for a lifetime, and if you have what you want for a little while, you will be deprived for a long time. There is no day of happiness but it is followed by a day of pain.

3) It should be noted that panicking will not make the calamity go away, and in fact, it makes it worse.

4) It should be noted that missing out on the reward for patience and surrender, which is mercy and guidance that Allah has granted as the reward for patience and turning to Him by saying, *Inna Lillaahi wa inna ilayhi raaji'oon* (Verily to Allah we belong and unto Him is our return) is worse than the calamity itself.

5) It should be noted that panicking makes one's enemy rejoice and makes one's friend feel sad; it makes Allah angry and makes the Shaytan happy; it destroys reward and weakens resolve. If he is patient, seeks reward, strives to please Allah, to make his friend happy and to make his enemy sad, and seeks to relieve his brothers of their burdens and to console them before they console him, this is steadfastness and a sign of perfection – not slapping one's cheeks, rending one's garment, wishing for death and being discontent with the Divine Decree.

6) It should be noted that what comes after being patient and seeking reward is pleasure and joy that is many times greater than what he could have got from keeping what he lost. Sufficient for him is the "house of praise" that will be built for him in Paradise as a reward for his praising his Lord and turning to Him (by saying *Inna Lillaahi wa inna ilayhi raaji'oon* (Verily to Allah we belong and unto Him is our return)). So, let him decide which of the two calamities is greater: a calamity in this world or the calamity of missing out on the house of praise in eternal Paradise.

Narrated Jabir: The Prophet (peace and blessings be upon him) said: "On the Day of Judgment, when the people who were tried (in this world) are given their rewards, the people who were pardoned (in life), will wish that their skins had been cut off with scissors while they were in the world." (Tirmidhi)

One of the salaf said:

"Were it not for the calamities of this world, we would come empty-handed on the Day of Resurrection."

7) It should be noted that the One Who is testing him is the Most Wise and the Most Merciful, and that He, may He be Glorified, did not send this calamity in order to destroy him or cause him pain, or finish him off, rather He is checking on him, testing his patience, acceptance and faith; it is so that He may hear his Du'a and supplication, so that He may see him standing before Him, seeking protection, filled with humility and complaining to Him.

8) It should be noted that were it not for the trials and tribulations of this world, a person could develop arrogance, self-admiration, a pharaonic attitude and hardheartedness which would lead to his doom in this world and in the Hereafter. It is a sign of the Mercy of the Most Merciful that He checks on him from time to time with the remedy of calamity, so as to protect him from these diseases, to keep his submission and servitude sound, and to eliminate all bad elements that may lead to his doom. Glory be to the One Who shows mercy by means of testing, and tests by means of blessing.

9) It should be noted that the bitterness of this world is the essence of sweetness in the Hereafter, as Allah will turn the former into the latter. Similarly, the sweetness of this world is the essence of bitterness in the Hereafter. It is better to move from temporary bitterness to eternal sweetness than the other way round. (7)

Anas b. Malik reported: "The Paradise is surrounded by hardships and the Hellfire is surrounded by temptations." (Muslim)

The patient believer will come to know that his adversity became many blessings.

Allah, the Exalted, says:

"You may dislike something although it is good for you, or like something, although it is bad for you." (Qur'an, Al-Baqarah 2:216)

"For indeed, with hardship (will be) ease." (Qur'an, Ash-Sharh 94:5)

1.5. Martyr will be in Paradise

A Shahid (Martyr) is considered one whose place in Paradise is promised:

From the Qur'an:

"And never think of those who have been killed in the cause of Allah as dead. Rather, they are alive with their Lord, receiving provision, Rejoicing in what Allah has bestowed upon them of His bounty, and they receive good tidings about those (to be martyred) after them who have not yet joined them - that there will be no fear concerning them, nor will they grieve." (Qur'an, Ali 'Imran 3:169-170)

"Verily, Allah has purchased of the believers their lives and their properties; for the price that theirs shall be the Paradise. They fight in Allah's Cause, so they kill (others) and are killed. It is a promise in truth which is binding on Him in the Tawrat (Torah) and the Injeel (Gospel) and the Quran. And who is truer to his covenant than Allah? Then rejoice in the bargain which you have concluded. That is the supreme success." (Qur'an, At-Tawbah 9:111)

"Those who emigrated in the Cause of Allah and after that were killed or died, surely, Allah will provide a good provision for them. And verily, it is Allah Who indeed is the Best of those who make provision. Truly, He will make them enter an entrance with which they shall be well-pleased, and verily, Allah indeed is All-Knowing, Most Forbearing." (Qur'an, Hajj 22:58-59)

From the Hadith:

1. Narrated Abu Hurairah: Allah's Messenger (peace and blessings be upon him) said, "Five are regarded as martyrs: They are those who die because of Plague, Abdominal disease, drowning or a falling building etc., and the martyrs in Allah's Cause." (Bukhari)
2. Narrated Abu Hurairah: The Messenger of Allah (peace and blessings be upon him) said: "Whom do you consider to be a martyr among you?" They (the Companions) said: 'Messenger of Allah, one who is slain in the way of Allah is a martyr.' He said: 'Then (if this is the definition of a martyr) the martyrs of my Umma will be small in number.' They asked: 'Messenger of Allah, who are they?' He said: 'One who is slain in the way of Allah is a martyr; one who dies in the way of Allah, is a

martyr; one who dies of Plague is a martyr; one who dies of Cholera is a martyr.' Ibn Miqsam said: 'I testify the truth of your father's statement (with regard to this tradition) that the Prophet (peace and blessings be upon him) said: 'One who is drowned is a martyr.'" (Muslim)
3. Narrated Abu Hurairah: The Prophet (peace and blessings be upon him) said, "He (a Muslim) who dies of an Abdominal disease is a martyr, and he who dies of Plague is a martyr." (Bukhari)
4. Narrated Aisha: "I asked Allah's Messenger (peace and blessings be upon him) about the Plague. He said, "That was a means of torture which Allah used to send upon whomsoever He wished, but He made it a source of Mercy for the believers, for anyone who is residing in a town in which this disease is present, and remains there and does not leave that town, but has patience and hopes for Allah's reward, and knows that nothing will befall him except what Allah has written for him, then he will get such reward as that of a martyr." (Bukhari)

    Narrated Abu Hurairah: "I heard Allah's Messenger (peace and blessings be upon him) saying "By Him in Whose Hands my life is! Were it not for some men who dislike to be left behind and for whom I do not have means of conveyance, I would not stay away (from any Holy Battle), I would love to be martyred in Allah's Cause and come to life and then get, martyred and then come to life and then get martyred and then get resurrected and then get martyred." (Bukhari)
5. Narrated Anas b. Malik that the Messenger of Allah (peace and blessings of Allah be upon him) said: "Who seeks martyrdom with sincerity shall get its reward, though he may not achieve it." (Muslim)
6. Narrated Anas bin Malik: The Prophet (peace and blessings be upon him) said: "Nobody who enters Paradise likes to go back to the world even if he got everything on the earth, except a Mujahid who wishes to return to the world so that he may be martyred ten times because of the dignity he receives (from Allah)." (Bukhari)

II. Disease is an Expiation of Sins

Allah, the Exalted, says:

"…whosoever works evil, will have the recompense thereof, and he will not find any protector or helper besides Allah." (Qur'an, An-Nisa 4:123)

"And verily, We will make them taste of the near torment (i.e. the torment in the life of this world, i.e. disasters, calamities, etc.) prior to the supreme torment (in the Hereafter), in order that they may (repent and) return (i.e. accept Islam)." (Qur'an, As-Sajdah 32:21)

"…and whoever shall incline therein to wrong unjustly, We will make him taste of a painful chastisement." (Qur'an, Al-Hajj 22:25)

Other Verse: Ar-Rum 30:41.

Universal Law of "Cause and Effect" and "Action and Reaction"

Sins (disobedience to God) cause diseases, calamities, disasters, hardships, difficulties (effect).

Abdullah ibn 'Abbas (May Allah be pleased with him) reported that the Prophet (May Allah's peace and blessings be upon him) visited a Bedouin while he was sick, and whenever he visited a sick person he would say: "No harm, it will be purification from sins if Allah wills." (Bukhari) (https://hadeethenc.com/en/browse/hadith/6009)

Narrated Abu Sa`id Al-Khudri and Abu Hurairah (May Allah be pleased with them): The Prophet (peace and blessings be upon him) said, "No fatigue, nor disease, nor sorrow, nor sadness, nor hurt, nor distress befalls a Muslim, even if it were the prick he receives from a thorn, but that Allah expiates some of his sins for that." (Bukhari) (https://hadeethenc.com/en/browse/hadith/3701)

Narrated 'Abdullah: "I visited Allah's Apostle while he was suffering from a high fever. I said, "O Allah's Apostle! You have a high fever." He said, "Yes, I have as much fever as two men of you." I said, "Is it because you will have a double reward?" He said, "Yes, it is so. No Muslim is afflicted with any harm, even if it were the prick of a thorn, but that Allah expiates his sins because of that, as a tree sheds its leaves." (Bukhari)

Epidemics are the Jinn Possession because of Humanity's Sins

Abu Musa (May Allah be pleased with him) reported that the Messenger of Allah (May Allah's peace and blessings be upon him) said: "The death of my Ummah is by stabbing and the Plague." It was said: "O Messenger of Allah, as for stabbing, we know it, but what is the Plague?" He said: "Jabbing by your enemies from among the Jinn. In both cases, there are martyrs." (Ahmad) (https://hadeethenc.com/en/browse/hadith/10568)

Aisha (May Allah be pleased with her) reported that she asked the Messenger of Allah (May Allah's peace and blessings be upon him) about the Plague. He told her that it was a torment that Allah would send upon whom He willed. Then Allah made it a mercy for the believers, so anyone in an area afflicted with Plague who stays therein patiently hoping for Allah's reward and believing that nothing will befall him except what Allah has foreordained for him will get a reward similar to that of a martyr." (Bukhari) (https://hadeethenc.com/en/browse/hadith/3161)

Narrated Abdullah bin Umar: The Messenger of Allah (peace and blessings be upon him) said: "O Muhajirun, there are five things with which you will be tested, and I seek refuge with Allah lest you live to see them: Immorality never appears among a people to such an extent that they commit it openly, but Plagues and Diseases that were never known among the predecessors will spread among them.

They do not cheat in weights and measures but they will be stricken with famine, severe calamity and the oppression of their rulers. They do not withhold the Zakah of their wealth, but rain will be withheld from the sky, and were it not for the animals, no rain would fall on them. They do not break their covenant with Allah and His Messenger, but Allah will enable their enemies to overpower them and take some of what is in their hands. Unless their leaders rule according to the Book of Allah and seek all good from that which Allah has revealed, Allah will cause them to fight one another." (Ibn Majah)

Disease is a Wake-Up Call

Allah by sending calamities remind people the purpose of human creation which is to worship Him.

Allah, the Exalted, says:

"And verily, We will make them taste the near torment (i.e. the torment in the life of this world, i.e. disasters, calamities, etc.) prior to the supreme torment (in the Hereafter), in order that they may (repent and) return (i.e. accept Islam)." (Qur'an, As-Sajdah 32:21)

Disease is a Blessing for the Disbelievers if they Repent

Allah, the Exalted, says:

"And those who invoke not any other ilah (god) along with Allah, nor kill such person as Allah has forbidden, except for just cause, nor commit illegal sexual intercourse and whoever does this shall receive the punishment. The torment will be doubled to him on the Day of Resurrection, and he will abide therein in disgrace; Except those who repent and believe (in Islamic Monotheism), and do righteous deeds; for those, Allah will change their sins into good deeds, and Allah is Oft-Forgiving, Most Merciful. And whosoever repents and does righteous good deeds; then verily, he repents towards Allah with true repentance." (Qur'an, Al-Furqan 25:68-71)

Abu Hurairah reported Allah's Messenger (peace be upon him) as saying: "Allah, the Exalted and Glorious, said: 'I live in the thought of My servant and I am with him as he remembers Me.' (The Holy Prophet) further said: 'By Allah, Allah is more pleased with the repentance of His servant than what one of you would do on finding the lost camel in the waterless desert.' 'When he draws near Me by the span of his hand. I draw near him by the length of a cubit and when he draws near Me by the length of a cubit. I draw near him by the length of a fathom and when he draws near Me walking, I draw close to him hurriedly." (Muslim)

Narrated Abdullah b. Masud that some people said to the Messenger of Allah (peace and blessings be upon him): "Messenger of Allah, would we be held responsible for our deeds committed in the state of ignorance (before embracing Islam)?" Upon this, he (the Holy Prophet) remarked: 'He who amongst you performed good deeds in Islam, he would not be held responsible for them (misdeeds which he committed in ignorance) and he who committed evil (even after embracing Islam) would be held responsible or his misdeeds that he committed in the state of ignorance as well as in that of Islam." (Muslim)

Narrated Ibn Shamasa Mahri: "We went to Amr b. al-As and he was about to die. He wept for a long time and turned his face towards the wall. His son said: 'Did the Messenger of Allah (peace be upon him not give you tidings of this? Did the Messenger of Allah (peace be upon him) not give you tidings of this?' He (the narrator) said: 'He turned his face (towards the audience) and said: 'The best thing which we can count upon is the testimony that there is no god but Allah and that Muhammad is the Apostle of Allah. Verily I have passed through three phases. (The first one) in which I found myself averse to none else more than I was averse to the Messenger of Allah (peace be upon him) and there was no other desire stronger in me than the one that I should overpower him and kill him. Had I died in this state, I would have been definitely one of the denizens of Fire.' He (the Holy Prophet) observed: 'Are you not aware of the fact that Islam wipes out all the previous (misdeeds)? Verily migration wipes out all the previous (misdeeds), and verily the pilgrimage wipes out all the (previous) misdeeds…'" (Muslim)

Narrated Ibn 'Abbas that some people amongst the polytheist had committed a large number of murders and had excessively indulged in fornication. Then they came to Muhammad (peace be upon him) and said: 'Whatever you assert and whatever you call to is indeed good. But if you inform us that there is atonement of our past deeds (then we would embrace Islam). Then it was revealed:
"And those who invoke not any other ilah (god) along with Allah, nor kill such life as Allah has forbidden, except for just cause, nor commit illegal sexual intercourse and whoever does this shall receive the punishment. The torment will be doubled to him on the Day of Resurrection, and he will abide therein in disgrace; Except those who repent and believe (in Islamic Monotheism), and do righteous deeds, for those, Allah will change their sins into good deeds, and Allah is Oft-Forgiving, Most Merciful." (Qur'an, Al-Furqan 25:68-70) "Say: "O 'Ibadi (My slaves) who have transgressed against themselves (by committing evil deeds and sins)! Despair not of the Mercy of Allah, verily Allah forgives all sins. Truly, He is Oft-Forgiving, Most Merciful." (Qur'an, Az-Zumar 39:53) (Muslim)

The new Muslim convert is being given the opportunity to have all of his previous sins converted into good deeds while possibly still being rewarded for good that he did before embracing Islam. This is part of Allah's Grace and Mercy. It is conditional though. The convert must take his Islam seriously, practice it properly and be a true Muslim while keeping himself from falling into the evils that he practiced before. If he somehow allows himself to fall back into his evil practices of old, he then loses a great opportunity that Allah has graciously offered him. (8)

Narrated Ibn Abbas (May Allah be pleased with him): The Messenger of Allah (peace and blessings of Allah be upon him) has related from his Lord: "Verily Allah, the Exalted, has written down the good deeds and the evil deeds, and then explained it (by saying): "Whosoever intended to perform a good deed, but did not do it, then Allah writes it down with Himself as a complete good deed. And if he intended to perform it and then did perform it, then Allah writes it down with Himself as from ten good deeds up to seven hundred times, up to many times multiplied. And if he intended to perform an evil deed, but did not do it, then Allah writes it down with Himself as a complete good deed. And if he intended it (i.e.

the evil deed) and then performed it, then Allah writes it down as one evil deed." (Bukhari and Muslim)

Allah, the Exalted, says:

"And whatsoever blessing you have, it is from Allah ..." (Qur'an, An-Nahl 16:53)

When they succeed at work, school or career, they think that it is because of their super intelligence, physical capacity, power. To humble the arrogant person, Allah, out of Mercy, put hardship, so they may come back to Allah.

This Temporary Life is Imperfect and the Enjoyment of Delusion

Allah, the Exalted, says:

"And the worldly life is not but amusement and diversion but the home of Hereafter is best for those who fear Allah. Will you not then reason?" (Qur'an, Al-An'am 6:32)

If you are looking for any perfection, whether a perfect health, job, spouse or husband, children… you are not going to find any of these things in this deluded world.

Narrated Mujahid: 'Abdullah bin 'Umar said, "Allah's Messenger (peace and blessings be upon him) took hold of my shoulder and said, 'Be in this world as if you were a stranger or a traveler.' The sub-narrator added: Ibn 'Umar used to say, "If you survive till the evening, do not expect to be alive in the morning, and if you survive till the morning, do not expect to be alive in the evening, and take from your health for your sickness, and (take) from your life for your death." (Bukhari)

Allah the Almighty created this temporary world only to pass the tests (faith, patience, morality, manners…) and attain the perfection in Paradise. This life is not meant to be perfect for relaxation. In this life we should struggle to attain our permanent residence in Paradise made from gold. For Muslims who follow the Glorious Qur'an and Sunnah, Allah prepared eternal Paradise, a peaceful, lovely place, with perfect weather. Muslims in Paradise wear gold, pearls, diamonds and garments made of the finest silk, and they recline on raised thrones. In Paradise, there is no hatred, jealousy, temptation, pain, sorrow, fatigue or death—there is only joy, happiness and pleasure. Allah promised the righteous the Garden of Paradise—where the trees are without thorns, where flowers and fruits are piled on top of each other, where clear and cool water flows constantly, and where companions have big, beautiful eyes. Where everything is free and *"There will circulate among them (servant) boys (especially) for them, as if they were pearls well-protected."* (Qur'an, At-Tur 52:24)

III. Disease is a Punishment

Allah, the Exalted, says:

"See they not that they are tried once or twice every year (with different kinds of calamities, disease, famine, etc.)? Yet, they turn not in repentance, nor do they learn a lesson (from it)." (Qur'an, At-Tawbah 9:126)

"Go to Fir'aun (Pharaoh), verily, he has transgressed all bounds (in crimes, sins, polytheism, disbelief, etc.)." (Qur'an, An-Nazi'at 79:17)

"And if the people of the towns had believed and had the Taqwa (piety), certainly We should have opened for them blessings from the heaven and the earth, but they belied (the Messengers). So, We took them (with punishment) for what they used to earn (polytheism and crimes, etc.)." (Qur'an, Al-A'raf 7:96)

Other Verses: *Al-'Ankabut 29:40, Ar-Ra'd 13:14 and 13:33-34, Al-Mu'minun 23:76, Al-An'am 6:43, Al-A'raf 7:130, 7:133 and 7:136.*

Calamity for the rebellious disbelievers cannot be to raise him in status, because the kaafir will have no weight before Allah on the Day of Resurrection. But there may be a lesson and a reminder for others in that, not to do what he did. And it may be an immediate punishment for him in this world, in addition to what is stored up for him in the Hereafter.

Table 1. Disease is a Test, Expiation of Sins or Punishment

SINS cause		
Diseases, Calamities, Disasters, Hardships		
Pious Muslims (Strict Qur'an and Sunnah)	Muslims committing Sins	Disbelievers (All non-Muslims)
Calamity is a Test to Raise Status if patient (e.g. The Prophet Ayub)	Calamity is a Blessing as expiates Sins and Raise of Status for many.	Calamity is Wake Up Call: 1. Calamity is Blessing if Repentance 2. Calamity is Punishment if Persistence with Sins

DISEASES ARE CAUSED BY POSITIVE IONS

Diseases are caused by Positive Ions:

1. Diseases caused by Decreased Oxygen Utilization
2. Diseases caused by Evil Jinn (Demons)

1. Diseases caused by Decreased Oxygen Utilization

Positive Ions

Positive Ions (Cautions) are formed by losing an electron. Positive Ions cause diseases, infertility, sick building syndrome, fatigue, headache, lack of energy, poor concentration, low immunity, sleep disorder, etc. Positive Ions are abundant in cities, industrial areas and produced by air conditioning, electrical (artificial lights, signboards, microwave, etc.) and electronic (internet, laptop, television, phone, etc.) devices, building and furniture materials, paint, carpets, upholstery, smoking, unhealthy environment, lifestyle, food and drinks, medications, medical devices, etc.
The Prophet Muhammad didn't recommend medical treatment in the diseases caused by Decreased Oxygen Utilization.

Hadith of Black Woman of Paradise

Abdullah ibn 'Abbas (May Allah be pleased with them said to 'Ata' ibn Abi Rabah: "Shall I show you a woman of the people of Paradise?" 'Ata' said: 'Yes.' He said: "This black woman came to the Messenger of Allah (May Allah's peace and blessings be upon him) and said: 'I suffer from Epilepsy and, as a result, my body becomes uncovered. So, please supplicate to Allah for me.' The Messenger of Allah (May Allah's peace and blessings be upon him) said to her: 'If you wish, be patient and you will enter Paradise; or, if you wish, I will supplicate to Allah to cure you.' She said: 'I will remain patient.' She then said: 'But I become uncovered, so please invoke Allah that I do not become uncovered.' So, he supplicated for her." (Bukhari and Muslim) (https://hadeethenc.com/en/browse/hadith/3160)

2. Diseases caused by Evil Jinn (Demons)

95% of diseases are caused by the Evil Jinn. Almighty Allah gave me this knowledge and confirmed by answering to my Istikhara prayer and Du'a.

Here are the proofs from the Noble Qur'an and Ahadith.

From the Qur'an:

"And remember Our slave Ayub (Job), when he invoked his Lord (saying): "Verily! Shaitan (Satan) has touched me with distress (by losing my health) and torment (by losing my wealth)!" (Qur'an, Sad 38:41)

"Shall I inform you (O people!) upon whom the Shayateen (Devils) descend? They descend on every lying (one who tells lies), sinful person." (Qur'an, Ash-Shu'ara 26:221)

"When the disbelievers listen to you reciting the Qur'an, they almost try to destroy you with their piercing eyes. Then they say, "He is certainly insane." (Qur'an, Al-Qalam 68:51-52)

The Verse refers to an Evil Eye. This meant that they want to make Muhammad sick and die with a special kind of look. It also suggests that the Verse is a metonymy for 'very angry glances', as they looked very furiously as if they wanted to kill Muhammad. (9)

Other Verses: Al-Baqarah 2:275, Al-Anbya 21:35, Al-Furqan 25:19, Al-Anfal 8:11, Al-Falaq 113:5, An-Nas 114:4-6, Taha 20:124, Ash-Shu'ara 26:227, Maryam 19:83, Az-Zukhruf 43:36, Al-A'raf 7:27, Al-Kahf 18:63.

From Ahadith:

1. Hadith on Disease: Seek refuge in Allah from physical, mental illness

Anas reported: The Prophet (peace and blessings be upon him) would say, "O Allah, I seek refuge in You from leprosy, madness, degenerative diseases and evil sicknesses." (Abu Dawud) (https://www.abuaminaelias.com/dailyhadithonline/2020/03/01/refuge-physical-mental-illness)

2. Narrated Aisha (May Allah be pleased with her): "When the Messenger of Allah (peace and blessings be upon him) came to a sick person, he would make supplication for him, and would say: Adhhibil-bas, Rabban-nas, washfi Antash-Shafi, la shifa'a illa shifa'uka shifa'an la yughadiru saqama (Take away the pain, O Lord of mankind, and grant healing, for You are the Healer, and there is no healing but Your healing that leaves no trace of sickness)." (Ibn Majah)

3. "Aisha reported that when Allah's Messenger (peace and blessings be upon him) fell ill, he recited over his body Mu'awwidhatan and blew over him and when his sickness was aggravated, I used to recite over him and rub him with his band with the hope that it was more blessed." (Muslim)

4. Aisha (May Allah be pleased with her) said, "If one of his family fell sick, the Messenger of Allah (peace and blessings be upon him) would blow over him and recite al Mu'awwidhaat (the three Quls)." (Bukhari and Muslim)

5. Narrated Umm Salama: "The Prophet (peace and blessings be upon him) saw in her house a girl whose face had a black spot. He said. "She is under the effect of an Evil Eye; so, treat her with a Ruqyah." (Bukhari)

6. Narrated Ash-Shifa', daughter of Abdullah: "The Messenger of Allah (peace and blessings be upon him) entered when I was with Hafsah, and he said to me: "Why do you not teach this one the spell for skin eruptions as you taught her writing." (Abu Dawud)

7. "There was an old woman who used to enter upon us and perform Ruqyah from Erysipelas: Contagious disease which causes fever and leaves a red coloration of the skin…" (Ibn Majah)

8. The Prophet (peace and blessings be upon him) used to seek refuge for al-Hasan and al-Husayn and say: "I seek refuge for you both in the perfect Words of Allah, from every Devil and every poisonous reptile, and from every Evil Eye)." (Tirmidhi, Abu Dawud. And he would say, "Thus Ibrahim used to seek refuge with Allah for Ishaq and Ismail, peace be upon them both." (Bukhari)

9. Epidemics are the Jinn Possession diseases because of Humanity's Sins

Abu Musa (May Allah be pleased with him) reported that the Messenger of Allah (May Allah's peace and blessings be upon him) said: "The death of my Ummah is by stabbing and the Plague." It was said: "O Messenger of Allah, as for stabbing, we know it, but what is the Plague?" He said: "Jabbing by your enemies from among the Jinn. In both cases, there are martyrs." (Ahmad)

The Messenger of Allah (peace and blessings be upon him) said: "The Plague is a calamity (or a punishment) that was sent upon the Children of Israel, or upon those who came before you. If you hear of it in some land, do not go there, and if it breaks out in a land where you are, do not leave, fleeing from it." (Bukhari and Muslim)

The word Taa'oon (translated as Plague) is also refers to any widespread disease (Epidemic) that spreads quickly and leads to the death of many people.

Al-Nawawi said in Sharh Saheeh Muslim:

"Taa'oon (plague) refers to boils that appear on the body. As for waba' (Epidemic), al-Khaleel and others said that it refers to the Plague. Others said that it refers to any widespread disease. The correct view, as noted by the scholars, is that it is any sickness that affects many people in one part of the land, but not all of it; differs from ordinary diseases in the large number of people affected and in other ways; and where they are all affected by the same kind of sickness, unlike at other times, when people suffer from different kinds of sickness." (Muslim)

10. Abu Sa'id reported: "The Messenger of Allah (peace and blessings be upon him) would seek refuge from Jinn and the Evil Eye of man, until the two chapters of refuge were revealed, Surahs Al-Falaq and An-Nas. After they were revealed, he took both of them and left everything else." (Tirmidhi)

Wathilah Ibn al-Asqa (May Allah be pleased with him) said: "A man complained of throat pain to the Messenger of Allah (peace and blessings of Allah be upon him) and he said to him: 'Recite the Qur'an upon yourself." (Bayhaqi)

11. Talha Ibn Masrif said: "It is said that indeed when the Qur'an is recited near a patient, he/she finds recovery." I visited Khaythamah when he was ill and I said: "I see that you are absolutely well today!". He said: "The Qur'an has been recited on me (i.e. it is through its blessings)." (Bayhaqi)

12. Satan causes Watering Eye

Narrated Zainab: "…and my eye began to water on the side nearest him. When I recited Ruqyah for it, it stopped, but if I did not recite Ruqyah it watered again.' He said: 'That is Satan, if you obey him, he leaves you alone but if you disobey him, he pokes you with his finger in your eye. But if you do what the Messenger of Allah (peace and blessings be upon him) used to do, that will be better for you and more effective in healing. Sprinkle water in your eye and say: Adhhibil-bas Rabban-nas, washfi Antash-Shafi, la shifa'a illa shafi'uka, shafi'an la yughadiru saqaman (Take away the pain, O Lord of mankind, and grant healing, for You are the Healer, and there is no healing but Your healing that leaves no trace of sickness)." (Ibn Majah) (https://sunnah.com/urn/1275750)

13. Evil Eye

Yahya related to me from Malik that Muhammad ibn Abi Umama ibn Sahl ibn Hunayf heard his father say, "My father, Sahl ibn Hunayf did a Ghusl at al-Kharrar. He removed the jubbah he had on while Amir ibn Rabia was watching, and Sahl was a man with beautiful white skin. Amir said to him, 'I have never seen anything like what I have seen today, not even the skin of a virgin.' Sahl fell ill on the spot, and his condition grew worse. Somebody went to the Messenger of Allah (peace and blessings be upon him) and told him that Sahl was ill, and could not go with him. The Messenger of Allah (peace and blessings be upon him) came to him, and Sahl told him what had happened with Amir. The Messenger of Allah, (peace and blessings be upon him) said, 'Why does one of you kill his brother? Why did you not say, "May Allah bless you?" (ta baraka-llah) The Evil Eye is true. Do Wudu from it.' Amir did

Wudu from it and Sahl went with the Messenger of Allah (peace and blessings be upon him) and there was nothing wrong with him." (https://sunnah.com/urn/417730)

14. Jinn Possessed Boy/Epilepsy

"Ya'la ibn Murah said: "I saw Allah's Messenger (peace and blessings be upon him) do three things which no one before or after me saw. I went with him on a trip. On the way, we passed by a woman sitting at the roadside with a young boy. She called out, "O Messenger of Allah, this boy is afflicted with a trial, and from him we have also been afflicted with a trial. I don't know how many times per day he is seized by fits." He (peace and blessings be upon him) said: "Give him to me." So, she lifted him up to the Prophet. He (peace and blessings be upon him) then placed the boy between himself and the middle of the saddle, opened the boy's mouth and blew in it three times, saying, "In the Name of Allah, I am the slave of Allah, get out, enemy of Allah!" Then he gave the boy back to her and said: 'Meet us on our return at this same place and inform us how he has managed." We then went. On our return, we found her in the same place with three sheep. When he said to her, "How has your son fared?" She replied: 'By the One who sent you with the truth, we have not detected anything (unusual) in his behavior up to this time..." (Ahmad vol.4, p.170, and al-Hakim, who declared it authentic, in Ibn Kathir's Al bidaya wal nihaya vol.6, p.146)

15. Hadith: Aphasia by Jinn Possession

Narrated Umm Jundub: "I saw the Messenger of Allah (peace and blessings be upon him) stoning the 'Aqabah Pillar from the bottom of the valley on the Day of Sacrifice, then he went away. A woman from Khath'am followed him, and with her was a son of hers who had been afflicted, he could not speak. She said: 'O Messenger of Allah! This is my son, and he is all I have left of my family. He has been afflicted and cannot speak.' The Messenger of Allah (peace be upon him) said: 'Bring me some water.' So, it was brought, and he washed his hands and rinsed out his mouth. Then he gave it to her and said: 'Give him some to drink, and pour some over him, and seek Allah's healing for him.'" She (Umm Jundub) said: "I met that woman and said: 'Why don't you give me some?' She said: 'It is only for the sick one.' I met that woman one year later and asked her about the boy. She said: 'He recovered and became (very) smart." (Ibn Majah) (https://sunnah.com/ibnmajah:3532)

16. Nine-tenths of sorceries by rebellious Jinn causing diseases which doctors cannot cure

Malik related to me that he heard that Umar ibn al-Khattab wanted to go to Iraq, and Kab al-Ahbar said to him, "Do not go there, amir al-muminin. There is nine-tenths of sorceries there and it is the place of the rebellious Jinn and the disease which the doctors are unable to cure." (Malik's Muwatta)

17. Sorcery - Black Magic - caused by Devils

Narrated Aisha: "Magic was worked on Allah's Messenger (peace and blessings be upon him) so that he used to think that he had sexual relations with his wives while he actually had not (Sufyan said: 'That is the hardest kind of Magic as it has such an effect'). Then one day he said, "O Aisha do you know that Allah has instructed me concerning the matter I asked Him about? Two men came to me and one of them sat near my head and the other sat near my feet. my head asked the other: 'What is wrong with this man?' The latter replied: 'he is under the effect of Magic.' The first one asked: 'Who has worked Magic on him?' The other replied: 'Labid bin Al-A'sam, a man from Bani Zuraiq who was an ally of the Jews and was a hypocrite.' The first one asked, 'What material did he use?' The other replied, 'A comb and the hair stuck to it.' The first one asked: 'Where (is that)?' The other replied: 'In a skin of pollen of a male date palm tree kept under a stone in the well of Dharwan.' So, the Prophet (peace and blessings be upon him) went to that well and took out those things and said: "That was the well which was shown to me (in a dream), Its water looked like the infusion of Henna leaves and its date-palm trees looked like the heads of Devils.' The Prophet (peace be upon him) added: 'Then that thing was taken out.' I said (to the Prophet, peace be upon him): 'Why do you not treat yourself with Nashra?' He said, 'Allah has cured me; I dislike to let evil spread among my people.'" (Bukhari)

18. Abu Umamah said he heard Allah's Messenger (peace and blessings be upon him) say: "Recite the Qur'an, for on the Day of Resurrection it will come as an intercessor for those who recite It. Recite the two bright ones, Al-Baqarah and Surah Ali 'Imran, for on the Day of Resurrection they will come as two clouds or two shades, or two flocks of birds in the ranks, pleading for those who recite them. Recite Surah Al-Baqarah, for to take recourse to it is a blessing and to give it up is a cause of grief, and the magicians cannot confront it." (Mu'awiya said: It has been conveyed to me that here Batala means magicians.) (Muslim)

19. Satan causes Blood Clots – many diseases!

Anas ibn Malik (May Allah be pleased with him) reported: Jibreel came to the Messenger of Allah (May Allah's peace and blessings be upon him) while he was playing with his playmates. He took hold of him, laid him on the ground, split open his chest, took the heart out and then extracted a **blood clot** out of it and said: "That was **the Devil's share** in you." Then he washed it with Zamzam water in a golden basin and then joined the wounded parts together after he restored the heart to its place. The boys came running to his mother, i.e. his wet nurse, and said: "Muhammad has been killed." They rushed to him and found his color was changed. Anas said: "I used to see the scar of this stitching on his chest." (Muslim)

20. The newborn child is attacked by Satan at birth

Narrated Zuhri with the same chain of transmitters (and the words are): "The newborn child is touched by the Satan (when he comes in the world) and he starts crying because of the touch of Satan." (Muslim)

21. Satan will not harm your child if you say this Du'a before the intercourse

Narrated Ibn 'Abbas: The Prophet (peace and blessings be upon him) said, "If anyone of you, on having sexual relationship with his wife, says: 'O Allah! Protect me from Satan, and prevent Satan from approaching the offspring you are going to give me,' and if it happens that the lady conceives a child, Satan will neither harm it nor be given power over it. (Bukhari)

22. The child cries when Satan pricks him

Abu Hurairah reported Allah's Messenger (peace and blessings be upon him) as saying: "The crying of the child (starts) when the Satan begins to prick him." (Muslim)

23. Keep your children close to you at sunset for the Devils spread out at that time

Narrated Jabir bin 'Abdullah: Allah's Messenger (peace and blessings be upon him) said, "When night falls (or it is evening), keep your children close to you for the Devils spread out at that time. But when an hour of the night elapses, you can let them free. Close the doors and mention the Name of Allah, for Satan does not open a closed door." (Bukhari)

24. Whenever a man is alone with a woman the Devil makes a third

Umar reported the Prophet (peace and blessings be upon him) as saying, "Whenever a man is alone with a woman the Devil makes a third." (Tirmidhi)

25. The Devil flows in a man like his blood

Anas reported God's Messenger (peace and blessings be upon him) as saying, "The Devil flows in a man like his blood." (Bukhari and Muslim)

26. The Devils among the Jinn and mankind

Narrated Abu Dharr: "I entered the Masjid and the Messenger of Allah (peace and blessings be upon him) was there, so I came and sat before him and he said: 'O Abu Dharr, seek refuge with Allah from the evils of the Devils among the Jinn and mankind.' I said: 'Are there Devils among mankind?' He said: 'Yes.'" (An-Nasa'i)

27. Nightmares and bad dreams are from Satan

Narrated Abu Qatada: The Prophet (peace be upon him) said, "A good dream that comes true is from Allah, and a bad dream is from Satan, so if anyone of you sees a bad dream, he should seek refuge with Allah from Satan and should spit on the left, for the bad dream will not harm him." (Bukhari)

28. Afflictions from Satan

Narrated Salim's father: The Prophet (peace and blessings be upon him) stood up beside the pulpit (and pointed with his finger towards the east) and said, "Afflictions are there!

Afflictions are there, from where the side of the head of Satan comes out" or said, "the side of the sun." (Bukhari)

29. Anger is from Satan

'Atiyyah reported: The Messenger of Allah (peace be and blessings be upon him) said, **"Verily, anger comes from Satan…"** (Abu Dawud) (https://sunnah.com/abudawud:4784)

30. Satan runs away from the house in which Surah Baqarah is recited

Abu Hurairah (May Allah be pleased with him) reported that the Messenger of Allah (May Allah's peace and blessings be upon him) said: "Do not turn your houses into graves. Indeed, Satan runs away from the house in which Surah Al-Baqarah is recited." (Muslim) (https://hadeethenc.com/en/browse/hadith/6208)

31. Reciting ten Verses from Surah Al-Baqarah at Night – The Shaytan will not enter the house that evening until the morning. When recited over a mentally ill person, he will be recovered

Narrated Abdullah bin Masud (May Allah be pleased with him): "Whoever recites ten Verses from Surah Al-Baqarah at night time the Shaytan will not enter the house that evening until the morning, (also) the first four verses of Surah Al-Baqarah, Ayatul Kursi and the two Verses after it, in addition to the three last Verses of Surah Al-Baqarah beginning with: *"…To Allah belongs what is in the heavens…"* (al-Darimi)
And in another narration: "…Shaytan or anything he dislikes will not come near him nor his family that day, and it is not recited over a mentally ill person except that he will recover from his illness." *Tabarani related it in his Kabeer, and al-Haythami said in his Majma': "The men of this narration are the narrators of the Saheeh except that ash-Sha'bee did not hear directly from Ibn Masud." (https://authentic-dua.com/2011/11/19/reciting-ten-verses-from-soorat-ul-baqarah)

32. Devils live in the toilets - seek refuge in Allah from male and female Devils

Narrated Zayd Ibn Arqam: The Messenger of Allah (peace and blessings be upon him) said: "These privies are frequented by the Jinns and Devils. So, when anyone amongst you goes there, he should say: 'I seek refuge in Allah from male and female Devils." (Abu Dawud)

33. Satan is present with any one of you in everything he does
Jabir reported: "I heard Allah's Apostle (peace and blessings be upon him) as saying: 'The Satan is present with any one of you in everything he does; he is present even when he eats food; so if any one of you drops a mouthful he should remove away anything filthy on it and eat it and not leave for the devil; and when he finishes (food) he should lick his fingers, for he does not know in what portion of his food the blessing lies.'" (Muslim) (https://sunnah.com/muslim:2033d)

Hippocrates and Jinn (Demonic) Possession

Hippocrates, the father of western medicine, described the Jinn (Demonic) Possession. Hippocrates didn't recommend medical treatment in diseases caused by Evil Jinn.

"And I see men become mad and demented from no manifest cause, and at the same time doing many things out of place; and I have known many persons in sleep groaning and crying out, some in a state of suffocation, some jumping up and fleeing out of doors, and deprived of their reason until they awaken, and afterward becoming well and rational as before, although they be pale and weak; and this will happen not once but frequently." (On the Sacred Disease (Classics Revisited), https://www.proquest.com/docview/1500818590)

Ibn Taymiyah (May Allah hve mercy on him) said:

"It is well known that Hippocrates was reported to have said the following with regard to certain potions. "It is useful for convulsions. I do not mean the type treated by temple priests, but I mean the convulsions treated by doctors." (10)

Prophet Jesus and Jinn (Demonic) Possession

Jesus, Allah's Messenger, made the connection "sins cause diseases" in the stories of two men paralyzed by Jinn Possession because of sins in Bethesda and Capernaum. (11, 12)

The exorcism of a boy possessed by a Demon, or a boy with a mute spirit, is one of the miracles attributed to Jesus. (13)
Jesus is surrounded by a crowd, one of whom asks for help for his son, who 'has a spirit that makes him unable to speak'. He explains that the spirit makes him foam at the mouth, grind his teeth, and become rigid. He tells Jesus that he had asked the disciples to cure the boy, but they had been unable to do so. Jesus responds by describing the crowd and his followers as a 'faithless generation'.
When he is brought to Jesus, the boy immediately experiences an epileptic seizure. Jesus asks the boy's father how long this has affected the child; the father replies that this had been since his childhood and asks Jesus to help if he can. Jesus tells him that everything is possible to one who believes, and the man responds, 'I believe; help my unbelief!'

Jesus emphasized the importance of faith in Allah, the One Who cures, and avoidance of sins.

"Then Jesus rebuked the demon, and it came out of the boy, and he was healed from that moment. Afterward the disciples came to Jesus privately and asked, "Why couldn't we drive it out?"
"Because you have so little faith," He answered. "For truly I tell you, if you have faith the size of a mustard seed, you can say to this mountain, 'Move from here to there', and it will move. Nothing will be impossible for you..." (Matthew 18-20)

"When the disciples of Jesus asked him (Jesus) how to cast the evil spirits away, he (Jesus) is reported to have said, *"But this kind never comes out except by prayer and fasting." (Matthew 17:21)*

All miracles which Jesus did, in fact, were performed by Almighty Allah.

Prophet Muhammad and Jinn (Demonic) Possession

The Prophet Muhammad didn't recommend medical treatment in diseases caused by Evil Jinn.

Hadith: Epilepsy by Jinn Possession

"Ya'la ibn Murah said: 'I saw Allah's Messenger (peace and blessings be upon him) do three things which no one before or after me saw. I went with him on a trip. On the way, we passed by a woman sitting at the roadside with a young boy. She called out, 'O Messenger of Allah, this boy is afflicted with a trial, and from him we have also been afflicted with a trial. I don't know how many times per day he is seized by fits.' He (peace and blessings be upon him) said: 'Give him to me.' So, she lifted him up to the Prophet. He (peace and blessings be upon him) then placed the boy between himself and the middle of the saddle, opened the boy's mouth and blew in it three times, saying, 'In the Name of Allah, I am the slave of Allah, get out, enemy of Allah!' Then he gave the boy back to her and said: 'Meet us on our return at this same place and inform us how he has managed.' We then went. On our return, we found her in the same place with three sheeps. When he said to her, 'How has your son fared?' She replied: 'By the One Who sent you with the truth, we have not detected anything (unusual) in his behavior up to this time… '" (Ahmad vol.4, p.170, and al-Haakim, who declared it authentic, in Ibn Kathir's Al bidaya wal nihaya vol.6, p.146)

Hadith: Aphasia by Jinn Possession

Narrated Umm Jundub: "I saw the Messenger of Allah (peace and blessings be upon him) stoning the 'Aqabah Pillar from the bottom of the valley on the Day of Sacrifice, then he went away. A woman from Khath'am followed him, and with her was a son of hers who had been afflicted, he could not speak. She said: 'O Messenger of Allah! This is my son, and he is all I have left of my family. He has been afflicted and cannot speak.' The Messenger of Allah (peace be upon him) said: 'Bring me some water.' So, it was brought, and he washed his hands and rinsed out his mouth. Then he gave it to her and said: 'Give him some to drink, and pour some over him, and seek Allah's healing for him.'" She (Umm Jundub) said: "I met that woman and said: 'Why don't you give me some?' She said: 'It is only for the sick one.' I met that woman one year later and asked her about the boy. She said: 'He recovered and became (very) smart.'" (Ibn Majah) (https://sunnah.com/ibnmajah:3532)

Hadith: Epidemics are Jinn Possession because of Sins

Abu Musa (May Allah be pleased with him) reported that the Messenger of Allah (May Allah's peace and blessings be upon him) said: "The death of my Ummah is by stabbing and the Plague." It was said: "O Messenger of Allah, as for stabbing, we know it, but what is the Plague?" He said: "Jabbing by your enemies from among the Jinn. In both cases, there are martyrs." (Ahmad)
(https://hadeethenc.com/en/browse/hadith/10568)

Ibn Taymiyah's Essay on Jinn (Demons) treatise provides a very clear, concise and authentic view of this intriguing and sinister world of Jinn based on the Qur'an, the Sunnah, the interpretation and experience of the Sahabah (companions of the Prophet and the early scholars of Islam). (10)

Jinn Possession Reasons

Allah, the Exalted, says:

"Surely, Shaitan (Satan) is an enemy to you, so take (treat) him as an enemy. He only invites his Hizb (followers) that they may become the dwellers of the blazing Fire." *(Qur'an, Fatir 35:6)*

The Jinn Possession is widespread.

Table. 2 JINN POSSESSION REASONS

		JINN POSSESSION REASONS
1	DESIRE	Desire of Power, Desire of Control of human life Attraction or Love
2	REVENGE	When unintentionally harming Jinn throwing hot water, stone, jumping, urinating on them or even killing)
3	JINN ARE EVIL	Create discomfort, mischief, harm, confusion
4	SINS	*"And whoever among you does wrong, We shall make him taste a great torment." (Qur'an, Al-Furqan 25:19)*
5	MISGUIDANCE	*"Then I will come to them from before them and behind them, from their right and from their left, and You will not find most of them as thankful ones (i.e. they will not be dutiful to You)." (Qur'an, Al-A'raf 7:17)*
6	SORCERY	Jinn Possession by Black Magic
7	EVIL EYE	Evil Eye is caused by Jealousy and/or Admiration
8	MAN WEAKNESS	Extreme Anger, Fear, Sadness and Ecstasy

WHY DO SINLESS CHILDREN SUFFER?

Allah, the Exalted, says:

"And know that your possessions and your children are but a trial and that surely with Allah is a mighty reward." (Qur'an, Al-Anfal 8:28)

"Allah does not charge a soul except (with that within) its capacity." (Qur'an, Al-Baqarah 2:155)

"Surely! Allah wrongs not even of the weight of an atom (or a small ant), but if there is any good (done), He doubles it, and gives from Him a great reward." (Qur'an, An-Nisa 4:40)

Other Verse: *Al-A'raf 7:156.*

Usama ibn Zayd ibn Harithah (May Allah be pleased with him) reported: The Prophet's daughter sent for him to come over because her son was dying. The Prophet (May Allah's peace and blessings be upon him) sent her the greeting of peace and this message: "To Allah belongs what He takes, and to Him belongs what He gives, and for everything He sets a specific term. So, she should have patience and seek the reward from Allah." She sent back urging him to come to her. So, he, along with Sa'd ibn 'Ubadah, Mu'adh ibn Jabal, Ubayy ibn Ka'b, Zayd ibn Thabit and other men (May Allah be pleased with them) went. The boy was given to the Messenger of Allah (May Allah's peace and blessings be upon him) and his breath was disturbed in his chest, which made the eyes of the Messenger of Allah overflow with tears. Thereupon, Sa'd said: "O Messenger of Allah, what is that?" He said: "That is mercy which Allah, the Exalted, puts in the hearts of His slaves." In another version: "In the hearts of those He wills of His slaves. Indeed, Allah is Merciful only to those of His slaves who are merciful." (Bukhari and Muslim)
(https://hadeethenc.com/en/browse/hadith/3290)

Abu Musa al-Ashari reported: The Messenger of Allah (peace and blessings be upon him) said, "When the child of a servant dies, Allah says to the angels: 'Have you taken the life of My servant's child?' They say: "Yes.' Allah says: 'Have you taken the fruit of his heart?' They say: 'Yes.' Allah says: 'What has My servant said?' They say: 'He has praised You and said: 'To Allah we belong and to Allah we return.' Allah says: "Build a house for My servant in Paradise and name it the House of Praise." (Tirmidhi)

Abu Ad-Darda' 'Uwaymir (May Allah be pleased with him) reported that the Prophet (May Allah's peace and blessings be upon him) said: "Help me seek the weak ones, for you are being granted victory and sustenance only because of your weak ones." (Tirmidhi) (https://hadeethenc.com/en/browse/hadith/3367)

Allah, the Exalted, says:

"…and whatsoever you spend of anything (in Allah's Cause), He will replace it. And He is the Best of providers." (Qur'an, Saba 34:39)

Narrated Aisha (May Allah be pleased with her) that the Prophet (peace and blessings be upon him) said: "The pen has been lifted from three: from the sleeper until he wakes up, from the minor until he grows up, and from the insane until he comes back to his senses or recovers." (An-Nasa'i)

Undoubtedly, in Allah's allowing children to suffer there is great wisdom which may be hidden from some people, thus they object to the Divine Decree and the Shaytan takes advantage of this issue to turn him away from the truth and right guidance.

Among the reasons why children suffer are the following:

1 - Free will: You get what you choose

Allah, the Exalted, says:

"Have you not considered those who exchanged the Favor of Allah for disbelief and settled their people (in) the home of ruin?" (Qur'an, Ibrahim 14:28)

When parents choose Satan as their lord, they choose to walk away from Allah's Kingdom. They remove their families from Allah's Protection *(Qur'an, 14:28)* and place it in Satan's care. Satan's incompetence guarantees large number of people remain in suffering. Satan's incompetence as a god ensures that evil, bloodshed and misery are spread through the earth. *(Qur'an, 2:30)*.

Free will is a double-edged sword. You get what you choose.

Should the parent's choices affect their children (for better or for worse)?

If people choose God's Kingdom and Protection and worship Him Alone, they can be assured of protection from harm and suffering night and day. If the people choose disbelief and transgression of Allah's Laws, the children suffer.

Allah, the Exalted, says:

"Whoever works righteousness, whether male or female, while he (or she) is a true believer (of Islamic Monotheism) verily, to him We will give a good life (in this world with respect, contentment and lawful provision), and We shall pay them certainly a reward in proportion to the best of what they used to do (i.e. Paradise in the Hereafter). So, when you want to recite the Qur'an, seek refuge with Allah from Shaitan (Satan), the outcast (the cursed one). Verily! He has no power over those who believe and put their trust only in their Lord (Allah). His power is only over those who obey and follow him (Satan), and those who join partners with Him (Allah) [i.e. those who are Mushrikun - polytheists - see Verse 6:121]." (Qur'an, An-Nahl 16:97-100)

"For each (person), there are angels in succession, before and behind him. They guard him by the Command of Allah. Verily! Allah will not change the good condition of a people as long as they do not change their state of goodness themselves (by committing sins and by being ungrateful and disobedient to Allah). But when Allah wills a people's punishment, there can be no turning back of it, and they will find besides Him no protector." (Qur'an, Ar-R'ad 13:11)

And of guaranteed Happiness, now and forever*.
"No doubt! Verily, the Auliya' of Allah [i.e. those who believe in the Oneness of Allah and fear Allah much (abstain from all kinds of sins and evil deeds which he has forbidden), and love Allah much (perform all kinds of good deeds which He has ordained)], no fear shall come upon them nor shall they grieve. Those who believed (in the Oneness of Allah - Islamic Monotheism), and used to fear Allah much (by abstaining from evil deeds and sins and by doing righteous deeds). For them are glad tidings, in the life of the present world (i.e. righteous dream seen by the person himself or shown to others), and in the Hereafter. No change can there be in the Words of Allah, this is indeed the supreme success." (Qur'an, Yunus 10:62-64)

*Happiness: Now and Forever**

*10:62-64 Most people think that they have to wait until the Day of Resurrection before they receive their rewards for righteousness or the retribution for wickedness. But the Qur'an repeatedly assures the believers that they are guaranteed perfect Happiness here in this world, now and forever. At the end of their interim here, they go directly to Paradise. (14)

2 - Learning lessons: the family of this child may be committing prohibited actions and neglecting obligatory duties, but when they see the suffering of their child, that prompts them to give up those haram actions such as not praying, consuming riba, alcohol, committing zina, smoking, especially if the child's suffering is due to an illness that they caused, as happens in the case of some of the haram things mentioned above.

3 - Thinking about the Hereafter, for there is no true happiness and peace except in Paradise; there is no suffering and pain there, only good health, well-being and happiness. And thinking about Hell, for that is the abode of eternal and never-ending pain and suffering.

So, one will do that which will bring him nearer to Paradise and take him further away from Hell.

4 - Mentally disabled people

One of the basic principles of Islam is to believe in the Wisdom of the Lord in what He creates and commands, and in what He wills and decrees, in the sense that He does not create anything in vain and He does not decree anything in which there is not some benefit for His slaves. So, everything that exists is His Will and Decree. Allah, the Exalted, says:

"Allah is the Creator of all things." *(Qur'an, Ar-Ra'd 13:16)*

His perfect Wisdom decrees that He creates opposites, so He has created Angels and Devils, night and day, purity and impurity, good and ugly, and He has created good and evil. He created His slaves with differences in their bodies and minds, and in their strengths. He has made some rich and some poor, some healthy and some sickly, some wise and some foolish. By His Wisdom, He tests them, and He tests some by means of others, to show who will be grateful and who will be ungrateful.

Allah, the Exalted, says:

"Verily, We have created man from Nutfah (drops) of mixed semen (sexual discharge of man and woman), in order to try him, so We made him hearer and seer. Verily, We showed him the way, whether he be grateful or ungrateful." *(Qur'an, Al-Insan 76:2)*

"Who has created death and life that He may test you which of you is best in deed." *(Qur'an, Al-Mulk 67:2)*

When the sound believer sees disabled people, he recognizes the blessing that Allah has bestowed upon him, so he gives thanks for His blessing, and he asks Him for good health. He knows that Allah is Able to do all things. People are incapable of comprehending Allah's Wisdom. He, Glorified and Exalted be He, cannot be questioned as to what He does, while they will be questioned. Whatever you understand of His Wisdom, believe in it, and whatever you cannot understand, say, "Allah knows best, and we know nothing except that which He have taught us, and He is the All-Knowing, Most Wise." (15)

Caring about disabled person is your chance to earn Paradise. (16, 17)

5 - Allah creates a child then causes him to die, perhaps if that child lived, he would have committed Major sins such as those that doom a person to Hell, and that would have condemned him to remain in Hell for eternity, or for a very long time, or he may have caused others such as his parents to deviate from the Path of Allah – as mentioned in the story of the boy whom al-Khidr killed, as told in the story of al-Khidr and Moosa in the Surah Al-Kahf. Alternatively, if this child lives, he may face such difficulties that in his case death is a Mercy from Allah.

Allah, the Exalted, says:

"And as for the boy, his parents were believers, and we feared that he would overburden them by transgression and disbelief." (Qur'an, Al-Kahf 18:80)

"So, we intended that their Lord should substitute for them one better than him in purity and nearer to mercy." (Qur'an, Al-Kahf 18:81)

Al-Nawawi (May Allah have mercy on him) said:

"The reliable Muslim scholars agreed that any Muslim child who dies, will be among the people of Paradise, because he was not responsible (i.e. had not yet reached the age of account). (Sharh Muslim, 16/207) (18)

6 - If Allah creates a child handicapped, perhaps this handicap will prevent him from committing many sins which, if he did them, would lead to his being punished on the Day of Resurrection.

7 - It is a means to show that the child is sick or in pain.

Ibn Qayyim al-Jawziyyah (May Allah have mercy on him) said:

"These pains are one of the inherent features of man's development from which no man or animal can be free. If man were free of pain, he would not be a man, rather he would be an angel or some other creature. Children's pain is not more difficult than the pain experienced by grownups, but grownups have become accustomed to pain so it is no longer a big issue for them. What a great difference there is between what a child suffers and what a rational adult suffers. All of that is one of the main aspects of the human condition. If man were not created like that, he would be a different creature. What do you think if a child gets hungry or thirsty, or cold, or tired – is it something that he was singled out for and tested with that the grownups are not tested with? Man – and indeed animals – have been created on this basis. They said: "If someone were to ask: Why has man been created thus? Why was he not created without this vulnerability to pain and suffering? This is a flawed question, because Allah has created him in a world of trials from a weak substance. So, he is vulnerable to diseases and suffering, and Allah has created him in such a way that he is vulnerable to all kinds of pain… The fact that these pains and pleasures coexist is one of the signs of the Hereafter, for Divine Wisdom has decreed that there should be two abodes: an abode that is devoted fully to pleasure, in which there is no pain at all, and an abode that is devoted fully to pain in which there is no pleasure at all. The former abode is Paradise and the latter abode is Hell." (Miftaah Daar al-Sa'aadah, 2/230, 231) (18, 19)

8 - The crying that is caused by the pain brings great benefits to the child's body.

Ibn Qayyim al-Jawziyyah (May Allah have mercy on him) said:

"Then think about the Wisdom of Allah in causing children to cry a lot, and the benefits that that brings to them. The doctors and naturalists have attested to the benefits of that and the wisdom behind it. They said: There is moisture in children's brains which, if it were to remain in their brains, would cause a great deal of harm. So, crying draws that moisture out and drains it from their brains, which makes them stronger and healthier. Moreover, crying and yelling widens the breathing passages and veins, and strengthens them, and it strengthens the nerves. How greatly do children benefit from the crying and yelling that we hear from them. If this is the wisdom with regard to crying that is caused by pain and the wisdom behind this never crossed your mind, the same applies to the suffering of children and its causes and good consequences. There is a great deal of wisdom that may be hidden from most of the people and they are greatly confused about it." (Miftaah Daar al-Sa'aadah, 2/228) (19)

9 - Children can be afflicted by the Evil Jinn (Jinn Possession, Sorcery, Evil Eye).

Ibn Taymiyah (May Allah have mercy on him) said:

"The occasional possession of man by the Jinn may be due to sensual desires on the part of the Jinn, capricious whims or even love, just as it may be among humans. Jinn and humans may also have intercourse with each other and beget children.

Many monks and nuns of medieval Europe reported that they were visited and ravished by voluptuous female Demons which were officially called Succubi and equally seductive and alluring fallen angels called incubi. Subsequently, many nuns became pregnant and killed their children at birth, burying them outside the nunneries." (10)

10 -Calamity may be a Mercy from Allah

The calamities that befall those who are innocent, and indeed happen to all people, and are not necessarily a punishment, rather they may be Mercy from Allah. (19)

The fate of Muslim children - if they die after the soul has been breathed in and before reaching puberty - is Paradise, as an Honor from Allah, may He be Exalted, to them and their parents and as a Mercy from Him, Whose Mercy encompasses all things. (20)

When Allah deprives a person of a certain physical ability or cause an illness, He, Almighty, will compensate him for it, by bestowing upon him some other gifts in a greater measure. Or He will compensate him in the Hereafter. Most assuredly, He will reward the Muslim in the Hereafter for all the hardships, pain and diseases he suffered in this world. Those who were not tested in this world, may wish that they had suffered calamities when they see the high status attained by those who bore calamities with patience.

The measures for protecting children from the accursed Satan

Before Conception

Narrated Ibn 'Abbas (May Allah be pleased with him): The Prophet (peace and blessings be upon him) said, "If anyone of you, when having sexual intercourse with his wife, says: Bismillah, Allahumma jannibni-Sh-Shaitan wa jannib-ish-Shaitan ma razaqtana (In the Name of Allah. O Allah, keep the Shaytan away from us and keep the Shaytan away from what You have blessed us with.) and if it is destined that they should have a child, then Satan will never be able to harm him." (Bukhari)

'Aqeeqah on the 7th day after the birth as a protection from Satan

Samurah (May Allah be pleased with him) reported that the Messenger of Allah (May Allah's peace and blessings be upon him) said: "A child is held in pledge for his 'Aqeeqah which should be slaughtered on his behalf on the seventh day after his birth, and he should be given a name, and his head should be shaved." (Ibn Majah, Abu Dawud) (https://hadeethenc.com/en/browse/hadith/64668)

Righteous Parents – Protected Children

Father should strive hard to obey Allah, the Most High, and obey His Messenger (peace and blessings of Allah be upon him) in word and deed, to fear Allah, may He be Glorified and Exalted, in secret and in public, and to seek halal earnings, whilst constantly remembering Allah and reading or reciting Qur'an. All of that will guarantee - by the Grace of Allah - that a person himself and his wife and children will be protected.

Narrated Ibn 'Abbas (May Allah be pleased with him) said, concerning the Verse in which Allah says: *"and their father was a righteous man." (Al-Kahf 18:82)*: They were protected because their father was righteous; there is no mention of whether his children were righteous. (classed by al-Hakim as Saheeh according to the conditions of al-Bukhari and Muslim; adh-Dhahabi agreed with him)

Ibn Kathir (May Allah have mercy on him) said:

"The words (interpretation of the meaning), *"and their father was a righteous man." (Al-Kahf 18:82)* indicate that the progeny of a righteous man will be protected, and the barakah (blessing) of his worship will benefit them in this world and the Hereafter, and by virtue of his intercession for them, they will be raised to the highest degrees in Paradise so that he may have the joy of the company, as it says in the Qur'an and is mentioned in the Sunnah." (End quote. Tafsir Ibn Kathir (5/186-187) (21)

Supplication (Du'a) is a means of protecting children

Allah, the Exalted, says:

"And those who say: 'Our Lord! Bestow on us wives and offspring who will be the comfort of our eyes, and make us leaders for the Muttaqoon (pious).'" (Qur'an, Al-Furqan 25:74)

Ruqyah is a means of protecting children

Narrated Ibn 'Abbas: The Prophet (peace and blessings be upon him) used to seek refuge with Allah for Al-Hasan and Al-Husain and say: "Your forefather (i.e. Abraham) used to seek refuge with Allah for Ishmael and Isaac by reciting the following: 'O Allah! I seek refuge with Your Perfect Words from every Devil and from poisonous pests and from every Evil, harmful, Envious Eye.'" (Bukhari)

Children should be prevented from going out after sunset

Narrated Jabir ibn 'Abdullah (May Allah be pleased with him) that the Prophet (peace and blessings of Allah be upon him) said: "When the wings of the night spread - or when evening comes - keep your children in, for the Devils come out at that time. Then when part of the night has passed, let them go. And close the doors and mention the Name of Allah, for the Shaytan does not open a closed door. And tie up your waterskins and mention the Name of Allah, and cover your vessels and mention the Name of Allah, even if you only put something over them, and extinguish your lamps." (Bukhari and Muslim)

Early teaching of the Qur'an and Sunnah for Protection from the Jinn

Children should say "Bismillah" before entering home, eating and drinking, dressing and undressing going under the tree, throwing hot water, stone or jump, before doing anything. They should know the Du'a before entering toilet, etc. They should learn the Du'as for the protection in the morning, evening and before sleeping. Should learn the Quranic Verses for the protection. (22, 23)

Children are accountable for their deeds from the puberty

Narrated Abdullah ibn Amr ibn al-'As: The Messenger of Allah (peace and blessings be upon him) said: "Command your children to pray when they become seven years old, and beat them for it (prayer) when they become ten years old; and arrange their beds (to sleep) separately." (Abu Dawud)

TYPES OF SINS

1. Against Allah, the Creator of the Universe
2. Ascribing a Partner or Rival to Allah
3. Any other religion (including Atheism) than Islam
4. Against Allah's Prophets
5. Against Ahl-Bayt
6. Against the Companions of the Prophet Muhammad
7. Innovations in Religion of Islam (Bid'ah)
8. Against Muslims
9. Against Humanity
10. Against Parents
11. Disrespect of Rulings on Marriage, Divorce, Family Life
12. Inheritance Laws
13. Against Neighbours
14. Preoccupation with the Worldly Life
15. Desires, Lust, Immorality
16. Lying and Listening to lies
17. Sins of the Tongue
18. Forbidden Business Transactions
19. Malpractices of Traders and Commercial organizations
20. Unlawful Clothing for men and women
21. Wanton Display of one's Beauty
22. Bad Manners and Behavior
23. Unlawful (Haram) Food and Income
24. Consumption of Haram
25. Music, Musical Instruments, Singing, Dancing
26. Celebrations of all Festivities except Al-Firt and Al-Adha
27. Wasting Allah's money
28. Strike, Democracy, Freedom
29. Injustice
30. Not Forbiding Evil
31. Disrespect of Islamic Rules of War
32. Against Animals and other Allah's Creations
33. Against Natural Environment
34. Sorcery, Fortune telling, Divination, Horoscope, Astrology, Superstition
35. Sport as a Profession (Football, Boxing, Fighting sports, etc.)
36. All kinds of games (chess, dice, duels, etc.)

37. Medicine Not Following the Qur'an and Prophetic Medicine
38. Vaccination
39. Disbelief in Destiny
40. Disbelief in Judgment Day
41. Disbelief in Paradise and Hellfire
42. Disrespect of Allah's commands and prohibitions in the Qur'an and Sunnah

MAJOR AND MINOR SINS

Allah, the Exalted, says:

"Those who break Allah's Covenant after ratifying it, and sever what Allah has ordered to be joined (as regards Allah's Religion of Islamic Monotheism, and to practice its legal Laws on the earth and also as regards keeping good relations with kith and kin), and do mischief on earth, it is they who are the losers." (Qur'an, Al-Baqarah 2:27)

"Whoever seeks as religion other than Islam, (which is the standard Religion conveyed by all the Prophets during history, and is based on complete submission to God, Allah) it will never be accepted from him, and in the Hereafter, he will be among the losers." (Qur'an, Ali 'Imran 3:85)

The Glorious Qur'an clarifies that Haram (unlawful) is harmful. Sins are acts which have been forbidden by Allah in the Qur'an and Sunnah. When God says "Do not", He means "do not hurt yourself". Anything that leads to it is also considered a Haram act. The sin is not limited to the person who engages in the prohibited activity, but the sin also extends to others who support the person in the sinful activity.
Allah, the Exalted, says:

"...whoever follows My Guidance shall neither go astray, nor fall into distress and misery." (Qur'an, Taha 20:163)

The person does an action and he will receive the fruit of this action, be it bitter or sweet.

Abu Hurairah reported: The Messenger of Allah (peace and blessings be upon him) said, "When the believer commits sin, a black spot appears on his heart. If he repents and gives up that sin and seeks forgiveness, his heart will be polished. But if (the sin) increases, (the black spot) increases. That is the Ran that Allah mentions in His Book: *"Nay! But on their hearts is the covering of sins which they used to earn." (Qur'an, Al-Mutaffifin 83:14)* (Ibn Majah)

Narrated Malik: Abdullah Ibn Masud used to say, "The slave continues to lie and a black spot grows in his heart until all his heart becomes black. Then he is written, in Allah's sight, among the liars." (Malik Muwatta)

Narrated An-Numan bin Bashir: "I heard Allah's Apostle (peace and blessings be upon him) saying, "…Beware! There is a piece of flesh in the body if it becomes good (reformed), the whole body becomes good but if it gets spoilt, the whole body gets spoilt and that is the heart." (Bukhari)

MAJOR SINS

Allah, the Exalted, says:

"Verily, Allah forgives not that partners should be set up with him in worship, but He forgives except that (anything else) to whom He pleases, and whoever sets up partners with Allah in worship, he has indeed invented a tremendous sin." (Qur'an, An-Nisa 4:48)

Every sin is a disobedience to Allah, the Creator.
Major sins are those acts which have been forbidden by Almighty Allah in the Qur'an and by His Messenger (peace and blessings be upon him); they are subject to a Curse, Divine Wrath or warning of Hell.

MINOR SINS

Minor sins are those actions, which displease Allah, the Exalted, for which there is no Hadd punishment in this world and no warning of punishment in the Hereafter, except when they are not repeated or done in certain circumstances.

WHEN MINOR SIN BECOMES MAJOR SIN AND SHIRK

Narrated Aisha (May Allah be pleased with her): "The Messenger of Allah (peace and blessings be upon him) said to me: 'O Aisha, beware of (evil) deeds that are regarded as insignificant, for they have a pursuer from Allah (i.e. accountability)." (Ibn Majah)

Abdullah ibn Masud reported: The Messenger of Allah, peace and blessings be upon him, said, "Beware of Minor sins. Verily, they pile upon a man until he is ruined." (Ahmad)

Narrated Sahl ibn Sa`d (May Allah be pleased with him): The Messenger of Allah (peace and blessings be upon him) said: "Beware of Minor sins, like a people who camped in the bottom of a valley, and one man brought a stick, another brought a stick, and so on, until they managed to bake their bread. There are some insignificant sins which, once (they accumulate) and a person is questioned about them, they lead to his doom." (Ahmad)

Ibn Taymiyah (May Allah have mercy on him) said:

"Adultery is a Major sin, but looking and touching are lamam (Minor sins) which may be forgiven if one avoids Major sin. But if a person persists in looking or touching, that becomes a Major sin, and persisting in that may be worse than a small amount of Major sin, for persisting in looking with desire, along with the connected feelings of mixing and touching, may be much worse than the evil of an isolated act of Zina. Hence the fuqaha' said concerning the witness of good character: he does not commit a Major sin or persist in a Minor sin… Indeed, looking and touching may lead a man to Shirk as Allah says: *"And of mankind are some who take (for worship) others besides Allah as rivals (to llaah). They love them as they love Allah." (Qur'an, Al-Baqarah 2:165)* The one who is in love, becomes a slave to the one he loves." (End quote from Majmoo' al-Fataawa (15/293) (24)

Stealing less than the threshold amount [that is, less than the value of stolen goods at which the hadd punishment of amputating the hand becomes due] is a Minor sin, but if the one from whom it is stolen possesses nothing else and losing it will lead to him becoming vulnerable, then it becomes a Major sin. (End quote from al-Haafiz) (25)

Sheikh Ibn 'Uthaymeen (May Allah have mercy on him) said:

"If a person persists in a Minor sin and that becomes his habit, then it becomes a Major sin because of persisting in it, not because of the deed in and of itself. Talking to a woman on the phone for the purpose of pleasure is Haram, but it is not a Major sin. However, if a person persists in doing that and it becomes his main focus to call these women and talk to them, then it becomes a Major sin. Persisting in a Minor sin makes it a Major sin because of persisting in it, because persisting in a Minor sin indicates that one is heedless of Allah, may He be Glorified and Exalted, or that one does not care about the prohibitions of Allah. End quote." (Liqa' al-Baab al-Maftooh (5/172) (25)

715 SINS

1. Religion Other than Islam

Our Creator, the Exalted, said

"And I (Allah) created not the Jinns and humans except they should worship Me (Alone)." (Qur'an, Adh-Dhariyat 51:56)

"This day, I have perfected your religion for you, completed My Favor upon you, and have chosen for you Islam as your religion." (Qur'an, Al-Ma'idah 5:3)

"And whoever seeks a religion other than Islam, it will never be accepted of him, and in the Hereafter, he will be one of the losers." (Qur'an, Ali 'Imran 3:85)

Other Verses: Al-An'am 6:125, Al-Bayyinah 98:5.

Allah gave the freedom to choose between Paradise and Hellfire in the next eternal life.

"There is no compulsion in religion. Verily, the Right Path has become distinct from the wrong path. Whoever disbelieves in Taghut and believes in Allah, then he has grasped the most trustworthy handhold that will never break. And Allah is All-Hearer, All-Knower." (Qur'an, Al-Baqarah 2:256)

"Whoever chooses to follow the Right Path follows it but for his own good; and whoever goes astray, goes but astray to his own loss; and no bearer of burdens shall be made to bear another's burden." (Qur'an, Al-Isra 17:15)

Other Verses: Al-Kahf 18:29, Ali 'Imran 3:85, At-Tawbah 9:33 and 9:72, Yunus 10:3, Ar-Rum 30:30.

The basic criterion for salvation in the Hereafter is the belief in Allah (the Oneness of God (*Tawheed*), His Angels, Books, Messengers, Predestination, as well as repentance to God, giving up sins, repairing the past, following the Glorious Qur'an and Sunnah, doing good deeds.

Salvation can only be attained through Allah's Judgment.

1.1. Islam is a Deen, Not to be Confused with Religion

Allah, the Exalted, says:

"Verily, the religion (Deen) of God (Allah) is Islam…" (Qur'an, Ali 'Imran 3:19)

The root of the Arabic word *Din is D-y-n*. This root has four primary meanings: mutual obligation, submission or acknowledgment, judicial authority and natural inclination or tendency. For example, the word *dana*, which comes from *din*, means "being indebted"; this term conveys an entire group of meanings related to the idea of debt. The word *dain*, depending on the way in which it is used, can mean either "debtor" or "creditor," words that have opposite meanings but are based on the same concept. To be *dain* means that one is obliged to follow all of the laws, customs and ordinances covering indebtedness. Being in debt also implies obligation, which is expressed in Arabic by the term *dayn*, another word that comes from the same root. Indebtedness may also involve formal judgment (*daynunak*) or conviction (*idanah*), terms that relate to one's obligation to pay or otherwise fulfill a debt or a contract… When one considers the four primary meanings of the root *dyn*, one realizes that in Islam, religion (*Deen*) is natural to the human condition. Religion conveys the idea of obligation or indebtedness, the acknowledgment of indebtedness, and the requirement to repay one's debts. (26, 27)

1.1.1. Deen is a Debt

Allah, the Exalted, says:

"O mankind! it is you who stand in need of Allah, but Allah is Rich (Free of all wants and needs), Worthy of all praise." (Qur'an, Fatir 35:15)

People owe debt of obedience to Allah, the Creator. The human beings are indebted to Allah for creating them, providing for them and maintaining their existence. All human beings are created in a state of absolute neediness of Allah, the One Who is absolutely Free from all needs. The mere fact of existence places man in a state of debt the moment he is created. As Allah is the Master, Creator and Sustainer of the Universe – man cannot utilize material things to repay this debt as he is not their proper owner. The only way man can ever repay his momentous debt to his Creator is by engaging in khidmah (service) to others and humbly submitting his very self to His pronouncements. Man was once nothing and did not exist, and now he is.

"And indeed, We created man (Adam) out of an extract of clay (water and earth)." (Qur'an, Al-Mu'minun 23:12)

"Thereafter We made him (the offspring of Adam) as a Nutfah (mixed drops of the male and female sexual discharge) (and lodged it) in a safe lodging (womb of the woman)." (Qur'an, Al-Mu'minun 23:13)

"Then We made the sperm-drop into a clinging clot, and We made the clot into a lump (of flesh), and We made (from) the lump, bones, and We covered the bones with flesh; then We developed him into another creation. So, Blessed is Allah, the Best of creators." (Qur'an, Al-Mu'minun 23:14)

Man's existence cannot really be directed to his parents, for he knows equally well that his parents too are subject to the same process by the same Creator and Provider. Man does not himself cause his own growth and development from the state of a clot of congealed blood to the one that now stands mature and perfect. He knows that even in his mature and perfect state he is not able to create for himself his sense of sight or hearing, or other – and let alone move himself in conscious growth and development in his helpless embryonic stage. The human being cannot create a race of new beings or maintain an entire Universe. According to the Qur'an, every human being acknowledges a debt to God at the core of his or her being. This debt is expressed as a covenant, established between humanity and its Creator even before the human race was placed on earth.

Allah, the Exalted, says:

"And (remember) when your Lord brought forth from the Children of Adam, from their loins, their seed (or from Adam's loin his offspring) and made them testify as to themselves (saying): "Am I not your Lord?" They said: "Yes! We testify," lest you should say on the Day of Resurrection: "Verily, we have been unaware of this." (Qur'an, Al-A'raf 7:172)

The rightly guided man realizes that his very self, his soul, has already acknowledged Allah as his Lord, even before his existence as a man, so that such a man recognizes his Creator and Cherisher, and Sustainer. The nature of the debt of creation and existence is so tremendously total that man, the moment he is created and given existence, is already in a state of utter loss, for he possesses really nothing himself, seeing that everything about him and in him and from him is what the Creator owns, Who owns everything. And this is the purpose of the Words in the Holy Qur'an:

"Indeed, mankind is in loss…" (Qur'an, Al-'Asr 103:2)

Seeing that he owns absolutely nothing to 'repay' his debt, except his own consciousness of the fact that he is himself the very substance of the debt, so must he 'repay' with himself, so must he 'return' himself to Him Who owns him absolutely. He is himself the debt to be returned to the Owner, and 'returning the debt' means to give himself up in service, or khidmah, to his Lord and Master; to abase himself before Him and so, the rightly guided man sincerely and consciously enslaves himself for the sake of God in order to fulfill His commands and prohibitions and ordinances, and thus to live out the dictates of His Law." (28)

1.1.2. Submission to the Divine Will and Decree of Allah

The word **Islam** means voluntary "Submission" or "Surrender" to the Will of God. It derives from the root of three letters: S-L-M.
What words come from the S-L-M root?

- **Salam** and **Islam**, peace and surrender, are familiar Arabic words.
- **Salama** (the infinitive form) derives from a word referring to the stinging of a snake. (sound peaceful?)
- **Aslim Taslam** (Arabic أسلم تسلم) means meaning "submit (to God) by accepting Islam and you will *get salvation*" (Abidullah Ghazi and Tasneema K Ghazi, Teachings of Our Prophet: A selection of Hadith for Children, IQRA International Education, p.3, Wikipedia and elsewhere)

Islam recognizes that humankind has free choice in whether to obey or disobey God, but ultimately, will be accountable to God on Judgment Day.

Allah, the Exalted, says:

"But whosoever turns away from My Reminder (i.e. neither believes in this Qur'an nor acts on its teachings) verily, for him is a life of hardship, and We shall raise him up blind on the Day of Resurrection. He will say: 'O my Lord! Why have you raised me up blind, while I had sight (before).'

(Allah) will say: 'Like this: Our Ayat (proofs, evidences, verses, lessons, signs, revelations, etc.) came unto you, but you disregarded them (i.e. you left them, did not think deeply in them, and you turned away from them), and so this Day, you will be neglected (in the Hellfire, away from Allah's Mercy).'

And thus, do We requite him who transgresses beyond bounds [i.e. commits the great sins and disobeys his Lord (Allah) and believes not in His Messengers, and His revealed Books, like this Qur'an], and believes not in the Ayat (proofs, evidences, verses, lessons, signs, revelations, etc.) of his Lord; and the torment of the Hereafter is far more severe and more lasting." (Qur'an, Taha 20:124-127)

Once you have understood this, then you will know that Allah has not created this Universe, with the earth and the heavens, the seas and the rivers, the mountains and plains, the oases and the deserts, fruit and vegetables, fish and birds, cattle except for your sake. (29)

"He it is Who created for you all that is on earth." (Qur'an, Al-Baqarah 2:29)

Then you will realize that the great purpose for which you exist is to worship your Creator. (30)

Allah created life and death to test His slaves in their performance of this duty of worship.

"Who has created death and life that He may test you which of you is best in deed. And He is the All-Mighty, the Oft-Forgiving." (Qur'an, Al-Mulk 67:2)

Allah promised those who do good in this world that in the Hereafter theirs will be Paradise as vast as the heavens and the earth, in which is that which no eye has ever seen, no ear has ever heard, nor has it ever entered the mind of man. He has warned those who do evil and neglect His rights over them that theirs will be a blazing Fire, in which they will neither live nor die, in which He has created all kinds of punishments and torments, hearing of which would turn a child's hair white, let alone seeing them and suffering them. Once you know this with certainty, then you will know that succeeding in this test is a serious matter which can only be achieved with a measure of effort and hardship which requires patience and forbearance. But this is hardship which passes swiftly and difficulty which soon comes to an end, because it is followed by eternal rest and happiness. So, what is an hour of hardship and a moment of pain when compared to that eternal delight. Allah in His Wisdom increases the reward of the sincere believers who remain steadfast in adhering to the Truth, those who give precedence to pleasing Him over everything else and sacrifice that which is most precious to them for the sake of Allah.

"Say, 'Indeed, my prayer, my rites of sacrifice, my living and my dying are for Allah, Lord of the worlds.'" (Qur'an, Al-An'am 6:162)

"And indeed, We have written in Az-Zabur [i.e. all the revealed Holy Books the Tawrat (Torah), the Injeel (Gospel), the Psalms, the Qur'an] after (We have already written in) Al-Lawh Al-Mahfuz (the Book that is in the heaven with Allah) that My righteous slaves shall inherit the land (i.e. the land of Paradise)." (Qur'an, Al-Anbya 21:105)

Narrated Abu Hurairah: Allah's Apostle (peace and blessings be upon him) said, "Every child is born with a true faith of Islam (i.e. to worship none but Allah Alone) but his parents convert him to Judaism, Christianity or Magainism, as an animal delivers a perfect baby animal. Do you find it mutilated?" Then Abu Hurairah recited the Holy Verses: *"The pure Allah's Islamic nature (True Faith of Islam) (i.e. worshipping none but Allah) with which He has created human beings. No change let there be in the religion of Allah (i.e. joining none in worship with Allah). That is the Straight Religion (Islam) but most of men know not." (30.30)* (Bukhari)

1.1.3. Deen Means Day of Judgment, Yawm al-Qiyamah or Yawm ad-Deen

Allah, the Exalted, says:

"In the Name of Allah, the Most Beneficent, the Most Merciful. All the praises and thanks be to Allah, the Lord of the 'Alamin (mankind, Jinns and all that exists). The Most Beneficent, the Most Merciful. The Only Owner (and the Only Ruling Judge) of the Day of Recompense (i.e. the Day of Resurrection)…" (Qur'an, Al-Fatihah 1:1-4)

"Verily, to Us will be their return, then verily, for Us will be their Reckoning." (Qur'an, Al-Ghashiyah 88:25-26)

The Messenger of Allah (peace and blessings be upon him) said: "A person's feet will not move on, on the Day of Resurrection, until he is questioned about his life and how he spent it, about his knowledge and what he did with it, about his wealth, from where he acquired it and on what he spent it, and about his body and for what he wore it out." (Tirmidhi)

1.1.4. Deen Means Disciplining Yourself

Allah, the Exalted, says:

"There is none in the heavens and the earth but comes unto the Most Beneficent (Allah) as a slave.
Verily, He knows each one of them, and has counted them a full counting. And every one of them will come to Him alone on the Day of Resurrection (without any helper or protector, or defender)." (Qur'an, Maryam 19:93-95)

Acknowledging your shortcomings is one of the first steps in disciplining yourself. Whoever tries to change for the sake of Allah, Allah will help him to change.

Two Prophets, Noah and Lot, strove to guide their respective wives, and how much guidance their wives received, but there was no interest on their part, so it was said to both of them:

"Enter the Fire along with those who enter!" (Qur'an, At-Tahrim 66:10)

Whereas the wife of Pharaoh – even though she was a member of the household of one of the greatest evildoers – was presented by Allah as an example to those who believe because she disciplined herself.
<u>Muslim should discipline himself:</u>

1 - Establishing the obligatory acts of worship well and on time, and cleansing the heart of any attachment to anybody and anything other than Allah.
2 - Reading Qur'an regularly and with understanding it.
3 - Reading beneficial books, for example, the biographies of the Prophets, their attitude and behavior.
4 - Attending Islamic educational programs such as classes and lectures.
5 - Remembering Allah at all times and conditions is the basis of submission to Allah.
6 - Keeping company only with righteous Muslims, they will pray for you.
7 - Acting upon the knowledge of Truth.
8 - Checking closely on yourself.
9 - Having confidence in yourself, whilst relying on Allah.
10 - Despising yourself for not doing enough for the sake of Allah. Man has to strive hard.
11 - Practicing isolation to have time to understand the Qur'an and Sunnah, to study Arabic language, to learn Allah's Names and Attributes. (31)

1.1.5. Islam is the Complete Code of Life for Humanity

Allah, the Exalted, says:

"Whoever works righteousness - whether male or female - while he (or she) is a true believer (of Islamic Monotheism) verily, to him We will give a good life (in this world with respect, contentment and lawful provision), and We shall pay them certainly a

reward in proportion to the best of what they used to do (i.e. Paradise in the Hereafter)."
(Qur'an, An-Nahl 16:97)

"Verily, those who say: 'Our Lord is (only) Allah,' and thereafter stand firm (on the Islamic Faith of Monotheism), on them shall be no fear, nor shall they grieve. Such shall be the dwellers of Paradise, abiding therein (forever) a reward for what they used to do."
(Qur'an, Al-Ahqaf 46:13-14)

Allah, the Exalted, says about His Prophet:

"And by the Mercy of Allah, you dealt with them gently. And had you been severe and harsh hearted, they would have broken away from about you; so, pass over (their faults), and ask (Allah's) Forgiveness for them; and consult them in the affairs. Then when you have taken a decision, put your trust in Allah, certainly, Allah loves those who put their trust (in Him)." (Qur'an, Ali 'Imran 3:159)

Narrated Imam Malik: "Yahya related to me from Malik that he had heard that the Messenger of Allah, (peace and blessings be upon him) said, "I was sent to perfect good character." (Malik Muwatta)

Islam instructs the Muslim to be honest, truthful, sincere, modest, merciful, just, respectful and abiding in his promise. And Islam prohibits all adjectives opposed to the previous and also prohibits the envy, hatred, hypocrisy, flattery, mockery, evil-speaking, lying, slander, vanity, showing off, etc.

The best Muslims are those who have the best character. The meaning of 'character' here is a good character towards Allah, towards other people, and towards society at large. It encompasses all of the Islamic virtues such justice, compassion, humility and truthfulness. (32)

1.1.6. Deen Means Rain

Allah, the Exalted, says:

"And put forward to them the example of the life of this world, it is like the water (rain) which We send down from the sky, and the vegetation of the earth mingles with it, and becomes fresh and green. But (later) it becomes dry and broken pieces, which the winds scatter. And Allah is Able to do everything." (Qur'an, Al-Kahf 18:45)

Rain, which carries great importance for all living and non-living things, is mentioned in various Verses of the Qur'an. Rain is "giving life to a dead land" and the Qur'an revives the dead heart.

1.1.7. Angel Jibreel Said: "O Muhammad, Tell me About Islam"

Narrated Umar bin Al-Khattab (May Allah have mercy on him): "One day when we were with the Messenger of Allah (peace and blessings be upon him), there appeared before us a man whose clothes were exceedingly white and his hair was exceedingly black, and there were no signs of travel on him. No one among us recognized him. He came and sat down by the Prophet (peace and blessings be upon him) and rested his knees against his and placed the palms on his hands on his thighs. He said: "O Muhammad, tell me about Islam." The Messenger of Allah (peace and blessings be upon him) said:

"Islam is to testify that there is none worthy of worship except Allah and that Muhammad is the Messenger of Allah, to establish regular prayer, to pay Zakah, to fast Ramadan and to go on pilgrimage to the House if you are able to." He said: "You have spoken the Truth." And we were amazed at his asking that and saying that he had spoken the Truth. Then he said: "Tell me about Iman (faith, belief)." He (peace and blessings be upon him) said: "It means believing in Allah, His Angels, His Books, His Messengers, and the Last Day, and believing in al-Qadar (the Divine Will and Decree), both good and bad." He said: "You have spoken the Truth." He said: "Tell me about Ihsan." He (peace and blessings be upon him) said: "It means worshipping Allah as if you can see Him, and although you cannot see Him, He can see you." (Muslim)

1.1.8. Islam is a Justice

Allah, the Exalted, says:

"Verily, Allah enjoins Al-Adl (i.e. justice and worshipping none but Allah Alone - Islamic Monotheism) and Al-Ihsan [i.e. to be patient in performing your duties to Allah, totally for Allah's sake and in accordance with the Sunnah (legal ways) of the Prophet SAW in a perfect manner], and giving (help) to kith and kin (i.e. all that Allah has ordered you to give them e.g. wealth, visiting, looking after them or any other kind of help, etc.): and forbids Al-Fahisha' (i.e. all evil deeds, e.g. illegal sexual acts, disobedience of parents, polytheism, to tell lies, to give false witness, to kill a life without right, etc.), and Al-Munkar (i.e. all that is prohibited by Islamic Law: polytheism of every kind, disbelief and every kind of evil deeds, etc.), and Al-Baghy (i.e. all kinds of oppression), He admonishes you, that you may take heed. God commands justice and fair dealing..." (Qur'an, An-Nahl 16:90)

"And whosoever does not judge by what Allah has revealed (then) such (people) are the Fasiqoon (the rebellious i.e. disobedient (of a lesser degree) to Allah." (Qur'an, Al-Ma'idah 5:47)

"O you who believe! Stand out firmly for justice, as witnesses to Allah, even though it be against yourselves or your parents, or your kin, be he rich or poor, Allah is a Better Protector to both (than you). So, follow not the lusts (of your hearts), lest you may avoid

justice, and if you distort your witness or refuse to give it, verily, Allah is Ever Well Acquainted with what you do." (Qur'an, An-Nisa 4:135)

1.2. Why is this Religion Called Islam?

In Arabic language dictionaries the meaning of the word Islam is submission to Allah's Will and Decrees, humbling oneself, sincerely believing in Allah and worshipping Allah alone. For all other religions, for which Almighty Allah didn't give authority, they are called by various names, either the name of a specific man or a specific nation, or creation.

Christianity takes its name from Christ and they worship man, Jesus, instead of God.

Buddhism takes its name from its founder, the Buddha. The Buddha (also known as Siddhartha Gotama or Siddhartha Gautama) was a philosopher, mendicant, meditator, religious leader.

Zoroastrians became well known by this name because their founder and standard-bearer was Zoroaster, an ancient Iranian spiritual leader.

Judaism took its name from a tribe known as Yehudah (Judah), so it became known as Judaism.

Except for Islam, for it is not attributed to any specific man or to any specific nation, rather its name refers to the meaning of the word Islam. What this name indicates is that the establishment and founding of this Religion was not the work of one particular man and that it is not only for one particular nation to the exclusion of all others. (30)

The human beings are God's viceroys on this earth. They possess a Divinely delegated power (by Allah's Grace) to civilize the earth and they are commanded not to corrupt it. Since human beings are directly accountable to God, their submission to God necessarily means that they submit to no other. Every person must exercise his or her conscience and mind and be fully responsible for his or her deeds.

Genuine submission must be guided by a longing and love for union with our Creator Who sends countless blessings upon us. Therefore, those who submit, do not find fulfillment simply in obedience but in love—a love for the One Who is a Provider, Protector, Nourisher, Cherisher, the Most Merciful and the Oft-Forgiving.

Allah said of Noah:

"And recite to them the news of Nooh (Noah). When he said to his people: 'O my people, if my stay (with you), and my reminding (you) of the Ayat (proofs, evidences, verses, lessons, signs, revelations, etc.) of Allah is hard on you, then I put my trust in Allah. So, devise

your plot, you and your partners, and let not your plot be in doubt for you. Then pass your sentence on me and give me no respite.

'But if you turn away (from accepting my doctrine of Islamic Monotheism, i.e. to worship none but Allah), then no reward have I asked of you, my reward is only from Allah, and I have been commanded to be of the Muslims (i.e. those who submit to Allah's Will).'" (Qur'an, Yunus 10:71-72)

Allah said of Ibrahim:

"And who turns away from the religion of Ibrahim (Abraham) (i.e. Islamic Monotheism) except him who befools himself? Truly, We chose him in this world and verily, in the Hereafter he will be among the righteous. When his Lord said to him, 'Submit (i.e. be a Muslim)!' He said, 'I have submitted myself (as a Muslim) to the Lord of the 'Alamin (mankind, Jinns and all that exists).' And this (submission to Allah, Islam) was enjoined by Ibrahim (Abraham) upon his sons and by Ya'qoob (Jacob) (saying), 'O my sons! Allah has chosen for you the (true) religion, then die not except in the Faith of Islam (as Muslims - Islamic Monotheism).'" (Qur'an, Al-Baqarah 2:130-132)

Allah said of Moosa:

"And Moosa (Moses) said: 'O my people! If you have believed in Allah, then put your trust in Him if you are Muslims (those who submit to Allah's Will).'" (Qur'an, Yunus 10:84)

Allah said of the Messiah:

"And when I (Allah) inspired Al-Hawariyyoon (the disciples) [of 'Eesa (Jesus)] to believe in Me and My Messenger, they said: 'We believe. And bear witness that we are Muslims.'" (Qur'an, Al-Ma'idah 5:111)

Allah said of the previous Prophets:

"…by which the Prophets, who submitted themselves to Allah's Will …" (Qur'an, Al-Ma'idah 5:44)

Bilqeez said:

"My Lord! Verily, I have wronged myself, and I submit [in Islam, together with Sulaymaan (Solomon)] to Allah, the Lord of the 'Aalameen (mankind, jinn and all that exists)." (Qur'an, An-Naml 27:44)

Islam is the religion from the creation of the first man. All the Prophets were Muslims starting from Adam, and their followers who adhered to their true religion, before it was distorted or abrogated, were Muslims. (33)

2. Ascribing Associates to Allah (Shirk)

Allah, the Exalted, says:

"Surely, Allah does not forgive associating anything with Him, and He forgives whatever is other than that to whomever He wills." (Qur'an, An-Nisa 4:48)

"Verily! Allah forgives not (the sin of) setting up partners in worship with Him, but He forgives whom He pleases sins other than that, and whoever sets up partners in worship with Allah, has indeed strayed far away." (Qur'an, An-Nisa 4:116)

"Who has made the earth a resting place for you, and the sky as a canopy, and sent down water (rain) from the sky and brought forth therewith fruits as a provision for you. Then do not set up rivals unto Allah (in worship) while you know (that He Alone has the right to be worshipped)." (Qur'an, Al-Baqarah 2:22)

Other Verses: Al-Baqarah 2:163, Ash-Shu'ara 26:96-97, Al-Ahqaf 46:5-6, Al-Muminoon 23:117, Fatir 35:13-14, Az-Zumar 39:65.

Narrated Abu Bakra: The Prophet (peace and blessings be upon him) said thrice, "Should I inform you out the greatest of the great sins?" They said, "Yes, O Allah's Apostle!" He (peace and blessings be upon him) said, "To join others in worship with Allah, and to be undutiful to one's parents." The Prophet (peace and blessings be upon him) then sat up after he had been reclining (on a pillow) and said, "And I warn you against giving a false witness, and he kept on saying that warning till we thought he would not stop." (Bukhari)

Allah, the Exalted, says:

"Say, "He is Allah, (the) One. Allah As-Samad (the Self-Sufficient Master, Whom all creatures need, He neither eats nor drinks). "He begets not, nor was He begotten; "And there is none co-equal or comparable unto Him." (Qur'an, Al-Ikhlas 112)

Allah, the Owner of all things, negates partnership with Him in every sense, whether it concerns Himself, His Names and Attributes or His Decree. It also demonstrates the distinctiveness of God in His Perfection, Magnificence and Majesty. The word *Ahad* is not used in affirmation for anyone besides God.

The *Tafsir* (commentary, exegesis) of Ibn Abbas for the Verse "Allah! As-Samad (i.e. the Eternally Besought of all)": The Chief Who is best in His Nobility. The Great One Who is best in His Greatness. The Tolerant One Who is best in His toleration. The Omnipotent Who is the best in His omnipotence, the All-Knowing Who is best in His Knowledge. The Self which is Perfect in all types of Nobility and Greatness - that Self is only Allah - the Most Revered and the Most Powerful. Allah Alone has these qualities for they do not apply to anyone save Him. No one is equal to Him and no one is like Him. Affirmation in the

Oneness negates all forms of polytheism and similitude. Affirmation of all the meanings of *As-Samad* includes all the Noble Names and the most exalted Attributes. This is the Tawheed of Affirmation.

The Tawheed of Purity is in the statement:

"He does not beget not nor is He begotten. And there is none comparable to Him". This statement can also be understood from the general statement: "Say! He is God! The One". Nothing came out of Him nor did He come out of anything. God has no son, no daughter, no wife, no family. He is One! He has no equal, no likeness and no similarity. Domination of the concept of Tawheed in this Surah. The affirmation of Oneness for the Lord in total and absolute contradiction to all forms of polytheism. His character of being "Eternally Besought of all", which proves all His Attributes, that He cannot suffer from any defect, negation of father and son which is an implication of Him being in no need and that all is in need of Him. All is characterized in the statement of His being besought and His Oneness.

Negation of an equal which includes negation of similarity, resemblances and likeness. This Surah includes all of these matters and is therefore rightly deserving of being called equal to a third of the Qur'an. (34)

MAJOR SHIRK

This means ascribing to someone other than Allah something that belongs only to Allah, such as Lordship (rububiyyah), Divinity (uluhiyyah) and the Divine Names and Attributes (al-asma' wa'l-sifat).

Types of Major Shirk

1. Shirk may sometimes take the form of beliefs.

Such as the belief that there is someone else who creates, gives life and death, reigns or controls the affairs of the universe along with Allah.

Or the belief that there is someone else who must be obeyed absolutely besides Allah, so they follow him in regarding as permissible or forbidden whatever he wants, even if that goes against the religion of the Messengers.

Or they may associate others with Allah in love and veneration, by loving a created being as they love Allah.

Allah, the Exalted, says:

"And of mankind are some who take (for worship) others besides Allah as rivals (to Allah). They love them as they love Allah." (Qur'an, Al-Baqarah 2:165)

Or the belief that there are those who know the Unseen as well as Allah. This is very common among some of the deviant sects such as the Rafidis (Shi'ah), extreme Sufis and Batinis (esoteric sects) in general. The Rafidis believe that their imams have knowledge of the Unseen, and the Batinis and Sufis believe similar things about their awliya ("saints"), and so on.

It is also Shirk to believe that there is someone who bestows mercy in a manner that is befitting only for Allah, so he shows mercy as Allah does and forgives sins and overlooks the bad deeds.

2. Shirk may sometimes take the form of words

Such as those who make Du'a or pray to someone other than Allah, or seek his help, or seek refuge with him with regard to matters over which no one has control except Allah, whether the person called upon is a Prophet, a wali ("saint"), an angel or a Jinn, or some other created being.

Or such as those who make fun of religion or who liken Allah to His creation, or say that there is another creator, provider or controller besides Allah.

3. Shirk may sometimes take the form of actions

Such as one who sacrifices, prays or prostrates to somebody or something other than Allah, or who promulgates laws to replace the Rulings of Allah and makes that the law to which people are obliged to refer for judgement; or one who supports the kafirs and helps them against the believers, and other acts that go against the basic meaning of Faith.

MINOR SHIRK

This includes everything that may lead to Major Shirk, or which is described in the texts as being Shirk, but does not reach the extent of being Major Shirk.

Types of Minor Shirk

1. It may also take the form of beliefs:

The belief that something may be a cause of bringing benefit or warding off harm, when Allah has not made it so; or believing that there is barakah (blessing) in a thing, when Allah has not made it so.

2. It sometimes takes the form of words:

Such as when they said, "We have been given rain by such and such a star," without believing that the stars could independently cause rain to fall; or swearing by something other than Allah, without believing in venerating the thing sworn by or regarding it as equal with Allah; or saying, "Whatever Allah wills and you will", and so on.

3. It sometimes takes the form of actions:

Such as hanging up Amulets or wearing a Talisman or String to dispel or ward off calamity, because everyone who attributes powers to a thing when Allah has not made it so, has associated something with Allah. This also applies to one who touches a thing seeking its barakah (blessing), when Allah has not created any barakah in it, such as kissing the doors of the Mosques, touching their thresholds, seeking healing from their dust, knocking the wood for protection, etc.

The Prophet Ibrahim (May Allah have mercy on him) said:

"…and keep me and my sons away from worshipping idols." (Qur'an, Ibrahim 14:35)

The Prophet (peace and blessings be upon him) taught the great Du'a to seek Protection of Allah from committing Shirk: "Shirk among you will be more subtle than the footsteps of an ant, but I will teach you something which, if you do it, both Minor and Major Shirk will be kept away from you.
Say: "Allaahumma 'innee 'a'oothu bika 'an 'ushrika bika wa 'ana 'a'lam, wa 'astaghfiruka lima la 'a'lam"
"O Allah, I seek refuge with You lest I should commit Shirk with You knowingly and I seek Your Forgiveness for what I do unknowingly." to repeat three times in the morning and evening." (Ahmad)

Major Shirk puts a person beyond the pale of Islam, so he is a kaafir and an apostate.

Shirk is a Major sin and transgression against the unique rights of Allah, which are to be worshipped and obeyed Alone, with no partner or associate. (35, 36)

Allah, the Exalted, says:

"And verily! This your religion (of Islamic Monotheism) is one religion, and I am your Lord, so keep your duty to Me." (Qur'an, Al-Mu'minun 23:52)

Allah created and fashioned (the noble shape) man and preferred man over other creations.

Allah, the Exalted, says:

"And We have certainly honored the children of Adam and carried them on the land and sea and provided for them of the good things and preferred them over much of what We have created, with (definite) preference." Qur'an, Al-Isra 17:70)

"And surely, We created you (your father Adam) and then gave you shape (the noble shape of a human being); then We told the angels, 'Prostrate yourselves to Adam.'" (Qur'an, Al-A'raf 7:11)

"O man! What has made you careless about your Lord, the Most Generous? Who created you, fashioned you perfectly, and gave you due proportion. In whatever form He willed, He put you together." (Qur'an, Al-Infitar 82:6-8)

Allah mentioned in His previous Books, the Torah and Gospel, the arrival of the last Prophet (Ahmad means Muhammad) that everybody should follow him.

Allah, the Exalted, says:

"And mix not Truth with falsehood, nor conceal the Truth [i.e. Muhammad, peace be upon him, is Allah's Messenger and his qualities are written in your Scriptures, the Taurat (Torah) and the Injeel (Gospel)] while you know (the Truth)." (Qur'an, Al-Baqarah 2:42)

Worshipping Other gods than Allah is Worshipping the Devil

Allah, the Exalted, says:

"So, set you (O Muhammad SAW) your face towards the religion of pure Islamic Monotheism Hanifa (worship none but Allah Alone) Allah's Fitrah (i.e. Allah's Islamic Monotheism), with which He has created mankind. No change let there be in Khalqillah (i.e. the Religion of Allah Islamic Monotheism), that is the Straight Religion, but most of men know not." [Tafsir At-Tabari, vol.21, p.41] (Qur'an, Ar-Rum 30:30)

'Iyad bin Himar reported that Allah's Messenger (peace and blessings be upon him), while delivering a sermon one day, said: "Behold, my Lord commanded me that I should teach you which you do not know and which He has taught me today. (He has instructed thus): 'The property which I have conferred upon them is lawful for them. I have created My servants as one having a natural inclination to the worship of Allah but it is Satan who turns them away from the right religion and he makes unlawful what has been declared lawful for them and he commands them to ascribe partnership with Me, although he has no justification for that…'" (Muslim)

Narrated Anas bin Malik: The Prophet (peace and blessings be upon him) said: "Allah, the Exalted, will say to the least tormented person among the people of Hell on the Day of Resurrection: 'Do you have anything on earth that you would give as a ransom (to protect yourself against the torment of Fire)?' He will say: 'Yes.' Then Allah will say: 'While you were in the backbone of Adam, I had demanded you much less than that, i.e. to associate nothing with Me; but you declined and worshipped others besides Me.'" (Bukhari and Muslim)

Narrated Abu Hurairah: Allah's Apostle (peace and blessings be upon him) said, "Every child is born with a true faith of Islam (i.e. to worship none but Allah Alone) but his parents convert him to Judaism, Christianity or Magainism, as an animal delivers a perfect baby animal. Do you find it mutilated?" Then Abu Hurairah recited the Holy Verse: *"The pure Allah's Islamic nature (true faith of Islam) (i.e. worshipping none but Allah) with which He has created human* beings. *No change let there be in the religion of Allah (i.e. joining none in worship with Allah). That is the Straight Religion (Islam) but most of men know, not." (30.30)* (Bukhari)

SOME OF IDOL WORSHIP FORMS

The Qur'an cites many forms of Idol worship, the unforgivable sin. (37)

1. <u>Jesus as an Idol</u>

Christians went astray worshipping Jesus, Muslim man and Allah's Messenger, instead of God, Allah.

Allah, the Exalted, says:

"Surely, they have disbelieved who say: "Allah is the Messiah ['Iesa (Jesus)], son of Maryam (Mary)." But the Messiah ['Iesa (Jesus)] said: "O Children of Israel! Worship Allah, my Lord and your Lord." Verily, whosoever sets up partners in worship with Allah, then Allah has forbidden Paradise for him, and the Fire will be his abode. And for the Zalimun (polytheists and wrongdoers) there are no helpers." (Qur'an, Al-Ma'idah 5:72)

"Verily, the likeness of 'Eesa (Jesus) before Allah is the likeness of Adam. He created him from dust, then (He) said to him: 'Be!' - and he was. (This is) the Truth from your Lord, so be not of those who doubt. Then whoever disputes with you concerning him ['Eesa (Jesus)] after (all this) knowledge that has come to you [i.e. 'Eesa (Jesus) being a slave of Allah, and having no share in Divinity], say (O Muhammad): 'Come, let us call our sons and your sons, our women and your women, ourselves and yourselves - then we pray and invoke (sincerely) the Curse of Allah upon those who lie.'" (Qur'an, Ali 'Imran 3:59-61)

"Surely, disbelievers are those who said: 'Allah is the third of the three (in a Trinity).' But there is no ilah (god) (none who has the right to be worshipped) but One Ilah (God - Allah). And if they cease not from what they say, verily, a painful torment will befall the disbelievers among them." (Qur'an, Al-Ma'idah 5:73)

Narrated Abu Hurairah (May Allah be pleased with him): The Prophet (peace and blessings be upon him) said: "There is no Prophet between me and him, that is, Jesus (peace be upon him). He will descent (to the earth). When you see him, recognize him: a man of medium height, reddish fair, wearing two light yellow garments, looking as if drops were falling down from his head though it will not be wet. He will fight the people for the cause of Islam. He will break the cross, kill swine and abolish jizyah. Allah will perish all religions except Islam. He will destroy the Antichrist and will live on the earth for forty years and then he will die. The Muslims will pray over him." (Abu Dawud)

2. <u>Worshipping the sons of Allah</u>

Allah, the Exalted, says:

"And they (Jews, Christians and pagans) say: Allah has begotten a son (children or offspring). Glory be to Him (Exalted be He above all that they associate with Him). Nay, to Him belongs all that is in the heavens and on earth, and all surrender with obedience (in worship) to Him." (Qur'an, Al-Baqarah 2:116)

The Jews said that 'Uzayr is a son of God, and the Christians said that the Messiah was a son of God. (38)

Allah, the Exalted, says:

"O people of the Scripture (Jews and Christians)! Do not exceed the limits in your religion, nor say of Allah aught but the Truth. The Messiah 'Iesa (Jesus), son of Maryam (Mary), was (no more than) a Messenger of Allah and His Word, ("Be!" - and he was) which He bestowed on Maryam (Mary) and a spirit (Ruh) created by Him; so, believe in Allah and His Messengers. Say not: "Three (trinity)!" Cease! (it is) better for you. For Allah is (the only) One Ilah (God), Glory be to Him (Far Exalted is He) above having a son. To Him belongs all that is in the heavens and all that is in the earth. And Allah is All-Sufficient as a Disposer of affairs." (Qur'an, An-Nisa 4:171)

"And the Jews say: 'Uzair (Ezra) is the son of Allah, and the Christians say: Messiah is the son of Allah. That is a saying from their mouths. They imitate the saying of the disbelievers of old. Allah's Curse be on them, how they are deluded away from the Truth!" (Qur'an, At-Tawbah 9:30)

"Allah has not taken any son, nor has there ever been with Him any deity. (If there had been), then each deity would have taken what it created, and some of them would have sought to overcome others. Exalted is Allah above what they describe (concerning Him)." (Qur'an, Al-Mu'minun 23:91)

Allah favored the Children of Israel, saved them from death, offered them a land. Jews knew the Truth but turned away from the Creator, except few of them. Allah's Book, Torah, was modified by Jewish rabbis, as Allah, the Exalted, says:

"O Children of Israel, remember My Favor that I have bestowed upon you and that I preferred you over the worlds. And fear a Day when no soul will suffice for another soul at all, nor will intercession be accepted from it, nor will compensation be taken from it, nor will they be aided. And (recall) when We saved your forefathers from the people of Pharaoh, who afflicted you with the worst torment, slaughtering your (newborn) sons and keeping your females alive. And in that was a great trial from your Lord." (Qur'an, Al-Baqarah 2:47-49)

"Do you (faithful believers) covet that they will believe in your religion in spite of the fact that a party of them (Jewish rabbis) used to hear the Word of Allah [the Taurat (Torah)], then they used to change it knowingly after they understood it?" (Qur'an, Al-Baqarah 2:75)

Narrated Abu Musa Al-Ashari: The Prophet (peace and blessings be upon him) said, "None is more patient than Allah against the harmful and annoying words He hears (from the people): They ascribe children to Him, yet He bestows upon them health and provision." (Bukhari)

3. Worshipping the daughters of Allah

Allah, the Exalted, says:

"Have you considered El-Lat and El-'Uzza And Manat (another idol of the pagan Arabs), the other third? Is it for you the males and for Him the females? That indeed is a division most unfair!" (Qur'an, An-Najm 53:19-22)

"And they assign daughters unto Allah! Glorified (and Exalted) be He above all that they associate with Him! And unto themselves what they desire." (Qur'an, An-Nahl 16:57)

"Then, has your Lord chosen you for (having) sons and taken from among the angels daughters? Indeed, you say a grave saying." (Qur'an, Al-Isra 17:40)

Other Verses: *As-Saffat 37:149.*

4. Worshipping female gods

Allah, the Exalted, says:

"They (all those who worship others than Allah) invoke nothing but female deities besides Him (Allah), and they invoke nothing but Shaitan (Satan), a persistent rebel!" (Qur'an, An-Nisa 4:117)

5. Statues as an Idol

Allah, the Exalted, says:

"And the people of Musa (Moses) made in his absence, out of their ornaments, the image of a calf (for worship). It had a sound (as if it was mooing). Did they not see that it could neither speak to them nor guide them to the way? They took it for worship and they were Zalimun (wrongdoers)." (Qur'an, Al-A'raf 7:148)

"And (remember) when We appointed for Musa (Moses) forty nights, and (in his absence) you took the calf (for worship), and you were Zalimun (polytheists and wrongdoers, etc.)." (Qur'an, Al-Baqarah 2:51)

"So, shun the abomination (worshipping) of idol, and shun lying speech (false statements)." (Qur'an, Al-Hajj 22:30)

Narrated Ibn Abbas (May Allah be pleased with him): "When Allah's Apostle (peace and blessings be upon him) came to Makkah, he refused to enter the Ka'bah with idols in it. He ordered idols to be taken out. So, they were taken out. The people took out the pictures of Abraham and Ishmael holding Azlams in their hands. Allah's Apostle (peace and blessings be upon him) said, 'May Allah curse these people. By Allah, both Abraham and Ishmael never did the game of chance with Azlams.' Then he entered the Ka'bah and said Takbir at its corners but did not offer the prayer in it." (Bukhari)

6. Worshipping Animal

Allah, the Exalted, says:

"Allah, it is He Who has made cattle for you, that you may ride on some of them and of some you eat." (Qur'an, Al-Ghafir 40:79)

"And verily! In the cattle, there is a lesson for you. We give you to drink of that which is in their bellies, from between excretions and blood, pure milk; palatable to the drinkers." (Qur'an, An-Nahl 16:66)

7. Jinn as Idols

Allah, the Exalted, says:

"And verily, there were men among mankind who took shelter with the males among the Jinns, but they (Jinns) increased them (mankind) in sin and transgression." (Qur'an, Al-Jinn 72:6)

"Yet, they join the Jinns as partners in worship with Allah, though He has created them (the Jinns), and they attribute falsely without knowledge sons and daughters to Him. Be He Glorified and Exalted above (all) that they attribute to Him." (Qur'an, Al-An'am 6:100)

When a human seeks the help of the Jinn to cause harm to someone or to protect him from the evil of one whose evil he fears, all of this is Shirk, and his prayers and fasting are not accepted. (39)

8. Children as Idols

Allah, the Exalted, says:

"But when He gave them a Salih (good in every aspect) child, they ascribed partners to Him (Allah) in that which He has given to them. High be Allah, the Exalted above all that they ascribe as partners to Him. (Tafsir At-Tabari, vol.9, p.148)." (Qur'an, Al-A'raf 7:190)

"Say: If your fathers, your sons, your brothers, your wives, your kindred, the wealth that you have gained, the commerce in which you fear a decline, and the dwellings in which you delight ... are dearer to you than Allah and His Messenger, and striving hard and fighting in His Cause, then wait until Allah brings about His Decision (torment). And Allah guides not the people who are Al-Fasiqun (the rebellious, disobedient to Allah)." (Qur'an, At-Tawbah 9:24)

When we love our kids more than we love God, that is Idolatry.

9. Humans as Idols

Allah, the Exalted, says:

"Verily, those whom you call upon besides Allah are slaves like you. So, call upon them and let them answer you if you are truthful." *(Qur'an, Al-A'raf 7:194)*

The veneration of Mary, Mother of Jesus.
Jesus was wrongly taken for god or son of God.
Uzair was revered by the Jews as *"the son of God" (At-Tawbah 9:30).*

Allah, the Exalted, says:

"So, because of their breach of their covenant, We cursed them and made their hearts grow hard. They change the words from their (right) places." (Qur'an, Al-Ma'idah 5:13)

Pharaoh, the king of Ancient Egypt, considered himself as a god.

Hindu deities: Vishnu, Lakshmi, Shiva, Parvati, Brahma, Saraswati, Vaishnavism, Shaivism, Shaktism, Smartism, Deva, Devi, Ishvara, Ishvari, Bhagavān, Bhagavati, etc. Gautama Buddha. Jehovah Wanyonyi, a self-proclaimed god who lived in Kenia. There are many other false deities. (40-42)

10. "Intercessors" as Idols

Allah, the Exalted, says:

"And they worship other than Allah that which neither harms them nor benefits them, and they say, "These are our intercessors with Allah" Say, "Do you inform Allah of something He does not know in the heavens or on the earth?" Exalted is He and High above what they associate with Him." (Qur'an, Yunus 10:18)

11. Property as an Idol

Love of things (money, goods, commodities, etc.) is a form of Idolatry.

Allah, the Exalted, says:

"And put forward to them the example of two men; unto one of them We had given two gardens of grapes, and We had surrounded both with date-palms; and had put between them green crops (cultivated fields, etc.). Each of those two gardens brought forth its produce, and failed not in the least therein, and We caused a river to gush forth in the midst of them. And he had property (or fruit) and he said to his companion, in the course of mutual talk: 'I am more than you in wealth and stronger in respect of men.' And he went into his garden while in a state (of pride and disbelief) unjust to himself. He said: 'I think not that this will ever perish. And I think not the Hour will ever come, and if indeed I am brought back to my Lord, (on the Day of Resurrection), I surely shall find better than this when I return to Him.'" (Qur'an, Al-Kahf 18:32-36)

"So, his fruits were encircled (with ruin). And he remained clapping his hands with sorrow over what he had spent upon it, while it was all destroyed on its trellises, he could only say: 'Would I had ascribed no partners to my Lord!'" (Qur'an, Al-Kahf 18:42)

12. The Prophets, Messengers and saints as Idols

Allah, the Exalted, says:

"It is not (possible) for any human being to whom Allah has given the Book and Al-Hukma (the knowledge and understanding of the Laws of religion, etc.) and Prophethood to say to the people: "Be my worshippers rather than Allah's." On the contrary (he would say): "Be you Rabbaniyun (learned men of religion who practice what they know and also preach others), because you are teaching the Book, and you are studying it." (Qur'an, Ali 'Imran 3:79)

Narrated Aisha (May Allah be pleased with her): Allah's Apostle (peace and blessings be upon him) in his fatal illness said, "Allah cursed the Jews and the Christians, for they built the places of worship at the graves of their prophets." And if that had not been the case, then the Prophet's grave would have been made prominent before the people. So, (the Prophet) was afraid or the people were afraid that his grave might be taken as a place for worship." (Bukhari)

13. God's servants as Idols

Allah, the Exalted, says:

"Do then those who disbelieve think that they can take My slaves [i.e. the angels, Allah's Messengers, 'Iesa (Jesus), son of Maryam (Mary), etc.] as Auliya' (lords, gods, protectors,

etc.) besides Me? Verily, We have prepared Hell as an entertainment for the disbelievers (in the Oneness of Allah Islamic Monotheism)." *(Qur'an, Al-Kahf 18:102)*

14. Ego as an Idol

Allah, the Exalted, says:

"Have you seen the one whose god is his own ego? Will you be his advocate?" (Qur'an, Al-Furqan 25:43)

"Have you noted the one whose god is his ego? Consequently, God sends him astray, despite his knowledge, seals his hearing and his mind, and places a veil on his eyes. Who then can guide him, after such a decision by God? Would you not take heed?" (Qur'an, Al-Jathiyah 45:23)

This is a common form of Idolatry. Most humans, because of their ego and desires, cannot bring themselves to worship Allah, nor can they make their opinion subordinate to God's opinion.

If we disobey God and His Messenger, we are committing Idol worship even though there is no image in front of us. This is because we would be giving our opinion more importance than God's Words.

The opinion is said by the obstinate sinner, sometimes, to be the justification for the refusal to do what Allah proscribed. But this isn't true. It is a lie. There is something behind the opinion. A refusal to accept Allah's Laws. This is what is meant by the sin of 'My Opinion' – when it is set up as a rival to Allah's Own Words. Pharaoh is on the same page as Iblees.

15. Upholding religious sources other than God's Words as an Idol

Allah, the Exalted, says:

"Say (O Muhammad SAW): "What thing is the most great in witness?" Say: "Allah (the Most Great!) is Witness between me and you; this Qur'an has been revealed to me that I may therewith warn you and whomsoever it may reach. Can you verily bear witness that besides Allah there are other aliha (gods)?" Say "I bear no (such) witness!" Say: "But in Truth He (Allah) is the Only One Ilah (God). And truly I am innocent of what you join in worship with Him." (Qur'an, Al-An'am 6:19)

16. Religious leaders and scholars as Idols

Allah, the Exalted, says:

'They (Jews and Christians) took their rabbis and their monks to be their lords besides Allah (by obeying them in things which they made lawful or unlawful according to their own desires without being ordered by Allah), and (they also took as their lord) Messiah, son of Maryam (Mary), while they (Jews and Christians) were commanded [in the Taurat (Torah) and the Injeel (Gospel)) to worship none but One Ilah (God - Allah) La ilaha illa Huwa (none has the right to be worshipped but He). Praise and glory be to Him, (far above is He) from having the partners they associate (with Him)." (Qur'an, At-Tawbah 9:31)

17. <u>Creating sects in religion is an Idol worship</u>

Allah, the Exalted, says:

"(Always) Turning in repentance to Him (only), and be afraid and dutiful to Him; and perform As-Salat (Iqamat as-Salat) and be not of Al-Mushrikun (the disbelievers in the Oneness of Allah, polytheists, idolaters, etc.). Of those who split up their religion (i.e. who left the true Islamic Monotheism), and became sects, [i.e. they invented new things in the religion (Bid'ah), and followed their vain desires], each sect rejoicing in that which is with it." (Qur'an, Ar-Rum 30:31-32)

18. <u>Dividing believers and providing comfort to those who oppose God and His Messengers is practicing Idol worship</u>

Allah, the Exalted, says:

"And (there are) those (hypocrites) who took for themselves a Mosque for causing harm and disbelief and division among the believers and as a station for whoever had warred against Allah and His Messenger before. And they will surely swear, "We intended only the best." And Allah testifies that indeed they are liars." (Qur'an, At-Tawbah 9:107)

19. <u>Secret Shirk – Showing Off</u>

Allah, the Exalted, describes the hypocrites:

"Verily, the hypocrites seek to deceive Allah, but it is He Who deceives them. And when they stand up for As-Salat (the prayer), they stand with laziness and to be seen of men, and they do not remember Allah but little." (Qur'an, An-Nisa 4:142)

Narrated Mahmud bin Labid: Allah's Messenger (peace and blessings be upon him) said: "The most dreadful thing which I fear about you is minor polytheism (Minor Shirk).' The companions asked: 'What is the minor polytheism?' He (peace and blessings be upon him) said: 'It is hypocrisy' and he (peace and blessings be upon him) added that on the Day of Judgment, when rewarding people for their deeds, Allah, the Most High, will say to the hypocrites: 'Go to those for the sake of whom you used to perform good deeds; and see whether you can get any reward from them.'" (Ahmad)

20. Swear by Anybody and Anything Other than Allah

Narrated Abdullah: The Prophet (peace and blessings be upon him) said, "Whoever has to take an oath should swear by Allah or remain silent." (i.e. he should not swear by other than Allah) (Bukhari)

Narrated Shaddad bin Aws: The Messenger of Allah (peace and blessings be upon him) said: "The thing that I fear most for my nation is associating others with Allah. I do not say that they will worship the sun or the moon, or idols, but deeds done for the sake of anyone other than Allah, and hidden desires." (Ibn Majah)

21. Worshipping Sun, Moon and Stars

Allah, the Exalted, says:

"And from among His Signs are the night and the day, and the sun and the moon. Prostrate not to the sun nor to the moon, but prostrate to Allah Who created them, if you (really) worship Him." (Qur'an, Fussilat 41:37)

"And that He (Allah) is the Lord of Sirius (the star which the pagan Arabs used to worship)." (Qur'an, An-Najm 53:49)

CONCLUSION:

The Idols do not speak and cannot judge

Allah, the Exalted, says:

"And Allah judges with Truth, while those to whom they invoke besides Him, cannot judge anything. Certainly, Allah! He is the All-Hearer, the All-Seer." (Qur'an, Al-Ghafir 40:20)

The Idols cannot create anything and are powerless

Allah, the Exalted, says:

"Say (O Muhammad SAW): "Who is the Lord of the heavens and the earth?" Say: "(It is) Allah." Say: "Have you then taken (for worship) Auliya' (protectors, etc.) other than Him, such as have no power either for benefit or for harm to themselves?" Say: "Is the blind equal to the one who sees? Or darkness equal to light? Or do they assign to Allah partners who created the like of His creation, so that the creation (which they made and His creation) seemed alike to them." Say: "Allah is the Creator of all things, He is the One, the Irresistible." (Qur'an, Ar-Ra'd 13:16)

"Say (O Muhammad SAW to these pagans): "Think! All that you invoke besides Allah show me! What have they created of the earth? Or have they a share in (the creation of) the heavens? Bring me a Book (revealed before this), or some trace of knowledge (in support of your claims), if you are truthful!" (Qur'an, Al-Ahqaf 46:4)

The Idols do not bring us closer to God

Allah, the Exalted, says:

"Surely, the religion (i.e. the worship and the obedience) is for Allah only. And those who take Auliya' (protectors and helpers) besides Him (say): "We worship them only that they may bring us near to Allah." Verily, Allah will judge between them concerning that wherein they differ. Truly, Allah guides not him who is a liar and a disbeliever." (Qur'an, Az-Zumar 39:3)

"And on the Day when We shall gather them all together, We shall say to those who joined partners in worship (with Us): "Where are your partners (false deities) whom you used to assert (as partners in worship with Allah)?" (Qur'an, Al-An'am 6:22)

The Idols cannot help us

Allah, the Exalted, says:

"And those whom you call upon besides Him (Allah) cannot help you nor can they help themselves." (Qur'an, Al-A'raf 7:197)

Humans and Jinn die, Allah is Eternal

Narrated Ibn 'Abbas: The Prophet (peace and blessings be upon him) used to say, "I seek refuge (with You) by Your 'Izzat, none has the right to be worshipped but You Who does not die while the Jinn and the human beings die." (Bukhari)

The disbelievers in Allah will be placed in eternal Hellfire

Allah, the Exalted, says:

"And indeed, it has been revealed to you (O Muhammad SAW), as it was to those (Allah's Messengers) before you: "If you join others in worship with Allah, (then) surely (all) your deeds will be in vain, and you will certainly be among the losers." (Qur'an, Az-Zumar 39:65)

Narrated Abdullah (May Allah be pleased with him): Allah's Apostle (peace and blessings be upon him) said, "Anyone who dies worshipping others along with Allah will definitely enter the Fire." I said, "Anyone who dies worshipping none along with Allah will definitely enter Paradise." (Bukhari)

'Iyad ibn Himar al-Mujashi'i (May Allah be pleased with him) reported that the Messenger of Allah (May Allah's peace and blessings be upon him) said while delivering his sermon one day: "Verily, my Lord has commanded me to teach you that which you do not know of what He has taught me today: 'Whatever wealth which I have conferred upon my slave is lawful for him. And I have created all My slaves with a natural predisposition to worship Allah Alone, but the Devils came to them and turned them away from their religion. They made unlawful for them what I have made lawful for them and commanded them to associate with Me in worship that for which I did not send down any authority.' And verily, Allah looked at the people of the earth and He hated them, both the Arabs and the non-Arabs among them, with the exception of some remnants from the People of the Book. And He said: 'I have sent you (Muhammad) in order to test you, and to test (others) through you. And I revealed to you a Book that cannot be washed away by water, to recite it while you are asleep or awake.' Indeed, Allah commanded me to burn down the Quraysh, to which I said: 'O My Lord, they would break my head like (breaking dry) bread.' Allah said: 'Turn them out as they turned you out, fight against them and We shall give you victory, spend and you shall be spent upon, and send an army and We shall send an army five times its size. Fight with those who obey you those who disobey you.' And He said: 'The inhabitants of Paradise are three (categories of people): He who possesses authority yet is just, charitable, and guided (to doing good), he who is merciful and tender-hearted towards his kin and every Muslim, and he who does not ask others despite having dependents to provide for.' He also said: 'The inhabitants of Hellfire are five (categories of people): The weak who lacks intellect (to prevent him from evil), who is subordinate to you, who does not seek to have family or wealth; and the dishonest whose greed cannot be concealed even in the case of minor things; and one who spends his entire day deceiving you with regards to your family and wealth; and (he mentioned) the miser or the liar and the ill-mannered who uses obscene and foul language." (Muslim) (https://hadeethenc.com/en/browse/hadith/10409)

WHY ARE THE MOST OF PEOPLE DISBELIEVERS

Allah, the Exalted, says:

"O children of Adam, let not Satan tempt you as he removed your parents from Paradise, stripping them of their clothing to show them their private parts. Indeed, he sees you, he and his tribe, from where you do not see them. Indeed, We have made the Devils allies to those who do not believe." *(Qur'an, Al-A'raf 7:27)*

Sheikh Muhammad Saalih al-Munajjid answered to the question:

"Why are most of the people on earth disbelievers, and why does Allah want them to enter Hell?"

Firstly:

Allah, the Exalted, does not love the transgressors, evildoers, disbelievers, so how can it be affirmed that Allah, may He be Exalted, loves all of His creation when the vast majority of them are these types of people? Rather Allah, may He be Exalted, loves those who do good, and He loves the pious, and He loves those who repent, and He loves those who purify themselves, and He loves those who are patient, and He loves those who put their trust in Him, and He loves those who are fair and just. These types of people are the ones for whom Allah, may He be Exalted, affirmed His love and they – naturally – cannot be any but those who affirm His Oneness and not those who associate others with Him.

But despite all that, among the Names of Allah, may He be Glorified, are the Names Ar-Rahman (the Most Gracious), Ar-Raheem (the Most Merciful); His Mercy precedes His Wrath, and His Pardon precedes His Punishment, and He is more Merciful to His slaves than a mother to her child.

There is a difference between mercy and love. Allah, may He be Glorified and Exalted, has sent down a share of His Mercy by virtue of which people show compassion towards one another, He grants provision to His slaves, gives them more time, is forbearing towards them and bears patiently their disbelief and offensive words. All of that is in this world; but in the Hereafter, His Mercy will be only for those who believed in Him and submitted to Him.

Secondly:
Most people on earth are non-Muslims because they are the ones who have chosen disbelief over Islam. Exception are those who didn't receive the message.

Allah, the Exalted, says:

"And who is more unjust than one who is reminded of the Verses of his Lord but turns away from them and forgets what his hands have put forth? Indeed, We have placed over their hearts coverings, lest they understand it, and in their ears deafness. And if you invite them to Guidance - they will never be guided, then - ever." (Qur'an, Al-Kahf 18:57)

They saw the clear signs that point to the truthfulness of the Prophet (peace and blessings of Allah be upon him) and the truthfulness of his call, and the truthfulness and miraculous nature of the Qur'an, and they heard the debates in which the enemies of Islam were defeated and their specious arguments refuted – yet despite all of that, and much more besides, they did not believe in Islam and they did not accept it as their religion; rather billions of them were content to worship a cross that they made or an idol that they carved, or a grave that they built up, or a cow that they worshipped instead of Allah. There is no power and no strength except with Allah.

The Truth is obvious and clear; the signs that point to the greatness of Islam are too many to be counted; no wise person can argue against the evidence that what these disbelievers are doing is false; sound human nature and reasoning reject those (false) acts of worship and the taking of other gods as lords instead of Allah, the One True God. Allah, the Exalted, has highlighted the evidence and has established proof against them.

Thirdly:

As for the answer to the question, So, why does Allah want the majority of His creation to enter Hell? The answer is that Allah, may He be Exalted, does not approve of the disbelief of these people and He does not like it, but they liked it for themselves.

Allah, the Exalted, says:

"If you disbelieve, then verily, Allah is not in need of you, He likes not disbelief for His slaves. And if you are grateful (by being believers), He is pleased therewith for you. No bearer of burdens shall bear the burden of another. Then to your Lord is your return, so He will inform you what you used to do. Verily, He is the All-Knower of that which is in (men's) breasts." (Qur'an, Az-Zumar 39:7)

Allah, the Exalted, does not force anyone to become a Muslim or to become a disbeliever; rather He, may He be Glorified and Exalted, has explained the paths of Truth and falsehood, right and wrong, Islam and disbelief, then He has given people the choice, along with His promise to the Muslims of reward and His warning to the disbelievers of Hell.

Allah, the Exalted, says:

"And say: 'The Truth is from your Lord.' Then whosoever wills, let him believe; and whosoever wills, let him disbelieve. Verily, We have prepared for the Zaalimoon (polytheists and wrongdoers) a Fire whose walls will be surrounding them (disbelievers in the Oneness of Allah). And if they ask for help (relief, water), they will be granted water like boiling oil, that will scald their faces. Terrible is the drink, and an evil Murtafaq (dwelling, resting place)! Verily, as for those who believed and did righteous deeds, certainly We shall not make the reward of anyone who does his (righteous) deeds in the most perfect manner to be lost. These! For them will be 'Adn (Eden) Paradise (everlasting Gardens); wherein rivers flow underneath them; therein they will be adorned with bracelets of gold, and they will wear green garments of fine and thick silk. They will recline therein on raised thrones. How good is the reward, and what an excellent Murtafaq (dwelling, resting place)!" (Qur'an, Al-Kahf 18:29-31)

"Verily, We have created man from Nutfah (drops) of mixed semen (sexual discharge of man and woman), in order to try him, so We made him hearer and seer. Verily, We showed him the way, whether he be grateful or ungrateful. Verily, We have prepared for the disbelievers iron chains, iron collars, and a blazing Fire. Verily, the Abraar (the pious believers of Islamic Monotheism) shall drink of a cup (of wine) mixed with (water from a spring in Paradise called) Kaafoor. A spring wherefrom the slaves of Allah will drink, causing it to gush forth abundantly." (Qur'an, Al-Insan 76:2-6)

Allah offered Guidance to people by sending Messengers with clear signs, yet they chose disbelief.

They were the people of Thamood.

Allah, the Exalted, says:

"And as for Thamood, We showed and made clear to them the Path of Truth (Islamic Monotheism) through Our Messenger (i.e. showed them the way of success), but they preferred blindness to Guidance; so, the Saa'iqah (a destructive awful cry, torment, hit, thunderbolt) of disgracing torment seized them because of what they used to earn. And We saved those who believed and used to fear Allah, keep their duty to Him and avoid evil." (Qur'an, Fussilat 41:17-18)

These modern disbelievers have a precedent; Messengers brought the Truth from their Lord to them. Allah, may He be Exalted, made the Messenger to their own people, so that they would recognize his truthfulness and honesty, and He gave each one of them a sign that is enough proof for people, yet despite that, they said that their Messengers were sorcerers or madmen.

The disbelievers of Quraysh demanded a sign from the Prophet (peace and blessings of Allah be upon him) so, that they would believe. He showed them the splitting of the moon, and they said that it was sorcery. So, the Words of Allah concerning them are true:

"and even if they see every one of the Ayat (signs) they will not believe therein." (Qur'an, Al-An'am 6:25)

The disbelievers did not stop at rejecting the Messengers of God, they conspired against them, to kill them or expel them from their lands.

Allah, the Exalted, says:

"And those who disbelieved, said to their Messengers: 'Surely, we shall drive you out of our land, or you shall return to our religion.' So, their Lord revealed to them: 'Truly, We shall destroy the Zaalimoon (polytheists, disbelievers and wrongdoers).'" (Qur'an, Ibrahim 14:13)

Allah, the Exalted, said about the people of Ibrahim (peace be upon him):

"So, nothing was the answer of [Ibrahim's (Abraham's)] people except that they said: 'Kill him or burn him.' Then Allah saved him from the fire. Verily, in this are indeed signs for a people who believe." (Qur'an, Al-'Ankabut 29:24)

Allah, the Exalted, said concerning the Prophet Muhammad (peace and blessings be upon him):

"And (remember) when the disbelievers plotted against you (O Muhammad SAW) to imprison you or to kill you, or to get you out (from your home, i.e. Makkah)." (Qur'an, Al-Anfal 8:30)

If this was the case with regard to those to whom the Messenger, whom they knew, brought the Message from his Lord, and they saw the signs with their own eyes, then what about those Indians, Chinese and Europeans, if the Arabian Prophet Muhammad (peace and blessings of Allah be upon him) came to them as a bringer of glad tidings and a warner?

When some of the polytheists claimed that Allah, may He be Exalted, approved of their disbelief and that if that was not the case, He would have diverted them from it, our Lord, may He be Blessed and Exalted, showed them to be liars and explained that they were only following their whims and desires and their forefathers who had gone astray.

Allah, the Exalted, said:

"And those who joined others in worship with Allah said: 'If Allah had so willed, neither we nor our fathers would have worshipped aught but Him, nor would we have forbidden anything without (Command from) Him.'" (Qur'an, An-Nahl 16:35)

"And verily, We have sent among every Ummah (community, nation) a Messenger (proclaiming): 'Worship Allah (Alone), and avoid (or keep away from) Taghoot (all false deities, i.e. do not worship Taghoot alongside Allah).' Then of them were some whom Allah guided and of them were some upon whom the straying was justified." (Qur'an, An-Nahl 16:36)

Fourthly:
No one will enter Paradise except a Muslim, because Islam abrogated all the previous religions. Allah, the Exalted, commanded all His creation to enter the religion of Islam and stated that He will never accept any other religion from anyone.

Allah, the Exalted, says:

"And whoever seeks a religion other than Islam, it will never be accepted of him, and in the Hereafter, he will be one of the losers." (Qur'an, Ali 'Imran 3:85)

With regard to the previous nations, everyone who believed in his Prophet and Messenger will enter Paradise; they were the Muslims of their time.

Allah, the Exalted, says:

"Verily, those who believe and those who are Jews and Christians, and Sabians, whoever believes in Allah and the Last Day and does righteous good deeds shall have their reward with their Lord, on them shall be no fear, nor shall they grieve." (Qur'an, Al-Baqarah 2:62)

Fifthly:
Ibn Taymiyah (May Allah have mercy on him) said:

"The Khaarijis were the first ones to regard the Muslims as disbelievers, saying that they become disbelievers because of committing sins. They also regarded as disbelievers those who disagreed with their innovation and regarded it as permissible to kill them and take their wealth. This is how the innovators are: they introduce an innovation and regard as disbelievers those who differ with them, concerning it. Ahl as-Sunnah wa'l-Jamaa'ah follow the Qur'an and Sunnah, and obey Allah and His Messenger; they follow the Truth and show compassion to all people. End quote." (Majmoo' al-Fataawa, 3/279)

Sixthly:
By the Mercy of Allah, the Exalted, to His slaves, He will not punish with Hell those whom the call of Islam did not reach. For those who are alive at the present, or who lived before, whom news of Islam did not reach, they will be tested on the Day of Resurrection. (43)

FINAL DESTINATION OF MUSLIMS AND NON-MUSLIMS

Table 3. Final Destination of Muslims and Non-Muslims

ALLAH has chosen Islam for all mankind "This day, I have perfected your religion for you, completed My Favor upon you, and have chosen for you Islam as your religion." (Qur'an, Al-Ma'idah 5:3)	
Muslims	All non-Muslims including atheists
Follow Allah The Creator of all that exists The Judge of Judgment Day	Follow Satan temporary god on earth "And whoever follows the footsteps of Satan - indeed, he enjoins immorality and wrongdoing." (Qur'an, An-Nur 24:21)
Muslims Follow the Truth: Qur'an and Sunnah "O you who have believed, obey Allah and obey the Messenger and those in authority among you." (Qur'an, An-*Nisa 4:59*)	**Non-Muslims** Follow the Falsehood, own whims and desires "Do you not see that We have sent the Devils upon the disbelievers, inciting them to (evil) with (constant) incitement?" (Qur'an, Maryam 19:83)

Blissful life	Depressed life
"Successful indeed are the believers." (Qur'an, Al-Mu'minun 23:1)	*"And whoever turns away from My remembrance - indeed, he will have a depressed life, and We will gather him on the Day of Resurrection blind." (Qur'an, Taha 20:124)*
ETERNAL PARADISE	ETERNAL HELLFIRE
"Indeed, for the righteous with their Lord are the Gardens of Pleasure." (Qur'an, Al-Qalam 68:34)	*"Indeed, Allah will gather the hypocrites and disbelievers in Hell all together." (Qur'an, An-Nisa 4:140)*

3. Bowing to Someone is Shirk

Bowing in Islam is almost entirely reserved for prayer. Even Muhammad (peace and blessings of Allah be upon him) would not allow people to bow to him. Bowing in reverence to another human is considered Shirk which is a very serious sin in Islam. (44)

4. Insulting Others' False Gods

Allah, the Exalted, says:

"And insult not those whom they (disbelievers) worship besides Allah, lest they insult Allah wrongfully without knowledge. Thus, We have made fair-seeming to each people its own doings; then to their Lord is their return and He shall then inform them of all that they used to do." (Qur'an, Al-An'am 6:108)

5. Making Idols

Allah, the Exalted, says:

"You worship besides Allah only idols, and you only invent falsehood. Verily, those whom you worship besides Allah have no power to give you provision, so seek your provision from Allah (Alone), and worship Him (Alone), and be grateful to Him. To Him (Alone) you will be brought back." (Qur'an, Al-'Ankabut 29:17)

"Do they hear you when you supplicate? Or do they benefit you, or do they harm?"
(Qur'an, Ash-Shu'ara 26:72-73)

The sin of making statues involves the sculptor, the buyer, the worshipper and deifiers. Making idols (Indian gods, Buddha, Jesus, calf, etc.) is forbidden.

Islam prescribes that idols should be destroyed and smashed, not made and repaired. (45)

1 – Batil (Falsehood, i.e. Satan or Polytheism, etc.) is Ever Bound to Vanish

Narrated Abdullah bin Masud: "The Prophet (peace and blessings be upon him) entered Makkah and (at that time) there were three hundred-and-sixty idols around the Ka'bah. He started stabbing the idols with a stick he had in his hand and reciting: *"And say: "Truth (i.e. Islamic Monotheism or this Qur'an or Jihad against polytheists) has come and Batil (falsehood, i.e. Satan or polytheism, etc.) has vanished. Surely! Batil is ever bound to vanish."* (Qur'an, Al-Isra 17:81)* (Bukhari)

2 – Prohibition of Trade of Idols

Narrated Jabir bin Abdullah: "I heard Allah's Apostle (peace and blessings be upon him), in the year of the Conquest of Makkah, saying, 'Allah and His Apostle made illegal the trade of alcohol, dead animals, pigs and idols.' The people asked, 'O Allah's Apostle! What about the fat of dead animals, for it was used for greasing the boats and the hides; and people use it for lights?' He (peace and blessings be upon him) said, 'No, it is illegal.' Allah's Apostle further said, 'May Allah curse the Jews, for Allah made the fat (of animals) illegal for them, yet they melted the fat and sold it and ate its price.'" (Bukhari)

3 – Do Not Leave an Image Without Obliterating it

Abu'l-Hayyaj al-Asadi told that 'Ali Ibn Abu Talib said to him: "Should I not send you on the same mission as Allah's Messenger (peace and blessings be upon him) sent me? Do not leave an image without obliterating it or a high grave without levelling It." This Hadith has been reported by Habib with the same chain of transmitters and he said: "(Do not leave) a picture without obliterating it." (Muslim)

4 – The Prophet Was Sent to Break Idols

Amr b. 'Abasa Sulami reported: "In the state of the Ignorance (before embracing Islam), I used to think that the people were in error and they were not on anything (which may be called the right path) and worshiped the idols. Meanwhile, I heard of a man in Makkah who was giving news (on the basis of his Prophetic knowledge); so, I sat on my ride and went to him. The Messenger of Allah (peace be upon him) was at that time hiding as his people had made life hard for him. I adopted a friendly attitude (towards the Makkans and thus managed) to enter Makkah and go to him (the Holy Prophet) and I said to him: 'Who are you?' He said: 'I am a Prophet (of Allah).' I again said: 'Who is a Prophet?' He said: '(I am a Prophet in the sense that) I have been sent by Allah.' I said: 'What is that which you have been sent with?' He said: 'I have been sent to join ties of relationship (with kindness and affection), to break the idols and to proclaim the Oneness of Allah (in a manner that) nothing is to be associated with Him.'" (Muslim)

5 – The Idols were Dismantled and Burnt in Dhul-Khalasa

Narrated Jarir: Allah's Messenger (peace and blessings of Allah be upon him) said to me, "Will you relieve me from Dhul-Khalasa? Dhul-Khalasa was a house (of an idol) belonging to the tribe of Khath'am called Al-Ka'ba Al-Yama-niya. So, I proceeded with one hundred and fifty cavalry men from the tribe of Ahmas, who were excellent knights. It happened that I could not sit firm on horses, so the Prophet (peace and blessings be upon him) stroke me over my chest till I saw his fingermarks over my chest, he said, 'O Allah! Make him firm and make him a guiding and rightly guided man.' Jarir proceeded towards that house, and dismantled and burnt it. Then he sent a man to Allah's Apostle informing him of that. Then the Messenger said, "By Him Who has sent you with the Truth, I did not come to you till I had left it like an emancipated or gabby camel (i.e. completely marred and spoilt)." Jarir added, "The Prophet (peace and blessings be upon him) asked for Allah's blessings for the horses and the men of Ahmas five times." (Bukhari)

6 – Prohibition of Worshipping and Making Pictures at the Grave

Narrated Aisha (May Allah be pleased with her): "Umm Habiba and Umm Salamah mentioned about a church they had seen in Ethiopia in which there were pictures. They told the Prophet about it, on which he (peace and blessings be upon him) said, "If any religious man dies amongst those people, they would build a place of worship at his grave and make these pictures in it. They will be the worst creature in the sight of Allah on the Day of Resurrection." (Bukhari)

6. Atheism

Allah, the Exalted, says:

"Were they created by nothing, or were they themselves the creators?" (Qur'an, At-Tur 52:35)

"Or did they create the heavens and the earth? Nay, but they have no firm Belief." (Qur'an, At-Tur 52:36)

Atheism is a complete disbelief in God, it is Greater sin than Shirk because it denies the position of Allah as the Unique Creator and Sustainer of the Universe. Atheist thinks that the Universe appeared by chance or existed from eternity, without beginning and end. (46)

There is One, supreme Creator and that everything else is merely a creation of the Creator with no share in Divinity. Allah has decreed all things from eternity and knows that they will happen at times that are known to Him, and in specific ways, and that He has written that and willed it, and they happen according to what He has decreed. It is only by knowing the Greatness of the Creator, man can realize his weakness, powerless, limitation. We are nobody and nothing without our Creator. We exist as Allah exists. We breathe, see, hear, speak, walk, healthy, wealthy…; all by Allah's Grace. This means that the one who does not acknowledge this Truth is an atheist and it is the worst deviation. There is no value in any good deed that he does, it is good only in his own eyes. The one who neglects the Creator, there cannot be any good in his actions, no blessings of Allah, and he has no share in the Hereafter.

Allah, the Exalted, says:

"How can you disbelieve in Allah? Seeing that you were dead and He gave you life. Then He will give you death, then again will bring you to life (on the Day of Resurrection) and then unto Him you will return." (Qur'an, Al-Baqarah 2:28)

7. Darwinism

Allah, the Exalted, says:

"(And mention) when your Lord said to the angels, "Indeed, I am going to create a human being from clay. So, when I have proportioned him and breathed into him of My (created) soul, then fall down to him in prostration." (Qur'an, Sad 38:71-72)

Other Verse: *As-Sajdah 32:4.*

Charles Darwin's theory of biological evolution, stating that all species of organisms arise and develop through the natural selection of small, inherited variations that increase the individual's ability to compete, survive and reproduce; it is a complete disbelief in Allah, the Creator of all that exists!

Allah, the Omnipotent, created all mankind:

- Adam without mother and father,
- Hawwa (Eve), Adam's wife, from the ribs of Adam,
- Jesus without father,
- All other people from two drops of water (from mother and father).

Allah is capable to do everything, just by saying "Be".

The embryology steps described in the Qur'an. The human body and soul are Allah's miracles.

Allah transformed some of Children of Israel into monkeys as a punishment for their disobedience.

Allah, the Exalted, says:

"And indeed, you knew those amongst you who transgressed in the matter of the Sabbath (i.e. Saturday). We said to them: 'Be you monkeys, despised and rejected.' So, We made this punishment an example to their own and to succeeding generations and a lesson to those who are Al-Muttaqoon (the pious)." (Qur'an, Al-Baqarah 2:65-66)

The transformation from the human beings into the monkeys was a punishment from Allah for their wrongdoing. This punishment was not exclusively for the Children of Israel, rather the Prophet (peace and blessings be upon him) told us that the Hour will not begin until such transformation happens among the Ummah too.

Narrated Abu Malik Ash'ari: The Messenger of Allah (peace and blessings be upon him) said: "People among my nation will drink wine, calling it by another name, and musical instruments will be played for them and singing girls (will sing for them). Allah will cause the earth to swallow them up, and will turn them into monkeys and pigs." (Ibn Majah)

8. Speaking about Allah Without Knowledge

Allah, the Exalted, says:

"And of the people is he who disputes about Allah without knowledge and follows every rebellious Devil." (Qur'an, Al Hajj 22:3)

"And among men is he who disputes about Allah, without knowledge or Guidance, or a Book giving light (from Allah)." (Qur'an, Al-Haj 22:8)

"Say (O Muhammad SAW): "(But) the things that my Lord has indeed forbidden are AlFawahish (great evil sins, every kind of unlawful sexual intercourse, etc.) whether committed openly or secretly, sins (of all kinds), unrighteous oppression, joining partners (in worship) with Allah for which He has given no authority, and saying things about Allah of which you have no knowledge." (Qur'an, Al-A'raf 7:33)

9. Disbelieving in Allah

Allah, the Exalted, says:

"Allah is the Creator of all things, and He is the Wakil (Trustee, Disposer of affairs, Guardian, etc.) over all things. To Him belong the keys of the heavens and the earth. And those who disbelieve in the Ayat (proofs, evidences, verses, signs, revelations, etc.) of Allah, such are they who will be the losers." (Qur'an, Az-Zumar 39:62-63)

"How is it that you deny Allah, while you were lifeless and He gave you life; then He will make you die, and then He will make you live again, and then to Him you will be returned?" (Qur'an, Al-Baqarah 2:28)

"Verily, those who disbelieve, and die while they are disbelievers, it is they on whom is the Curse of Allah and of the angels and mankind, combined." (Qur'an, Al-Baqarah 2:161)

Other Verses: Fatir 35:3, Al-Baqarah 2:39, Taha 20:126-128, Az-Zumar 39:67, Al-Anfal 8:52.

Narrated Abu Hurairah (May Allah be pleased with him): The Messenger of Allah (peace and blessings be upon him) said: "Allah Almighty has said: 'The son of Adam denied Me and he had no right to do so. And he reviled Me and he had no right to do so. As for his denying Me, it is his saying: 'He will not remake me as He made me at first' (1) - and the initial creation (of him) is no easier for Me than remaking him. As for his reviling Me, it is his saying: Allah has taken to Himself a son, while I am the One, the Everlasting Refuge. I begot not nor was I begotten, and there is none comparable to Me. (1) i.e. bring me back to life after death.'" (Bukhari)

10. Thinking Negative about Allah

Abu Hurairah (May Allah be pleased with him) reported that the Prophet (May Allah's peace and blessings be upon him) said: "Allah, Glorified and Exalted, said: 'I am as My slave thinks of Me, and I am with him wherever he remembers Me.' By Allah, Allah is more pleased with the repentance of His servant than one of you would be upon finding his lost camel in a barren desert. 'Whoever draws nearer to Me by a hand span, I draw nearer to him by a cubit; and whoever draws nearer to Me by a cubit, I draw nearer to him by a fathom; and whoever comes towards Me walking, I go to him running'" (Bukhari and Muslim; this is the wording of one of the narrations of Imam Muslim)
(https://hadeethenc.com/en/browse/hadith/3636)

Abu Muhammad al-Maqdisī in his book "Reflections: Expecting the Best from Allah" wrote:

"In accordance with how good your expectations of and hope in Allah are and how truthful your reliance and trust are in Him, Allah will not betray your hopes in the least, as He does not betray the hopes of those who hope and does not cause any effort to go to waste." (47)

Narrated Jabir (May Allah be pleased with him): "I heard the Prophet (peace and blessings of Allah be upon him) say, three days before he died: "No one of you should die except thinking positively of Allah." (Muslim)

11. Neglecting any Obligatory Act Ordered by our Creator

Allah, the Exalted, says:

"Do you then believe in a part of the Book and disbelieve in the other? What then is the reward of such among you as do this but disgrace in the life of this world and on the day of resurrection they shall be sent back to the most grievous chastisement and Allah is not at all heedless of what you do." (Qur'an, Al-Baqarah 2:85)

"Those are the ones who disbelieve in the Verses of their Lord and in (their) meeting Him, so their deeds have become worthless; and We will not assign to them on the Day of Resurrection any weight (i.e. importance)." (Qur'an, Al-Kahf 18:105)

"And for those who did wrong there is another punishment before that, but most of them do not know." (Qur'an, At-Tur 52-47)

Other Verse: *Az-Zumar 39:47.*

The Five Pillars of Islam

The most important Muslim practices are the Five Pillars of Islam.

The Five Pillars of Islam are the five obligations that every Muslim must satisfy in order to live a good and responsible life according to Islam.

The Five Pillars consist of:

- **Shahadah**: Ashhadu alla ilaha illallah wa ashhadu anna Muhammadarrasulullah "I bear witness that there is no deity but Allah, and I bear witness that Muhammad is the Messenger of Allah."
- **Salat**: performing prayers in the proper way five times each day
- **Zakat**: paying alms (or charity) tax to benefit the poor and the needy
- **Sawm**: fasting during Ramadan
- **Hajj**: pilgrimage to Makkah

12. Questioning Allah for What He Does

Allah, the Exalted, says:

"He cannot be questioned as to what He does, while they will be questioned." (Qur'an, Al-Anbya 21:23)

"But stop them, verily they are to be questioned." (Qur'an, As-Saffat 37:24)

"So, by your Lord (O Muhammad SAW), We shall certainly call all of them to account. For all that they used to do." (Qur'an, Al-Hijr 15:92-93)

Other Verse: *Al-Ma'idah 5:101.*

One of the frightening events that will take place on that Day is that Allah will place a seal on the hearts of the disbelievers and hypocrites, and their hands and feet will speak of what they used to do. They will not be questioned at that time; rather their bodies will be questioned and will bear witness against them, speaking of their sins. (48)

And there are other Verses that indicate the opposite of that, such as the following:

Allah, the Exalted, says:

"So, on that Day no question will be asked of man or Jinn as to his sin." (Qur'an, Ar-Rahman 55:39)

"But the Mujrimoon (criminals, disbelievers, polytheists, sinners, etc.) will not be questioned of their sins." (Qur'an, Al-Qasas 28:78)

"The Mujrimoon (polytheists, criminals, sinners, etc.) will be known by their marks." (Qur'an, Ar-Rahman 55:41)

13. Not Remembering Allah

Allah, the Exalted, says:

"Therefore remember Me (by praying, glorifying). I will remember you." (Qur'an, Al-Baqarah 2:152)

"And remember your Rubb by your tongue and within yourself, humbly and with fear and without loudness in words, in the mornings and in the afternoons, and be not of those who are neglectful." (Qur'an, Al-A'raf 7:205)

"And remember Allah much, that you may be successful." (Qur'an, Al-Jumu'ah 62:10)

Other Verse: Al-Ahzab 33:35 and 33:41-42, Al-'Ankabut 29:45.

<u>For the Disbelievers in Allah: Miserable Life Unavoidable</u>

"But whosoever turns away from My Reminder (i.e. neither believes in this Quran nor acts on its orders, etc.) verily, for him is a life of hardship, and We shall raise him up blind on the Day of Resurrection." (Qur'an, Taha 20:124)

"And thus, do We requite him who transgresses beyond bounds [i.e. commits the great sins and disobeys his Lord (Allah) and believes not in His Messengers, and His revealed Books, like this Qur'an, etc.], and believes not in the Ayat (proofs, evidences, verses, lessons, signs, revelations, etc.) of his Lord, and the torment of the Hereafter is far more severe and everlasting." (Qur'an, Taha 20:127)

Abu Hurairah (May Allah be pleased with him) reported that the Prophet (May Allah's peace and blessings be upon him) said: "Anyone who relieves a hardship for a believer in this world, Allah will relieve one of his hardships on the Day of Resurrection. Anyone who makes things easy for a hard-pressed person, Allah will make things easy for him in this world and in the Hereafter. Anyone who covers up the faults and sins of a Muslim, Allah will cover up his faults and sins in this world and in the Hereafter. Allah supports His slave as long as the slave supports his brother. Anyone who travels a path in search of knowledge, Allah will make an easy path for him to Paradise. There are no people who gather in one of the houses of Allah, reciting the Book of Allah, learning it and teaching it, except tranquility descends upon them, mercy covers them, the angels flock and hover around them, and Allah mentions them in the presence of those near Him (in the Heavens). And anyone who lags behind in doing good deeds, his noble lineage will not advance him any faster." (Muslim) (https://hadeethenc.com/en/browse/hadith/4801)
Abu Hurairah (May Allah be pleased with him) reported that the Prophet (May Allah's peace and blessings be upon him) said: "Verily, this world is cursed, and everything in it is cursed, except the remembrance of Allah in all what is relevant to it; a scholar and a seeker of knowledge." (Ibn Majah and Tirmidhi) (https://hadeethenc.com/en/browse/hadith/3788)

Abu Ad-Darda (May Allah be pleased with him) reported that the Messenger of Allah (May Allah's peace and blessings be upon him) said: "Shall I not inform you of the best of your deeds which are the most praiseworthy in the sight of your Lord, and the highest in rank, and better for you than spending gold and silver in charity, and better for you than encountering your enemies in battle so they strike your necks and you strike theirs?" They said: 'Certainly.' He said: "Remembrance of Allah, the Exalted."
(Ibn Majah) (https://hadeethenc.com/en/browse/hadith/3575)

Narrated Abu Musa Al-Ash'ari (May Allah be pleased with him): The Prophet (peace and blessings be upon him) said, "The similitude of one who remembers his Rubb and one who does not remember Him, is like that of the living and the dead." (Bukhari and Muslim)

Narrated Abu Hurairah (May Allah be pleased with him): The Messenger of Allah (peace and blessings be upon him) said, "There are two statements that are light for the tongue to remember, heavy in the scales and are dear to the Merciful: 'Subhan-Allahi wa bihamdihi, Subhan-Allahil-Azim (Glory be to Allah and His is the Praise, (and) Allah, the Greatest is free from imperfection).'" (Bukhari and Muslim)

Narrated Abu Hurairah (May Allah be pleased with him): The Messenger of Allah (peace and blessings be upon him) said, "The uttering of the words: "Subhan-Allah (Allah is free from imperfection), Al-hamdu lillah (all praise is due to Allah), La ilaha illallah (there is no true god except Allah) and Allahu Akbar (Allah is the Greatest)' is dearer to me than anything over which the sun rises." (Muslim)

Narrated Abu Hurairah (May Allah be pleased with him): The Messenger of Allah (peace and blessings be upon him) said, "He who utters a hundred times in a day these words: 'La ilaha illallahu, wahdahu la sharika lahu, lahul-mulku wa lahul-hamdu, wa Huwa 'ala kulli sha'in Qadir (there is no true god except Allah. He is One and He has no partner with Him; His is the Sovereignty and His is the Praise, and He is Omnipotent)', he will have a reward equivalent to that for emancipating ten slaves, a hundred good deeds will be recorded to his credit, hundreds of his sins will be blotted out from his scroll, and he will be safeguarded against the Devil on that day till the evening; and no one will exceed him in doing more excellent good deeds except someone who has recited these words more often than him. And he who utters: 'Subhan-Allahi wa bihamdihi (Allah is free from imperfection and His is the Praise)' one hundred times a day, his sins will be obliterated even if they are equal to the extent of the foam of the ocean." (Bukhari and Muslim)

Narrated Abu Hurairah (May Allah be pleased with him): The Messenger of Allah (peace and blessings be upon him) said, "He who recites after every prayer: Subhan-Allah (Allah is free from imperfection) thirty-three times; Al-hamdu lillah (Praise be to Allah) thirty-three times; Allahu Akbar (Allah is Greatest) thirty-three times; and completes the hundred with: La ilaha illallahu, wahdahu la sharika lahu, lahul-mulku wa lahul-hamdu, wa Huwa 'ala kulli shai'in Qadir (there is no true god except Allah. He is One and He has no partner with Him. His is the Sovereignty and His is the Praise, and He is Omnipotent), will have all his sins pardoned even if they may be as large as the foam on the surface of the sea." (Muslim)

Narrated Juwairiyah bint Al-Harith (May Allah be pleased with her), the Mother of the Believers:

"The Prophet (peace and blessings be upon him) came out from my apartment in the morning as I was busy in performing the dawn prayer. He (peace and blessings be upon him) came back in the forenoon and found me sitting there. The Prophet (peace and blessings be upon him) said, 'Are you still in the same position as I left you.' I replied in the affirmative. Thereupon, the Prophet (peace and blessings be upon him) said, 'I recited four words three times after I had left you. If these are to be weighed against all you have recited since morning, these will be heavier. These are: Subhan-Allahi wa bihamdihi, 'adada khalqihi, wa rida nafsihi, wa zinatah 'arshihi, wa midada kalimatihi [Allah is free from imperfection and I begin with His Praise, as many times as the number of His creatures, in accordance with His Good Pleasure, equal to the weight of His Throne and equal to the ink that may be used in recording the words (for His Praise)].'" (Muslim)

Narrated Jabir (May Allah be pleased with him): The Prophet (peace and blessings be upon him) said,
"For him who says: 'Subhan-Allahi wa bi hamdihi (Allah is free from imperfection, and I begin with praising Him, and to him, a palm-tree will be planted in Jannah." (Tirmidhi)

Narrated Abu Musa (May Allah be pleased with him): The Messenger of Allah (peace and blessings be upon him) said to me, "Shall I not guide you to a treasure from the treasures of Jannah?" I said: 'Yes, O Messenger of Allah!' Thereupon he (peace and blessings be upon him) said, '(Recite) 'La hawla wa la quwwata illa billah' (There is no change of a condition nor power except by Allah).'" (Bukhari and Muslim)

14. Feeling Secure from the Plot of Allah

Allah, the Exalted, says:

"(They took to fight because of their) arrogance in the land and their plotting of evil. But the evil plot encompasses only him who makes it. Then, can they expect anything (else), but the Sunnah (way of dealing) of the peoples of old? So, no change will you find in Allah's Sunnah (way of dealing), and no turning off will you find in Allah's Sunnah (way of dealing)." (Qur'an, Fatir 35:43)
"And (remember) when the disbelievers plotted against you (O Muhammad) to imprison you or to kill you, or to get you out (from your home, i.e. Makkah); they were plotting and Allah too was plotting; and Allah is the Best of those who plot." (Qur'an, Al-Anfal 8:30)

"Verily, they are but plotting a plot (against you O Muhammad, peace be upon him). And I (too) am planning a plan." (Qur'an, At-Tariq 86:15-16)

Other Verse: *At-Tur 52:42, An-Nisa 4:108.*

15. Despair of the Mercy of Allah

Allah, the Exalted, says:
"Say, "O My servants who have transgressed against themselves (by sinning), do not despair of the Mercy of Allah. Indeed, Allah forgives all sins. Indeed, it is He Who is the Forgiving, the Merciful." (Qur'an, Az-Zumar 39:53)

"And who despairs of the Mercy of his Lord except those who are astray?" (Qur'an, Al-Hijr 15:56)

"Certainly no one despairs of Allah's Mercy, except the people who disbelieve." (Qur'an, Yusuf 12:87)

Other Verses: Al-Baqarah 2:214, Al-A'raf 7:156, Al-Mu'minun 23:118.

Narrated Abu Dharr (May Allah be pleased with him): The Prophet (peace and blessings be upon him) said, "Allah the Almighty says: 'Whosoever does a good deed, will have (reward) ten times like it and I add more; and whosoever does an evil, will have the punishment like it or I will forgive (him); and whosoever approaches Me by one span, I will approach him by one cubit; and whosoever approaches Me by one cubit, I approach him by one fathom, and whosoever comes to Me walking, I go to him running; and whosoever meets Me with an earth-load of sins without associating anything with Me, I meet him with Forgiveness like that." (Muslim)

Narrated Abu Hurairah (May Allah be pleased with him): "I heard Messenger of Allah (peace and blessings be upon him) saying, "When Allah created the creatures, He wrote in the Book, which is with Him over His Throne: 'Verily, My Mercy prevailed over My Wrath." (Bukhari and Muslim)

Narrated Abu Hurairah (May Allah be pleased with him): The Prophet (peace and blessings be upon him) said, "Allah, the Exalted and Glorious, said: "A slave committed a sin and he said: 'O Allah, forgive my sin', and Allah said: 'My slave committed a sin and then he realized that he has a Rubb Who forgives the sin or punishes for the sin.' He then again committed a sin and said: 'My Rubb, forgive my sin', and Almighty Allah said: 'My slave committed a sin and then realized that he has a Rubb Who forgives his sin or punishes for the sin.' He again committed a sin and said: 'My Rubb, forgive my sin', and Almighty Allah said: 'My slave has committed a sin and then realized that he has a Rubb Who forgives the sin or takes (him) to account for sin, I have granted Forgiveness to my slave. Let him do whatever he likes." (Muslim) 'Abd al-A'la said: "I do not know whether he said thrice or four times to do "what you desire". The Hadlth has been narrated on the authority of 'Abd al-A'la b. Hammad with the same chain of transmitters.

Narrated Abu Musa (May Allah be pleased with him): The Prophet (peace and blessings be upon him) said, "Allah, the Exalted, stretches His Hand during the night, so that those who commit sins by day may repent, and He stretches His Hand in the day, so that those who commit sins by night may repent. He keeps doing so until the sun rises from the west." (Muslim)

Commentary: Allah's stretching of His Hands is one of His Attributes, and as Muslims we have to believe in this without reasoning, as is the case with His other Attributes. This has been the stand of our pious predecessors (As-Salaf-us-Salih). The process of acceptance of penitence by Allah will continue until the Day of Resurrection when the sun will rise from the west and repenting or accepting Islam will not avail. Therefore, one should not make any delay in penitence. (49)

Anas ibn Malik (May Allah be pleased with him) reported that the Prophet (May Allah's peace and blessings be upon him) said: "When a disbeliever does a good deed, he is rewarded for it in this world. As to the believer, Allah the Almighty saves his good deeds to reward him in the Hereafter and provides him with sustenance in this life as a reward for his obedience." (Muslim)
(https://hadeethenc.com/en/browse/hadith/10105)

Abu Hurairah (May Allah be pleased with him) reported: The Messenger of Allah (peace and blessings be upon him) said, "Allah has divided Mercy into one hundred parts; and He retained with Him ninety-nine parts, and sent down to earth one part. Through this one-part creatures deal with one another with compassion, so much so that an animal lifts its hoof over its young lest it should hurt it." (Bukhari and Muslim)

Narrated Jabir bin 'Abdullah (May Allah be pleased with him): "I heard the Prophet (peace and blessings be upon him) saying three days before his death: "Let none of you die unless he has good expectations from Allah." (Muslim)

Narrated Anas (May Allah be pleased with him): "I heard the Messenger of Allah (peace and blessings be upon him) say: "Allah, the Exalted, said: 'O son of Adam, so long as you call upon Me and ask of Me, I shall forgive you for what you have done, and I shall not mind. O son of Adam, were your sins to reach the clouds of the sky and were you then to ask Forgiveness of Me, I would forgive you. O son of Adam, were you to come to Me with sins nearly as great as the earth and were you then to face Me, ascribing no partner to Me, I would bring you Forgiveness nearly as great as it.'" (Tirmidhi and Ahmad)

Commentary:
1. What it really means is that if sins of a Muslim, committed in ignorance and carelessness, become so numerous that in stacks touch the heights of skies, he should not lose hope in Allah's Mercy. If he repents wholeheartedly for his sins, makes penitence for them and begs Allah's Forgiveness, he will certainly find Allah's Mercy open for him.
2. Shirk (polytheism) is an absolutely unpardonable sin. All other sins, how many and how grave they may be, can be forgiven by Allah. He will pardon them if He likes and send the sinful persons straight to Jannah, or keep them for a while in Hell and then shift them to Jannah. In any case, the punishment of Hell will not be eternal for them, as it is for the Mushriks (polytheist). (50)

Jacob (Ya'qub, peace be upon him), after he lost two children, he did not despair, rather he said:

"He [Ya'qub (Jacob)] said: "Nay, but your own selves have beguiled you into something. So, patience is most fitting (for me). May be Allah will bring them (back) all to me. Truly He! only He is All-Knowing, All-Wise." (Qur'an, Yusuf 12:83)

Zakariah (peace be upon him) did not despair even with old age from having children:

"Saying: "My Lord! Indeed, my bones have grown feeble, and grey hair has spread on my head, And I have never been unblest in my invocation to You, O my Lord!" (Qur'an, Maryam 19:4)

Despairing of the Mercy of Allah is one of the traps of Shaytan.
Despondency is tougher than despair of the Mercy of Allah.
Disappointment literally means hopelessness of good, depression, melancholy, dejection.

Four Promises from Allah, the Exalted:

1) *"So, Remember Me, I Will Remember You." (Qur'an, Al-Baqarah 2:152)*

2) *"If you are grateful, I will surely increase you." (Qur'an, Ibrahim 14:7)*

3) *"Call upon Me and I will respond to you." (Qur'an, Ghafir 40:60)*

4) *"Allah will not punish them while they seek Forgiveness." (Qur'an, Al-Anfal 8:33)*

16. Seeking Help of Other than Allah is Shirk

Allah, the Exalted, says:

"And when My slaves ask you (O Muhammad SAW) concerning Me, then (answer them), I am indeed near (to them by My Knowledge). I respond to the invocations of the supplicant when he calls on Me <u>(without any mediator or intercessor)</u>. So, let them obey Me and believe in Me, so that they may be led aright." (Qur'an, Al-Baqarah 2:186)

"And invoke not besides Allah, any that will neither profit you, nor hurt you, but if (in case) you did so, you shall certainly be one of the Zalimun (polytheists and wrongdoers). And if Allah touches you with hurt, there is none who can remove it but He; and if He intends any good for you, there is none who can repel His Favour which He causes it to

reach whomsoever of His slaves He will. And He is the Oft-Forgiving, Most Merciful."
(Qur'an, Yunus 10:106-107)

"Verily, those whom you worship besides Allah have no power to give you provision, so seek your provision from Allah (Alone), and worship Him (Alone), and be grateful to Him. To Him (Alone) you will be brought back." (Qur'an, Al-'Ankabut 29:17)

Other Verses: An-Naml 27:62, Al-Anfal 8:45.

Allah calls Himself Al-Musta'an— The One whose help is sought— on two occasions in the Qur'an. Al-Musta'an is the One whose assistance and support are sought and in whom refuge is taken. Any help the creation provides to each other, is through His help Alone!
Musta'an comes from the root *'ayn-waaw-noon* which points to two main meanings. The first main meaning is to seek or ask for help and assistance and the second is to aid, cooperate and help one another. A third meaning is to be middle-aged.
This root appears 11 times in the Qur'an in five derived forms. Examples of these forms are *wa a'aanahu* ("and helped him"), *ta'aawanoo* ("help one another"), *nasta'eenu* "(we ask for help") and *'awaanun* ("middle-aged"). (51)

In each prayer you say: *"You (Alone) we worship, and You (Alone) we ask for help (for each and everything)." (Qur'an, Al-Fatihah 1:5)*

Seek Al-Musta'an first and foremost.

Focus less on people, don't fear the effect of anyone's decisions and know that even if people seem to benefit you, the true source is Al-Musta'an.

Limit yourself in asking others.

Hadith on Independence: Paradise for one who never asks people for anything
Thawban reported: The Messenger of Allah (peace and blessings be upon him) said, "Who will guarantee for me that he will not ask people for anything, and I will guarantee for him Paradise?" Thawban said, "I will," and after that he would not ask anyone for anything. (Abu Dawud)
https://www.abuaminaelias.com/dailyhadithonline/2012/10/21/jannah-never-ask-people

Even though in cases it is permissible to ask others, limiting yourself in seeking aid from others is a characteristic of the pious and takes courage and strength and truly reliance on Allah; the promise for those people is no less than Paradise.

"Allah is sufficient for me. La ilaha illa Huwa (none has the right to be worshipped but He), in Him I put my trust and He is the Lord of the Mighty Throne." (Qur'an, At-Tawbah 9:129)

Ḥasbiyallahu la ilaha illa huwa `alayhi tawakkalt, wa huwa Rabbu 'l-`Arshi 'l-`Aẓīm.
Allah is sufficient for me. There is none worthy of worship but Him. I have placed my trust in Him, He is Lord of the Majestic Throne. (Recite seven times in Arabic in the morning and evening)
Reference: Allah will grant whoever recites these seven times in the morning or evening whatever he desires from this world or the next. (Ibn As-Sunni, Abu Dawud) (https://sunnah.com/hisn/84)

Abu Abbas Abdullah bin Abbas (May Allah be pleased with him) said: "One day I was behind the Prophet (peace and blessings of Allah be upon him) riding on the same mount and he said, "O young man, I shall teach you some words of advice: "Be mindful of Allah and Allah will protect you. Be mindful of Allah and you will find Him in front of you. If you ask, then ask Allah Alone; and if you seek help, then seek help from Allah Alone. And know that if the nation were to gather together to benefit you with anything, they would not benefit you except with what Allah had already prescribed for you. And if they were to gather together to harm you with anything, they would not harm you except with what Allah had already prescribed against you. The pens have been lifted and the pages have dried…" (Tirmidhi)

The Qur'an says:

"I put my trust in Allah, my Lord and your Lord! There is not a moving (living) creature but He has grasp of its forelock. Verily, my Lord is on the Straight Path (the Truth)." (Qur'an, Hud 11:56)

"He is my Lord! La ilaha illa Huwa (none has the right to be worshipped but He)! In Him is my trust, and to Him will be my return with repentance." (Qur'an, Ar-R'ad 13:30)

"And it is Allah (Alone) Whose help can be sought against that which you assert." (Qur'an, Yusuf 12:18)

"Our Lord is the Most Beneficent, Whose Help is to be sought against that which you attribute…" (Qur'an, Al-Anbya 21:112)

17. Abomination of Saying "Forgive me if You Wish, O Allah!"

Narrated Abu Hurairah (May Allah be pleased with him) said: The Messenger of Allah (peace and blessings be upon him) said, "You must not supplicate: 'O Allah! forgive me if You wish; O Allah bestow Mercy on me if You wish.' But beg from Allah with certitude for no one has the power to compel Allah." (Bukhari and Muslim)

Narrated Anas (May Allah be pleased with him): The Messenger of Allah (peace and blessings be upon him) said, "When one of you supplicates, let him be decisive and he should not say:

'O Allah, bestow upon me such and such if You wish' because no one has the power to compel Him." (Bukhari and Muslim)

Commentary: One should pray to Allah will full confidence that He will answer his prayers. One should also persist in praying and never give in to despair. (52)

18. To Have No Fear of Allah

Allah, the Exalted, says:

"Therefore, fear not men but fear Me." (Qur'an, Al-Ma'idah 5:44)

"So, fear Allah and adjust all matters of difference among you, and obey Allah and His Messenger (Muhammad), if you are believers." (Qur'an, Al-Anfal 8:1)

"And Allah warns you against Himself (His Punishment)." (Qur'an, Ali 'Imran 3:30)

Other Verses: *Al-Baqarah 2:40, Al-Hujurat 49:1, Al-Hajj 22:1-2, Al-Buruj 85:12, Hud 11:102-106, 'Abasa 80:34-37, Ar-Rahman 55:46, At-Tur 52:25-28, An-Nisa 4:1, Al-Ahzab 33:70-71.*

Narrated Anas bin Malik (May Allah be pleased with him): The Messenger of Allah (peace and blessings be upon him) delivered a Khutbah to us the like of which I had never heard from him before. He said,
"If you knew what I know, you would laugh little and weep much." Thereupon those present covered their faces and began sobbing." (Bukhari and Muslim)

Narrated Abu Dharr (May Allah be pleased with him): The Messenger of Allah (peace and blessings be upon him) said, "I see what you do not see and I hear what you do not hear; heaven has squeaked, and it has right to do so. By Him, in Whose Hand my soul is, there is not a space of four fingers in which there is not an angel who is prostrating his forehead before Allah, the Exalted. By Allah, if you knew what I know, you would laugh little, weep much, and you would not enjoy women in beds, but would go out to the open space beseeching Allah." (Tirmidhi)

Abu Barzah (May Allah be pleased with him) reported: The Messenger of Allah (peace and blessings be upon him) said, "Man's feet will not move on the Day of Resurrection before he is asked about his life, how did he consume it, his knowledge, what did he do with it, his wealth, how did he earn it and how did he dispose of it, and about his body, how did he wear it out." (Tirmidhi)

Narrated Aisha (May Allah be pleased with her): "I heard Messenger of Allah (peace and blessings be upon him) saying, 'The people will be assembled on the Day of Resurrection barefooted, naked and uncircumcised.' I said, 'O Messenger of Allah! Will the men and the women be together on that Day; looking at one another?' Upon this Messenger of Allah (peace and blessings be upon him) said, 'O Aisha, the matter will be too serious for them to look at one another.'" (Bukhari and Muslim)

Commentary: This Hadith mentions the horrors and torments of the Day of Resurrection which makes its connection with this chapter obvious. What this chapter and Ahadith mentioned in it, make clear is that a Muslim should never be unmindful of the preparations for the Hereafter nor should he ever lose sight of the fact that he has to appear before Allah on the Day of Resurrection and account for all his actions. In order to save himself from the humiliation on that Day, he should lead a life of Faith and fear of Allah. Those who do not do so and lead a life free from fear of Allah and torments of the Hereafter, will have no hesitation in disobeying Allah, which will inevitably lead them to humiliation, disgrace and heavy punishment in the Hereafter. (53)

Narrated Abu Dhar Jundub bin Junadah and Muadh bin Jabal: The Messenger of Allah (peace and blessings be upon him) said, "Fear Allah wherever you are, and follow up a bad deed with a good one and it will wipe it out, and behave well towards people." (Tirmidhi)

Abu Khalid Al-Walibi narrated from Abu Hurairah and he (one of the narrators) said: "I do not know except that he attributed it to the Prophet (peace and blessings be upon him): 'Allah says, 'O son of Adam, devote yourself to My worship, and I will fill your heart with contentment and take care of your poverty; but if you do not do that, then I will fill your heart with worldly concerns and will not take care of your poverty.'" (Ibn Majah)

Abu Hurairah (May Allah be pleased with him) reported: The Messenger of Allah (May Allah's peace and blessings be upon him) was asked about the foremost deed that leads people to Paradise, and he replied: "Fear of Allah and good character." Then, he was asked about the most things that lead people into Hellfire, and he said: "The tongue and the private parts." (Ibn Majah, Tirmidhi and Ahmad)
(https://hadeethenc.com/en/browse/hadith/5812)

19. Saying "Don't Judge me!" or "Only God Can Judge me!"

Allah, the Exalted, says:

"You [true believers in Islamic Monotheism, and real followers of Prophet Muhammad SAW and his Sunnah (legal ways, etc.)] are the best of peoples ever raised up for mankind..." (Qur'an, Ali 'Imran 3:110)

"...We said, "O Zul-Qarnain! Either punish them or treat them kindly." (Qur'an, Al-Kahf 18:86)

"...Whoever does wrong will be punished by us, then will be returned to their Lord, Who will punish them with a horrible torment." (Qur'an, Al- Kahf 18:87)
Other Verse: At-Tawbah 9:71.

Many Muslims today are using statements like "Don't judge me!" or "Only God can judge me!", mostly by those wanting to find a loophole to justify their questionable actions and to run away from advice. The Sahabah, when advised to fear Allah, would thank the person who had just reminded them - with tears in their eyes. Today if someone questions our behavior, we feel, we are being accused - or worse insulted! Instead, we start to retort by finding fault with the person advising us and saying, "Hey! You aren't perfect, you can't tell me what to do." Well, if that were the case, no one on the face of the earth across the stretch of time, could advise anyone else save the Prophet of Allah (peace and blessings of Allah be upon him) himself. By the standards of Prophet Muhammad (peace and blessings of Allah be upon him), these are feeble excuses fit to be given only by the immature. (54)
We need to embrace the concept that we could have done something wrong; we should actually be thankful that we have someone who has taken time to advise us and acting according the Qur'an and Sunnah – forbidding evil – it is a communal and individual obligation.

Why should we bother as to what others do?

Firstly, Allah, the Exalted, says:

"Let there arise out of you a group of people inviting to all that is good (Islam), enjoining Al-Ma'ruf (i.e. Islamic Monotheism and all that Islam orders one to do) and forbidding Al-Munkar (polytheism and disbelief and all that Islam has forbidden). And it is they who are the successful." (Qur'an, Ali 'Imran 3:104)

Secondly, if my fellow Muslim sins, then yes it does have an impact on me. If one part of the body is infected, it weakens the whole body. We have the story of how the people of Musa were denied rain just because of the sinful actions of one man.

Allah, the Exalted, says:

"Evil (sins and disobedience of Allah, etc.) has appeared on land and sea because of what the hands of men have earned (by oppression and evil deeds, etc.), that Allah may make them taste a part of that which they have done, in order that they may return (by repenting to Allah, and begging His Pardon)." (Qur'an, Ar-Rum 30:41)

If the Ummah fails to do its duty of enjoining what is good and forbidding what is evil or wrong, or corrupt, then it will spread throughout the Ummah, and it will deserve the Curse of Allah. For Allah cursed those among the Children of Israel who disbelieved because they failed in this important duty.

Allah, the Exalted, says:

"Those among the Children of Israel who disbelieved were cursed by the tongue of Dawood (David) and Isa (Jesus), son of Maryam (Mary). That was because they disobeyed (Allah and the Messengers) and were ever transgressing beyond bounds. They used not to forbid one another from Al–Munkar (wrong, evildoing, sins, polytheism, disbelief) which they committed. Vile indeed was what they used to do." (Qur'an, Al-Ma'idah 5:78-79)

Abu Bakr (May Allah be pleased with him) said: "O people, you recite this Verse: *"O you who believe, upon you is responsibility for yourselves. Those who have gone astray will not harm you when you have been guided." (Surah Al-Ma'idah 5:105)*, but I have heard Messenger of Allah (May Allah's peace and blessings be upon him) say: 'When people see an oppressor but do not prevent him committing sin, it is likely that Allah will punish them all.'" (Ibn Majah, Tirmidhi) (https://hadeethenc.com/en/browse/hadith/3470)

Imam Ibn Qayyim (May Allah have mercy on him) said:

"The Shaitan has misled most people by beautifying for them the performance of certain voluntary acts of worship such as voluntary prayers and voluntary fasting while neglecting other obligatory acts of worship such as enjoining the good and eradicating the evil, to the extent that they do not even make the intention of performing them….For the essence of our religion is to perform what Allah, the Exalted, ordered us to do. The one who does not perform his obligations is actually worse than the one who performs sins. Anyone having some knowledge about the Revelation of Allah, the guidance of the Prophet (peace and blessings of Allah be upon him) and the life of the companions would see that those who are pointed at today as the most pious people are in fact the least pious… Indeed, what deen and what good is there in a person who witnesses the sanctity of Allah, the Exalted, being violated, His Hudud not applied, His religion abandoned, the Sunnah of His Messenger (peace and blessings be upon him) shunned, and yet remains still with a cold heart and a silent tongue - a dumb Shaitan. In the same way the one who talks falsehood is a speaking Shaitan. Isn't the misfortune of Islam due only to those who whenever their food and positions are secure, would not care about what happens to the religion? The best among them would offer a sorry face. But if there was a shortcoming in one of the things their heart is attached to like their rank or money, they would sacrifice and strive, and strain, and struggle, and use the three levels of prevention (their hands, tongues and hearts, as mentioned in Hadith 49) according to their capability. These people, besides deserving the Anger of Allah, are afflicted with the greatest calamity without even knowing it: They have a dead heart. Indeed, the more alive a person's heart is, the stronger its anger for the sake of Allah and the more complete his support to Islam and Muslims." (55)

Abu Sa'id Al-Khudri reported: The Messenger of Allah (peace and blessings be upon him) said: "Whoever among you sees evil, should change it with his hand. If he is unable to do so, then with his tongue. If he is unable to do so, then with his heart and that is the weakest level of faith." (Muslim)

Ibn Masud (May Allah be pleased with him) reported: The Messenger of Allah (May Allah's peace and blessings be upon him) said: "No Prophet had been sent before me by Allah to his people but he had, among his people, disciples and companions, who followed his ways and

obeyed his command. Then, there came after them successors who claimed what they did not practice and practiced what they were not commanded to do. Whoever strives against them with his hand is a believer; whoever strives against them with his heart is a believer; and whoever strives against them with his tongue is a believer. Beyond that there is no mustard seed's weight of faith." (Muslim)
(https://hadeethenc.com/en/browse/hadith/3480)

Abu Sa'id (May Allah be pleased with him) said that the Messenger of Allah (peace and blessings be upon him) said: "Let not any one of you belittle himself." They said: 'O Messenger of Allah, how can any one of us belittle himself?" He said: "He finds a matter concerning Allah about which he should say something, and he does not say (it), so Allah (Mighty and Sublime be He) says to him on the Day of Resurrection: "What prevented you from saying something about such-and-such and such-and-such?" He says: (It was) out of fear of people." Then He says: "Rather, it is I whom you should more properly fear." (Ibn Majah)

Can we judge?

We have numerous examples throughout our history of giving *nasiha* and judging people based on their actions. Many of the collectors of Hadith like Imam Bukhari used to judge the reliability of the person narrating the Hadith by their outward actions and not by "What's in the heart, Allah knows."
Abdullah ibn 'Utbah ibn Masud reported: "I heard 'Umar ibn al-Khattab (May Allah be pleased with him) say: "People were judged by the Divine Revelation during the lifetime of the Messenger of Allah (May Allah's peace and blessings be upon him) but the Divine Revelation has ceased. Now, we only judge you by what is apparent to us from your deeds. Whoever appears to be good, we trust and honor him, and what he does in secret is no concern of ours, for Allah will judge him for what he does in secret. Whoever appears to be evil, we will not trust or believe him, even if he says that his intentions are good." (Bukhari) (https://hadeethenc.com/en/browse/hadith/4234)

Abdullah ibn 'Umar (May Allah be pleased with him) said: "When we noticed that a man was not present at Fajr and 'Isha' prayer, we would think badly of him." (Haakim in al-Mustadrak, 764, and elsewhere; he classed it Saheeh according to the conditions of the two Sheikhs (Bukhari and Muslim), and al-Dhahabi and al-Albaani agreed with him.

How to Judge?

Allah, the Exalted, says:

"But no, by your Lord, they can have no Faith, until they make you (O Muhammad SAW) judge in all disputes between them, and find in themselves no resistance against your decisions, and accept (them) with full submission." (Qur'an, An-Nisa 4:65)

"Whatever of good reaches you, is from Allah, but whatever of evil befalls you, is from yourself. And We have sent you (O Muhammad SAW) as a Messenger to mankind, and Allah is Sufficient as a Witness." (Qur'an, An-Nisa 4:79)

"And so, judge (you O Muhammad SAW) between them by what Allah has revealed and follow not their vain desires, but beware of them lest they turn you (O Muhammad SAW) far away from some of that which Allah has sent down to you. And if they turn away, then know that Allah's Will is to punish them for some sins of theirs. And truly, most of men are Fasiqun (rebellious and disobedient to Allah)." (Qur'an, Al-Ma'idah 5:49)

Other Verse: *Al-Kahf 18:86-88, Al-A'la 87:9-11.*

The criterion by which we are supposed to judge is what Allah has revealed and His Prophet (peace and blessings be upon him). We don't let personal bias or hidden grudges take precedence over our advice and actions in enjoining good and forbidding evil based on the Qur'an and Sunnah.

There are also those who just question and judge unnecessarily without any intention of helping, but rather just to show themselves as superior or it's like. But you should care for the one you are advising - just as if they were your own brother or sister.

Some say that they have good intentions, yet their actions are quite contrary to what they say. Don't accept that the ends justify the means. No, good intentions - when joined with reprehensible actions - are deficient, insufficient. It doesn't work - simply saying something - we have to walk the talk.

True, proper intentions are the first requisite for pleasing Allah, and we know that He will judge our deeds starting from our intentions. But among our brethren we judge by deeds while allowing them the possibility that we have misread them. However, their improper deeds warrant our gentle counsel to them.

<u>Here is what we MUST DO:</u>

- Make as many excuses as possible for the sake of your brother/sister by giving them the benefit of the doubt. Understand the scenario of the action and the situation of the doer whilst he was committing that action.
- Practice extreme patience.

As my grandmother says, "People who start practicing the Deen anew are generally very strict and go to extremes. They forget that they themselves were once sinners and at the edge of the cliff. Had not Allah saved them, where would they be? How would they feel if they themselves were so harshly reprimanded?" (54)

- Keep a calm tone, that doesn't sound accusatory - and with a smile on the face. Take them aside and make it clear that you do this only out of love and care for the person.
- Speak to their parents or someone close to them whom they trust or whom they at least respect enough to take advice from.
- Advise privately first but if the person keeps committing sin and inviting people to it in public, then such people deserve to be spoken to more openly and warned against. Exhaust yourself in advising privately and having *husn al-dhan* (good thoughts and excuses) first before even thinking of going to the next step.

Here is what we MUST NOT DO:

- We DON'T tell them, "You are going to HELL!" or "Allah will not forgive you!"

Hey, did Allah tell you His Judgment?

We don't single out people marking them for Hell or Heaven. That is solely up to Allah. What we say in advice is that these actions or continuing them without repentance, may set them up for Hell using the Qur'an Verses and Ahadith.

- We DON'T shame or call people out in public for their sins unless a host of criteria are met. For all we know, the person didn't know that what they were doing is wrong or were just plain ignorant that they even committed that wrong.
- We DON'T become accusatory and take the 'holier than thou' route because then that would be of no help other than just putting the person into defensive mode. And then all your well-intended *nasiha* would fall on deaf ears. Humility needs to be learnt and with it the *adab* of giving *nasiha,* or even how to differ over something might be what is called for.

The most hated speech to Allah

'Abdullah ibn Masud (May Allah have mercy on him) narrated: The Prophet (peace and blessings be upon him) said: "The most hated speech to Allah is when a man says to another man, 'Fear Allah!' And he replies, 'Worry about your own self!'" (An-Nasa'i ('Amalul Yawmi Wal Laylah, Hadith: 849 -As Sunanul Kubra, Hadith: 10619) and Bayhaqi and Abul Qasim Al Isbahani (Shu'abul Iman, Hadith: 621 and At Targhib Wat Tarhib, Hadith: 766) (https://hadithanswers.com/the-most-hated-speech-in-the-sight-of-allah-taala)

20. Lying about Allah and the Prophet

Allah, the Exalted, warns:

"So, who does more wrong than he who forges a lie against Allah or denies His Ayat (proofs, evidences, verses, lessons, signs, revelations, etc.)? Surely, the Mujrimoon (criminals, sinners, disbelievers and polytheists) will never be successful!" (Qur'an, Yunus 10:17)

"And say not concerning that which your tongues put forth falsely: "This is lawful and this is forbidden," so as to invent lies against Allah. Verily, those who invent lies against Allah will never prosper." (Qur'an, An-Nahl 16:116)

"Say: 'Verily, those who invent lies against Allah will never be successful.'" (Qur'an, Yunus 10:69)

Other Verses: *Al-Ma'idah 5:33, An-Nisa 4:49-50.*

Narrated `Abdullah (May Allah be pleased with him): The Prophet (peace and blessings be upon him) said, "Truthfulness leads to righteousness, and righteousness leads to Paradise. And a man keeps on telling the truth until he becomes a truthful person. Falsehood leads to Al-Fajur (i.e. wickedness, evildoing), and Al-Fajur (wickedness) leads to the Hellfire, and a man may keep on telling lies till he is written before Allah, a liar." (Bukhari)

Narrated Ali (May Allah be pleased with him): The Prophet (peace and blessings of Allah be upon him) said: "Do not tell a lie against me, for whoever tells a lie against me (intentionally) then he will surely enter the Hellfire." (Bukhari)
Lying upon Allah's Messenger (peace and blessings be upon him) is indirectly lying upon Allah the Almighty.

21. Exchanging the Signs of Allah for a Small Price

Allah, the Exalted, says:

"And believe in what I have sent down confirming that which is (already) with you, and be not the first to disbelieve in it. And do not exchange My Signs for a small price, and fear (only) Me." (Qur'an, Al-Baqarah 2:41)

"So, woe to those who write the 'scripture' with their own hands, then say, 'This is from Allah,' in order to exchange it for a small price. Woe to them for what their hands have written and woe to them for what they earn." (Qur'an, Al-Baqarah 2:79)

"Indeed, they who conceal what Allah has sent down of the Book and exchange it for a small price – those consume not into their bellies except the Fire. And Allah will not speak to them on the Day of Resurrection, nor will He purify them. And they will have a painful punishment." (Qur'an, Al-Baqarah 2:174)

22. Prohibiting the Invocation of Allah in Mosques

Allah, the Exalted, says:

"And who are more unjust than those who prevent the Name of Allah from being mentioned in His Mosques and strive toward their destruction. It is not for them to enter them except in fear. For them in this world is disgrace, and they will have in the Hereafter a great Punishment." (Qur'an, Al-Baqarah 2:114)

23. Believing that Allah is Everywhere

Allah, the Exalted, says:

"The Most Beneficent (Allah) Istawa (rose over) the (Mighty) Throne (in a manner that suits His Majesty)." (Qur'an, Taha 20:5)

"Surely, your Lord is Allah Who created the heavens and the earth in six days and then rose over (istawa) the Throne (in a manner that suits His Majesty), disposing the affair of all things." (Qur'an, Yunus 10:3)

"To Him ascend (all) the goodly words, and the righteous deeds exalt it (i.e. the goodly words are not accepted by Allah unless and until they are followed by good deeds)." (Qur'an, Fatir 35:10)

Other Verses: *As-Sajdah 32:4, Al-Hadid 57:3.*

Allah is with His slaves wherever they are with His Knowledge while being above His Throne.

"Have you not seen that Allah knows whatsoever is in the heavens and whatsoever is on the earth? There is no najwa (secret counsel) of three but He is their fourth (with His Knowledge, while He Himself is over the Throne, over the seventh heaven), — nor of five but He is their sixth (with His Knowledge), — nor of less than that or more but He is with them (with His Knowledge) wheresoever they may be." (Qur'an, Al-Mujadilah 58:7)

"He it is Who created the heavens and the earth in six days and then rose over (istawa) the Throne (in a manner that suits His Majesty). He knows what goes into the earth and what comes forth from it, and what descends from the heaven and what ascends thereto. And He is with you (by His Knowledge) wheresoever you may be." (Qur'an, Al-Hadid 57:4)

"And We are nearer to him than his jugular vein (by Our Knowledge)." (Qur'an, Qaf 50:16)

Sheikh Ibn 'Uthaymeen (May Allah have mercy on him) said:

"This view has implications that are very, very false, because if you say that Allah is everywhere, this implies that He is in lavatories – Allah forbid – and in other places that filled with impurities and filth, and who would describe his Lord in such terms? It is not possible for any believer to describe his Lord in such terms." (End quote from Fataawa Noor 'ala ad-Darb by Ibn 'Uthaymeen) (56)

Narrated Mu'adh bin Jabal: The Messenger of Allah (peace and blessings be upon him) said: "Whoever fasts Ramadan, performs the Salat, performs Hajj to the House" - I do not know whether he mentioned Zakat or not - "except that it is binding on Allah that He forgives him, whether he emigrated in the cause of Allah, or remained in his land in which he was born." Mu'adh said: "Should I not inform the people of this?" The Messenger of Allah (peace and blessings of Allah be upon him) said, "Leave the people to do deeds, for verily in Paradise there are a hundred levels, what is between every two levels is like what is between the heavens and the earth. Al-Firdaus is the highest of Paradise and its most expansive, and above that is the Throne of Ar-Rahman (the Most Merciful), and from it the rivers of Paradise are made to flow forth. So, when you ask Allah, ask Him for Al-Firdaus." (Tirmidhi)

24. Believing that Allah is Without Image and is Formless and Disbelieving in His Attributes

Allah, the Exalted, says:

"And He is the Most High, the Most Great." (Qur'an, Al-Baqarah 2:255)

"Blessed is He in Whose Hand is the dominion, and He is Able to do all things." (Qur'an, Al-Mulk 67:1)

"He (may He be Exalted) also says: 'Do you feel secure that He, Who is over the heaven, will not cause the earth to sink with you, and then it should quake? Or do you feel secure that He, Who is over the heaven, will not send against you a violent whirlwind?" (Qur'an, Al-Mulk 67:16-17)

The Qur'an describes Allah as speaking, sitting on a Throne, having a Face, Two Eyes, Two Hands, Two Feet. Allah has described Himself and His Messenger (peace be upon him) has described Him, i.e. being High above His Creatures, rising over His 'Arsh (Throne), being Distinct from His Creation, and being Incomparable in any respect to His Creatures and other attributes. (57)

Narrated Abu Sa'id Al-Khudri: "…The Prophet (peace be upon him) said: "Don't you trust me though I am the trustworthy man of the One in the Heavens, and I receive the news of

Heaven (i.e. Divine Inspiration) both in the morning and in the evening..." (Bukhari) (https://sunnah.com/bukhari:4351)

Allah, the Exalted, has a Face

Allah, the Exalted, says:

"And the Face of your Lord full of Majesty and Honor will abide forever." (Qur'an, Ar-Rahman 55:27)

"Everything will perish except His Face." (Qur'an, Al-Qasas 28:88)

Allah, the Exalted, has Two Hands

Allah, the Exalted, says:
"(Allah) said: "O Iblis (Satan)! What prevents you from prostrating yourself to one whom I have created with Both My Hands. Are you too proud (to fall prostrate to Adam) or are you one of the high exalted?" (Qur'an, Sad 38:75)

"Nay, Both His Hands are widely outstretched. He spends (of His Bounty) as He wills." (Qur'an, Al-Ma'idah, 5:64)

Allah, the Exalted, has Two Feet

Narrated Abu Hurairah (May Allah be pleased with him): The Prophet (peace and blessings of Allah be upon him) said: "Hell and Paradise disputed, and Hell said: 'I have been favored with the arrogant and proud.' Paradise said: 'What is the matter with me, that no one will enter me except the weak, humble and downtrodden?' Allah, may He be Blessed and Exalted, said to Paradise: 'You are My Mercy by which I will show Mercy to whomsoever I will of My slaves.' And He said to Hell: 'You are My Punishment with which I will punish whomsoever I will of My slaves. And each of you will be full.' As for Hell, it will not be full until Allah, may He be Blessed and Exalted, places His Foot on it and it says, 'Enough, enough.' Then it will be full and all its parts will be integrated together, and Allah will not treat any of His creation unjustly. As for Paradise, Allah will create a creation just for it." (Bukhari and Muslim)

Ibn 'Abbas (May Allah be pleased with him) said: "The Kursi (footstool) is the place of the Two Feet, and the size of Throne cannot be known." (Ibn Khuzaymah in at-Tawheed, 1/248, no.154; Ibn Abi Shaybah in al-'Arsh, 61; ad-Daarimi in ar-Radd 'ala al-Muraysi; 'Abdullah ibn al-Imam Ahmad in as-Sunnah; and al-Haakim in al-Mustadrak, 2/282 – he classed it as Saheeh according to the conditions of the two sheikhs (al-Bukhari and Muslim), and adh-Dhahabi agreed with him. It was also classed as Saheeh by al-Albaani in Mukhtasar al-'Uluw, p.102; and by Ahmad Shaakir in 'Umdat at-Tafseer, 2/163.

Allah, the Exalted, has Two Eyes

Allah, the Exalted, says:

"In order that you may be brought up under My Eye." (Qur'an, Taha 20:39)

"Floating under Our Eyes." (Qur'an, Al-Qamar 54:14)

Narrated People: The Prophet (peace and blessings be upon him) said, "Allah did not send any Prophet but that he warned his nation of the one-eyed liar (Ad-Dajjal). He is one-eyed while your Lord is not one-eyed, the word 'Kafir' (unbeliever) is written between his two eyes." (Bukhari)

Allah, the Exalted, has a Shin

Allah, the Exalted, says:

"(Remember) the Day when the Shin shall be laid bare (i.e. the Day of Resurrection) and they shall be called to prostrate themselves (to Allah), but they (hypocrites, and those who pray to show off or to gain good reputation) shall not be able to do so." (Qur'an, Al-Qalam 68:42)

Narrated Abu Sa'id Al-Khudri: "We said, "O Allah's Messenger! Shall we see our Lord on the Day of Resurrection?" He (peace and blessings be upon him) said, "Do you have any difficulty in seeing the sun and the moon when the sky is clear?"... 'Do you know any sign by which you can recognize Him?' They will say. 'The Shin,' and so Allah will then uncover His Shin whereupon every believer will prostrate before Him and there will remain those who used to prostrate before Him just for showing off and for gaining good reputation. These people will try to prostrate but their backs will be rigid like one piece of a wood (and they will not be able to prostrate) …" (Bukhari)

The Divine Essence

The traits of the Divine Essence are exclusive to Allah and necessary to Him. Meaning, no other being may have these qualities, and it is impossible for Him to be without them. (58)

1. **Existence (*wujud*)** – Allah's existence is necessarily known from the existence of anything else. In other words, since creation exists, the Creator must exist. In this way, He is the necessary Existent (*wajib al-wujud*). This holds for all periods, places and possible Universes. The opposite of this attribute would be non-existence, which is a logically impossible scenario as it would entail that nothing else exists.
2. **Pre-eternality (*qidam*)** – After understanding that all creation depends on Allah for its existence, then also understand that Allah has always existed. Time is Allah's creation. Thus, His existence was "before" time. He is neither confined nor affected by it. If it were to end, His necessary existence would continue unchanged.
3. **Ever-lasting (*baqa'*)** – There can never be a situation whether before, during or after the creation of time in which Allah does not exist.

4. **He is unlike creation (*mukhalafah li al-ḥawadith*)** – Everything other than Allah came into existence from non-existence due to dependency on Him. All things other than Allah have some deficiency. He, the Most High, is free of any imperfections. Thus, He is unlike anything and also unlike whatever the imagination can conjure up about Him.
5. **Self-Subsistence (*qiyam bi nafsihi*)** – Allah depends on nothing else for His existence, be that a creator, place, time or anything else. Meaning, He exists on His own (*al-ṣamad*).
6. **One (*waḥdaniyyah*)** – Three different meanings applying to Allah's Essence and Attributes are necessary here. He is Alone without a second, Unique without a similar, and One without division.

Allah's Attributes

Allah, the Exalted, says:

"There is nothing like Him; and He is the All-Hearer, the All-Seer." (Qur'an, Ash-Shuraa 42:11)

"Say: He is Allah, the One and Only; Allah As-Samad (The Self-Sufficient Master, Whom all creatures need, He neither eats nor drinks). He begets not, nor was He begotten; And there is none co-equal or comparable unto Him." (Qur'an, Al-Ikhlas 112)

Some of Allah's Attributes:

1. Life (*ḥayah*) – He is Alive; and its opposite, death, is impossible for Him.

Allah states about Himself:

"And put your trust (O Muhammad SAW) in the Ever Living One Who dies not, and glorify His Praises, and Sufficient is He as the All-Knower of the sins of His slaves." (Qur'an, Al-Furqan 25:58)

2. Power (*qudrah*) – He is Omnipotent, Possessing Infinite and Irresistible Power. His awesome Power is on display from the grandiosity of the Universe to the intricacies of the cell. The opposite is weakness or inability, and this is impossible for Him.

"Allah creates what He wills. Verily! Allah is Able to do all things." (Qur'an, An-Nur 24:45)

3. Knowledge (`*ilm*) – He knows everything – all that existed, exists, will exist and will not exist. He knows it to the smallest and most minute detail. Creation is a testament to the limitless Perfect Knowledge with Him. The opposite is ignorance, an impossibility for Him in every way.

"And with Him are the keys of the unseen; none knows them except Him. And He knows what is on the land and in the sea. Not a leaf falls but that He knows it. And no grain is there within the darknesses of the earth and no moist or dry [thing] but that it is [written] in a Clear Record." (Qur'an, Al-An'am 6:59)

4. Will (*iradah*) – He has willed in pre-eternity that which was and which is to be (*mā kāna wa mā yakūn*). Whatever He desires is, and what He does not is not. There is no one to repulse His Will, nor anyone to defer His command. His Will is absolute, and He cannot be compelled to do anything.

Allah, the Exalted, says:

"He does what He wills." (Qur'an, Al-Buruj 85:16)

5. Hearing (*sam'*) – He hears all sounds without reliance on any organs, sound waves, propagating particles or the like for it.

Allah, the Exalted, says:

"Verily, Allah is All-Hearer, All-Knower." (Qur'an, Al-Anfal 8:17)

Abu Masa al-Ash'ari (May Allah be pleased with him) reported: "We were on a journey with the Prophet (May Allah's peace and blessings be upon him) and whenever we ascended from a valley we would say "there is no god but Allah" and "Allah is the Greatest" and we would raise our voices. So, the Prophet (May Allah's peace and blessings be upon him) said: "O people, do not trouble yourselves too much. He Whom you are calling is not deaf or absent. Verily, He is with you, He is All-Hearing and Ever Near." (Bukhari and Muslim. This is the wording of Bukhari)
(https://hadeethenc.com/en/browse/hadith/6207)

6. Seeing (*baṣr*) – He sees all forms and colors without reliance on organs, light waves or the like for it.

"Surely, it is Allah who is Hearing, Seeing." (Qur'an, Ghafir 40:20)

7. Speech (*kalam*) – Similar to His Hearing and Seeing, His speech does not rely on any organs, sound waves, letters or interpretation. It is through this Attribute that He communicated. The Qur'an being a communication from Allah, His *kalam* as well.

"Musa came at Our appointed time and his Lord spoke to him." (Qur'an, Al-A'raf 7:143)

8. Originating (*takwīn*) – To bring something into existence from non-existence. With His Will, Knowledge and Power, He brings everything into existence.

"When He decides a matter, He simply says to it: "Be," and it comes to be." (Qur'an, Al-Baqarah 2:117)

Aisha (May Allah be pleased with her) reported: "One night I did not find the Prophet (May Allah's peace and blessings be upon him). As I groped in search of him, I found him bowing – or prostrating – and saying: "Glory and Praise be to You. There is no god but You." In another narration: "My hand fell over his feet while he was in prostration, with his feet erect. He was supplicating: 'O Allah, I seek refuge in Your Pleasure from Your Wrath and in Your Pardon from Your Punishment, and I seek refuge in You from You. I am not capable of enumerating Praise of You. You are as You have praised Yourself.'" (Muslim) (https://hadeethenc.com/en/browse/hadith/3566)

25. Reciting the Names of Allah in Certain Combinations

Sheikh 'Abd-Allaah ibn Munayyi' said regarding reciting Allah's Names in certain conditions:

"This is not permissible, and if he believes in it, it is Bid'ah. Every Zhikr that involves reciting a certain number of times, or in a certain place, or at a certain time, or in a certain manner, that is not prescribed in Shariah, is Bid'ah. With regard to the Most Beautiful Names of Allah, the way to use these in worship is to call upon Allah by these Names, as He says: *"And (all) the Most Beautiful Names belong to Allah, so call on Him by them…" (Al-A'raf 7:180)*. Merely reciting them in certain combinations is not a prescribed form of worship. (59)

26. Calling Allah by the names which are not in the Qur'an or Ahadith

Allah, the Exalted, says:

"And to Allah belong the best Names, so invoke Him by them. And leave (the company of) those who practice deviation concerning His Names. They will be recompensed for what they have been doing." (Qur'an, Al-Isra 7:180)

Narrated Abu Hurairah (May Allah be pleased with him): The Messenger of Allah (peace and blessings of Allah be upon him) said: "Allah has ninety-nine Names, one hundred less one. Whoever learns them will enter Paradise." (Bukhari and Muslim)

The Names of Allah, may He be Exalted, are a tawqeefi matter, i.e. they can only be known through Divine Revelation, the Qur'an and Ahadith. The names like Ar-Rashid, Al-Wajud (the Existent), Ad-Dahr (time), Al-Wajid (One that gives existence to others), Hannan, As-Saboor are not the Names of Allah. (60-66)

27. Repeating the Name of Allah on its Own or the Pronoun Huwa (He) is a Sufi Bid'ah

Allah, the Exalted, says:

"They (the Jews, Quraish pagans, idolaters, etc.) did not estimate Allah with an estimation due to Him when they said: "Nothing did Allah send down to any human being (by inspiration)." Say (O Muhammad SAW): "Who then sent down the Book which Musa (Moses) brought, a light and a guidance to mankind which you (the Jews) have made into (separate) paper sheets, disclosing (some of it) and concealing (much). And you (believers in Allah and His Messenger Muhammad SAW), were taught (through the Qur'an) that which neither you nor your fathers knew." Say: "Allah (sent it down)." Then leave them to play in their vain discussions." (Tafsir Al-Qurtubi, vol.7, p.37) (Qur'an, Al-An'am 6:91)

There is no doubt that it is Bid'ah to mention the Name of Allah on its own or - even worse - to repeat the pronoun "Huwa" ("He"). There is no proof of remembering Allah by saying a single Name such as "Allah" repeatedly from the Prophet (peace and blessings of Allah be upon him) or from any of his companions. (67)

The Standing Committee was asked about someone who remembers Allah by saying "Ya Lateef" repeatedly. They replied:

"That is not permissible because it was not narrated from the Prophet (peace and blessings of Allah be upon him). Rather it was proven that he said: "Whoever innovates something in this matter of ours (i.e. Islam) that is not part of it, will have it rejected." According to another version: "Whoever does any action that is not part of this matter of ours will have it rejected." (Fataawa al-Lajnah al-Daa'imah, 2/379)

"With regard to the questioner saying that they say, "Hu, Hu, Hu" – those people are adding to their Bid'ah because they are calling Allah by a word by which He did not call Himself. "Hu" is not one of the
names of Allah. (See Fataawa al-Lajnah al-Daa'imah, 2/185)

Ibn Taymiyah (May Allah have mercy on him) said:

"The Name of Allah on its own, either as a noun ("Allah") or a pronoun ("Huwa") is not a complete phrase or meaningful sentence. It has no implications to do with Iman (Faith) or kufr (disbelief), commands or prohibitions. This was not mentioned by anyone from the Salaf (early generations) of this Ummah, and it was not prescribed by the Messenger of Allah (peace and blessings of Allah be upon him). It does not bring any knowledge to the heart or bestow any kind of benefit upon it. All it does is give an unclear idea which is not defined by any negation or affirmation. Unless there is previous knowledge in a person's mind or he is in a state of mind where he could benefit from this, he gains no benefit at all. Islam prescribes Adhkar which in and of themselves bring benefit to the heart, without any such need for anything else. Some of those who persisted in this kind of "Dhikr" ended up in various kinds of heresies and ideas of "wahdat al-wujood" (unity of all that exists, pantheism), as has been explained in detail elsewhere. It was mentioned that one of the sheikhs said: "I am afraid of dying between negation and affirmation", but this is not an example to be followed, because it is obviously erroneous. If a person were to die in this state, he would die according to his intention, because actions are judged by intention. It was reported that the Prophet (peace and blessings of Allah be upon him) commanded us to tell the dying person to say "Laa ilaaha ill-Allah", and he said, "Anyone whose last words are Laa ilaaha ill-Allah will enter Paradise." If this word (Laa ilaaha ill-Allah) was something which required caution, why should we tell the dying person to say something which, if he dies in the middle of saying it, will lead to an improper death? Rather, if this were the case, he would be told to say "Allah, Allah" or "Huwa, Huwa." Mentioning the pronoun on its own is further removed from the Sunnah and is a worse kind of Bid'ah, which is closer to the misguidance of the Shaytan. If a person says "Yaa Huwa, yaa Huwa (O He, O He)" or "Huwa, Huwa (He, He)" and so on, the pronoun does not refer to anything except whatever his heart imagines, and hearts may be guided or misguided. Some sheikhs use as evidence to support saying "Allah" (the Name on its own) the Ayah: *"Say: 'Allah (sent it down).' Then leave them..." (Al-An'am 6:91).* They think that Allah commanded His Prophet to say His Name on its own, but this is a mistake according to the consensus of the scholars, because the meaning of the phrase "Say: 'Allah'" is that it is Allah Who sent down the Book which was brought by Moosa. This is in response to the question: *"Say (O Muhammad): 'Who then sent down the Book which Moosa (Moses) brought, a light and a guidance to mankind which you (the Jews) have made into (separate) paper sheets, disclosing (some of it) and concealing (much). And you (believers in Allah and His Messenger Muhammad) were taught (through the Qur'an) that which neither you nor your fathers knew.' Say: 'Allah (sent it down).'" (Al-An'am 6:91),* i.e. Allah is the One Who revealed the Book which was brought by Moosa. This is a refutation of the view of those who said, *"Nothing did Allah send down to any human being (by Revelation)." (Al-An'am 6:91).* Allah says: *"Who then sent down the Book which Moosa brought?"* Then He says: *"Say: "Allah sent it down, then leave these liars to play in their vain discussions." (Al-An'am 6:91)* (Tafsir Al-Qurtubi, vol.7, p.37)

What we have said above is further explained by the comments of Seebawayh and other grammarians, who noted that when the Arabs say "Qaala" (or other forms of the verb meaning "to say"), they do not quote verbatim, rather they state what was said, giving a complete meaning. So what follows is a sentence with a complete meaning, or a nominal sentence, or a verbal sentence. Hence after saying "qaala" they give a kasrah to the particle "anna" (making it "inna"); "qaala" cannot be followed by a noun standing alone. Allah did not command anyone to mention His Name on its own, and it is not prescribed for the Muslims to say His Name on its own. Saying His Name on its own does not enhance Faith or explain anything about the religion, according to the consensus of the scholars of Islam; it is not enjoined in any act of worship or in any case where Allah addresses them." (Majmoo' al-Fataawa, 10/226-229)

And he (May Allah have mercy on him) also said:

"Repeating the Name of Allah on its own, such as saying "Allah, Allah," or the pronoun, such as "Huwa, Huwa" is not prescribed in either the Qur'an or the Sunnah. It is not reported that any of the salaf of this ummah or any of the righteous scholars who are taken as examples did this. It is only spoken by misguided people of the later generations. Perhaps, they are following a sheikh who had no control over himself in this regard, such as al-Shubli who, it was narrated, used to say 'Allah, Allah.' It was said to him, 'Why do you not say Laa ilaaha ill-Allah?' He said, "I am afraid of dying between the negation [saying La ilaaha (there is no god)] and the affirmation (ill-Allah (except Allah)]!" This is one of the mistakes made by al-Shubli, who may be forgiven for it because of the sincerity of his faith and the strength of his emotions which overwhelmed him. Sometimes he would go crazy and would be taken to the asylum, and he would shave off his beard. There are other instances of this type in his case, which are not to be taken as examples, even if he may be excused or rewarded for them. If a person intends to say Laa ilaaha ill-Allah, and he dies before completing it, that will not harm him at all, because actions are judged by intentions, and what he intended to do is what will be written down for him. Some of them go to extremes in this matter, and say that saying the Name of Allah is for the 'elite' whilst saying La ilaaha ill-Allah is for the 'masses.' Some of them say that saying Laa ilaaha ill-Allah is for the mu'mineen (believers), saying 'Allah' is for the 'aarifeen and saying 'Huwa' is for the muhaqqiqeen. One of them may restrict himself to saying, when alone or in a gathering, 'Allah, Allah, Allah' or 'Huwa' or 'Yaa Huwa', or even 'La Huwa illa Huwa (there is no He except He)'! Some of those who have written about spiritual matters have expressed approval of this, quoting some known figures who, however, were in a state of overwhelming emotion at the time, or quoting opinions, or quoting false reports – for example, some of them reported that the Prophet (peace and blessings of Allah be upon him) told 'Ali ibn Abi Talib to say 'Allah, Allah, Allah.' The Prophet (peace and blessings of Allah be upon him) said it three times, then he told 'Ali to say it three times, so he said it three times. This Hadith is fabricated (mawdoo'), according to the consensus of the scholars of Hadith. It is narrated that the Prophet (peace and blessings of Allah be upon him) taught people various Adhkar to say, and the best of Dhikr is Laa ilaaha ill-Allah. This is what he urged his paternal uncle Abu Talib to say when he was dying. He said, "O uncle, say Laa ilaaha ill-Allah and I will defend you thereby before Allah." And he said: "I know of a word which no one says when he is dying but his soul finds rest in it." And he said, "Anyone whose last words are Laa ilaaha ill-Allah will enter Paradise." And he said, "Whoever dies knowing that there is no god except Allah will enter Paradise." And he said: "I have been commanded to fight people until they bear witness that there is no god except Allah and that Muhammad is the Messenger of Allah. If they do that, their blood and wealth will be safe from me, except for what is due from them (e.g. Zakah, etc.), and their reckoning is with Allah." And there are many similar Ahadith." (Majmoo' al-Fataawa, 10/556-558) (68)

28. Writing the Name of Allah on the Cars

Allah, the Exalted, says:

"And (all) the Most Beautiful Names belong to Allah, so call on Him by them, and leave the company of those who belie or deny (or utter impious speech against) His Names. They will be requited for what they used to do." (Qur'an, Al-A'raf 7:180)

It is not permissible for calligraphers, painters or others to write the Allah's Magnificent Names and Attributes on the back of the car or whatsoever. This is an act of Bid'ah (innovation in religion) that has no origin in the Qur'an or Sunnah, and Allah did not prescribe it as an act of worship. Moreover, writing Qur'an in this way involves insulting the Names and Attributes of Allah and not keeping them away from inappropriate things. Perhaps, this leads the person to Shirk (associating others with Allah in His Divinity or worship) when he uses it as an amulet that brings about good and wards off evil merely by writing it. Allah does not teach us His Names and Attributes to be written on sets, placards or cars. Rather, Allah, Glorified and Exalted be He, revealed His Names and Attributes to teach His slaves about Himself, so that they may affirm them as He revealed them in the Qur'an or to His Messenger (peace and blessings be upon him) and believe in all the Perfection and Majesty they convey. A Muslim should acknowledge them as belonging to Allah without Tahrif (distortion of the meaning), Ta'til (negation of the meaning or function of Allah's Attributes), Tamthil (likening Allah's Attributes to those of His Creation), Takyif (descriptive designation of Allah's Attributes), or Tashbih (comparison), and guard their sanctity against abuse and inappropriate things. (69)

29. Comparing the Creator to His creation

Allah, the Exalted, says:

*"Say (O Muhammad (peace be upon him)): "He is Allah, (the) One. Allah As-Samad (The Self-Sufficient Master, Whom all creatures need, He neither eats nor drinks). He begets not, nor was He begotten;
And there is none co-equal or comparable unto Him."* (Qur'an, Al-Ikhlas 112:1-4)

"The Creator of the heavens and the earth. He has made for you mates from yourselves, and for the cattle (also) mates. By this means He creates you (in the wombs). There is nothing like unto Him, and He is the All-Hearer, the All-Seer." (Qur'an, Ash-Shuraa 42:11)

"No vision can grasp Him, but His Grasp is over all vision. He is the Most Subtle and Courteous, Well-Acquainted with all things." (Qur'an, Al-An'am 6:103)

Other Verses: Muhammad 47:19, Al-Hajj 22:75, Al-Hadid 57:3, Al-Hijr 15:23, Al-Baqarah 2:164, Al-Hashr 59:23-24, Yasin 36:82, As-Sajdah 32:4, An-Nahl 16:40.

30. Belief in Pantheism

Allah, the Exalted, says:

"He is the First (nothing is before Him) and the Last (nothing is after Him), the Most High (nothing is above Him) and the Most Near (nothing is nearer than Him). And He is the All-Knower of everything." (Qur'an, Al-Hadid 57:3)

"And there is none co-equal or comparable unto Him." (Qur'an, Al-Ikhlas 112:4)

There is no any evidence for those who believe in pantheism that God is one with His creation and is present inside them. This belief is blasphemous, and Allah is far Exalted above such claims. Indeed, this is disbelief, we seek refuge with Allah against it, of which Allah and His Messenger (May Allah's peace and blessings be upon him) are innocent of. (https://hadeethenc.com/en/browse/hadith/6337)

Narrated Abu Hurairah (May Allah be pleased with him): The Messenger of Allah (peace and blessings of Allah be upon him) said: "Verily Allah, may He be Exalted, says: 'Whosoever shows enmity to a close friend of Mine, I shall declare war on him. My slave draws not close to Me with anything more loved by Me than the obligatory religious duties I have enjoined upon him, and My slave continues to draw close to Me with supererogatory works, so that I will love him. So, when I love him, I will be his hearing with which he hears, his vision with which he sees, his hand with which he strikes and his foot with which he walks. Were he to ask (something) of Me, I would surely give it to him, and were he to seek refuge in Me, I would surely grant him it." (Bukhari)

The pantheists (al-ittihaadiyyah) quote this Hadith as evidence for their false belief. They said that this Hadith is indicative of the union between the Creator and the created being, if the latter draws close to Allah, may He be Exalted, by doing obligatory religious duties, whereupon the slave – we seek refuge with Allah from such notions – becomes part of the essence of God, and hears with the Hearing of Allah and sees with His Vision! In other words, the Creator becomes one with the created being, and they become one and the same! Undoubtedly, this is kufr (disbelief) that puts one beyond the pale of Islam. The Hadith that they quoted as evidence is in fact evidence against them, because it affirms that there are two separate entities, namely the Creator and the created being, and highlights the difference between them; it affirms that there is a worshipper and an object of his worship, and highlights the difference between them; it affirms that there is a lover and a beloved, one who asks and One Who responds. There is nothing in it to indicate that the two become one. (70)

Ibn Taymiyah (May Allah have mercy on him) said:

"The heretics and pantheists quote it as evidence for their belief because Allah says (in this Hadith Qudsi): "I will be his hearing, his vision, his hand and his foot." But the Hadith constitutes evidence against them in numerous ways, including the following: Allah says: "Whoever shows enmity to a close friend of Mine is declaring war on Me." Thus, it affirms that there is someone who is challenging Allah, and a close friend of Allah who is someone other than the challenger, and in it Allah, may He be Glorified, affirms for Himself that He has one who is close to Him and one who is challenging Him.

He says: "My slave draws not close to Me with anything more loved by Me than the obligatory religious duties I have enjoined upon him." This affirms that there is a slave who seeks to draw close to his Lord, and there is a Lord Who enjoined those obligatory religious duties.

He says: "and My slave continues to draw close to Me with supererogatory works, so that I shall love him." Thus, He affirms that there is one who seeks to draw close and one to Whom closeness is sought; there is One Who loves and a beloved who is distinct from him. All of this contradicts their view that all existence is one.

He says: "So when I love him, I will be his hearing with which he hears, his vision with which he sees…" Allah grants these things to His slave after He loves him, but in the view of the pantheists this is the case both before and after He loves him." (End quote from Majmooʻ al-Fataawa (2/371-372)

And he (May Allah have mercy on him) said:

"Then Allah says: "Were he to ask (something) of Me, I would surely give it to him, and were he to seek refuge in Me, I would surely grant him it." Thus, He differentiated between the one who asks and the One Who is asked, between the one who seeks refuge and the One Who grants him it. He describes the slave as asking of his Lord and seeking refuge with Him. This Hadith combines many sublime meanings." (End quote from Majmooʻ al-Fataawa (17/134) (70)

Pantheism is the belief that reality is identical with Divinity, that God is equal to the Universe. Many of the religious traditions and spiritual writings are marked by pantheistic ideas and feelings. For example, in Hinduism of the Advaita Vedanta school, in some varieties of Kabbalistic Judaism, in Celtic spirituality, and in Sufi mysticism.

31. Rejection or Denial of what Allah Has Revealed to Prophet

Allah, the Exalted, says:

"Those who follow the Messenger, the unlettered Prophet, whom they find written in what they have of the Torah and the Gospel, who enjoins upon them what is right and forbids them what is wrong and makes lawful for them the good things and prohibits for them the evil and relieves them of their burden and the shackles which were upon them. So, they who have believed in him, honored him, supported him and followed the light

which was sent down with him – it is those who will be the successful." (Qur'an, Al-A'raf 7:157)

"O you who believe! Obey Allah and obey the Messenger (Muhammad SAW), and those of you (Muslims) who are in authority. (And) if you differ in anything amongst yourselves, refer it to Allah and His Messenger (SAW), if you believe in Allah and in the Last Day. That is better and more suitable for final determination." (Qur'an, An-Nisa 4:59)

"But no, by your Lord, they can have no Faith, until they make you (O Muhammad (peace and blessings of Allah be upon him)) judge in all disputes between them, and find in themselves no resistance against your decisions, and accept (them) with full submission." (Qur'an, An-Nisa 4:65)

Other Verses: *An-Nisa 4:136 and 4:150-151, An-Nur 24:63, Al-Muddaththir 74:35-36, Al-An'am 6:34, An-Nahl 16:44, Al-Hadid 57:9, Ali 'Imran 3:31.*

Narrated Jabir bin Abdullah: The Prophet (peace and blessings be upon him) said, "I have been given five things which were not given to anyone else before me. 1. Allah made me victorious by awe, (by His frightening my enemies) for a distance of one month's journey, 2. The earth has been made for me (and for my followers) a place for praying and a thing to perform Tayammum, therefore anyone of my followers can pray wherever the time of a prayer is due, 3. The booty has been made Halal (lawful) for me yet it was not lawful for anyone else before me, 4. I have been given the right of Intercession (on the Day of Resurrection), 5. Every Prophet used to be sent to his nation only but I have been sent to all mankind." (Bukhari)

Abu Musa (May Allah be pleased with him) reported: The Messenger of Allah (peace and blessings be upon him) said, "The guidance and knowledge with which Allah has sent me are like abundant rain which fell on a land. A fertile part of it absorbed the water and brought forth profuse herbage and pasture; and solid ground patches which retained the water by which Allah has benefited people, who drank from it, irrigated their crops and sowed their seeds; and another sandy plane which could neither retain the water nor produce herbage. Such is the similitude of the person who becomes well-versed in the religion of Allah and receives benefit from the Message entrusted to me by Allah, so he himself has learned and taught it to others; such is also the similitude of the person who has stubbornly and ignorantly rejected Allah's Guidance with which I have been sent." (Bukhari and Muslim)

Narrated Abdullah bin Umar: The Messenger of Allah (peace and blessings be upon him) said: "I have been ordered to fight against people until they testify that there is no god but Allah and that Muhammad is the Messenger of Allah and until they perform the prayers and pay the Zakat, and if they do so, they will have gained protection from me for their lives and property, unless they do acts that are punishable in accordance with Islam, and their reckoning will be with Allah the Almighty." (Bukhari and Muslim)

32. Claiming that the Story of the Isra' and Mi'raj is a Myth

Allah, the Exalted, says:

"Glorified (and Exalted) be He (Allah) (above all that (evil) they associate with Him), Who took His slave (Muhammad (blessings and peace of Allah be upon him)) for a journey by night from Al-Masjid-al-Haram (at Makkah) to the farthest Mosque (in Jerusalem), the neighbourhood whereof We have blessed, in order that We might show him (Muhammad (peace and blessings of Allah be upon him)) of Our Ayat (proofs, evidences, lessons, signs, etc.). Verily, He is the All-Hearer, the All-Seer." (Qur'an, Al-Isra 17:1)

"And they say: 'We shall not believe in you (O Muhammad (peace and blessings be upon him), until you cause a spring to gush forth from the earth for us; 'Or you have a garden of date-palms and grapes, and cause rivers to gush forth in their midst abundantly; 'Or you cause the heaven to fall upon us in pieces, as you have pretended, or you bring Allah and the angels before (us) face to face; 'Or you have a house of adornable materials (like silver and pure gold, etc.), or you ascend up into the sky, and even then, we will put no faith in your ascension until you bring down for us a Book that we would read.' Say (O Muhammad (peace and blessings be upon him)): 'Glorified and Exalted be my Lord (Allah) above all that evil they (polytheists) associate with Him! Am I anything but a man, sent as a Messenger?" (Qur'an, Al-Isra 17:90-93)

"Nay, every one of them desires that he should be given pages spread out (coming from Allah with a writing that Islam is the Right Religion, and Muhammad (peace and blessings be upon him) has come with the Truth from Allah the Lord of the heavens and earth, etc.)." (Qur'an, Al-Muddaththir 74:52)

Narrated Malik bin Sasaa: The Prophet (peace and blessings be upon him) said, "While I was at the House in a state midway between sleep and wakefulness, (an angel recognized me) as the man lying between two men. A golden tray full of wisdom and belief was brought to me and my body was cut open from the throat to the lower part of the abdomen and then my abdomen was washed with Zamzam water and (my heart was) filled with wisdom and belief. Al-Buraq, a white animal, smaller than a mule and bigger than a donkey was brought to me and I set out with Gabriel. When I reached the nearest heaven. Gabriel said to the heaven gate-keeper, 'Open the gate.' The gatekeeper asked, 'Who is it?' He said, 'Gabriel.' The gate-keeper asked, 'Who is accompanying you?' Gabriel said, 'Muhammad.' The gate-keeper said, 'Has he been called?' Gabriel said, 'Yes.' Then it was said, 'He is welcomed. What a wonderful visit his is!' Then I met Adam and greeted him and he said, 'You are welcomed O son and a Prophet.' Then we ascended to the second heaven. It was asked, 'Who is it?' Gabriel said, 'Gabriel.' It was said, 'Who is with you?' He said, 'Muhammad.' It was asked, 'Has he been sent for?' He said, 'Yes.' It was said, 'He is welcomed. What a wonderful visit his is!' Then I met Jesus and Yahya (John) who said, 'You are welcomed, O brother and a Prophet.' Then we ascended to the third heaven. It was asked, 'Who is it?' Gabriel said, 'Gabriel.' It was asked, 'Who is with you? Gabriel said, 'Muhammad.' It was asked, 'Has he been sent for?' 'Yes.' said Gabriel. 'He is welcomed. What a wonderful visit his is!' (The Prophet added:) 'There I met

Joseph and greeted him', and he replied, 'You are welcomed, O brother and a Prophet!' Then we ascended to the 4th heaven and again the same questions and answers were exchanged as in the previous heavens. 'There I met Idris and greeted him.' He said, 'You are welcomed. O brother and Prophet.' Then we ascended to the 5th heaven and again the same questions and answers were exchanged as in previous heavens. 'There I met and greeted Aaron', who said, 'You are welcomed. O brother and a Prophet.' Then we ascended to the 6th heaven and again the same questions and answers were exchanged as in the previous heavens. 'There I met and greeted Moses', who said, 'You are welcomed. O brother and a Prophet.' When I proceeded on, he started weeping and on being asked why he was weeping, he said, 'O Lord! Followers of this youth who was sent after me will enter Paradise in greater number than my followers.' Then we ascended to the seventh heaven and again the same questions and answers were exchanged as in the previous heavens. 'There I met and greeted Abraham', who said, 'You are welcomed. O son and a Prophet.' Then I was shown Al-Bait-al-Ma'mur (i.e. Allah's House). I asked Gabriel about it and he said, 'This is Al Bait-ul-Ma'mur where 70,000 angels perform prayers daily and when they leave, they never return to it (but always a fresh batch comes into it daily).' Then I was shown Sidrat-ul-Muntaha (i.e. a tree in the seventh heaven) and I saw its Nabk fruits which resembled the clay jugs of Hajr (i.e. a town in Arabia), and its leaves were like the ears of elephants, and four rivers originated at its root, two of them were apparent and two were hidden. I asked Gabriel about those rivers and he said, 'The two hidden rivers are in Paradise, and the apparent ones are the Nile and the Euphrates.' Then fifty prayers were enjoined on me. I descended till I met Moses who asked me, 'What have you done?' I said, 'Fifty prayers have been enjoined on me.' He said, 'I know the people better than you, because I had the hardest experience to bring Bani Israel to obedience. Your followers cannot put up with such obligation. So, return to your Lord and request Him (to reduce the number of prayers.' I returned and requested Allah (for reduction) and He made it forty. I returned and (met Moses) and had a similar discussion, and then returned again to Allah for reduction and He made it thirty, then twenty, then ten, and then I came to Moses who repeated the same advice. Ultimately Allah reduced it to five. When I came to Moses again, he said, 'What have you done?' I said, 'Allah has made it five only.' He repeated the same advice but I said that I surrendered (to Allah's Final Order)" Allah's Apostle was addressed by Allah, "I have decreed My obligation and have reduced the burden on My slaves, and I shall reward a single good deed as if it were ten good deeds." (Bukhari) (71)

33. Celebrating the Night of Ascension the Isra' and Mi'raj

Allah, the Exalted, says:

"Glorified (and Exalted) be He (Allah) [above all that (evil) they associate with Him] Who took His slave (Muhammad) for a journey by night from Al-Masjid Al-Haram (at Makkah) to Al-Masjid Al-Aqsa (in Jerusalem), the neighbourhood whereof We have blessed, in order that We might show him (Muhammad) of Our Ayat (proofs, evidences, lessons, signs, etc.). Verily, He is the All-Hearer, the All-Seer." (Qur'an, Al-Isra 17:1)

With regard to this night on which the Isra' and Mi'raj took place, there is nothing in the Saheeh Hadith to indicate that it is in Rajab or in any other month. Everything that has been narrated concerning a specific date for these events cannot be proven to have come from the Prophet (peace and blessings of Allah be upon him) according to the scholars of Hadith. (72)

34. Forgetting Sending Salat to the Prophet Muhammad

Allah, the Exalted, says:

"Allah sends His Salat (Graces, Honors, Blessings, Mercy, etc.) on the Prophet (Muhammad SAW) and also His angels too (ask Allah to bless and forgive him). O you who believe! Send your Salat on (ask Allah to bless) him (Muhammad SAW), and (you should) greet (salute) him with the Islamic way of greeting (salutation i.e. As-Salamu Alaikum)." (Qur'an, Al-Ahzab 33:56)

"And whatsoever the Messenger (Muhammad (blessings and peace of Allah be upon him)) gives you, take it, and whatsoever he forbids you, abstain (from it), and fear Allah. Verily, Allah is Severe in punishment." (Qur'an, Al-Hashr 57:9)

Narrated 'Abdur-Rahman bin Abi Laila: "Ka'b bin 'Ujra met me and said, 'Shall I give you a present?' Once the Prophet (peace and blessings be upon him) came to us and we said, 'O Allah's Messenger! send 'Salat' upon you?' He said, 'Say: Allahumma Salli ala Muhammadin wa 'ala 'Ali Muhammadin, kama sal-laita 'ala all Ibrahima innaka Hamidun Majid. ala all Ibrahima, innaka Hamidun Majid.

(O Allah, send prayers upon Muhammad and upon the family of Muhammad, as You sent prayers upon Ibrahim and upon the family of Ibrahim; You are indeed worthy of Praise, full of Glory. O Allah, send blessings upon Muhammad and upon the family of Muhammad as You sent blessings upon Ibrahim and upon the family of Ibrahim; You are indeed worthy of Praise, full of Glory)." (Bukhari)

Narrated Abu Humaid As-Saidi: The people said, "O Allah's Messenger (peace be upon him)! How may we send Salat on you?" He said, "Say: Allahumma Salli 'ala- Muhammadin wa azwajihi wa dhurriyyatihi kama sal-laita 'ala 'Ali Ibrahim; wa barik 'ala Muhammadin wa azwajihi wa dhurriyyatihi kamabarakta 'ala 'Ali Ibrahim innaka hamidun majid. (O Allah, send Your salah (Grace, Honor and Mercy) upon Muhammad and upon his wives and offspring, as You sent Your salah upon Ibrahim, and send Your blessings upon Muhammad and upon his wives and offspring, as You sent Your blessings upon the family of Ibrahim. You are indeed Praiseworthy, Most Glorious)." (Bukhari)

Narrated Abu Hurairah: The Messenger of Allah (peace and blessings be upon him) said, "Whoever sends blessings upon me once, Allah send blessings upon him ten times." (Muslim)

Narrated Ibn Masud: The Prophet (peace and blessings be upon him) said: "The closest of people to me on the Day of Resurrection will be those who send the most blessings on me." (Tirmidhi)

Abdallah b. 'Amr b. al-'As reported: God's Messenger (peace and blessings be upon him) as saying, "When you hear the mu'adhdhin repeat what he says, then invoke a blessing on me, for everyone who invokes one blessing on me will receive ten blessings from God. Then ask God to give me the wasila, which is a rank in Paradise fitting for only one of God's servants, and I hope that I may be the one. If anyone asks that I be given the wasila, he will be assured of my Intercession." (Muslim)

Narrated 'Umar ibn al-Khattab (May Allah be pleased with him): "Du'a is suspended between heaven and earth and none of it is taken up until you send blessings upon your Prophet (peace and blessings of Allah be upon him)." (Tirmidhi)

35. Visiting Places and Mosques in which the Prophet Prayed (apart from Quba', Uhud, al-Baqee)

The Prophet (peace and blessings of Allah be upon him) said: "No journey should be made to visit Mosques except for three: this Mosque of mine in Madinah, al-Masjid al-Haram [in Makkah] and al-Masjid al-Aqsa (in al-Quds/Jerusalem). (Bukhari and Muslim; this version narrated by Muslim).

Other places which it is prescribed to visit without travelling expressly for that purpose are the grave of the Prophet (peace and blessings of Allah be upon him), the graves of his two companions (Abu Bakr and 'Umar), the graves of the people of al-Baqee' (the cemetery of Madinah), the graves of the martyrs of Uhud, and finally, the Mosque of Quba. With regard to visiting other Mosques and historical sites and claiming that they are "places which a person should visit", there is no basis for doing this… Visits to these places should be disallowed as a preventative measure. This is indicated by the actions of the righteous salaf, above all the rightly-guided khaleefah 'Umar ibn al-Khattab (May Allah be pleased with him).

It was narrated that al-Ma'roor ibn Suwayd (May Allah have mercy on him) said: "We went out with 'Umar ibn al-Khattab and we came across a Mosque on our route. The people rushed to pray in that Mosque, and 'Umar said, 'What is the matter with them?' They said, 'This is a Mosque in which the Messenger of Allah (peace and blessings of Allah be upon him) prayed.' 'Umar said: 'O people, those who came before you were destroyed because they followed such (practices) until they made them places of worship. Whoever happens to be there at the time of prayer, let him pray there, and whoever is not there at the time of prayer, let him continue his journey.'" (Ibn Waddah in his book al-Bida' wa'l-Nahiy 'anhaa; classed as Saheeh by Ibn Taymiyah in al-Majmoo', 1/281)

Ibn Taymiyah (May Allah have mercy on him) said, commenting on this story:

"The Prophet (peace and blessings of Allah be upon him) had not singled out that place for prayer; he prayed there only because he happened to be staying there. Hence 'Umar thought that imitating him outwardly without having the same reason for doing, so did not count as following the Prophet (peace and blessings of Allah be upon him). Singling out that place for prayer was like the innovations of the People of the Book which had led to their doom, so he forbade the Muslims to imitate them in this manner. The one who did that was imitating the Prophet (peace and blessings of Allah be upon him) in outward appearances, but he was imitating the Jews and Christians in his intention, which is the action of the heart. The action of the heart is what counts, because following in one's intention is more serious than following in outward appearances." (Majmoo' al-Fataawa, 1/281)

Sheikh 'Abd al-'Azeez ibn Baaz (May Allah have mercy on him) said, after mentioning the places which it is prescribed to visit in Madinah:

"With regard to the seven Mosques, Masjid al-Qiblatayn (the Mosque of the Two Qiblahs), and other places which some authors who wrote about the rituals of Hajj include among the places to be visited, there is no basis for doing that, and there is no evidence for doing so. What is prescribed for the believer at all times is to follow (the Sunnah), not to innovate." (Fataawa Islamiyyah, 2/313) (73)

36. Denying the Rights of the Ahl Al-Bayt

Allah, the Exalted, says:

"Our Lord! Send amongst them a Messenger of their own (and indeed Allah answered their invocation by sending Muhammad, peace be upon him), who shall recite unto them Your Verses and instruct them in the Book (this Qur'an) and Al-Hikmah (full knowledge of the Islamic Laws and jurisprudence or wisdom, or Prophethood, etc.), and sanctify them. Verily! You are the All-Mighty, the All-Wise." (Qur'an, Al-Baqarah 2:129)

Ahl al-Bayt (Arabic: "People of the House") designation in Islam for the family of the Prophet Muhammad, particularly his daughter Fāṭima, her husband Ali (who was also Muhammad's cousin), their sons al-Ḥusayn and Ḥasan and their descendants. The members of Ahl Al-Bayt are the members of the Prophet's family: his wives, his children, Banu Hashim, Banu al-Muttalib and their freed slaves. Denying the rights of Ahl Al-Bayt is Major sin; it means denying whatever Allah has revealed. (74)

The Wives of the Prophet

Allah, the Exalted, says:

"O wives of the Prophet! You are not like any other women. If you keep your duty (to Allah), then be not soft in speech, lest he in whose heart is a disease (of hypocrisy, or evil desire for adultery, etc.) should be moved with desire, but speak in an honorable manner. And stay in your houses, and do not display yourselves like that of the times of Ignorance, and perform As-Salat (Iqamat as-Salat), and give Zakat and obey Allah and His Messenger. Allah wishes only to remove Ar-Rijs (evil deeds and sins, etc.) from you, O members of the family (of the Prophet SAW), and to purify you with a thorough purification." (Qur'an, Al-Ahzab 33:32-33)

Banu Hashim and Banu al-Muttalib

Narrated Jubair bin Mut'im: 'Uthman bin Affan went (to the Prophet) and said, "O Allah's Apostle! You gave property to Bani Al-Muttalib and did not give us, although we and they are of the same degree of relationship to you." The Prophet (peace and blessings of Allah be upon him) said, "Only Bani Hashim and Bani Al Muttalib are one thing (as regards family status)." (Bukhari)

Narrated Wathilah bin Al-Asqa': The Messenger of Allah (peace and blessings of Allah be upon him) said: "Indeed Allah has chosen Isma'il from the children of Ibrahim, and He has chosen Banu Kinah from the children of Isma'il, and He has chosen the Quraish from Banu Kinanah, and He has chosen Banu Hashim from Quraish, and He has chosen me from Banu Hashim." (Tirmidhi)

The family of Ali, the family of 'Aqil, the family of Ja'far and the family of Abbas

Yazid bin Haiyan reported: "...The Prophet (peace and blessings be upon him) said: "I am about to receive a messenger (the angel of death) from my Rubb and I will respond to Allah's Call, but I am leaving with you two weighty things: the first is the Book of Allah, in which there is Right Guidance and Light, so hold fast to the Book of Allah and adhere to it.' He exhorted (us to hold fast) to the Book of Allah and then said, 'The second is the members of my household, I remind you (to be kind) to the members of my family. I remind you (to be kind) to the members of my family.' Husain said to Zaid, 'Who are the members of his household, O Zaid? Aren't his wives the members of his family?' Thereupon Zaid said, 'His wives are the members of his family. (But here) the members of his family are those for whom Zakat is forbidden.' He asked, 'Who are they?' Zaid said, Ali and the offspring of Ali, 'Aqil and the offspring of 'Aqil and the offspring of Ja'far and the offspring of 'Abbas. Husain said: 'These are those for whom the acceptance of Zakat is forbidden.' Zaid said: 'Yes.'" (Muslim) (https://sunnah.com/riyadussalihin:346)

Aisha reported that Allah's Apostle (peace and blessings of Allah be upon him) went out one morning wearing a striped cloak of the black camel's hair that there came Hasan b. Ali. He wrapped him under it, then came Husain and he wrapped him under it along with the other one (Hasan). Then came Fatima and he took her under it, then came Ali and he also took him under it and then said: *"Allah only desires to take away any uncleanliness from you, O people of the household, and purify you (thorough purifying)."* (Al-Ahzab 33:33) (Muslim)

Narrated Urwa b. Zubair who narrated from Aisha that she informed him that Fatima, daughter of the Messenger of Allah (peace and blessings of Allah be upon him), sent someone to Abu Bakr to demand from him her share of the legacy left by the Messenger of Allah (peace and blessings of Allah be upon him) from what Allah had bestowed upon him at Madinah and Fadak, and what was left from one-fifth of the income (annually received) from Khaibar. Abu Bakr said: "The Messenger of Allah (peace and blessings of Allah be upon him) said: 'We (Prophets) do not have any heirs; what we leave behind is (to be given in) charity.' The household of the Messenger of Allah (peace and blessings of Allah be upon him) will live on the income from these properties, but, by Allah, I will not change the charity of the Messenger of Allah (peace and blessings of Allah be upon him) from the condition in which it was in his own time. I will do the same with it as the Messenger of Allah (peace be upon him) himself used to do.' So, Abu Bakr refused to hand over anything from it to Fatima who got angry with Abu Bakr for this reason. She forsook him and did not talk to him until the end of her life. She lived for six months after the death of the Messenger of Allah (peace and blessings of Allah be upon him). When she died, her husband, Ali b. Abu Talib, buried her at night. He did not inform Abu Bakr about her death and offered the funeral prayer over her himself. During the lifetime of Fatima, Ali received (special) regard from the people. After she had died, he felt estrangement in the faces of the people towards him. So, he sought to make peace with Abu Bakr and offer his allegiance to him. He had not yet owed allegiance to him as Caliph during these months. He sent a person to Abu Bakr requesting him to visit him unaccompanied by anyone (disapproving the presence of Umar). 'Umar said to Abu Bakr: 'By Allah, you will not visit them alone.' Abu Bakr said: 'What will they do to me? By Allah, I will visit them.' And he did pay them a visit alone. All recited Tashahhud (as it is done in the beginning of a religious sermon), then said: 'We recognize your moral excellence and what Allah has bestowed upon you. We do not envy the favor (i.e. the Caliphate) which Allah has conferred upon you but you have done it (assumed the position of Caliph) alone (without consulting us), and we thought we had a right (to be consulted) on account of our kinship with the Messenger of Allah (peace and blessings of Allah be upon him).' He continued to talk to Abu Bakr (in this vein) until the latter's eyes welled up with tears. Then Abd Bakr spoke and said: 'By Allah, in Whose Hand is my life, the kinship of the Messenger of Allah (peace and blessings of Allah be upon him) is dearer to me than the kinship of my own people. As regards the dispute that has arisen between you and me about these properties, I have not deviated from the right course and I have not given up doing about them what the Messenger of Allah (peace and blessings of Allah be upon him) used to do.' So, Ali said to Abu Bakr: 'This afternoon is (fixed) for (swearing) allegiance (to you).' So, when Abu Bakr had finished his Zuhr prayer, he ascended the pulpit and recited Tashahhud, and described the status of Ali, his delay in swearing allegiance and the excuse which lie had offered to him (for this delay). (After this) he asked for God's Forgiveness. Then Ali b. Abu Talib recited the Tashahhud. extolled the merits of Abu Bakr and (said that) his action was not prompted by any jealousy of Abu Bakr on his part or his refusal to accept the high position which Allah had conferred upon him, (adding:) but we were of the opinion that we should have a share in the government, but the matter had been decided without taking us into confidence, and this displeased us. Hence the delay in offering allegiance.' The Muslims were pleased with this (explanation) and they said: 'You have done the right thing.' The Muslims were (again) favorably inclined to Ali since he adopted the proper course of action." (Muslim)

37. Cursing the Companions of the Prophet

Allah, the Exalted, says:

"Muhammad (peace be upon him) is the Messenger of Allah, and those who are with him are severe against disbelievers, and merciful among themselves. You see them bowing and falling down prostrate (in prayer), seeking Bounty from Allah and (His) Good Pleasure. The mark of them (i.e. of their Faith) is on their faces (foreheads) from the traces of (their) prostration (during prayers). This is their description in the Taurat (Torah). But their description in the Injeel (Gospel) is like a (sown) seed which sends forth its shoot, then makes it strong, it then becomes thick, and it stands straight on its stem, delighting the sowers that He may enrage the disbelievers with them. Allah has promised those among them who believe (i.e. all those who follow Islamic Monotheism, the religion of Prophet Muhammad SAW till the Day of Resurrection) and do righteous good deeds, Forgiveness and a mighty reward (i.e. Paradise)." (Qur'an, Al-Fath 48:29)

Narrated al-Bara' (May Allah be pleased with him): "I heard the Prophet (peace and blessings be upon him) say: "The Ansar: none loves them but a believer and none hates them but a hypocrite. So, Allah will love him who loves them, and He will hate him who hates them." (Bukhari)

38. Claiming that Ali Was Given Specific knowledge of Khilafah (Caliphate), which Was Not Given to Anybody else

Narrated Yazid bin Sharik bin Tariq (May Allah be pleased with him): "I saw Ali (May Allah be pleased with him) giving a Khutbah (sermon) from the pulpit and I heard him saying: "By Allah, we have no book to read except Allah's Book and what is written in this scroll. He unrolled the scroll which showed a list of what sorts of camels to be given as blood money, and other legal matters relating to killing game in the sanctuary of Makkah and the expiation thereof. In it was also written: The Messenger of Allah (peace and blessings be upon him) said: 'Al-Madinah is a sanctuary from 'Air to Thaur (mountains). He who innovates in this territory new ideas in Islam, commits a sin therein, or shelters the innovators, will incur the Curse of Allah, the angels and all the people, and Allah will accept from him neither repentance nor a ransom on the Day of Resurrection. The asylum (pledge of protection) granted by any Muslim (even of the) lowest status is to be honored and respected by all other Muslims, and whoever betrays a Muslim in this respect (by violating the pledge) will incur the Curse of Allah, the angels and all the people; and Allah will accept from him neither repentance nor a ransom on the Day of Resurrection. Whoever attributes his fatherhood to someone other than his (real) father, and takes someone else as his master other than his (real) master without his permission, will incur the Curse of Allah, the angels and all the people, and Allah will accept from him neither repentance nor a ransom on the Day of Resurrection.'" (Bukhari and Muslim)

Commentary: Air is a small mountain near Al-Madinah and Thaur is also a small mountain behind the famous Mount Uhud. The area between these two mountains is the forbidden area. It means that like the Haram of Makkah, no game should be killed, no trees or plants of this area should be cut and no disbeliever or polytheists should enter its boundary. The words "a'dl" and "sarf" translated here as 'repentance' and 'ransom' respectively also mean obligatory and voluntary (Nafl) acts of worship.

It has been established here that any act of disobedience or sin committed in Al-Madinah becomes a greater sin than if it is committed anywhere else. This Hadith also establishes that the claim that Ali (May Allah be pleased with him) was given some specific knowledge of Khilafah (caliphate), which was not given to anybody else, is also false. (75)

39. Disrespect of the Noble Qur'an

Allah, the Exalted, says:
"(This is) a Book (the Qur'an) which We have sent down to you, full of blessings, that they may ponder over its Verses, and that men of understanding may remember." (Qur'an, Sad 38:29)

"Verily, this Qur'an guides to that which is most just and right." (Qur'an, Al-Isra 17:90)

"Say: It is for those who believe, a Guide and a Healing." (Qur'an, Fussilat 41:44)

Other Verses: *Al-Baqarah 2:2, Yunus 10:57, Al-A'raf 7:204.*

Abu Malik at-Ash'ari reported: The Messenger of Allah (peace and blessings of Allah be upon him) said: "Cleanliness is half of faith and al-Hamdu Lillah (all praise and gratitude is for Allah Alone) fills the scale, and Subhan Allah (Glory be to Allah) and al-Hamdu Lillah fill up what is between the heavens and the earth, and prayer is a light, and charity is proof (of one's faith) and endurance is a brightness and the **Holy Qur'an is a proof on your behalf or against you**. All men go out early in the morning and sell themselves, thereby setting themselves free or destroying themselves." (Muslim)

Abu Umama said he heard Allah's Messenger (peace and blessings be upon him) say: "Recite the Qur'an, for on the Day of Resurrection it will come as an intercessor for those who recite It. Recite the two bright ones, Al-Baqarah and Surah Ali 'Imran, for on the Day of Resurrection they will come as two clouds or two shades, or two flocks of birds in the ranks, pleading for those who recite them. Recite Surah Al-Baqarah, for to take recourse to it is a blessing and to give it up is a cause of grief, and the magicians cannot confront it." (Mu'awiya said: It has been conveyed to me that here Batala means magicians) (Muslim)

'Umar bin Al-Khattab (May Allah be pleased with him) reported: The Prophet (peace and blessings be upon him) said, "Verily, Allah elevates some people with this Qur'an and abases others." (Muslim)

Narrated 'Uthman bin 'Affan: The Prophet (peace and blessings be upon him) said, "The most superior among you (Muslims) are those who learn the Qur'an and teach it." (Bukhari) Mu'awiyah (May Allah be pleased with him) reported: The Messenger of Allah (peace and blessings be upon him) said, "When Allah wishes good for someone, He bestows upon him the understanding of Deen." (Bukhari and Muslim)

Ibn Abbas reported: The Messenger of Allah (peace and blessings be upon him) said: "Whoever speaks on the Qur'an without knowledge, let him take his seat in Hellfire." (Tirmidhi)

'Abdullah bin 'Amr bin Al-'As (May Allah be pleased with him) reported: The Prophet (peace and blessings of Allah be upon him) said, "The one who was devoted to the Qur'an will be told on the Day of Resurrection: 'Recite and ascend (in ranks) as you used to recite when you were in the world. Your rank will be at the last Ayah you recite.'" (Abu Dawud and Tirmidhi)

Narrated 'Amr ibn Hazm (May Allah be pleased with him): The Prophet (peace and blessings of Allah be upon him) wrote to the people of Yemen: "No one should touch the Qur'an except one who is tahir (pure)." This is a jayyid Hadith which has a number of other isnads which strengthen it. (76)
The Qur'an should be recited in a pleasant tone, slowly and with thinking upon the meaning.

It is forbidden to handover Qur'an to the disbeliever, if he is going to cause disrespect to it.

It is not allowed to bring the Qur'an into the toilet, the place of Devils.

Concealing any part of the Qur'an is a Major sin.

The Fortune tellers harm people by Black Magic using the Taweez and Amulets with the Qur'anic Verses written in impurities like menstrual blood, etc., or some Qur'anic Words written backwards. They may walk on the Qur'an, bring the Qur'an to toilet at the request of Devils.

40. Reciting Verses of the Qur'an a Specific Number of Times and with Specific Intention

It is not permissible to single out certain Verses of the Qur'an to recite for specific purposes, unless there is specific Shariah evidence such as if there is a Saheeh Hadith from the Prophet (peace and blessings of Allah be upon him) concerning the virtues of a certain Surahs or Verses, which the Muslim may recite with the aim of attaining those virtues and benefits. (77)

The entire Qur'an is a blessing and reward, and goodness, but claiming that a certain Verse has a certain effect, especially in the case of these claims that they can relieve difficulty and financial hardships, is something that requires evidence.

41. Distributing and Selling the Verses of the Qur'an for the Protection

Distributing and selling the specific Surahs or Ayats of the Qur'an to a number of people, each of whom reads a Surah in order to say Du'a after that asking for abundant provision or protection and so on is an innovation (Bid'ah), because that is not proven from the Prophet (peace and blessings of Allah be upon him) in word or in deed, or from any of the Sahabah (May Allah be pleased with them), or from the imams of the salaf (May Allah have mercy on them). (78)

42. Hanging Verses of the Qur'an and/or Allah's Name on Walls

Hanging plaques and cloths containing Ayats of the Qur'an in home, school, social club and places of business involves a number of reservations and prohibitions according to Islam, such as the following:

1) In most cases, hanging such things on the wall is done for purposes of decoration and adornment, as the Ayats are written in calligraphy and colourful brocade. This is an inappropriate use of the Qur'an. The Qur'an was revealed to guide all mankind and to be read regularly.
2) Some people hang up such things for blessing which is a form of Bid'ah. The blessing comes from reading or reciting the Qur'an, not from hanging it up or placing it on shelves, or turning it into artwork.
3) This is contrary to the practice of the Prophet (peace and blessings of Allah be upon him) and the rightly-guided khaleefahs (May Allah be pleased with them) who never did such a thing.
4) Hanging up such pictures or plaques could lead to Shirk, because some people think that these things are amulets that will protect the house and its people from evil and disease. The One Who really offers protection is Allah, may He be Glorified, and one of the means of gaining His Protection is sincere recitation of the Qur'an and Du'as taught in the Qur'an and Sunnah.
5) There is the risk that the Qur'an may be used, in such cases, as ways of promoting business and increasing one's earnings. The Qur'an should be protected from being used for such purposes.

6) Many of these plaques are painted with real gold, which makes using and hanging them up even more haram. The production and sale of these pictures and plaques involves extravagance and wasting Allah's money.
7) Many of these plaques involve a kind of carelessness, because the letters are twisted into complex designs that are of no benefit to anyone because they are barely legible. Some words are fashioned into the shape of a bird or a man prostrating, and similarly forbidden pictures of animate beings.
8) Ayats and Surahs of the Qur'an are exposed to misuse and abuse by this practice. For example, when moving house, they are piled up with the rest of the furniture and belongings, and other objects may be placed on top of them. This also happens when they are taken down so that the wall may be painted or cleaned.
9) Some Muslims whose observance of Islam is lacking put these plaques and pictures up so that they can feel that they are doing something religious, in order to reduce their feelings of guilt in spite of the fact that this practice does not help them in any way.

We must close the doors of evil and follow the Glorious Qur'an and the last Messenger of Allah who was sent as the best example to follow the Straight Path. The Muslims must turn to the Book of Allah, read it and recite it, and act in accordance with it. (78, 79)

43. Swearing or Taking an Oath by Placing Hand on the Mushaf

An oath is not binding unless it is sworn by one of the Names of Allah or by one of His Attributes.

Swearing on the Qur'an is swearing by the Word of Allah which is one of His Attributes. As for swearing by the Mushaf, if what is meant is the Word of Allah contained therein, then it is an Islamically acceptable oath, but if what is meant is the paper and ink, then it is an oath by something other than Allah, which is Shirk, as the Prophet (peace and blessings of Allah be upon him) said: "Whoever swears by something other than Allah has committed an act of kufr or Shirk." (Tirmidhi and Abu Dawud)

The word *Muṣḥaf* is meant to distinguish between Muhammad's recitations and the physical, written Qur'an. This term does not appear in the Qur'an itself, though it does refer to itself as a K*itab* or Book, in many Verses. Hence it is better not to swear by the Mushaf, because the Mushaf contains the Word of Allah and it contains paper and ink. As for putting one's hand on the Mushaf or inside it, this is an innovated thing (Bid'ah) which some people do for emphasis to warn the one who is swearing the oath against lying. (80, 81)

44. Leaving the Broadcast of the Holy Qur'an Playing at the Places of Business and at Home

Sheikh 'Abd al-'Azeez ibn Baaz (May Allah have mercy on him) was asked:

"What is the ruling on having a radio or cassette recorder playing the Holy Qur'an in the house, when going out of the house to visit family or relatives?" He replied: "There is nothing wrong with that, so long as there is no idle talk going on around it. If there is someone nearby who is engaging in idle talk and speaking and arguing, then that is not right; it is better not to leave the radio on in that case, and it should be turned off, because that is a kind of showing disrespect towards the Qur'an. But if the radio is on when there is no one around or there is someone who is listening or keeping quiet, or sleeping, then there is nothing wrong with it. End quote." (82)

45. Arguing About the Qur'an

Allah, the Exalted, says:

"And argue with them in the fairest manner." (Qur'an, An-Nahl 16:125)

Abdullah ibn 'Amr (May Allah be pleased with him) reported: The Prophet (peace and blessings be upon him) said: "Do not argue about the Qur'an, for arguing about it constitutes disbelief." (Abu Dawud)
(https://hadeethenc.com/en/browse/hadith/10854)

46. Rejection of the Qur'an as the Word of God

Allah, the Exalted, says:

"Or they say, "He (Prophet Muhammad SAW) forged it (the Qur'an)." Say: "Bring you then ten forged Surah (Chapters) like unto it, and call whomsoever you can, other than Allah (to your help), if you speak the Truth!" (Qur'an, Hud 11:13)

"If you are in doubt about what We have revealed to Our servant, then bring a Surah similar to this, and do call your supporters other than Allah, if you are true…" (Qur'an, Al-Baqarah 2:23)

"But if you do not - and you will never be able to - then guard yourselves against the Fire, the fuel of which will be men and stones. It has been prepared for disbelievers." (Qur'an, Al-Baqarah 2:24)

Other Verses: Al-Baqarah 2:41, Al-Hijr 15:9, Al-An'am 6:34, Al-Kahf 18:27, Fussilat 41:42.

All of the Attributes of Allah, the Exalted, are uncreated; they are eternal, with no beginning. Therefore, the scholars said that the Qur'an is not created, because it is the Word of Allah, and that is one of His Attributes.

Ibn Taymiyah (May Allah have mercy on him) said:

"When we recite the Qur'an, we recite it with our voices that are created, that cannot resemble the voice of the Lord. The Qur'an that we recite is the Word of Allah, conveyed from Him and not heard directly from Him. Rather we recite it with our voices. The words are the Words of the Creator, but the voice is the sound of the reciter, as is indicated by the Qur'an and Sunnah, as well as common sense. Allah, may He be Exalted, says: *"And if anyone of the Mushrikoon (polytheists, idolaters, pagans, disbelievers in the Oneness of Allah) seeks your protection then grant him protection, so that he may hear the Word of Allah (the Qur'an), and then escort him to where he can be secure."* (At-Tawbah 9:6)
And the Prophet (peace and blessings of Allah be upon him) said: "Make the Qur'an beautiful with your voices." (End quote from Majmoo' al-Fataawa (12/98). See also: Majmoo' al-Fataawa (12/53) (83)

With regard to people's actions, they are created.
Allah, the Exalted, says:

"While Allah has created you and what you do (or make)." (Qur'an, As-Saffat 37:96)

47. Reciting the Qur'an During the Funeral, at the Grave and During the Days of Condolence on the Death Anniversary of the Person

When the news of death in the family reaches the relatives and friends, the first thing that they should say is the following Qur'anic Verse:

"Who, when afflicted with calamity, say: "Truly! To Allah we belong and truly, to Him we shall return." (Qur'an, Al-Baqarah 2:156)

In the case of the husband or wife, he (or she) should add *"Allahumma ajirni fi musibati wakhluf li khayran minha (or minhu if it is the wife saying it)."* (O Allah grant me refuge in my affliction and replace her (or him) with someone better).

Reading the Qur'an during the funeral, at the grave or on the day of condolence is an innovation (Bid'ah). There is no evidence that the reward for the recitation of the Qur'an will reach the deceased person. The Messenger (peace and blessings of Allah be upon him) did not do that for the Muslims who died, such as his daughters who died during his lifetime. So, it is better for the believer not to do that and not to read Qur'an for either the dead or the living, or to offer Salah, or fast voluntarily on their behalf, because there is no evidence for any of these things. The basic principle regarding acts of worship is to refrain from everything except that which is proven to be enjoined by Allah or by His Messenger (peace and blessings of Allah be upon him). (84)

Abu Hurairah (May Allah be pleased with him) reported: The Messenger of Allah (peace and blessings of Allah be upon him) said, "When a man dies, his deeds come to an end except for three things: Sadaqah Jariyah (ceaseless charity), a knowledge which is beneficial or a virtuous descendant who prays for him (for the deceased)." (Muslim)

Charity, Du'as, obligatory missed fasting, Hajj or Umrah on behalf of the dead or one who is incapable will all benefit both the living and the dead. (85)

48. Prohibition of Carrying the Qur'an into the Land of Enemy

Allah, the Exalted, says:

"Verily, as for those whom the angels take (in death) while they are wronging themselves (as they stayed among the disbelievers even though emigration was obligatory for them), they (angels) say (to them): "In what (condition) were you?" They reply: "We were weak and oppressed on the earth." They (angels) say: "Was not the earth of Allah spacious enough for you to emigrate therein?" Such men will find their abode in Hell - what an evil destination!" (Qur'an, An-Nisa 4:97)

"Except the weak ones among men, women and children who cannot devise a plan, nor are they able to direct their way." (Qur'an, An-Nisa 4:98)

Ibn 'Umar (May Allah be pleased with him) said: "The Messenger of Allah (peace and blessings be upon him) forbade travelling to the land of the enemy carrying the Qur'an." (Bukhari and Muslim)

Commentary: This prohibition is out of fear that the disbelievers might abase and demean the Qur'an and will not give it due respect. It is, however, permissible to take it to places where there is no such fear. (86)

Narrated Jarir ibn Abdullah: The Messenger of Allah (peace and blessings of Allah be upon him) sent an expedition to Khath'am. Some people sought protection by having recourse to prostration, and were hastily killed. When the Prophet (peace and blessings of Allah be upon him) heard that, he ordered half the blood-wit to be paid for them, saying: "I am not responsible for any Muslim who stays among polytheists." They asked: "Why, Messenger of Allah?" He said: "Their fires should not be visible to one another." (Abu Dawud)

49. Saying "Sadaqa Allaah al-'Azeem" (Allah has spoken the Truth)

There is no basis in the Qur'an and Sunnah for adding these words - "Sadaqa Allaah al-'Azeem" - when finishing reading Qur'an. It is a Bid'ah. (87)

50. Disrespect of Ka'bah

Allah, the Exalted, says:
"I swear by this city, Makkah." (Qur'an, Al-Balad 90:1)

"Verily, the first House (of worship) appointed for mankind was that at Bakkah (Makkah), full of blessing, and a guidance for al-'aalameen (mankind and Jinns)." (Qur'an, Ali 'Imran 3:96)

"And whoever respects the sacred ordinances of Allah, it is better for him with his Lord." (Qur'an, Al-Hajj 22:30)

Other Verses: *Al-Ma'idah 5:2, Al-Fil 105:1-5, Ad-Dukhan 44:37.*

In Ka'bah, Sacred House, even bad intentions are punishable.

"Tubba, King of Yemen, Abu Karab As'ad intended in his heart to destroy Ka'bah and kill its people who did not welcome him without informing anybody about his plan. Suddenly, he was hit with a painful headache, and stinky fluid burst from his eyes, ears, nose and mouth. Everybody resisted away from him as a result of his bad odour. His minister then gathered the doctors, but they could not come near him to treat him due to his bad smell. At night one of the scholars came to the minister and informed him that he may know the cause of Tuba's sickness and that he knows its cure. The minister was delighted at hearing the news and he took him to see the King. The scholar said to the King: "Tell me the truth, did you intend to do something bad to this House (meaning the Ka'bah)." To that the King said: "Yes, I intended to destroy it and to kill its people." The scholar then said: **"Know that your pain and affliction is the result of your bad intentions."** He then said to him: "The Lord (Owner) of this House has the complete Power and nothing happens in His dominion except what He willed, He knows about the secrets and about the hidden things." That scholar, who was a follower of Prophet Ibrahim (Abraham), then taught the King about the Religion of Islam. **The King embraced Islam immediately and was cured from his sickness."** (1, 2)

The Golden Ratio of the earth, the Miracle of Allah the Almighty, is Ka'bah, the House of Allah. The Golden Ratio proves that Islam is a True Religion, the belief in One Supreme God "Allah" and Qur'an is the true Word of God. Phi What is this Golden ratio? It is the Constant - 1.618. The proportion of distance between Makkah and North Pole to the distance between Makkah and South Pole is exactly 1.618 which is the Golden Ratio. Moreover, the proportion of the distance between South Pole and Makkah a to the distance between both poles is again 1.618. The proportion of Eastern distance to the Western distance of Makkah's solstice line is again 1.618. The proportion of the distance from Makkah to the solstice line from the west side and perimeter of world at that latitude is also surprisingly equal to the Golden Ratio, 1.618.

Allah, the Exalted, says:

"Verily, the first House (of worship) appointed for mankind was that at Makkah, full of blessing, and a Guidance for the mankind." (Qur'an, Ali 'Imran 3:96)

The 47 letters from the Verse = 19980 km between North and South Poles, then 29 letters from the beginning of the Verse till the word Makkah and substitute it with 12348 km. Then, if we divide both of the values, we get: 47/29 = 1.620, which is very close to 1.618

The same Golden Ratio 1.618 is found in the Universe, galaxies, nature, human creation, human organs, teeth, beauty, heart pulses, DNA spiral, plants, snow flake crystals, architectural structures, including Pyramids in Egypt, etc. (88)

51. Reciting Specific Supplications in Each Circuit of Tawaf or Lap of Sa'i during Hajj and 'Umrah

There are no specific supplications in each circuit of Tawaf (circumambulation of the Ka'bah) or Lap of Sa'i (going between as-Safa and al-Marwah) during Hajj and 'Umrah.

Sheikh Muhammad ibn Saalih al-'Uthaymeen (May Allah have mercy on him) said:

"There is no specific Du'a for each circuit (of Tawaf); rather specifying a particular Du'a for each circuit is a kind of innovation (Bid'ah) because that was not narrated from the Prophet (peace and blessings of Allah be upon him). All that has been narrated is to say Takbeer when touching the Black Stone and to say *"Rabbana aatina fi'd-dunya hasanatan wa fi'l-aakhirati hasanah wa qina 'adhaab an-naar (Our Lord! Give us in this world that which is good and in the Hereafter that which is good, and save us from the torment of the Fire)."* (Al-Baqarah 2:201) between ar-Rukn al-Yamaani (the Yemeni Corner) and the Black Stone. As for the rest, it is Dhikr, recitation of Qur'an and Du'a in general terms, and there is nothing specific to be recited in one circuit and not another." (Majmoo' Fataawa ash-Shaykh al-'Uthaymeen (22/336) (89)

In the supplication for the last day, there is something that is reprehensible and contrary to Islamic teaching: namely Tawassul (seeking to draw closer to Allah) in the supplication by virtue of the Prophet (peace and blessings of Allah be upon him) and by virtue of the members of his household. (90)

52. Doing Mischief in the Masjid Al-Haram in Makkah

Allah, the Exalted, says:

"Verily! Those who disbelieve and hinder (men) from the Path of Allah, and from Al-Masjid Al-Haram (at Makkah) which We have made (open) to (all) men, the dweller in it and the visitor from the country are equal there [as regards its sanctity and pilgrimage (Hajj and 'Umrah)]. And whoever inclines to evil actions therein or to do wrong (i.e. practice polytheism and leave Islamic Monotheism), him We shall cause to taste a painful torment." (Qur'an, Al-Hajj 25:22)

"Indeed, those who have disbelieved and avert (people) from the way of Allah and (from) Al-Masjid Al-Haram, which We made for the people - equal are the resident therein and one from outside; and (also) whoever intends (a deed) therein of deviation (in religion) or wrongdoing - We will make him taste of a painful punishment." (Qur'an, Al-Hajj 22:25)

"Whoever brings a good deed (Islamic Monotheism and deeds of obedience to Allah and His Messenger SAW) shall have ten times the like thereof to his credit, and whoever brings an evil deed (polytheism, disbelief, hypocrisy, and deeds of disobedience to Allah and His Messenger SAW) shall have only the recompense of the like thereof, and they will not be wronged." (Qur'an, Al-An'am 6:160)

Committing a sin in the Sacred Mosque in Makkah is very heinous and grave; and even having an intention to do wrong in Al-Haram entails a great punishment. (1, 2, 91)

Committing an evil deed in Al-Haram Mosque is graver but not counted as more than one sin but it is the degree that increases, not the number. On the other hand, good deeds are doubled in terms of degree and number. (91)

53. Disbelieving in Destiny (Qadar)

Allah, the Exalted, says:

"No disaster strikes except by Allah's Permission, and whoever believes in Allah, He guides his heart, Allah is the Knower of all things." (Qur'an, At-Taghabun 64:11)

"Say: "Nothing shall ever happen to us except what Allah has ordained for us. He is our Maula (Lord, Helper and Protector)." And in Allah let the believers put their trust." (Qur'an, At-Tawbah 9:51)

"So, Exalted is He in Whose Hand is the realm of all things, and to Him you will be returned." (Qur'an, Yasin 36:83)

Other Verses: Al-Qalam 68:47, Al-An'am 6:59, Az-Zumar 39:62, Al-Furqan 25:2, Al-Zalzalah 99:7-8, Ar-Ra'd 13:39)

Ibn Ad-Daylami reported: "I went to Ubayy ibn Ka'b and said: 'There is something in my heart about Predestination, so tell me something in the hope that Allah will remove it from my heart.' He said: 'If you spend the like of Uhud in gold, Allah will not accept it from you until you believe in Predestination, and know that what has befallen you, would not have missed you, and what has missed you, would not have befallen you. If you die on other than this, you will be among the people of Hellfire.' He added: 'Then, I went to Abdullah ibn Masud, Hudhayfah ibn al-Yaman and Zayd ibn Thabit, and each of them told me the same thing on the authority of the Prophet (May Allah's peace and blessings be upon him).'" (Ibn Majah) (https://hadeethenc.com/en/browse/hadith/5954)

'Ubadah ibn As-Samit (May Allah be pleased with him) said to his son: "O Son, you will not taste true faith until you know that whatever has come to you, would never have missed you, and that whatever has missed you, would never have come to you. I heard the Messenger of Allah (May Allah's peace and blessings be upon him) say: 'The first thing Allah created was the Pen. He commanded it to write. It said: 'My Lord, what shall I write?' He said: 'Write down what has been ordained for all things until the establishment of the Hour.' O Son, I heard the Messenger of Allah (May Allah's peace and blessings be upon him) say: 'Whoever dies believing otherwise, does not belong to me.'"
In a narration by Imam Ahmad: "Verily, the first thing Allah the Almighty created was the Pen. He said to it: 'Write.' So, in that very hour it wrote down all what was to occur up to the Day of Judgment."

In a narration by Ibn Wahb, the Messenger of Allah (May Allah's peace and blessings be upon him) said: "So, whoever disbelieved in fate, the good and the bad thereof, Allah will burn him with the Hellfire." (Ibn Wahb in Al-Qadar, Tirmidhi, Abu Dawud, Ahmad) (https://hadeethenc.com/en/browse/hadith/5979)

Narrated Abdullah bin Masud: The Messenger of Allah (peace and blessings be upon him), the most truthful, the most trusted, told us: "Verily the creation of any one of you takes place when he is assembled in his mother's womb; for forty days he is as a drop of fluid, then it becomes a clot for a similar period. Thereafter, it is a lump looking like it has been chewed for a similar period. Then an angel is sent to him, who breathes the ruh (spirit) into him. This angel is commanded to write Four Decrees: that he writes down his provision (rizq), his life span, his deeds, and whether he will be among the wretched or the blessed. I swear by Allah - there is no God but He - one of you may perform the deeds of the people of Paradise till there is naught but an arm's length between him and it, when that which has been written will outstrip him, so that he performs the deeds of the people of the Hellfire; one of you may perform the deeds of the people of the Hellfire, till there is naught but an arm's length between him and it, when that which has been written will overtake him, so that he performs the deeds of the people of Paradise and enters therein." (Bukhari and Muslim)

"As a man looks around himself and looks to his own self and within himself, he finds that there are hundred and one things in shaping and reshaping of which he has no hand, e. g. in determining the climate of the land in which he is born, in canalizing the courses of rivers which flow therein and in determining the nature of the soil thereof. He finds himself absolutely powerless. As he looks to himself, he finds that there are so many things in him which are beyond his control, viz. the measure of intellect he has been endowed with, the shape and form of his physical structure with which he has been sent to this world, and the inclinations, and so many other qualities of head and heart which are embedded in his very nature. In all these aspects of life he finds himself helpless before the Great and Mighty Power that created him. On the other hand, there are so many things in which man finds himself quite empowered. As he looks to the marvelous achievements of man despite all odds, he finds it difficult to believe that he is a mere puppet in the mighty hand of Nature. This problem of Predestination and free will, in which man finds his life hanging, has been adequately solved by the Qur'an and the Sunnah. We give below a brief summary of their elucidations. The first principle which Islam lays down in regard to Taqdir is that man is neither completely the master of his fate nor is he bound to the blind law of Predestination. So far as the Sovereignty of Allah's Will is concerned, it is all-pervading and nothing falls outside its orbit. Not even a leaf, therefore, stirs without His Will. It is His Will that prevails everywhere. To God belongs the sovereignty of heavens and the earth. He created what He pleaseth, giving to whom He pleaseth females and to whom He pleaseth males, or conjoining them males and females, and He maketh whom He pleaseth barren, verify He hath Knowledge and Power (xlii. 48). Men are, therefore, completely subordinate to the Overruling Power of God, they cannot do anything unless God wills so. His mighty grasp is, therefore, over everything. The Almighty Lord, Who has created everything and has determined its nature and course, has in His infinite Wisdom and Mercy conferred upon man a limited autonomy according to which a man is free to do or not to do a certain thing. It is because of this autonomy enjoyed by man that he is hold accountable for his deeds. The concept of human responsibility and that of his answerability for his deeds and misdeeds becomes meaningless if he is supposed to be deprived of this autonomy." (Muslim)

Predestination (Qadar) is one of the six pillars of Faith. Qadar means that Allah has decreed everything that happens in the Universe according to His Knowledge and Wisdom. (92)

There are two types of Qadar.

1. **Definite Qadar**

    This is the type of Decree which Allah, the Creator, has written in the Mother of the Book, Preserved tablet (Al-Lawh Al-Mahfuz) and this Decree will never change.

2. **Indefinite Qadar**

    This is the type of Decree which Allah made and make it known to angels.

    The Decrees contained in the books of the angels, such as lifespan and provisions, may increase or decrease according to various circumstances, thereafter, the angels will re-write a person's provision and lifespan. This type of Qadar may change if Allah wills.

Ibn Taymiyah (May Allah have mercy on him) wrote:

"There are two types of provision and lifespan:

1. The first type has already been decreed and is written in Umm al-Kitaab (Al-Lawh Al-Mahfuz), and cannot be changed or altered.
2. The second type of Qadar, Allah has informed His angels of His Decrees.

This is the type where provisions and lifespan may increase or decrease.

However, the Decrees contained in the books of the angels, such as lifespan and provisions, may increase or decrease according to various circumstances; thereafter, the angels will re-write a person's provision and lifespan. If a person upholds the ties of kinship, his provisions and lifespan will be extended, otherwise they will decrease." (Majmoo'al-Fataawa 8/540)

Belief in al-Qadar includes four things:

1. The belief that Allah knows all things, in general and in detail, from eternity to eternity, whether that has to do with His actions or the actions of His slaves.
2. The belief that Allah has written all matters that would ever occur in a Preserved tablet (Al-Lawh Al-Mahfuz, the Book of Decrees).

3. The belief that whatever happens only happens by the Will of Allah – whether that has to do with His actions or the actions of created beings.
4. The belief that all things that happen are created by Allah in their essence, their attributes and their movements.

Allah says concerning His actions:

"And your Lord creates whatsoever He wills and chooses." (Qur'an, Al-Qasas 28:68)

"..and Allah does what He wills." (Qur'an, Ibrahim 14:27)

"He it is Who shapes you in the wombs as He wills." (Qur'an, Ali 'Imran 3:6)

Other Verse: Ali 'Imran 3:26-27.

Allah says concerning the actions of created human beings:

"And you did not kill them, but it was Allah who killed them. And you threw not, [O Muḥammad], when you threw, but it was Allah who threw that He might test the believers with a good test. Indeed, Allah is Hearing and Knowing." (Qur'an, Al-Anfal 8:17)

"To whomsoever among you who wills to walk straight. And you cannot will unless (it be) that Allah wills, the Lord of the 'Alamin (mankind, Jinns and all that exists)." (Qur'an, At-Takwir 81:28-29)

"If your Lord had so willed, they would not have done it." (Qur'an, Al-An'am 6:112)

Other Verses: Fatir 35:2, At-Taghabun 64:11, Al-A'raf 7:179.

Narrated Abdullah bin Abbas: "One day I was riding (a horse/camel) behind the Prophet (peace be upon him) when he said: "Young man, I shall teach you some words (of advice): Be mindful of Allah, and Allah will take care of you. Be mindful of Allah, and you shall find Him at your side. If you ask, ask of Allah;
if you need help, seek it from Allah. Know that if the whole world were to gather together to in order to help you, they would not be able to help you except if Allah had written so. And if the whole world were to gather together in order to harm you, they would not harm you except if Allah had written so. The pens have been lifted, and the pages are dry.'" (Tirmidhi)

Almighty Allah says concerning man's will:

"That is (without doubt) the True Day. So, whosoever wills, let him seek a place with (or a way to) His Lord (by obeying Him in this worldly life)!" (Qur'an, An-Naba 78:39)

"But you cannot will unless Allah wills; Allah is Knowing, Wise." (Qur'an, Al-Insan 76:30)

Almighty Allah says concerning man's ability:

"So, keep your duty to Allah and fear Him as much as you can." (Qur'an, At-Taghabun 64:16)

"Allah burdens not a person beyond his scope. He gets reward for that (good) which he has earned, and he is punished for that (evil) which he has earned." (Qur'an, Al-Baqarah 2:286)

Man has a will and the ability to do what he wants and not to do what he does not want.

But the will and ability of man are subject to the Will and Decree of Allah.

Ibn Taymiyah (May Allah have mercy on him) said with regard to man's deeds:

"People act in a real sense, and Allah is the Creator of their actions. A person may be a believer or a kaafir, righteous or immoral, he may pray and fast. People have control over their actions, and they have their own will, and Allah is the Creator of their control and will, as Allah says: *"To whomsoever among you who wills to walk straight. And you cannot will unless (it be) that Allah wills, the Lord of the 'Aalameen (mankind, Jinns and all that exists)."* (Qur'an, At-Takwir 81:28-29) (al-Waasitiyyah ma'a Sharh Harraas, p.65)

Ali (May Allah have mercy on him) reported: "We were in a funeral in the graveyard of Gharqad that Allah's Messenger (peace and blessings be upon him) came to us and we sat around him. He had a stick with him. He lowered his head and began to scratch the earth with his stick, and then said: 'There is not one amongst you whom a seat in Paradise or Hell has not been allotted and about whom it has not been written down whether he would be an evil person or a blessed person.' A person said: 'Allah's Messenger, should we not then depend upon our destiny and abandon our deeds?' Thereupon, he said: 'Acts of everyone will be facilitated in, that which has been created for him so that whoever belongs to the company of the blessed, will have good works made easier for him, and whoever belongs to the unfortunate ones, will have evil acts made easier for him. He then recited this Verse from the Qur'an:
"Then, who gives to the needy and guards against evil, and accepts the excellent (the Truth of Islam and the Path of righteousness it prescribes), We shall make easy for him the easy end, and who is miserly and considers himself above need, We shall make easy for him the difficult end." (XCii. 5-10) (Muslim)

Allah states the wisdom behind pre-ordainment that the slave should neither despair if calamity afflicts, nor become proud and haughty on achieving good; because every calamity that befalls him was previously designated and all blessings are due to Allah's Favor and Mercy.

Abu Hurairah reported Allah's Messenger (peace and blessings be upon him) as saying: "A strong believer is better and is more lovable to Allah than a weak believer, and there is good in everyone, (but) cherish that which gives you benefit (in the Hereafter) and seek help from

Allah and do not lose heart, and if anything (in the form of trouble) comes to you, don't say: 'If I had not done that, it would not have happened so and so, but say: Allah did that what He had ordained to do and your "if" opens the (gate) for the Satan." (Muslim)

Like our Salaf would say, "There is no protection from the Qadr of Allah, except with Allah." What some people say, that we have the choice to follow whatever path we want but at the end of this path you will find what Allah has decreed for you, is a correct view. (93)

Benefits of Believing in Qadr

1. It grants its believer the peace of mind and sense of relaxation to know, that which has befallen him, was never meant to pass him by and that which has passed him was never meant to befall him;
2. It gives its believer the will and determination to do righteous deeds and grants him the knowledge of the fact that nothing can harm him or stop him except that which Allah has willed;
3. Teaches its believer not to be arrogant and vain but rather to be modest and humble because he realizes that his actions are created by Allah and that such and such an event occurred, not because he was rich or was given beauty and good lineage but rather because it was the Will of Allah.
4. Teaches its believer to do as much as is in his capability and then leave the rest up to Allah, and then to be satisfied with the result as he did as much as his ability permitted him to do so.

What can change the destiny, it is a Du'a

Abu Hurairah, Ali and Jabir (May Allah have mercy on them) reported: The Messenger of Allah (peace and blessings be upon him) said: "Du'a is the weapon of the believer, the pillar of the religion, and the light of the heavens and earth." (Mustadrak Hakim, vol.1 p.492 and Musnad Abi Ya'la, Hadith: 439) https://hadithanswers.com/dua-is-the-weapon-of-believerpillar-of-din-and-light-of-heavens-and-earth/

Du'a is a powerful weapon of the believer, it can change the Divine Decree. Du'a is from the most beneficial types of healing, it is the enemy of illness and affliction – repressing it and treating it, preventing its occurrence, removing it or at least alleviating it. It is beneficial with regard to what has been decreed and what has not been decreed. (94)

54. Saying: "If Only I Had Done Such-and-Such"

Abu Hurairah (May Allah be pleased with him) reported that the Prophet (May Allah's peace and blessings be upon him) said: "Strive for that which will benefit you, seek Allah's help and do not lose heart or determination. If anything befalls you, do not say: 'If only I had done such-and-such'; rather, say: 'Allah has decreed and whatever He wills, He does.' Saying 'if' opens (the door to) the deeds of the Devil." (Muslim) (https://hadeethenc.com/en/browse/hadith/5929)

55. Using Allah's Decree (Qadar) as an Excuse for Your Sin

Allah, the Exalted, says:

"Messengers as bearers of good news as well as of warning in order that mankind should have no plea against Allah after the (coming of) Messengers. And Allah is Ever All-Powerful, All-Wise." (Qur'an, An-Nisa 4:165)

"Those who took partners (in worship) with Allah will say: 'If Allah had willed, we would not have taken partners (in worship) with Him, nor would our fathers, and we would not have forbidden anything (against His Will).' Likewise belied those who were before them, (they argued falsely with Allah's Messengers), till they tasted Our Wrath. Say: 'Have you any knowledge (proof) that you can produce before us? Verily, you follow nothing but guess and you do nothing but lie.'" (Qur'an, Al-An'am 6:14)

"Had we but listened or used our intelligence, we would not have been among the dwellers of the blazing Fire!" (Qur'an, Al-Mulk 67:10)

Other Verses: *At-Taghabun 64:16, Al-Muddaththir 74:43.*

Narrated Abu Hurairah: The Prophet (peace and blessings be upon him) said, "Adam and Moses argued with each other. Moses said to Adam. 'O Adam! You are our father who disappointed us and turned us out of Paradise.' Then Adam said to him, 'O Moses! Allah favored you with His talk (talked to you directly) and He wrote (the Torah) for you with His Own Hand. Do you blame me for action which Allah had written in my fate forty years before my creation?' So, Adam confuted Moses, Adam confuted Moses," the Prophet (peace be upon him) added, repeating the Statement three times." (Bukhari)

It is not permissible using al-Qadar as an excuse for committing sin or not doing obligatory actions. (95, 96)

56. Talking About Future Without "In Shaa Allah"

Allah, the Exalted, says:

"And never say of anything, "I shall do such and such thing tomorrow." Except (with the saying), "If Allah will!" And remember your Lord when you forget and say: "It may be that my Lord guides me unto a nearer way of Truth than this." (Qur'an, Al-Kahf 18:23-24)

Other Verses: *Al-Qalam 68:17-19.*

In shaa Allah is an Arabic language expression meaning "if God wills" or "God willing".

Abu Hurairah (May Allah be pleased with him) reported that the Prophet (May Allah's peace and blessings be upon him) said: "Sulayman ibn Dawud (peace be upon him) said: 'I will indeed have sexual intercourse with seventy women at night, and each one of them will give birth to a child who will fight in the Cause of Allah.' It was said to him: 'Say: Allah willing!' But he did not do so. He had intercourse with them all, but none of them gave birth, except for one woman who gave birth to half a person." Upon this, the Messenger (May Allah's peace and blessings be upon him) said: "If he had said, 'Allah willing,' he would not have failed in his oath, and his desire would have been fulfilled." (Bukhari and Muslim)
(https://hadeethenc.com/en/browse/hadith/2977)

57. Abomination of Saying- "What Allah Wills and so-and-so Wills"

Narrated Hudhaifah bin Yaman (May Allah be pleased with him): The Prophet (peace and blessings be upon him) said, "Say not: 'What Allah wills and so-and-so wills', but say: 'What Allah wills, and then what so-and-so wills.'" (Abu Dawud)

Commentary: The first form mentioned in this Hadith is prohibited for the reason that it combines the will of someone with the Will of Allah, which is utterly wrong and against the factual position. In the second form, the Will of Allah comes first, which is the correct position, and the will of someone else comes later which is subject to the Will of Allah. The later form is quite fair.
It is as if someone says to a person, "I have only Allah's Support and yours". In this statement Allah and man (the person addressed) are given the same status, which is the most unfair and unjust. It would, however, be all right to say "We have the support of Allah and then yours", because this statement does not have any trace of Shirk, which the former statement has. (97)

58. Ruling on one who Rejects a Saheeh Hadith

Allah, the Exalted, says:

"Nor does he speak of (his own) desire. It is but a Revelation revealed." (Qur'an, An-Najm 53:3-4)

"But no, by your Lord, they can have no Faith, until they make you (O Muhammad (peace and blessings be upon him)) judge in all disputes between them, and find in themselves no resistance against your decisions, and accept (them) with full submission." (Qur'an, An-Nisa 4:65)

Ibn Taymiyah (May Allah have mercy on him) said:

"Whatever the Messenger (peace and blessings of Allah be upon him) narrates from his Lord, it is obligatory to believe in it, whether we understand its meaning or not, because he is the most truthful one [namely the Prophet (peace and blessings of Allah be upon him)]. Whatever it says in the Qur'an and Sunnah, every believer must believe in it, even if he does not understand its meaning." (End quote. Majmoo' al-Fataawa (3/41)

It says in Fataawa al-Lajnah ad-Daa'imah: "The one who denies that we should follow the Sunnah is a disbeliever, because he is expressing disbelief in Allah and His Messenger, and rejecting the consensus of the Muslims." (End quote. Fataawa al-Lajnah ad-Daa'imah (vol.2, 3/194) (98)

59. Not Making Room in the Assemblies

Allah, the Exalted, says:

"O you who believe! When you are told to make room in the assemblies, (spread out and) make room. Allah will give you (ample) room (from His Mercy). And when you are told to rise up [for prayers, Jihad (holy fighting in Allah's Cause), or for any other good deed], rise up. Allah will exalt in degree those of you who believe, and those who have been granted knowledge. And Allah is Well-Acquainted with what you do." (Qur'an, Al-Mujadilah 58:11)

60. Excessive Questioning and Disagreement (in Disputed Religious Matters)

Allah, the Exalted, says:

"O you who have believed, do not ask about things which, if they are shown to you, will distress you. But if you ask about them while the Qur'an is being revealed, they will be shown to you. Allah has pardoned that which is past; and Allah is Forgiving and Forbearing." (Qur'an, Al-Ma'idah 5:101)

Narrated Abu Hurairah: "I heard the Messenger of Allah (peace and blessings be upon him) say: "Avoid that which I forbid you to do and do that which I command you to do to the best of your capacity. Verily, the people before you were destroyed only because of their excessive questioning and their disagreement with their Prophets." (Bukhari and Muslim)

Narrated Al-Mughira bin Shuba: The Prophet (peace and blessings be upon him) said, "Allah has forbidden for you: 1) to be undutiful to your mothers, 2) to bury your daughters alive, 3) do not to pay the rights of the others (e.g. charity, etc.) and 4) to beg of men (begging). And Allah has hated for you: 1) Qil and Qal (useless talk or that you talk too much about others), 2) to ask too many questions (in disputed religious matters) and 3) to waste the wealth (by extravagance with lack of wisdom and thinking)." (Bukhari)

61. Not Performing the Prayers

Allah, the Exalted, says:

"And I (Allah) created not the Jinns and humans except they should worship Me (Alone)." (Qur'an, Adh-Dhariyat 51:56)

"Guard strictly (five obligatory) As-Salawat (the prayers) especially the middle Salat (i.e. the best prayer 'Asr). And stand before Allah with obedience [and do not speak to others during the Salat (prayers)]. And if you fear (an enemy), perform Salat (pray) on foot or riding. And when you are in safety, offer the Salat (prayer) in the manner He has taught you, which you knew not (before)." (Qur'an, Al-Baqarah 2:238-239)

"Recite, [O Muhammad], what has been revealed to you of the Book and establish prayer. Indeed, prayer prohibits immorality and wrongdoing, and the remembrance of Allah is greater. And Allah knows that which you do." (Qur'an, Al-'Ankabut 29:45)

Jabir bin 'Abdullah (May Allah be pleased with him) narrated: Allah's Messenger (peace and blessings be upon him) said: "The key to Paradise is Prayer, and the key to Prayer is Wudu." (Tirmidhi)

Narrated Abu Hurairah: The Prophet (peace and blessings be upon him) said: "Allah, Mighty and Sublime be He, says: 'The first of his actions for which a servant of Allah will be held accountable on the Day of Resurrection will be his prayers.' If they are in order, then he will have prospered and succeeded; and if they are wanting, then he will have failed and lost. If there is something defective in his obligatory prayers, the Lord, Glorified and Exalted be He, will say: 'See if My servant has any supererogatory prayers with which may be completed that which was defective in his obligatory prayers.' Then the rest of his actions will be judged in like fashion." (Tirmidhi, Abu Dawud, An-Nasa'i, Ibn Majah and Ahmad)

Narrated Abu Darda: "My close friend (peace and blessings of Allah be upon him) advised me: "Do not associate anything with Allah, even if you are cut and burned. Do not neglect any prescribed prayer deliberately, for whoever neglects it deliberately no longer has the protection of Allah. And do not drink wine, for it is the key to all evil." (Ibn Majah)

The Merits of Ablution (Wudu or Ghusl)

Allah, the Exalted, says:

"Truly, Allah loves those who turn unto Him in repentance and loves those who purify themselves (by taking a bath and cleaning, and washing thoroughly their private parts, bodies, for their prayers, etc.)." (Qur'an, Al-Baqarah 2:222)

"O you who believe! When you intend to offer As-Salat (the prayer), wash your faces and your hands (forearms) up to the elbows, wipe (by passing wet hands over) your heads, and (wash) your feet up to the ankles. If you are in a state of Janaba (i.e. after a sexual discharge), purify yourselves (bathe your whole body). But if you are ill or on a journey, or any of you comes from responding to the call of nature, or you have been in contact with women (i.e. sexual intercourse) and you find no water, then perform Tayammum with clean earth and rub therewith your faces and hands. Allah does not want to place you in difficulty, but He wants to purify you, and to complete His Favor to you that you may be thankful." (Qur'an, Al-Ma'idah 5:6)

1. The Believers will be Recognized by their Traces of Wudu on the Day of Judgment

Narrated Abu Hurairah (May Allah be pleased with him): "I heard the Messenger of Allah (peace and blessings be upon him) saying: 'On the Day of Resurrection, my followers (or Ummah) will be summoned 'Al-Ghurr Al-Muhajjalun' from the traces of Wudu. Whoever can increase the area of his radiance should do so.'" (Bukhari and Muslim)

2. The Adornment of a Believer in Jannah will Reach up to where the Water Reached his Body

Narrated Abu Hurairah (May Allah be pleased with him): "I heard my Khalil (the Messenger of Allah, peace and blessings be upon him) as saying, 'The adornment of the believer (in Jannah) will reach the places where the water of Wudu reaches (his body).'" (Muslim)

3. Expiation of Sins even Under the Nails

Narrated 'Uthman bin 'Affan (May Allah be pleased with him): The Messenger of Allah (peace and blessings be upon him) said, "He who performs the Wudu perfectly (i.e. according to Sunnah), his sins will depart from his body, even from under his nails." (Muslim)

4. Expiation of Sins and Supererogatory Act of Worship

Narrated 'Uthman bin 'Affan (May Allah be pleased with him): "I saw the Messenger of Allah (peace and blessings be upon him) performing Wudu the way I have just done it and said, 'He who performs Wudu like this, his previous sins will be forgiven and his Salat and walking to the Mosque will be considered as supererogatory act of worship.'" (Muslim)

5. Expiation of Sins Committed by Eyes, Hands and Feet

Narrated Abu Hurairah (May Allah be pleased with him): The Messenger of Allah (peace and blessings be upon him) said, "When a Muslim or a believer, washes his face (in the course of Wudu), every sin which he committed with his eyes, will be washed away from his face with water, or with the last drop of water; when he washes his hands, every sin which is committed by his hands will be effaced from his hands with the water, or with the last drop of water; and when he washes his feet, every sin his feet committed will be washed away with the water, or with the last drop of water; until he finally emerges cleansed of all his sins." (Muslim)

6. Bright Faces and White Limbs

Narrated Abu Hurairah (May Allah be pleased with him): "The Messenger of Allah (peace and blessings be upon him) went to the (Baqi') cemetery and said, "May you be secured from punishment, O dwellers of abode of the believers! We, if Allah wills, will follow you. I wish we see my brothers." The Companions said, "O Messenger of Allah! Are not we your brothers?" He (peace and blessings be upon him) said, "You are my Companions, but my brothers are those who have not come into the world yet." They said; "O Messenger of Allah! How will you recognize those of your Ummah who are not born yet?" He (peace and blessings be upon him) said, "Say, if a man has white-footed horses with white foreheads among horses which are pure black, will he not recognize his own horses?" They said; "Certainly, O Messenger of Allah!" He (peace and blessings be upon him) said, "They (my followers) will come with bright faces and white limbs because of Wudu; and I will arrive at the Haud (Al-Kawthar) ahead of them." (Muslim)

7. Performing Wudu in Hardship Removes Sins and Elevates Ranks

Narrated Abu Hurairah (May Allah be pleased with him): The Messenger of Allah (peace and blessings be upon him) said, "Shall I not tell you something by which Allah effaces sins and elevates ranks (in Paradise)?" The Companions said: "Certainly, O Messenger of Allah." He (peace and blessings be upon him) said, "Performing the Wudu properly even in difficulty, increasing attendance of prayer in the Mosque, and waiting for the next prayer after observing one prayer; and this is Jihad." (Muslim) (99)

The Prophet (May Allah's peace and blessings be upon him) used to present issues as questions so that the people would pay more attention to what was coming. So, the Prophet (May Allah's peace and blessings be upon him) said: "Shall I not tell you something by which Allah effaces sins and elevates ranks (in Paradise)?" The Companions said: "Certainly, O Messenger of Allah." In other words: tell us as we would love to know about what will increase our ranks and erase our sins. He said: "Firstly: Performing the ablution properly even in difficulty, as during the days of winter, when the water is cold. So, if a person completes his ablution given this hardship, this is proof of his completeness of faith. Thereby, Allah will raise his rank and erase his sins. Secondly: Attending the five daily prayers in the Mosque, even if it is far. Thirdly: Having the desire to pray. Every time he finishes a prayer, his heart is attached to the next one. This is proof of his faith, love and desire to pray more of these great prayers. If he awaits prayer after prayer, this is among the reasons for which Allah raises his rank and erases his sins. Then the Prophet informed that constant commitment to purification (ablution), prayer and worship is like Jihad for the sake of Allah. (https://hadeethenc.com/en/browse/hadith/3574)

8. Purification is Half of Faith

Abu Malik at-Ash'ari reported: The Messenger of Allah (peace and blessings be upon him) said: "Cleanliness is half of Faith and Al-Hamdu Liliah (Praise be to Allah) fills the scale, and Subhan Allah (Glory be to Allah) and Al-Hamdu Liliah (Praise be to Allah) fill up what is between the heavens and the earth, and prayer is a light, and charity is proof (of one's Faith) and endurance is a brightness and the Holy Qur'an is a proof on your behalf or against you. All men go out early in the morning and sell themselves, thereby setting themselves free or destroying themselves." (Muslim)

9. The Eight Gates of Paradise are Opened if after Ablution you Testify Shahada

Narrated 'Umar bin Al-Khattab (May Allah be pleased with him): The Messenger of Allah (peace and blessings be upon him) said, "Whoever of you performs Wudu carefully and then affirms: 'Ash-hadu an la ilaha illallahu Wahdahu la sharika Lahu, wa ash-hadu anna Muhammadan 'abduhu wa Rasuluhu [I testify that there so no true god except Allah Alone, Who has no partners and that Muhammad (peace and blessings be upon him) is His slave and Messenger]', the eight gates of Jannah are opened for him. He may enter through whichever of these gates he desires (to enter)." (Muslim)

10. Ablution Removes Satan from the Nose

Abu Hurairah reported: The Prophet (peace and blessings be upon him) said, "When one of you awakens from his sleep, then let him perform ablution and sniff water into his nose three times. Verily, Satan spends the night in the upper part of his nose." (Bukhari)

11. Satan's three knots at the back of the head of anyone when he sleeps are undone with Wudu and Prayer

Narrated Abu Hurairah: Allah's Messenger (peace and blessings be upon him) said, "During your sleep, Satan ties three knots at the back of the head of each one of you, and he seals each knot with the following words: 'The night is long, so keep on sleeping.' When that person wakes up and remembers Allah, one knot is undone; when he makes ablution the second knot is undone; and when he prays, all his knots are undone, and he gets up in the morning active and in good spirits, otherwise he gets up in bad spirits and sluggish." (Bukhari and Muslim) (https://hadeethenc.com/en/browse/hadith/3731)

12. Satan urinates in the ear(s) of man who slept the night till morning (after sunrise)

Narrated 'Abdullah: "It was mentioned before the Prophet that there was a man who slept the night till morning (after sunrise). The Prophet (peace and blessings be upon him) said, "He is a man in whose ears (or ear) Satan had urinated." (Bukhari)

13. Angel will Seek Forgiveness for you

Ibn 'Abbas (May Allah have mercy on him): The Messenger of Allah (peace and blessings be upon him) said, "Purify these bodies and Allah will purify you, for there is no slave who goes to sleep in a state of purity but an Angel spends the night with him, and every time he turns over, (the Angel) says, 'O Allah! Forgive Your slave, for he went to bed in a state of purity." (Tabarani)

14. Rewards for Ghusl on Friday

Abu Sa'id reported that the Prophet (peace and blessings be upon him) said, "Ghusl on Friday is obligatory (wajib) on every adult, as is using a toothbrush and applying some perfume." (Bukhari and Muslim) https://www.iium.edu.my/deed/lawbase/fiqh_us_sunnah/vol1/fsn_vol1b.html.

Narrated Aws ibn Aws al-Thaqafi: The Messenger of Allah (peace and blessings be upon him) said:
"Whoever does Ghusl on Friday and causes (his wife) to do Ghusl, and sets out early, and comes close to the imam and listens, and keeps quiet, for every step he takes he will have the reward of fasting and praying Qiyaam for one year." (Tirmidhi)

Abu Hurairah (May Allah be pleased with him) reported: The Messenger of Allah (May Allah's peace and blessings be upon him) said: "It is due upon every Muslim to take a bath once in every seven days, where he should wash his head and body." (Bukhari and Muslim) (https://hadeethenc.com/en/browse/hadith/65084)

15. Previous Sins will be Forgiven if Two Ra'kahs Performed After Wudu

Narrated Humran bin Aban: "I saw Uthman bin Affan (May Allah be pleased with him) performing Wudu. He poured water on his hands three times and washed them, then he rinsed his mouth and his nose, then he washed his face three times, then he washed right arm to the elbow three times, then the left likewise. Then he wiped his head, then he washed his right foot three times, then the left likewise. Then he said: 'I saw the Messenger of Allah (peace and blessings be upon him) performing Wudu like I have just done.' Then he said: 'Whoever performs Wudu as I have done, then prays two Rak'ahs without letting his thoughts wander, his previous sins will be forgiven.'" (An-Nasai)

16. Preserving Wudu is a Sign of Iman

Narrated Abdullah bin Amr: The Messenger of Allah (peace and blessings be upon him) said: "Adhere to righteousness even though you will not be able to do all acts of virtue. Know that among the best of your deeds is prayer and that no one maintains his ablution except a believer." (Ibn Majah)

17. Wudu should be done in the manner prescribed by the Prophet

Umar ibn al-Khattab (May Allah be pleased with him) reported: "A man performed ablution and left a small part on his foot equal to the space of a nail unwashed. The Messenger of Allah (May Allah's peace and blessings be upon him) saw that and said: "Go back and perform ablution properly." He performed it again and prayed." (Muslim) (https://hadeethenc.com/en/browse/hadith/8386)

The Excellence of Adhan

1. The Blessings of Pronouncing Adhan

Narrated Abu Hurairah (May Allah be pleased with him): The Messenger of Allah (peace and blessings be upon him) said: "Were people to know the blessing of pronouncing Adhan and the standing in the first row, they would even draw lots to secure these privileges. And were they to realize the reward of performing Salah early, they would race for it; and were they to know the merits of Salah after nightfall ('Isha') and the dawn (Fajr) Salah, they would come to them even if they had to crawl." (Bukhari and Muslim)

2. The Caller to Prayer will have Abundant Rewards on Judgment Day

Mu'awiyah (May Allah be pleased with him) reported: The Messenger of Allah (May Allah's peace and blessings be upon him) said: "The Muezzins will have the longest necks of all the people on the Day of Judgment." (Muslim) (https://hadeethenc.com/en/browse/hadith/10115)

3. Whoever Hears the Adhan, will Testify for you on Judgment Day

Narrated 'Abdullah bin 'Abdur-Rahman: Abu Sa'id Al-Khudri (May Allah be pleased with him) said to me: "I see that you like living among your sheep in wilderness. So, whenever you are with your sheep or in wilderness and you want to call Adhan, you should raise your voice because whoever hears the Adhan, whether a human or Jinn, or any other creature, will testify for you on the Day of Resurrection." Abu Sa'id added: "I heard this from the Messenger of Allah (peace and blessings be upon him)." (Bukhari)

4. Satan Cannot Tolerate Adhan

Abu Hurairah (May Allah be pleased with him) reported that the Prophet (May Allah's peace and blessings be upon him) said: "When the call to prayer is announced, the Devil takes to his heels and breaks wind with noise so as not to hear the call. When the call to prayer is over, he returns. When the Iqamah is announced, he takes to his heels, and after it is over, he returns again to distract the attention of the worshiper and make him remember things which were not on his mind before the prayer, saying: 'Remember such-and-such, and remember such-and-such,' until the worshiper forgets how many units of prayer he performed." (Bukhari and Muslim) (https://hadeethenc.com/en/browse/hadith/10109)

5. Intercession of the Prophet on Judgment Day

Narrated Jabir (May Allah be pleased with him): The Messenger of Allah (peace and blessings be upon him) said, "He who says upon hearing the Adhan: 'Allahumma Rabba hadhihid-da'wati-ttammati, was-salatil-qa'imati, ati Muhammadanil-wasilata wal-fadhilata, wab'athu maqaman mahmuda nilladhi wa 'adtahu [O Allah, Rubb of this perfect call (Da'wah) and of the established prayer (As-Salah), grant Muhammad the Wasilah and superiority, and raise him up to a praiseworthy position which You have promised him]', it becomes incumbent upon me to intercede for him on the Day of Resurrection." (Bukhari)

6. Sins will be Forgiven

Narrated Sa'd bin Abu Waqqas (May Allah be pleased with him): The Prophet (peace and blessings be upon him) said, "He who says after the Adhan: 'Ash-hadu an la ilaha illallah Wah-dahu la sharika Lahu; wa ash-hadu anna Muhammadan 'abduhu wa Rasuluhu, radhitu Billahi Rabban, wa bi Muhammadin Rasulan, wa bil Islami Dinan (I testify that there is no true god except Allah Alone; He has no partners and that Muhammad (peace and blessings be upon him) is His slave and Messenger; I am content with Allah as my Rubb, with Muhammad as my Messenger and with Islam as my Deen), his sins will be forgiven." (Muslim)

7. Du'a Between the Adhan and the Iqamah is Never Rejected

Narrated Anas (May Allah be pleased with him): The Messenger of Allah (peace and blessings be upon him) said: "The supplication made between the Adhan and the Iqamah is never rejected." (Tirmidhi)

8. Adhan is an Invitation towards Meeting with Allah, the Creator

It serves a great purpose of achieving the highest state of morality and uprightness of heart and soul because of its direct link with the Prayer. (100)

9. Adhan Glorifies the Lord and His Messenger

Saying "Allah is the Greatest" is to testify the Ultimate Power of the Creator of the Universe, Who controls every phenomenon happening in this world and heavens. Second phrase "There is none worthy of worship except Allah" fulfills the very first criterion of Muslim faith, i.e. to believe in One God`s Supremacy and comparing no one to Him.

10. The Expression "Come to Success" means Attainment of many of God`s Blessings

11. Adhan in the Ear of Newborn (Sunnah)

Narrated Abu Rafi` (a Companion): "I saw the Messenger of Allah (peace and blessings be upon him) give Adhan in the ear of al-Hasan, the son of Ali, when Fatima gave birth to him." (Tirmidhi)

The Excellence of Proceeding towards the Mosque Walking

Abu Hurairah (May Allah be pleased with him) reported that the Messenger (May Allah's peace and blessings be upon him) said: "He who goes to the Mosque in the morning or in the evening, Allah prepares an honorable abode for him in Paradise, every time he goes to the Mosque; in the morning or in the evening." (Bukhari and Muslim)

Abu Hurairah (May Allah be pleased with him) reported: The Prophet (peace and blessings be upon him) said, "He who purifies (performs Wudu) himself in his house and then walks to one of the houses of Allah (Mosque) for performing an obligatory Salah, one step of his will wipe out his sins and another step will elevate his rank (in Jannah)." (Muslim)

Buraidah (May Allah be pleased with him) reported: The Messenger of Allah (peace and blessings be upon him) said, "Convey glad tidings to those who walk to the Mosque in the darkness. For they will be given full light on the Day of Resurrection." (Tirmidhi and Abu Dawud)

Abu Hurairah (May Allah be pleased with him) reported: The Messenger of Allah (peace and blessings be upon him) said, "Shall I not tell you something by which Allah effaces the sins and elevates the ranks (in Jannah)." The Companions said: "Yes (please tell us), O Messenger of Allah." He said, "Performing the Wudu' properly in spite of difficult circumstances, walking with more paces to the Mosque, and waiting for the next Salah (prayer) after observing Salah; and that is Ar-Ribat, and that is Ar-Ribat." (Muslim)

Commentary: One who goes to the Mosque again and again to perform Salat in congregation deserves that one bears witness to his faith. This Hadith also brings into prominence the merit and distinction of those who have an attachment to Mosque, a passion for worship and remembrance of Allah, and fondness for the construction and maintenance of the Mosque. This Hadith is weak in authenticity but correct in its meanings and significance. (101)

The Excellence of Waiting for As-Salah (The Prayer)

Abu Hurairah (May Allah be pleased with him) reported: The Messenger of Allah (peace and blessings be upon him) said, "Everyone among you will be deemed to be occupied in Salah (prayer) constantly so long as Salah (the prayer) detains him (from worldly concerns), and nothing prevents him from returning to his family but Salah." (Bukhari and Muslim)

Anas (May Allah be pleased with him) reported: "Once the Messenger of Allah (peace and blessings be upon him) delayed the night prayer ('Isha') till midnight. He (peace and blessings be upon him) turned to us after Salah (prayer) and said, "The people slept after performing their Salah, but you who waited, will be accounted as engaged in Salah throughout the period of your waiting." (Bukhari)

Commentary: We learn from this Hadith that it is an act of merit and reward to sit and wait for the Imam and the Jama'ah (congregation) and one who does so will be treated as one who is engaged in Salah. We also learn from this Hadith that if a person performs Salah when its time is due, it is quite fair, although in that case he will not get the reward of waiting for the Imam and the Jama'ah. (102)

The Excellence of As-Salah (The Prayer)

Allah, the Exalted, says:

"Verily, As-Salah (the prayer) prevents from Al-Fahisha' (i.e. great sins of every kind, unlawful sexual intercourse, etc.) and Al-Munkar (i.e. disbelief, polytheism, and every kind of evil wicked deed, etc.) and the remembering (praising, etc.) of (you by) Allah (in front of the angels) is greater indeed [than your remembering (praising, etc.) Allah in prayers, etc.]. And Allah knows what you do." (Qur'an, Al-'Ankabut 29:45)

"And perform As-Salat (Iqamat As-Salah), at the two ends of the day and in some hours of the night [i.e. the five compulsory Salah (prayers)]. Verily, the good deeds remove the evil deeds (i.e. small sins). That is a reminder (an advice) for the mindful (those who accept advice)." (Qur'an, Hud 11:114)

"But there came after them an evil generation, who neglected prayers and followed sensual desires, so they will meet perdition." (Qur'an, Maryam 19:59)

Other Verses: *An-Nisa 4:102, Al-Muddaththir 74:42-48.*

"Prayer is the soul of religion. Where there is no prayer, there can be no purification of the soul. The non-praying man is rightly considered to be a soulless man. Take prayer out of the world, and it is all over with religion because it is with prayer that man has the consciousness of God and selfless love for humanity and inner sense of piety. Prayer is, therefore, the first, the highest and the most solemn phenomenon and manifestation of religion." (Muslim)

Abu Hurairah (May Allah be pleased with him) reported: "I heard the Messenger of Allah (peace and blessings be upon him) saying, "Say, if there were a river at the door of one of you in which he takes a bath five times a day, would any soiling remain on him?" They replied, "No soiling would leave on him." He (peace and blessings be upon him) said, "That is the five (obligatory) Salah (prayers). Allah obliterates all sins as a result of performing them." (Bukhari and Muslim)

Ibn Masud (May Allah be pleased with him) reported: "A man kissed a woman. So, he came to the Messenger of Allah (peace and blessings be upon him) and informed him about it. Then Allah revealed this Ayah: *"And perform the Salah, between the two ends of the day and in some hours of the night. Verily, the good deeds efface the evil deeds (i.e. Minor sins)." (11:114)* The man asked the Messenger of Allah (peace and blessings be upon him) whether this applies to him only. The Messenger of Allah (peace and blessings be upon him) said, "It applies to all of my Ummah." (Bukhari and Muslim)

Abu Hurairah (May Allah be pleased with him) reported: The Messenger of Allah (peace and blessings be upon him) said, "The five (daily) Salah (prayers) and the Friday (prayer) to the Friday (prayer) expiate whatever (Minor sins) may be committed in between, so long as Major sins are avoided." (Muslim)

Commentary: This Hadith elucidates that the Minor sins committed during the interval of the five prescribed Salah and in the period intervening between one Jumu'ah and the other are pardoned with the performance of the five-time prescribed Salah and the Jumu'ah prayer, provided one does not commit Major sins which are not forgiven without repentance. Sins like Shirk (associating someone with Allah in worship), disobedience of parents, false oath, false evidence, encroachment on an orphan's property, calumny against chaste women, etc., fall in the category of Major sins and will not be forgiven by means of Salah only. (103)

Prayer is the First Thing to be Judged on Judgment Day

Huraith bin Qabisah narrated: "I arrived in Al-Madinah and said: 'O Allah! Facilitate me to be in a righteous gathering.'" He said: "I sat with Abu Hurairah and said: 'Indeed I asked Allah to provide me with a righteous gathering. So, narrate a Hadith to me which you heard from Allah's Messenger (peace and blessings be upon him) so that perhaps Allah would cause me to benefit from it.' He said: 'I heard Allah's Messenger (peace and blessings be upon him) say: "Indeed the first deed by which a servant will be called to account on the Day of Resurrection is his Salat. If it is complete, he is successful and saved, but if it is defective, he has failed and lost. So, if something is deficient in his obligatory (prayers) then the Lord, Mighty and Sublime says: 'Look! Are there any voluntary (prayers) for my worshipper?' So, with them, what was deficient in his obligatory (prayers) will be completed. Then the rest of his deeds will be treated like that." (Tirmidhi)

Prayer is Expiation of Sins and Increase in Good Deeds

Abu Hurairah (May Allah be pleased with him) reported that the Messenger of Allah (May Allah's peace and blessings be upon him) said: "Shall I not tell you something by which Allah erases sins and elevates ranks (in Paradise)?" The Companions said: "Certainly, O Messenger of Allah." He said: "Performing the ablution properly even in difficulty, increasing attendance of prayer in the Mosque, and waiting for the next prayer after observing one prayer; and this is Jihad." (Muslim)

Prayer is Light

Narrated Abu Malik Al-Harith bin Asim Al-Ashari (May Allah have mercy on him): The Messenger of Allah (peace and blessings be upon him) said: "Cleanliness is half of Faith. The phrase Al-Hamdulillah ('All praise be to Allah') fills the scale. The phrases Subhanallah ('High is Allah above every imperfection and need; He is pure and perfect') and Al-Hamdulillah ('All praise be to Allah') together fill – or each fill – what is between the heavens and the earth. Prayer is a light. Charity is a proof. Patience is brightness. The Qur'an is either an argument for or against you. And everyone goes in the morning and sells himself, thereby setting himself free or destroying himself." (Muslim)

Two Rak'ahs Before the Dawn (Fajr) Prayer are Better than Whole this World

Narrated Aisha (May Allah be pleased with her): The Prophet (peace and blessings be upon him) said,
"The two Rak'ahs before the dawn (Fajr) prayer are better than this world and all it contains." (Muslim)

In Prostration the Person is the Closest to His Lord

Narrated Abu Hurairah (May Allah be pleased with him): The Messenger of Allah (peace and blessings be upon him) said, "A slave becomes nearest to his Rubb when he is in prostration. So, increase supplications while prostrating." (Muslim)

Narrated 'Ubadah bin Samit: The Messenger of Allah (peace and blessings be upon him) said: "No one prostrates to Allah but Allah will record one Hasanah (good reward) for him, and will erase thereby one bad deed and raise him in status one degree. So, prostrate a great deal." (Ibn Majah)

Praying After Wudu – his sins are forgiven

Humran, the freed slave of 'Uthman, reported that he saw 'Uthman call for water to perform ablution, then he poured the water on his hands from the vessel and washed them three times. Then he put his right hand in the water and rinsed his mouth and his nose. Then he washed his face three times and his arms up to the elbow three times. Then he wiped his head and washed each of his feet three times. Then he said: "I saw the Messenger of Allah (May Allah's peace and blessings be upon him) perform ablution like I have just done." Then he said: "Whoever performs ablution as I have done and then stands and prays two Rak'ahs without letting his thoughts wander, his previous sins will be forgiven." (Bukhari and Muslim) (https://hadeethenc.com/en/browse/hadith/3313)

Angels pray for one so long as he remains in the place where he has performed prayer

Narrated Abu Hurairah (May Allah be pleased with him): The Messenger of Allah (peace and blessings be upon him) said, "The angels supplicate in favor of one of you so long as he remains in the place where he has performed Salat (prayer) in a state of Wudu. They (the angels) say: 'O Allah, forgive him, O Allah, have mercy on him.'" (Bukhari)

Prayer is a Shield Against Satan, Evil Deeds and Bad Temper

Abu Hurairah (May Allah be pleased with him) reported that the Messenger of Allah (May Allah's peace and blessings be upon him) said: "When the son of Adam recites a Verse of prostration and then falls down in prostration, the Devil retreats, weeps and says: 'Woe unto him!" In the narration of Abu Kurayb the words are: "Woe unto me – the son of Adam was commanded to prostrate, and he prostrated, so Paradise is for him. However, I was commanded to prostrate, but I refused to, so the Fire is for me.'" (Muslim)

The Excellence of Morning (Fajr) and Afternoon ('Asr) Prayers

Abu Musa (May Allah be pleased with him) reported: Messenger of Allah (peace and blessings be upon him) said, "He who observes Al-Bardan (i.e. Fajr and 'Asr prayers) will enter Jannah." (Bukhari and Muslim)

Jundub bin Sufyan (May Allah be pleased with him) reported: The Messenger of Allah (peace and blessings be upon him) said, "He who offers the dawn (Fajr) prayers will come under the Protection of Allah. O son of Adam! Beware, lest Allah should call you to account in any respect from (for withdrawing) His Protection." (Muslim)

Abu Hurairah (May Allah be pleased with him) reported: The Messenger of Allah (peace and blessings be upon him) said, "There are angels who take turns in visiting you by night and by day, and they all assemble at the dawn (Fajr) and the afternoon ('Asr) prayers. Those who have spent the night with you, ascend to the heaven and their Rabb, Who knows better about them, asks: 'In what condition did you leave My slaves?' They reply: 'We left them while they were performing Salah and we went to them while they were performing Salat.'" (Bukhari and Muslim)

Commentary: The angels for the night come at the time of 'Asr when the angels for the morning are present. This is how the angels of the two shifts assemble at this time. The angels of the shift of 'Asr leave their duty in the morning, and the angels of the morning shift resume their duty when the pious persons are engaged in Fajr prayer. This is how the two groups assemble again at that time. Thus, when the angels come or go, the people who are punctual in their prayer are engaged in Fajr and 'Asr. Almighty Allah knows everything but even then,

He asks the angels about his pious slaves so that the piousness of the believers and their merit and distinction become evident to them. (104)

Shurouq Prayer 15 minutes after Sunrise Bring the Rewards of Hajj and Umrah

Narrated Anas ibn Malik (May Allah be pleased with him): The Prophet (peace and blessings be upon him) said: "Whoever prays Fajr in congregation, then sits remembering Allah until the sun rises, then prays two Rak'ahs, will have a reward like that of Hajj and 'Umrah, complete, complete, complete." (Tirmidhi)

The Excellence of Fajr and Isha Prayers in the Mosque

Narrated Abu Hurairah (May Allah be pleased with him): The Messenger of Allah (peace and blessings be upon him) said, "He who goes to the Mosque in the morning or in the evening, Allah prepares for him a place an honorable abode for him in Paradise, every time he goes to the Mosque; in the morning or in the evening." (Bukhari and Muslim)

Fajr and Isha Prayers in Congregation Bring the Reward of Praying the Whole Night

Narrated Uthman bin Affan: Allah's Messenger (peace and blessings be upon him) said: "Whoever attends Isha (prayer) in congregation, then he has (the reward as if he had) stood half of the night. And whoever prays Isha and Fajr in congregation, then he has (the reward as if he had) spend the entire night standing (in prayer)." (Tirmidhi)

Fajr and Isha Prayers Safeguard from Hypocrisy
Narrated Abu Hurairah: The Prophet (peace and blessings be upon him) said, "No prayer is harder for the hypocrites than the Fajr and the 'Isha' prayers, and if they knew the reward for these prayers at their respective times, they would certainly present themselves (in the Mosques) even if they had to crawl." The Prophet (peace and blessings be upon him) added, "Certainly, I decided to order the Mu'adh-dhin (Call maker) to pronounce Iqamah and order a man to lead the prayer, and then take a fire flame to burn all those who had not left their houses, so far for the prayer along with their houses." (Bukhari)

Abandoning the Prayer is Disbelief

Narrated Jabir: The Prophet (peace and blessings be upon him) said: "Verily between man and between polytheism and unbelief is the negligence of prayer." (Muslim)
Man means here faith.

No Good Deeds will be Accepted from One who Does Not Pray

Allah, the Exalted, warned:

"...let not your wealth and your children divert you from remembrance of Allah. And whoever does that - then those are the losers." (Qur'an, Al-Munafiqun 63:9)

Prayer is the Best Medicine
Narrated Abu Hurairah: "The Prophet (peace and blessings be upon him) set out in the early morning and I did likewise. I prayed, then I sat. The Prophet (peace and blessings be upon him) turned to me and said: 'Do you have a stomach problem?' I said: 'Yes, O Messenger of Allah.' He said: 'Get up and pray, for in prayer there is Healing.'" (Ibn Majah)

62. Praying Without Intention, Ablution, Mentioning the Name of Allah and Seeking the Refuge with Allah from the Accursed Satan

'Umar bin Al-Khattab (May Allah be pleased with him) reported: The Messenger of Allah (peace and blessings be upon him) said, "The deeds are considered by the intentions, and a person will get the reward according to his intention. So, whoever emigrated for Allah and His Messenger, his emigration will be for Allah and His Messenger; and whoever emigrated for worldly benefits or for a woman to marry, his emigration would be for what he emigrated for." (Bukhari and Muslim)

The intention turns permissible deeds into the acts of worship, if free from showing off. (105)

Abu Hurairah reported that the Messenger of Allah (May Allah's peace and blessings be upon him) said: "The prayer of a person who does not perform ablution is invalid, and the ablution of a person who does not mention the Name of Allah is invalid." (Ibn Majah, Abu Dawud, Ahmad)
(https://hadeethenc.com/en/browse/hadith/8384)

63. Actions by Intentions

Allah, the Exalted, says:

"And when you have completed the prayer, remember Allah standing, sitting or (lying) on your sides. But when you become secure, re-establish (regular) prayer. Indeed, prayer has been decreed upon the believers a decree of specified times." (Qur'an, An-Nisa 4:103)

'Umar ibn al-Khattab (May Allah be pleased with him) reported that the Prophet (May Allah's peace and blessings be upon him) said: "Verily, the reward of deeds depends on the intentions, and each person will be rewarded according to what he intended. So, he whose migration is for the sake of Allah and His Messenger, then his migration is for the sake of Allah and His Messenger, and he whose migration is to achieve some worldly gain or to take some woman in marriage, then his migration is for that for which he migrated." (Bukhari and Muslim) (https://hadeethenc.com/en/browse/hadith/4560)

For righteous actions have two conditions: sincerity and following the Sunnah of the Prophet (peace and blessings be upon him). This Hadith speaks about the first condition of sincerity. The Prophet (peace and blessings be upon him) said: "Everyone will have what they have intended." Some may falsely be led to believe that there is a repetition. The first phrase, as mentioned previously, indicates that only the actions that have intentions are regarded. The second phrase: "Everyone will be rewarded according to their intention", indicates that the intention is the basis for either a reward or punishment. Whatever is for Allah the Exalted and in accordance to the Sunnah, then the person will earn a reward, and whatever is for other than Allah the Exalted, then the person will be punished. The Prophet (peace and blessings be upon him) said: "Whoever's migration was to Allah and His Messenger, then their migration is to Allah and His Messenger. The Prophet repeated "migration is to Allah and His Messenger" to honor it and highlight its importance. But whoever's migration was for some parts of worldly life that they wished to acquire, or for a woman to marry, then their migration was for whatever they migrated for. Neither of these cases are migrants for the sake of Allah. The Prophet (peace and blessings be upon him) said: "Their migration was for whatever they migrated for" and did not repeat the specific aim of the migration as a means of showing its insignificance and lack of importance. While they may attain the worldly matter that they sought, they will not earn reward for their migration.

This Hadith has many lessons and we will just consider a few of them:

- Intentions are conditions for the correctness of actions. Intentions are what distinguish between ordinary actions and acts of worship. Intentions are also the basis for distinguishing between different acts of worship. For example, although Zuhr and Asr are both 4 Rak'aks, it is the intention that distinguishes between them.
- If one does not intend something for the sake of Allah, then they are not rewarded for it even if it is the same outwardly action. For example, a person may perform intermittent fasting from Fajr and Maghreb only intending a physical benefit such as losing weight. Although technically he fasted the same period of time as prescribed for a voluntary fasting, he would not be rewarded for it because he did not intend to fast for the sake of Allah.
- Whoever intends something and takes concrete steps but is not able to do the action due to factors outside their control, then they will still be rewarded for the intention. For example, if someone intended to perform Umrah and took concrete steps such as saving money, buying a ticket and making a reservation but in the end was prevented from going due to a factor outside his control such as a debilitating illness then he will be still rewarded for the intention.
- Based on intentions, ordinary actions can become acts of worship. For example, all humans need to eat, drink and sleep simply to survive. However, if someone has the intention of eating in order to make his body stronger for worship then his eating

in itself becomes an act of worship. The same can be said for other ordinary aspects of life such as working and earning a living. If one intends to seek Allah's Pleasure, then these ordinary actions become actions of worship that one is rewarded for.

Putting this Hadith into Action

We need to put this Hadith into action.

1. Monitor and safeguard our intentions
   - One needs to monitor what drives them to do actions. Is it so that people can say how kind they are? Or how generous they are? Or thoughtful and caring they are? If that is the case, certainly people will praise them and but they will not earn a reward for their actions.
   - Sometimes people advertise their actions without even realizing it. For example, a person may announce that they can't eat on a particular day because they are fasting. Or they may go out of their way to broadcast an act of kindness that they did in response to seeing a needy person.
   - We should be cautious were possible to hide our actions like the pious predecessors who would hide that they were fasting from their own family and friends. When leaving the house, they would give the meal to a poor person along the way. Their family thought that they had breakfast. When they went to the market, their friends there assumed that they already ate at home.
2. We should make a habit of transforming the customary acts into acts of worships
   - For example, when eating and sleeping intend that the primary driver is to get stronger for worship.
   - For example, when earning money – intend to support family and help poor people etc. (106, 107)

Narrated Sad bin Abi Waqqas: Allah's Apostle (peace and blessings be upon him) said, "You will be rewarded for whatever you spend for Allah's sake even if it were a morsel which you put in your wife's mouth." (Bukhari)

Uttering the Intention (Niyyah) in Acts of Worship is a Bid'ah (innovation).

The intention is not spoken out loud. The intention is the will and intent of the heart. It was not narrated that the Messenger of Allah (peace and blessings of Allah be upon him) or his Sahabah did it, or that he commanded anyone among his ummah to utter the intention. Indeed, uttering the intention is a of irrational thinking and falling short in religious commitment. In terms of falling short in religious commitment, that is because it is Bid'ah (innovation). In terms of irrational thinking, that is because it is like a person who wants to eat some food saying, "I intend to put my hand in this vessel, take out a morsel of food, put it in my mouth and chew it, then swallow it, and eat until I have had my fill." This is sheer foolishness and ignorance. (108)

64. Washing Mouth and Nose Separately During Wudu

Narrated 'Abd-Allaah ibn Zayd that he demonstrated for them the Wudu of the Prophet (peace and blessings of Allah be upon him): "He rinsed his mouth and nose using one handful (of water), and he did that three times." (Bukhari and Muslim)

This Hadith indicates that the Sunnah is not to separate the rinsing of the mouth and nose, and to rinse both the mouth and nose from a single handful of water, then rinse the mouth and nose from a single handful, then rinse the mouth and nose from a single mouthful. (109)

65. Prayer Without Recitation of the Surah Al-Fatihah

'Ubadah ibn As-Samit (May Allah be pleased with him) reported that the Prophet (May Allah's peace and blessings be upon him) said: "The prayer of someone who did not recite Surah Al-Fatihah is invalid." (Bukhari and Muslim) (https://hadeethenc.com/en/browse/hadith/5378)

Abu Hurairah (May Allah be pleased with him) reported: The Prophet (May Allah's peace and blessings be upon him) said: "Whoever offers a prayer in which he does not recite Umm al-Qur'an (Surah Al-Fatihah), it is deficient, it is deficient, it is deficient, incomplete." It was said to Abu Hurairah: "O Abu Hurairah, we sometimes pray behind the Imam." He said: "Recite it to yourself, for I heard the Messenger of Allah (May Allah's peace and blessings be upon him) say: 'Allah Almighty said: 'I have divided prayer between Myself and My servant into two halves, and My servant shall have what he has asked for.' When the servant says: 'All praise be to Allah, the Lord of the worlds', Allah Almighty says: 'My servant has praised Me.' And when he says 'The Most Compassionate, the Most Merciful', Allah Almighty says: 'My servant has extolled Me.' And when he says 'Master of the Day of Judgment', Allah Almighty says: 'My servant has glorified Me' - And He also says: 'My servant entrusted his affairs to Me' - And when he says, 'You Alone we worship, and You Alone we ask for help', He says: 'This is between Me and My servant, and My servant shall have what he has asked for.' And when he says 'Guide us to the Straight Path, the path of those whom You have blessed; not of those who incurred Your Wrath, or of those who went astray', He says: 'This is for My servant, and My servant shall have what he has asked for.'" (Muslim) (https://hadeethenc.com/en/browse/hadith/65099)

66. Closing the Eyes while Praying

Allah, the Exalted, says:

"Successful indeed are the believers. Those who offer their Salah (prayers) with all solemnity and full submissiveness." (Qur'an, Al-Mu'minun 23:1-2)

Closing the eyes while praying is not Sunnah. (110, 111)

67. Ruling on Tahiyyat Al-Masjid - Greeting the Mosque

Abu Qatadah as-Salami (May Allah be pleased with him) reported that the Prophet (May Allah's peace and blessings be upon him) said: "When anyone of you enters the Mosque, let him offer two Rak'ahs before he sits down." (Bukhari and Muslim) (https://hadeethenc.com/en/browse/hadith/65091) (112)

68. Omitting Prayer Intentionally

Allah, the Exalted, says:

"...and keep up prayer and be not of the polytheists..." (Qur'an, Ar-Rum 30:31)

69. The Severity of Punishment for Missing the Asr Prayer

Allah, the Exalted, says:

"Guard strictly (five obligatory) As-Salawat (the prayers) especially the middle Salat (i.e. the best prayer – 'Asr)." (Qur'an, Al-Baqarah 2:238)

Buraydah ibn al-Husayb (May Allah be pleased with him) reported that the Messenger of Allah (May Allah's peace and blessings be upon him) said: "If anyone abandons the Asr prayer (deliberately) their deeds will be rendered null and void." (Bukhari) (https://hadeethenc.com/en/browse/hadith/6261)

Narrated Ibn Umar (May Allah be pleased with him): The Prophet (peace and blessings be upon him) said: "Whoever misses the 'Asr prayer (intentionally) then it is as if he lost his family and property." (Bukhari)

Ali ibn Abi Talib (May Allah be pleased with him) reported that the Messenger of Allah (May Allah's peace and blessings be upon him) said: "May Allah fill their graves and houses with fire, as they distracted us from the middle prayer until the sunset." In another narration: "They distracted us from the middle prayer", meaning: the Asr prayer. Then he offered it between the Maghrib and the Isha. Ibn Masud (May Allah be pleased with him) reported: "The polytheists distracted the Messenger of Allah (May Allah's peace and blessings be upon him) from observing the Asr prayer till the sun became red or yellow. So, the Messenger of Allah (May Allah's peace and blessings be upon him) said: "May Allah fill their bellies and graves with fire!" (Muslim) (https://hadeethenc.com/en/browse/hadith/3538)

70. Disapproval of Delaying the Prayer from its Prescribed Time

Allah, the Exalted, says:

"So, woe to those performers of prayers who delay their prayer from their stated fixed times." (Qur'an, Al-Ma'un 107:3-4)

"Verily the prayer is enjoined on the believers at fixed times." (Qur'an, An-Nisa 4:103)
"Guard strictly (five obligatory) As-Salawat (the prayers) especially the middle Salat (i.e. the best prayer 'Asr)." (Qur'an, Al-Baqarah 2:238)

Other Verse: *Maryam 19:59.*

Narrated 'Abdullah: "I asked the Prophet (peace and blessings be upon him) "Which deed is the dearest to Allah?" He (peace and blessings be upon him) replied, "To offer the prayers at their early stated fixed times." I asked, "What is the next (in goodness)?" He replied, "To be good and dutiful to your parents"
I again asked, "What is the next (in goodness)?" He replied, 'To participate in Jihad (religious fighting) in Allah's Cause." 'Abdullah added, "I asked only that much and if I had asked more, the Prophet (peace and blessings be upon him) would have told me more." (Bukhari)

71. Excellence of Congregational Prayers and Warning for Missing it

Allah, the Exalted, says:

"When you (O Messenger Muhammad) are among them and lead them in As-Salah (the prayer), let one party of them stand up [in Salah (prayer)] with you taking their arms with them; when they finish their prostrations, let them take their positions in the rear

and let the other party come up which have not yet prayed, and let them pray with you." (Qur'an, An-Nisa 4:102)

"And perform As-Salah (Iqamat As-Salah) and give Zakat, and bow down (or submit yourselves with obedience to Allah) along with Ar-Raaki'oon (those who bow)." (Qur'an, Al-Baqarah 2:43)

"O Maryam! Submit yourself with obedience to your Lord (Allah, by worshipping none but Him Alone) and prostrate yourself, and bow down along with Ar-Raaki'oon (those who bow down)." (Qur'an, Ali 'Imran 3:43)

Ibn 'Umar (May Allah be pleased with him) reported: The Messenger of Allah (peace and blessings be upon him) said, "Salat in congregation is twenty-seven times more meritorious than a Salat performed individually." (Bukhari and Muslim)

Abu Hurairah (May Allah be pleased with him) reported: The Messenger of Allah (peace and blessings be upon him) said, "A man's Salah in congregation is twenty-five times more rewarding than his Salah at home or in his shop, and that is because when he performs his Wudu' properly and proceeds towards the Mosque with the purpose of performing Salah in congregation, he does not take a step without being raised a degree (in rank) for it and having a sin remitted for it, till he enters the Mosque. When he is performing Salah, the angels continue to invoke blessings of Allah on him as long as he is in his place of worship in a state of Wudu'. They say: 'O Allah! Have mercy on him! O Allah! Forgive him.' He is deemed to be engaged in Salah as long as he waits for it." (Bukhari and Muslim)

Abu Hurairah (May Allah be pleased with him) reported: "A blind man came to the Messenger of Allah (peace and blessings be upon him) and said: "O Messenger of Allah! I have no one to guide me to the Mosque." He, therefore, sought his permission to perform Salah (prayer) in his house. He (peace and blessings be upon him) granted him permission. When the man turned away, he called him back, and said, "Do you hear the Adhan (Call to prayer)?" He replied in the affirmative. The Messenger of Allah (peace and blessings be upon him) then directed him to respond to it." (Muslim)

Abu Hurairah (May Allah be pleased with him) reported: The Messenger of Allah (peace and blessings be upon him) said, "By Him in Whose Hand my life is, I sometimes thought of giving orders for firewood to be collected, then for proclaiming the Adhan for Salah. Then I would appoint an Imam to lead Salah, and then go to the houses of those who do not come to perform Salah in congregation, and set fire to their houses on them." (Bukhari and Muslim)

Ibn Masud (May Allah be pleased with him) reported: "He who likes to meet Allah tomorrow (i.e. on the Day of Requital) as a Muslim, should take care and observe the Salah when the Adhan is announced for them. Allah has expounded to your Prophet (peace and blessings be upon him) the ways of Right Guidance, and these (the prayers) are part of the Right Guidance. If you have to perform Salah in your houses, as this man who stays away (from the Mosque) and performs Salah in his house, you will abandon the Sunnah (practice) of your Prophet (peace and blessings be upon him), and the departure from the Sunnah of your Prophet (peace and blessings be upon him) will lead you astray. I have seen the time when no one stayed behind except a well-known hypocrite. I also saw that a man was brought swaying (on account of weakness) between two men till he was set up in a row (in the Mosque)." (Muslim)

Abud-Darda' (May Allah be pleased with him) reported: "I heard the Messenger of Allah (peace and blessings be upon him) saying, "If three men in a village or in the desert, make no arrangement for Salah in congregation, Satan must have certainly overcome them. So, observe Salah in congregation, for the wolf eats up a solitary sheep that stays far from the flock." (Abu Dawud)

Commentary: This Hadith also stresses the importance of offering Salah in congregation and mentions the disadvantages of offering it individually. One who remains aloof from the congregation, is like the sheep which is separated from its herd and becomes a victim of the wolf. One who lives alone is easily overpowered by satanic doubts. (113)

Narrated Abu Hurairah: The Prophet (peace and blessings be upon him) said, "Martyrs are those who die because of drowning, Plague, an abdominal disease, or of being buried alive by a falling building." And then he added, "If the people knew the reward for the Zuhr prayer in its early time, they would race for it. If they knew the reward for the 'Isha' and the Fajr prayers in congregation, they would join them even if they had to crawl. If they knew the reward for the first row, they would draw lots for it." (Bukhari)

Abd al-Rahman b. Abd 'Amr reported: "Uthman b. 'Affan narrated in the Mosque after evening prayer and sat alone. I also sat alone with him, so he said: '0, son of my brother, I heard the Messenger of Allah (peace and blessings be upon him) say: 'He who observed the 'Isha' prayer in congregation, it was as if he prayed up to midnight, and he who prayed the morning prayer in congregation, it was as if he prayed the whole night.'" (Muslim)

Here is a story of Sheikh Barsisa who prayed 70 years but he is in Hellfire: https://www.youtube.com/watch?v=sOjSzCkp4Xk

72. Du'a After Iqamah

Narrated Anas ibn Malik (May Allah be pleased with him): The Prophet (peace and blessings be upon him) said: "Straighten your rows as the straightening of rows is essential for a perfect and correct prayer." (Bukhari and Muslim)

After Iqamah, the imam addresses to the worshipers to straighten the rows and stand close together.

Raising hands and make Du'a after Iqamah and before the Imam says "Allahu Akbar" is not a Sunnah.

73. Obligation to Straighten the Rows

An-Nu'man bin Bashir (May Allah be pleased with him) reported: "I heard the Messenger of Allah (peace and blessings be upon him) saying, "Straighten your rows; otherwise, Allah will create dissension among you." (Bukhari and Muslim)

An-Nu'man bin Bashir (May Allah be pleased with him) said: "The Messenger of Allah (peace and blessings be upon him) directed us to keep our rows as straight as arrows. He continued stressing this until he realized that we had learnt it from him (recognized its significance). One day he came into the Mosque and stood up. He was just about to say Takbir (Allah is Greater) when he noticed a man whose chest was projected from the row, so he said, "O slaves of Allah, you must straighten your rows or Allah will certainly put your faces in opposite directions." (Muslim)

Al-Bara' bin 'Azib (May Allah be pleased with him) reported: "The Messenger of Allah (peace and blessings be upon him) used to pass between the rows from one end to the other, touching our chest and shoulders (i.e. arranging the rows) in line and saying, "Do not be out of line; otherwise your hearts will be in disagreement." He would add, "Allah and His angels invoke blessings upon the first rows." (Abu Dawud)

Ibn 'Umar (May Allah be pleased with him) reported: The Messenger of Allah (peace and blessings be upon him) said, "Arrange the rows in order, stand shoulder to shoulder, close the gaps, be accommodating to your brothers, and do not leave gaps for Satan. Whoever joins up a row, he will be joined to Allah (i.e. to the Mercy of Allah); and whoever cuts off a row, he will be cut off from Allah (i.e. from His Mercy)." (Abu Dawud)

Anas (May Allah be pleased with him) reported: The Messenger of Allah (peace and blessings be upon him) said, "Stand close together in your rows, keep nearer to one another, and put your necks in line, for by Him in Whose Hands my soul is, I see the Satan entering through the opening in the row like Al-hadhaf (i.e. a type of small black sheep found in Yemen)." (Abu Dawud)

Anas (May Allah be pleased with him) reported: The Messenger of Allah (peace and blessings be upon him) said, "Fill (complete) the first row, then the one next to it; and if there is any deficiency (incompleteness), it should be in the last row." (Abu Dawud)

Al-Bara' (May Allah be pleased with him) reported: "Whenever we performed Salah behind the Messenger of Allah (peace and blessings be upon him), we liked to be on his right side so that his face might turn towards us (at the end of the Salah). One day, I heard Messenger of Allah (peace and blessings be upon him) supplicating, "O my Rubb! Shield me from Your Torment on the Day when You will gather (or said, 'resurrect') Your slaves." (Muslim)

Commentary: This Hadith describes the merit of standing on the right side of the Imam and tells us that for the Imam it is Sunnah of the Prophet (peace and blessings be upon him) to sit after the congregational Salah with his face towards his followers. (114)

Narrated An-Nu'man bin 'Bashir: The Prophet (peace and blessings be upon him) said, "Straighten your rows or Allah will alter your faces." (Bukhari)

Narrated Anas bin Malik: The Prophet (peace and blessings be upon him) said, "Straighten your rows for I see you from behind my back." Anas added, "Every one of us used to put his shoulder with the shoulder of his companion and his foot with the foot of his companion." (Bukhari)

Narrated Abu Masud (May Allah be pleased with him): The Messenger of Allah (peace and blessings be upon him) used to touch our shoulders when we were praying and he would say: "Make the rows straight and do not differ, lest your hearts differ." (Muslim)

74. Undesirability of Observing Nafl Prayer when the Mu'adhdhin Begins Iqamah

Abu Hurairah reported the Apostle of Allah (peace and blessings be upon him) as saying: "When the prayer commences then there is no prayer (valid), but the obligatory prayer." (Muslim)

Abdullah b. Malik b. Buhaina reported: The Messenger of Allah (peace and blessings be upon him) happened to pass by a person who was busy in praying while the (Fard of the) dawn prayer had commenced. He said something to him, which we do not know what it was. When we turned back, we surrounded him and said: "What is it that the Messenger of Allah (peace be upon him) said to you?" He replied: "He (the Holy Prophet) had said to me that he perceived as if one of them was about to observe four (Rak'ahs) of the dawn prayer." (Muslim)

Ibn Buhaina reported: The dawn prayer had commenced when the Messenger of Allah (peace and blessings be upon him) saw a person observing prayer, whereas the Mu'adhdhin had pronounced the Iqamah. Upon this he (the Holy Prophet) remarked: "Do you say four (Rak'ahs) of Fard in the dawn prayer?" (Muslim)

'Abdullah b. Sarjis reported: "A person entered the Mosque, while the Messenger of Allah (peace be upon him) was leading the dawn prayer. He observed two Rak'ahs in a corner of the Mosque, and then joined the Messenger of Allah (peace and blessings be upon him) in prayer. When the Messenger of Allah (peace be upon him) had pronounced salutations (he had concluded the prayer), he said: "O, so and so, which one out of these two prayers did you count (as your Fard prayer), the one that you observed alone or the prayer that you observed with us?" (Muslim)

75. Regular Recitation of the Qunut During the Fajr Prayer

Abu Malik al-Ashjaʻi Saʻd ibn Tariq (May Allah be pleased with him) reported: "I said to my father: "O father, you prayed behind the Messenger of Allah (May Allah's peace and blessings be upon him), Abu Bakr, ʻUmar, ʻUthmān and ʻAli here in Kufah for about five years. Did they use to recite the Qunut in the Fajr prayer?" He said: "O son, this is an innovation in religion." (Ibn Majah, Tirmidhi and Ahmad) (https://hadeethenc.com/en/browse/hadith/10935)

76. Missing the Friday Prayer Without Valid Excuse

Allah, the Exalted, says:

"O you who believe (Muslims)! When the call is proclaimed for the Salat (prayer) on the day of Friday (Jumu'ah prayer), come to the remembrance of Allah [Jumu'ah religious talk (Khutbah) and Salat (prayer)] and leave off business (and every other thing), that is better for you if you did but know!" (Qur'an, Al-Jumu'ah 62:9)

"Then when the (Jumu'ah) Salat (prayer) is finished, you may disperse through the land and seek the Bounty of Allah (by working, etc.), and remember Allah much, that you may be successful. And when they see some merchandise or some amusement [beating of Tambur (drum), etc.] they disperse headlong to it, and leave you (Muhammad SAW) standing [while delivering Jumu'ah's religious talk (Khutbah)]. Say "That which Allah has is better than any amusement or merchandise! And Allah is the Best of providers." (Qur'an, Al-Jumu'ah 62:10-11)

Why Friday is called Jumu'ah?

Many reasons have been given by the scholars about calling Friday as Jumu'ah. Some are as follows:

1. The word Jumu'ah is derived from al-Jam', literally 'to gather' or 'gathering'. Since the Muslims gather on this day in the grand Mosques, it is called as Jumu'ah.

2. It was during Friday when Allah finished the creation, the sixth day, during which Allah created the heavens and the earth. In other words, the whole creation was gathered on this day and therefore it was named Jumu'ah.
3. Adam (May peace be upon him) was created on this day i.e. he was assembled and therefore it is called Jumu'ah. (115)

A. EXCELLENCE OF FRIDAY

1. Friday is the Best Day of the Year

Narrated Abu Hurairah: The Apostle of Allah (peace and blessings be upon him) said: "The best day on which the sun has risen is Friday; on it Adam was created, on it he was made to enter Paradise, on it he was expelled from it. And the last Hour will take place on no day other than Friday." (Muslim)

Narrated Aws ibn Aws: The Prophet (peace and blessings of Allah be upon him) said: "Among the most excellent of your days is Friday; on it Adam was created, on it he died, on it the last trumpet will be blown, and on it the shout will be made, so invoke more blessings on me that day, for your blessings will be submitted to me." The people asked: 'Messenger of Allah, how can it be that our blessings will be submitted to you while your body is decayed?' He replied: 'Allah, the Exalted, has prohibited the earth from consuming the bodies of Prophets.'" (Abu Dawud)

Narrated Abu Hurairah: "I heard Allah's Apostle (peace and blessings be upon him) saying, 'We (Muslims) are the last (to come) but (will be) the foremost on the Day of Resurrection though the former nations were given the Holy Scriptures before us. And this was their day (Friday) the celebration of which was made compulsory for them but they differed about it. So, Allah gave us the Guidance for it (Friday) and all the other people are behind us in this respect: the Jews' (holy day is) tomorrow (i.e. Saturday) and the Christians' (is) the day after tomorrow (i.e. Sunday).'" (Bukhari)

2. The Best Friday, on the Day of Arafat, Allah Has Chosen Islam for Humanity

Narrated Tariq bin Shihaab: "A Jew said to 'Umar, 'O Chief of the Believers, if this Verse: *'This day, I have perfected your religion for you, completed My Favor upon you, and have chosen for you Islam as your religion.' (Qur'an, Al-Ma'idah 5:3)* had been revealed upon us, we would have taken that day as an 'Eid (festival) day." 'Umar said, "I know definitely on what day this Verse was revealed; it was revealed on the Day of 'Arafah, on a Friday." (Bukhari)

3. Friday is the Witnessing Day and Arafah's Day is the Witnessed Day

Allah, the Exalted, says:

"And by the witnessing day (i.e. Friday), and by the witnessed day [i.e. the day of 'Arafat (Hajj) the ninth of Dhul-Hijjah]" *(Qur'an, Al-Buruj 85:3)*

"And (remember) when your Lord brought forth from the Children of Adam, from their loins, their seed (or from Adam's loin his offspring) and made them testify as to themselves (saying): "Am I not your Lord?" They said: "Yes! We testify," lest you should say on the Day of Resurrection: "Verily, we have been unaware of this." (Qur'an, Al-A'raf 7:172)

Narrated Abu Hurairah (May Allah be pleased with him): The Messenger of Allah (peace and blessings be upon him) said: "Al-Yawmul-Maw'ud (the Promised Day) is the Day of Resurrection, and Al-Yawmul-Mashhud (the Attended Day) is the Day of Arafah, and Ash-Shahid (the witness) is Friday." He said: "The sun does not rise nor set, upon a day that is more virtuous than it. In it, there is an hour in which no believing worshiper makes a supplication to Allah for good, except that Allah answers it for him, and he does not seek Allah's aid for something, except that He aids him in it." (Tirmidhi)

Dr Zaik Nakir explains the seven Virtues of the Day of Arafah. (116)

4. On the Day of 'Arafah, Allah Release the People Abundantly from Fire

Narrated Jabir (May Allah be pleased with him): Allah's Messenger (peace and blessings be upon him) said: "No other days are better to Allah than the first ten days of Hajj Month. The narrator said: "A man asked: "0 Allah's Messenger! Are these days better or the similar number of days of fighting in the Cause of Allah?" The Prophet (peace and blessings be upon him) said: "These days are better than the same number of days of fighting for the sake of Allah. And no other day is better to Allah than the day of Arafah when Allah, the Exalted, descends to the lowest heaven (world's sky) and boasts of the people on earth to the inhabitants of heaven (angels) and says: "Look at My slaves who have corne with grown hair covered with dust to perform Hajj. They have come from all directions hoping for My Mercy though they haven't seen My Punishment. So, there is no other day than the Day of 'Arafah when the people are released abundantly from Fire." (Ibn Hibban)

5. Friday Is Greater than the Days of 'Eid

Narrated Abu Lubaabah ibn 'Abd al-Mundhir: The Prophet (peace and blessings of Allah be upon him) said: "Friday is the Master of days, and the greatest of them before Allah. It is greater before Allah than the day of Al-Adha and the day of Al-Fitr. It has five characteristics: on this day Allah created Adam, on it He sent Adam down to the earth, on it Allah caused Adam to die, on it there is a time when a person does not ask Allah for anything but He gives it to him, so long as he does not ask for anything haram, and on it the Hour will begin. There is no angel who is close to Allah, no heaven, no earth, no wind, no mountain and no sea that does not fear Friday." (Ibn Majah)

6. Friday is a Celebration

Ibn Abbas reported: The Messenger of Allah (peace and blessings be upon him) said, "Verily, Allah has made this day of Friday a celebration for the Muslims. Whoever comes to Friday prayer, let him bathe himself, apply perfume if he has it, and use the tooth stick." (Ibn Majah)

7. Friday Recitation of the Surah Al-Kahf

Narrated Abu Sa'id al-Khudri (May Allah be pleased with him): The Prophet (peace and blessings be upon him) said, "Whoever reads Surah Al-Kahf on the day of Jumu'ah, will have a light that will shine from him from one Friday to the next." (al-Hakim and al-Bayhaqi)

Narrated Abu Sa'id al-Khudri (May Allah be pleased with him): The Prophet (peace be upon him) said:
"Whoever reads Surah Al-Kahf on the night of Jumu'ah, will have a light that will stretch between him and the Ancient House (the Ka'bah)." (al-Darimi)

Abu Darda reported: The Prophet (peace and blessings be upon him) said, "One who memorized the first ten Verses of Surah Al-Kahf will be secure against the Dajjal (Anti-Christ)." (Muslim)

8. Sending a lot of Blessings upon the Prophet (peace be upon him)

Allah, the Exalted, says:

"Allah sends His Salat (Graces, Honors, Blessings, Mercy, etc.) on the Prophet (Muhammad SAW) and also His angels too (ask Allah to bless and forgive him). O you who believe! Send your Salat on (ask Allah to bless) him (Muhammad SAW), and (you should) greet (salute) him with the Islamic way of greeting (salutation i.e. As-Salamu 'Alaikum)." (Qur'an, Al-Ahzab 33:56)

Aws bin Aws (May Allah be pleased with him) reported: The Messenger of Allah (peace and blessings of Allah be upon him) said, "Among the best of your days is Friday. On that day pray to Allah to exalt my mention frequently, for your such supplications are presented to me." (Abu Dawud)

Commentary: This Hadith brings forth the following three points:
1. The auspiciousness of time further enhances the merits of virtuous deeds, as is evident from the stress on reciting more and more salutations on the Prophet (peace be upon him) on Friday.
2. On Jumu'ah, salutation is presented to the Prophet (peace and blessings of Allah be upon him). This statement goes to prove that he does not hear salutation of anyone directly, either from near or from far. There is a famous Hadith which says that he hears it from near but this is not "Saheeh" technically. Therefore, the truth of the matter is that he does not hear it directly. It is the angels who convey it to him.
3. The most well-worded is "Ibrahimi salutation" because the Prophet (peace and blessings be upon him) himself taught it to his Companions. The salutation is: Allahumma salli

'ala Muhammadin wa 'ala ali Muhammadin, kama sallaita 'ala Ibrahima, wa 'ala ali Ibrahima, innaka Hamidun Majeed. Allahumma barik 'ala Muhammadin wa 'ala ali Muhammadin, kama barakta 'ala Ibrahima, wa 'ala ali Ibrahima, innaka Hamidun Majeed. (117)

Another salutation is "Allaahumma salli 'ala Muhammadin wa 'ala azwaajihi wa dhurriyyatihi kama salayta 'ala Ibraaheem, wa baarik 'ala Muhammadin wa 'ala azwaajihi wa dhurriyyatihi kama baarakta 'ala aali Ibraaheem, innaka hameedun majeed." (O Allah, send Your salah (Grace, Honor and Mercy) upon Muhammad and upon his wives and offspring, as You sent Your salah upon Ibrahim, and send Your blessings upon Muhammad and upon his wives and offspring, as You sent Your blessings upon the family of Ibrahim. You are indeed Praiseworthy, Most Glorious.) (Bukhari and Muslim)

The Virtue of Sending a Great Deal of Blessings Upon the Prophet

Allah, the Exalted, says:

"Allah sends His Salat (Graces, Honors, Blessings, Mercy, etc.) on the Prophet (Muhammad SAW) and also His angels too (ask Allah to bless and forgive him). O you who believe! Send your Salat on (ask Allah to bless) him (Muhammad SAW), and (you should) greet (salute) him with the Islamic way of greeting (salutation i.e. As-Salamu 'Alaikum)." (Qur'an, Al-Ahzab 33:56)

'Amr bin Malik Al-Janbi narrated that he heard Fadalah bin 'Ubaid saying: "The Prophet (peace and blessings be upon him) heard a man supplicating in his Salat but he did not send Salat upon the Prophet (peace and blessings be upon him), so the Prophet (peace and blessings be upon him) said: 'This one has rushed.' Then he called him and said to him, or to someone other than him: 'When one of you performs Salat, then let him begin by expressing gratitude to Allah and praising Him. Then, let him send Salat upon the Prophet (peace be upon him), then let him supplicate after that, whatever he wishes.'" (Tirmidhi)

Ali (May Allah be pleased with him) reported: The Messenger of Allah (peace and blessings be upon him) said, "The miser is the one in whose presence I am mentioned but he does not supplicate for me." (Tirmidhi)

Narrated Anas ibn Malik (May Allah be pleased with him): The Prophet (peace and blessings be upon him) said: "Whoever sends blessings upon me once, Allah will send blessings upon him tenfold and ten bad deeds of his will be erased, and he will be raised ten degrees in status." (An-Nasa'i)

Abu Hurairah (May Allah be pleased with him) reported: The Messenger of Allah (peace and blessings be upon him) said: "He who blesses me once, Allah would bless him ten times." (Muslim)

Jabir (May Allah be pleased with him) reported that the Prophet (May Allah's peace and blessings be upon him) said: "Whoever says on hearing the call to prayer: 'O Allah, Lord of this perfect call and the prayer that is to be offered, grant Muhammad the Wasilah (the highest position of Paradise) and the Fadilah (the degree of superiority), and resurrect him to the praiseworthy station that You have promised him,' He will definitely be granted my intercession on the Day of Judgment." (Bukhari) (https://hadeethenc.com/en/browse/hadith/10635)

Ibn Masud reported: The Messenger of Allah (peace and blessings be upon him) said: "The closest of the people to me on the Day of Resurrection are those who most often invoked blessings upon me." (Tirmidhi)

Narrated Ubayy ibn Ka'b (May Allah be pleased with him): "I said: "O Messenger of Allah, I send a great deal of blessings upon you; how much of my Du'as should be sending blessings upon you?" He said: "Whatever you wish." I said: "One quarter?" He said: "Whatever you wish, and if you do more, that will be better for you." I said: "One half?" He said: "Whatever you wish and if you do more, that will be better for you." I said: "Two thirds? He said: "Whatever you wish and if you do more, that will be better for you." I said: "I will make all of my Du'as for you." He said: "Then your concerns will be taken care of and your sins will be forgiven." (Tirmidhi, al-Mundhiri, al-Haafiz) (118)

9. Friday Hour is the Best Hour of the Year

Narrated Abu Hurairah (May Allah be pleased with him): The Messenger of Allah (peace and blessings be upon him) mentioned Friday and said: "On this day there is an hour when no Muslim slave stands and prays, and asks Allah for something, but Allah will give it to him," and he gestured with his hand to indicate that whatever he asks for, is as nothing to Allah." (Bukhari)

Abu Hurairah (May Allah be pleased with him) reported: The Messenger of Allah (peace and blessings be upon him) said while talking about the merits of Friday, "There is a time on Friday at which a Muslim, while he (or she) is performing Salat and is supplicating, will be granted whatever he (or she) is supplicating for." And he (peace be upon him) pointed with his hand to indicate that this period of time is very short." (Bukhari and Muslim)

Commentary: This Hadith mentions another distinction of Jumu'ah, namely a moment in which every prayer that a person then makes is granted with the condition that what one is asking for is good and lawful. It is a very short moment and its time has also not been revealed. For this reason, one should remember Allah frequently and prayed to Him on Jumu'ah, so that one attains that moment when prayers are answered. Prayers can also be answered outside Salat if one happens to be supplicating at the specified moment. (117)

Narrated Jabir ibn 'Abd-Allah: The Messenger of Allah (peace and blessings of Allah be upon him) said: "Friday is twelve hours in which there is no Muslim who asks Allah for something but He will give it to him, so seek the last hour after 'Asr." (Abu Dawud and An-Nasa'i)

10. Blessings of Sadaqah on a Friday

With all the amazing virtues of Friday, it is no wonder that the act of making Sadaqah on Master day is just as blessed.

11. Do Not Single out Friday for Qiyam Al-Layl Prayer and for Fasting

Abu Hurairah (May Allah be pleased with him) said: "I heard the Prophet (peace and blessings of Allah be upon him) say, 'None of you should fast on a Friday unless he fasts the day before or the day after.'" (Bukhari and Muslim)

12. The Hour of Qiyamah (Judgment Day) will Be on a Friday

Allah, the Exalted, says:

"I swear by the Day of Resurrection." (Qur'an, Al-Qiyamah 75:1)

Narrated Abu Hurairah: The Prophet (peace and blessings be upon him) said: "The best day on which the sun has risen is Friday; on it Adam was created. on it he was made to enter Paradise, on it he was expelled from it. And the last Hour will take place on no day other than Friday." (Muslim)

13. The People of Paradise will Have a Gathering with their Lord Every Friday

Allah, the Exalted, says:
"Some faces that Day shall be Nadirah (shining and radiant). Looking at their Lord (Allah)." (Qur'an, Al-Qiyamah 75:22-23)

Anas ibn Malik said: The Messenger of Allah (peace and blessings of Allah be upon him) said: "Jibreel came to me with something like a white mirror in his hand, on which there was a black spot. I said: 'What is this, O Jibreel?' He said: 'This is Jumu'ah (Friday); it is the Master of days and we call it Yawm al-Mazeed (the day of more – cf.) *"There they will have all that they desire, and We have more (for them, i.e. a glance at the All-Mighty, All-Majestic)."* (Qaf 50:35) I said: 'O Jibreel, what does "more" mean?' He said: 'That is because your Lord has allocated a valley in Paradise that is more fragrant than white musk. When Friday comes, among the days in the Hereafter, the Lord, may He be Blessed and Exalted, will descend from His Throne ('Arsh) to His Kursi, and the Kursi will be surrounded with seats of light on which the Prophets will sit. These seats will be surrounded with footstools of gold on which the martyrs will sit. The people of the chambers will come down from the chambers and sit on sand hills of musk, and those who sit on the sand hills will not think that those who sit on the footstools and seats are any better off than them. Then the Owner of Majesty and Honor will appear and say: 'Ask of Me.' They will say: 'We ask for Your good Pleasure, O Lord.' He will say: 'It is because I am pleased with you that you are in My Paradise, and you are honored.' Then He will say (again): 'Ask of Me.' They will say all together: 'We ask for Your good Pleasure.' He will ask them to testify that He is pleased with them. Then He will say (once more): 'Ask of Me,' and they will ask of Him until each one of them is finished. Then He will grant them that which no eye has seen, no ear has heard, and it has not crossed the mind of any human."

It was also narrated by Ibn Abi'd-Dunya in Sifat al-Jannah (88) via another isnaad; he added: "… there is nothing that they are more eager for than Friday; the more they gaze more upon their Lord, the more they will increase in honor." (Tabarani in al-Mu'jam al-Kabeer (6717) Al-Mundhiri (May Allah have mercy on him) said: "It was narrated by Ibn Abi'd-Dunya and by at-Tabarani in al-Awsat with two isnaads, one of which is jayyid qawiy. A shorter version was also narrated by Abu Ya'la; the men of its isnaad are the men of as-Saheeh. And it was also narrated by al-Bazzaar. End quote" (at-Targheeb wa't-Tarheeb, 4/311; classed as Hasan by al-Albaani in Saheeh at-Targheeb, 3761)

Narrated Anas ibn Malik: The Messenger of Allah (peace and blessings of Allah be upon him) said: "In Paradise there is a market to which they will come every Friday. Then the north wind will blow and will blow on their faces and garments, and increase them in beauty. Then they will return to their families having increased in beauty and their families will say to them: "By Allah, you have increased in beauty", and they will say: "By Allah, you too have increased in beauty." (Muslim)

14. Whoever Dies on Friday Is Protected from the Trial of the Grave

Narrated 'Abd-Allaah ibn 'Amr (May Allah be pleased with him): The Messenger of Allah (peace and blessings be upon him) said: "Whoever passes away on a Friday, will be saved from the punishment of the grave." (Ahmad)

B. FRIDAY PRAYER IS THE BEST OF PRAYERS

I. Friday Fajr Prayer in Congregation

Narrated Abu Hurairah (May Allah be pleased with him): "The Prophet (peace and blessings be upon him) used to recite the following in the Fajr prayer of Friday, "Alif, Lam, Mim, Tanzil…" (Surah As- Sajdah, 32) and "Hal-ata-ala-l-Insani…" (i.e. Surah Ad-Dahr, 76) (Bukhari)

II. Friday (Jumu'ah) Prayer

1. Ghusl for Jumu'ah Prayer

Narrated 'Abdullah bin 'Umar: "I heard Allah's Messenger (peace and blessings of Allah be upon him) saying, "Anyone of you coming for the Jumu'ah prayer should take a bath." (Bukhari)

Narrated Abu Sa'id Al-Khudri: Allah's Messenger (peace and blessings be upon him) said, "The taking of a bath on Friday is compulsory for every Muslim who has attained the age of puberty." (Bukhari)

2. Putting on One's Best Cloth, Using Perfume and Miswak on Friday

Narrated Abu Said: "I testify that Allah's Apostle (peace and blessings be upon him) said, "The taking of a bath on Friday is compulsory for every male Muslim who has attained the age of puberty and (also) the cleaning of his teeth with Siwak, and the using of perfume if it is available." Amr (a sub-narrator) said, "I confirm that the taking of a bath is compulsory, but as for the Siwak and the using of perfume, Allah knows better whether it is obligatory or not, but according to the Hadith it is as above." (Bukhari)

Narrated Salma Al-Farsi: The Prophet (peace and blessings be upon him) said, "Whoever takes a bath on Friday, purifies himself as much as he can, then uses his (hair) oil or perfumes himself with the scent of his house, then proceeds (for the Jumu'ah prayer) and does not separate two persons sitting together (in the Mosque), then prays as much as (Allah has) written for him and then remains silent while the Imam is delivering the Khutbah, his sins in-between the present and the last Friday would be forgiven." (Bukhari)

A woman is not to wear perfume in public which can attract the attention of men.

3. Excellence of Going out Early and Walking to Jumu'ah Prayer in the Mosque

Abu Hurairah (May Allah have mercy on him) reported: The Prophet (peace and blessings be upon him) said: "When one performs Wudu at home thoroughly and leaves for the Masjid solely to offer salah (in congregation), for every step taken towards the Masjid (in this state of Wudu), one stage is elevated in the Hereafter and one sin is forgiven." (Bukhari and Muslim) (https://hadithanswers.com/the-virtue-of-walking-to-the-masjid-for-salah)

4. Prohibition of Buying and Selling Once Jumu'ah Adhan is Proclaimed

Allah, the Exalted, says:

"O you who believe (Muslims)! When the call is proclaimed for the Salah (prayer) on Friday (Jumu'ah prayer), come to the remembrance of Allah [Jumu'ah religious talk (Khutbah) and Salah (prayer)] and leave off business (and every other thing). That is better for you if you did but know!" (Qur'an, Al-Jumu'ah 62:9)

5. On Friday the Angels at Every Gate of the Mosque Write the Names of the Worshippers Chronologically (the time of arrival)

Narrated Abu Hurairah: The Prophet (peace and blessings be upon him) said, "On every Friday the angels take their stand at every gate of the Mosques to write the names of the people chronologically (i.e. according to the time of their arrival for the Friday prayer) and when the Imam sits (on the pulpit) they fold up their scrolls and get ready to listen to the sermon." (Bukhari)

Narrated Abu Hurairah (May Allah be pleased with him): The Prophet (peace and blessings be upon him) said, "Any person who takes a bath on Friday like the bath of Janabah and then goes for the prayer (in the first hour, i.e. early), it is as if he had sacrificed a camel (in Allah's

Cause); and whoever goes in the second hour it is as if he had sacrificed a cow; and whoever goes in the third hour, then it is as if he had sacrificed a horned ram; and if one goes in the fourth hour, then it is as if he had sacrificed a hen; and whoever goes in the fifth hour then it is as if he had offered an egg. When the Imam comes out (i.e. starts delivering the Khutbah), the angels present themselves to listen to the Khutbah." (Bukhari)

Commentary: This Hadith mentions the merits of going early for Salah Al-Jumu'ah and narrates inducements provided for it. The earlier a person goes for it, the greater his reward will be. In fact, the reward for it goes on diminishing in proportion to the delay that he makes in reaching the Mosque for this purpose so much so that he who reaches the Masjid after the Khutbah, will be totally deprived of the benefits which go with it because his name does not figure in the register which shows men of merits. (117)

6. Reward of One Year's Fasting and Praying Qiyam for Jumu'ah Prayer in the Mosque

Narrated Aws ibn Aws (May Allah be pleased with him): The Prophet (peace and blessings be upon him) said: "Whoever does Ghusl on Friday and causes (his wife) to do Ghusl, and sets out early, and comes close to the imam and listens and keeps quiet, for every step he takes he will have the reward of fasting and praying Qiyam for one year." (Tirmidhi)

7. Sit Close to the Imam - Two Shares of Reward

Ali ibn Abi Talib delivered a Khutbah in Kufah and said in his Khutbah: "If a man sits in a place where he can hear and see (the imam) and listens attentively, and does not engage in idle speech or fidgeting, he will have two shares of reward. If he stays far away and sits in a place where he cannot hear but he listens attentively and does not engage in idle speech or fidgeting, he will have one share of reward. If he sits in a place where he can hear and see but he engages in idle speech or fidgets, and does not listen attentively, then he will have one share of sin." And at the end of that he said: "I heard the Messenger of Allah (peace and blessings of Allah be upon him) say that." (Abu Dawud)

8. Prohibition of Separating Two People Sitting Together in the Mosque

Narrated Salma Al-Farsi: The Prophet (peace and blessings of Allah be upon him) said, "Whoever takes a bath on Friday, purifies himself as much as he can, then uses his (hair) oil or perfumes himself with the scent of his house, then proceeds (for the Jumu'ah prayer) and does not separate two persons sitting together (in the Mosque), then prays as much as (Allah has) written for him and then remains silent while the Imam is delivering the Khutbah, his sins in-between the present and the last Friday would be forgiven." (Bukhari)

9. Keep Silent and Listen Attentively the Khutbah

Abu Hurairah (May Allah be pleased with him) reported: Messenger of Allah (peace and blessings be upon him) said, "He who performs his Ghusl perfectly and comes to Jumu'ah prayer and listens (to the Khutbah) silently, the sins which he has committed since the previous Friday plus three more days (i.e. 10 days) will be forgiven for him. One who distracts himself with pebbles during the Khutbah will not get the (Jumu'ah) reward." (Muslim)

Narrated Abu Hurairah: The Messenger of Allah (peace and blessings be upon him) said: "If you say to your companion, 'Listen attentively on a Friday, when the imam is delivering the khutbah, then you have engaged in idle speech." (Bukhari and Muslim)

10. Speaking or Playing with Anything like Pebbles, Phone During the Khutbah

Narrated Abu'l-Darda' (May Allah be pleased with him) said: The Prophet (peace and blessings of Allah be upon him) sat on the minbar and addressed the people, and he recited a Verse. Ubayy ibn Ka'b was next to me, so I said to him: "O Ubayy, when was this Verse revealed?" But he refused to speak to me, so I asked him again and he refused to speak to me, until the Prophet (peace and blessings of Allah be upon him) came down (from the minbar). Then Ubayy said to me: "You have gained nothing from your Jumu'ah except idle talk." When the Messenger of Allah (peace and blessings be upon him) had finished (the prayer), I went to him and told him (what had happened). He said: "Ubayy was right. When you hear your imam speaking, then keep quiet and listen attentively until he has finished." (Ahmad and Ibn Majah)

Abu Hurairah (May Allah be pleased with him) reported: The Messenger of Allah (peace and blessings be upon him) said, "If anyone performs Ghusl properly, then comes to the Friday prayer, listens to the Khutbah (religious talk) attentively and keeps silent, his (Minor) sins between that Friday and the following Friday will be forgiven, with the addition of three more days; but he who touches pebbles* has caused an interruption." (Muslim)

Abu Hurairah (May Allah be pleased with him) reported that the Prophet (May Allah's peace and blessings be upon him) said: "He who performs ablution properly, then comes to the Friday prayer and listens to it attentively and keeps silent, his sins between that Friday and the following Friday will be forgiven, with the addition of three more days; but he who touches a pebble has engaged in idle activity." (Muslim) (https://hadeethenc.com/en/browse/hadith/5433)

*Speaking or touching anything (the Qur'an, pebbles, mobile, devices to count, etc.) during Khutbah will cancel the Jumu'ah reward.

Exception

A Non-Arab Muslim can read the translation of Khutbah in his language on phone during the Khutbah.

Sheikh 'Abd ar-Rahmaan al-Barraak (May Allah preserve him) said:

"There is nothing wrong with that, and this does not come under the heading of fidgeting that is prohibited, because it is done for a need, and not by way of missing about. End quote." (119)

11. Jumu'ah Qur'an Verses

Narrated Ubaidullah bin Abdullah: "Dahhak bin Qais wrote to Nu'man bin Bashir, saying: 'Tell us what the Messenger of Allah (peace and blessings of Allah be upon him) used to recite on Friday along with Surah Al-Jumu'ah.' He said: 'He used to recite: *"Has there come to you the narration of the overwhelming (i.e. the Day of Resurrection)?"' (Al-Ghashiyah 88)* (Ibn Majah)

It is a Sunnah to recite in the Jumu'ah Prayer Surahs Al-A`la, Al-Ghashiyah, Al-Jumu`ah and Al-Munafiqun, or Surah Al-Insan which starts by: *"Has there not been over man a period of time"* after reciting Surah Al-Fatihah.

12. Expiation of Sins from the Present and the Last Friday

Narrated Salman-Al-Farsi (May Allah be pleased with him): The Prophet (peace and blessings of Allah be upon him) said, "Whoever takes a bath on Friday, purifies himself as much as he can, then uses his (hair) oil or perfumes himself with the scent of his house, then proceeds (for the Jumu'ah prayer) and does not separate two persons sitting together (in the Mosque), then prays as much as (Allah has) written for him and then remains silent while the Imam is delivering the Khutbah, his sins in-between the present and the last Friday would be forgiven." (Bukhari)

Narrated Abu Hurairah (May Allah be pleased with him): The Prophet (peace and blessings be upon him) said, "He who took a bath and then came for Jumu'ah prayer and then prayed what was fixed for him, then kept silence till the Imam finished the sermon, and then prayed along with him, his sins between that time and the next Friday would be forgiven, and even of three days more." (Muslim)

Narrated Abu Hurairah (May Allah be pleased with him): The Prophet (peace and blessings be upon him) said: "The five (daily) prayers, and Friday prayer to the next Friday prayer, and Ramadan to the next Ramadan, are expiation of sins committed in between them, so long as Major sins are avoided." (Muslim)

Commentary: This Hadith makes it clear that the good actions mentioned in it are means of forgiveness of sins but only if one saves oneself from Major sins. Thus, it is abundantly clear that the sins which are pardoned through these good actions are Minor sins. Major sins will not be forgiven by means of Salat and Saum (fasting). Sincere repentance for them is indispensable. (117)

13. Allah Will Seal the Hearts of Those who Miss the Friday Prayers

Ibn 'Umar and Abu Hurairah (May Allah be pleased with them) reported: "We heard the Messenger of Allah (peace and blessings be upon him) saying (while delivering Khutbah on his wooden pulpit), "Either some people (i.e. hypocrites) stop neglecting the Friday prayers or Allah will seal their hearts and they will be among the heedless." (Muslim)

Commentary: "They will be among the heedless" means those who will become utterly unmindful of the remembrance of Allah and His Orders. Such people are Munafiqun (hypocrites), whose abode will be Hell. It means that negligence of Jumu'ah for a long time is such a serious offence that it can even seal a man's heart, which finishes all hopes and chances of one's improvement. (117)

Narrated Abu Al-Ja'd Ad-Damri: The Prophet (peace and blessings be upon him) said: "He who leaves the Friday prayer (continuously) for three Fridays on account of slackness, Allah will print a stamp on his heart." (Abu Dawud)

Narrated Mujahid: "Sayyidina Ibn Abbas (May Allah have mercy on him) was asked about a man who kept fast during day time and offered salah all night but did not attend Jumu'ah (Friday) or any congregation. He said, "He will go to Hell." Hannad reported it. He heard from Maharabi who from Layth who from Mujahid. The Hadith means to say that the man did not attend Friday and other congregational salah intentionally or because of arrogance, or because he regarded the congregation as lowly." (Tirmidhi)

77. Prayers Before and After Jumu'ah

Nawafil Prayers before Khutbah

Narrated Salman al-Faarisi: The Prophet (peace and blessings of Allah be upon him) said: "Whoever does Ghusl on Friday, purifies himself as much as he can, uses (hair) oil or perfumes himself with the perfume of his house, then goes out (for the Jumu'ah prayer) and does not separate between two (persons sitting together in the Mosque), then prays as much as is decreed for him, then remains silent whilst the imam is speaking, his sins between the present and the last Friday will be forgiven for him." (Bukhari and Muslim)

The prayers mentioned in the Hadith are Nawafil prayers and intention should be done for Nawafil prayers (Not for Sunnah) and can be prayed unlimited number until Khutbah. (120)

It is not valid to pray the regular Sunnah prayer of Zuhr on Friday, because Jumu'ah is not Zuhr; rather it is a prayer with its own rulings. Performing regular Sunnah Zuhr prayers on Jumu'ah is a Bid'ah.

Sunnah Prayers After Khutbah

Ibn 'Umar (May Allah be pleased with him) reported: "The Prophet (peace and blessings be upon him) would not perform any Salat (in the Mosque) after the Friday prayer till he had returned to his house. He would then perform two Rak'ahs there." (Muslim)

'Abdullah bin 'Umar (May Allah be pleased with them) reported: I performed along with the Prophet (peace and blessings be upon him) two Rak'ah (Sunnah prayer) after the Jumu'ah prayer." (Bukhari and Muslim)

Abu Hurairah (May Allah be pleased with him) reported: The Messenger of Allah (peace and blessings of Allah be upon him) said, "If anyone of you performs the Friday prayer, he should perform four Rak'ah (Sunnah) after it." (Muslim)

Commentary: In one Hadith, there is mention of four Rak'ahs, while in the other it is mentioned as two Rak'ahs. It can be deduced that both of these are acceptable. 'Ulama' are of the opinion that one who performs them in the Mosque, should perform four Rak'ahs; Whereas the one performing them at home, should perform two Rak'ahs with one Taslim. It is better to perform them in twos as the Prophet (peace be upon him) is reported to have said, "Perform the Nawafil of the day and night in twos." (Bukhari) (121)

78. Using Anything to Count Adhkar Other than the Fingers

Abu Hurairah (May Allah be pleased with him) reported that the Prophet (May Allah's peace and blessings be upon him) said: "He who performs ablution properly, then comes to the Friday prayer and listens to it attentively and keeps silent, his sins between that Friday and the following Friday will be forgiven, with the addition of three more days; but he who touches a pebble has engaged in idle activity." (Muslim)

Ibn Taymiyah said in al-Fataawa (22/187):

"Some of them might show off by putting their prayer-mats over their shoulders and carrying their masbahahs in their hands, making them symbols of religion and prayer. It is known from the mutawatir reports (reports in such large numbers that they couldn't be forged) that neither the Prophet (peace and blessings of Allah be upon him) nor his Companions used these as symbols. They used to recite Tasbeeh and count on their fingers, as the Hadith says: "**Count on your fingers, for they will be asked, and will be made to speak**." Some of them may count their Tasbeeh with pebbles or date stones. Some people say that doing Tasbeeh with the masbahah is makrooh (disliked), and some allow it, but no one says that Tasbeeh with the masbahah is better than Tasbeeh with the fingers." Then he (May Allah have mercy on him) goes on to discuss the issue of showing off with the masbahah, saying that it is showing off with regard to something that is not prescribed by Islam, which is worse than showing off with regard to something that is prescribed. (122)

79. Prohibition on Stepping over People when Coming to Jumu'ah Prayer

Narrated 'Abd-Allaah ibn Busr (May Allah be pleased with him) said: "A man came and started stepping over the people one Friday when the Messenger of Allah (peace and blessings be upon him) was delivering the Khutbah, and the Prophet (peace and be upon him) said to him: "Sit down, for you have annoyed (people)." (Abu Dawud and Ibn Majah)

80. Undesirability of Sitting with Legs Drawn Up to Belly During Friday Sermon

Mu'adh bin Anas Al-Juhani (May Allah be pleased with him) said: "The Prophet (peace and blessings be upon him) forbade (us) from sitting with our legs drawn up to our belly (Ihtiba') during the Friday Khutbah (religious talk before the prayer)." (Abu Dawud and Tirmidhi)

Commentary: Habut is the root word of Ihtiba' which means to sit in such a position that the two knees are joined by means of the hand or some cloth with one's belly. To sit in this style during the Friday sermon is not desirable because it causes drowsiness which in turn interrupts the sermon. It must be remembered that listening to the Friday sermon is obligatory and drowsiness during the course of the sermon is likely to disturb it and can also spoil Wudu which is a prerequisite for the validation of Salat. (123)

It is preferable not to sit with the legs drawn up when the imam is delivering the Khutbah on Friday, but if a person does sit with his legs drawn up and there is no risk of his 'awrah becoming uncovered or of him falling asleep, then there is nothing wrong with it in that case. And Allah knows best. (124)

Sheikh 'Abd-Allaah ibn Humayd (May Allah have mercy on him) was asked about pointing one's feet in the direction of the Qiblah. He replied:

"There is nothing to say that this is not allowed, but some of the scholars regarded it as makrooh (disliked) to stretch the feet out towards the Ka'bah if one is close to it; they regarded this as makrooh but not emphatically so. But if there is a Mosque somewhere else and there is a Muslim there who points his feet towards the Qiblah, there is no harm in that and he is not doing anything forbidden in sha Allah, as the scholars stated. And Allah knows best." (See Fataawa al-Shaykh Ibn Humayd, p.144) (125)

81. Deal or Sale During Friday's Prayers

Allah, the Exalted, says:

"O you who believe (Muslims)! When the call is proclaimed for the Salah (prayer) on Friday (Jumu'ah prayer), come to the remembrance of Allah [Jumu'ah religious talk (Khutbah) and Salah (prayer)] and leave off business." (Qur'an, Al-Jumu'ah 62:9)

"The Words mean: stop dealing with trade, and come and listen to the Khutbah, and perform Jumu'ah prayer in the Mosque with the imam. This means that it is haram to buy and sell after the second Adhan which comes when the khateeb sits on the minbar, until the prayer ends, unless there is a case of necessity which calls for buying or selling, such as buying water for the purpose of purification or a garment to cover one's 'awrah for prayer. End quote." (Fataawa al-Lajnah al-Daa'imah, 13/101-102) (126)

Narrated Abu Hurairah (May Allah be pleased with him): The Messenger of Allah (peace and blessings be upon him) said: "What if one of you were to take a flock of sheep and look for grass for them one or two miles away, but he cannot find any at that distance, so he goes further away? Then (the time for) Friday comes but he does not attend it, then (another) Friday comes but he does not attend it, and (another) Friday comes but he does not attend it, until Allah places a seal on his heart." (Ibn Majah)

82. Congratulating "Jumu'ah Mubarak"

Narrated Ibn Abbas (May Allah be pleased with him): The Messenger of Allah (peace and blessings of Allah be upon him) said: "This is a day of 'Eid that Allah has ordained for the Muslims, so whoever comes to Jumu'ah, let him do Ghusl, and if he has any perfume let him put some on, and you should use the miswak." (Ibn Majah)

As for congratulating one another on the occasion of Friday, what seems to us to be the case is that it is not prescribed because the fact that Friday is an Eid was known to the Sahabah (May Allah be pleased with them), and they were more knowledgeable than us about its virtues, and they were keen to respect it and give it its due, but there is no report to suggest that they used to congratulate one another on Fridays. (127, 128)

83. A Man Should Not Make his Brother Get up to Sit in his Place

Narrated Ibn Juraij: "I heard Nazi' saying, "Ibn 'Umar said, 'The Prophet (peace and blessings be upon him) forbade that a man should make another man to get up to sit in his place'". I said to Nafi`, 'Is it for Jumu'ah prayer only?' He replied, "For Jumu'ah prayer and any other (prayer)." (Bukhari)

84. Rushing when Reciting Qur'an and Praying

Allah, the Exalted, says:

"And recite the Qur'an (aloud) in a slow, (pleasant tone and) style." (Qur'an, Al-Muzzammil 73:4)

"(This is) a Book (the Qur'an) which We have sent down to you, full of blessings, that they may ponder over its Verses, and that men of understanding may remember." (Qur'an, Sad 38:29)

Narrated Abu Hurairah: "A man entered the Mosque and performed prayer, and the Prophet (peace and blessings be upon him) was in a corner of the Mosque. The man came and greeted him, and he said: "And also upon you. Go back and repeat your prayer, for you have not prayed." So, he went back and repeated his prayer, then he came and greeted the Prophet (peace and blessings be upon him). He said: "And also upon you. Go back and repeat your prayer, for you have not prayed." On the third occasion, the man said: "Teach me, O Messenger of Allah!" He said: "When you stand up to offer the prayer, perform ablution properly, then stand to face the prayer direction and say Allahu Akbar. Then recite whatever you can of Qur'an, and then bow until you can feel at ease bowing. Then stand up until you feel at ease standing, then prostrate until you feel at ease prostrating. Then raise your head until you are sitting up straight. Do that throughout your prayer." (Ibn Majah)

Why rush your prayer when you are offering your salah to the Creator of the Time?

The Sunnah is for the one who is reciting to recite at a measured pace (tarteel) and not to rush, so that he may ponder and think about what he is reciting. The Sunnah is to ponder, think. Reading so fast that some letters or Verses are not pronounced properly is not permissible; rather the worshipper should recite slowly and not be hasty, so that the recitation will be correct and clear, and he can ponder and think about (what he is reciting). If he omits or changes some of the letters, this is a kind of recitation that is not permissible. Rather he has to recite carefully and at a measured pace, so that the letters and words are pronounced in full. The same applies to prayer: he should not rush when bowing or prostrating, or when sitting between the two prostrations, or when standing after bowing. Rather he should move with deliberation and calmly. This is what is required. Moving calmly is an essential obligation; "pecking" and moving hastily in prayer invalidates the prayer.

The believer should not rush when prostrating; rather he has to settle in the position, as this is one of the essential parts of prayer and is necessary. Yet it is prescribed not to pause too long (in any position) and not to rush, and he should offer Du'a' whilst prostrating and repeat the words Subhaana. (129, 130)

85. Not Separating the Obligatory and Voluntary Prayers

Narrated Abu Hurairah (May Allah be pleased with him): The Prophet (peace and blessings of Allah be upon him) said: "Is any one of you incapable, when he prays, of stepping forwards or backwards, or to his right or left?" – meaning in order to offer a nafil prayer, i.e. a nafil prayer after an obligatory prayer. (Abu Dawud and Ibn Majah)

One of the companions of the Prophet (peace and blessings be upon him) reports that the Prophet prayed the afternoon prayer and right afterward a man stood up to pray. 'Umar saw him and told him: "Sit, the People of the Book were destroyed because they did not differentiate between their prayers." The Prophet said: "Well said, Ibn al-Khattab (i.e. 'Umar)." (Ahmad)

Narrated Mu'awiyah ibn Abu Sufyan: Umar ibn Ata ibn Abu Khuwar said that Nafi ibn Jubayr sent him to as-Sa'ib the son of Namir's sister with a view to asking him about what he had seen in the prayer of Mu'awiyah. He said: "Yes, I observed the Jumu'ah prayer along with him in Maqsura and when the imam pronounced salutation I stood up at my place and observed (Sunnah Rak'ahs). As he entered (the apartment) he sent for me and said: "Do not repeat what you have done. Whenever you have observed the Jumu'ah prayer, do not observe (optional Sunnah/Nafl prayers) till you have talked or (moved), or got out, for the Messenger of Allah (peace and blessings be upon him) had ordered us to do this and not to combine two (types of) prayers without talking or moving, or going out." (Muslim)

An-Nawawi (May Allah have mercy on him) said in his commentary on Saheeh Muslim:

"This offers proof for the view of our companions – i.e. the Shaafa'i fuqaha' – that in the case of nafil prayer, both those that are offered regularly (Sunnah prayers) and others, it is mustahabb to move from where one offered the obligatory prayer to another spot, and the best is to move to one's home; otherwise one may move to another spot in the Mosque or elsewhere, so as to increase the number of places in which one prostrates, and so as to separate the nafil prayer from the obligatory one. The words "until we spoke" indicate that separating the prayers may also be done by speaking, but doing it by moving is preferable, because of what we have mentioned. And Allah knows best." (131)

86. Putting Two Prayers Together Without any Excuse

Allah, the Exalted, says:

"Verily, the prayer is enjoined on the believers at fixed hours" (Qur'an, An-Nisa 4:103)

Narrated 'Abdullah: "I asked the Prophet (peace and blessings be upon him): "Which deed is the dearest to Allah?" He replied, "To offer the prayers at their early stated fixed times." I asked, "What is the next (in goodness)?" He replied, "To be good and dutiful to your parents" I again asked, "What is the next (in goodness)?" He replied, 'To participate in Jihad (religious fighting) in Allah's Cause." 'Abdullah added, "I asked only that much and if I had asked more, the Prophet would have told me more." (Bukhari)

87. Ruling on Joining and Shortening Prayers for Travelers

The meaning of shortening prayers is that the four-Rak'ahs prayers become two Rak'ahs when traveling.

As for joining prayers, it means that the worshipper joins two prayers, Zuhr and 'Asr, or Maghrib and 'Isha', at the time of the earlier or later of the two prayers.

Ibn 'Umar (May Allah be pleased with him) said: "I accompanied the Messenger of Allah (peace and blessings of Allah be upon him) and he did not do more than two Rak'ahs whilst travelling, and the same applies to Abu Bakr, 'Umar and 'Uthman (May Allah be pleased with them)." (Bukhari)

As for joining prayers, the scholars are not agreed on its permissibility except in the case of the pilgrim in 'Arafah and Muzdalifah. Some scholars said that it is not permissible to join prayers anywhere except in these two places. The correct view is that of the majority of scholars, which is that it is permissible to join prayers if there is an excuse for doing so, because it is proven that the Prophet (peace and blessings of Allah be upon him) did that in places other than 'Arafah and Muzdalifah. The reasons which make it permissible to join prayers are broader than those which make it permissible to shorten them. Joining prayers is permissible for every traveler, and for the non-traveler if it is too difficult for him to offer every prayer on time, such as one who is sick, or if there is rain, or he is busy with some work that he cannot delay in order to pray, such as a student taking an exam or a doctor who is doing surgery and so on. With regard to shortening prayers, that is only permissible when travelling. (132-134)

88. Preventing Women from Praying in the Mosque

Allah, the Exalted, ordered to the mother of Jesus (May Allah have mercy on them) to bow down with those who bow down (i.e. in congregation).

"And (remember) when the angels said: "O Maryam (Mary)! Verily, Allah has chosen you, purified you (from polytheism and disbelief), and chosen you above the women of the 'Aalameen (mankind and Jinns) (of her lifetime). O Mary! "Submit yourself with obedience to your Lord (Allah, by worshipping none but Him Alone) and prostrate yourself, and bow down along with Ar-Raaki'oon (those who bow down)." (Qur'an, Ali 'Imran 3:42-43)

Narrated Aisha (May Allah be pleased with her): "Allah's Apostle used to offer the Fajr prayer and some believing women covered with their veiling sheets used to attend the Fajr prayer with him and then they would return to their homes unrecognized." (Bukhari)

Zainab, the wife of Abdullah (b.'Umar), reported: The Messenger of Allah (peace and blessings of Allah be upon him) said to us: "When any one of you comes to the Mosque, she should not apply perfume." (Muslim)

The benefit of praying in the Mosque or at home depends upon the circumstances

For example, a wife who cares for multiple children would find it difficult to attend the Mosque for prayers. She cannot leave them alone. She might have trouble waking them up from sleeping, making them Wudu and dressing or preventing her children from disrupting other worshipers, or she might have other obligations at home, or it might be dangerous for her to travel to the Mosque alone or with children, that make it better for her to pray in her house.

Ibn 'Umar reported: The Messenger of Allah (peace and blessings be upon him) said: "Do not prevent your women from visiting the Mosque; even though their houses are better for them (for praying)." (Abu Dawud)

If woman is not prevented by her children or other problematic factors, she may benefit from praying in the Mosque (rewards from every step walking to the Mosque, for praying in congregation (rewards for Jumu'ah prayer in congregation are very high), for staying in the Mosque between two prayers, etc.).

Allah Almighty sent a man to me who said: "You should pray in the Mosque Jumu'ah prayer!"

The women should never abandon the Mosque completely.

The fact that the Prophet (peace and blessings be upon him) prohibited men from preventing women from praying in the Mosque which proves that there are the benefits to be earned by their attendance.

Narrated Salim from his father ('Abdullah b. Umar): The Messenger of Allah (peace and blessings be upon him) said: "When women ask permission for going to the Mosque, do not prevent them." (Muslim)

Narrated Ibn Umar: The Messenger of Allah (peace and blessings be upon him) said: "Prayer in congregation is better than prayer alone by twenty-seven degrees." (Bukhari and Muslim)

The benefit of the Mosque is not simply from prayer, but also from women's fellowship with other sisters, from attending the Qur'an classes, etc.
Narrated Abu Hurairah: The Messenger of Allah (peace and blessings be upon him) said: "The best rows for men are the front rows and the worst are the back rows. The best rows for women are the back rows and the worst are the front rows." (Muslim)

Umm Salamah reported: "The Prophet (peace and blessings be upon him) would end prayer with salutations of peace and remain in his place for a while. The Prophet would end prayer and the women would depart to enter their homes before he would depart." (Bukhari)

All of these evidences and more demonstrate that women regularly prayed in congregation with the Prophet (peace and blessings be upon him). Thus, if women have the proper intention and adhere to Islamic etiquette, they benefit from praying in the Mosque. (135)

Nowadays, the majority of Mosques have separated entrance and hall for women.

After the passing of the Prophet (peace and blessings be upon him), Aisha criticized the women who violated the sanctity and solemnity of worship in the Mosque.

Narrated Aisha (May Allah be pleased with her): "Were the Messenger of Allah (peace and blessings be upon him) to see what women are doing now, he would have prevented them from attending the Mosque, just as the women of the Children of Israel were prevented from attending." (Muslim)

89. Women Praying Differently from Men

Allah, the Exalted, says:

"O Mary! "Submit yourself with obedience to your Lord (Allah, by worshipping none but Him Alone) and prostrate yourself, and Irka'i (bow down, etc.) along with Ar-Raki'un (those who bow down, etc.)." (Qur'an, Ali 'Imran 3:43)

Malik ibn al-Huwayrith reported: The Prophet (peace and blessings be upon him) said, "Pray as you have seen me praying..." (Bukhari and Muslim)
Following are the differences between men and women prayers:

1) woman do not have to give Adhan or Iqamah, because it requires raising the voice, which women are not permitted to do.

2) The imam (or the leader of the prayer) of a group of women stands in the middle of the first row.
3) woman should keep her limbs close to her body during rukoo' and sujood, and not spread them out, because this is more modest and covering. (Al-Mughni 2/258).
4) woman leading the prayer should read aloud as long as no non-Mahram man can hear her.
5) If one woman and one man are praying, she should stand behind him, not next to him.
6) If women are praying in rows behind men, the back rows are better for them than the front rows.
7) for women praying at home, Allah Almighty and His Prophet (peace and blessings be upon him) ordered praying in congregation.

Umm Waraqah bint 'Abdullah ibn al-Harith al-Ansari reported that she had memorized the Qur'an, and the Prophet (May Allah's peace and blessings be upon him) ordered her to lead her household in prayers. There was a Muezzin for her, and she used to lead her household in prayer. (Abu Dawud) (https://hadeethenc.com/en/browse/hadith/11307)

8) Praying in the Mosque is encouraged for those who can leave children at home or can take them in the Mosque (if they are not noisy) or don't have other responsibilities at home (looking after sick or old person, etc.) as the wives of the Prophet (peace and blessings be upon him) were regularly praying in the Mosque. Nowadays, the prayer rooms and the entrance door for men and women are separated to avoid mixing.
9) Women should attend Jumu'ah prayer as Almighty Allah sent to me a man who said: "You should pray in the Mosque on Friday." The rewards for Jumu'ah prayer in the Mosque: the sacrifice of the camel for those who arrive first in the Mosque, the reward of a year of fasting and standing in night prayer, angels asking for forgiveness of the worshippers on the first row, etc.

Narrated Abu Hurairah: The Prophet (peace and blessings be upon him) said, "When it is a Friday, the angels stand at the gate of the Mosque and keep on writing the names of the persons coming to the Mosque in succession according to their arrivals. The example of the one who enters the Mosque in the earliest hour is that of one offering a camel (in sacrifice). The one coming next is like one offering a cow and then a ram and then a chicken and then an egg respectively. When the Imam comes out (for Jumu'ah prayer) they (i.e. angels) fold their papers and listen to the Khutbah." (Bukhari)

Abu Hurairah (May Allah be pleased with him) reported: The Messenger of Allah (peace and blessings be upon him) said, "If anyone performs Wudu properly, then comes to the Friday prayer, listens to the Khutbah (religious talk) attentively and keeps silent, his (Minor) sins between that Friday and the following Friday will be forgiven, with the addition of three more days; but he who touches pebbles has caused an interruption." (Muslim)

Aws bin Aws (May Allah have mercy on him) narrated: "Allah's Messenger (peace and blessings be upon him) said to me: 'Whoever performs Ghusl on Friday, and bathes completely, and goes early, arriving early, gets close and listens and is silent, there will be for him in every step he takes the reward of a year of fasting and standing in prayer.'" (Tirmidhi)

All other differences in women prayers are Bid'ah, e.g. women bowing about 30 degrees instead of 90, prostrating like a dog, counting Tasbeen between Rak'ahs, etc.

90. Breaking the Ruling in the Mosque

Allah, the Exalted, says:

"And that the Mosques are Allah's." (Qur'an, Al-Jinn 72:18)

"And who is more unjust than he who prevents (men) from the Masjid of Allah, that His Name should be remembered in them and strives to ruin them?" (Qur'an, Al-Baqarah 2:114)

Amr bin Shu'aib narrated from his father, from his grandfather (Abdullah bin Amr Al-As): "Allah's Messenger (peace and blessings be upon him) prohibited the recitation of poetry in the Masjid, and from selling and buying in it, and (he prohibited) the people from forming circles in it on Friday before the Salat." (Tirmidhi)

Disrespect of the Ruling of the Mosque, like demolishing it or making it impure, is a Major sin. Entering the Mosque in a state of impurity (menstruation, post-partum bleeding, dirty clothes, etc.) is not permitted. Makruh (disliked, detestable) are the following acts: sleeping in the Mosque, raising one's voice, announcing lost property loudly, asking something from a person, reciting poetry, discussing worldly matters. We must not go to the Mosque after eating onion, garlic or anything that creates a foul breath as the angels will not enter.

91. Prohibition of Raising one's Head Before the Imam

Narrated Abu Hurairah (May Allah be pleased with him): The Prophet (peace and blessings be upon him) said, "Does he who raises up his head before the imam not fear that Allah will make his head that of a donkey or make his appearance similar to that of donkey?" (Bukhari and Muslim)

Commentary: This Hadith has a stern warning for those who take precedence over the imam in the course of Salat. The faces of such will be turned by Allah into those of donkeys, and that is least difficult for Him. (136)

Abu Hurairah (May Allah be pleased with him) reported that the Prophet (May Allah's peace and blessings be upon him) said: "The imam is appointed so that he should be followed; so, do not act differently from him. When he makes Takbir, all of you should say it after him; bow when he bows; say 'O our Lord, all Praise be to You' when he says: Allah hears the one who praises Him; prostrate when he prostates; and all of you should pray sitting when he prays sitting." (Bukhari and Muslim) (https://hadeethenc.com/en/browse/hadith/6029)

92. Prohibition of Raising one's Eyes Towards the Sky During Prayer

Narrated Anas bin Malik (May Allah be pleased with him): The Messenger of Allah (peace and blessings be upon him) said, "How is it that some people raise their eyes towards the sky during As-Salat (the prayer)?" He stressed (this point) and added, "People must refrain from raising their eyes towards heaven in Salat (prayer), or else their sights will certainly be snatched away." (Bukhari)

Commentary: Looking towards the sky during prayer disturbs the concentration in Salat and there is a stern warning against this bad habit. (137)

93. Undesirability of Glancing in One Direction of the Other During Prayer

Narrated Aisha (May Allah be pleased with her): "I asked the Messenger of Allah (peace and blessings be upon him) about random looks in Salat (prayer), and he replied, "It is something which Satan snatches from the slave's Salat." (Bukhari)

Narrated Anas (May Allah be pleased with him): The Messenger of Allah (peace and blessings be upon him) said to me, "Beware of looking around in Salat (prayer), because random looks in Salat are a cause of destruction. If there should be no help from it, it is permissible in the voluntary and not in obligatory Salat." (Tirmidhi)

Commentary: Seeing here and there even in voluntary Salat is not permissible. However, if at all looking is inevitable, one can slightly turn his face because if one turns the whole body, his Salat would become invalid as he would not be facing the Qiblah which is essential for Salat. (138)

94. Prohibition of Placing the Hands on the Sides During Prayer

Abu Hurairah (May Allah be pleased with him) said: "We are prohibited from placing the hand on the side during As-Salat (the prayer)." (Bukhari and Muslim)

Commentary: There are two sides of everyone, the left and the right. Since keeping hands on one of them is a sign of arrogance, this is prohibited in Salat. (139)

95. Prohibition of Praying with one's Hands on one's Waist

Abu Hurairah (May Allah be pleased with him) reported: "The Prophet (May Allah's peace and blessings be upon him) forbade praying with one's hands on one's waist." (Bukhari and Muslim)

96. Prohibition of Sitting with Left Hand Behind the Back and Leaning on the Fleshy Part of it

'Amr ibn 'Al Sharid quoted his father Sharid as saying: "The Prophet (peace and blessings be upon him) came upon me when I was sitting thus: having my left hand behind my back and leaning on the fleshy part of it, and said: 'Are you sitting in the manner of those with whom Allah is angry?'" (Abu Dawud, Ahmad, Ibn Hibban, Mustadrak Hakim)

Sheikh Sabuni (May Allah have mercy on him) explains,

"This is the posture of the Jews. They sit leaning on the palms of the right hand while placing the left hand behind their backs, just as donkeys do when laying down." (Sharhu Riyad as Saliheen, Hadith: 822) (140)

97. Ruling on Raising the Hands in the Prayer

Malik ibn al-Huwayrith reported: The Prophet (peace and blessings be upon him) said, "Pray as you have seen me praying. When the time of prayer arrives, let one of you announce the Call to prayer for you and then let the older of you leader the prayer." (Bukhari and Muslim)

Narrated 'Abd-Allaah ibn 'Umar (May Allah be pleased with him), who said that the Messenger of Allah (peace and blessings of Allah be upon him) used to raise his hands to shoulder level when he started to pray, when he said "Allaahu akbar" before bowing in rukoo', and when he raised his head from rukoo." (Bukhari and Muslim)

Imam al-Bukhari (May Allah have mercy on him) wrote a separate book on this issue which he called Juz' fi Raf' al-Yadayn (Section on Raising the Hands), in which he proved that the hands should be raised at these two points on the prayer, and he strongly denounced those who go against that. He narrated that al-Hasan said: "The Companions of the Messenger of Allah (peace and blessings of Allah be upon him) used to raise their hands during prayer when they bowed and when they stood up (from bowing)." Al-Bukhari said, "Al-Hasan did not exclude any of the Sahabah from that, and it was not proven that any one among the Sahabah did not raise his hands." (al-Majmoo' by al-Nawawi, 3/399-406)

Hence 'Ali ibn al-Madeeni, the sheikh of al-Bukhari, said: "It is the duty of the Muslims to raise their hands when they bow in rukoo' and when they stand up from rukoo'." Al-Bukhari said: "'Ali was the most knowledgeable of the people of his time."

There is a fourth place where it is mustahabb to raise the hands during prayer; that is when standing up after the first Tashahhud for the third Rak'ah. (141)

It is proven in the Sunnah that the Prophet (peace and blessings of Allah be upon him) used to raise his hands at four points in the prayer:

1. When saying the opening takbeer (takbeerat al-ihram),
2. Before bowing,
3. When rising from bowing,
4. When standing up for the third Rak'ah, i.e. after reciting the first Tashahhud. (142, 143)

Narrated Naafi that when Ibn 'Umar started to pray, he would say takbeer and raise his hands; and before he bowed he would raise his hands; and when he said, 'Sami'a Allahu liman hamidah (Allah hears those who praise Him)' he would raise his hands; and when he stood up following the (first) two Rak'ahs he would raise his hands. Ibn 'Umar attributed that to the Prophet of Allah (peace and blessings of Allah be upon him)." (Bukhari)

Narrated Muhammad ibn 'Amr ibn 'Ata' that Abu Humayd al-Saa'idi said: "I heard him when he was among ten of the companions of the Messenger of Allah (peace and blessings of Allah be upon him), one of whom was Abu Qataadah ibn Rib'i, saying, 'I am the most knowledgeable of you about the prayer of the Messenger of Allah (peace and blessings be upon him).' They said: 'You are not among the seniors of us in terms of companionship and you are not among those who met him often.' He said: 'Yes, I was.' They said: 'Then tell us.' He said: 'When the Messenger of Allah (peace and blessings of Allah be upon him) stood up to pray, he stood up straight and raised his hands until they were in line with his shoulders. When he wanted to bow in rukoo', he raised his hands until they were in line with his shoulders, then he said "Allaahu akbar" and bowed, and he made his backbone straight, neither raising his head nor lowering it, and he put his hands on his knees. Then he said "Sami'a Allaahu liman hamidah (Allah hears those who praise Him)," and raised his hands and stood up straight until every bone went back to its place. Then he went down in prostration, then he said "Allaahu akbar" and held his upper arms away from his body and spread out his toes. Then he would tuck his foot under his body and sit on it. Then he sat upright until every bone has returned to its place. Then he went down in prostration. Then he said "Allaahu akbar" and tucked his foot under his body and sat on it. Then he sat upright until every bone has returned to its place. Then he got up, then he did likewise in the second Rak'ah, and when he stood up after two Rak'ahs, he said takbeer and raised his hands until they were in line with his shoulders, as he did when he started the prayer, then he did likewise until, in the Rak'ah with which he ended his prayer, he pushed back his right foot and sat on his left buttock mutawarrikan (with the left upper thigh on the ground and both feet protruding from one (i.e. the right) side), then he said the salaam." (Tirmidhi, Abu Dawud, An-Nasa'i and Ibn Majah)

98. Prohibition of Passing in Front of a Worshipper While he is Praying

Narrated Abul-Juhaim 'Abdullah bin Al-Harith (May Allah be pleased with him): The Messenger of Allah (peace and blessings be upon him) said, "If the person who passes in front of a praying person, realizes the enormity of the sinfulness of this act, it will have been better for him to wait forty than to pass in front of him." (Bukhari and Muslim) (The narrator was not sure whether the Prophet (peace and blessings be upon him) said forty days, months or years)

Commentary: We learn from this Hadith that it is a great sin to pass before a person who is offering Salat. People should also take care that they do not offer Salat without placing a Sutrah in front of them. (144)

Abu Sa'id al-Khudri (May Allah be pleased with him) reported that the Prophet (May Allah's peace and blessings be upon him) said: "If anyone of you is praying behind something that conceals him from people and somebody tries to pass in front of him, he should push him away; if he refuses, the praying person should use force against him for he is a Devil." Another narration reads: "If anyone of you is praying, he should not let anyone pass in front of him; if he refuses then use force, for he has a (Devil) companion with him." (Muslim) (https://hadeethenc.com/en/browse/hadith/10871)

99. Prohibition to Recite Qur'an when Bowing and Prostrating

Ibn 'Abbas (May Allah be pleased with him) reported: The Messenger of Allah (May Allah's peace and blessings be upon him) drew the curtain (of his chamber) aside to see the people standing in rows behind Abu Bakr in prayer. He then said: "O people, there is nothing remaining of the glad tidings of Prophethood except a good vision that a Muslim sees or someone else sees it for him. Verily, I have been forbidden to recite the Qur'an while bowing or prostrating. So, while bowing, glorify the Lord, and while prostrating, engage in supplication diligently, for it is most likely that your supplications would be answered." (Muslim) (https://hadeethenc.com/en/browse/hadith/10922)

100. Not Settling his Spine when Bowing and Prostrating

Narrated Rifaa bin Rafi Az-Zuraqi: "One day we were praying behind the Prophet (peace and blessings be upon him). When he raised his head from bowing, he said, "Sami'a-l-lahu Liman hamida." A man behind him said, "Rabbana walaka-l hamd hamdan Kathiran taiyiban mubarakan fihi" (O our Lord! All the Praises are for You, many good and blessed Praises). When the Prophet completed the prayer, he asked, "Who has said these words?" The man replied, "I." The Prophet said, "I saw over thirty angels competing to write it first." Prophet rose (from bowing) and stood straight till all the vertebrae of his spinal column came to a natural position." (Bukhari)

Narrated Abu Masud Al-Ansari: Allah's Messenger (peace and blessings be upon him) said, "Prayer is of no merit to one who does not keep his back straight in ruku and sajdah." (Tirmidhi)

101. Ruling on Forgetting a Prostration of Forgetfulness

If a worshipper deliberately omitted the prostration of forgetfulness for omitting an obligatory part of the prayer, then his prayer is invalid, just as if he deliberately omitted any obligatory part of the prayer. But if he forgot to do the prostration of forgetfulness, if he remembers it after saying the salam, he should do it, unless a long time has passed or he has left the Mosque, in which case he does not have to do anything, and his prayer is valid.

Sheikh Ibn 'Uthaymeen was asked about a man who forgot the first tashahhud, and he knew that he had to do the prostration of forgetfulness before the salam, but he forgot and said the salam. What is the ruling?" He replied:

"If he remembers within a short time, he should do the prostration, but if a long time has passed, then it is waived, such as if he did not remember until after a long time, if he had left the Mosque then he does not have to go back to the Mosque, and it is waived in his case." (End quote. Fataawa Ibn 'Uthaymeen (14/50).

If the imam forgets to do the prostration of forgetfulness, the person praying behind him should not do it on his own. Rather he should say the salam with the imam, then remind him after the salam to do the prostration of forgetfulness, then the imam should prostrate and the person praying behind him should prostrate too. (145, 146)

102. Prostrating for the Sake of Du'a is an Innovation

The fact that prostration is an act of worship within prayer does not necessarily mean that it is an act of worship outside of prayer. As for prostration for the sake of Du'a, there is nothing in Shariah to indicate that it is permissible or mustahabb. (147-149)

103. Prohibition of Putting the Forearms on the Ground (in the Prostration) Like a Dog

Narrated Anas bin Malik: The Prophet (peace and blessings be upon him) said, "Be straight in the prostrations and none of you should put his forearms on the ground (in the prostration) like a dog." (Bukhari)

Narrated Muhammad bin Amr bin Ata: "I was sitting with some of the companions of Allah's Apostle and we were discussing about the way of praying of the Prophet (peace and blessings be upon him). Abu Humaid As-Saidi said, 'I remember the prayer of Allah's Apostle (peace and blessings be upon him) better than any one of you. I saw him raising both his hands up to the level of the shoulders on saying the takbeer, and on bowing he placed his hands on both knees and bent his back straight, then he (peace and blessings be upon him) stood up straight from bowing till all the vertebrate took their normal positions. In prostrations, he (peace and blessings be upon him) placed both his hands on the ground with the forearms away from the ground and away from his body, and his toes were facing the Qiblah. On sitting in the second Rak'ah, he sat on his left foot and propped up the right one; and in the last Rak'ah he (peace and blessings be upon him) pushed his left foot forward and kept the other foot propped up and sat over the buttocks." (Bukhari)

104. Saying "Taqabbal Allah (May Allah accept it)" after Prayer

Abu Najeeh al-'Irbaad ibn Saariyah (May Allah be pleased with him): The Messenger of Allah (peace and blessings of Allah be upon him) gave us a sermon by which our hearts were filled with fear and tears came to our eyes. So, we said, "O Messenger of Allah! It is as though this is a farewell sermon, so counsel us." He (peace and blessings of Allah be upon him) said, "I counsel you to have taqwa (fear) of Allah, and to listen and obey (your leader), even if a slave were to become your ameer. Verily, he among you who lives long, will see great controversy, so you must keep to my Sunnah and to the Sunnah of the Khulafa ar-Rashideen (the rightly guided caliphs), those who guide to the right way. Cling to it stubbornly (literally: with your molar teeth). Beware of newly invented matters (in the religion), for verily every Bid'ah (Innovation) is misguidance." (Abu Dawud)

Sheikh Ibn 'Uthaymeen (May Allah have mercy on him) was asked:

"What is your opinion on shaking hands and saying "Taqabbal Allah (May Allah accept it)" immediately after finishing the prayer?" He replied:

"There is no basis for shaking hands or saying "Taqabbal Allah (May Allah accept it)" after finishing the prayer; that was not narrated from the Prophet (peace and blessings of Allah be upon him) or from his Companions (May Allah be pleased with them)." (Majmu' Fataawa wa Rasail Ibn 'Uthaymeen, 13/171)

He was also asked:

"There are some people who add things to the Adhkar following the prayer, such as when some of them say "Taqabbal Allah (May Allah accept it)"; or after doing Wudu, they say "Zamzam." What do you think?" He replied: "This does not come under the heading of Dhikr; rather this is a kind of Du'a, when a person finishes (the prayer) and says "Taqabbal Allah mink (May Allah accept it from you)." Nevertheless, we do not think that people should do this, either after Wudu or after the prayer, or after drinking Zamzam water, because if you do such things, it may become something that people do regularly and think it is prescribed, for lack of knowledge." (Majmu' Fataawa wa Rasail Ibn 'Uthaymeen, 13/211) (150)

105. Praying Witr with Three Rak'ahs Like Maghrib

The Prophet (peace and blessings of Allah be upon him) prayed Witr in different ways. He prayed one Rak'ah and three, and five, and seven, and nine. And he prayed three Rak'ahs in two different ways, either continuously with one Tashahhud, or saying salam after two Rak'ahs and praying one Rak'ah and saying salam after it. He did not pray it like Maghrib, with two Tashahhuds and one salam. Rather he forbade doing that and said: "Do not pray Witr with three Rak'ahs like Maghrib." (al-Hakim, al-Bayhaqi, al-Daaraqutni. Al-Haafiz ibn Hajar said in Fath al-Baari (4/301): Its isnaad fulfils the conditions of the two Sheikhs (Bukhari and Muslim) (151, 152)

106. Prohibition of Spitting in the Mosque

Narrated Anas bin Malik (May Allah be pleased with him): The Messenger of Allah (peace and blessings be upon him) said, "Spitting in the Mosque is a sin, and its expiation is that the spittle should be buried in earth." (Bukhari and Muslim)

Aisha (May Allah be pleased with her) said: "The Messenger of Allah (peace and blessings be upon him) saw spittle or snot, or sputum, sticking to the wall towards Qiblah and scratched it off." (Bukhari and Muslim)

Anas (May Allah be pleased with him) reported: The Prophet (peace and blessings be upon him) noticed spittle in the Mosque in the direction of the Qiblah. The signs of disgust were perceived on his face. Then, he stood up and scraped it away with his own hand and said, "When you stand in Salat, you hold communion with your Rubb and He is between you and the Qiblah. Let no one therefore cast out his spittle in that direction, but only to his left or under his foot." Then he caught hold a corner of his sheet, spat into it and folded it up and said, "Or he should do like this." (Bukhari and Muslim)

Commentary: Worshippers are under obligation to observe certain manners in the Mosque with the most important being abstinence from spitting towards Qiblah (Ka'bah). (153)

107. Using the Mosque for Urinating or Easing Oneself

Anas (May Allah be pleased with him) said: The Messenger of Allah (peace and blessings be upon him) said, "It is not proper to use the Mosque for urinating or easing oneself. They are merely built for the remembrance of Allah and the recitation of the Qur'an" or as he stated." (Muslim)

Anas b. Malik reported: "While we were in the Mosque with Allah's Messenger (peace and blessings be upon him), a desert Arab came and stood up and began to urinate in the Mosque. The Companions of Allah's Messenger (peace be upon him) said: 'Stop, stop.' but the Messenger of Allah (peace and blessings be upon him) said: 'Don't interrupt him; leave him alone.' They left him alone, and when he finished urinating, Allah's Messenger (peace be upon him) called him and said to him: 'These Mosques are not the places meant for urine and filth, but are only for the remembrance of Allah, prayer and the recitation of the Qur'an', or Allah's

Messenger said something like that. He (the narrator) said that he (the Holy Prophet) then gave orders to one of the people who brought a bucket of water and poured It over." (Muslim)

Commentary:
1. The Prophet (peace and blessings be upon him) said this on the urination of a Bedouin in the Mosque. He made him understand very politely and prudently that Mosques are meant for worship, remembrance of Allah, recitation of the Qur'an and similar other acts of piety, and one should not do anything that violates their sanctity.
2. The narrator has added the words "or as he stated." (154)

Narrated by Abu Aiyub Al-Ansari: The Prophet (peace and blessings be upon him) said, "While defecating, neither face nor turn your back to the Qiblah but face either east or west." Abu Aiyub added. "When we arrived in Sham we came across some lavatories facing the Qiblah; therefore we turned ourselves while using them and asked for Allah's Forgiveness." (Bukhari)

Salman (May Allah be pleased with him) reported that it was said to him: "Your Prophet taught you everything, even how to relieve yourself." Salman replied: "Yes, he did. He prohibited us from facing the Qiblah when defecating or urinating, and from using the right hand, using less than three stones, and using dung and bones in Istinja'." (Muslim) (https://hadeethenc.com/en/browse/hadith/10048)

It is prohibited to face towards the Qiblah or turn one's back towards it when relieving oneself out in the open (urinating or defecating), but that is permissible inside buildings or where there is a screen between oneself and the Ka'bah, close in front if one is facing towards the Qiblah and close behind if one has one's back to it, such as a saddle, a tree, a mountain and so on. (154)

108. Undesirability of Quarrelling or Raising Voices in the Mosque

Allah, the Exalted, says:

"Guard strictly (five obligatory) As-Salawat (the prayers) especially the middle Salat (i.e. the best prayer 'Asr). And stand before Allah with obedience [and do not speak to others during the Salat (prayers)]." (Qur'an, Al-Baqarah 2:238)

Narrated Abu Hurairah (May Allah be pleased with him): The Messenger of Allah (peace and blessings be upon him) said, "If anyone hears a man inquiring in the Mosque about something he has lost, he should say: 'La raddaha Allahu 'alaika (May Allah not restore it to you)', for Mosques are not built for this purpose." (Muslim)

Narrated Abu Hurairah (May Allah be pleased with him): The Messenger of Allah (peace and blessings be upon him) said, "When you see someone buying or selling in the Mosque, say to him: 'La arbaha-Allahu tijarataka (May Allah not make your bargain profitable)!' When you see someone announcing something lost in it, say: 'May Allah not restore it to you!'" (Tirmidhi)

Narrated Buraidah (May Allah be pleased with him): "A man announced (the loss of his camel) in the Mosque, uttering these words: "Has any one seen my red camel?" Upon this the Messenger of Allah (peace and blessings be upon him) said, "May it not be restored to you! The Mosques are built for what they are meant to be (i.e. prayer, remembrance of Allah, acquiring knowledge, etc.)." (Muslim)

Narrated 'Amr bin Shu'aib on the authority of his grandfather (May Allah be pleased with him):
"The Messenger of Allah (peace and blessings be upon him) prohibited (us) from buying and selling in the Mosque; (he also prohibited us from) making announcement in it about something lost and from reciting poems in it." (Abu Dawud and Tirmidhi)

Commentary:
1. Some 'Ulama' have stated that the prohibition in the above stated Ahadith is in the nature of aversion and disgust if the acts mentioned in the Hadith do not lead to disturbing those engaged in worship (be it Salat, recitation of the Qur'an or similar good acts) in the Mosque. If they do disturb the worshippers, then the prohibition would be absolute.
2. Recitation of such poems is prohibited which relate to love stories and romantic tales. There is no harm in reciting such poems in Mosques which relate to the Oneness of Allah, obedience of His Prophet (peace and blessings be upon him), and other subjects meant for the reformation of Muslims.
3. It is permissible to talk about the problems of Muslims and any other issues which are concerned with the welfare of community at large.
4. It is prohibited to hold Qawwali (singing spiritual topics) in Mosques because it is accompanied by music and musical instruments. The Verses recited in Qawwali are largely based on exaggeration and go beyond the limits prescribed by the Shariah. Such things unnecessarily pacify the sentiments of the public and incline them to inaction. It is a pity that many people regard Qawwali permissible, which is sheer ignorance. (155)

Narrated As-Sa'ib bin Yazid (May Allah be pleased with him): "While I was in the Mosque, someone threw a pebble at me, and when I looked up, I saw that it was 'Umar bin Al-Khattab, who said: "Go and call me these two men." I brought them and 'Umar (May Allah be pleased with him) asked them: "Where are you from?" On their replying that they belonged to At-Taif, he said: "Had you been the inhabitants of Al-Madinah, I would have given you a beating for raising your voices in the Mosque of the Messenger of Allah (peace and blessings be upon him)." (Bukhari)

Zayd ibn Arqam (May Allah be pleased with him) reported: "We used to speak during the prayer; a man would talk with his companion at his side in the prayer until (this Verse) was revealed: *"...And stand before Allah in devout obedience." (Qur'an, Al-Baqarah 2:238)* So, we were commanded to keep silent, such that we were forbidden to talk (to each other during prayer)." (Bukhari and Muslim) (https://hadeethenc.com/en/browse/hadith/5204)

109. Undesirability of Entering the Mosque After Eating Raw Onion or Garlic

Ibn 'Umar (May Allah be pleased with them) said: The Prophet (peace and blessings be upon him) said, "He who has eaten garlic should not come to our Mosque." (Bukhari and Muslim)

Narrated Anas (May Allah be pleased with him): The Prophet (peace and blessings be upon him) said, "He who has eaten from this plant (i.e. garlic) should not approach us and should not offer Salat (prayer) along with us." (Bukhari and Muslim)

Narrated Jabir (May Allah be pleased with him): The Prophet (peace and blessings be upon him) said, "He who has eaten garlic or onion should keep away from us or our Mosques." (Bukhari and Muslim)

The narration in Muslim is: "He who has eaten onion or garlic or leek should not approach our Mosque, because the angels are also offended by the strong smells) that offend the children of Adam." (Muslim)

Everything that has an offensive odor, such as radish, leeks, tobacco and cigarettes are included here. Onions and garlic are mentioned in particular because they are eaten often. Leeks are stipulated in a Hadith reported by Jabir ibn 'Abdullah (May Allah be pleased with him) and narrated by Muslim. So, if anyone smelled of onion or garlic in the Mosque, they would be ordered to be taken out as far as Al-Baqī', because it offends not only people but also the angels, as was related in an authentic Hadith. In Ibn Majah, we read: "At the time of the Messenger of Allah (May Allah's peace and blessings be upon him) if a foul odor was detected on a man, I would see him seized by the arm and taken out to Al-Baqī'." "So, anyone who (wants to) eat them, let them eliminate (their odor) by cooking." This is because cooking eliminated the odor and if the odor is eliminated, one may enter the Mosque because the reason for the prohibition no longer exists. Cooking onion and garlic thoroughly is required if someone wishes to enter the Mosque for prayer or any other purpose. (https://hadeethenc.com/en/browse/hadith/8953)

Narrated 'Umar (May Allah be pleased with him) in the sermon of Friday prayer: "O you people! You eat garlic and onion. I think the odour of these to be very offensive. I saw that if the Messenger of Allah (peace and blessings be upon him) happened to find a man with such offensive odour in the Mosque, he would order him to be taken out of the Mosque and sent to Al-Baqi'. He who wants to eat any of these, should cook them till their odour dies out. (Muslim)

We also learn from this Hadith that Mosques should be kept free from every kind of filth and odorous things. (156)

110. Forbiddance to Go out of the Mosque After the Adhan Has Been Announced

Once Call for the Prayer was announced, it is not permissible to leave the Mosque, except for the ablution (if outside of the Mosque), valid emergency or going to pray in another Mosque, where Imam has better voice, etc.

111. Building Lofty Mosques

Ibn 'Abbas (May Allah be pleased with him) reported that the Messenger of Allah (May Allah's peace and blessings be upon him) said: "I have not been ordered to build lofty Mosques." Ibn 'Abbas added: "You will surely adorn them as the Jews and Christians did (with their synagogues and churches)." (Abu Dawud) (https://hadeethenc.com/en/browse/hadith/10898)

112. Praying at Forbidden Times

Narrated Ibn 'Umar: Allah's Apostle (peace and blessings be upon him) said, "None of you should try to pray at sunrise or sunset." (Bukhari)

Narrated Abu Hurairah: "Allah's Apostle forbade two kinds of sales, two kinds of dresses and two prayers. He forbade offering prayers after the Fajr prayer till the rising of the sun and after the 'Asr prayer till its setting. He also forbade "Ishtimal-Assama" and "al-Ihtiba" in one garment in such a way that one's private parts are exposed towards the sky. He also forbade the sales called "Munabadha" and "Mulamasa." (Bukhari) (https://www.iium.edu.my/deed/hadith/bukhari/010)

Narrated Qaza'a slave of Ziyad: Abu Sa`id who participated in twelve Ghazawat with the Prophet (peace and blessings be upon him) said, "I heard four things from Allah's Messenger (peace be upon him) (or I narrate them from the Prophet, peace be upon him) which won my admiration and appreciation. They are: 1) "No lady should travel without her husband or without a Dhu-Mahram for a two-days' journey. 2) No fasting is permissible on two days: 'Eid Al-Fitr and 'Eid Al-Adha, 3) No prayer after two prayers, after the 'Asr prayer till the sunset and after the morning prayer till the sunrise 4) Not to travel (for visiting) except for three Mosques, i.e. Al-Masjid Al-Haram (in Makkah), my Mosque (in Madina) and Masjid al-Aqsa (in Jerusalem)." (Bukhari) (https://sunnah.com/bukhari:1864)

Forbidden times to pray are as follows:

1. from dawn until the sun has risen to the height of a spear,
2. when it is directly overhead at noon until it has passed its zenith,
3. from 'Asr prayer until the sun has set completely.

Narrated Musa bin Ali bin Rabah: "I heard my father say: 'I heard Uqbah bin Amir Al-Juhani say: "There are three times during which the Messenger of Allah (peace and blessings be upon him) forbade us to pray in or bury our dead: When the sun has clearly started to rise, until it is fully risen; when it is directly overhead at noon, until it has passed its zenith; and when it is close to its setting, until it has fully set.'" (An-Nasa'i)

"Ibn 'Umar (May Allah be pleased with him) reported: The Messenger of Allah (peace and blessings be upon him) said: "When the edge of the sun rises, avoid prayer until it becomes prominent; and if the edge of the sun disappears, avoid prayer until it sets. And do not offer your prayer at the time of sunrise or sunset, for it rises between two horns of a Devil – or the Devil." (Bukhari)

There is no forbidden time for Tahiyyat al-Masjid ("Greeting the Mosque"), missed prayer (if forgets or sleeps), prayer for a reason (see below).

Abu Qataadah (May Allah be pleased with him) said: The Prophet (peace and blessings of Allah be upon him) said: "When one of you enters the Mosque, let him not sit down until he has prayed two Rak'ahs." (Bukhari and Muslim)

Narrated Anas (May Allah have mercy on him): The Prophet (peace and blessings of Allah be upon him) said, "If anyone forgets a prayer, he should pray that prayer when he remembers it. There is no expiation except to pray the same." Then he recited: *"Establish prayer for My (i.e. Allah's) remembrance." (20.14)* (Bukhari)

Sheikh al-Islam Ibn Taymiyah said:
"Prayers which are done for a reason, such as the prostration of recitation, greeting the Mosque, the Eclipse prayer, prayer immediately after purifying oneself, as mentioned in the Hadith of Bilal, and Istikhara prayer should not be delayed if the reason comes up at a time when prayer is disallowed, because delaying them may cause one to miss them, such as if the one who is praying Istikhara may miss the thing concerning which he is seeking guidance, if he delays the prayer. The same applies to the prayer of repentance. If a person commits a sin, then it is obligatory to repent straight away, and it is recommended for him to pray two Rak'ahs, then repent, as it says in the Hadith of Abu Bakr al-Siddeeq." (End quote from Majmoo' al-Fataawa (23/215) (156)

113. Praying in the Bathroom

Abu Sa'id Al-Khudri narrated: Allah's Messenger (peace and blessings be upon him) said: "All of the earth is a Masjid except for the graveyard and the washroom." (Tirmidhi)

114. Prayer in a House Taken Illegally

Allah, the Exalted, says:

"And eat up not one another's property unjustly (in any illegal way, e.g. stealing, robbing, deceiving." (Qur'an, Al-Baqarah 2:18)

Narrated Abu Salama: "That there was a dispute between him and some people (about a piece of land). When he told Aisha about it, she said, "O Abu Salama! Avoid taking the land unjustly, for the Prophet (peace and blessings be upon him) said, 'Whoever usurps even one span of the land of somebody, his neck will be encircled with seven earths (on the Day of Resurrection)." (Bukhari)

115. Preventing from Praying

Abu Hurairah (May Allah be pleased with him) reported that Abu Jahl asked (the people of Makkah): "Does Muhammad place his face on the ground in your presence?" It was said to him: 'Yes.' He said: "By Al-Lāt and Al-'Uzza! If I were to see him do that, I would trample his neck or I would smear his face with dust." He went to the Messenger of Allah (May Allah's peace and blessings be upon him) as he was engaged in prayer and thought of trampling his neck (and the people say) that he came near him but turned upon his heels and tried to ward off something with his hands. It was said to him: "What is the matter with you?" He said: "There is a ditch of fire and horror, and wings between me and him." Thereupon, Allah's Messenger (May Allah's peace and blessings be upon him) said: "If he had come near me, the angels would have torn him to pieces." Then Allah, the Exalted, revealed this Verse. (The narrator) said: "We do not know whether it is the Hadith transmitted by Abu Hurairah or something conveyed to him from another source: *"Nay! Verily, man does transgress all bounds (in disbelief and evil deed, etc.). Because he considers himself self-sufficient. Surely! Unto your Lord is the return. Have you (O Muhammad (peace be upon him)) seen him (i.e. Abu Jahl) who prevents, A slave (Muhammad (peace be upon him)) when he prays? Tell me, if he (Muhammad (peace be upon him)) is on the Guidance (of Allah)? Or enjoins piety? Tell me if he (the disbeliever, Abu Jahl) denies (the Truth, i.e. this Qur'an), and turns away? Knows he not that Allah does see (what he does)? Nay! If he (Abu Jahl) ceases not, We will catch him by the forelock, A lying, sinful forelock! Then, let him call upon his council (of helpers), We will call the guards of Hell (to deal with him)! Nay! (O Muhammad (peace be upon him)! Do not obey him (Abu Jahl). Fall prostrate and draw near to Allah!" (Qur'an, Al-'Alaq 96:6-19)*

'Ubaydullah (a sub-narrator) made this addition: "And He ordered him (to do what is mentioned in the Verse)." Ibn 'Abd al-A'la also added that by "Nadiyah" (in the Verse: associates), he meant his people.
(Muslim) (https://hadeethenc.com/en/browse/hadith/10558)

116. Prohibition to Pray Istikhara on Behalf of Someone Else

Sheikh Ibn 'Uthaymeen (May Allah have mercy on him) said:

"Istikhara can only be done by the person who wants to do something or is thinking of doing it. It is not valid to pray Istikhara on behalf of another person, even if he delegates him to do that and says: 'Pray Istikhara to Allah for me (and ask Him to guide me concerning this matter)', because the Messenger (peace and blessings of Allah be upon him) said: "'If any one of you is deliberating about a decision he has to make, then let him pray two Rak'ahs..." By the same token, if two people enter the Mosque and one of them says to the other: 'Pray two Rak'ahs for me to 'greet the Mosque' (Tahiyyat Al-Masjid), and I am going to sit down', that is not valid. Istikhara prayer is connected to the person who is seeking guidance concerning the thing he wants to do. End quote." (Liqa' al-Baab al-Maftooh, no. 89) (157)

It is not permissible to pay someone to pray the Istikhara Prayer on your behalf. (158)

117. Abomination of Holding Conversation After Isha (Night) Prayer

Narrated Abu Barzah (May Allah be pleased with him): "The Messenger of Allah (peace and blessings be upon him) disliked going to bed before the 'Isha' (night) prayer and indulging in conversation after it." (Bukhari and Muslim)

Commentary: The prohibition of going to bed before 'Isha' prayer is that if one sleeps late at night, it becomes difficult for him to get up for Tahajjud prayer or Fajr prayer. Moreover, if a person goes to sleep soon after 'Isha' prayer, all his activities of the day will end at 'Isha', which is the most meritorious act. (159)

118. Ruling on Making up of Missed Prayer and Fast

Allah, the Exalted, says:

"Verily, As-Salah (the prayer) is enjoined on the believers at fixed hours." (Qur'an, An-Nisa 4:103)

Firstly:

With regard to missing prayers, one of the following three scenarios must apply:

1 – When you miss a prayer unintentionally, for a legitimate Shariah excuse, such as forgetting or sleeping, although you are basically very keen to perform the prayer on time. In this case you are excused but you have to make it up as soon as you remember it.

Anas ibn Malik (May Allah be pleased with him) reported that the Prophet (May Allah's peace and blessings be upon him) said: "Whoever forgets a prayer, should perform it once he remembers it, and there is no expiation for it except this." (Bukhari and Muslim) (https://hadeethenc.com/en/browse/hadith/65088)

This does not mean that a person should sleep deliberately when a prayer is due, until he misses it, then use sleep as an excuse, or neglect a means that would help him to do the prayer, and then take that as an excuse. Rather he must make use of all the means he can, as the Messenger (peace and blessings of Allah be upon him) did in this case, when he appointed one person to stay awake and wake them up to pray, but that person was overcome by drowsiness, so he did not wake them up. This is the case in which a person may be excused.

2 – When you miss a prayer deliberately. This is a Major sin, and it is so serious that some of the scholars stated that the one who does this is a kaafir. (Majmoo' Fataawa wa Maqaalaat Samaahat al-Sheikh Ibn Baaz, 10/374).

The one who does this has to repent sincerely, according to scholarly consensus. With regard to making up the prayer, there was a difference of opinion among the scholars as to whether or not it would be accepted from him if he makes it up afterwards. Most of the scholars said that he should make it up and that his prayer is valid, although he is a sinner (i.e. if he does not repent – and Allah knows best), as Sheikh Ibn 'Uthyameen quoted from them in al-Sharh al-Mumti', 2/89.

The view favored by Sheikh al-Islam Ibn Taymiyah (May Allah have mercy on him) is that it is not valid, and that it is not prescribed for him to make it up. He said in al-Ikhtiyaaraat (34):

"It is not prescribed for the one who misses a prayer deliberately to make it up, and the prayer, if he makes it up, is not valid; rather he should do a lot of voluntary (naafil) prayers. This is the view of a group among the Salaf." One of the contemporary scholars who regarded this view as more correct is Sheikh Ibn 'Uthaymeen (May Allah have mercy on him); he quoted as evidence for that the words of the Prophet (peace and blessings of Allah be upon him), "Whoever does an action that is not in accordance with this matter of ours (i.e. Islam), will have it rejected." (Bukhari and Muslim)

Sheikh 'Abd al-'Azeez ibn Baaz (May Allah have mercy on him) was asked:

"I did not pray until the age of twenty-four. Now with every Fard (obligatory prayer) I offer another Fard. Is it permissible for me to do that? Should I carry on doing that, or is there something else I have to do?" He replied:

"The one who missed prayers deliberately does not have to make them up, according to the correct scholarly view. Rather he has to repent to Allah, because prayer is the foundation of Islam, and failing to pray is the greatest of sins. In fact, failing to pray constitutes major kufr according to the more correct of the two scholarly opinions, because it is narrated that."

Buraida reported: God's Messenger (peace and blessings be upon him) as saying, "The covenant between us and them is prayer, so if anyone abandons it, he has become an infidel." (Ahmad, Tirmidhi, Nasa'i and Ibn Majah)

The Prophet (peace and blessings of Allah be upon him) said: "Between a man and Shirk and kufr there stands his giving up prayer." (Muslim)

3 - He omitted the prayer for a reason but he was not aware of it, such as unconsciousness. In this case the prayer is waived for him and he does not have to make it up.

The scholars of the Standing Committee were asked:

"If a person remains unconscious for a month and does not pray throughout that period, then he regains consciousness after that, does he have to repeat the missed prayers?" They replied:

"He does not have to make up the prayers that he missed during that period, because he comes under the same ruling as one who is insane, and the Pen is lifted from one who is insane (i.e. his deeds are not recorded). End quote." (Fataawa al-Lajnah al-Daa'imah, 6/21)

Secondly:

With regard to making up missed fasts, if you did not fast during the time when you did not pray, then you do not have to make up those fasts, because the one who does not pray is a kaafir in the sense of major kufr that puts him beyond the pale of Islam – as stated above. When a kaafir becomes Muslim, he is not obliged to make up acts of worship that he did not do when he was a kaafir.

But if you did not fast at a time when you were praying, then one of the following two scenarios must apply:

1. Either you did not form the intention to fast from the night before, and you decided rather that you would not fast. In this case making up the fasts would not be valid in your case, because you failed to do the act of worship at the time prescribed for it by Islam, with no excuse.

2. Or you started to fast then you broke the fast during the day. In this case you have to make it up, because when the Prophet (peace and blessings of Allah be upon him) commanded the one who had had intercourse during the day in Ramadan to offer expiation for that, he said to him: "It doesn't matter; fast another day in its stead.'" (Abu Dawud and Tirmidhi)

Sheikh Ibn 'Uthaymeen (May Allah have mercy on him) was asked about the ruling on breaking the fast during the day in Ramadan with no excuse. He replied:

"Breaking the fast during the day in Ramadan with no excuse is a Major sin, which makes a person a faasiq (disobedient, evildoer) who has to repent to Allah and make up the day when he broke his fast. i.e. if he fasted then during the day, he broke his fast with no excuse, then he has sinned, and he has to make up the day when he broke the fast, because when he started it, it became binding upon him, so he has to make it up, like a vow. But if he did not fast at all, deliberately, with no excuse, then it is most likely that he does not have to make it up, because that will not benefit him at all, for it will never be accepted from him. The basic principle with regard to every act of worship which is to be done at a specific time is that if it is delayed beyond that time with no excuse, it will not be accepted, because the Prophet (peace and blessings of Allah be upon him) said: "Whoever does any action that is not in accordance with this matter of ours, will have it rejected." And he has transgressed the limits set by Allah, and transgressing the limits set by Allah is zulm (wrongdoing), and good deeds are not accepted from the wrongdoer. If he had done this act of worship ahead of time – i.e. before the time for it began – it would not have been accepted of him, and by the same token, if he does it after that it will not be accepted from him, unless he has an excuse." (End quote. Majmoo' Fataawa al-Sheikh Ibn 'Uthaymeen (19, question no. 45)

Allah, the Exalted, says:

"Salah, indeed, is a duty enjoined upon the faithful at the appointed times." *(Qur'an, An-Nisa 4:103)*

The majority of scholars and imams are of the opinion that one must make up for all of the prayers one has missed in life, no matter how many they are. One of the best ways to do this—as has been suggested by one scholar—is to pray with each Fard that you perform another Fard in lieu of what you missed in the past.

The eminent Muslim scholar, Dr. Su`ad Salih, professor of Fiqh at Al-Azhar University, states: "Brother in Islam, bear in mind that in Islam, takleef (accountability) depends on maturity and sound mind. The Prophet (peace and blessings be upon him) stated that three people are not accountable for their actions: 1) the child until he becomes mature, 2) the insane until he is of sound mind, and 3) the sleeping person until he wakes up. Accordingly, scholars of Islam state that being sane and mature are conditions for accountability. There are some reasons that could suspend the person's accountability such as forgetfulness and compulsion. Then, a sane and mature Muslim should carry out his duties — such as prayer — as long as there is nothing that hinders him from doing so. Prayer is one of the most important pillars of Islam. As for the prayers you have missed, you should make up for them at their due times. You can pray each prayer twice: one for the current prayer and the other for making up for the missed one." In the light of the above fatwas, it is clear that the one who missed prayers for many years may count the missed prayers and make up for them in the hope that Almighty Allah will forgive him.

However, the above view has been rejected by scholars such as ibn Taymiyah, Shawkani and Ibn Hazm. They are of the view that a person who has deliberately missed his prayers can never make up for them. Therefore, the only option left for him is to repent, ask Forgiveness of Allah, and do lots of good works; by doing so he can hope to receive Allah's Mercy.

Ibn Taymiyah (May Allah have mercy on him), while advancing this point of view, further states:

"To insist that a person who has strayed away from Islam for a number of years and then returns to the fold of Islam must make qadha' of all his missed prayers serves only as a deterrent against his repentance, and thus it amounts to limiting the infinite Mercy of Allah." He, therefore, dismisses this view and rules that it is sufficient for him to repent, make lots of Istighfar (asking forgiveness) and good works. (160)

Al-Shawkani (May Allah have mercy on him) said:

"Ibn Taymiyah said: Those who disagree – i.e. those who say that he should make up the prayer – do not have any proof to support their argument. Most of them say that he does not have to make it up unless there is a clear command (based on evidence), but there is no such command in this case. We do not disagree that it is obligatory to make it up; rather we disagree as to whether the made-up prayer will be accepted from him and whether prayer offered at the wrong time is valid. He discussed this matter at length and he favoured the view that was mentioned by Dawud and those who agreed with him, and the matter is as he puts it, because I made a thorough study of this matter and I did not see any reliable evidence that obliges the one who misses a prayer deliberately to make it up." (161)

119. Disrespect of the Ruling of Ramadan

Allah, the Exalted, says:

"The month of Ramadan in which was revealed the Qur'an, a Guidance for mankind and clear proofs for the Guidance and the Criterion (between right and wrong). So, whoever of you sights (the crescent on the first night of) the month (of Ramadan i.e. is present at his home), he must observe Saum (fasts) that month…" (Qur'an, Al-Baqarah 2:185)

Narrated Abu Hurairah: Allah's Messenger (peace and blessings of Allah be upon him) said, "Fasting is a shield (or a screen, or a shelter). So, the person observing fasting should avoid sexual relation with his wife, and should not behave foolishly and impudently, and if somebody fights with him or abuses him, he should tell him twice, 'I am fasting." The Prophet (peace and blessings be upon him) added, "By Him in Whose Hands my soul is, the smell coming out from the mouth of a fasting person is better in the sight of Allah than the smell of musk. (Allah says about the fasting person), 'He has left his food, drink and desires for My sake. The fast is for Me. So, I will reward (the fasting person) for it and the reward of good deeds is multiplied ten times." (Bukhari)

Narrated Talha bin 'Ubaid-Ullah: "A Bedouin with unkempt hair came to Allah's Apostle and said, "O Allah's Apostle! Inform me what Allah has made compulsory for me as regards the prayers." He replied: "You have to offer perfectly the five compulsory prayers in a day and night (24 hours), unless you want to pray Nawafil." The Bedouin further asked, "Inform me what Allah has made compulsory for me as regards fasting." He replied, "You have to fast during the whole month of Ramadan, unless you want to fast more as Nawafil." The Bedouin further asked, "Tell me how much Zakat Allah has enjoined on me." Thus, Allah's Apostle informed him about all the rules (i.e. fundamentals) of Islam. The Bedouin then said, "By Him Who has honored you, I will neither perform any Nawafil nor will I decrease what Allah has enjoined on me." Allah's Apostle said, "If he is saying the truth, he will succeed (or he will be granted Paradise)." (Bukhari)

Narrated Sahl: The Prophet (peace and blessings of Allah be upon him) said, "There is a gate in Paradise called Ar-Raiyan, and those who observe fasts will enter through it on the Day of Resurrection and none except them will enter through it. It will be said, 'Where are those who used to observe fasts?' They will get up, and none except them will enter through it. After their entry the gate will be closed and nobody will enter through it." (Bukhari)

Narrated Abu Hurairah: Allah's Messenger (peace and blessings of Allah be upon him) said, "Allah said, 'All the deeds of Adam's sons (people) are for them, except fasting which is for Me, and I will give the reward for it.' Fasting is a shield or protection from the fire, and from committing sins. 'By Him in Whose Hands my soul is, the unpleasant smell coming out from the mouth of a fasting person is better in the sight of Allah than the smell of musk. There are two pleasures for the fasting person, one at the time of his fast, and the other at the time when he will meet his Lord; then he will be pleased because of his fasting." (Bukhari)

Narrated Abu Hurairah (May Allah have mercy on him): The Prophet (peace and blessings of Allah be upon him) said, "Whoever does not give up forged speech and evil actions, Allah is not in need of his leaving his food and drink (i.e. Allah will not accept his fasting)." (Bukhari)

Ramadan and Fasting have multiples virtues and rewards. (162)

Ramadan Rulings:

1. Sins are to be avoided as they may render one's fasting futile.
2. Deliberate eating and drinking, making oneself vomit, injection containing nourishment nullify the fast.
3. Sexual intercourse nullifies the fast.
4. Zakat Al-Fitr is prescribed by Allah as a purification for some sins and to feed the poor Muslims.

120. Breaking One's Fast During Ramadan Without Valid Excuse

Allah, the Exalted, says:

"O you who believe! Observing As-Sawm (the fasting) is prescribed for you as it was prescribed for those before you, that you may become Al-Muttaqoon (the pious). [Observing Saum (fasts)] for a fixed number of days, but if any of you is ill or on a journey, the same number (should be made up) from other days. And as for those who can fast with difficulty, (e.g. an old man), they have (a choice either to fast or) to feed a Miskeen (poor person) (for every day). But whoever does good of his own accord, it is better for him. And that you fast is better for you if only you know." (Qur'an, Al-Baqarah 2:183-184)

Narrated Abu Hurairah: Allah's Messenger (peace and blessings of Allah be upon him) said, "Whoever observes fasts during the month of Ramadan out of sincere faith, and hoping to attain Allah's rewards, then all his past sins will be forgiven." (Bukhari)

For those who intentionally break the fast by eating or drinking, they have to make up for that and also repent.
For breaking fast by having sexual intercourse, they should offer expiation (kafaarah) for that day as well as making up the fast and repent:

1. Free a slave, and if that is not possible.
2. Fast for two consecutive Hijri (moon) months, and if that's not possible.
3. Feed sixty poor people.

If there is a delay in making up the fasts until after the following Ramadan, they feed one poor person for each of the delayed days. (163)

121. Singling out the first third of Ramadan to pray for mercy, the second third to pray for forgiveness and the last third to pray for ransom from Hell is an innovation

Singling out the first third of Ramadan to pray for Mercy, the second third to pray for Forgiveness and the last third to pray for ransom from Hell is an innovation for which there is no basis in Islamic teachings. There is also no justification for singling out these times for these supplications, because all the days of Ramadan are equal in that regard. Rather the Muslim may pray for whatever he wants of goodness in this world and the Hereafter throughout Ramadan; that includes asking Allah for Mercy, Forgiveness, ransom from the Fire and admission to Paradise. The entire month of Ramadan is Mercy from Allah; the entire month is also Forgiveness and ransom from the Fire. None of these blessings is restricted to any one part of the month to the exclusion of any other part, and this is a reflection of the vastness of Allah's Mercy. (164)

122. There is No Specific Du'a for Each Day and Night of Ramadan

The basic principle with regard to acts of worship is Tawqeef; it is not permissible to worship Allah, may He be Exalted, through any act of worship unless this act of worship is proven in the Qur'an and Sunnah to be an act of worship prescribed by Allah. Therefore, it is not permissible to invent acts of worship or to limit them to a particular time or occasion, unless the Islamic teachings indicate that. (165)

It is good for the one who offers Du'a to follow proper etiquette and to recite many of the Du'as that have been narrated from the Prophet (peace and blessings of Allah be upon him):

"Our Lord, give us that which is good in this world and that which is good in the Hereafter, and protect us from the torment of the Fire)." (Qur'an, Al-Baqarah 2:201)

"Our Lord! Bestow on us from our wives and our offspring who will be the comfort of our eyes, and make us leaders for the Muttaqoon (the pious)." (Qur'an, Al-Furqan 25:74)

"O my Lord! Make me one who performs As-Salat (Iqamat as-Salat), and (also) from my offspring, our Lord! And accept my invocation. Our Lord! Forgive me and my parents, and (all) the believers on the Day when the reckoning will be established)." (Qur'an, Ibrahim 14:40-41)

Aisha (May Allah be pleased with her) reported: "I asked: 'O Messenger of Allah! If I realize Lailat-ul-Qadr (Night of Decree), what should I supplicate in it?" He (peace and blessings be upon him) replied, "You should supplicate: Allahumma innaka 'afuwwun, tuhibbul-'afwa, fa'fu' anni (O Allah, you are Most Forgiving, and you love forgiveness; so, forgive me).'" (Tirmidhi)

Narrated Aisha (May Allah be pleased with her): The Messenger of Allah (peace and blessings of Allah be upon him) taught her this supplication: "Allahumma inni as'aluka minal-khayri kullihi, 'ajilihi wa ajilihi, ma 'alimtu minhu wa ma la a'lam. Wa a'udhu bika minash-sharri kullihi, 'ajilihi wa ajilihi, ma 'alimtu minhu wa ma la a'lam. Allahumma inni as'aluka min khayri ma sa'alaka 'abduka wa nabiyyuka, wa a'udhu bika min sharri ma 'adha bihi 'abduka wa nabiyyuka. Allahumma inni as'alukal-jannatah wa ma qarrab ilayha min qawlin aw 'amalin, wa a'udhu bika minan-nari wa ma qarraba ilayha min qawlin aw 'amalin, wa as'aluka an taj'al kulla qada'in qadaytahuli khayran (O Allah, I ask You for all that is good in this world and in the Hereafter, what I know and what I do not know. O Allah, I seek refuge with You from all evil in this world and in the Hereafter, what I know and what I do not know. O Allah, I ask You for the good that Your slave and Prophet has asked You for, and I seek refuge with You from the evil from which Your slave and Prophet sought refuge. O Allah, I ask You for Paradise and for that which brings one closer to it in word and deed, and I seek refuge in You from Hell and from that which brings one closer to it in word and deed. And I ask You to make every Decree that You decree concerning me good)." (Ibn Majah)

Narrated Ibn 'Umar: "The Messenger of Allah (peace and blessings of Allah be upon him) never abandoned these supplications, every morning and evening: Allahumma inni as'alukal-'afwa wal-'afiyah fid-dunya wal-akhirah. Allahumma inni as'alukal-'afwa wal-'afiyah fi dini wa dunyaya wa ahli wa mali. Allahum-mastur 'awrati, wa amin raw'ati wahfazni min bayni yadayya, wa min khalfi, wa 'an yamini wa 'an shimali, wa min fawqi, wa 'audhu bika an ughtala min tahti (O Allah, I ask You for Forgiveness and well-being in this world and in the Hereafter. O Allah, I ask You for Forgiveness and well-being in my religious and my worldly affairs. O Allah, conceal my faults, calm my fears and protect me from before me and behind me, from my right and my left, and from above me, and I seek refuge in You from being taken unaware from beneath me)." Waki' (one of the narrators, explaining) said: "Meaning Al-Khasf (disgrace)." (Ibn Majah)

Narrated 'Umar: The Messenger of Allah (peace and blessings of Allah be upon him) used to say when breaking his fast: "Dhahaba al-zama' wa abtalat al-'urooq wa thabata al-ajr in shaa Allah (Thirst is gone, the veins are moistened and the reward is confirmed, if Allah wills)." (Abu Dawud)

Similarly, it is recommended to recite general Du'as from the Qur'an and Sunnah.

123. Ruling on I'tikaaf

I'tikaf is prescribed according to the Quran and Sunnah. (166)
Allah, the Exalted, says:

"and We commanded Ibrahim (Abraham) and Isma'il (Ishmael) that they should purify My House (the Ka'bah at Makkah) for those who are circumambulating it or staying (I'tikaf), or bowing, or prostrating themselves (there, in prayer)." (Qur'an, Al-Baqarah 2:125)

"And do not have sexual relations with them (your wives) while you are in I'tikaf (i.e. confining oneself in a Mosque for prayers and invocations leaving the worldly activities) in the Mosques." (Qur'an, Al-Baqarah 2:187)

The Prophet (peace and blessings of Allah be upon him) used to order that a kind of tent be pitched for him in the Mosque, and he would stay in it, keeping away from people and turning to his Lord, so he could be on his own with his Lord in a true sense of the word.

Abu Hurairah (May Allah be pleased with him) reported: The Prophet (peace and blessings of Allah be upon him) used to observe I'tikaf every year (during Ramadan) for ten days; in the year in which he passed away, he observed I'tikaf for twenty days. (Bukhari)

Aisha (May Allah be pleased with her) reported that the Messenger of Allah (peace and blessing be upon him) used to observe I'tikif in the last ten days of Ramadan till Allah called him back (to his heavenly home). Then his wives observed I'tikaf after him. (Muslim)

The basic principle is that I'tikaf is Sunnah, not obligatory, unless one made a vow to do it, in which case it becomes obligatory.

Aisha reported: The Prophet (peace and blessings be upon him) said, "Whoever vows to obey Allah, let him obey Him. Whoever vows to disobey Allah, he must not disobey Him." (Bukhari)

Things to avoid during I'tikaf

The Sunnah is for the mu'takif not to visit any sick person during his I'tikaf, or to accept any invitation, attend to his family's needs, attend any funeral or go to work outside the Mosque.

Aisha (May Allah be pleased with her) said: "The Sunnah for the mu'takif is not to visit any sick person or attend any funeral, or touch, or be intimate with any woman, or go out for any reason except those which cannot be avoided." (Abu Dawud)

Yahya related to me from Malik from Ibn Shihab from Amra bint Abd ar-Rahman that when Aisha was doing I'tikaf she would only ask after sick people if she was walking and not if she was standing still.
Malik said, "A person doing I'tikaf should not carry out obligations of his, nor leave the Mosque for them, nor should he help anyone. He should only leave the Mosque to relieve himself. If he were able to go out to do things for people, visiting the sick, praying over the dead and following funeral processions would be the things with the most claim on his coming out."

Malik said, "A person doing I'tikaf is not doing I'tikaf until he avoids what some one doing I'tikaf should avoid, namely, visiting the sick, praying over the dead, and entering houses, except to relieve himself." (Malik Muwatta)

Marriage contract in I'tikaf

Malik said, "There is no harm in someone who is in itikaf entering into a marriage contract as long as there is no physical relationship. A woman in itikaf may also be betrothed as long as there is no physical relationship. What is haram for someone in itikaf in relation to his womenfolk during the day is haram for him during the night."
Yahya said that Ziyad said that Malik said, "It is not halal for a man to have intercourse with his wife while he is in itikaf, nor for him to take pleasure in her by kissing her, or whatever. However, I have not heard anyone disapproving of a man, or woman, in itikaf getting married as long as there is no physical relationship. Marriage is not disapproved of for someone fasting."
"There is, however, a distinction between the marriage of someone in itikaf and that of someone who is muhrim, in that some one who is muhrim can eat, drink, visit the sick and attend funerals, but cannot put on perfume, whilst a man or woman in itikaf can put on oil and perfume and groom their hair, but cannot attend funerals or pray over the dead or visit the sick. Thus, their situations with regard to marriage are different."
"This is the sunnah as it has come down to us regarding marriage for those who are muhrim, doing itikaf, or fasting." (Malik Muwatta)

124. Ruling of Zakat Al-Fitr

Allah, the Exalted, says:

"Take, (O, Muhammad), from their wealth a charity by which you purify them and cause them increase, and invoke (Allah 's blessings) upon them." (Qur'an, At-Tawbah 9:103)

"Zakah expenditures are only for the poor and for the needy, and for those employed to collect (Zakah), and for bringing hearts together (for Islam), and for freeing captives (or slaves), and for those in debt, and for the Cause of Allah, and for the (stranded) traveller - an obligation (imposed) by Allah. And Allah is Knowing and Wise." (Qur'an, At-Tawbah 9:60)

"Those who do not give Zakah, and in the Hereafter they are disbelievers." (Qur'an, Fussilat 41:7)

Other Verse: *Ali 'Imran 3:180.*

Zakat Al-Fitr is obligatory on (capable) Muslim which is given at the end of Ramadan before Eid Prayer, and to be paid on his own behalf and on behalf of those on whose maintenance he is obliged to spend, on every member of the household, if he has wealth surplus to his and his dependents' needs for the day and night of 'Eid: one sa' of food. Zakah al-Fitr charity is something exclusive to the MUSLIM poor and needy. (167, 168)

Ibn 'Umar (May Allah be pleased with him) said: "The Messenger of Allah (peace and blessings of Allah be upon him) made Zakat Al-Fitr, one saa' of dates or one saa' of barley, obligatory on the Muslims, slave and free, male and female, young and old, and commanded that it should be given before the people went out to (Eid) pray." (Bukhari)

Ibn 'Abbas said: "The Messenger of Allah (peace and blessings of Allah be upon him) made Zakat Al-Fitr obligatory as a means of purifying the fasting person from idle talk and foul language, and to feed the poor. Whoever pays it before the (Eid) prayer, it is an accepted Zakah, and whoever pays it after the (Eid) prayer, it is just a kind of charity (sadaqah)." (Abu Dawud)

Abu Sa'id al-Khudri (May Allah be pleased with him) said: "At the time of the Prophet (peace and blessings of Allah be upon him) we used to give it in the form of a saa' of food…" (Bukhari)

As for giving Zakat Al-Fitr in the form of money, this is not permissible at all, because the Prophet (peace and blessings of Allah be upon him) said that it must be given in the form of food, not money.

Shaykh Ibn 'Uthaymeen (May Allah have mercy on him) said:

With regard to one who knows that it must be in the form of food, but he gives it in the form of cash because it is easier for him, that is not acceptable. But in the example mentioned by the questioner, if we cannot find anyone who will accept food, i.e., there is no one who will accept the rice or dates or wheat, and they will not accept anything but cash, in that case we may give it in the form of cash. So we should work out the cash value of a saa' of average quality food and give it to them." (End quote from Fataawa Noor 'ala al-Darb) (169)

The travelers have to pay Zakat Al-Fitr in the town where they are at the time it becomes obligatory.

The scholars of the Standing Committee for Issuing Fatwas (al-Lajnah ad-Daa'imah li'l-Ifta, 9/386) were asked: "What is the ruling on someone who was able to give Zakat Al-Fitr but did not?" They replied:

"The one who did not give Zakat Al-Fitr must repent to Allah, may He be Glorified and Exalted, and ask Him for forgiveness, because he has sinned by withholding it. He must also give it to those who are entitled to it, although after the Eid prayer it is regarded as ordinary charity. End quote." (170)

125. Ruling on One Who Does Not Pay Zakah on Wealth

Allah, the Exalted, says:

"And establish prayer and give zakah and bow with those who bow (in worship and obedience)." (Quran, Al-Baqarah 2:177)

"It is not Al-Birr (piety, righteousness, and each and every act of obedience to Allah, etc.) that you turn your faces towards east and (or) west (in prayers); but Al-Birr is (the quality of) the one who believes in Allah, the Last Day, the Angels, the Book, the Prophets and gives his wealth, in spite of love for it, to the kinsfolk, to the orphans, and to Al-Masakin (the poor), and to the wayfarer, and to those who ask, and to set slaves free, performs As-Salat (Iqamat-as-Salat), and gives the Zakat, and who fulfill their covenant when they make it, and who are As-Sabirin (the patient ones, etc.) in extreme poverty and ailment (disease) and at the time of fighting (during the battles). Such are the people of the truth and they are Al-Muttaqun (pious - see V.2:2)." (Qur'an, Al-Baqarah 2:177)

Zakat: purifying and blessing your wealth. It is considered in Islam as a religious obligation, as one of the Five Pillars of Islam, and by Quranic ranking, is next after Prayer (*Salat*) in importance.
So much is the importance of Zakat in Islam that it has been mentioned at eighty-two places in the Qur'an in close connection with Prayer. (Muslim)
Zakah is due on wealth if it reaches the nisaab (minimum threshold at which Zakah becomes due) and one full Hijri year has passed since it reached the nisaab. The nisaab is the equivalent of 85 grams of gold or 595 grams of silver. The rate that must be paid for Zakah is one quarter of one tenth (2.5%). (171)

According the Qur'an, there are eight categories of people who qualify to benefit from Zakat funds.

"Zakah expenditures are only for the poor and for the needy and for those employed to collect (Zakah) and for bringing hearts together (for Islam) and for freeing captives (or slaves) and for those in debt and for the cause of Allah and for the (stranded) traveler - an obligation (imposed) by Allah. And Allah is Knowing and Wise." (Qur'an, At-Tawbah 9:60)

Charity does not decrease wealth; rather it increases it.

Allah, the Exalted, says:

"…and whatsoever you spend of anything (in Allah's Cause), He will replace it. And He is the Best of providers." (Qur'an, Saba 34:39)

Sheikh Ibn 'Uthaymeen (May Allah have mercy on him) said concerning Zakah:

"It is obligatory according to the consensus of the Muslims. Whoever denies that it is obligatory is a kaafir, unless he is new in Islam or grew up in a remote area far from knowledge and scholars, in which case he is excused, but he should be told. If after he is told about it, he still denies it, then he is a kaafir and an apostate. As for the one who withholds it out of stinginess and carelessness, there is a difference of opinion among the scholars. Some of them said that he is a kaafir, and this was one of the two views narrated from Imam Ahmad. Others said that he is not a kaafir, and this is the correct opinion, but he has committed a Major sin. The evidence that he is not a kaafir is the Hadith of Abu Hurairah (May Allah be pleased with him), according to which the Prophet (peace and blessings of Allah be upon him) mentioned the punishment of the one who withholds Zakah on gold and silver, then he said: "… until judgement has been passed among all people, then he will be shown his path, either to Paradise or to Hell." If it is possible that he may be shown his path to Paradise, then he is not a kaafir, because the kaafir cannot be shown his path to Paradise. But the one who withholds it out of stinginess or carelessness is committing a great sin which Allah mentions in the Verses:

"And let not those who covetously withhold of that which Allah has bestowed on them of His Bounty (wealth) think that it is good for them (and so they do not pay the obligatory Zakah). Nay, it will be worse for them; the things which they covetously withheld, shall be tied to their necks like a collar on the Day of Resurrection. And to Allah belongs the heritage of the heavens and the earth; and Allah is Well-Acquainted with all that you do." (Qur'an, Ali 'Imran 3:180)

"And those who hoard up gold and silver (Al-Kanz: the money, the Zakah of which has not been paid) and spend them not in the way of Allah, announce unto them a painful torment. On the Day when that (Al-Kanz: money, gold and silver, the Zakah of which has not been paid) will be heated in the fire of Hell and with it will be branded their foreheads, their flanks, and their backs, (and it will be said unto them:) 'This is the treasure which you hoarded for yourselves. Now taste of what you used to hoard.'"
(Qur'an, At-Tawbah 9:34-35) (End quote from Majmoo' Fataawa al-Shaykh Ibn 'Uthaymeen (918/14). (172)

Narrated Abu Aiyub: "A man said to the Prophet (peace and blessings of Allah be upon him) "Tell me of such a deed as will make me enter Paradise." The people said, "What is the matter with him? What is the matter with him?" The Prophet (peace and blessings be upon him) said, "He has something to ask. (What he needs greatly). The Prophet (peace and blessings of Allah be upon him) said: '(In order to enter Paradise) you should worship Allah and do not ascribe any partners to Him, offer prayer perfectly, pay the Zakat and keep good relations with your kith and kin.'" (Bukhari)

Abu Hurairah reported Allah's Messenger (peace and blessings be upon him) as saying: "There is no owner of treasure who does not pay his Zakah, but it will be heated in the Fire of Hell and made into plates with which his sides and forehead will be branded until Allah passes judgement between His slaves on a Day the length of which will be like fifty thousand years, then he will see his path and whether it leads to Paradise or to Hell. And there is no owner of camels who does not pay Zakah on them, but a soft sandy plain will be prepared for him and they will be made to step on him. Every time the last of them has gone the first of them will return, until Allah passes judgement between His slaves on a Day the length of which will be like fifty thousand years, then he will see his path and whether it leads to Paradise or to Hell. And there is no owner of sheep who does not pay Zakah on them but a soft sandy plain will be prepared for him, and he will find none of them missing, with twisted horns or without horns or with broken horns, and they will be made to gore him with their horns and trample him with their hooves…" (Muslim)

Jabir b. 'Abdullah al-Ansari reported Allah's Messenger (peace be upon him) as saying: "The owner of a camel who does not pay what is due on it (would be punished in this way) that on the Day of Resurrection many more (along with his camel) would come and the owner would be made to sit on a soft sandy ground and they would trample him with their feet and hooves. And no owner of the cattle who does not pay what is due on them (would be spared the punishment) but on the Day of Resurrection, many more would come and he (the owner) would be made to sit on the soft sandy ground and would be gored by their horns and trampled under their feet. And no owner of the goats and sheep who does not pay what is due on them (would be spared of punishment) but many more would come on the Day of Resurrection and he (the owner) would be made to sit on a soft sandy ground and they would gore him with their horns and trample him under their hooves. And there would be more (among this flock of sheep and goat) without horns or with broken horns. And no owner of the treasure who does not pay its due but his treasure would come on the Day of Resurrection like a bald snake and would pursue him with its mouth open, and when it would come near, he would run away from it, and he would be called thus: "Take your treasure which you concealed, for I do not need it…" (Muslim)

Narrated Abu Hurairah: Allah's Apostle (peace and blessings of Allah be upon him) said, "Whoever is made wealthy by Allah and does not pay the Zakat of his wealth, then on the Day of Resurrection his wealth will be made like a bald-headed poisonous male snake with two black spots over the eyes. The snake will encircle his neck and bite his cheeks and say, 'I am your wealth, I am your treasure.' "Then the Prophet recited the holy Verses: *'Let not those who withhold . . .' (to the end of the Verse). (3.180).*" (Bukhari)

Narrated Ibn Abbas: The Prophet (peace and blessings of Allah be upon him) sent Mu'adh to Yemen and said, "Invite the people to testify that none has the right to be worshipped but Allah and I am Allah's Messenger (peace and blessings of Allah be upon him), and if they obey you to do so, then teach them that Allah has enjoined on them five prayers in every day and night (in twenty-four hours), and if they obey you to do so, then teach them that Allah has made it obligatory for them to pay the Zakat from their property, and it is to be taken from the wealthy among them and given to the poor." (Bukhari)

126. Not Paying Khums

Allah, the Exalted, says:

"What Allah gave as booty (Fai') to His Messenger (Muhammad SAW) from the people of the townships, - it is for Allah, His Messenger (Muhammad SAW), the kindred (of Messenger Muhammad SAW), the orphans, Al-Masakin (the poor), and the wayfarer, in order that it may not become a fortune used by the rich among you. And whatsoever the Messenger (Muhammad SAW) gives you, take it, and whatsoever he forbids you, abstain (from it), and fear Allah. Verily, Allah is Severe in punishment." (Qur'an, Al-Hashr 59:7)

"And know that whatever you gain, a fifth of it is for Allah and for the Apostle and for the near of kin, and the orphans, and the needy, and the wayfarer, if you believe in Allah and in that which We revealed to Our servant, or the day of distinction, the day on which the two parties met; and Allah has power over all things." (Qur'an, Al-Anfal 8:41)

Narrated Ibn 'Abbas: "The delegates of the tribe of 'Abdul-Qais came and said, "O Allah's Messenger! We are from the tribe of Rabi'a, and there are the infidels of the tribe of Mudar intervening between you and us, so we cannot come to you except in the Sacred Months. So please order us some instructions that we may apply it to ourselves and also invite our people whom we left behind us to observe as well." The Prophet (peace and blessings of Allah be upon him) said, "I order you (to do) four (things) and forbid you (to do) four: I order you to believe in Allah, that is, to testify that none has the right to be worshipped but Allah (the Prophet (peace and blessings of Allah be upon him) pointed with his hand); to offer prayers perfectly; to pay Zakat; to fast the month of Ramadan, and to pay the Khumus (i.e. one-fifth) of the war booty to Allah and I forbid you to use Ad-dubba', An-Naqir, Al-Hantam and Al-Muzaffat (i.e. utensils used for preparing alcoholic drinks)." (Bukhari)

127. Not Performing the Hajj When Able to

Allah, the Exalted, says:

"And Hajj (pilgrimage to Makkah) to the House (Ka'bah) is a duty that mankind owes to Allah, those who can afford the expenses (for one's conveyance, provision and residence); and whoever disbelieves [i.e. denies Hajj (pilgrimage to Makkah), then he is a disbeliever of Allah], then Allah stands not in need of any of the 'Alamin (mankind, Jinns and all that exists)." (Qur'an, Ali 'Imran 3:97)

"And whoever is blind in this, he shall (also) be blind in the Hereafter and more erring from the way." (Qur'an, Al-Isra 17:72)

Narrated Ibn 'Umar (May Allah be pleased with him): The Messenger of Allah (peace and blessings be upon him) said, "(The superstructure of) Islam is based on five pillars, testifying the fact that La ilaha illallah wa anna Muhammad-ar-Rasul-ullah (There is no true god except Allah, and Muhammad (peace and blessings be upon him) is the Messenger of Allah), establishing As-Salat (the prayers), paying Zakat (poor due), the pilgrimage to the House of Allah (Ka'bah), and the Saum (fasting) during the month of Ramadan." (Bukhari and Muslim)

Narrated Abu Hurairah (May Allah be pleased with him): The Messenger of Allah (peace and blessings be upon him) delivered a Khutbah and said, "O people! Hajj (pilgrimage to the House of Allah) has been made incumbent upon you, so perform Hajj." A man inquired: "O Messenger of Allah, is it prescribed every year?" He (peace and blessings be upon him) remained silent till the man repeated it thrice. Then he (peace and blessings be upon him) said, "Had I replied in the affirmative, it would have surely become obligatory, and you would not have been able to fulfill it." Afterwards, he said, "Do not ask me so long as I do not impose anything upon you, because those who were before you were destroyed on account of their frequent questioning and their disagreement with their Prophets. So, when I order you to do something, do it as far as you can; and when I forbid you from doing anything, eschew it." (Muslim)

Narrated Abu Hurairah (May Allah be pleased with him): The Messenger of Allah (peace and blessings be upon him) said, "Whoever performs Hajj (pilgrimage) and does not have sexual relations (with his wife), nor commits sin, nor disputes unjustly (during Hajj), then he returns from Hajj as pure and free from sins as on the day on which his mother gave birth to him." (Bukhari and Muslim)

Narrated Abu Hurairah (May Allah be pleased with him): The Messenger of Allah (peace and blessings be upon him) said, "(The performance of) 'Umrah is an expiation for the sins committed between it and the previous 'Umrah; and the reward of Hajj Mabrur (i.e. one accepted) is nothing but Jannah." (Bukhari and Muslim)

Narrated Aisha (May Allah be pleased with her): "I said: "O Messenger of Allah! We consider Jihad as the best deed, should we not then go for Jihad?" The Messenger of Allah (peace and blessings be upon him) said, "The best Jihad for you women is Hajj Mabrur (i.e. one accepted by Allah)." (Bukhari)

Narrated Aisha (May Allah be pleased with her): The Messenger of Allah (peace and blessings be upon him) said, "There is no day on which Allah sets free more slaves from Hell than He does on the Day of 'Arafah." (Muslim)

Narrated Ibn 'Abbas (May Allah be pleased with him): The Prophet (peace and blessings be upon him) said, "(The performance of) 'Umrah during Ramadan is equal to Hajj (pilgrimage)." Or said, "Equal to the performance of Hajj with me." (Bukhari and Muslim)

Commentary: "Equal to the performance of Hajj" means the return and reward to which Hajj is eligible. It does not mean that it will serve as a substitute for Hajj and absolve one from the need to perform it. (173)

128. Disrespect of Ihram Clothes

Narrated Abdullah bin Umar: "A person stood up and asked, "O Allah's Apostle! What clothes may be worn in the state of Ihram?" The Prophet replied, "Do not wear a shirt or trousers, or any headgear (e.g. a turban), or a hooded cloak; but if somebody has no shoes he can wear leather stockings provided they are cut short off the ankles, and also do not wear anything perfumed with Wars or saffron, and the Muhrima (a woman in the state of Ihram) should not cover her face or wear gloves." (Bukhari)

129. Prohibition of Having a Hair Cut or Paring one's Nail During the First Ten Days of Dhul-Hijjah for one Who Intends to Sacrifice an Animal

Narrated Umm Salamah (May Allah be pleased with her): The Messenger of Allah (peace and blessings be upon him) said, "When anyone of you intends to sacrifice the animal and enter in the month of Dhul-Hijjah, he should not get his hair cut or nails pared till he has offered his sacrifice." (Muslim)

Commentary: According to this Hadith, one who intends to sacrifice animal on 'Eid Al-Adha, should abstain from paring nails, having a haircut, and shaving the armpits and the private parts so that his sacrifice is in accordance with the Sunnah. One should have a haircut on the tenth of Dhul-Hijjah after having offered the sacrifice. Some Ahadith tell us that if a person who does not sacrifice an animal on 'Eid Al-Adha but pares his nails and has his haircut on the tenth Dhul-Hijjah will be given by Allah the reward of sacrifice. (174)

Narrated Abdullah ibn Amr ibn al-'As: The Prophet (peace and blessings be upon him) said: "I have been commanded to celebrate festival ('Eid) on the day of sacrifice, which Allah, Most High, has appointed for this community." A man said: "If I do not find except a she-goat or a she-camel borrowed for milk or other benefits, should I sacrifice it?" He said: "No, but you should clip your hair and nails, trim your moustaches and shave your pubes. This is all your sacrifice in the Eyes of Allah, Most High." (Abu Dawud)

130. Disrespect of Rulings of Udhiyah (Sacrifice)

Allah, the Exalted, says:

"Therefore, turn in prayer to your Lord and sacrifice (to Him only)." (Qur'an, Al-Kawthar 108:2)

"Say (O Muhammad SAW): "Verily, my Salat (prayer), my sacrifice, my living and my dying are for Allah, the Lord of the 'Alamin (mankind, Jinns and all that exists). He has no partner. And of this I have been commanded, and I am the first of the Muslims." (Qur'an, Al-An'am 6:162-163)

"And for every nation We have appointed religious ceremonies, that they may mention the Name of Allah over the beast of cattle that He has given them for food. And your Ilah (God) is One Ilah (God Allah), so you must submit to Him Alone (in Islam)…" (Qur'an, Al-Hajj 22:34)

Narrated Abu Hurairah: The Messenger of Allah (peace and blessings be upon him) said: "Whoever can afford it, but does not offer a sacrifice, let him not come near our prayer place." (Ibn Majah)

Narrated Mikhnaf bin Sulaim: "We were standing with the Prophet (peace and blessings be upon him) at Arafat and he said: 'O people, each family each year must offer Udhiyah and 'Atirah.'" (Ibn Majah)

Conditions of Udhiyah

1. The intention of offering sacrifice for the sake of Allah.

2. Udhiyah refers to the animal (camel, cattle or sheep) that is sacrificed as an act of worship to Allah.

3. The animal should have reached the required age, which is six months for a lamb, one year for a goat, two years for a cow and five years for a camel.

Narrated Sulaiman bin Abdur-Rahman: "I heard Ubaid bin Fairuz say: 'I said to Bara' bin 'Azib: "Tell us of the sacrificial animals that the Messenger of Allah (peace and blessings be upon him) disliked or forbade." He said: "Allah's Messenger (peace and blessings be upon him) said like this with his hand. And my hand is shorter than his hand: 'There are four that will not be accepted as sacrifices: The one-eyed animal that is obviously blind in one eye; the sick animal that is obviously sick; the lame animal with an obvious limp; and the animal that is so emaciated that it is as if there is no marrow in its bones.'" He said: "And I dislike that the animal should have some fault in its ears." He said: "What you dislike, forget about it and do not make it forbidden to anyone." (Ibn Majah)

4. It is not permissible to sell any part of selected animal or give it away, except in exchange for one that is better. It is permissible to ride it if necessary. If an animal gives birth, its offspring should be sacrificed along with it.

Narrated Anas: The Prophet (peace be upon him) saw a man driving a Badana (i.e. camel for sacrifice) and said to him, "Ride on it." The man said, "O Allah's Apostle (peace and blessings be upon him)! It is a Badana." The Prophet (peace and blessings be upon him) repeated his order and on the third or fourth time he said, "Ride it ("woe to you" or said: "May Allah be merciful to you)." (Bukhari)

5. The specified time for sacrifice.

Udhiyah is done during the period from after the prayer on the Day of Nahr (Eid al-Adha) until before sunset on the last of the Days of Tashreeq (the 13th day of Dhu'l-Hijjah).

Narrated Al-Bara: "I heard the Prophet (peace and blessings be upon him) delivering a Khutbah saying, "The first thing to be done on this day (first day of Eid Al-Adha) is to pray; and after returning from the prayer we slaughter our sacrifices (in the Name of Allah) and whoever does so, he acted according to our Sunnah (traditions)." (Bukhari)

Narrated Jundub: "On the day of Nahr the Prophet (peace and blessings be upon him) offered the prayer and delivered the Khutbah and then slaughtered the sacrifice and said, "Anybody who slaughtered (his sacrifice) before the prayer should slaughter another animal in lieu of it, and the one who has not yet slaughtered should slaughter the sacrifice mentioning Allah's Name on it." (Bukhari)

6. Perfection in Slaughtering Animal.

Abu Ya'la Shaddad bin Aws (May Allah be pleased with him) said: The Messenger of Allah (peace and blessings of Allah be upon him) said: "Verily Allah has prescribed ihsan (proficiency, perfection) in all things. So, if you kill then kill well; and if you slaughter, then slaughter well. Let each one of you sharpen his blade and let him spare suffering to the animal he slaughters." (Muslim)

A halal slaughter involves a sharp knife that the animal does not see before slaughtering; the animal must be well-rested and fed before and the slaughtering shouldn't not take place in front of other animals. To reduce pain and suffering of the animal it should be a single quick cut across the throat.

7. Allah's Name should be recited, by saying "Bismillah" before slaughtering.

Narrated 'Abaya bin Rafa'a bin Raft' bin Khadij: The Prophet (peace and blessings be upon him) said, "Use whatever causes blood to flow, and eat the animals if the Name of Allah has been mentioned on slaughtering them." (Bukhari)

8. Before slaughtering, he should say, *"Allaahumma haadha 'anni wa 'an aali bayti."* "O Allah, this is on behalf of myself and the members of my household" and he may include in the reward for it whoever he wishes, living or dead. He does not have to make a separate sacrifice on behalf of deceased person.

9. Blood must be drained out of the carcass.

10. Distribution of meat.

It is recommended to divide the meat into three:

1/3 part for the person who supplied the animal,
1/3 part to be shared out among their family, friends or neighbours,
1/3 part to be given to those who are poor or in need.

Narrated Ali (May Allah have mercy on him): "The Prophet ordered me to supervise the (slaughtering) of Budn (Hadi camel) and to distribute their meat, skins and covering sheets in charity and not to give anything (of their bodies) to the butcher as wages for slaughtering." (Bukhari)

11. Prohibition on removing hair and nails regards only the person who is going to offer a sacrifice, whether he or she delegates someone else to do the actual slaughter or not. The prohibition does not apply to the person who is doing the sacrifice on behalf of another.

If a person deliberately takes something (from his hair or nails), he must seek the Forgiveness of Allah, but he does not have to pay any fidyah (penalty), and his Udhiyah is still valid. Whoever needs to remove some of his hair or nails because leaving it will cause him harm, such as a torn nail or a wound in a site covered by hair, should remove it, and there is no sin on him if he does so. (175)

Punishment for neglecting Udhiyah

It is mentioned in *Jawaahir al-Ikleel Sharh Mukhtasar Khaleel* that if people neglect Udhiyah, they should be fought, because it is one of the rituals of Islam. (*Rasaa'il Fiqhiyyah* by Sheikh Ibn 'Uthaymeen, p.46)

131. Congratulating the Pilgrim after he Returns and Decorating the House for him

There is no report in the Sunnah about decorating the house with plants and lights for the pilgrim's arrival, and there is no report that the Sahabah did that. Some contemporary scholars have issued fatwas stating that it is not permissible to do that, and they mentioned several reasons:

1. That this action was not narrated from the Prophet (peace and blessings of Allah be upon him) or his companions, so it is a Bid'ah (an innovation).
2. It is a kind of showing off.
3. It is a waste of money.

But this action is a custom and tradition, not an act of worship. Decorating the house for the pilgrim's arrival if done with simple things, without any great expense, seems permissible. These actions do not necessarily imply showing off. Congratulating the pilgrim who has returned from Hajj, and making food for him or the pilgrim makes food himself and invites people to a meal, that is also permissible.

Narrated Ibn 'Abbas (May Allah be pleased with him): "When the Prophet (peace and blessings be upon him) came to Makkah – during the conquest – the children of Banu 'Abd al-Muttalib met him and he carried one of them in front of him (on his mount) and another behind him." (Bukhari, in Kitaab al 'Umrah; the chapter: "Chapter on welcoming arriving pilgrims, and three men on one mount.")

Al-Nawawi (May Allah have mercy on him) said:

"It is mustahabb to offer naqee'ah, which is a type of food that is made to welcome a traveler, and the word may also refer to what is done by the arriving traveler or what others do for him … among the evidence that is quoted for that is the Hadith of Jabir (May Allah be pleased with him) which says that when the Messenger of Allah (peace and blessings of Allah be upon him) came to Madinah from a journey, he would slaughter a camel or a cow." (Bukhari) (Al-Majmoo' (4/400) (176)

132. Violation of the Ruling of Four Sacred Months

Allah, the Exalted, says:

"O you who believe! Violate not the sanctity of the Symbols of Allah, nor of the Sacred Month, nor of the animals brought for sacrifice, nor the garlanded people or animals, etc. [Marked by the garlands on their necks made from the outer part of the tree stems (of Makkah) for their security], nor the people coming to the Sacred House (Makkah) seeking the Bounty and good Pleasure of their Lord. But when you finish the Ihram (of Hajj or 'Umrah), you may hunt, and let not the hatred of some people in (once) stopping you from Al-Masjid Al-Haram (at Makkah), lead you to transgression (and hostility on your part). Help you one another in Al-Birr and At-Taqwa (virtue, righteousness and piety); but do not help one another in sin and transgression. And fear Allah. Verily, Allah is Severe in punishment." (Qur'an, Al-Ma'idah 5:2)

"They ask you concerning fighting in the Sacred Months (i.e. 1st, 7th, 11th and 12th months of the Islamic calendar). Say, "Fighting therein is a great (transgression) but a greater (transgression) with Allah is to prevent mankind from following the way of Allah, to disbelieve in Him, to prevent access to Al-Masjid Al-Haram (at Makkah), and to drive out its inhabitants, and Al-Fitnah is worse than killing. And they will never cease fighting you until they turn you back from your religion (Islamic Monotheism) if they

can. And whosoever of you turns back from his religion and dies as a disbeliever, then his deeds will be lost in this life and in the Hereafter, and they will be the dwellers of the Fire. They will abide therein forever." (Qur'an, Al-Baqarah 2:217)

"Verily, the number of months with Allah is twelve months (in a year), so it was ordained by Allah on the day when He created the heavens and the earth; of them, four are sacred. That is the Right Religion, so wrong not yourselves therein..." (Qur'an, At-Tawbah 9:36)

Qutaadah said concerning this phrase *"so wrong not yourselves therein..."* that wrongdoing during the sacred months is more serious and more sinful that wrongdoing at any other time. Wrongdoing at any time is a serious matter, but Allah gives more weight to whichever of His commands He will. Allah has chosen certain ones of His creation. He has chosen from among the angels Messengers and from among mankind Messengers. He chose from among speech the remembrance of Him (Zhikr). He chose from among the earth the Mosques, from among the months Ramadan and the sacred months, from among the days Friday, and from among the nights Laylat al-Qadr, so, venerate that which Allah has told us to venerate. (Tafsir of Surah al-Tawbah, Ayah 36 of Ibn Kathir) (177)

Narrated Abdur Rahman bin Abi Bakras father: "Once the Prophet was riding his camel and a man was holding its rein. The Prophet asked, "What is the day today?" We kept quiet, thinking that he might give that day another name. He said, "Isn't it the day of Nahr (slaughtering of the animals of sacrifice)?" We replied, "Yes." He further asked, "Which month is this?" We again kept quiet, thinking that he might give it another name. Then he said, "Isn't it the month of Dhul-Hijjah?" We replied, "Yes." He said, "Verily! Your blood, property and honor are sacred to one another (i.e. Muslims) like the sanctity of this day of yours, in this month of yours and in this city of yours. It is incumbent upon those who are present to inform those who are absent because those who are absent might comprehend (what I have said) better than the present audience." (Bukhari)

133. Rajab Month Innovations

The following innovations are commonly practiced in Rajab:

1 - Salat al-Ragha'ib.

2 - Rajab major events but none of these reports are true.

The reports that the Prophet (peace and blessings be upon him) was born on the first night of Rajab and that he received his Mission on the twenty-seventh (or twenty-fifth) of this month are false.

3 - Celebrating Prophet's Night Journey.

There is no Saheeh report that the Prophet's Night Journey (al-Isra) took place on the twenty-seventh of Rajab. The recitation of the story of the Miraj and celebrations to commemorate it on the twenty-seventh of Rajab or singling out this night to perform extra acts of worship such as Qiyam al-Layl or fasting are Bid'ah. (178)

4 - Salat Umm Dawood halfway through Rajab.

5 - Specific Du'as which are recited during Rajab are all fabrications and innovations.

6 - Visiting graves specifically in Rajab is Bid'ah because graves are to be visited at any time.

7 - Koonday - Distributing special type of breads after reciting some Verses and Prayers.

8 - Fasting in Rajab.

Al-Hafiz ibn Hajar said in Tabayyun al-'Ajab bima wurida fî Fadl Rajab:
"No Saheeh Hadith that may be used as evidence has been narrated concerning the virtues of the month of Rajab or fasting this month, or fasting in any specific part of it, or observing Qiyam al-Layl specifically during this month. Imam Abu Isma'il al-Harawi al-Hafiz has already stated this before me, and we have narrated this from others also." (https://sunnahonline.com/ilm/sunnah/0042.htm)

9 - Umrah in Rajab.

Narrated 'Urwa bin Az-Zubair: "I asked 'Aisha (whether the Prophet (peace be upon him) had performed 'Umrah in Rajab). She replied, "Allah's Messenger (peace and blessings be upon him) never performed any 'Umrah in Rajab." (Bukhari)

10 - Al-'Atirah (a kind of sacrifice).

During the Jahiliyyah, the Arabs used to slaughter a sacrifice as an act of Idols worship. When Islam came, Allah, the Exalted, and His Messenger commanded that sacrifices were to be offered only to Allah.

The fuqaha' differed as to the rulings on offering sacrifices during Rajab. The majority of the Hanafis, Malikis and Hanbalis stated that the sacrifice of al-'Atirah was abrogated. Their evidence was the Hadith, "There is no Fir' and no 'Atirah", narrated from Abu Hurairah (Bukhari and Muslim). The Shafi'is and Ibn Sirin said that al-'Atirah had not been abrogated.

Narrated Mikhnaf ibn Sulaym: "We were staying with the Apostle of Allah (peace and blessings be upon him) at Arafat. He said: "O people, every family must offer a sacrifice and an Atirah. Do you know what the Atirah is? It is what you call the Rajab sacrifice." Abu Dawud said: 'Atriah has been abrogated, and this tradition is an abrogated one.'" (Abu Dawud)

Narrated Nubayshah: "A man called out to the Messenger of Allah (peace and blessings of Allah be upon him): 'We used to offer the sacrifice of al-'Atirah during the Jahiliyyah in the month of Rajab. What do you command us to do? He said, "Offer sacrifices, no matter which month is it …" (Abu Dawud, An-Nasa'i and Ibn Majah)

Ibn Hajar said: "The Messenger of Allah (peace and blessings of Allah be upon him) did not abolish it in principle, but he abolished the idea of making this sacrifice especially in Rajab." (https://sunnahonline.com/ilm/sunnah/0042.htm)

11. The Hadith "Whoever says in Rajab 'I ask Allah for Forgiveness, there is no god but He Alone, with no partner or associate, and I repent to Him one hundred times, and ends it with charity, Allah will decree for him Mercy and Forgiveness. And whoever says it four hundred times, Allah will decree for him the reward of one hundred martyrs, and when he meets Allah on the Day of Resurrection, He will say to him: 'You affirmed My Sovereignty, so wish for whatever you want so that I may give it to you, for there is none who prevails but Me." is fabricated. (179)

134. Shaban Month Innovations

The following innovations are commonly practiced in Shaban:

1 - Specifying the 15th of Sha'ban by fasting or reciting the Qur'an, or performing voluntary prayers

Fasting the 15th of Sha'ban or specifying it with reciting the Qur'an, or making (particular) supplications has no basis. (Sheikh Ibn 'Uthaymeen, al-Bid'u wal-Muhdathaat wa maa laa Asla lahu, p.612, Fataawa Sheikh Muhammad Ibn Saalih al-'Uthaymeen, vol.1, p.190) (180)

2 - Laylat al-Nisf (mid-Sha'ban)

Muhammad 'Abd al-Salam al-Shuqayri said:

"Imam al-Fatni said in Tadhkirat al-Mawdu'at: 'Among the innovations that have been introduced on "Laylat an-Nisf" (mid-Sha'ban) is al-Salat al-Alfiyyah, which is one hundred Rak'ahs in which Surah Al-Ikhlas is recited ten times in each Rak'ah offered in congregation; they pay more attention to this than to Jumu'ah and 'Eid prayers, although there is no report concerning it, except da'if (weak) and mawdu' (fabricated) reports, and we should not be deceived by the fact that these reports were quoted by the authors of al-Qut and al-Ihya and others, nor should we be deceived by what was mentioned in Tafsir al-Tha'labi, that it is Laylat al-Qadr.'"

Al-'Iraqi said:

"The Hadith about the prayer on Laylat al-Nisf (mid-Sha'ban) is false. Ibn al-Jawzi narrated it in al-Mawdu'at (which is a compilation of fabricated Ahadith): Chapter on the Hadith, prayer and supplication on Laylat al-Nisf: "The Hadith, "When the night of 'Nisf Sha'ban' (mid-Shaban) comes, spend the night in prayer and fast on that day" was narrated by Ibn Majah from 'Ali. Muhashiyyah said: (It was also narrated) in al-Zawaid. Its isnad is da'if (weak) because of the weakness of Ibn Abi Basrah, of whom Ahmad and Ibn Ma'in said: 'He fabricates Hadith.'"

Praying six Rak'ahs on Laylat al-Nisf with the intention of warding off calamity, having a long life and being independent of people, and reciting Yasin and offering Du'a in between that — there is no doubt that this is something that has been introduced into the religion and is contrary to the Sunnah of the Messenger of Allah (peace and blessings of Allah be upon him). The commentator on al-Ihya said: 'This prayer is well known in the books of later Sufi masters, but I have not seen any Saheeh report in the Sunnah to support it and the connected Du'a. Rather, this is the action of some sheikhs.' Our companions said: 'It is makruh to gather on any of the nights mentioned in the Mosques or elsewhere.' Al-Najm al-Ghayti said, describing spending the night of al-Nisf (mid-Shaban) praying in congregation: 'That was denounced by most of the scholars of the Hijaz, including 'Ata and Ibn Abi Mulaykah, the fuqaha of Madinah and the companions of Malik. They said: 'All of that is an innovation (Bid'ah) and there is no report to suggest that the Prophet spent that night in praying in congregation or that his Companions did that either.' Al-Nawawi said: 'The prayers of Rajab and Sha'ban are two reprehensible innovations." (Al-Sunan wa'l-Mubtada'at, p.144)

3 - Alfiyah prayer

The prayer was dubbed alfiyah prayer because there are 1000 times recitation of chapter Al-Ikhlas, in 100 Rak'ahs is an innovation.

4 - Shab e Barat in Islam

Some people use the word al-Sha'baniyyah to refer to the last days of Sha'ban and say, "These are the days of bidding farewell to food", and they take advantage of these days to eat a lot before Ramadan begins. Some scholars say that this idea was originally taken from the Christians, who used to do that as their fasting period (Lent) approached. (181)

5 - Giving sadaqah specifically on the night of 15th of Sha'ban

6 - Performing the tradition of 'Ruwahan-sadranan'

This tradition mostly spread in Java region, particularly in Central Java and Yogyakarta. The followers used the Sha'ban as a special month particularly for visiting the graves and performing an event to invoke salvation for the village. Basically, this is a tradition of the Hindus, animism and dynamism. Hence, we can firmly state that the ruling for such act is forbidden, since we are prohibited to conserve the tradition of unbelievers. (182)

135. Muharram Month Innovations

Abu Qatadah Al-Ansari (May Allah have mercy on him) narrated, 'The Messenger of Allah (peace and blessings of Allah be upon him) was asked about fasting on the day of Arafah (the 9th of the month of Dhul Hijjah). He replied, "Fasting on the day of Arafah is an expiation for the preceding year and the following year." He was also asked about fasting on the Day of Ashura (the 10th of the month of Muharram). He replied, "Fasting on the Day of Ashura is an expiation for the preceding year." The Messenger of Allah (peace and blessings of Allah be upon him) was also asked about fasting on Monday, and he replied, "This is the day on which I was born and the day on which I was sent (with the Message of Islam) and the day on which I received Revelation." (Muslim)

The Shia (rafidah) took the month of Muharram as a time of mourning and sorrow as they remember the death of Husayn (May Allah be pleased with him). Celebrating that day is an innovation (Bid'ah), and making it an anniversary for mourning is also an innovation. (183)

Narrated 'Abdullah ibn Masud (May Allah be pleased with him): The Prophet (peace and blessings of Allah be upon him) said: "He is not one of us who strikes his cheeks, rends his garment or cries with the cry of the Jaahiliyyah." (Bukhari and Muslim)

Ibn Taymiyah (May Allah have mercy on him) was asked about the things that people do on 'Ashura', such as wearing kohl, taking a bath (Ghusl), wearing henna, shaking hands with one another, cooking grains (hubub), showing happiness and so on. Was any of these reported from the Prophet (peace and blessings of Allah be upon him) in a Saheeh Hadith or not? If nothing to that effect was reported in a Saheeh Hadith, is doing these things Bid'ah or not? Is there any basis for what the other group do, such as grieving and mourning, going without anything to drink, eulogizing and wailing, reciting in a crazy manner and rending their garments?" His reply was:

"Praise be to Allah, the Lord of the worlds. Nothing to that effect has been reported in any Saheeh Hadith from the Prophet (peace and blessings of Allah be upon him) or from his Companions. None of the Imams of the Muslims encouraged or recommended such things, neither the four Imams, nor any others. No reliable scholars have narrated anything like this, neither from the Prophet (peace and blessings of Allah be upon him), nor from the Sahabah, nor from the Tabi'een; neither in any Saheeh report or in a da'if (weak) report; neither in the books of Saheeh, nor in al-Sunan, nor in the Musnads. No Hadith of this nature was known during the best centuries, but some of the later narrators reported Ahadith like the one which says, "Whoever puts kohl in his eyes on the day of 'Ashura' will not suffer from eye disease in that year, and whoever takes a bath (does Ghusl) on the day of 'Ashura' will not get sick in that year," and so on. They also reported a fabricated Hadith that is falsely attributed to the Prophet (peace and blessings of Allah be upon him), which says, "Whoever is generous to his family on the day of 'Ashura', Allah will be generous to him for the rest of the year." Reporting all of this from the Prophet (peace and blessings of Allah be upon him) is tantamount to lying."

Then he [Ibn Taymiyah (May Allah have mercy on him)] discussed in brief the tribulations that had occurred in the early days of this Ummah and the killing of al-Husayn (May Allah be pleased with him), and what the various sects had done because of this. Then he said:

"An ignorant, wrongful group – who were either heretics and hypocrites, or misguided and misled – made a show of allegiance to him and the members of his household, so they took the day of 'Ashura' as a day of mourning and wailing, in which they openly displayed the rituals of jahiliyyah such as slapping their cheeks and rending their garments, grieving in the manner of the Jahiliyyah...The Shaytan made this attractive to those who are misled, so they took the day of 'Ashura' as an occasion of mourning, when they grieve and wail, recite poems of grief and tell stories filled with lies. Whatever truth there may be in these stories serves no purpose other than the renewal of their grief and sectarian feeling, and the stirring up of hatred and hostility among the Muslims, which they do by cursing those who came before them… The evil and harm that they do to the Muslims cannot be enumerated by any man, no matter how eloquent he is. Some others – either Nasibis who oppose and have enmity towards al-Husayn and his family or ignorant people who try to fight evil with evil, corruption with corruption, lies with lies and Bid'ah with Bid'ah – opposed them by fabricating reports in favor of making the day of 'Ashura' a day of celebration, by wearing kohl and henna, spending money on one's children, cooking special dishes and other things that are done on Eids and special occasions. These people took the day of 'Ashura' as a festival like Eid, whereas the others took it as a day of mourning. Both are wrong, and both go against the Sunnah, even though the other group (those who take it as a day of mourning) are worse in intention and more ignorant, and more plainly wrong… Neither the Prophet (peace and blessings of Allah be upon him) nor his successors (the khulafa' al-rashidun) did any of these things on the day of 'Ashura', they neither made it a day of mourning nor a day of celebration…As for the other things, such as cooking special dishes with or without grains, or wearing new clothes, or spending money on one's family, or buying the year's supplies on that day, or doing special acts of worship such as special prayers or deliberately slaughtering an animal on that day, or saving some of the meat of the sacrifice to cook with grains, or wearing kohl and henna, or taking a bath (Ghusl), or shaking hands with one another, or visiting one another, or visiting the Mosques and mashhads (shrines) and so on… all of this is reprehensible Bid'ah and is wrong. None of it has anything to do with the Sunnah of the Messenger of Allah (peace and blessings of Allah be upon him) or the way of the Khulafa' al-Rashidun. It was not approved of by any of the Imams of the Muslims, not Malik, not al-Thawri, not al-Layth ibn Sa'd, not Abu Hanifah, not al-Uzaa'i, not al-Shafa'i, not Ahmad ibn Hanbal, not Ishaq ibn Rahwayh, not any of the Imams and scholars of the Muslims." (Fataawa al-Kubra by Ibn Taymiyah) (184)

136. Salat al-Hajah is Innovation Worship Allah the Prophet's way

It is prescribed for the Muslim to worship Allah in the ways that He has prescribed in His Book, and in the ways that have been proven from the Prophet (peace and blessings of Allah be upon him).

What is Salat al-Hajah?

Salat al-Hajah was narrated in da'eef (weak) or munkar (denounced) Ahadith - as far as we know - which cannot be used as proof and which are not fit to base acts of worship on. (*Fatawa al-Lajnah al-Daimah*, 8/162). Salat al-Hajah is mentioned in four Ahadith, two of which are fabricated. In one Hadith Salat al-Hajah has twelve Rak'ahs and in the other it has two. The third Hadith is da'eef jiddan (very weak) and the fourth Hadith is da'eef (weak). In the last two Ahadith the prayer has two Rak'ahs.

It is narrated from Ibn Masud (May Allah be pleased with him) that the Prophet (peace and blessings of Allah be upon him) said: "Twelve Rak'ahs that you pray by night or day and recite the Tashahhud between each two Rak'ahs. When you recite Tashahhud at the end of the prayer, then praise Allah and send peace and blessings upon the Prophet, and recite the Opening of the Book seven times whilst you are prostrating and say: 'Laa ilaaha ill-Allah wahdahu laa shareeka lah, lahu'l-mulk wa lahu'l-hamd was huwa 'ala kulli shay'in qadeer (There is no god but Allah Alone with no partner or associate, His is the Dominion, to Him be Praise, and He has power over all things) ten times.' Then say: "O Allah, I ask You by the Glory of Your Throne and the Mercy of Your Book and Your greatest Names and Your highest Majesty and Your perfect Words,' Then ask for what you need, then raise your head and say salam right and left. Do not teach it to the foolish for they will pray and will be answered." Narrated Ibn al-Jawzi in al-Mawdoo'aat (2/63) via 'Aamir ibn Khadaash from 'Amr ibn Haroon al-Balkhi. Ibn al-Jawzi narrated from Ibn Ma'een that 'Amr al-Balkhi was a liar, and he said: It is narrated in Saheeh reports that it is forbidden to recite Qur'an when prostrating. See: al-Mawdoo'aat (2/63) and Tadreeb al-Mawdoo'aat by al-Dhahabi (p.167).

Sheikh al-Albaani (May Allah have mercy on him) said:

"I say: But the report referred to is false and is not Saheeh (sound). It was narrated by Ibn al-Jawzi in al-Mawdoo'aat and he said: 'This is undoubtedly a fabricated (mawdoo') Hadith, and al-Haafiz al-Zayla'i agreed with him in Nasab al-Raayah (273). So, it cannot be taken as evidence…" (185)

'Abdullah ibn Abi Awfa al-Aslami said: The Messenger of Allah (peace and blessings of Allah be upon him) came out to us and said: "Whoever has need of something from Allah or any one of His creation, let him do Wudu and pray two Rak'ahs, then let him say, 'There is no god but Allah, the Forbearing, the Most Generous. Glory be to Allah, Lord of the mighty Throne. Praise be to Allah, the Lord of the worlds. O Allah, I ask You for Your Mercy and Forgiveness and I ask You for all good things and for safety from all sins. I ask You not to leave any sin without forgiving it or any distress without relieving it, or any need which it pleases You to fulfil without fulfilling it for me.' Then let him ask Allah for whatever matter of this world or the Hereafter that he wishes, for it will be fulfilled." (Ibn Majah, Iqamat al-Salah wa'l-Sunnah, 1374) Al-Tirmdihi said: "This is a ghareeb (strange) Hadith, and concerning its isnad it was said: Faid ibn 'Abd al-Rahman is weak in Hadith.

The author of al-Sunan wa'l-Mubtada'at said, after mentioning what al-Tirmidhi said concerning Faid ibn 'Abd al-Rahman: Ahmad said: "He is matruk (left, i.e. his Hadith is not to be accepted), and Ibn al-'Arabi described him as da'eef (weak). And he said: "You know what is said concerning this Hadith. It is better and more perfect and safer for you to make Du'a to Allah in the depths of the night and between the Adhan and Iqamah and at the end of every prayer before the Taslim; and on Fridays, for then there are times when Du'a is answered; and when breaking one's fast. For your Lord says: *"Invoke Me [i.e. believe in My Oneness (Islamic Monotheism) and ask Me for anything] I will respond to your (invocation)." (Qur'an, Fussilat 40:60) "And when My slaves ask you (O Muhammad) concerning Me, then (answer them), I am indeed near (to them by My Knowledge). I respond to the invocations of the supplicant when he calls on Me (without any mediator or intercessor)." (Qur'an, Al-Baqarah 2:186) "And (all) the Most Beautiful Names belong to Allah, so call on Him by them"* (Qur'an, Al-A'raf 7:180) (Al-Sunan wa'l-Mubtada'at by al-Shuqayri, p.124) (185)

137. Prohibition of Heresies in Religion

Allah, the Exalted, says:

"For that is Allah, your Lord, the Truth. And what can be beyond Truth except error? So how are you averted?" (Qur'an, Yunus 10:32)

"O you who have believed, obey Allah and obey the Messenger and those in authority among you. And if you disagree over anything, refer it to Allah and the Messenger, if you should believe in Allah and the Last Day. That is the best (way) and best in result." (Qur'an, An-Nisa 4:59)

"And verily, this is My Straight Path, so follow it, and follow not (other) paths, for they will separate you away from His Path." (Qur'an, Al-An'am 6:153)

Other Verse: Ali 'Imran 3:31.

Narrated Aisha (May Allah be pleased with her): The Messenger of Allah (peace and blessings be upon him) said, "If anyone introduces in our matter something which does not belong to it, will be rejected." (Bukhari and Muslim)

Commentary: This Hadith lays down a very important principle. Unfortunately, Muslims have not attached any importance to this Hadith and the principle given in it with the result that innovations in the Deen have become so common that they have been taken for true Deen; our people act upon them and are made to practice them. One reason for this is their lack of education and ignorance about Deen. The second reason is their lack of understanding of the principle prescribed in this Hadith although it is stated in very explicit terms. The principle that we learn from this Hadith is that every such action or activity is innovation which is done as a virtue and to gain the Pleasure of Allah but is not consonant with the teachings of the Qur'an and Sunnah, or which does not agree with the interpretation of the Nuss (text) given by the Companions of the Prophet (peace and blessings be upon him) or their successors (Tabi'un). The reason being that the period of the Companions and the Tabi'un is the Khair-ul-Qurun (the best of all generations). Thus, any action or activity that is deprived of the support of these generations falls in the category of heresies. (186)

Narrated Jabir (May Allah be pleased with him): "Whenever the Messenger of Allah (peace and blessings be upon him) delivered a Khutbah, his eyes would become red, his tone loud and he showed anger as if he were warning us against an army. He (peace and blessings be upon him) would say, "The enemy is about to attack you in the morning and the enemy is advancing against you in the evening." He would further say, "I am sent with the final Hour like these two fingers of mine." Messenger of Allah (peace and blessings be upon him) held up his index finger and the middle finger together to illustrate. He used to add: "To proceed, the best speech is the Book of Allah and the best guidance is the guidance of Muhammad (peace and blessings be upon him), the worst practice is the introduction of new practices in Islam and every Bid'ah is a misguidance." He would also say, "I am, in respect of rights, nearer to every believer than his own self. He who leaves an estate, it belongs to his heirs, and he who leaves a debt, it is my responsibility to pay it off." (Muslim)

138. Religious Excessiveness

Allah, the Exalted, says:

"Allah intends for you ease and does not intend for you hardship." (Qur'an, Al-Baqarah 2:185)

"Say (O Muhammad SAW): "Who has forbidden the adoration with clothes given by Allah, which He has produced for his slaves, and At-Taiyibat [all kinds of Halal (lawful) things] of food?" Say: "They are, in the life of this world, for those who believe, (and) exclusively for them (believers) on the Day of Resurrection (the disbelievers will not share them)." Thus, We explain the Ayat (Islamic Laws) in detail for people who have knowledge." (Qur'an, Al-A'raf 7:32)

"Allah burdens not a person beyond his scope. He gets reward for that (good) which he has earned, and he is punished for that (evil) which he has earned." (Qur'an, Al-Baqarah 2:286)

Juwairiyah bint Al-Harith (May Allah be pleased with her), the Mother of the Believers, reported: The Prophet (peace and blessings be upon him) came out from my apartment in the morning as I was busy in performing the dawn prayer. He came back in the forenoon and found me sitting there. The Prophet (peace and blessings be upon him) said, "Are you still in the same position as I left you." I replied in the affirmative. Thereupon the Prophet said, "I recited four words three times after I had left you. If these are to be weighed against all you have recited since morning, these will be heavier. These are: Subhan-Allahi wa bihamdihi, 'adada khalqihi, wa rida nafsihi, wa zinatah 'arshihi, wa midada kalimatihi [Allah is free from imperfection and I begin with His Praise, as many times as the number of His creatures, in accordance with His good Pleasure, equal to the weight of His Throne and equal to the ink that may be used in recording the words (for His Praise)]." (Muslim)

Narrated Anas bin Malik: The Prophet (peace and blessings be upon him) said, "Facilitate things to people (concerning religious matters), and do not make it hard for them and give them good tidings and do not make them run away (from Islam)." (Bukhari)

Narrated Anas bin Malik: "A group of three men came to the houses of the wives of the Prophet (peace and blessings be upon him) asking how the Prophet (peace and blessings be upon him) worshiped (Allah), and when they were informed about that, they considered their worship insufficient and said, "Where are we from the Prophet (peace be upon him) as his past and future sins have been forgiven." Then one of them said, "I will offer the prayer throughout the night forever." The other said, "I will fast throughout the year and will not break my fast." The third said, "I will keep away from the women and will not marry forever." Allah's Messenger (peace and blessings be upon him) came to them and said, "Are you the same people who said so-and-so? By Allah, I am more submissive to Allah and more afraid of Him than you; yet I fast and break my fast, I do sleep and I also marry women." (Bukhari)

Narrated 'Abdullah bin 'Amr bin Al-'As: Allah's Messenger (peace and blessings be upon him) said, "O 'Abdullah! Have I not been informed that you fast all the day and stand in prayer all night?" I said, "Yes, O Allah's Messenger!" He (peace and blessings be upon him) said, "Do not do that! Observe the fast sometimes and also leave them (the fast) at other times; stand up for the prayer at night and also sleep at night. Your body has a right over you, your eyes have a right over you and your wife has a right over you." (Bukhari)

Narrated 'Aisha (May Allah have mercy on her): Once the Prophet (peace and blessings be upon him) came while a woman was sitting with me. He said, "Who is she?" I replied, "She is so and so," and told him about her (excessive) praying. He said disapprovingly, "Do (good) deeds which is within your capacity (without being overtaxed) as Allah does not get tired (of giving rewards) but (surely) you will get tired and the best deed (act of worship) in the sight of Allah is that which is done regularly." (Bukhari)

Narrated Abu Hurairah: The Messenger of Allah (peace and blessings be upon him) said: "Be moderate and adhere to moderation, for there is no one among you who will be saved by his deeds." They said: "Not even you, O Messenger of Allah?" He said: "Not even me. Unless Allah encompasses me with Mercy and Grace from Him." (Ibn Majah)

139. Prohibition of Monasticism

Allah, the Exalted, says:

"Then, We sent after them, Our Messengers, and We sent 'Iesa (Jesus) son of Maryam (Mary), and gave him the Injeel (Gospel). And We ordained in the hearts of those who followed him, compassion and Mercy. But the Monasticism which they invented for themselves, We did not prescribe for them, but (they sought it) only to please Allah therewith, but that they did not observe it with the right observance.

140. Avoiding Jihad

Allah, the Exalted, says:

"O you who believe! When you meet those, who disbelieve marching for war, then turn not your backs to them. And whoever shall turn his back to them on that day - unless he turns aside for the sake of fighting or withdraws to a company then he, indeed, becomes deserving of Allah's Wrath and his abode is Hell; and an evil destination shall it be." (Qur'an, Al-Anfal 8:15-16)

"Jihad (holy fighting in Allah's Cause) is ordained for you (Muslims) though you dislike it, and it may be that you dislike a thing which is good for you and that you like a thing which is bad for you. Allah knows but you do not know." (Qur'an, Al-Baqarah 2:216)

"Remember` when you were running far away` in panic`—not looking at anyone—while the Messenger was calling to you from behind! So, Allah rewarded your disobedience with distress upon distress. Now, do not grieve over the victory you were denied or the injury you suffered. And Allah is All-Aware of what you do." Qur'an, Ali 'Imran 3:153)

Other Verse: At-Tawbah 9:111, As-Saf 61:10-13.

Narrated Ibn Masud (May Allah be pleased with him): "I asked the Messenger of Allah (peace and blessings be upon him): "Which action is dearest to Allah?" He (peace and blessings be upon him) replied, "Performing As-Salat (the prayer) at its earliest fixed time." I asked, "What is next (in goodness)?" He (peace and blessings be upon him) said, "Kindness towards parents." I asked, "What is next (in goodness)?" He (peace and blessings be upon him) said, "To participate in Jihad in the Cause of Allah." (Bukhari and Muslim)

Narrated Abu Sa'id Al-Khudri (May Allah be pleased with him): "A man came to the Messenger of Allah (peace and blessings be upon him) and said, "Who is the best among men?" He (peace and blessings be upon him) replied, "A believer who strives in the way of

Allah with his wealth and life." The man asked again, "Who is next to him (in excellence)?" He (peace and blessings be upon him) said, "Next to him is a man who is engaged in worshipping his Rubb in a mountain valley, leaving the people secure from his mischief." (Bukhari and Muslim)

Sahl bin Sa'd (May Allah be pleased with him) reported: The Messenger of Allah (peace and blessings be upon him) said, "Observing Ribat (e.g. guarding the Islamic frontier for the sake of Allah) for a single day is far better than the world and all that it contains. A place in Jannah as small as the whip of your horse is far better than the world and all that it contains. An endeavor (fighting) in the Cause of Allah in the evening or in the morning is far better than the world and all that it contains." (Bukhari and Muslim)

Fadalah ibn 'Ubayd, Salman Al-Farisi and 'Uqbah ibn 'Amir al-Juhani (May Allah be pleased with them) reported that the Prophet (May Allah's peace and blessings be upon him) said: "The actions of every dead person come to a halt except the one who is garrisoned on the frontier in the way of Allah. His deeds will keep growing till the Day of Judgment, and he will be secure from the trial in the grave." (Tirmidhi, Abu Dawud and Ahmad) (https://hadeethenc.com/en/browse/hadith/2756)
Salman al-Farisi (May Allah be pleased with him) reported: "I heard the Messenger of Allah (peace and blessings be upon him) as saying, "Observing Ribat (guarding the Muslim frontiers) in the way of Allah for a day and a night is far better than observing Saum (fasting) for a whole month and standing in Salat (prayer) in all its nights. If a person dies (while performing Ribat), he will receive the reward for his righteous deeds perpetually, will receive his provision and will be saved from the trials of the grave." (Muslim)

Commentary: Good deeds of a Muslim who dies or is martyred on the frontier will perpetuate and will be credited to his account till the Day of Resurrection; and like all other martyrs, sustenance will be provided to him even after his death. As Allah says: *'Think not of those as dead who are killed in the way of Allah. Nay, they are alive, with their Rubb, and they have provision." (3:169)* (187)

Abu Hurairah (May Allah be pleased with him) reported: The Messenger of Allah (peace and blessings be upon him) said, "Allah guarantees that he who goes out to fight in His way believing in Him and affirming the Truth of His Messenger, will either be admitted to Jannah or will be brought back to his home (safely) from where he has set out, with whatever reward or share of booty he may have gained. By Him in Whose Hand Muhammad's soul is, if a person is wounded in the way of Allah, he will come on the Day of Resurrection with his wound in the same condition as it was on the day when he received it; its colour will be the colour of blood but its smell will be the smell of musk. By Him in Whose Hand Muhammad's soul is, if it were not to be too hard upon the Muslims, I would not lag behind any expedition to fight in the Cause of Allah, but I have neither abundant means to provide them conveyance (horses) nor all other Muslims have it, and it will be hard on them to remain behind when I go forth (for Jihad). By Him in Whose Hand Muhammad's soul is, I love to fight in the way of Allah and get killed, to fight again and get killed and to fight again and get killed." (Muslim)

Abu Hurairah (May Allah be pleased with him) reported: "One of the Prophet's Companions came upon a valley containing a rivulet of fresh water and was delighted by it. He reflected: 'I wish to withdraw from people and settle in this valley; but I won't do so without the permission of the Messenger of Allah (peace and blessings be upon him). This was mentioned to the Messenger of Allah (peace and blessings be upon him) and he said (to the man), "Do not do that, for when any of you remains in Allah's way, it is better for him than performing Salah (prayer) in his house for seventy years. Do you not wish that Allah should forgive you and admit you to Jannah? Fight in Allah's way, for he who fights in Allah's Cause as long as the time between two consecutive turns of milking a she-camel, will be surely admitted to Jannah." (Tirmidhi)

Abu Sa'id Al-Khudri (May Allah be pleased with him) reported: The Messenger of Allah (peace and blessings be upon him) said, "If anyone is pleased with Allah as his Rubb, with Islam as his religion and with Muhammad (peace and blessings be upon him) as (Allah's) Messenger, surely, he will be entitled to enter Jannah." Abu Sa'id was delighted with this and requested the Messenger of Allah (peace and blessings be upon him) to repeat it. He (peace and blessings be upon him) repeated it again and then said, "There is also another act by which Allah will elevate the position of a (pious believing) slave in Jannah to a grade one hundred degrees higher. And the distance between any two grades is equal to the distance between heaven and earth." He asked the Messenger of Allah (peace and blessings be upon him) what it was and he (peace and blessings be upon him) replied, "Jihad in the way of Allah; Jihad in the way of Allah." (Muslim)

Abu Bakr bin Abu Musa Al-Ash'ari reported: "I heard my father saying in the presence of the enemy: "The Messenger of Allah (peace and blessings be upon him) said, "The gates of Jannah are under the shades of the swords." A man with a shaggy appearance got up and said, "O Abu Musa! Did you hear the Messenger of Allah (peace and blessings be upon him) say that in person?" Abu Musa replied in the affirmative; so, he returned to his companions and said: "I tender you farewell greetings." Then he broke the scabbard of his sword and threw it away. He rushed towards the enemy with his sword and fought with it till he was martyred. (Muslim)

Narrated Abu 'Abs 'Abdur-Rahman bin Jabr (May Allah be pleased with him): The Messenger of Allah (peace and blessings be upon him) said, "It will not happen that the feet soiled with dust while (doing Jihad) in the way of Allah, will be touched by the Fire (of Hell)." (Bukhari)

Abu Umamah (May Allah be pleased with him) reported: The Messenger of Allah (peace and blessings be upon him) said, "The best of charities is to provide canopy in the Cause of Allah, to pay wages to a servant in the way of Allah, and to provide a camel in the way of Allah (to be used by a Mujahid)." (Tirmidhi)

Narrated Anas (May Allah be pleased with him): The Prophet (peace and blessings be upon him) said,
"No one who has entered Jannah will desire to return to this world even if he should be given all that the world contains, except a martyr. For he will learn that he should return to the

world and be killed ten times on account of the dignity that he will experience by virtue of his martyrdom."

Narrated 'Abdullah bin 'Amr bin Al-'As (May Allah be pleased with him): The Messenger of Allah (peace and blessings be upon him) said, "Allah forgives every sin of a martyr, except his debt." (Muslim)

Abu Qataadah (May Allah be pleased with him) reported: "The Messenger of Allah (peace and blessings be upon him) stood up among his Companions and said, "Jihad in the way of Allah and belief in Allah (with all His Attributes) are the most meritorious of actions." A man stood up and said: "O Messenger of Allah! Inform me if I am killed in the way of Allah, will my sins be blotted out?" The Messenger of Allah (peace and blessings be upon him) said, "Yes, in case you are killed in the way of Allah and you remained patient, hopeful of reward, and advancing forward without retracing back (i.e. while fighting)." Then he said, "What was your question?" He inquired again: "Inform me, if I am killed in the way of Allah, will all my sins be blotted out?" The Messenger of Allah (peace and blessings be upon him) replied, "If you remained patient, hopeful of reward and always fought without turning your back upon enemy, everything, except debt, will be forgiven. Jibreel has told me this." (Muslim)

Anas (May Allah be pleased with him) reported: "My uncle Anas bin An-Nadr (May Allah be pleased with him) was absent from the battle of Badr. He said: "O Messenger of Allah! I was absent from the first battle you fought against the pagans. (By Allah!) if Allah gives me a chance to fight against the pagans, no doubt, Allah will see how (bravely) I will fight." On the Day of Uhud, when the Muslims turned their backs and fled, he said, "O Allah! I apologize to You for what these (i.e. his companions) have done, and I denounce what these (i.e. the pagans) have done." Then he advanced and Sa'd bin Mu'adh met him. He said: "O Sa'd bin Mu'adh! By the Rubb of An-Nadr, Jannah! I am smelling its aroma coming from before (the mountain of) Uhud." Later on, Sa'd said: "O Messenger of Allah! I cannot achieve or do what he (i.e. Anas bin An-Nadr) did. We found more than eighty wounds by swords, spears and arrows on his body. We found him dead and his body was mutilated so badly that none except his sister could recognize him by his finger." We used to think that the following Ayah was revealed concerning him and other men of his sort: *"Among the believers are men who have been true to their covenant with Allah (i.e. they have gone out for Jihad, and showed not their backs to the disbelievers), of them some have fulfilled their obligations (i.e. have been martyred)." (33:23)* (https://sunnah.com/riyadussalihin:1317)

Narrated Samurah (May Allah be pleased with him): The Messenger of Allah (peace and blessings be upon him) said, "Last night two men (angels) came to me (in a dream) and made me ascend a tree and then admitted me into a nice and excellent house, the like of which I have never seen before. One of them said: 'This house is the house of martyrs.'" (Bukhari)

Narrated 'Abdullah bin Abu Aufa (May Allah be pleased with him): "On one occasion the Messenger of Allah (peace and blessings be upon him) was confronting the enemy. He waited until the sun had declined. Then he stood up to address the people and said, "O people! Do not wish for an encounter with the enemy. Pray to Allah to grant you safety; (but) when you encounter them, show patience and know that Jannah is under the shades of the swords." Then he (peace and blessings be upon him) said: "Allahumma munzilal-kitab, wa mujriyas-sahab, wa hazimal-Ahzab, ihzimhum wansurna alaihim (O Allah, Revealer of the Book, Disperser of the clouds, Defeater of the Confederates, put our enemy to rout and support us against them)." (Bukhari and Muslim)

As-Sa'ib bin Yazid (May Allah be pleased with him) reported: "When the Prophet (peace and blessings be upon him) returned from the battle of Tabuk, people went out from Al-Madinah to meet him and I also met him with other children at Thaniyah-tul-Wada."(Abu Dawud)

Abu Umamah (May Allah be pleased with him) reported: The Prophet (peace and blessings be upon him) said, "He who neither takes part in fighting nor equips a warrior, nor looks after his (the warrior's) family, will be afflicted by severe calamities before the Day of Resurrection." (Abu Dawud)

Anas (May Allah be pleased with him) reported: The Prophet (peace and blessings be upon him) said,
"Fight the polytheists with your wealth, lives and tongues." (Abu Dawud)

Narrated Abu Hurairah (May Allah be pleased with him): The Messenger of Allah (peace and blessings be upon him) said, "Whoever dies without having fought in the Cause of Allah or without having thought of fighting (in the Cause of Allah), will die with one characteristic of hypocrisy in him." (Muslim)
(https://hadeethenc.com/en/browse/hadith/6404)

Abu Hurairah (May Allah be pleased with him) reported that the Messenger of Allah (May Allah's peace and blessings be upon him) said: "No one is wounded in the way of Allah except that he comes on the Day of Judgment with his wound bleeding; the color is that of blood, and the smell is that of musk."
(Bukhari and Muslim) (https://hadeethenc.com/en/browse/hadith/2991)

141. Islamic Rules of War

Allah, the Exalted, says:

"And fight in the Way of Allah those who fight you, but transgress not the limits. Truly, Allah likes not the transgressors. [This Verse is the first one that was revealed in connection with Jihad, but it was supplemented by another (V.9:36)]." (Qur'an, Al-Baqarah 2:190)

"Those who believe, fight in the Cause of Allah, and those who disbelieve, fight in the cause of Taghut (Satan, etc.). So, fight you against the friends of Shaitan (Satan); Ever feeble indeed is the plot of Shaitan (Satan)." (Qur'an, An-Nisa 4:76)

"O you who believe! When you meet (an enemy) force, take a firm stand against them and remember the Name of Allah much (both with tongue and mind), so that you may be successful. And obey Allah and His Messenger, and do not dispute (with one another) lest you lose courage and your strength depart, and be patient. Surely, Allah is with those who are As-Sabirin (the patient ones, etc.)." (Qur'an, Al-Anfal 8:45-46)

Other Verses: *Al-Hajj 22:39-41, An-Nisa 4:75, Al-Insan 76:8-9, At-Tawbah 9:6)*
The Muslims have been exhorted to observe five principles of war:

1. Be steadfast in the face of the enemy.
2. Have full reliance on the help of Allah and remember Him much.
3. Have the unity of purpose and solidarity of corporate life always before your eyes.
4. Be fully aware of the lofty purpose before you in fighting.
5. Don't be proud and boastful in your attitude and behavior. (Muslim)

Abu Bakr (May Allah be pleased with him) gave to his army while sending her on the expedition to the Syrian borders is permeated with the noble spirit with which the war in Islam is permitted. He said: "Stop, O people, that I may give you ten rules for your guidance in the battlefield. Do not commit treachery or deviate from the Right Path. You must not mutilate dead bodies. Neither kill a child, nor a woman, nor an aged man. Bring no harm to the trees, nor burn them with fire, especially those which are fruitful. Slay not ary of the enemy's flock. save for your food. You are likely to pass by people who have devoted their lives to monastic services; leave them alone" (Muslim)
'Umar, the Second Caliph, addressed to Sa'd b. Abu Waqqas, "Always search your minds and hearts and stress upon your men the need of perfect integrity and sincerity in the Cause of Allah. There should be no material end before them in laying down their lives but they should deem it a means whereby they can please their Lord and entitle themselves to His favor: such a spirit of selflessness should be inculcated in the minds of those who unfortunately lack it. Be firm in the thicket of the battle as Allah helps man according to the perseverance that he shows in the cause of His faith and he would be rewarded in accordance with the spirit of sacrifice which he displays for the sake of the Lord. Be careful that those who have been entrusted to your care receive no harm at your hands and are never deprived of any of their legitimate rights." (Muslm) (https://www.iium.edu.my/deed/hadith/muslim/019_smt.html)
Abu Hurairah (May Allah have mercy on him) reported: The Messenger of Allah (peace and blessings be upon him) said: "When any one of you fights with his brother, he should avoid his face for Allah created Adam in His own Image." (Muslim)

Abu Hurairah and Jabir (May Allah be pleased with them) reported: The Prophet (peace and blessings be upon him) said, "War is deception." (Bukhari and Muslim)

Islam is the Religion of mercy and justice. Islamic Law prohibits the use of force for material gain or revenge.

142. Prohibition of Killing Women and Children in War

Narrated 'Abdullah that a woman was found killed in one of the battles fought by the Messenger of Allah (peace and blessings be upon him). He disapproved of the killing of women and children. (Muslim)

Abu Bakr (May Allah be pleased with him) gave to his army while sending her on the expedition to the Syrian borders is permeated with the noble spirit with which the war in Islam is permitted. He said: "Stop, O people, that I may give you ten rules for your guidance in the battlefield. Do not commit treachery or deviate from the Right Path. You must not mutilate dead bodies. Neither kill a child, nor a woman, nor an aged man…" (Muslim) (https://www.iium.edu.my/deed/hadith/muslim/019)

143. Treatment of Prisoners of War in Islam

Allah, the Exalted, says

"And they give food, in spite of their love for it (or for the love of Him), to the Miskeen (the poor), the orphan and the captive, (Saying): 'We feed you seeking Allah's Countenance only. We wish for no reward, nor thanks from you.'" (Qur'an, Al-Insan 76:8-9)

War in Islam should not be waged for the sole purpose of shedding blood or seeking vengeance. If the Muslims capture the prisoners of war and take them to a place that has been prepared for them, they should not harm them or torture them with beatings, depriving them of food and water, leaving them out in the sun or the cold, burning them with fire or putting covers over their mouths, ears and eyes and putting them in cages like animals. Rather they should treat them with kindness and mercy, feed them well and encourage them to enter Islam.

Narrated Abu Hurairah: The Prophet (peace and blessings of Allah be upon him) sent some cavalry towards Najd and they brought a man from the tribe of Banu Hanifa who was called Thumama bin Uthal. They fastened him to one of the pillars of the Mosque. The Prophet went to him and said, "What have you got, O Thumama?" He replied," I have got a good thought, O Muhammad! If you should kill me, you would kill a person who has already killed somebody, and if you should set me free, you would do a favor to one who is grateful, and if you want property, then ask me whatever wealth you want." He was left till the next day when the Prophet (peace and blessings of Allah be upon him) said to him, "What have you got, Thumama? He said, "What I told you, i.e. if you set me free, you would do a favor to one who is grateful." The Prophet (peace and blessings of Allah be upon him) left him till the day after, when he said, "What have you got, O Thumama?" He said, "I have got what I told you. "On that the Prophet (peace and blessings of Allah be upon him) said, "Release Thumama." So, he (i.e. Thumama) went to a garden of date-palm trees near to the Mosque, took a bath (Ghusl) and then entered the Mosque and said, "I testify that None has the right to be worshipped except Allah, and also testify that Muhammad is His Apostle! By Allah, O Muhammad! There was no face on the surface of the earth most disliked by me than yours, but now your face has become the most beloved face to me. By Allah, there was no religion most disliked by me than yours, but now it is the most beloved religion to me. By Allah, there was no town most disliked by me than your town, but now it is the most beloved town to me. Your cavalry arrested me (at the time) when I was intending to perform the 'Umrah. And now what do you think?" The Prophet (peace and blessings of Allah be upon him) gave him good tidings (congratulated him) and ordered him to perform the 'Umrah. So, when he came to Makkah, someone said to him, "You have become a Sabian?" Thumama replied, "No! By Allah, I have embraced Islam with Muhammad, Apostle of Allah. No, by Allah! Not a single grain of wheat will come to you from Yamamah unless the Prophet gives his permission." (Bukhari)

The ruling on tying up prisoners:

It is well known that if prisoners are able to escape, they will not hesitate to do so, because they may be afraid of dying and they do not know what awaits them. Hence the Muslims were commanded to tie up their prisoners and to tie their hands to their necks, lest they run away. This is something that still happens and is well known to all people. The wisdom behind permitting the taking of prisoners is so as to weaken the enemy and ward off his evil by keeping him away from the battlefield so that he cannot be effective or play any role; it also creates a means of freeing Muslim prisoners by trading the prisoners whom we are holding.

Detaining prisoners

Prisoners should be detained until it is decided what is the best move. The ruler of the Muslims should detain prisoners until he decides what is in the Muslims' best interests. He may ransom them for money, or exchange them for Muslim prisoners, or release them for nothing in return, or distribute them among the Muslims as slaves, or kill the men, but not the women and children, because the Prophet (peace and blessings of Allah be upon him) forbade killing the latter. The purpose behind detaining prisoners is so that the Muslims may be protected from their evil. The Prophet (peace and blessings of Allah be upon him) used to enjoin the Muslims to treat prisoners well, whereas the Romans and those who came before them the Assyrians and Pharaohs, all used to put out their prisoners' eyes with hot irons, and flay them alive, feeding their skins to dogs, such that the prisoners preferred death to life. (188)

144. Misappropriation of Spoils of War, Muslim Funds or Zakah

Allah, the Exalted, says:

"It is not for any Prophet to take illegally a part of booty (Ghulul), and whosoever deceives his companions as regards the booty, he shall bring forth on the Day of Resurrection that

which he took (illegally). Then every person shall be paid in full what he has earned, - and they shall not be dealt with unjustly." (Qur'an, Ali 'Imran 3:161)

"Is then one who follows (seeks) the good Pleasure of Allah (by not taking illegally a part of the booty) like the one who draws on himself the Wrath of Allah (by taking a part of the booty illegally - Ghulul)? - his abode is Hell - and worst, indeed is that destination!" (Qur'an, Ali 'Imran 3:162)

"No Prophet could ever act dishonestly. If any person acts dishonestly, he shall, on the Day of Judgment, restore what he misappropriated, then shall every soul receive its due whatever it earned." (Qur'an, Al-Baqarah 2:161)

Narrated Simak bin Harb, that Mus'ab bin Sa'd said: "Abdullah bin 'Umar came to visit Ibn 'Amir when he was sick and he said: 'Won't you supplicate to Allah for me, O Ibn 'Umar?' He said: 'I heard the Messenger of Allah (peace and blessings be upon him) say: "No Salah is accepted without Wudu (purification), and no charity (is accepted) that comes from Ghulul (1)" and you were the governor of Al-Basrah.' (1) Goods pilfered from the spoils of war prior to their authorized distribution." (Muslim)

145. Impatience

Allah, the Exalted, says:

"So, wait patiently (O Muhammad SAW) for the decision of your Lord, for verily, you are under Our Eyes, and glorify the Praises of your Lord when you get up from sleep." (Qur'an, At-Tur 52:48)

"O you who believe! Seek help in patience and As-Salah (the prayer). Truly! Allah is with As-Sabirin (the patient ones, etc.)." (Qur'an, Al-Baqarah 2:153)

"And seek help in patience and As-Salat (the prayer) and truly it is extremely heavy and hard except for Al-Khashi'un [i.e. the true believers in Allah - those who obey Allah with full submission, fear much from His Punishment, and believe in His Promise (Paradise, etc.) and in His Warnings (Hell, etc.)]." (Qur'an, Al-Baqarah 2:45)

Other Verses: *Taha 20:130, Al-Baqarah 2:155–157 and 2:177, Al-'Asr 103:2-3, An-Nahl 16:126-127, Al-Ma'arij 70:19-23.*

Abu Hurairah (May Allah be pleased with him) reported that the Prophet (May Allah's peace and blessings be upon him) said: "The supplication of one of you is answered, as long as he is not in haste, saying: 'I have supplicated to my Lord, but He did not answer me.'" In another narration by Muslim: "The supplication of a slave will continue to be answered, as long as he does not ask for a sin or sever a tie of kinship, and is not hasty." It was said: "O Messenger of Allah, what is hastiness?" He said: "It is to say: 'I have supplicated and supplicated, but I have not seen it has been answered.' He would then lose hope and stop supplicating." (Bukhari and Muslim) (https://hadeethenc.com/en/browse/hadith/3232)

Narated Abu Said Al-Khudri: Some Ansari persons asked for (something) from Allah's Apostle (peace and blessings be upon him) and he gave them. They again asked him for (something) and he again gave them. And then they asked him and he gave them again till all that was with him finished. And then he said, "If I had anything, I would not keep it away from you. (Remember) Whoever abstains from asking others, Allah will make him contented, and whoever tries to make himself self-sufficient, Allah will make him self-sufficient. And whoever remains patient, Allah will make him patient. Nobody can be given a blessing better and greater than patience." (Bukhari)

Narrated Anas bin Malik: "The Prophet (peace and blessings be upon him) passed by a woman who was weeping beside a grave. He told her to fear Allah and be patient. She said to him, 'Go away, for you have not been afflicted with a calamity like mine.' And she did not recognize him. Then she was informed that he was the Prophet (peace and blessings be upon him). So, she went to the house of the Prophet (peace and blessings be upon him) and there she did not find any guard. Then she said to him, 'I did not recognize you.' He (peace and blessings be upon him) said, 'Verily, the patience is at the first stroke of a calamity.'" (Bukhari)

Narrated 'Ata bin Abi Rabah: "Ibn 'Abbas said to me, 'Shall I show you a woman of the people of Paradise?' I said, "Yes." He said, "This black lady came to the Prophet and said, 'I get attacks of epilepsy and my body becomes uncovered; please invoke Allah for me.' The Prophet (peace and blessings be upon him) said (to her), 'If you wish, be patient and you will have (enter) Paradise; and if you wish, I will invoke Allah to cure you.' She said, 'I will remain patient,' and added, 'but I become uncovered, so please invoke Allah for me that I may not become uncovered.' So, he invoked Allah for her.'" (Bukhari)

NO ONE IS MORE PATIENT THAN ALLAH IN BEARING OFFENSIVE THINGS

Abu Musa al-Ash'ari (May Allah be pleased with him) reported that the Prophet (May Allah's peace and blessings be upon him) said: "None or nothing is more patient about the offensive statements he hears than Allah. Verily, they ascribe a son to Him, yet He still grants them good health and sustenance."
(Bukhari and Muslim) (https://hadeethenc.com/en/browse/hadith/8299)

146. Fighting when Enemy Asked for a Peace

Allah, the Exalted, says:

"But if they incline to peace, you also incline to it, and (put your) trust in Allah. Verily, He is the All-Hearer, the All-Knower." (Qur'an, Al-Anfal 8:61)

147. Fighting Among the Believers Without Making Reconciliation

Allah, the Exalted, says:

"And if two parties or groups among the believers fall to fighting, then make peace between them both, but if one of them rebels against the other, then fight you (all) against the one that which rebels till it complies with the Command of Allah; then if it complies, then make reconciliation between them justly, and be equitable. Verily! Allah loves those who are equitable." (Qur'an, Al-Hujurat 49:9)

148. Frowning, Turning Away or Neglecting Those who Come to you Seeking Knowledge

Allah, the Exalted, says:

"(The Prophet (peace be upon him)) frowned and turned away, Because there came to him the blind man (i.e. 'Abdullah bin Umm-Maktum, who came to the Prophet (peace be upon him) while he was preaching to one or some of the Quraish chiefs). But what could tell you that per chance he might become pure (from sins)? Or that he might receive admonition, and that the admonition might profit him?" (Qur'an, 'Abasa 80:1-4)

149. Learning Sacred Knowledge for the Sake of this World or Concealing It

Allah, the Exalted, says:

"Indeed, those who conceal what We sent down of clear proofs and Guidance after We made it clear for the people in the Scripture - those are cursed by Allah and cursed by those who curse." (Qur'an, Al-Baqarah 2:159)
Abu Hurairah reported: The Messenger of Allah (peace and blessings be upon him) said: "Whoever is asked for knowledge and he conceals it, Allah will clothe him with a bridle of Fire on the Day of Resurrection." (Abu Dawud and Tirmidhi)

150. Killing Muslim

Allah, the Exalted, says:

"And whoever kills a believer intentionally, his recompense is Hell to abide therein; and the Wrath and the Curse of Allah are upon him, and a great punishment is prepared for him." (Qur'an, An-Nisa 4:93)

"The punishment of those who wage war against Allah and His Apostle and strive to make mischief in the land is only this, that they should be murdered or crucified, or their hands and their feet should be cut off on opposite sides, or they should be exiled; this shall be as a disgrace for them in this world, and in the Hereafter they shall have a grievous chastisement, Except those who repent before you have them in your power; so know that Allah is Forgiving, Merciful." (Qur'an, Al-Ma'idah 5:33-34)

"Because of that We ordained for the Children of Israel that if anyone killed a person not in retaliation of murder, or (and) to spread mischief in the land - it would be as if he killed all mankind, and if anyone saved a life, it would be as if he saved the life of all mankind. And indeed, there came to them Our Messengers with clear proofs, evidences and signs, even then after that many of them continued to exceed the limits (e.g. by doing oppression unjustly and exceeding beyond the limits set by Allah by committing the Major sins) in the land!" (Qur'an, Al-Ma'idah 5:32)

Other Verse: Al-'Alaq 96:6-19.

Narrated 'Abdullah (May Allah have mercy on him): The Prophet (peace and blessings be upon him) said,
"Abusing a Muslim is Fusuq (an evil doing) and killing him is Kufr (disbelief)." (Bukhari)

Narrated Abdullah bin Masud (May Allah have mercy on him): The Messenger of Allah (peace and blessings be upon him) said: "It is not permissible to spill the blood of a Muslim except in three (instances): the married person who commits adultery, a life for a life and the one who forsakes his religion and separates from the community." (Bukhari and Muslim)

151. Supplying Weapons to Disbelievers which Shall be Used Against Muslims

Abu Hurairah (May Allah be pleased with him) said: The Messenger of Allah (peace and blessings be upon him) said, "He who takes up arms against us, is none of us; and he who cheats us, is none of us." (Muslim)

152. Prohibition of Reviling a Muslim Without any Cause

Allah, the Exalted, says:

"And those who annoy believing men and women undeservedly, bear on themselves the crime of slander and plain sin." (Qur'an Al-Ahzab 33:58)

"And make yourself gentle to the believers." (Qur'an, Al-Hijr 15:88)

Ibn Masud (May Allah be pleased with him) reported: The Messenger of Allah (peace and blessings be upon him) said, "Reviling a Muslim is Fusuq (disobedience of Allah) and killing him is (tantamount to) disbelief." (Bukhari and Muslim)

Abu Dharr (May Allah be pleased with him) reported: "I heard the Messenger of Allah (peace and blessings be upon him) saying, "When any Muslim accuses another Muslim of sin or of disbelief, the reproach rebounds upon the one who utters it, if the other person is not deserving of it." (Bukhari)

Commentary: What this Hadith stresses is that one should never say about a Muslim that he is sinful (Fasiq) or disbeliever (Kafir) when he is not so. The reason is that in that case, one who says it, will be held Fasiq or Kafir. (189)

Abu Hurairah (May Allah be pleased with him) said: The Messenger of Allah (peace and blessings be upon him) said, "When two persons indulge in abusing each other, the beginner will be the sinner so long as the oppressed does not transgress the limits." (Muslim)

Abu Hurairah (May Allah be pleased with him) said: "A drunkard was brought to the Prophet (peace be upon him). He said, "Give him a beating." Then some beat him with their hands, some with their shoes, and some with (a folded) piece of cloth. When he left, someone said to him: "May Allah disgrace you!" The Prophet (peace be upon him) said, "Do not help Satan overcome him by uttering such words." (Bukhari)

Abu Hurairah (May Allah be pleased with him) said: "I heard the Messenger of Allah (peace and blessings be upon him) saying, "He who accuses his slave of Zina will receive the punishment (Hadd) of slander on the Day of Resurrection, unless the accusation of Zina was true." (Bukhari and Muslim)

153. Prohibition of Spying on Muslims and to be Inquisitive About Others

Allah, the Exalted, says:

"And do not spy." *(Qur'an, Al-Hujurat 49:12)*

"And those who annoy believing men and women undeservedly, bear on themselves the crime of slander and plain sin." *(Qur'an, Al-Ahzab 33:58)*

Narrated Abu Hurairah (May Allah be pleased with him): The Messenger of Allah (peace and blessings be upon him) said, "Beware of suspicion, for suspicion is the worst of false tales. Do not look for other's faults. Do not spy one another, and do not practice Najsh (means to offer a high price for something in order to allure another customer who is interested in the thing). Do not be jealous of one another and do not nurse enmity against one another. Do not sever ties with one another. Become the slaves of Allah, and be brothers to one another as He commanded. A Muslim is the brother of a Muslim. He should neither oppress him nor humiliate him. The piety is here! The piety is here!" While saying so he pointed towards his chest. "It is enough evil for a Muslim to look down upon his Muslim brother. All things of a Muslim are inviolable for his brother in Faith: his blood, his wealth and his honor. Verily, Allah does not look to your bodies nor to your faces but He looks to your hearts and your deeds."

Narrated Muawiyah (May Allah be pleased with him): "I heard the Messenger of Allah (peace and blessings be upon him) saying, "If you find faults with Muslims, you will corrupt them." (Abu Dawud)

Commentary: If a Muslim looks for the defects of another and hunts for his weaknesses, other Muslims will also adopt the same attitude towards him, and this situation will create dissension and conflict in society. This also will make them fall prey to sins and make them persistent in committing them. For this reason, spying and finding faults with Muslims has been prohibited by Shariah. (190)

It has been reported that a man was brought before Abdullah bin Masud (May Allah be pleased with him) because his beard was giving out smell of wine. Ibn Masud said: "We have been prohibited from spying (on Muslims) and finding faults (with them). But we can take to task only and only if the sin is overt." (Abu Dawud)

Salamah ibn al-Akwa' (May Allah be pleased with him) said: "A spy from among the polytheists came to the Prophet (May Allah's peace and blessings be upon him) while he was on a journey. The spy stayed with the Prophet's Companions (May Allah be pleased with them) and talked to them, and then he left. Thereupon, the Prophet (May Allah's peace and blessings be upon him) said: 'Go in pursuit of him and kill him.' I killed him, and the Prophet (May Allah's peace and blessings be upon him) gave me his belongings (as an extra share)." According to another Hadith, the Prophet (May Allah's peace and blessings be upon him) said: "Who killed the spy?" They (the Companions) said: "Ibn al-Akwa'" He said: "All the belongings of the killed man are for him (Salamah)." (Muslim - Bukhari and Muslim) (https://hadeethenc.com/en/browse/hadith/2939)

154. Prohibition of Despising Muslims

Allah, the Exalted, says:

"O you who believe! Let not a group scoff at another group, it may be that the latter are better than the former; nor let (some) women scoff at other women, it may be that the latter are better than the former, nor defame one another, nor insult one another by nicknames. How bad is it, to insult one's brother after having Faith [i.e. to call your Muslim brother (a faithful believer) as: "O sinner", or "O wicked", etc.]. And whosoever does not repent, then such are indeed Zalimun (wrongdoers, etc.)." (Qur'an, Al-Hujurat 49:11)

Narrated Abu Hurairah (May Allah be pleased with him): The Messenger of Allah (peace and blessings be upon him) said, "It is enough evil for a Muslim to look down upon his (Muslim) brother." (Muslim)

Narrated Ibn Masud (May Allah be pleased with him): The Prophet (peace and blessings be upon him) said, "The haughty, even with pride equal to a mustard seed in his heart, will not enter Jannah." A man enquired: "What about that a person likes fine dress and fine shoes?" He said: "Allah is Beautiful and likes beauty. Pride amounts to disclaiming Truth out of self-esteem and despising people." (Muslim)

Narrated Jundub bin 'Abdullah (May Allah be pleased with him): The Messenger of Allah (peace and blessings be upon him) said, "Once someone said: 'By Allah! Allah will not forgive such and such (a person).'" Thereupon Allah, the Exalted and the Glorious, said: "Who is he who takes an oath in My Name that I will not grant pardon to so-and-so? fruitless." (Muslim)

Commentary: Some people become self-conceited as a result of their excessive worship to the point that they start disparaging and making low estimates of their fellow Muslims and their deeds, little knowing that God, Glorious is He, is of vast Forgiveness. They do not realize that if Allah so wills, He can destroy all their deeds and consign them to Hell and send the other people who have been disparaged and underestimated to Jannah. Therefore, one should never become proud of his piety nor should one consider others of little value or good deeds, as only Allah Alone knows what is inside our hearts. (191)

155. Harming and Insulting Muslims

Allah, the Exalted, says:

"And never think that Allah is unaware of what the wrongdoers do. He only delays them for a Day when eyes will stare (in horror)." (Qur'an, Ibrahim 14:42)

"And those who harm believing men and believing women for (something) other than what they have earned have certainly born upon themselves a slander and manifest sin." (Qur'an, Al-Ahzab 33:58)

"That is because Allah is the Protector of those who believe." (Qur'an, Muhammad 47:11)

Other Verses: Al-Bayyinah 98:7, Al-Munafiqun 63:8, Al-'Alaq 96:6-19.

Abu Barzah reported: "I said, 'O Prophet of Allah, teach me something that will benefit me." The Prophet (peace and blessings be upon him) said, **"Remove harmful things from the roads of the Muslims."** (Muslim)

Abdullah ibn Masud reported: The Messenger of Allah (peace and blessings be upon him) said: "The believer does not taunt others, he does not curse others, he does not use profanity, and he does not abuse others." (Tirmidhi)

Answer to Insults: No better punishment for fools than to be silent

Al-Qurtubi reported: "A man insulted Qanbar, who was under the patronage of Ali ibn Abi Talib (May Allah be pleased with him). Ali called out to him, "O Qanbar! Leave one who insults you and ignore him. It will please the Merciful, displease Satan, and punish your insulter. No punishment for the fool is like refusing to answer him." (Tafsir al-Qurṭubi 41:33) Narrated Abu Dharr that he heard the Prophet (peace and blessings be upon him) saying, "If somebody accuses another of Fusuq (by calling him 'Fasiq' i.e. a wicked person) or accuses him of Kufr, such an accusation will revert to him (i.e. the accuser) if his companion (the accused) is innocent." (Bukhari)

Abu Sirmah (May Allah be pleased with him) reported that the Prophet (May Allah's peace and blessings be upon him) said: "Whoever harms others, Allah will harm him, and whoever causes hardship to others Allah will cause hardship to him." (Ibn Majah) (https://hadeethenc.com/en/browse/hadith/5375)

Narrated Abu Sa'id al-Khudri: The Messenger of Allah (peace and blessings be upon him) said: "There should be neither causing harm nor reciprocating harm. Whoever harms others, Allah will harm him, and whoever causes hardship to others, Allah will cause hardship to him." (al-Hakim and al-Bayhaqi)

Narrated Abu Hurairah (May Allah be pleased with him) that the Messenger of Allah (peace and blessings of Allah be upon him) said: "Do you know what bankrupt means?" They said: 'Among us, the one who is bankrupt is the one who has no money or wealth.' He said: 'The one who is bankrupt among my Ummah is the one who will come on the Day of Resurrection with prayer, fasting and Zakah, but he will come having insulted this one, slandered that one, consumed the wealth of this one, shed the blood of that one and beaten this one. They will each be given from his good deeds, and if his good deeds run out before the scores have been settled, some of their bad deeds will be taken and cast upon him, then he will be thrown into Hell." (Muslim)

Hastening of punishment in this world, like the punishment of sin for Muslims in the Hereafter, is a matter that is subject to the Will of Allah, may He be Glorified and Exalted. If He wills, He will punish a person for that in this world; or if He wills, He will delay his punishment until the Hereafter; or if He wills, He will pardon the person and will compensate the one who was wronged for what he suffered of harm with something that will please him, if the one who caused harm and hardship repents. Harm may befall a person in this world at the end of his life, so he is sent back to a feeble age, his children defiantly disobey him, his wife leaves him, his wealth is lost and the like. So today you see him well off, but Allah will make things difficult for him and cause harm to befall him at the end of his life. But people are hasty in seeking vengeance against those who have wronged them, and if they see such a person in a state of well-being today, they think that he will remain like that all his life. (192)

Narrated Abu Hurairah (May Allah be pleased with him): The Prophet (peace and blessings be upon him) said: "There are three whose supplication will not be rejected: a just ruler, a fasting person until he breaks his fast and the supplication of one who has been wronged, which is carried on the clouds, and the gates of the heavens are opened for it, and the Lord, may He be Glorified and Exalted, says: 'By My Might, I shall surely support you, even if it is after a while.'" (Ahmad)

Abu Hurairah (May Allah be pleased with him) reported that Abu Jahl asked (the people of Makkah): "Does Muhammad place his face on the ground in your presence?" It was said to him: 'Yes.' He said: "By Al-Lāt and Al-'Uzza! If I were to see him do that, I would trample his neck, or I would smear his face with dust." He went to the Messenger of Allah (May Allah's peace and blessings be upon him) as he was engaged in prayer and thought of trampling his neck (and the people say) that he came near him but turned upon his heels and tried to ward off something with his hands. It was said to him: "What is the matter with you?" He said: "There is a ditch of fire and horror and wings between me and him." Thereupon, Allah's Messenger (May Allah's peace and blessings be upon him) said: "If he had come near me, the angels would have torn him to pieces." Then Allah, the Exalted, revealed this Verse: "*No! (But) indeed, man transgresses, because he sees himself self-sufficient. Indeed, to your Lord is the return. Have you seen the one who forbids a servant when he prays? Have you seen if he is upon Guidance or enjoins righteousness? Have you seen if he (Abu Jahl) denies and turns away? Does he not know that Allah sees? No! If he does not desist, We will surely drag him by the forelock - a lying, sinful forelock. Then let him call his associates; We will summon the guards of Hell. No! Do not obey him.*" (Surah Al-'Alaq 96:6-19) (Muslim) (https://hadeethenc.com/en/browse/hadith/10558)

156. Rights and Obligations of Muslim Over Another Muslim

Allah, the Exalted, says:

"The believers are nothing else than brothers (in Islamic religion). So, make reconciliation between your brothers, and fear Allah, that you may receive Mercy." (Qur'an, Al-Hujurat 49:10)

"When those who believe in Our Ayat (proofs, evidences, verses, lessons, signs, revelations, etc.) come to you, say: "Salamun 'Alaikum" (peace be on you)." (Qur'an, An'am 6:54)

"When you are greeted with a greeting, greet in return with what is better than it or (at least) return it equally. Certainly, Allah is Ever a Careful Account Taker of all things." (Qur'an, An-Nisa 4:86)

Narrated Al-Bara bin Azib: Allah's Apostle (peace and blessings be upon him) ordered us to do seven things and forbade us to do other seven. He ordered us: to follow the funeral procession, to visit the sick, to accept invitations, to help the oppressed, to fulfill the oaths, to return the greeting and to reply to the sneezer: (saying, "May Allah be Merciful on you," provided the sneezer says, "All the Praises are for Allah"). He forbade us to use silver utensils and dishes, and to wear golden rings, silk (clothes), Dibaj (pure silk cloth), Qissi and Istabraq (two kinds of silk cloths)." (Bukhari)

1. The Greeting of Salam

Narrated Abu Hurairah (May Allah be pleased with him): The Messenger of Allah (peace and blessings be upon him) observed: "You shall not enter Paradise so long as you do not affirm belief (in all those things which are the articles of Faith) and you will not believe as long as you do not love one another. Should I not direct you to a thing which, if you do, will foster love amongst you: (i. e.) give currency to (the practice of paying salutation to one another by saying) 'As-salamu Alaikum.'" (Muslim)

Abdullah ibn Salam (May Allah be pleased with him) reported: "I heard the Messenger of Allah (May Allah's peace and blessings be upon him) say: 'O people, spread the greeting of peace profusely, maintain kinship ties, feed others and pray at night when people are asleep, you will enter Paradise in peace.'" (Ibn Majah, Tirmidhi, Ahmad, Ad-Daarimi) (https://hadeethenc.com/en/browse/hadith/5520)

2. Visiting the sick it is a communal obligation

Narrated Ali (May Allah be pleased with him): "I heard the Messenger of Allah (peace and blessings be upon him) say: 'Whoever comes to his Muslim brother and visits him (when he is sick), he is walking among the harvest of Paradise until he sits down, and when he sits down, he is covered with mercy. If it is morning, seventy thousand angels will send blessings upon him until evening, and if it is evening, seventy thousand angels will send blessings upon him until morning.'" (Ibn Majah)

3. Attending funerals is a communal obligation

Abdullah ibn Abbas (May Allah be pleased with him) reported: The Messenger of Allah (peace and blessings be upon him) said, "A Muslim man does not die while forty men pray over him, who do not associate any partners with Allah, but that Allah will accept their intercession for him." (Muslim)

Aisha (May Allah be pleased with her) reported: Allah's Apostle (peace and blessings be upon him) as saying: "If a company of Muslims numbering one hundred pray over a dead person, all of them interceding for him, their intercession for him will be accepted." (Muslim)

Abu Hurairah (May Allah be pleased with him) reported: "The Messenger of Allah (May Allah's peace and blessings be upon him) said: "Whoever attends a funeral until he offers the funeral prayer will get a reward equal to one Qirat; and whoever attends it until the dead person is buried will get a reward equal to two Qirats." It was asked: "What are the two Qirats?" He replied: "Like two huge mountains." In a narration by Muslim: "The smallest of them is like Mount Uhud." (Bukhari and Muslim) (https://hadeethenc.com/en/browse/hadith/5397)

4. With regard to accepting invitations

If the invitation is to a wedding feast, then the majority of scholars are of the view that it is obligatory to accept unless there is a legitimate reason not to do so. If it is for something other than a wedding feast, the majority are of the view that it is mustahabb. But there are conditions for accepting invitations in general terms. (193)

5. Saying "Yarhamuk Allah" (May Allah have mercy on you)

Narrated Abu Hurairah (May Allah be pleased with him): The Prophet (peace and blessings be upon him) said: "Allah likes the act of sneezing and dislikes the act of yawning, so if any one of you sneezes and praises Allah (says 'Al-hamdu Lillaah'), it is a duty on every Muslim who hears him to say to him, 'Yarhamuk Allah (May Allah have mercy on you).'" (Bukhari)

6. Offering Advice

Al-Mullah 'Ali al-Qaari (May Allah have mercy on him) said: "If he asks you for advice" means if he asks you for advice, then give it to him; it is obligatory. It is also obligatory to give advice even if he did not ask for it. End quote." (Mirqaat al-Mafaateeh, 5/213) (193)

7. Muslim Should Not Oppress Another, nor should he hand him over to an oppressor.

Narrated Abu Hurairah: The Messenger of Allah (peace and blessings be upon him) said: "The Muslim is the one from whose tongue and hand the people are safe, and the believer is the one from whom the people's lives and wealth are safe." (An-Nasa'i)

Abdullah ibn 'Amr and Jabir ibn 'Abdullah (May Allah be pleased with them) reported that the Prophet (May Allah's peace and blessings be upon him) said: "The true Muslim is the one from whose tongue and hand the Muslims are safe, and the Muhajir (emigrant) is the one who abandons what Allah has forbidden." Abu Musa (May Allah be pleased with him) reported that he said: "O Messenger of Allah, who is the best among Muslims?" He said: "The one from whose tongue and hand the Muslims are safe." (Bukhari and Muslim) (https://hadeethenc.com/en/browse/hadith/10101)

Narrated Abdullah bin Umar: Allah's Apostle (peace and blessings of Allah be upon him) said, "A Muslim is a brother of another Muslim, so he should not oppress him, nor should he hand him over to an oppressor. Whoever fulfilled the needs of his brother, Allah will fulfill his needs; whoever brought his (Muslim) brother out of a discomfort, Allah will bring him out of the discomforts of the Day of Resurrection, and whoever screened a Muslim, Allah will screen him on the Day of Resurrection." (Bukhari)

8. Muslim must love for his brother what he loves for himself

Narrated Anas bin Malik: The Prophet (peace and blessings be upon him) said: "None of you truly believes (in Allah and in His religion) until he loves for his brother what he loves for himself." (Bukhari and Muslim)

Narrated Abu Darda: The Prophet (peace and blessings be upon him) said, "Whoever protects the honor of his brother in his absence, Allah will protect his face from the Fire on the Day of Judgment." (Tirmidhi and Ahmad) (https://hadeethenc.com/en/browse/hadith/5514)

Abu Hurairah (May Allah be pleased with him) reported that the Prophet (May Allah's peace and blessings be upon him) said: "Do not envy one another, do not raise prices by overbidding against one another, do not hate one another, do not turn your backs on each other, and do not undercut one another in trade; but be, O slaves of Allah, as brothers. A Muslim is the brother of a Muslim; he does not wrong him, he does not fail him (when he needs him), he does not lie to him, and he does not show contempt for him. Piety lies here - and he pointed to his chest three times. It is enough evil for a Muslim to hold his Muslim brother in contempt. All of a Muslim is inviolable to another Muslim: his blood, his property and his honor." (Muslim) (https://hadeethenc.com/en/browse/hadith/4706)

Narrated Abu Musa: The Prophet (peace and blessings be upon him) said, "A believer to another believer is like a building whose different parts enforce each other." The Prophet (peace and blessings be upon him) then clasped his hands with the fingers interlaced (while saying that). (Bukhari)

'Abdullah bin 'Amr bin Al-'As (May Allah be pleased with him) reported: The Messenger of Allah (peace and blessings be upon him) said, "A (true) Muslim is one from whose tongue and hand the Muslims are safe; and a Muhajir (Emigrant) is he who leaves the deeds which Allah has prohibited." (Bukhari and Muslim)

'Abdullah bin 'Amr bin Al-'As (May Allah be pleased with him) said: The Messenger of Allah (peace and blessings be upon him) said, "He who desires to be rescued from the Fire of Hell and to enter Jannah, should die in a state of complete belief in Allah and the Last Day, and should do unto others what he wishes to be done unto him." (Muslim)

Umm Ad-Darda (May Allah be pleased with her) reported that the Prophet (May Allah's peace and blessings be upon him) said: "The supplication of a Muslim for a fellow Muslim in his absence is answered. At his head, there is an entrusted angel. Whenever one invokes good for his brother, the entrusted angel says: 'Amen, and likewise to you.'" (Muslim) (https://hadeethenc.com/en/browse/hadith/3219)

Exception

Narrated Abdullah bin Masud: The Messenger of Allah (peace and blessings be upon him) said: "The blood of a man who is a Muslim is not lawful (i.e. cannot be lawfully shed), save if he belongs to one of three (classes): a married man who is an adulterer; life for a life (i.e. for murder); one who is a deserter of his religion, abandoning the community." (Bukhari and Muslim)

157. Shaking Hands with Both Hands

Narrated Al-Bara' ibn Azib: The Prophet (peace and blessings be upon him) said: "Two Muslims will not meet and shake hands having their sins forgiven them before they separate." (Abu Dawud)

Sheikh al-Albaani said in al-Silsilah al-Saheehah (1/22), mentioning what is to be learned from some Ahadith:

"Taking hold of one hand when shaking hands. This is mentioned in many Ahadith, and it is what is implied linguistically. Al-Mundhiri said (3/270): "It was narrated by al-Tabarani in al-Awsat and I do not know of anyone who is majrooh (unacceptable) among its narrators. I say: And it has corroborating evidence which raises it to the level of being Saheeh." These Ahadith all indicate that the Sunnah in shaking hands is to use just one hand. End quote."

As for the view of some Hanafi and Maliki fuqaha', that it is mustahabb to shake hands using both hands, putting the palm of the left hand over the back of one's brother's hand; this is not proven to be Sunnah from the Prophet (peace and blessings of Allah be upon him) or from his companions. Rather the most that can be said concerning some Ahadith that refer to it is that the Prophet (peace and blessings of Allah be upon him) took the hand of one of his companions in both of his hands as a sign of extra care in teaching, guiding and so on, as it says in Saheeh al-Bukhari and Saheeh Muslim that Ibn Masud (May Allah be pleased with him) said: 'The Messenger of Allah (peace and blessings of Allah be upon him) taught me the Tashahhud, holding my hand between both of his.' But that is not the usual habit, based on the evidence of the previous report which says that the basic principle is shaking hands with one hand, which is stated clearly in some reports. This Hadith indicates that too, because if the custom among the Sahabah had been to shake hands using both hands, Ibn Masud would not have mentioned that. The fact that he mentions it indicates that it was not the usual habit of the Prophet (peace and blessings of Allah be upon him) with his companions. Nevertheless, shaking hands using both hands should not be described as a Bid'ah (innovation), rather it is something that is permissible, but the Sunnah, which it is better to adhere to, is to shake hands using just one hand. (194)

158. Forsaking his Muslim Brother for More than Three Days

Allah, the Exalted, says:

"The believers are nothing else than brothers (in Islamic religion). So, make reconciliation between your brothers." (Qur'an, Al-Hujurat 49:10)

"There is no good in most of their secret talks save (in) him who orders Sadaqah (charity in Allah's Cause), or Ma'roof (Islamic Monotheism and all the good and righteous deeds which Allah has ordained), or conciliation between mankind; and he who does this, seeking the good Pleasure of Allah, We shall give him a great reward." (Qur'an, An-Nisa 4:114)

The Prophet (peace and blessings be upon him) said: "It is not permissible for a man to forsake his Muslim brother for more than three days, each of them turning away from the other when they meet. The better of them is the one who gives the greeting of salam first." (Bukhari and Muslim)

Abu Darda reported: The Messenger of Allah (peace and blessings be upon him) said: "Shall I not tell you of what is better in degree than extra fasting, prayer and charity?" They said, "Of course!" The Prophet (peace and blessings be upon him) said: "Reconciliation between people. Verily, corrupted relations between people is the razor." (Tirmidhi)

159. Causing Trouble Between Muslims

Allah, the Exalted, says:

"And hold fast, all of you together, to the Rope of Allah (i.e. this Qur'an), and be not divided among yourselves" (Qur'an, Ali 'Imran 3:103)

Abu Darda (May Allah be pleased with him) reported: The Messenger of Allah (peace and blessings be upon him) said: "Shall I not tell you of what is better in degree than extra fasting, prayer and charity?" They said, "Of course!" The Prophet said, "Reconciliation between people. Verily, corrupted relations between people is the razor." (Tirmidhi)

Narrated Abdullah ibn Masud (May Allah be pleased with him): The Prophet (peace and blessings of Allah be upon him) said: "The believer is not given to criticizing people or given to cursing, or foul-mouthed, or shameless." (Tirmidhi)

160. Prohibition of Calling a Muslim a Disbeliever

Allah, the Exalted, says:

"O you who believe! When you go (to fight) in the Cause of Allah, verify (the Truth), and say not to anyone who greets you (by embracing Islam): "You are not a believer"; seeking the perishable goods of the worldly life. There are much more profits and booties with Allah. Even as he is now, so were you yourselves before till Allah conferred on you His Favors (i.e. guided you to Islam), therefore, be cautious in discrimination. Allah is Ever Well Aware of what you do." (Qur'an, An-Nisa 4:94)

"And there is no sin on you concerning that in which you made a mistake, except in regard to what your hearts deliberately intend. And Allah is Ever Oft-Forgiving, Most Merciful." (Qur'an, Al-Ahzab 33:5)

Abu Dharr (May Allah be pleased with him) said: "I heard the Messenger of Allah (peace and blessings be upon him) saying, 'If somebody accuses another of disbelief or calls him the enemy of Allah, such an accusation will revert to him (the accuser) if the accused is innocent.'" (Bukhari and Muslim)

Commentary: This Hadith also tells us that to call without reason any Muslim a Kafir or enemy of Allah is strictly prohibited. (195)

161. Muslims Taking Non-Muslims as Auliya (friends, protectors, helpers, etc.)

Allah, the Exalted, says:

"Let not the believers take the disbelievers as Auliya (supporters, helpers, etc.) instead of the believers, and whoever does that will never be helped by Allah in any way, except if you indeed fear a danger from them. And Allah warns you against Himself (His Punishment), and to Allah is the final return." (Qur'an, Ali 'Imran 3:28)

"Verily! As for those whom the angels take (in death) while they are wronging themselves (as they stayed among the disbelievers even though emigration was obligatory for them), they (angels) say (to them): "In what (condition) were you?" They reply: "We were weak and oppressed on earth." They (angels) say: "Was not the earth of Allah spacious enough for you to emigrate therein?" Such men will find their abode in Hell - What an evil destination!" (Qur'an, An-Nisa 4:97)

"O you who believe! Take not the Jews and the Christians as Auliya' (friends, protectors, helpers, etc.), they are but Auliya' to one another. And if any amongst you takes them as Auliya', then surely he is one of them. Verily, Allah guides not those people who are the Zalimun (polytheists and wrongdoers, and unjust)." (Qur'an, Al-Ma'idah 5:51)

Other Verses: Al-Mumtahanah 60:8-9 and 60:13, An-Nisa 4:144, Al-Ma'idah 5:57-58.

Muslims should call non-Muslims to Islam

Anas (May Allah be pleased with him) reported: "A young Jewish boy who was in the service of the Prophet (peace and blessings be upon him) fell ill. The Prophet (peace and blessings be upon him) went to visit him. He sat down by his head and said to him, "Embrace Islam." The little boy looked at his father who was sitting beside him. He said: "Obey Abul-Qasim (i.e. the Messenger of Allah (peace and blessings be upon him)." So, he embraced Islam and the Prophet (peace and blessings be upon him) stepped out saying, "Praise be to Allah Who has saved him from Hellfire." (Bukhari)

Muslim should treat non-Muslim with kindness and justice

Narrated Asma bint Abu Bakr: "My mother came to me during the lifetime of Allah's Apostle (peace and blessings be upon him) and she was a Mushrikah (polytheist, pagan, idolatress). I said to Allah's Apostle (peace and blessings be upon him) (seeking his verdict), "My mother has come to me and she desires to receive a reward from me, shall I keep good relations with her?" The Prophet (peace and blessings be upon him) said, "Yes, keep good relation with her." (Bukhari)

The Prophet (peace and blessings be upon him) used to do business with non-Muslims

Narrated Aisha (May Allah have mercy on her): "Allah's Apostle (peace and blessings upon him) bought some foodstuff (barley) from a Jew on credit and mortgaged his iron armor to him (the armor stands for a guarantor)." (Bukhari)

Islam preserves the lives of non-Muslims who are given protection by Muslims

Narrated 'Abdullah bin 'Amr: The Prophet (peace and blessings be upon him) said, "Whoever kills a Mu'ahid (a person who is granted the pledge of protection by the Muslims) shall not smell the fragrance of Paradise though its fragrance can be smelt at a distance of forty years (of traveling)." (Bukhari)

(https://hadeethenc.com/en/browse/hadith/64637)

There is no problem with Muslims keeping casual friendships with non-Muslims as long as Muslims have influence on non-Muslims and as long as those people do not oppose or dislike Islam and Muslims, do not engage in or wrongly influence Muslims towards immoral behavior, and are not unjust and oppressive to anyone, especially Muslims. (196)

162. Greeting the Non-Muslims and Prohibition of Taking an Initiative

Abu Hurairah (May Allah be pleased with him) reported that the Messenger of Allah (May Allah's peace and blessings be upon him) said: "Do not initiate the greeting of peace to the Jews and Christians, and if you meet them on a road, force them to go to the narrowest part thereof." (Muslim)
(https://hadeethenc.com/en/browse/hadith/5347)

Anas (May Allah be pleased with him) reported: The Messenger of Allah (peace and blessings upon him) said, "When the people of the Book greet you (i.e. by saying 'As-Samu 'Alaikum,' meaning death be upon you), you should respond with: 'Wa 'alaikum' [The same on you (i.e. and death will be upon you, for no one will escape death)]." (Bukhari and Muslim)

Usamah bin Zaid (May Allah be pleased with him) reported: "The Prophet (peace and blessings upon him) passed by a mixed company of people which included Muslims, polytheists and Jews, and he gave them the greeting (i.e. saying As-Salamu 'Alaikum)." (Bukhari and Muslim)

Commentary: If there is a mixed assembly of Muslims and non-Muslims, one should utter greeting to it but consider Muslims as one's addressees. (197)

163. Greeting with a Gesture

Allah, the Exalted, says:

"...greet one another with a greeting from Allah (i.e. say: As-Salamu Alaikum - peace be on you) blessed and good." (Qur'an, An-Nur 24:61)

"When you are greeted with a greeting, greet in return with what is better than it or (at least) return it equally. Certainly, Allah is Ever a Careful Account Taker of all things." (Qur'an, An-Nisa 4:86)

"Their greeting on the Day they shall meet Him will be Salam: Peace (i.e. the angels will say to them: Salamu Alaikum)!" (Qur'an, Al-Ahzab 33:44)

Abu Hurairah (May Allah be pleased with him) reported: Messenger of Allah (peace and blessings of Allah be upon him) said, "By Him in Whose Hand my soul is! You will not enter Jannah until you believe, and you shall not believe until you love one another. May I inform you of something, if you do, you love each other. Promote greeting amongst you (by saying As-salamu 'alaikum to one another)." (Muslim)

Narrated 'Abdullah ibn 'Amr: The Messenger of Allah (peace and blessings of Allah be upon him) said: "He is not one of us who imitates others. Do not imitate the Jews or the Christians, for the greeting of the Jews is a gesture with the fingers and the greeting of the Christians is a gesture with the hand." (Tirmidhi)

Narrated Jabir ibn 'Abdullah: The Prophet (peace and blessings of Allah be upon him): "Do not greet one another with the greeting of the Jews; their greeting is with the head and the hand, and with gestures." (An-Nasa'i)

Nawawi (May Allah have mercy on him) said:

"This (the Hadith of Jabir) does not contradict the Hadith of Asmaa' bint Yazeed: "The Prophet (peace and blessings of Allah be upon him) passed through the Mosque where a group of women were sitting, and he greeted them with a wave of his hand. This Hadith is to be interpreted as meaning that he greeted them with both a gesture and the words of greeting. The prohibition on greeting with a gesture only is limited to those who are able – both physically and within the limits of Shariah – to speak the words of greeting. Otherwise it is permissible for the one who is doing something that prevents him from speaking to respond to a greeting with a gesture – such as when one is praying or when one is far away; it is also permissible to use gestures if one is unable to speak ("dumb") or when greeting the deaf." (198)

Greeting with a gesture and without speaking is an imitation of the Jews or Christians. The same applies to many military salutes.

The military salute that soldiers give to one another, in the form of a gesture with the hand, is a kind of greeting that is not allowed in Islam, it is a Bid'ah; rather the greeting of the Muslims is by saying "As-salamu 'alaykum (peace be upon you). (See: al-Lama' by al-Turkmaani, 1/285, 282) (199)

Greeting "namaste" means 'I bow to the divine in you' which is contrary to the Islamic belief as "namaste" seems to imply god resides in us or that god is everywhere, or that we are a part of god himself which is against Tawheed. Namaste is usually spoken with a slight bow and hands pressed together, palms touching and fingers pointing upwards, thumbs close to the chest.

Boxing greeting or greeting by elbow bumps are non-Islamic greeting.

164. Standing up for Someone to Venerate him

Allah, the Exalted, says:

"Allah has promised those among you who believe and do righteous good deeds, that He will certainly grant them succession to (the present rulers) in the earth, as He granted it to those before them, and that He will grant them the authority to practice their religion that which He has chosen for them (i.e. Islam). And He will surely give them in exchange a safe security after their fear (provided) they (believers) worship Me and do not associate anything (in worship) with Me. But whoever disbelieved after this, they are the Fasiqun (rebellious, disobedient to Allah)." (Qur'an, An-Nur 24:55)

Ibn Taymiyah (May Allah have mercy on him) said:

"It was not the custom of the salaf at the time of the Prophet (peace and blessings of Allah be upon him) and the Rightly-Guided Caliphs to stand up every time they saw him (the Prophet, peace and blessings of Allah be upon him), as many people do. Rather Anas ibn Malik said: "No person was dearer to them than the Prophet (peace and blessings of Allah be upon him), but when they saw him, they did not stand up for him because they knew that he disliked that." (Tirmidhi). But they may have stood up for one who was returning from away, in order to greet him, as it was narrated that the Prophet (peace and blessings of Allah be upon him) stood up for 'Ikrimah, and he said to the Ansar when Sa'd ibn Mu'aadh came: "Stand up for your chief." (Bukhari and Muslim) That was when he (Sa'd) came to pass judgement on Banu Qurayzah, because they said that would accept his verdict…" (200)

If a person stands up to welcome his guest and honour him or to shake hands with him, or greet him, this is something which is prescribed in Islam. But to remain standing when people are sitting by way of veneration, or standing at the door without greeting anyone or shaking hands with anyone, this should not be done. Even worse than that is standing up to venerate a person when he is sitting down, not for the sake of guarding him but only for the purpose of veneration.

165. Saluting the Flag, Standing up for it and Singing the National Anthem

Allah, the Exalted, says:

"greet one another with a greeting from Allah (i.e. say: As-Salamu Alaikum - peace be on you) blessed and good." (Qur'an, An-Nur 24:61)

"When you are greeted with a greeting, greet in return with what is better than it, or (at least) return it equally." (Qur'an, An-Nisa 4:86)

"Their greeting on the Day they shall meet Him will be Salam: Peace (i.e. the angels will say to them: Salamu Alaikum)!" (Qur'an, Al-Ahzab 33:44)

Sheikh 'Abdul-'Aziz ibn 'Abdullah ibn Baaz, Sheikh 'Abdur-Razaq 'Afeefi, Sheikh 'Abdullah ibn Ghadyan, Sheikh 'Abdullah ibn Qa 'ood (1/236) said:

"It is not permissible to salute the flag; it is obligatory to rule according to the Law of Islam and refer to it for judgment; it is not permissible for the Muslim to greet leaders and superiors with the greeting of non-Muslims, because of what has been narrated of the prohibition on resembling them, and because that is going to extremes in showing respect to them." (199)

The Prophet (peace and blessings of Allah be upon him) said: "By the One in Whose Hand is my soul, you will not enter Paradise until you believe, and you will not believe until you love one another. Shall I not tell you of something which, if you do it, you will love one another? Spread (the greeting of) peace among yourselves.'" (Ibn Majah)

166. Undesirability of Praising a Person in his Presence

Abu Musa Al-Ash`ari (May Allah be pleased with him) said: "The Prophet (peace and blessings be upon him) heard a person lauding another person or praising him too much. Thereupon he (peace and blessings be upon him) said, "You killed the man", or he said, "You ruined the man." (Bukhari and Muslim)

Abu Bakrah (May Allah be pleased with him) reported: "Mention of a man was made to the Prophet (peace and blessings be upon him) and someone praised him whereupon he (peace and blessings be upon him) said, 'Woe be to you! You have broken the neck of your friend!' He repeated this several times and added, 'If one of you has to praise his friend at all, he should say: 'I reckon him to be such and such and Allah knows him well', if you think him to be so-and-so, you will be accountable to Allah because no one can testify the purity of others against Allah.'" (Bukhari and Muslim)

Commentary: This Hadith prohibits us from praising anyone in his face. If at all one has to praise someone, he should say that "In my opinion, he is such and such", provided he really thinks as he says. The reason for this is that it is Allah Alone Who knows him thoroughly and none can claim to be innocent before Him. (201)

Hammam bin Al-Harith (May Allah be pleased with him) reported: "A person began to praise 'Uthman (May Allah be pleased with him), and Al-Miqdad (May Allah be pleased with him) sat upon his knees and began to throw pebbles upon the flatterer's face. 'Uthman (May Allah be pleased with him) said: 'What is the matter with you?" He said: 'Verily, the Messenger of Allah (peace and blessings be upon him) said, 'When you see those who shower undue praises upon others throw dust upon their faces.'" (Muslim)

167. Committing Evil After Embracing Islam

Narrated Abdullah bin Masud: "Some people said to the Messenger of Allah (peace and blessings be upon him): 'Messenger of Allah, would we be held responsible for our deeds committed in the state of ignorance (before embracing Islam)?' Upon this he (peace and blessings be upon him) remarked: 'He who amongst you performed good deeds in Islam, he would not be held responsible for them (misdeeds which he committed in ignorance), and he who committed evil (even after embracing Islam), would be held responsible for his misdeeds that he committed in the state of ignorance as well as in that of Islam. (Muslim)

168. Breach of Faith, Apostasy from Islam

Allah, the Exalted, says:

"And whosoever of you turns back from his religion and dies as a disbeliever, then his deeds will be lost in this life and in the Hereafter, and they will be the dwellers of the Fire. They will abide therein forever." (Qur'an, Al-Baqarah 2:217)

"And whoever turns away from My remembrance - indeed, he will have a depressed life, and We will gather him on the Day of Resurrection blind." (Qur'an, Taha 20:124)

"And recite to them, (O Muhammad), the news of him to whom We gave (knowledge of) Our signs, but he detached himself from them; so, Satan pursued him, and he became of the deviators." (Qur'an, Al-A'raf 7:175)

Other Verse: Ali 'Imran 3:90.

Narrated Jabir (May Allah be pleased with him): "I heard the Apostle (peace and blessings be upon him) saying, 'Verily between man and between polytheism and unbelief is the negligence of prayer.'" (Muslim)

Narrated Thawban that the Prophet (peace and blessings be upon him) said: "I certainly know people of my nation who will come on the Day of Resurrection with good deeds like the mountains of Tihamah, but Allah will make them like scattered dust." Thawban said: "O Messenger of Allah, describe them to us and tell us more, so that we will not become of them unknowingly." He said: "They are your brothers and from your race, worshiping at night as you do, but they will be people who, when they are alone, transgress the sacred limits of Allah." (Ibn Majah)

Narrated Abdullah bin Masud: The Messenger of Allah (peace and blessings be upon him) said:

"The blood of a man who is a Muslim is not lawful (i.e. cannot be lawfully shed), save if he belongs to one of three (classes): a married man who is an adulterer; life for a life (i.e. for murder); one who is a deserter of his religion, abandoning the community." (Bukhari and Muslim)

Narrated Ibn Abbas (May Allah have mercy on him): The Messenger of Allah (peace and blessings be upon him) said, "He who changes his religion (i.e. apostates) kill him." (Bukhari)

Narrated Asma': The Prophet (peace and blessings be upon him) said, "I will be at my Lake-Fount (Kawthar) waiting for whoever will come to me. Then some people will be taken away from me whereupon I will say, 'My followers!' It will be said, 'You do not know, they turned apostates as renegades (deserted their religion).'" (Ibn Abi Mulaika said, "Allah, we seek refuge with You from turning on our heels from the (Islamic) religion and from being put to trial"). (Bukhari)

Misdeeds remove him from Allah's Protection, so he becomes prey for the thieves and bandits.

169. Calling People to Misguidance

Allah, the Exalted, says:

"They will bear their own burdens in full on the Day of Resurrection, and also of the burdens of those whom they misled without knowledge. Evil indeed is that which they shall bear!" (Qur'an, An-Nahl 16:25)

"And verily, this (i.e. Allah's Commandments mentioned in the above two Verses 151 and 152) is My Straight Path, so follow it, and follow not (other) paths, for they will separate you away from His Path. This He has ordained for you that you may become Al-Muttaqun (the pious)" (Qur'an, Al-An'am 6:153)

"This (Qur'an) is a Message for mankind (and a clear proof against them), in order that they may be warned thereby, and that they may know that He is the Only One Ilah (God - Allah) - (none has the right to be worshipped but Allah) - and that men of understanding may take heed." (Qur'an, Ibrahim 14:52)

Other Verse: *Yusuf 12:108.*

The Muslims must follow the example and guidance of their Messenger and call others to Islam, bearing insults and harm with patience for the sake of Allah, as their Messenger (peace and blessings of Allah be upon him) did:

"Indeed, in the Messenger of Allah (Muhammad) you have a good example to follow for him who hopes for (the Meeting with) Allah and the Last Day, and remembers Allah much." (Qur'an, Al-Ahzab 33:21)

Jabir ibn 'Abdullah (May Allah be pleased with him) reported: "We were with the Messenger of Allah (May Allah's peace and blessings be upon him) shortly after dawn when there came to him some people clad in woolen rags or covered with sleeveless blankets; and with swords hanging down from their necks. Most of them, rather all of them, belonged to the Mudar tribe. The Prophet's face changed when he saw them starving. Then he went into his house and came out; then he commanded Bilal to proclaim the Adhan. So, he proclaimed the Adhan and recited Iqamah and the Prophet led the prayer. Then he delivered a sermon saying: *"O mankind, fear your Lord, Who created you from one soul and created from it its mate and dispersed from both of them many men and women. And fear Allah, through Whom you ask one another, and the wombs. Indeed, Allah is ever, over you, an Observer."*

(Surah An-Nisa 4:1) He also recited a Verse at the end of Surah Al-Hashr: *"O you who believe, fear Allah and keep your duty to Him. And let everyone look what he has sent forth for the tomorrow." (Surah, Al-Hashr 59:18)* Thereafter, every man gave in charity dinar, dirham, clothes, measure-full of wheat and measure-full of dates till he said: "Give in charity be it half a date." Then a man from the Ansar came with a bag which was difficult for him to hold in

his hand. Thereafter, the people came successively (with charity) till I saw two heaps of food and clothes. I noticed that the Messenger's face was glowing like that of the bright moon or glittering gold. Then he said: "Whosoever introduces a good practice in Islam, there is for him its reward and the reward of those who act upon it after him without anything being diminished from their rewards. And whosoever introduces an evil practice in Islam will shoulder its sin and the sins of all those who will act upon it, without diminishing in any way their burden." (Muslim)
(https://hadeethenc.com/en/browse/hadith/3506)

170. Condemnation of Double-Faced People - Hypocrisy

Allah, the Exalted, says:
"Verily, the hypocrites will be in the lowest depth (grade) of the Fire; no helper will you find for them." (Qur'an, An-Nisa 4:145)

"And when they meet those who believe, they say: "We believe," but when they are alone with their Shayateen (Devils - polytheists, hypocrites), they say: "Truly, we are with you; verily, we were but mocking. But Allah mocks at them and gives them increase in their wrongdoing to wander blindly." (Qur'an, Al-Baqarah 2:14-15)

"And when you look at them, their bodies please you; and when they speak, you listen to their words. They are as blocks of wood propped up. They think that every cry is against them. They are the enemies, so beware of them. May Allah curse them! How are they denying (or deviating from) the Right Path." (Qur'an, Al-Munafiqun 63:4)

Other Verse: *At-Tawbah 9:67.*

Narrated Abu Hurairah (May Allah be pleased with him): The Messenger of Allah (peace and blessings be upon him) said, "People are like ores. Those who were excellent in the Days of Ignorance are excellent in Islam provided they acquire the knowledge and understanding of the religion. You will find the best people in it (Islam) those who had a deep hatred (for leadership). You will find the worst among the people a double-faced person who appears to some people with one face and to others with another face." (Bukhari and Muslim)

Muhammad bin Zaid reported: "Some people said to my grandfather, 'Abdullah bin 'Umar (May Allah be pleased with him): 'We visit our rulers and tell them things contrary to what we say when we leave them.' 'Abdullah bin 'Umar (May Allah be pleased with him) replied: "In the days of the Messenger of Allah (peace and blessings be upon him), we counted this act as an act of hypocrisy." (Bukhari)

Commentary: This Hadith points out that to praise the rulers in their presence and to condemn them in their absence amounts to practical hypocrisy because what one has in his heart does not find expression in his speech, and what one expresses in his words does not agree with what one has in his heart. The conduct of a true Muslim should be that if a ruler is noble, just and pious, he should admire him even in his presence (when there arises a need for it, and not for the sake of flattering him) and he should also praise him in his absence. If the ruler is bad, he should warn him of the evil consequences of his bad conduct to his face, and the same attitude should be maintained when he is not present because this is the well-meaning attitude which has been ordained to every Muslim. (202)

Narrated Ammar: The Prophet (peace and blessings be upon him) said: "He who is two-faced in this world will have two tongues of fire on the Day of Resurrection." (Abu Dawud)

171. Condemnation and Prohibition of Falsehood

Allah, the Exalted, says:

"There is no compulsion in religion. Verily, the Right Path has become distinct from the wrong path. Whoever disbelieves in Taghut and believes in Allah, then he has grasped the most trustworthy handhold that will never break. And Allah is All-Hearer, All-Knower." (Qur'an, Al-Baqarah 2:256)

"Verily, it is the Truth from your Lord, but most of mankind believe not." (Qur'an, Hud 11:17)

"And say: "Truth (i.e. Islamic Monotheism or this Qur'an or Jihad against polytheists) has come and Batil (falsehood, i.e. Satan or polytheism, etc.) has vanished. Surely! Batil is ever bound to vanish." (Qur'an, Al-Isra 17:81)

Other Verse: An-Nahl 16:117.

Narrated Ibn Masud (May Allah be pleased with him): The Messenger of Allah (peace and blessings be upon him) said, "Truth leads to piety and piety leads to Jannah. A man persists in speaking the truth till he is recorded with Allah as a truthful man. Falsehood leads to transgression and transgression leads to the Hellfire. A man continues to speak falsehood till he is recorded with Allah as a great liar." (Bukhari and Muslim)

Commentary:
1. Whatever attitude one adopts becomes his special trait and then he becomes known by it. Therefore, one should always adopt virtues and good conduct so that he may attain a high esteem with Allah and be also remembered well by people.
2. Truth is the way to salvation while falsehood is the way to destruction. (203)

Narrated 'Abdullah bin 'Amr (May Allah be pleased with him) said: The Prophet (peace and blessings be upon him) said, "Whoever has the following four (characteristics) will be a pure hypocrite and whoever has one of the following four characteristics will have one characteristic of hypocrisy unless and until he gives it up.

1. Whenever he is entrusted, he betrays.
2. Whenever he speaks, he tells a lie.
3. Whenever he makes a covenant, he proves treacherous.
4. Whenever he quarrels, he behaves in a very imprudent, evil and insulting manner." (Bukhari)

Ibn 'Abbas (May Allah be pleased with him) said: The Prophet (peace and blessings be upon him) said, "He who narrates a dream which he has not seen will be put to trouble to join into a knot two barley seeds which he will not be able to do; and he who seeks to listen to the talk of a people (secretly) will have molten lead poured into his ears on the Day of Resurrection; and he who makes a picture (of people or other creatures with a soul, such as animals and insects) will be (severely punished), and he will be asked to infuse spirit therein, which he will not be able to do." (Bukhari)

Ibn 'Umar (May Allah be pleased with him) reported: The Prophet (peace and blessings be upon him) as saying: "The worst of lies is to pretend to have seen something which he has not seen." (Bukhari)

Sumurah bin Jundub (May Allah be pleased with him) said: The Messenger of Allah (peace and blessings be upon him) very often used to ask his Companions, "Do any one of you has seen a dream?" So, dreams would be narrated to him by those whom Allah willed to relate. One day he (peace and blessings be upon him) said, "Last night I had a vision in which two men (angels) came to me and woke me up and said to me, 'Proceed!' I set out with them and we came across a man lying down, and behold, another man was standing over his head, holding a big rock. Behold, he was throwing the rock at the man's head, smashing it. When he struck him, the stone rolled away and he went after it to get it, and no sooner had he returned to this man, his head was healed and restored to its former condition. The thrower (of the rock) then did the same as he had done before. I said to my two companions, 'Subhan-Allah! Who are these?' They said: 'Proceed, proceed.' So, we proceeded and came to a man lying in a prone position and another man standing over his head with an iron hook, and behold, he would put the hook in one side of the man's mouth and tear off that side of his face to the back (of the neck), and similarly tear his nose from front to back, and his eyes from front to back. Then he turned to the other side of the man's face and did just as he has done with the first side. He had hardly completed that (second) side when the first returned to its normal state. I said to my two companions, 'Subhan-Allah! Who are these?' They said, 'Proceed, proceed.' So, we proceeded and came across something like a Tannur (a kind of baking oven, a pit usually clay-lined for baking bread)." I (the narrator) think the Prophet (peace and blessings be upon him) said, "In that oven there was much noise and voices." The Prophet (peace and blessings be upon him) added, "We looked into it and found naked men and women, and behold, a flame of fire was reaching to them from underneath, and when it reached them, they cried loudly." I asked, 'Who are these?' They said to me, 'Proceed, proceed.' And so, we proceeded and came across a river." I (the narrator) think he said, "red like blood." The Prophet (peace and blessings be upon him) added, "And behold, in the river there was a man swimming, and on the bank, there was a man who had collected many stones. Behold, while the other man was swimming, he went near him. The former opened his mouth and the latter (on the bank) threw a stone into his mouth whereupon he went swimming again. Then again, he (the former) returned to him (the latter), and every time the former returned, he opened his mouth, and the latter threw a stone into his mouth, (and so on) the performance was repeated. I asked my two companions, 'Who are these?' They replied, 'Proceed, proceed.' And we proceeded till we came to a man with a repulsive appearance, the most repulsive appearance you ever saw a man having! Beside him there was a fire, and he was kindling it and running around it. I asked my two companions, 'Who is this (man).' They said to me, 'Proceed, proceed!' So, we proceeded till we reached a garden of deep green dense vegetation, having all sorts of spring colours. In the midst of the garden there was a very tall man, and I could hardly see his head because of his great height, and around him there were children in such a large number as I have never seen! I said to my two companions, 'Who is this?' They replied, 'Proceed, proceed.' So, we proceeded till we came to a majestic, huge garden, greater and better than any garden I have ever seen! My two companions said to me, 'Ascend up' and I ascended up." The Prophet (peace and blessings be upon him) added, "So we ascended till we reached a city built of gold and silver bricks, and we went to its gate and asked (the gatekeeper) to open the gate, and it was opened; and we entered the city and found in it men with one side of their bodies as handsome as the most handsome person you have ever seen, and the other side as ugly as the ugliest person you have ever seen! My two companions ordered those men to throw themselves into the river. Behold, there was a river flowing across (the city), and its water was like milk in whiteness. Those men went and threw themselves in it and then returned to us after the ugliness (of their bodies) had disappeared, and they came in the best shape." The Prophet (peace and blessings be upon him) further added, "My two companions said to me: 'This place is the 'Adn Jannah, and that is your place.' I raised up my sight, and behold, there I saw a palace like a white cloud! My two companions said to me, 'That palace is your place,' I said to them, 'May Allah bless you both! Let me enter it.' They replied, 'As for now, you will not enter it, but you shall enter it (one day).' I said to them, 'I have seen many wonders tonight. What does all that mean which I have seen?' They replied, 'We will inform you: As for the first man you came upon, whose head was being smashed with the rock, he is the symbol of the one who studies the Qur'an and then neither recites it nor acts on its orders, and sleeps, neglecting the enjoined prayers. As for the man you came upon, whose sides of mouth, nostrils and eyes were torn off from front to back, he is the symbol of the man who goes out of his house in the morning and tells lies that are spread all over the world. And those naked men and women whom you saw in a construction resembling an oven, they are the adulterers and the adulteresses. And the man who was given a stone to swallow is the eater of Ar-Riba (usury), and the bad-looking man whom you saw near the fire, kindling it and going around it, is Malik, the gatekeeper of Hell, and the tall man you saw in the garden is (Prophet) Abraham, and the children around him are those who died upon Al-Fitrah (the Islamic Faith of Monotheism).'" The narrator added: Some Muslims asked the Prophet (peace and blessings be upon him), "O Messenger of Allah! What about the children of Al-Mushrikun (i.e. polytheists, pagans, idolaters and disbelievers in the Oneness of Allah and in His Messenger Muhammad (peace and blessings be upon him)?" The Prophet (peace and blessings be upon him) replied, "And also the children of Al-Mushrikun." The Prophet (peace and blessings be upon him) added: "My two companions added, 'The men you saw half handsome and half ugly were these people who had mixed an act that was good with another that was bad, but Allah forgave them.'" (Bukhari)

171a. Falsehood that is Permissible

Allah, the Exalted, says:

"O you who believe! Fear Allah, and be with those who are true (in words and deeds)." (Qur'an, At—Tawbah 9:119)

Narrated Abdullah: The Prophet (peace and blessings be upon him) said, "Truthfulness leads to righteousness, and righteousness leads to Paradise. And a man keeps on telling the truth until he becomes a truthful person. Falsehood leads to Al-Fajur (i.e. wickedness, evildoing), and Al-Fajur (wickedness) leads to the Hellfire, and a man may keep on telling lies till he is written before Allah, a liar." (Bukhari)

Umm Kulthum bint 'Uqbah ibn Abi Mu'ayt (May Allah be pleased with her) reported that the Prophet (May Allah's peace and blessings be upon him) said: "The liar is not the one who seeks reconciliation between people, conveying good or saying good things." There is an addition in the narration of Muslim, saying: that I did not hear him giving permission of lying in anything except in three (things): the war, reconciliation between people, and what a man says to his wife and what a woman says to her husband." (Bukhari and Muslim) (https://hadeethenc.com/en/browse/hadith/3853)

172. Prohibition of Lying and Listening to Lies

Allah, the Exalted, says:
"Surely Allah does not guide him aright who is a liar, ungrateful." (Qur'an, Az-Zumar 39:3)

"... the Curse of Allah be on him if he is one of the liars." (Qur'an, An-Nur 24:8)

"Nay! If he (Abu Jahl) ceases not, We will catch him by the forelock." (Qur'an, Al-'Alaq 96:15)

Other Verses: An-Nahl 16:105, Ali 'Imran 3:61.

The Most Evil Kind of Lies are:

1. Prohibition of Lying about Allah and His Messenger

Allah, the Exalted, says:

"And who can be more unjust than he who invents a lie against Allah or says: "I have received inspiration", whereas he is not inspired in anything; and who says, "I will reveal the like of what Allah has revealed." And if you could but see when the Zalimun (polytheists and wrongdoers, etc.) are in the agonies of death, while the angels are stretching forth their hands (saying): "Deliver your souls! This day you shall be recompensed with the torment of degradation because of what you used to utter against Allah other than the truth. And you used to reject His Ayats (proofs, evidences, verses, lessons, signs, revelations, etc.) with disrespect!" (Qur'an, Al-An'am 6:93)

"Say: 'Verily, those who invent lies against Allah will never be successful.'" (Qur'an, Yunus 10:69)

Narrated 'Ali: The Prophet (peace and blessings be upon him) said, "Do not tell a lie against me for whoever tells a lie against me (intentionally) then he will surely enter the Hellfire." (Bukhari)

2. Prohibition of Lying in Buying and Selling

Hakim b. Hazim (May Allah be pleased with him) reported Allah's Messenger (peace and blessings be upon him) as saying: "Both parties in a business transaction have the right to annul it so long as they have not separated; and if they speak the truth and make everything clear, they will be blessed in their transaction; but if they tell a lie and conceal anything, the blessing on their transaction will be blotted out." (Muslim)

3. Prohibition of Lying About Visions and Dreams

Wāthilah ibn al-Asqa' (May Allah be pleased with him) reported that the Prophet (May Allah's peace and blessings be upon him) said: "From the gravest of lies is someone who ascribes himself to other than his biological father or claims to have seen something in a dream which he actually never saw, or ascribes something to the Messenger of Allah (May Allah's peace and blessings be upon him) which he did not say." (Bukhari) (https://hadeethenc.com/en/browse/hadith/3633)

Narrated Ibn 'Abbas: The Prophet (peace and blessings of Allah be upon him) said, "Whoever claims to have seen a dream which he did not see, will be ordered to make a knot between two barley grains which he will not be able to do; and if somebody listens to the talk of some people who do not like him (to listen) or they run away from him, then molten lead will be poured into his ears on the Day of Resurrection; and whoever makes a picture, will be punished on the Day of Resurrection and will be ordered to put a soul in that picture, which he will not be able to do." (Bukhari)

4. Prohibition of Speaking About Everything he Hears

Yahya bin Yahya narrated to us, Hushaym informed us, on authority of Sulayman at-Taymi, on authority of Abi Uthman an-Nahdi, he said, Umar bin ul-Khattab (May Allah be pleased with them) said: "It is enough of a lie for a man that he narrates everything he hears." (Muslim)

5. Prohibition of Lying in Jest and Pleasantry

Narrated Abu Umamah: The Prophet (peace and blessings be upon him) said: "I stand guarantee for a house in the middle of Jannah for the person who avoids lying even if he were joking/in jest." (Abu Dawud)

Narrated Mu'awiyah ibn Haydah: The Prophet (peace and blessings be upon him) said: "Woe to the one who speaks lies to make the people laugh. Woe to him! Woe to him!" (Tirmidhi and Abi Dawud)
For instance, telling that, "A certain lady wants to marry you," when actually there is no truth in it. Celebrating April Fools' Day (lie to make fun) is against the teachings of Islam.

Prohibition of Listening to a Lie

Allah, the Exalted, says:

"(They are) avid listeners to falsehood, devourers of (what is) unlawful." (Qur'an, Al-Ma'idah 5:42)

Punishment for Lying:

1. Hypocrisy in the Heart

Allah, the Exalted, says:

"And of them are some who made a covenant with Allah (saying): 'If He bestowed on us of His Bounty, we will verily, give Sadaqah (Zakah and voluntary charity in Allah's Cause) and will be certainly among those who are righteous.' Then when He gave them of His Bounty, they became niggardly [refused to pay the Sadaqah (Zakah or voluntary charity)], and turned away, averse. So, He punished them by putting hypocrisy into their hearts till the Day whereon they shall meet Him, because they broke that (covenant with Allah) which they had promised to Him and because they used to tell lies." (Qur'an, At-Tawbah 9:75-77)

Narrated 'Abdullah bin 'Amr: The Prophet (peace and blessings be upon him) said, "Whoever has the following four (characteristics) will be a pure hypocrite and whoever has one of the following four characteristics will have one characteristic of hypocrisy unless and until he gives it up: 1. Whenever he is entrusted, he betrays, 2. Whenever he speaks, he tells a lie, 3.

Whenever he makes a covenant, he proves treacherous, 4. Whenever he quarrels, he behaves in a very imprudent, evil and insulting manner." (Bukhari)

2. Guidance to Evildoing and to the Fire

Narrated Abdullah: The Prophet (peace and blessings be upon him) said, "Truthfulness leads to righteousness, and righteousness leads to Paradise. And a man keeps on telling the truth until he becomes a truthful person. Falsehood leads to Al-Fajur (i.e. wickedness, evildoing), and Al-Fajur (wickedness) leads to the Hellfire, and a man may keep on telling lies till he is written before Allah, a liar." (Bukhari)

3. His Testimony will be Rejected

Allah, the Exalted, says:

"Why did they not produce four witnesses? Since they (the slanderers) have not produced witnesses! Then with Allah they are the liars." (Qur'an, An-Nur 24:13)

The testimony of the evildoer and liar cannot be accepted, because Allah says:

"And take as witness two just persons from among you (Muslims)." (Qur'an, At-Talaq 65:2)

4. Blackening of the Face in this World and in the Hereafter

Allah, the Exalted, says:

"And on the Day of Resurrection you will see those who lied against Allah (i.e. attributed to Him sons, partners, etc.) their faces will be black. Is there not in Hell an abode for the arrogant ones?" (Qur'an, Az-Zumar 39:60)

5. The Liar will have the Flesh of his Cheeks Torn to the Back of his Head

Narrated Samura bin Jundab (May Allah have mercy on him): "…The Prophet (peace and blessings be upon him) said: "But I had seen (a dream) last night that two men came to me, caught hold of my hands, and took me to the Sacred Land (Jerusalem). There, I saw a person sitting and another standing with an iron hook in his hand pushing it inside the mouth of the former till it reached the jawbone, and then tore off one side of his cheek, and then did the same with the other side; in the meantime, the first side of his cheek became normal again and then he repeated the same operation again. I said, 'What is this?'…

'…Tell me all about that I have seen.' They said, 'Yes. As for the one whose cheek you saw being torn away, he was a liar and he used to tell lies, and the people would report those lies on his authority till they spread all over the world. So, he will be punished like that till the Day of Resurrection." (Bukhari)

(https://sunnah.com/riyadussalihin:1546)

6. Lying Causes forgetfulness

When lying changes memory for the truth. (204)

7. Lying Causes Diseases, Memory Loss

Allah, the Exalted, says:

"none but Shaitan (Satan) made me forget…" (Qur'an, Al-Kahf 18:63)

"Shall I inform you (O people!) upon whom the Shayateen (Devils) descend? They descend on every lying (one who tells lies), sinful person." (Qur'an, Ash-Shu'ara 26:221-222)

"In their hearts is disease, so Allah has increased their disease; and for them is a painful punishment because they (habitually) used to lie." (Quran, Al-Baqarah 2:10)

Qais said: Abu Bakr stood up and praised and glorified Allah, then he said: "O people, you recite this Verse: *"O you who believe! Take care of your own selves. If you follow the (Right) Guidance…" (Al-Ma'idah 5:105)*, but you do not interpret it properly. I heard the Messenger of Allah (peace and blessings be upon him) say: "If the people see evil and do not change it, soon Allah will send His Punishment upon them all." He (Qais) said: 'I heard Abu Bakr say: 'O people, beware of lying for lying is contrary to Faith.'" (Ahmad)

173. Defamation

Allah, the Exalted, says:

"O you who believe! Let not a group scoff at another group, it may be that the latter are better than the former; nor let (some) women scoff at other women, it may be that the latter are better than the former, nor defame one another, nor insult one another by nicknames. How bad is it, to insult one's brother after having Faith [i.e. to call your Muslim brother (a faithful believer) as: "O sinner" or "O wicked", etc.]. And whosoever does not repent, then such are indeed Zalimun (wrongdoers, etc.)." (Qur'an, Al-Hujurat 49:11)

The Messenger of Allah (peace and blessings be upon him) said: "Two matters are signs of disbelief on the part of those who indulge in them: defaming and speaking evil of a person's lineage, and wailing over the dead." (Muslim)

174. Speaking Without Knowledge

Allah, the Exalted, warns:

"So, do not argue about them except with an obvious argument." (Qur'an, Al-Kahf 18:22)

"And follow not (O man i.e. say not or do not, or witness not, etc.) that of which you have no knowledge (e.g. one's saying: "I have seen", while in fact he has not seen, or "I have heard," while he has not heard). Verily! The hearing and the sight, and the heart, of each of those you will be questioned (by Allah)." (Qur'an, Al-Isra 17:36)

"O you who believe! Fear Allah, and be with those who are true (in words and deeds)." (Qur'an, At-Tawbah 9:119)

Abu Umamah (May Allah be pleased with him) reported: The Messenger of Allah (peace and blessings be upon him) said, "The superiority of the learned over the devout worshipper is like my superiority over the most inferior amongst you (in good deeds)." He went on to say, "Allah, His angels, the dwellers of the heaven and the earth, and even the ant in its hole and the fish (in water) supplicate in favour of those who teach people knowledge." (Tirmidhi)

Abud-Darda (May Allah be pleased with him) reported: The Messenger of Allah (peace and blessings be upon him) said, "He who follows a path in quest of knowledge, Allah will make the path of Jannah easy to him. The angels lower their wings over the seeker of knowledge, being pleased with what he does. The inhabitants of the heavens and the earth, and even the fish in the depth of the oceans seek forgiveness for him. The superiority of the learned man over the devout worshipper is like that of the full moon to the rest of the stars (i.e. in brightness). The learned are the heirs of the Prophets who bequeath neither dinar nor dirham but only that of knowledge; and he who acquires it, has in fact acquired an abundant portion." (Abu Dawud and Tirmidhi)

Abu Hurairah (May Allah be pleased with him) reported: The Messenger of Allah (peace and blessings be upon him) said, "He who does not acquire knowledge with the sole intention of seeking the Pleasure of Allah but for worldly gain, will not smell the fragrance of Jannah on the Day of Resurrection." (Abu Dawud)

'Abdullah bin 'Amr bin Al-'As (May Allah be pleased with him) reported: "I heard the Messenger of Allah (peace and blessings be upon him) saying: "Verily, Allah does not take away knowledge by snatching it from the people, but He takes it away by taking away (the lives of) the religious scholars till none of the scholars stays alive. Then the people will take ignorant ones as their leaders, who, when asked to deliver religious verdicts, will issue them without knowledge, the result being that they will go astray and will lead others astray." (Bukhari and Muslim)

Narrated 'Abdullah ibn 'Amr ibn al-'Aas (May Allah be pleased with him) from the Prophet (peace and blessings of Allah be upon him) that he said: "The Qur'an was not revealed to contradict itself; rather parts of it confirmed other parts. Whatever you understand of it, act upon it, and whatever you do not understand of it, refer it to one who has knowledge of it." (Ahmad)

175. Following his Own Desire

Allah, the Exalted, says:

"Have you seen the one who takes as his god his own desire? Then would you be responsible for him?" (Qur'an, Al-Furqan 25:43)

"But there came after them successors who neglected prayer and pursued desires; so, they are going to meet evil." (Qur'an, Maryam 19:59)

"So do not let one avert you from it who does not believe in it and follows his desire, for you [then] would perish." (Qur'an, Taha 20:16)

Other Verses: *Sad 38:26, Al-A'raf 7:175-176, Al-Qasas 28:50.*

Narrated Abu Hurairah: Allah's Messenger (peace and blessings be upon him) said, "The Hellfire is surrounded by all kinds of desires and passions, while Paradise is surrounded by all kinds of disliked undesirable things." (Bukhari)

Sahl bin Sa'd As-Sa'idi (May Allah be pleased with him) reported: "A man came to the Prophet (peace and blessings be upon him) and said, "O Messenger of Allah, guide me to such an action which, if I do Allah will love me and the people will also love me." He (peace and blessings be upon him) said, "Have no desire for this world, Allah will love you; and have no desire for what people possess, and the people will love you." (Ibn Majah)

Qutbah ibn Malik (May Allah be pleased with him) reported that the Prophet (May Allah's peace and blessings be upon him) said: "O Allah, Keep me away from reprehensible morals, deeds, inclinations and illnesses." (Tirmidhi) (https://hadeethenc.com/en/browse/hadith/5329)

Sa'd ibn Abi Waqqas (May Allah be pleased with him) reported that the Prophet (May Allah's peace and blessings be upon him) said: "Verily, Allah loves the servant who is pious, free of wants and inconspicuous." (Muslim) (https://hadeethenc.com/en/browse/hadith/5545)

Abu Hurairah (May Allah be pleased with him) reported that the Prophet (May Allah's peace and blessings be upon him) said: "The son of Adam has been destined his share of fornication, which he will inevitably acquire. The eyes fornicate by looking, the ears fornicate by listening, the tongue fornicates by speaking, the hand fornicates by hitting, the foot fornicates by stepping. The heart loves and wishes. The genitals prove or disapprove that." (Bukhari and Muslim) (https://hadeethenc.com/en/browse/hadith/8898)

'Uqbah ibn 'Amir (May Allah be pleased with him) reported: The Messenger of Allah (May Allah's peace and blessings be upon him) said: "I fear two things for my Ummah: the Qur'an and milk. As for milk, they seek the countryside, follow desires and neglect the prayers. As for the Qur'an, the hypocrites learn it to argue with the believers by means of it." (Ahmad) (https://hadeethenc.com/en/browse/hadith/10856)

Abu Hurairah (May Allah be pleased with him) reported: The Messenger of Allah (peace and blessings be upon him) said, "Seven people Allah will give them His Shade on the Day when there would be no shade but the Shade of His Throne (i.e. on the Day of Resurrection): And they are: a just ruler, a youth who grew up with the worship of Allah, a person whose heart is attached to the Mosques, two men who love and meet each other and depart from each other for the sake of Allah, a man whom an extremely beautiful woman seduces (for illicit relation), but he (rejects this offer and) says: 'I fear Allah', a man who gives in charity and conceals it (to such an extent) that the left hand does not know what the right has given; and a man who remembers Allah in solitude and his eyes become tearful." (Bukhari and Muslim)

176. Preoccupation with this Life

'Abdullah ibn Masud (May Allah be pleased with him) reported: The Prophet (May Allah's peace and blessings be upon him) said: "Do not crave for property lest you should become consumed with desire for worldly life." (Tirmidhi and Ahmad) (https://hadeethenc.com/en/browse/hadith/6614)

Anas ibn Malik (May Allah be pleased with him) reported that the Prophet (May Allah's peace and blessings be upon him) said: "The wealthiest of people in this world, from among the dwellers of Fire, will be brought on the Day of Judgment and dipped once in the Fire then he will be asked: 'O son of Adam, Have you ever witnessed any goodness? Have you ever experienced any bliss?' He will say: 'O Lord, by Allah I have not.' Then, the most miserable of people in this world, from among the dwellers of Paradise, will be dipped once in Paradise then he will be asked: 'O son of Adam, have you ever witnessed any misery? Have you ever experienced any hardship?' He will say: 'No by Allah, I have never witnessed any misery nor have I experienced any hardship." (Muslim) (https://hadeethenc.com/en/browse/hadith/4248)

'Abdur-Rahman bin Aban bin 'Uthman bin 'Affan narrated that his father said: "Zaid bin Thabit departed from Marwan at mid-day. I said: 'He has not sent him out at this time of the day except for something he asked.' So, I asked him, and he said: 'He asked me about some things we heard from the Messenger of Allah (peace and blessings be upon him) say: "Whoever is focused only on this world, Allah will confound his affairs and make him fear poverty constantly, and he will not get anything of this world except that which has been decreed for him. Whoever is focused on the Hereafter, Allah will settle his affairs for him and make him feel content with his lot, and his provision and worldly gains will undoubtedly come to him." (Ibn Majah)

Abu Sa'id al-Khudri (May Allah be pleased with him) reported: The Messenger of Allah (May Allah's peace and blessings be upon him) once sat on the pulpit and we sat around him. He said: "Verily, among the things I fear the most for you is the splendor and pleasures of this worldly life when they become plentifully available to you." (Bukhari and Muslim) (https://hadeethenc.com/en/browse/hadith/4180)

177. Bad Character and Manners

Allah, the Exalted, says:

"And verily, you (O Muhammad (SAW)) are on an exalted (standard of) character." (Qur'an, Al-Qalam 68:4)

"And We have sent you (O Muhammad SAW) not but as a mercy for the 'Alamin (mankind, Jinns and all that exists)." (Qur'an, Al-Anbya 21:107)

"And tell My servants to say that which is best." (Qur'an, Al-Isra 17:53)

Other Verses: *Taha 20:44, Al-Baqarah 2:83, Ali 'Imran 3:134, Al-Furqan 25:63, Al-Balad 90:17-18, An-Nahl 16:125, Luqman 31:19.*

Ibn 'Abbas (May Allah be pleased with him) reported: The Messenger of Allah (peace and blessings be upon him) said to Ashaj Abdul-Qais (May Allah be pleased with him), "You possess two qualities that Allah loves. These are clemency and tolerance." (Muslim)

Commentary: This Hadith teaches us to adopt a patient, mild and discreet attitude towards others. (205)

Aisha (May Allah be pleased with her) reported: The Messenger of Allah (peace and blessings be upon him) said, "Allah is Forbearer and loves forbearance in all matters." (Bukhari and Muslim)

Narrated Aisha (May Allah be pleased with her): The Prophet (peace and blessings be upon him) said,

"Aisha, verily Allah is Kind and He loves kindness and confers upon kindness which He does not confer upon severity and does not confer upon anything else besides it (kindness)." (Muslim)

Narrated Anas bin Malik: The Prophet (peace and blessings be upon him) said, "Make things easy for the people, and do not make it difficult for them, and make them calm (with glad tidings) and do not repulse (them)." (Bukhari)

Narrated Jarir bin 'Abdullah (May Allah be pleased with him): Messenger of Allah (peace and blessings be upon him) said, "He who is deprived of forbearance and gentleness is, in fact, deprived of all good." (Muslim)

Narrated Aisha (May Allah be pleased with her): "Whenever the Prophet (peace and blessings be upon him) was given a choice between two matters, he would (always) choose the easier as long as it was not sinful to do so; but if it was sinful, he was most strict in avoiding it. He never took revenge upon anybody for his own sake; But when Allah's Legal Bindings were outraged, he would take revenge for Allah's sake." (Bukhari and Muslim)

Ibn Masud (May Allah be pleased with him) reported: The Messenger of Allah (peace and blessings be upon him) said, "Shall I not tell you whom the Hellfire is forbidden to touch? It is forbidden to touch a man who is always accessible, having polite and tender nature." (Tirmidhi)

Narrated Anas (May Allah have mercy on him): "The Messenger of Allah (peace and blessings be upon him) was the best of all the people in behavior." (Bukhari and Muslim)

Narrated Anas (May Allah be pleased with him): "I never felt any piece of velvet or silk softer than the palm of the Messenger of Allah (peace and blessings be upon him), nor did I smell any fragrance more pleasant than the smell of Messenger of Allah (peace and blessings be upon him). I served him for ten years, and he never said 'Uff' (an expression of disgust) to me. He never said 'why did you do that?' for something I had done, nor did he ever say 'why did you not do such and such' for something I had not done." (Bukhari and Muslim)

Narrated Nawwas bin Sam'an (May Allah be pleased with him): "I asked the Messenger of Allah (peace and blessings be upon him) about virtue and sin, and he said, "Virtue is noble behavior, and sin is that which creates doubt and you do not like people to know about it." (Muslim)

Narrated 'Abdullah bin 'Amr bin Al-'as: "The Messenger of Allah (peace and blessings be upon him) did not indulge in loose talk nor did he like to listen to it. He used to say, "The best of you is the best among you in conduct." (Bukhari and Muslim)

Commentary: This Hadith, apart from describing the refined behavior and sublime morality of Messenger of Allah (peace and blessings be upon him), tells us that a person with the highest moral sense is in fact the best among people. (206)

Narrated Abud-Darda: The Prophet (peace and blessings be upon him) said, "Nothing will be heavier on the Day of Resurrection in the scale of the believer than good manners. Allah hates one who utters foul or coarse language." (Tirmidhi)

Abdullah ibn Amr reported: The Messenger of Allah (peace and blessings be upon him) said, "Whoever would love to be delivered from Hellfire and admitted into Paradise, let him meet his end with faith in Allah and the Last Day, and let him treat people as he would love to be treated." (Muslim)

Abu Hamzah Anas bin Malik (May Allah be pleased with him) - the servant of the Messenger of Allah (peace and blessings of Allah be upon him) - said that the Prophet (peace and blessings of Allah be upon him) said: "None of you will believe until you love for your brother what you love for yourself." (Bukhari and Muslim)
Ibn 'Umar (May Allah be pleased with him) reported: The Messenger of Allah (peace and blessings be upon him) passed by a man of the Ansar who was admonishing his brother regarding shyness. The Messenger of Allah (peace and blessings be upon him) said, "Leave him alone, for modesty is a part of Iman." (Bukhari and Muslim)

'Imran bin Husain (May Allah be pleased with him) reported: The Messenger of Allah (peace and blessings be upon him) said, "Shyness does not bring anything except good." (Bukhari and Muslim)

Narrated Aisha (May Allah be pleased with her): "I heard the Messenger of Allah (peace and blessings be upon him) saying: 'A believer will attain by his good behavior the rank of one who prays during the night and observes fasting during the day.'" (Abu Dawud)

Narrated Abu Umamah Al-Bahili: The Messenger of Allah (peace and blessings be upon him) said, "I guarantee a house in Jannah for one who gives up arguing, even if he is in the right; and I guarantee a home in the middle of Jannah for one who abandons lying even for the sake of fun; and I guarantee a house in the highest part of Jannah for one who has good manners." (Abu Dawud)

Aisha (May Allah be pleased with her) reported: "I asked the Prophet (peace and blessings be upon him),
"Have you ever experienced a day harder than the day of the battle of Uhud?" He replied, "Indeed, I experienced them (dangers) at the hands of your people (i.e. the disbelievers from amongst the Quraish tribe). The hardest treatment I met from them was on the Day of 'Aqabah when I went to Ibn 'Abd Yalil bin 'Abd Kulal (who was one of the chiefs of Ta'if) with the purpose of inviting him to Islam, but he made no response (to my call). So, I departed with deep distress. I did not recover until I arrived at Qarn ath-Tha'alib. There, I raised my head and saw a cloud which had cast its shadow on me. I saw in it Jibreel (Gabriel) (peace be upon him) who called me and said: 'Indeed, Allah, the Exalted, heard what your people said to you and the response they made to you. And He has sent you the angel in charge of the mountains to order him to do to them what you wish.' Then the angel of the mountains called me, greeted me and said: 'O Muhammad, Allah listened to what your people had said

to you. I am the angel of the mountains, and my Rubb has sent me to you so that you may give me your orders. (I will carry out your orders). If you wish, I will bring together the two mountains that stand opposite to each other at the extremities of Makkah to crush them in between.'" But the Messenger of Allah (peace and blessings be upon him) said, "I rather hope that Allah will raise from among their descendants' people as will worship Allah the One, and will not ascribe partners to Him (in worship)." (Bukhari and Muslim)

Narrated Anas (May Allah be pleased with him): "I was walking with the Messenger of Allah (peace and blessings be upon him) who was wearing a Najrani cloak with a very thick border when a Bedouin happened to meet him. He took hold of the side of his cloak and drew it violently. I noticed that the violence of jerk had bruised the neck of Messenger of Allah (peace and blessings be upon him). The Bedouin said: "O Muhammad! Give me out of Allah's wealth that you possess." The Messenger of Allah (peace and blessings be upon him) turned to him and smiled, and directed that he should be given something." (Bukhari and Muslim)

Narrated Abu Hurairah: The Messenger of Allah (peace and blessings be upon him) observed: "He who intended to do good, but did not do it, one good was recorded for him, and he who intended to do good and also did it, ten to seven hundred good deeds were recorded for him. And he who intended evil but did not commit it, no entry was made against his name, but if he committed that, it was recorded." (Muslim)

Narrated Aisha (May Allah be pleased with her): The Messenger of Allah (peace and blessings be upon him) said: "Verily, the most complete of believers in faith are those with the best character and who are most kind to their families." (Tirmidhi)

Narrated Abu Hurairah: It was said, "O Messenger of Allah, pray against the idolaters!" The Messenger of Allah (peace and blessings be upon him) said: "Verily, I was not sent to invoke curses, but rather I was only sent as mercy." (Muslim)

Narrated Ibn Masud: The Messenger of Allah (peace and blessings be upon him) said: "The believer does not insult others, does not curse others, is not vulgar and is not shameless." (Tirmidhi)

Abu Hurairah reported Allah's Messenger (peace and blessings be upon him) as saying: "Verily Allah does not look to your faces and your wealth but He looks to your heart and to your deeds." (Muslim)

Anas Ibn Malik reported: The Messenger of Allah (peace and blessings be upon him) said: "The faith of a servant is not upright until his heart is upright, and his heart is not upright until his tongue is upright. A man will not enter Paradise if his neighbor is not secure from his evil." (Aḥmad)

'Abdullah ibn 'Amr and Jabir ibn 'Abdullah (May Allah be pleased with them) reported that the Prophet (May Allah's peace and blessings be upon him) said: "The true Muslim is the one from whose tongue and hand the Muslims are safe, and the Muhājir (emigrant) is the one who abandons what Allah has forbidden." Abu Musa (May Allah be pleased with him) reported that he said: "O Messenger of Allah, who is the best among Muslims?" He said: "The one from whose tongue and hand the Muslims are safe." (Bukhari and Muslim) (https://hadeethenc.com/en/browse/hadith/10101)

Abu Hurairah (May Allah be pleased with him) reported that the Prophet (May Allah's peace and blessings be upon him) said: "There is no servant who conceals the faults of another servant in this worldly life, except that Allah will conceal his faults on the Day of Resurrection." (Muslim)
(https://hadeethenc.com/en/browse/hadith/3777)

Al-Nu'man Ibn Bashir reported: The Messenger of Allah (peace and blessings be upon him) said: "The parable of the believers in their affection, mercy and compassion for each other is that of a body. When any limb aches, the whole body reacts with sleeplessness and fever." (Bukhari and Muslim)

'Iyad bin Himar (May Allah be pleased with him) said: The Messenger of Allah (peace and blessings be upon him) said, "Verily, Allah has revealed to me that you should adopt humility. So that no one may wrong another and no one may be disdainful and haughty towards another." (Muslim)

Abu Hurairah (May Allah be pleased with him) reported: The Messenger of Allah (peace and blessings be upon him) said, "Do you know who is the bankrupt?" They said: "The bankrupt among us is one who has neither money with him nor any property". He said, "The real bankrupt of my Ummah would be he who would come on the Day of Resurrection with Salat, Saum and Sadaqah (charity), (but he will find himself bankrupt on that Day as he will have exhausted the good deeds) because he reviled others, brought calumny against others, unlawfully devoured the wealth of others, shed the blood of others and beat others; so his good deeds would be credited to the account of those (who suffered at his hand). If his good deeds fall short to clear the account, their sins would be entered in his account and he would be thrown in the Hellfire." (Muslim)

Abu Hurairah (May Allah be pleased with him) reported: The Messenger of Allah (peace and blessings be upon him) said, "Seven people Allah will give them His Shade on the Day when there would be no shade but the Shade of His Throne (i.e. on the Day of Resurrection): And they are: a just ruler, a youth who grew up with the worship of Allah, a person whose heart is attached to the Mosques, two men who love and meet each other and depart from each other for the sake of Allah; a man whom an extremely beautiful woman seduces (for illicit relation), but he (rejects this offer and) says: 'I fear Allah'; a man who gives in charity and conceals it (to such an extent) that the left hand does not know what the right has given; and a man who remembers Allah in solitude and his eyes become tearful." (Bukhari)

Commentary: In order to win the Pleasure of Allah, he should be forgiving and tolerant with regard to the sufferings he experiences at the hands of people. Both, good behavior and the example of the Prophet (peace and blessings be upon him), call for such an attitude. (207)

'Abdullah ibn 'Amr (May Allah be pleased with him) reported that the Prophet (May Allah's peace and blessings be upon him) said: "Those who are merciful will be shown Mercy by the Most Merciful. Be merciful to those on the earth and the One in the heaven will be Merciful to you." (Tirmidhi, Abu Dawud and Ahmad) (https://hadeethenc.com/en/browse/hadith/8289)

Abu Dharr and Mu'adh ibn Jabal (May Allah be pleased with them) reported that the Prophet (May Allah's peace and blessings be upon him) said: "Fear Allah wherever you are, follow a bad deed with a good deed and it will erase it, and treat people with good morals." (Tirmidhi, Ahmad and Al-Darimi) (https://hadeethenc.com/en/browse/hadith/4302)

Abu 'Abdur-Rahman 'Abdullah ibn Masud (May Allah be pleased with him) said: "It is as though I am looking at Allah's Messenger as he tells the story of one of the Prophets (peace be upon them) as his people struck him and caused him to bleed, and he wiped the blood from his face, saying: 'Allah, forgive my people for they do not know.'" (Bukhari and Muslim) (https://hadeethenc.com/en/browse/hadith/3594)

178. Warning Against Persecution of the Pious, the Weak and the Indigent

Allah, the Exalted, says:

"And those who annoy believing men and women undeservedly, bear on themselves the crime of slander and plain sin." (Qur'an, Al-Ahzab 33:58)

"Therefore, treat not the orphan with oppression. And repulse not the beggar." (Qur'an, Ad-Duha 93:9-10)

Jundub bin Abdullah (May Allah be pleased with him) reported: The Messenger of Allah (peace and blessings be upon him) said, "He who performs the Fajr (dawn) prayer comes under the Protection of Allah, so beware lest Allah questions you about what you owe Him. For if He questions anyone of you and he falls short of fulfilling the duty which he owes Him, He will requite and then throw upon his face into the Hellfire." (Muslim)

Abu Hurairah (May Allah be pleased with him) reported that the Prophet (May Allah's peace and blessings be upon him) said: "Verily Allah said: 'Whoever shows enmity to a pious worshiper of Mine, I declare war against him. My slave does not draw near to Me with anything dearer to Me than what I have made obligatory for him. My slave continues to draw near to Me by doing supererogatory deeds until I love him. When I love him, I become his hearing with which he hears, his sight with which he sees, his hand with which he strikes, and his foot with which he walks. Were he to ask Me for something, I would surely give it to him, and were he to seek refuge with Me, I would surely grant him refuge, I do not hesitate to do anything as I hesitate to take the soul of the believer, for he hates death, and I hate to hurt him.'" (Bukhari) (https://hadeethenc.com/en/browse/hadith/6337)

179. Prohibition of Disobeying Parents and Severance of Relations

Allah, the Exalted, says:

"Worship Allah and join none with Him (in worship); and do good to parents…" (Qur'an, An-Nisa 4:36)

"Say (O Muhammad): Come, I will recite what your Lord has prohibited you from: Join not anything in worship with Him; be good and dutiful to your parents…" (Qur'an, Al-An'am 6:151)

"And We have enjoined on man (to be dutiful and good) to his parents. His mother bore him in weakness and hardship upon weakness and hardship, and his weaning is in two years, give thanks to Me and to your parents, unto Me is the final destination." (Qur'an, Luqman 31:14)

Other Verses: *Muhammad 47:22-23, Ar-Ra'd 13:25, Al-Isra 17:23-24.*
Abu Bakrah (May Allah be pleased with him) reported: The Prophet (May Allah's peace and blessings be upon him) said: "Shall I not inform you of the biggest of the Major sins?" Messenger of Allah (peace and blessings be upon him) asked this question thrice. We said, "Yes, O Messenger of Allah, please inform us." He said, "Ascribing partners to Allah and to be undutiful to your parents." The Messenger of Allah (peace and blessings be upon him) sat up from his reclining position and said, "And I warn you against giving forged statement and a false testimony; I warn you against giving forged statement and a false testimony." Messenger of Allah (peace and blessings be upon him) kept on repeating that warning till we wished he would stop." (Bukhari and Muslim) (https://hadeethenc.com/en/browse/hadith/2941)

Narrated Al-Walid bin 'Aizar: "I heard Abi 'Amr 'Ash-Shaibani saying, "The owner of this house", he pointed to `Abdullah's house, said, 'I asked the Prophet (peace and blessings be upon him): 'Which deed is loved most by Allah?' He replied, 'To offer prayers at their early (very first) stated times.'" `Abdullah asked, "What is the next (in goodness)?" The Prophet (peace and blessings be upon him) said, "To be good and dutiful to one's parents," `Abdullah asked, "What is the next (in goodness)?" The Prophet (peace and blessings be upon him) said, "To participate in Jihad for Allah's Cause." `Abdullah added, "The Prophet (peace and blessings be upon him) narrated to me these three things, and if I had asked more, he would have told me more." (Bukhari)

Narrated Abdullah bin 'Amr bin Al-'As (May Allah be pleased with him): The Prophet (peace and blessings be upon him) said, "(Of the) Major sins are: to ascribe partners to Allah, disobey parents, murder someone and to take a false oath (intentionally)." (Bukhari)

Narrated 'Abdullah bin 'Amr bin Al-'As (May Allah be pleased with him): The Messenger of Allah (peace and blessings be upon him) said, "It is one of the gravest sins to abuse one's parents." It was asked (by the people): "O Messenger of Allah, can a man abuse his own parents?" Messenger of Allah (peace and blessings be upon him) said, "He abuses the father of somebody who, in return, abuses the former's father; he then abuses the mother of somebody who, in return, abuses his mother." (Bukhari and Muslim)

Narrated Abu Muhammad Jubair bin Mut'im (May Allah be pleased with him): The Messenger of Allah (peace and blessings be upon him) said, "The person who severs the bond of kinship, will not enter Jannah." (Bukhari and Muslim)

Narrated Abu 'Isa Al-Mughirah bin Shu'bah (May Allah be pleased with him): The Prophet (peace and blessings be upon him) said, "Allah has forbidden you: disobedience to your mothers, to withhold (what you should give) or demand (what you do not deserve), and to bury your daughters alive. And Allah dislikes idle talk, to ask too many questions (for things which will be of no benefit to one), and to waste your wealth." (Bukhari and Muslim)

'Abdullah ibn 'Amr ibn al-'As (May Allah be pleased with him) reported: "A man came to the Prophet (May Allah's peace and blessings be upon him) and said: "I pledge allegiance to you to immigrate and fight for Allah's Cause seeking Allah's reward." He said: "Is either of your parents alive?" He replied: "Yes, both of them." The Prophet (May Allah's peace and blessings be upon him) asked him: "Do you seek reward from Allah?" He replied: 'Yes.' The Prophet (May Allah's peace and blessings be upon him) said: "Then return to your parents and accompany them in a best way." (Bukhari and Muslim) (https://hadeethenc.com/en/browse/hadith/3260)

Abu Hurairah (May Allah be pleased with him) reported that the Prophet (May Allah's peace and blessings be upon him) said: "May he be disgraced, may he be disgraced, may he be disgraced, he whose parents, one or both, reach old age in his life and he does not enter Paradise (because of his goodness towards them)." (Muslim) (https://hadeethenc.com/en/browse/hadith/3718)

Narrated Abdullah bin Amr: The Prophet (peace and blessings be upon him) said: "The Lord's Pleasure is in the parent's pleasure, and the Lord's Anger is in the parent's anger." (Tirmidhi)

Narrated Mu'awiyah bin Jahimah As-Sulami, that Jahimah came to the Prophet (peace and blessings be upon him) and said: "O Messenger of Allah! I want to go out and fight (in Jihad) and I have come to ask your advice." He said: "Do you have a mother?" He said: "Yes." He said: "Then stay with her, for Paradise is beneath her feet." (An-Nasa'i)

Narrated Abu Hurairah: "A man came to Allah's Messenger (peace and blessings be upon him) and said, "O Allah's Messenger (peace and blessings be upon him)! Who is more entitled to be treated with the best companionship by me?" The Prophet (peace and blessings be upon him) said, "Your mother." The man said. "Who is next?" The Prophet said, "Your mother." The man further said, "Who is next?" The Prophet (peace and blessings be upon him) said, "Your mother." The man asked for the fourth time, "Who is next?" The Prophet (peace and blessings be upon him) said, "Your father." (Bukhari)

IF PARENTS ARE THE DISBELIEVERS

Allah, the Exalted, says:

"When it is said to them: "Follow what Allah has sent down." They say: "Nay! We shall follow what we found our fathers following." (Would they do that!) Even though their fathers did not understand anything nor were they guided?" (Qur'an, Al-Baqarah 2:170)

"O you who believe! Take not for Auliya' (supporters and helpers) your fathers and your brothers if they prefer disbelief to belief. And whoever of you does so, then he is one of the Zalimun (wrongdoers, etc.)." (Qur'an, At-Tawbah 9:23)

"And We have enjoined upon man goodness to parents. But if they endeavor to make you associate with Me that of which you have no knowledge, do not obey them. To Me is your return, and I will inform you about what you used to do." (Qur'an, Al-'Ankabut 29:8)

Other Verses: Luqman 31:14-15, At-Tawbah 9:24.

The believing children should be very careful not to do things simply because their parents did it, especially if knowledge reaches them that their practices contradict the Qur'an and Sunnah.

Ali (May Allah have mercy on him) reported: The Prophet (peace and blessings be upon him) said, "There is no obedience to the creation (if it entails) the disobedience of the Creator." (Ibn Hibban; Al Ihsan, Hadith: 4568 and Ahmad, vol.1 p.31) (https://hadithanswers.com/there-is-no-obedience-to-the-creation-in-the-disobedience-of-the-creator)

Ali (May Allah have mercy on him) reported: The Prophet (peace and blessings be upon him) said: "…There is no obedience to anyone in sinful acts, obedience is only in meritorious acts." (Bukhari and Muslim) (https://hadithanswers.com/there-is-no-obedience-to-the-creation-in-the-disobedience-of-the-creator)

Narrated Asma' bint Abu Bakr: "My mother came to me, hoping (for my favor) during the lifetime of the Prophet. I asked the Prophet, "May I treat her kindly?" He replied, "Yes." Ibn 'Uyaina said, "Then Allah revealed: *'Allah forbids you not with regards to those who fought not against you because of religion, and drove you not out from your homes, that you should show them kindness and deal justly with them.'.......(60.8)* (Bukhari) (https://sunnah.com/bukhari:5978)

180. Responsibilities and Obligations of the Parents Forward their Children

Allah, the Exalted, says:

"And those who say: 'Our Lord! Bestow on us wives and offspring who will be the comfort of our eyes, and make us leaders for the Muttaqoon (pious).'" (Qur'an, Al-Furqan 25:74)

"No mother or father should be made to suffer for their child." (Qur'an, Al-Baqarah 2:233)

"O you who have believed, protect yourselves and your families from a Fire whose fuel is people and stones, over which are (appointed) angels, harsh and severe; they do not disobey Allah in what He commands them but do what they are commanded." (Qur'an, At-Tahrim 66:6)

Narrated Ibn Abbas (May Allah be pleased with him) said: The Messenger of Allah (peace and blessings of Allah be upon him) said: "If anyone of you on having sexual relations with his wife said (and he must say it before starting) 'In the Name of Allah. O Allah! Protect us from Satan and also protect what you bestow upon us (i.e. the coming offspring) from Satan, and if it is destined that they should have a child then, Satan will never be able to harm that offspring." (Bukhari)

Narrated Abu Hurairah (May Allah be pleased with him): The Prophet (peace and blessings of Allah be upon him) said, "When any human being is born. Satan touches him at both sides of the body with his two fingers, except Jesus, the son of Mary, whom Satan tried to touch but failed, for he touched the placenta-cover instead." (Bukhari)

Narrated Abu Rafi': "I saw the Messenger of Allah (peace and blessings of Allah be upon him) uttering the Call to prayer (Adhan) in the ear of al-Hasan ibn Ali when Fatima gave birth to him." (Abu Dawud)

Narrated Jabir (May Allah be pleased with him): The Prophet (peace and blessings of Allah be upon him) said, "When night falls, then keep your children close to you, for the Devil spread out then. An hour later you can let them free; and close the gates of your house (at night), and mention Allah's Name thereupon, and cover your utensils, and mention Allah's Name thereupon, (and if you don't have something to cover your utensil) you may put across it something (e.g. a piece of wood etc.)." (Bukhari)

Narrated Ibn Abbas (May Allah be pleased with him): The Prophet (peace and blessings of Allah be upon him) used to seek refuge with Allah for Al-Hasan and Al-Husayn and say: "Your forefather (i.e. Abraham) used to seek refuge with Allah for Ishmael and Isaac by reciting the following: 'O Allah! I seek refuge with Your Perfect Words from every Devil and from poisonous pests and from every evil, harmful Envious Eye.'" (Bukhari)

Narrated 'Abdullah (May Allah be pleased with him) that the Messenger of Allah (peace and blessings of Allah be upon him) said: "Each of you is a shepherd and is responsible for his flock. The ruler who is in charge of people is a shepherd and is responsible for them. The man is the shepherd of his household and is responsible for them. The woman is the shepherd of her husband's house and child, and is responsible for them. The slave is the shepherd of his master's wealth and is responsible for it. Each of you is a shepherd and each of you is responsible for his flock." (Bukhari and Muslim)

Narrated Anas bin Malik (May Allah be pleased with him): The Messenger of Allah (peace and blessings of Allah be upon him) said: "Be kind to your children and perfect their manners." (Ibn Majah)

Narrated Aisha (May Allah be pleased with her), the wife of the Prophet: "A lady along with her two daughters came to me asking me (for some alms), but she found nothing with me except one date which I gave to her and she divided it between her two daughters, and then she got up and went away. Then the Prophet (peace and blessings be upon him) came in and I informed him about this story. He said, "Whoever is in charge of (put to test by) these daughters and treats them generously, then they will act as a shield for him from the Hellfire." (Bukhari)

An-Nu'man ibn Bashir (May Allah be pleased with him) reported: "My father gave me some of his property as a gift. My mother 'Amrah bint Rawāha said: 'I shall not be satisfied until you make the Messenger of Allah (May Allah's peace and blessings be upon him) a witness to it.' My father went to the Messenger of Allah (May Allah's peace and blessings be upon him) in order to make him witness to the gift he has given me. The Messenger of Allah (May Allah's peace and blessings be upon him) asked him: "Have you done the same with all your children?" He said: 'No.' Thereupon, he said: "Fear Allah, and be just regarding your children." So, my father returned and took back the gift. According to another wording, the Prophet (May Allah's peace and blessings be upon him) said: "Then do not make me a witness to this, for indeed, I do not bear witness to injustice." According to a third wording, he said: "Then let someone other than me be a witness to this." (Bukhari and Muslim with multiple versions)
(https://hadeethenc.com/en/browse/hadith/6035)

Narrated Abu Hurairah: Allah's Messenger (peace be upon him) kissed Al-Hasan bin 'Ali while Al-Aqra' bin H'Abis at-Tamim was sitting beside him. Al-Aqra said, "I have ten children and I have never kissed anyone of them." Allah's Messenger (peace and blessings of Allah be upon him) cast a look at him and said, "Whoever is not merciful to others will not be treated mercifully." (Bukhari)

Anas said: "The Messenger of Allah (peace and blessings be upon him) was one of the best of men in character. One day he sent me to do something, and I said: I swore by Allah that I would not go. But in my heart, I felt that I should go to do what the Prophet of Allah (peace and blessings be upon him) had commanded me; so, I went out and came upon some boys who were playing in the street. All of a sudden, the Messenger of Allah (peace and blessings be upon him) who had come up behind caught me by the back of the neck, and when I looked at him, he was laughing.' He said: 'Go where I ordered you, little Anas.' I replied: 'Yes, I am going, Apostle of Allah!' Anas said: 'I swear by Allah, I served him for seven or nine years, and he never said to me about a thing which I had done: 'Why did you do such and such?' Nor about a thing which I left: 'Why did not do such and such?'" (Abu Dawud)

Abu Hurairah (May Allah be pleased with him) reported: The Messenger of Allah (peace and blessings be upon him) said, "When a man dies, his deeds come to an end except for three things: Sadaqah Jariyah (ceaseless charity); a knowledge which is beneficial, or a virtuous descendant who prays for him (for the deceased)." (Muslim)

181. Ruling for Naming Children

Allah, the Exalted, says:

"Do you know of any who is similar to Him?" (Qur'an, Maryam 19:65)

"Therefore, be patient (O Muhammad SAW) as did the Messengers of strong will and be in no haste about them (disbelievers). On the Day when they will see that (torment) with which they are promised (i.e. threatened, it will be) as if they had not stayed more than an hour in a single day. (O mankind! This Qur'an is sufficient as) a clear Message (or proclamation to save yourself from destruction). But shall any be destroyed except the people who are Al-Fasiqun (the rebellious, disobedient to Allah)." (Qur'an, Al-Ahqaf 45:36)

Ibn Umar (May Allah have mercy on him) reported that Allah's Messenger (peace and blessings be upon him) said: "The names dearest to Allah are 'Abdullah and 'Abd al-Rahman." (Muslim)
Abu Wahb, a Companion, reported that the Prophet (peace and blessings be upon him) said, "Name yourselves with the names of the Prophets. The names which Allah Almighty loves most are 'Abdullah and 'Abdu'r-Rahman. The most truthful names are Harith and Humam. The ugliest names are Harb and Murra." (Al-Adab Al-Mufrad, Bukhari)

Prohibition of Naming Children by:

- Names of Allah which are befitting only for Him, may He be Glorified, such as al-Khaliq (the Creator), al-Raziq (the Provider), al-Rabb (the Lord), al-Rahman

(the Most Merciful), etc. Names which describe Attributes which are true only of Allah, such as Malik al-Mulook (King of kings), al-Qaahir (the Subduer), etc. It is haram to call people by these Names, and they must be changed.
- Enslavement to or worship of anything other than Allah, including Prophets and angels. It is not permissible to be enslaved to or to worship anyone or anything other than Allah. Among the names which express enslavement to or worship of anything other than Allah are 'Abd al-Rasool ("slave of the Messenger"), 'Abd al-Nabi ("slave of the Prophet") and 'Abd al-Ameer (slave of the prince) and other names which imply worship of or submission to anything other than Allah. The person who has a name like this must change it.
- The great Sahaabi 'Abd al-Rahman ibn 'Awf (May Allah be pleased with him) said: "My name was 'Abd 'Amr – or according to one report, 'Abd al-Ka'bah – and when I became Muslim, the Messenger of Allah (peace and blessings of Allah be upon him) called me 'Abd al-Rahman." (Al-Hakim)
- Names that belong exclusively to the kuffaar and are not used by anyone else, such as 'Abd al-Maseeh ("slave of the Messiah"), Butrous (Peter), Jurjus (George) and other names which denote religions of kufr.
- Names of idols and false gods which are worshipped instead of Allah, such as naming someone after a Devil.

Disapproval of Giving Ugly Names and such Names as can be as Ill Omens

Samura b. Jundub reported: "Allah's Messenger (peace and blessings be upon him) forbade us to give names to our servants as these four names: Aflah (Successful), Rabdh (Profit), Yasar (Wealth) and Nafi' (Beneficial)." (Muslim)

Excellence of Changing Ugly Names to Good Names

Ibn 'Umar (May Allah have mercy on him) reported that Allah's Messenger (peace be upon him) changed the name of 'Asiya (Disobedient) and said: "You are Jamila (i.e. good and handsome)." Ahmad (one of the narrators) narrated it with a slight variation of wording." (Muslim)

Muhammad b. 'Amr b. 'Ata' reported: "I had given the name Barra to my daughter. Zainab, daughter of Abu Salama, told me that Allah's' Messenger (May peace and blessings be upon him) had forbidden me to give this name. (She said): "I was also called Barra, but Allah's Messenger (peace and blessings be upon him) said: "Don't hold yourself to be pious. It is God Alone Who knows the people of piety among you." They (the Companions) said: "Then, what name should we give to her?" He said: "Name her as Zainab." (Muslim)

Names which are Makrooh (Disliked)

- It is makrooh (disliked) to use names which have off-putting meanings, either because the meaning is ugly or because it will provoke others to make fun of the person. Such names also go against the teaching of the Prophet (peace and blessings

of Allah be upon him) who commanded us to give beautiful names. Examples of such (objectionable) names include Harb ("war"), Rashaash (sprinkles or drizzle), and Hiyaam – which is the name of a disease suffered by camels.
- It is makrooh to use names which have sexual or provocative meanings.
- It is makrooh to deliberately name someone after immoral people such as singers and actors/actresses, etc. If they have good names, it is permissible to use those names, but it must be because of the meaning of the name and not because of the desire to imitate those people.
- It is makrooh to give names which have meanings that refer to sin, such as Saariq ("thief") or Zaalim ("wrongdoer"); or to give the names of the sinners, such as Fir'awn (Pharaoh), Haamaan (the name of Pharaoh's minister) and Qaroon.
- It is makrooh to use the names of animals which are well-known for their undesirable characteristics, such as al-Himaar (donkey), al-Kalb (dog), al-Qird (monkey), etc.
- It is makrooh to use any name which is added to the words "al-Deen" or "al-Islam" (i.e. names which appear in idaafah – genitive construction – with these words), such as Noor al-Deen ("light of the religion"), Shams al-Deen ("sun of the religion"), Noor al-Islam ("light of Islam"), Shams al-Islam ("sun of Islam"), etc., because these names give a person more than he deserves. Imam al-Nawawi (May Allah have mercy on him) disliked his nickname of Muhiy al-Deen ("reviver of the religion"); Sheikh al-Islam Ibn Taymiyah (May Allah have mercy on him) also disliked his nickname of Taqiy al-Deen ("piety of the religion"), and he used to say, "But my family gave me this nickname and it became well-known."
- It is makrooh to add any word to the Name of Allah except the word 'Abd (slave), as in 'Abd-Allah (Abdullah). Example of this include Hasab-Allaah, Rahmat-Allaah (the Mercy of Allah), etc. It is similarly makrooh to add words to the word al-Rasool (the Messenger).
- It is makrooh to use the names of angels or to call people after the names of Surahs in the Qur'an, such as Taha, Yasin, etc. (See Tuhfat al-Mawdood by Ibn al-Qayyim, p.109)

There are Four Categories of Good Names:

The first (best) category is the names 'Abdullah and 'Abd al-Rahman.

The second category is all the names which express enslavement to and worship of Allah, such as 'Abd al-Azeez, 'Abd al-Raheem, 'Abd al-Malik, 'Abd al-Ilaah, 'Abd al-Salaam, etc.

The third category is the names of Prophets and Messengers (peace and blessings of Allah be upon them). The best and greatest of them is Muhammad (peace and blessings of Allah be upon him); the name Ahmad is also one of his names. It is mustahabb to use their names, following their example and hoping to reach a higher status.

Next come the names of the *"Messengers of strong will" (Al-Ahqaf 46:35)*, namely Ibrahim, Moosa, 'Eesa and Nooh, then the rest of the Prophets (peace and blessings of Allah be upon them).

The fourth category is any other good name which has a proper and pleasant meaning.

It is good to pay attention to a number of matters when giving names to our children:

1. Recognizing the fact that this name will stay with the person for his entire lifetime, and it could cause some embarrassment or problems for him which in turn could make him feel badly towards his father, mother or whoever gave him this name.

2. When looking at names in order to choose one, we should look at it from a number of angles. We should look at the name itself, and also think of how it will sound when this person is a child, a youth, an adult, an old man and a father, and how it will suit his father to be called "Abu" (Father of).

3. Choosing the name is the right of the father, because he is the one after whom the child will be named (son of or daughter of…). But it is mustahabb for the father to involve the mother in the decision and to ask for her opinion as to whether she thinks the name is good, so that she will feel happy.

4. The child must be named after his father even if the father is deceased or divorced, etc., even if he does not take care of the child or see him at all. It is utterly haram to name a child after anyone other than his father, except in one case, which is when the child is born as the result of adultery (Allah forbid). In this case the child should be named after his mother and it is not permissible to name him after his father. (208)

182. Not Commanding Your Children to Pray when they are Seven Years Old

Narrated Abdullah ibn Amr ibn al-'As: The Messenger of Allah (peace and blessings be upon him) said: "Command your children to pray when they become seven years old, and beat them for it (prayer) when they become ten years old; and arrange their beds (to sleep) separately." (Abu Dawud)

183. Stern Warning Against Disowning One's Child

Allah, the Exalted, says:

"Call them by (the names of) their fathers; it is more just in the sight of Allah. But if you do not know their fathers - then they are (still) your brothers in religion and those

entrusted to you. And there is no blame upon you for that in which you have erred but (only for) what your hearts intended. And ever is Allah Forgiving and Merciful." (Qur'an, Al-Ahzab 33:5)

Narrated Abu Hurairah that he heard the Messenger of Allah (peace and blessings be upon him) say when the Verse of Mula'anah (Li'an) was revealed: "Any woman who falsely attributes a man to people to whom he does not belong, has no share from Allah, and Allah will not admit her to His Paradise. Any man who denies his son while looking at him (knowing that he is indeed his son), Allah, the Mighty and Sublime, will cast him away, and disgrace him before the first and the last on the Day of Resurrection." (An-Nasa'i)

Aisha (May Allah be pleased with her) reported: Sa'd ibn Abi Waqqas and 'Abd ibn Zam'ah disputed over (the lineage of) a boy. Sa'd said: "O Messenger of Allah, this is the son of my brother 'Utbah ibn Abi Waqqas. He entrusted him to me saying that he was his own son. Just look at him and see how he resembles him." 'Abd ibn Zam'ah said: "O Messenger of Allah, he is my brother, as he was born on the bed of my father from his slave girl." The Messenger of Allah (May Allah's peace and blessings be upon him) looked at the boy and saw that he clearly resembled 'Utbah. Thereupon, he said: "He is yours, O 'Abd ibn Zam'ah. The child belongs to the owner of the bed, and the stone is for the one who commits illegal sexual intercourse. O Sawdah, cover yourself from him." So, that boy never saw Sawdah uncovered." (Bukhari and Muslim) (https://hadeethenc.com/en/browse/hadith/6160)

Li'an (Divorce by Curse, an Islamic procedure in which a man denies a child being his), because the basic principle is that the child belongs to the marital bed, as the Prophet (peace and blessings be upon him) said, "The child is for the bed and the adulterer gets nothing." (Bukhari and Muslim)

But if the husband is certain or thinks it most likely that the child is not his, then he may deny it, by means of the process of Li'an.

Li'an is done as described in the Verse in which Allah says:

"And for those who accuse their wives, but have no witnesses except themselves, let the testimony of one of them be four testimonies (i.e. testifies four times) by Allah that he is one of those who speak the truth. And the fifth (testimony should be) the invoking of the Curse of Allah on him if he be of those who tell a lie (against her). But it shall avert the punishment (of stoning to death) from her, if she bears witness four times by Allah, that he (her husband) is telling a lie. And the fifth (testimony) should be that the Wrath of Allah be upon her if he (her husband) speaks the truth." (Qur'an, An-Nur 24:6-9)

So, the husband should say four times, "I bear witness by Allah that I am telling the truth in my accusation of her committing adultery" or "I bear witness by Allah that you have committed adultery and this is not my child." And the fifth time he adds: "May the Curse of Allah be upon me if I am telling a lie."

And the woman – if she denies it – should say: "I bear witness by Allah that he is lying, and that this child is his child." And the fifth time she should pray that the Wrath of Allah should be upon her if he is telling the truth.

The Li'an should be done in the Mosque in the presence of a number of Muslims, along with the judge or his deputy, or whoever they agree to appoint from among the Muslims.

When two spouses engage in Li'an, a number of things happen as a result:

1 – The husband is not subject to the Hadd punishment for slander

2 – The wife is not subject to the Hadd punishment for adultery.

3 – Husband and wife are divorced automatically, and this divorce is not dependent upon a judge's ruling; rather divorce takes place as soon as the process of Li'an is completed, according to many scholars.

4 – They are forever forbidden to remarry.

5 – The child is not to be named after his father, rather he should be named after his mother. He and the husband cannot inherit from one another, and the husband is not obliged to spend on him because he is a stranger to him. (209)

184. Prohibition of Giving Preference to Children Over one Another in Giving Gifts, etc.

Narrated An-Nu'man bin Bashir (May Allah be pleased with him): "My father took me to the Messenger of Allah (peace and blessings be upon him) and said to him: "I have gifted one of my slaves to this son of mine." The Messenger of Allah (peace and blessings be upon him) said, "Have you given such gift to every son of yours?" He replied, "No." Thereupon he said, "Take this gift back."

Commentary: We learn from this Hadith the following important points:
1. In every matter, one should consult scholars and experts of Shariah. This was the practice of the Companions (May Allah be pleased with them).
2. Parents should deal with all their children with equity and justice. Preferential treatment with any child affects them adversely. Obviously, injustice creates tension for parents as well as children and eventually family ties are broken.
3. This Hadith is also advanced by those 'Ulama' in support of their contention that if a person wants to distribute his property among his children during his lifetime, he should not make any discrimination among his male and female children and should give an equal share to all of them. (210)

185. Child Abuse

Allah, the Exalted, says:

"O you who believe! Ward off yourselves and your families against a Fire (Hell) whose fuel is men and stones, over which are (appointed) angels stern (and) severe, who disobey not (from executing) the Commands they receive from Allah, but do that which they are commanded." (Qur'an, At-Tahrim 66:6)

"And warn your tribe (O Muhammad SAW) of near kindred." (Qur'an, Ash-Shu'ara 26:214)

Narrated 'Abdullah bin 'Umar: Allah's Messenger (peace and blessings be upon him) said, "Surely! Every one of you is a guardian and is responsible for his charges: The Imam (ruler) of the people is a guardian and is responsible for his subjects; a man is the guardian of his family (household) and is responsible for his subjects; a woman is the guardian of her husband's home and of his children, and is responsible for them; and the slave of a man is a guardian of his master's property and is responsible for it. Surely, everyone of you is a guardian and responsible for his charges." (Bukhari)

Anas bin Malik narrated that: "An older man came to talk to the Prophet (peace and blessings be upon him) and the people were hesitant to make room for him. The Prophet (peace and blessings be upon him) said: "He is not one of us who does not show mercy on our young and honnor our old." (Tirmidhi) (https://hadeethenc.com/en/browse/hadith/3083)

Narrated Abu Hurairah (May Allah be pleased with him): The Messenger of Allah (peace and blessings of Allah be upon him) kissed al-Hasan ibn 'Ali when al-Aqra' ibn Haabis al-Tameemi was sitting with him. Al-Aqra' said: "I have ten children and I have never kissed one of them." The Messenger of Allah (peace and blessings of Allah be upon him) said: "The one who does not show mercy will not be shown mercy." (Bukhari and Muslim)

Narrated Abu Hurairah (May Allah be pleased with him) said: The Messenger of Allah (peace and blessings of Allah be upon him) said: "Teach your children to pray when they are seven years old, and smack them (lightly) if they do not do so when they are ten, and separate them in their beds." (Abu Dawud)

186. Killing Your Children

Allah, the Exalted, says:

"And kill not your children for fear of poverty. We provide for them and for you. Surely, the killing of them is a great sin." (Qur'an, Al-Isra 17:31)

Narrated 'Abdullah: "During some of the Ghazawat of the Prophet (peace and blessings be upon him) a woman was found killed. Allah's Messenger (peace and blessings be upon him) disapproved the killing of women and children." (Bukhari)

Narrated Ubada bin As-Samit who took part in the battle of Badr and was a Naqib (a person heading a group of six persons), on the night of Al-'Aqaba pledge: Allah's Apostle said while a group of his companions were around him, "Swear allegiance to me for: not to join anything in worship along with Allah, not to steal, not to commit illegal sexual intercourse, not to kill your children, not to accuse an innocent person (to spread such an accusation among people), not to be disobedient (when ordered) to do good deed." The Prophet added: "Whoever among you fulfills his pledge will be rewarded by Allah. And whoever indulges in any one of them (except the ascription of partners to Allah) and gets the punishment in this world, that punishment will be an expiation for that sin. And if one indulges in any of them, and Allah conceals his sin, it is up to Him to forgive or punish him (in the Hereafter)." 'Ubada bin As-Samit added: "So we swore allegiance for these." (points to Allah's Apostle) (Bukhari)

187. Killing Your Daughters

Allah, the Exalted, says:

"And when the news of (the birth of) a female (child) is brought to any of them, his face becomes dark, and he is filled with inward grief!" (Qur'an, An-Nahl 16:58)

"He hides himself from the people because of the evil of that whereof he has been informed. Shall he keep her with dishonor or bury her in the earth? Certainly, evil is their decision." (Qur'an, An-Nahl 16:59)

"And when the female (infant) buried alive (as the pagan Arabs used to do) shall be questioned. For what sin she was killed?" (Qur'an, At-Takwir 81:8-9)

Narrated Abdullah ibn Abbas: The Prophet (peace and blessings be upon him) said: "If anyone has a female child, and does not bury her alive or slight her, or prefer his children (i.e. the male ones) to her, Allah will bring him into Paradise. Uthman did not mention "male children." (Abu Dawud)

Uqbah bin Amir said: "I heard the Messenger of Allah (peace and blessings be upon him) say:

"Whoever has three daughters and is patient towards them, and feeds them, gives them to drink, and clothes them from his wealth; they will be a shield for him from the Fire on the Day of Resurrection." (Ibn Majah)

Narrated Ibn Abbas that the Messenger of Allah (peace and blessings be upon him) said: "There is no man whose two daughters reach the age of puberty and he treats them kindly for the time they are together, but they will gain him admittance to Paradise." (Ibn Majah)

Narrated Asma bint Abi Bakr: "I saw Zaid bin Amr bin Nufail standing with his back against the Ka'bah and saying, "O people of Quraish! By Allah, none amongst you is on the religion of Abraham except me." He used to preserve the lives of little girls: If somebody wanted to kill his daughter, he would say to him, "Do not kill her for I will feed her on your behalf." So, he would take her, and when she grew up nicely, he would say to her father, "Now if you want her, I will give her to you, and if you wish, I will feed her on your behalf." (Bukhari)

Narrated Al-Mughira bin Shuba: The Prophet (peace and blessings be upon him) said, "Allah has forbidden for you: to be undutiful to your mothers, to bury your daughters alive, do not to pay the rights of the others (e.g. charity, etc.) and to beg of men (begging). And Allah has hated for you: Qil and Qal (useless talk or that you talk too much about others), to ask too many questions, (in disputed religious matters) and to waste the wealth (by extravagance with lack of wisdom and thinking)." (Bukhari)

188. Prohibition of Legal Adoption

Allah, the Exalted, says:
"...nor has He made your adopted sons your real sons. That is but your saying with your mouths. But Allah says the Truth, and He guides to the (Right) Way." (Qur'an, Al-Ahzab 33:4)

"Call them (adopted sons) by (the names of) their fathers, that is more just with Allah. But if you know not their father's (names, call them) your brothers in Faith and Mawalikum (your freed slaves). And there is no sin on you if you make a mistake therein, except in regard to what your hearts deliberately intend. And Allah is Ever Oft-Forgiving, Most Merciful." (Qur'an, Al-Ahzab 33:5)

Narrated 'Aisha (the wife of the Prophet): "Abu Hudhaifa, one of those who fought the battle of Badr, with Allah's Apostle adopted Salim as his son and married his niece Hind bint Al-Wahd bin 'Utba to him' and Salim was a freed slave of an Ansari woman. Allah's Messenger (peace and blessings be upon him) also adopted Zaid as his son. In the Pre-Islamic period of Ignorance the custom was that, if one adopted a son, the people would call him by the name of the adopted-father whom he would inherit as well, till Allah revealed: *"Call them (adopted sons) By (the names of) their fathers." (33:5)* (Bukhari)

Narrated Abu Dharr: The Prophet (peace and blessings be upon him) said, "If somebody claims to be the son of any other than his real father knowingly, he but disbelieves in Allah, and if somebody claims to belong to some folk to whom he does not belong, let such a person take his place in the Hellfire." (Bukhari)

Narrated Wathila bin Al-Asqa: Allah's Messenger (peace and blessings be upon him) said, "Verily, one of the worst lies is to claim falsely to be the son of someone other than one's real father, or to claim to have had a dream one has not had, or to attribute to me what I have not said." (Bukhari)

Adoption means that a man takes an orphan and makes him like one of his own children, calling him after him, so that the orphan is not allowed to marry one of the man's daughters, and so the sons of the adoptive father are regarded as brothers of the orphan and his daughters are regarded as his sisters, and his (the father's) sisters are regarded as his paternal aunts, and so on.

Allah has forbidden adoption and deems all its consequences invalid because it causes knowledge of people's lineage to be lost. (211)

Al-Nawawi said:

"This is clearly stating the emphatic prohibition of claiming to belong to anyone other than one's real father because this involves ingratitude and a denial of the rights of inheritance, as well as cutting family ties and undutifulness to parents." (al-Nawawi's statement ends) (212)

189. Ruling of Sponsoring Orphan

Allah, the Exalted, says:

"…And they ask you concerning orphans. Say: The best thing is to work honestly in their property, and if you mix your affairs with theirs, then they are your brothers. And Allah knows him who means mischief (e.g. to swallow their property) from him who means good (e.g. to save their property). And if Allah had wished, He could have put you into difficulties. Truly, Allah is All-Mighty, All-Wise." (Qur'an Al-Baqarah 2:220)

Raising a child who is not one's genetic child is allowed and, in the case of an orphan, even encouraged.

Narrated Sahl ibn Sa'd: The Messenger of Allah (peace and blessings be upon him) said: "Myself and the caretaker of an orphan will be in Paradise like this", and he held his two fingers together." (Bukhari)

Narrated Ibn 'Abbas: "Some people claim that the order in the above Verse is cancelled, by Allah, it is not cancelled, but the people have stopped acting on it. There are two kinds of guardians (who are in charge of the inheritance): One is that who inherits; such a person should give (of what he inherits to the relatives, the orphans and the needy, etc.), the other is that who does not inherit (e.g. the guardian of the orphans): such a person should speak kindly and say (to those who are present at the time of distribution), "I cannot give it to you (as the wealth belongs to the orphans)." (Bukhari)

Allah commanded that whoever sponsors an orphan child is not to attribute it to himself, but to its biological father if he is known; otherwise, the child should be called 'Mawla' or 'brother-in-religion'. In this way, Islam prevents people from changing truth and preserves the rights of heirs from loss or reduction, protects against mingling between the sexes, and being in the private company of a non-Mahram (person to whom marriage is legitimate) such as that between the male adoptee and the Maharem (persons to whom marriage is illegitimate) of his adoptive father as well as between a female adoptee and her adoptive father, his sons and male relatives. Such mingling spreads corruption, the evils of which are only known to Allah Almighty Who has knowledge of what He created—He is the Ever Kind and All-Knowing. When the orphans reach adolescence, they must be separated from the wives and daughters of the sponsor. The orphaned girl may be beautiful and may become attractive before adolescence, so the sponsor must watch his sons lest they fall into doing haram things with the orphans, because this could happen and be a means of causing mischief which it will be difficult to put right. Based on this, the responsibility of sponsoring an orphan in Islam includes all the responsibilities and duties of adoption except changing lineage, which Islam prohibits, and its ensuing consequences. (213)

The child does not become a true child of the "adoptive" parents. The child is named after the biological, not adoptive, father.

<u>The sponsored child can become a Mahram to his sponsoring family</u>:

1. If the child is breastfed by the sponsoring mother.

If that woman who adopted a child breastfed the adopted child five times before the age of two years, then he would become a son to her through breastfeeding, and her husband would become a father to him through breastfeeding, and their children would all become brothers and sisters to him through breastfeeding. The rule of milk kinship applies to sponsored and non-sponsored children, and is not specific to sponsored children, and does not confer the right to inheritance to the sponsored.

2. The child must maintain his/her original identity through either the middle or last name. He/she should know that they are adopted but not be treated differently and have full comfort at home.
Inheritance can only be assigned through the 1/3 portion. The child could even be given more through this process than one's natural children. Sponsoring an orphan means that a man brings the orphan to live in his house, or he sponsors him somewhere other than his house,

without giving him his name or forbidding that which is permitted or permitting that which is forbidden, as is the case with adoption. Rather the one who sponsors an orphan is doing a generous deed. So, there can be no comparison between one who sponsors an orphan and one who adopts a child, because of the great difference between them and because sponsoring orphans is something which is encouraged in Islam. (214)

190. Adoption Fraud

Adoption in its legal form is prohibited in Islam, but Islam allowed persons to cover needy, namely orphaned, children with protection and financial support.

Fraudulent adoptions can include adoption agencies, facilitators, birth mothers and, in some cases, potential adoptive parents.

Adoption agency may charge excessive fees. Adoption agency may take money for services that were never rendered. Adoption facilitator failing to provide adoptive families with known information about a child's physical, emotional or development problems or with critical background information about the child's birth family.

A pregnant woman promising multiple families her unborn child while accepting payments from the families with or without the intention to complete the adoption. A non-pregnant woman who poses as a birth mother while collecting money for living expenses, with no ability to complete the adoption process.

Buying and selling children are prohibited.

191. Elder Abuse

Meaning and Characteristics of Older Adults
The term 'Sheikh' means 'old person' in Arabic, but in the Qur'an and Hadith, it has two meanings: advanced in religious knowledge and advanced in age. The first interpretation of the word indicates knowledge and wisdom and is associated with experiences accumulated over a lifetime.
The word Sheikh as old age appears in four places in the Qur'an. One example is:

"She said (in astonishment): "Woe unto me! Shall I bear a child while I am an old woman, and here is my husband, an old man? Verily! This is a strange thing!" (Qur'an, Hud 11:72)

This Verse frames older age persons as those who can no longer procreate; thus, ageing in this Verse is linked to physical, not mental, disability.

Another example is:

"He, it is Who has created you (Adam) from dust, then from a Nutfah [mixed semen drops of male and female discharge (i.e. Adam's offspring)] then from a clot (a piece of coagulated blood), then brings you forth as children, then (makes you grow) to reach the age of full strength, and afterwards to be old (men and women), though some among you die before, and that you reach an appointed term, in order that you may understand."
(Qur'an Ghafir 40:67)

This Verse reflects how developmental stages are described in the Qur'an, where being an old adult is framed as closeness to death. (215)

Anas ibn Malik reported: The Messenger of Allah (peace and blessings be upon him) said, "No youth honors his elders but that Allah will appoint someone to honor him in his old age." (Tirmidhi)

Abu Musa (May Allah be pleased with him) reported: The Messenger of Allah (peace and blessings be upon him) said, "It is out of reverence to Allah in respecting an aged Muslim, and the one who commits the Qur'an to memory and does not exaggerate pronouncing its letters nor forgets it after memorizing, and to respect the just ruler." (Abu Dawud)
'Abdullah ibn 'Amr ibn al-'As (May Allah be pleased with him) reported that the Prophet (May Allah's peace and blessings be upon him) said: "He does not belong to us who does not show mercy to our young and honor our old." (Tirmidhi) (https://hadeethenc.com/en/browse/hadith/3083)

Narrated 'Ubadah ibn Samit: The Prophet (peace and blessings be upon him) said: "He who does not respect our elders, and does not have mercy on our children, and does not acknowledge the rights our scholars, is not of my Ummah." (Ahmad)

Abu Hurairah (May Allah be pleased with him) reported that the Prophet (May Allah's peace and blessings be upon him) said: "The young should greet the old, the passer-by should greet the one who is sitting, and the small group of people should greet the larger one." Another narration adds: "and the one who is riding should greet the one who is walking." (Bukhari and Muslim)
(https://hadeethenc.com/en/browse/hadith/5352)

"Neither kill a child, nor a woman, nor an aged man." (Muslim)
(https://www.iium.edu.my/deed/hadith/muslim/019)

192. Prohibition of Breaking Ties and Relationships

Allah, the Exalted, says:

"... and fear Allah through Whom you demand your mutual (rights), and (do not cut the relations of) the wombs (kinship)..." (Qur'an, An-Nisa 4:1)

"And give to the kindred his due and to the miskeen (poor)..." (Qur'an, Al-Isra 17:26)

"So, would you perhaps, if you turned away, cause corruption on earth and sever your (ties of) relationship? Those (who do so) are the ones that Allah has cursed, so He deafened them and blinded their vision." (Qur'an, Muhammad 47:22-23)

Other Verse: Ar-Ra'd 13:25.

Anas bin Malik (May Allah be pleased with him) said: The Messenger of Allah (peace and blessings be upon him) said, "Do not desert (stop talking to) one another, do not nurse hatred towards one another, do not be jealous of one another, and become as fellow brothers and slaves of Allah. It is not lawful for a Muslim to stop talking to his brother (Muslim) for more than three days." (Bukhari and Muslim)

Abu Ayyub Al-Ansari (May Allah be pleased with him) said: The Messenger of Allah (peace and blessings be upon him) said, "It is not lawful for a Muslim to desert (stop talking to) his brother beyond three nights, the one turning one way and the other turning to the other way when they meet, the better of the two is one who is the first to greet the other." (Bukhari and Muslim)

Abu Hurairah (May Allah be pleased with him) said: The Messenger of Allah (peace and blessings be upon him) said, "People's deeds are presented before Allah on Mondays and Thursdays, and then every slave (of Allah) is granted forgiveness (of Minor sins) if he does not associate anything with Allah in worship. But the person in whose heart there is rancor against his brother, will not be pardoned. With regard to them, it is said twice: 'Hold these two until they are reconciled.'" (Muslim)

Jabir (May Allah be pleased with him) said: "I heard the Messenger of Allah (peace and blessings be upon him) as saying, "The Satan has despaired of being worshipped by those who engage in prayer in the Arabian Peninsula but (has not lost hope) in creating dissension among them." (Muslim)

Commentary:
1. This Hadith is one of the proofs of Prophethood of Muhammad (peace and blessings be upon him). His prophecy has come true that Muslims will fight among themselves and, as a result of mutual conflicts, sever links with one another; and this situation will arise as a result of the mischief, provocation and evil suggestions made by Satan.

2. One of the benefits of Salat is to maintain and strengthen the feeling of brotherhood and fraternity between Muslims. (216)

Abu Hurairah (May Allah be pleased with him) said: The Messenger of Allah (peace and blessings be upon him) said, "It is not lawful for a Muslim to forsake his (Muslim) brother beyond three days; and whosoever does so for more than three days, and then dies, will certainly enter the Hell." (Abu Dawud)

Narrated Abu Khirash Hadrad bin Abu Hadrad Al-Aslami (May Allah be pleased with him): "I heard the Prophet (peace and blessings of Allah be upon him) saying, "Whosoever forsakes his brother for a year is like one who sheds his blood." (Abu Dawud)

Narrated Abu Hurairah (May Allah be pleased with him): The Messenger of Allah (peace and blessings of Allah be upon him) said, "It is not permissible for a believer to forsake his (Muslim) brother for more than three days. If three days have passed, he should meet him and greet him; and if other responds to it they will both share the reward; but if he does not respond, he will bear his sin and the one who (has taken the initiative to) greet (the other) will be absolved of the sin of forsaking (one's brother in Faith)." (Abu Dawud)

Anas ibn Malik (May Allah be pleased with him) reported: "I heard the Messenger of Allah (May Allah's peace and blessings be upon him) say: "Whoever loves to have his sustenance expanded and his term of life prolonged should maintain ties of kinship." (Bukhari and Muslim)
(https://hadeethenc.com/en/browse/hadith/5372)

Narrated Aisha, (May Allah be pleased with her), the wife of the Prophet: The Prophet (peace and blessings be upon him) said, "The word 'Ar-Rahm' (womb) derives its name from 'Ar-Rahman' (i.e. Allah). So, whosoever keeps good relations with it (womb i.e. kith and kin), Allah will keep good relations with him, and whosoever will sever it (i.e. severs his bonds of kith and kin) Allah too will sever His relations with him." (Bukhari)

Abu Hurairah (May Allah be pleased with him) said: "The Messenger of Allah (peace and blessings of Allah be upon him) said: "Allah created the Universe, and when He had finished, kinship (al-Rahm) stood up and said, "This is the standing up of one who seeks Your Protection from being cut off." Allah said, "Yes, would it please you if I were to take care of those who take care of you and cut off those who cut you off?" It said, "Of course." Allah said, "Then your prayer is granted." Then the Prophet (peace and blessings of Allah be upon him) said, "Recite, if you wish: *'Would you then, if you were given the authority, do mischief in the land, and sever your ties of kinship? Such are they whom Allah has cursed, so that He has made them deaf and blinded their sight. (Qur'an, Muhammad 47:22-23).'"* (Muslim)

Jubair b. Mutlim reported that his father narrated to him that Allah's Messenger (May peace be upon him) said: "The severer of the tie of kinship would not get into Paradise." (Muslim)

Abdullah ibn 'Amr ibn al-'As (May Allah be pleased with him) reported that the Prophet (May Allah's peace and blessings be upon him) said: "The one who upholds ties of kinship is not the one who recompenses the good done to him by his relatives; rather, he is the one who keeps good relations with those relatives who had severed the bond of kinship with him." (Bukhari) (https://hadeethenc.com/en/browse/hadith/3854)

193. Insult Families

Allah, the Exalted, says:

"…be dutiful and good to parents and to kindred…" (Qur'an, Al-Baqarah 2:83)

"…and speak good to people in the best manner (i.e. enjoin righteousness and forbid evil)…" (Qur'an, Al-Baqarah 2:83)

"The recompense for an evil is an evil like thereof, but whoever forgives and makes reconciliation, his reward is due from Allah. Verily, He likes not the Zalimun (oppressors, polytheists and wrongdoers, etc.)." (Qur'an, Ash-Shuraa 42:40)

Other Verse: Al-Hujurat 49:11.

'Abdullah bin 'Amr bin Al-'As (May Allah be pleased with him) reported: The Messenger of Allah (peace and blessings be upon him) said, "It is one of the gravest sins to abuse one's parents." It was asked (by the people): "O Messenger of Allah, can a man abuse his own parents?" Messenger of Allah (peace and blessings be upon him) said, "He abuses the father of somebody who, in return, abuses the former's father; he then abuses the mother of somebody who, in return, abuses his mother." (Bukhari and Muslim)

194. Prohibition of Deriding one's Lineage

Allah, the Exalted, says:

"And those who annoy believing men and women undeservedly, bear on themselves the crime of slander and plain sin." (Qur'an, Al-Azhab 33:58)

Narrated Abu Hurairah (May Allah be pleased with him): The Messenger of Allah (peace and blessings be upon him) said, "Two matters are signs of disbelief on the part of those who indulge in them: defaming and speaking evil of a person's lineage, and wailing over the dead." (Muslim)

Commentary: Both sins mentioned in this Hadith are such that if a Muslim thinks them lawful and still commits them, he will become a Kafir. To defame someone's lineage means to disgrace or humiliate somebody by saying to him or to her: "Your father belongs to such and such profession" or "Your mother is such and such / so-and-so" or "You are a weaver, blacksmith, launder, cobbler, etc." (217)

195. Prohibition of Attributing Wrong Fatherhood

Allah, the Exalted, says:

"Call them by (the names of) their fathers; it is more just in the sight of Allah. But if you do not know their fathers - then they are (still) your brothers in religion and those entrusted to you. And there is no blame upon you for that in which you have erred but (only for) what your hearts intended. And ever is Allah Forgiving and Merciful." (Qur'an, Al-Ahzab 33:5)

Narrated Sa`d bin Abu Waqqas (May Allah be pleased with him): The Prophet (peace and blessings be upon him) said, "He who (falsely) attributes his fatherhood to anyone besides his real father, knowing that he is not his father, will be forbidden to enter Jannah." (Bukhari and Muslim)

Narrated Abu Dharr (May Allah be pleased with him): The Prophet (peace and blessings be upon him) said: "There is no man who knowingly calls himself after someone other than his father but he has committed kufr. Whoever claims to belong to people to whom he has no ties of blood, let him take his place in Hell." (Bukhari and Muslim)

Narrated Abu Hurairah (May Allah be pleased with him): The Prophet (peace and blessings be upon him) said, "Do not turn away from your fathers, for he who turns away from his father, will be guilty of committing an act of disbelief." (Bukhari and Muslim)

Commentary: To attribute one's fatherhood to someone other than one's real father due to the latter's poverty or in order to live a life of ease and comfort under the care of the person to whom one wishes to attribute his fatherhood, knowing that it is not lawful, is an act of kufr (disbelief). (218)

Narrated Yazid bin Sharik bin Tariq (May Allah be pleased with him): "I saw Ali (May Allah be pleased with him) giving a Khutbah (sermon) from the pulpit and I heard him saying: "By Allah, we have no book to read except Allah's Book and what is written in this scroll. He unrolled the scroll which showed a list of what sorts of camels to be given as blood-money, and other legal matters relating to killing game in the sanctuary of Makkah and the expiation thereof. In it was also written: The Messenger of Allah (peace and blessings be upon him) said: 'Al-Madinah is a sanctuary from `Air to Thaur (mountains). He who innovates in this territory new ideas in Islam, commits a sin therein, or shelters the innovators, will incur the Curse of Allah, the angels and all the people, and Allah will accept from him neither repentance nor a ransom on the Day of Resurrection. The asylum (pledge of protection) granted by any Muslim (even of the) lowest status is to be honored and respected by all other Muslims, and whoever betrays a Muslim in this respect (by violating the pledge) will incur the Curse of Allah, the angels and all the people; and Allah will accept from him neither repentance nor a ransom on the Day of Resurrection. Whoever attributes his fatherhood to someone other than his (real) father, and takes someone else as his master other than his (real) master without his permission, will incur the Curse of Allah, the angels and all the people, and Allah will accept from him neither repentance nor a ransom on the Day of Resurrection." (Bukhari and Muslim)

196. Changing his Father's/Family Name

'Abdullah ibn 'Umar (May Allah be pleased with him) reported that the Prophet (May Allah's peace and blessings be upon him) said: "When Allah the Almighty gathers together (on the Day of Judgment) all the earlier and later generations of mankind, a banner will be raised for every betrayer, and it will be said: 'This is the betrayal of so-and-so, the son of so-and-so.'" (Bukhari and Muslim)
(https://hadeethenc.com/en/browse/hadith/2936)

Sheikh Bakr Abu Zayd (May Allah preserve him) said:

"This is one of the beauties of Shariah, because calling a person by his father's name is more appropriate for knowing who is who and telling people apart. The father is the protector and maintainer of the child and his mother both inside and outside the home. This is why the father mixes with people in the marketplaces and takes risks by travelling to earn a halal living and strive for their sakes. So, the child is given the name of the father, not of the mother who is hidden away and who is one of those whom Allah commanded: *"...And stay in your houses." (Qur'an, Al-Ahzab 33:33)* (Tasmiyat al-Mawlood, 30, 31)

On the basis of the above, there is no blood tie between the husband and wife, so how can she take his surname as if she is part of the same lineage? Moreover, she may get divorced, or her husband may die, and she may marry another man. Will she keep changing her surname every time she marries another man? Furthermore, there are rulings attached to her being named after her father, which have to do with inheritance, spending and who is a Mahram, etc. Taking her husband's surname overlooks all that. The husband is named after his own father, and what does she have to do with the lineage of her husband's father? This goes against common sense and true facts. The husband has nothing that makes him better than his wife so that she should take his surname, whilst he takes his father's name. (219)

197. Looking Inside the House Without Permission

Allah, the Exalted, says:

"O you who believe! Enter not houses other than your own, until you have asked permission and greeted those in them." (Qur'an, An-Nur 24:27)

"And when the children among you come to puberty, then let them (also) ask for permission, as those senior to them (in age)." (Qur'an, An-Nur 24:59)

Abu Musa Al-Ash'ari (May Allah be pleased with him) reported: The Messenger of Allah (peace and blessings be upon him) said, "Permission is to be sought thrice. If it is accorded, you may enter; otherwise, go back." (Bukhari and Muslim)

Sahl bin Sa'd (May Allah be pleased with him) reported: The Messenger of Allah (peace and blessings be upon him) said, "Seeking permission to enter (somebody's house) has been prescribed in order to restrain the eyes (from looking at something we are not supposed to look at)." (Bukhari and Muslim)

Commentary: Within the four walls of their homes, people are normally engaged in different types of domestic chores, or they rest in seclusion. Women understandably do things at home in a relaxed manner which is scarcely possible for them in the presence of a man not belonging to their household. We commit an intrusion upon others' privacy and also eye the Hijab-observing women by entering a house without permission. Both the things are prohibited and must be avoided. (220)

Rib'i bin Hirash (May Allah be pleased with him) reported: "A man of Banu 'Amir tribe has told us that he had asked the Prophet (peace and blessings be upon him) for permission to enter when he was at home. He said: "May I enter?" Messenger of Allah (peace and blessings be upon him) said to the servant, "Go out and instruct him about the manner of seeking permission. Tell him to say: As-Salamu 'Alaikum (may you be safe from evil). May I come in?" The man heard this and said: "As-Salamu 'Alaikum (may you be safe from evil). May I come in?" The Prophet (peace and blessings be upon him) then accorded permission to him and he entered in." (Abu Dawud)

198. Rights of Neighbours

Allah, the Exalted, says:

"Worship Allah and associate nothing with Him, and to parents do good, and to relatives, orphans, the needy, the near neighbor, the neighbor farther away, the companion at your

side, the traveler and those whom your right hands possess. Indeed, Allah does not like those who are self-deluding and boastful." (Qur'an, An-Nisa 4:36)

Ibn 'Umar and Aisha (May Allah be pleased with them) reported: The Messenger of Allah (peace and blessings be upon him) said, "Jibreel kept recommending treating neighbours with kindness until I thought he would assign a share of inheritance." (Bukhari and Muslim)

Abu Dharr (May Allah be pleased with him) reported: The Messenger of Allah (peace and blessings be upon him) commanded me thus, "O Abu Dharr! Whenever you prepare a broth, put plenty of water in it, and give some of it to your neighbours." (Muslim)

Abu Hurairah (May Allah be pleased with him) reported: The Prophet (peace and blessings be upon him) said, "By Allah, he is not a believer! By Allah, he is not a believer! By Allah, he is not a believer." It was asked, "Who is that, O Messenger of Allah?" He said, "One whose neighbour does not feel safe from his evil." (Bukhari and Muslim)

Commentary: This Hadith reveals that hurting or troubling a neighbour is such a serious offence that it causes Allah's Wrath, and thus Punishment in Hell. (221)

Abu Hurairah (May Allah be pleased with him) reported: The Messenger of Allah (peace and blessings be upon him) said, "O Muslim women! No one of you should consider insignificant (a gift) to give to her neighbour even if it is (a gift of) the trotters of a sheep." (Bukhari and Muslim)

Abu Hurairah (May Allah be pleased with him) reported: The Messenger of Allah (peace and blessings be upon him) said, "No one should prohibit his neighbour from placing a peg in his wall". Abu Hurairah (May Allah be pleased with him) added: "Now I see you turning away from this (Sunnah), but by Allah, I shall go on proclaiming it." (Bukhari and Muslim)

Abu Hurairah (May Allah be pleased with him) reported: Messenger of Allah (peace and blessings be upon him) said, "He who believes in Allah and the Last Day let him not harm his neighbour; and he who believes in Allah and the Last Day let him show hospitality to his guest; and he who believes in Allah and the Last Day let him speak good or remain silent." (Bukhari and Muslim)

Aisha (May Allah be pleased with her) reported: "I said, 'O Messenger of Allah (peace and blessings be upon him), I have two neighbours, to which of them should I send a present?'" He (peace and blessings be upon him) replied, "To the one whose door is nearer to you." (Bukhari)

Abdullah bin 'Umar (May Allah be pleased with him) reported: The Messenger of Allah (peace and blessings be upon him) said, "The best of companions with Allah is the one who is best to his companions, and the best of neighbours to Allah is the one who is the best of them to his neighbor." (Tirmidhi)

199. Inheritance Judgment by Any law Other than the Laws of Allah

Allah, the Exalted, says:

"Legislation is not but for Allah." (Qur'an, Yusuf 12:40)

"...and He makes none to share in His Decision and His Rule." (Qur'an, Al-Kahf 18:26)

The followers of those who promulgate human laws other than those which Allah has ordained, are associating others with Allah and it is a Shirk.

Narrated Sad bin Abi Waqqas: "The Prophet (peace and blessings be upon him) came visiting me while I was (sick) in Makkah, (Amir the sub-narrator said, and he disliked to die in the land, whence he had already migrated). He (i.e. the Prophet (peace and blessings be upon him) said, "May Allah bestow His Mercy on Ibn Afra (Sad bin Khaula)." I said, "O Allah's Apostle! May I will all my property (in charity)?" He said, "No." I said, "Then may I will half of it?" He said, "No." I said, "One third?" He said: "Yes, one third, yet even one third is too much. It is better for you to leave your inheritors wealthy than to leave them poor begging others, and whatever you spend for Allah's sake will be considered as a charitable deed even the handful of food you put in your wife's mouth. Allah may lengthen your age so that some people may benefit by you, and some others be harmed by you." At that time Sad had only one daughter." (Bukhari)

Narrated Ibn 'Abbas: The Prophet (peace and blessings be upon him) said, "Give the Fara'id (the shares of the inheritance that are prescribed in the Qur'an) to those who are entitled to receive it. Then whatever remains, should be given to the closest male relative of the deceased." (Bukhari)

When a Muslim dies, there are four duties which need to be performed. They are:

1. To pay funeral and burial expenses.
2. To pay debts of the deceased.
3. To determine the value / will of the deceased if any (which is capped to one third of the estate as the remainder is decided by Shariah Law).
4. To distribute the remainder of estate and property to the relatives of the deceased according to Shariah Law.

Muslims are also encouraged to give money to the orphans and poor if they are present during the division of property. (222)

200. Bringing Loss to the Bequest (Wasiyya)

Allah, the Exalted, says:

"It is prescribed for you, when death approaches any of you, if he leaves wealth, that he make a bequest to parents and next of kin, according to reasonable manners. (This is) a duty upon Al-Muttaqun (the pious - see V.2:2)." (Qur'an, An-Baqarah 2:180)

"After payment of legacies and debts: so that no loss is caused (to any)." (Qur'an, An-Nisa 4:12)

"And whosoever disobeys Allah and His Messenger (Muhammad SAW), and transgresses His limits, He will cast him into the Fire, to abide therein; and he shall have a disgraceful torment." (Qur'an, An-Nisa 4:14)

Ibn Umar (May Allah be pleased with him) reported Allah's Messenger (May peace and blessings be upon him) as saying: "It is the duty of a Muslim who has something which is to be given as a bequest not to have it for two nights without having his Will written down regarding it." (Muslim)
Wasiyya (The Will)

A bequest (Wasiyya) or Will is defined as a transfer to come into operation after the testator's death. The testator is called Musi, and the legatee or devisee is called Musa lahu, and the executor is called Wasi. It is a spiritual testament of a man enabling him to make up his shortcomings in the worldly life and securing rewards in the Hereafter. (Muslim)
"Again, the principle on which the legality of a testamentary disposition is based being in defiance pro tanto of the rights of heirs generally the Law requires that such disposition should be for the benefit of non-heirs alone." (Muslim)
"A further reason why a bequest in favour of an heir is not allowed is that it would amount to giving preference to some heirs over others, thus defeating the spirit of the Law which has fixed the portion of each in the inheritance and causing disputes among persons related to one another. If the other heirs consent to a bequest to one of them or to a bequest of more than one-third of the estate, the above reasons no longer hold good and the bequest as made will be valid." (Abdur Rahim, The Principles of Muhammadan jurisprudence, p.311-2) (Muslim)
Before dying, everyone leaving behind wealth and property should write or dictate a Will in which they may give away up to one-third of their wealth to those who would not inherit from them based on Islamic Inheritance Laws. According to the Shariah, one is entitled to make a Will for one-third of one's property and not beyond that so that the rights of the legal heirs are not adversely affected.
It is, however, preferable and most advisable not to will away the property if the legal heirs are poor, because it manifests benevolence to the heirs who have superior claim to it from the relations in which they stand. (Muslim)
This recommendation was instituted by Allah to protect the rights of non-inheriting relatives and friends. According to Islamic Law, wealth obtained by Wasiyya is not considered inheritance, but a gift. Under this Law Muslims may leave a portion of their wealth to

non-Muslim relatives and a Muslim may also receive a portion in a Will from a non-Muslim relative, because it is considered a gift. Otherwise "A Muslim cannot inherit from a disbeliever nor can a disbeliever inherit from a Muslim." (Bukhari and Muslim) According to the system of Islamic Inheritance Laws (Fara'id), non-Muslims are not classified as heirs to Muslims. Likewise, Muslims have no right to take portions of their dead non-Muslim relatives' wealth. That is, if the deceased non-Muslim relative does not write a Will (Wasiyya) and the non-Muslim state divides up his/her wealth according to its manmade laws, the Muslim relative is prohibited by Islamic Law to accept any share allotted to him/her by this process. (223, 224)
It is considered haram for a father to deprive his children, the women or the children of a wife who is not favorable to him an inheritance. (225)
In Shariah Law, only relatives with a legitimate blood relationship to the deceased are entitled to inherit.

In general, a full brother will exclude a half-brother who shares a common father ("consanguine" brother), but not a half-brother who shares a common mother.

It is not permissible to make a Will concerning one's heir, because he has a share by Shariah Law. But if the gift is being given to one of the children for a Shariah reason, such as the child being poor or in debt, or needing medical treatment, then there is nothing wrong with that. And Allah knows best.

201. Inheritance: Who Has the Right to Claim the Deceased's Estate?

Allah, the Exalted, says:

"There is a share for men and a share for women from what is left by parents and those nearest related, whether the property be small or large — a legal share." (Qur'an, An-Nisa 4:7)

"Allah commands you as regard your children's (inheritance): to the male, a portion equal to that of two females; if (there are) only daughters, two or more, their share is two-thirds of the inheritance; if only one, her share is a half. For parents, a sixth share of inheritance to each if the deceased left children; if no children, and the parents are the (only) heirs, the mother has a third; if the deceased left brothers or (sisters), the mother has a sixth. (The distribution in all cases is) after the payment of legacies he may have bequeathed or debts. You know not which of them, whether your parents or your children, are nearest to you in benefit; (these fixed shares) are ordained by Allah. And Allah is Ever All-Knower, All-Wise." (Qur'an, An-Nisa 4:11)

"And whosoever disobeys Allah and His Messenger (Muhammad) and transgresses His limits, He will cast him into the Fire, to abide therein; and he shall have a disgraceful torment." *(Qur'an, An-Nisa 4:14)*

Four persons cannot get inheritance:

(a) a fugitive slave who has fled away from his master,
(b) one who has murdered one's predecessor intentionally or unintentionally
(c) one who professes a religion other than Islam,
(d) one living in Dar-ul-Harb cannot inherit the property of one living in Dar-ul-Islam and vice versa.

According to Islam, the heirs have been divided into three classes.

A) Dhaw-u'l-Fara'id are those persons who have a right to definite shares in assets left by the deceased. These sharers are twelve in number; four males: father, grandfather, uterine brothers and husband; and eight females: mother, grandmother, uterine sister, wife, single daughter, son's daughter, full sister, consanguine sister.

1. Father's share is one-sixth when the deceased leaves a son or a son's son, but if the deceased is not survived by a son or grandson his father will, in addition to this share (one-sixth), also get a share of being 'Asabat.
2. The grandfather's share is like that of father's share but in three conditions:

    2.1. According to Imam Bukhari and Imam Muslim, the presence of father deprives even the brothers of their share in the inheritance but this is not the case with the grandfather. Imam Abu Hanifa is of the opinion that the presence of grandfather deprives the brother of his share in the inheritance.
    2.2. If the father of the deceased is alive, then the share of the mother is of what is left from the share of the wife of the deceased. The presence of grandfather does not reduce the share of the mother of the deceased.
    2.3. The grandmother of the deceased has no share in the presence of the father of the deceased but she has a share in the presence of the grandfather.

3. The third set of sharers are uterine brothers and sisters. They are entitled to one-sixth if their number is one, and one-third if they are more than one.
4. The husband's share is one-half of the property of the deceased wife if she has no children, but in case of children it is one-fourth.
5. The wife is entitled to one-fourth if the husband dies childless; otherwise it is one-eighth.
6. Real daughter: one-half when alone, and two-thirds if more than one. If the deceased is survived by a male child also, the daughters are then treated as Asabat and the male child would get double of what falls to the lot of daughters. The granddaughters stand on the same level as daughters. But in case the deceased is survived by one real daughter and one or more than one granddaughter they

would get one-sixth. The granddaughter is not entitled to any share if the deceased is survived by a son, but if he is survived by grandsons and granddaughters, they would be treated as 'Asabat and the male grandchild would get double of what goes to the female grandchild.
7. Full sister gets one-half if she is alone, and two-thirds if they are more than one.
8. Consanguine sister is entitled to one-half if one, and two thirds if more.
9. Mother is entitled to one-sixth when she has a child or grandchild, and in case of being childless she gets one-third of the share.
10. If the deceased is survived either by paternal grandmother or maternal grandmother, or even by both, they are entitled to one-sixth. The grandmother (maternal) is deprived of her share if the mother of the deceased is alive; and if father is alive the paternal grandmother is deprived of this share.

B) When the heirs of the first group have received the respective shares, the residue of the assets falls to the share of those relatives who are called Asabat which, according to the Shariah, implies those relatives in whose line of relationship no female enters. This is the second group of inheritors.

There is no fixed share of the 'Asabat. If the deceased is not survived by any Dhaw-u'l-Fara'id, the whole of the property falls to their share; and If Dhaw-u'l.Fara'id are there to get their due share, the residue will be taken by the Asabat. The following are the 'Asabat:

1. Son: He is the first to get the residue in order of succession. The daughters are entitled to half of the share as given to the son. The grandsons are not entitled to any share in the presence of the son. If the son is not living, then the grandson is entitled to a share in the inheritance. If there are more than one son, the inheritance will be distributed equally amongst them.
2. The father, grandfather and the great-grandfather are included in the category of Dhaw-u'l-Fara'id. If, however, the deceased is not survived by category of a son, grandson of great-grandson, then the father will fall under the category of 'Asabat, and, in the absence of the father, the grandfather assumes that position.
3. If the deceased is not survived by son or grandson, or father, or grandfather, i.e. none amongst the 'Asabat, then the brother, and in the absence of brother his son, and in the absence of son, his grandson will be entitled to share in the inheritance as 'Asabat and the female would also join them in share claiming half of the share as compared with male.
4. If unfortunately, the deceased is survived by none of the above-mentioned relatives amongst the 'Asabat, then consanguine brother will be entitled to share in the inheritance and he will be preferred to full brother's son.
5. Then comes the turn of full paternal uncle.

C) The last category of inheritors is known ad Dhaw-u'l Arham, i.e. relations connected through females, but it is in extremely rare cases that they get any share in the inheritance. The following relatives come under this category.

1. The son of the daughter and daughter of the daughter.
2. The son of the daughter of the son, and daughter of the daughter of the son and their children.
3. Maternal grandfather, maternal grandfather of the father, the grandfather of the mother, maternal grandfather of the mother, the grandmother of the mother, the children of the sisters, the sisters of the father and those of the mother, etc. (226)

202. Inheritance Division Among the Heirs of a Deceased Muslim

Allah, the Exalted, says:

"These are the limits (set by) Allah, and whoever obeys Allah and His Messenger will be admitted by Him to gardens (in Paradise) under which rivers flow, abiding eternally therein; and that is the great attainment." (Qur'an, An-Nisa 4:13)

Here are some examples of the Inheritance division in the Qur'an:

1. If the daughter is an only child, i.e. she has no brothers or sisters (i.e. heirs who are descendants), then she has a half of the legacy of the deceased.

Allah, the Exalted, says:

"…if only one, her share is a half…" (Qur'an, An-Nisa 4:11)

2. If there are more than one daughter – two or more – and the deceased has no male children, then their share is two-thirds.

Allah, the Exalted, says:

"…if (there are) only daughters, two or more, their share is two-thirds of the inheritance…" (Qur'an, An-Nisa 4:11)

3. If there are the children both males and females of the deceased then "to the male, a portion equal
to that of two females"

Allah, the Exalted, says:

"Allah has enjoined upon you with regards to your children that the (entitlement of) the male is twice that of the female." (Qur'an, An-Nisa 4:11)

One explanation of why a daughter is entitled to only half that of the son is that Islam decrees that women, upon marriage are entitled to a "Mahr" from the husband.

Almighty Allah bestows the responsibility and accountability on men to provide safety, protection and sustenance to women. The husband's obligation is to care for and maintain his wife and children.

4. Regarding Husband's Inheritance Part:

Allah, the Exalted, says:

"And for you is half of what your wives leave if they have no child. But if they have a child, for you is one fourth of what they leave, after any bequest they (may have) made or debt." *(Qur'an, An-Nisa 4:12)*

5. Regarding the Wife/Wives' Inheritance Part:

Allah, the Exalted, says:

"And for the wives is one fourth if you leave no child. But if you leave a child, then for them is an eighth of what you leave, after any bequest you (may have) made or debt." *(Qur'an, An-Nisa 4:12)*

6. If a Man or Woman Leaves Neither Ascendants nor Descendants:

6a. But Has a Brother or a Sister

Allah, the Exalted, says:

"If the man or woman whose inheritance is in question has left neither ascendants nor descendants but has left a brother or a sister, then for each one of them is a sixth." *(Qur'an, An-Nisa 4:12)*

"They ask you for a legal verdict. Say: "Allah directs (thus) about AlKalalah (those who leave neither descendants nor ascendants as heirs). If it is a man that dies, leaving a sister, but no child, she shall have half the inheritance. If (such a deceased was) a woman, who left no child, her brother takes her inheritance. If there are two sisters, they shall have two-thirds of the inheritance; if there are brothers and sisters, the male will have twice the share of the female. (Thus) does Allah makes clear to you (His Law) lest you go astray. And Allah is the All-Knower of everything." *(Qur'an, An-Nisa 4:176)*

6b. But if the Sisters and Brothers are More than Two

Allah, the Exalted, says:

"But if they are more than two, they share a third, after payment of legacies he (or she) may have bequeathed or debts, so that no loss is caused (to anyone). This is a Commandment from Allah; and Allah is Ever All-Knowing, Most Forbearing." (Qur'an, An-Nisa 4:12)

Aisha (May Allah be pleased with her) narrated that the Messenger of Allah (peace and blessings be upon him) said: "The maternal uncle inherits from the one who has no heirs." (Tirmidhi)

Failure to distribute the inheritance by Allah's Laws in the Qur'an constitutes a Major sin.

If a Muslim dies, the transferable rights will include all the rights pertaining to the property, usufruct and any other dependent rights like outstanding debts. It shall also cover the obligations of the deceased which can be paid off from his estate. Further, whatever is residue, post payment of funeral obligations, shall be divided among the heirs.

Following are the ways under which the property will be distributed:

A. One half (1/2) of the property will be given to:

- The husband, if the wife has no successor;
- The daughter, if the deceased has no other children;
- The daughter of the son or of his descendants, if the deceased has a child or a grandchild higher in degree with her;
- The sister, if she has no brother or sister, a successor of the deceased, father or grandfather;
- Consanguine sister, if she has no brother or germane sister or brother, a successor of deceased, father or grandfather.

B. One-fourth of the property will be given to:

- The husband, if the wife has a descendant;
- The wife, if the husband has no descendant.

C. One eight of the property will be given to:

- The wife, if the husband has a successor.

D. Two-third of the property will be given to:

- Two or more daughters, if deceased has no son;
- Two or more daughters of son, or his successors, if the deceased, has no son, grandson of the same degree;

- Two or more germane sisters, if there is no germane brother, successor, father or grandfather;
- Two or more consanguine sisters, if there is no consanguine brother, a germane brother or sister, a successor, father or grandfather.

E. One-third of the property will be given to:

- The mother, if the deceased has no successor or if there is no one else to succeed;
- Two or more of mother's children, if there is no successor or father, or grandfather, the property shall be divided equally;
- The paternal grandfather, if he concurs the estate of germane or consanguine brother and in the absence of forced heirs;

F. One-sixth of the property will be given to:

- The father upon concurring with succeeding descendent;
- The paternal grandfather, if the deceased has a successor, if the forced heir is present, if his share is less than one-sixth or one-third of the reminder, or if nothing is residual post taking his forced share;
- Mother, along with successor of deceased or with two or more brother and sisters;
- Grandmother, if she is not ineligible for an inheritance. (227)

203. No Inheritance Between Muslim and non-Muslim

Usamah ibn Zayd (May Allah be pleased with him) reported: The Prophet (May Allah's peace and blessings be upon him) said: "A Muslim cannot inherit from a disbeliever nor can a disbeliever inherit from a Muslim." (Bukhari and Muslim) (https://hadeethenc.com/en/browse/hadith/64716)

204. No Inheritance for Illegitimate Child

Narrated from 'Amr bin Shu'aib, from his father, from his grandfather that the Messenger of Allah (peace and blessings of Allah be upon him) said: "Whoever commits adultery with a slave woman or a free woman, his child is illegitimate, and he cannot inherit from him or be inherited from (i.e. this child cannot inherit from him)." (Ibn Majah)

Narrated 'Amr bin Shu'aib, from his father, from his grandfather, that the Messenger of Allah (peace and blessings of Allah be upon him) said: "Every child who is attributed to his father after his father to whom he is attributed has died, and his heirs attributed him to him after he died, he ruled that* whoever was born to a slave woman whom he owned at the time when he had intercourse with her, he should be named after the one to whom he was attributed, but he has no share of any inheritance that was distributed previously. Whatever inheritance he finds has not yet been distributed, he will have a share of it. But he cannot be named after his father if the man whom he claimed as his father did not acknowledge him. If he was born to a slave woman whom his father did not own, or to a free woman with whom he committed adultery, then he cannot be named after him and he does not inherit from him, even if the one whom he claims as his father acknowledges him. So, he is an illegitimate child who belongs to his mother's people, whoever they are, whether she is a free woman or a slave." (Ibn Majah)

*The illegitimate child, i.e. the child of Zina (adultery/fornication). (https://sunnah.com/ibnmajah:2746)

In Islamic Law, only relatives with a legitimate blood relationship to the deceased are entitled to inherit.

205. No Inheritance for Adopted Child

Legal adoption is prohibited. In the Islamic Law, the adoption of a child does not bring legal consequences in terms of blood relations and inheritance relationships with adoptive parents.

Islam allowed persons to cover needy, namely orphaned, children with protection and financial support. In other words, any parent can give the parental care and affection to a child without granting him any legal obligations such as inheritance.

206. No Inheritance for Murderer

Narrated Abu Hurairah: The Prophet (peace and blessings be upon him) said: "The murderer will not inherit." (Tirmidhi)

207. Prohibition of Celibacy

Allah, the Exalted, says:

"O you who believe! Make not unlawful the Tayyibaat (all that is good as regards foods, things, deeds, beliefs, persons) which Allah has made lawful to you, and transgress not. Verily, Allah does not like the transgressors." (Qur'an, Al-Ma'idah 5:87)

"And among His Signs is this, that He created for you wives from among yourselves, that you may find repose in them, and He has put between you affection and mercy. Verily, in that are indeed signs for a people who reflect." (Qur'an, Ar-Rum 30:21)

"O Prophet! Why do you ban (for yourself) that which Allah has made lawful to you, seeking to please your wives? And Allah is Oft-Forgiving, Most Merciful." (Qur'an, At-Tahrim 66:1)

Islam does not regard it as a union only for the gratification of sexual lust, but a social contract with wide and varied responsibilities and duties. The reason behind it is that, according to the Divine Faith, a woman is not a plaything in the hand of man, but a spiritual and moral being who is entrusted to him on the sacred pledge to which Allah is made a witness. The wife is, therefore, not meant, to provide sensuous pleasure only to the male, but to fully co-operate with him in making the life of the family and ultimately of the whole humanity significantly meaningful. (Muslim, Kitab Al-Nikah (The Book of Marriage)

Narrated Aisha (May Allah be pleased with her): "The Messenger of Allah (peace and blessings be upon him) forbade celibacy." (An-Nasa'i)

Narrated Ibn Abbas: The Messenger of Allah (peace and blessings be upon him) said: "There is nothing like marriage, for two who love one another." (Ibn Majah)

Narrated Aisha (May Allah be pleased with her): The Messenger of Allah (peace and blessings be upon him) said: "Marriage is part of my Sunnah, and whoever does not follow my Sunnah has nothing to do with me. Get married, for I will boast of your great numbers before the nations. Whoever has the means, let him get married, and whoever does not, then he should fast for it will diminish his desire." (Ibn Majah)

Narrated Sa'd ibn Abi Waqqas (May Allah be pleased with him): "The Messenger of Allah (peace and blessings be upon him) forbade 'Uthman ibn Maz'oon to be celibate. If he had given him permission, we would have gotten ourselves castrated." (Bukhari and Muslim)

Narrated Anas bin Malik: "A group of three men came to the houses of the wives of the Prophet (peace and blessings be upon him) asking how the Prophet (peace and blessings be upon him) worshiped (Allah), and when they were informed about that, they considered their worship insufficient and said, "Where are we from the Prophet (peace be upon him) as his past and future sins have been forgiven." Then one of them said, "I will offer the prayer throughout the night forever." The other said, "I will fast throughout the year and will not break my fast." The third said, "I will keep away from the women and will not marry forever." Allah's Messenger (peace and blessings be upon him) came to them and said, "Are you the same people who said so-and-so? By Allah, I am more submissive to Allah and more afraid of Him than you; yet I fast and break my fast, I do sleep and I also marry women." (Bukhari)

Narrated 'Abdullah: "We were with the Prophet (peace and blessings be upon him) while we were young and had no wealth. So, Allah's Messenger (peace and blessings be upon him) said, "O young people! Whoever among you can marry, should marry, because it helps him lower his gaze and guard his modesty (i.e. his private parts from committing illegal sexual intercourse, etc.), and whoever is not able to marry, he should fast, as fasting diminishes his sexual power." (Bukhari)

Some of the Sahabah wanted to be celibate and keep away from women, but the Prophet (peace and blessings of Allah be upon him) forbade them to do that, and Allah revealed this Verse *(Al-Ma'idah 5:87)* (228)

Islam encourages early marriage according Shariah Laws and prohibits immorality.

208. Ruling on Choosing Your Wife/Husband

Allah, the Exalted, says:

"And marry those among you who are single (i.e. a man who has no wife and the woman who has no husband) and (also marry) the Salihun (pious, fit and capable ones) of your (male) slaves and maid-servants (female slaves). If they be poor, Allah will enrich them out of His Bounty. And Allah is All-Sufficient for His creatures' needs, All-Knowing (about the state of the people)." (Qur'an, An-Nur 24:32)

"They (your wives) are as a garment to you, and you are as a garment to them." (Qur'an, Al-Baqarah 2:187)

"And those who say: "Our Lord! Bestow on us from our wives and our offspring who will be the comfort of our eyes, and make us leaders for the Muttaqun" (pious - see V.2:2 and the footnote of V.3:164)." (Qur'an, Al-Furqan 25:74)

Marry the Religious Woman/Man

Allah, the Exalted, says:

"Our Lord! And make them enter the 'Adn (Eden) Paradise (everlasting Gardens) which you have promised them, and to the righteous among their fathers, their wives and their offspring! Verily, You are the All-Mighty, the All-Wise." (Qur'an, Ghafir 40:8)

"And marry those among you who are single (i.e. a man who has no wife and the woman who has no husband) and (also marry) the Salihun (pious, fit and capable ones) of your (male) slaves and maid-servants (female slaves)..." (Qur'an, An-Nur 24:32)

Narrated Usamah bin Zaid (May Allah be pleased with him): The Prophet (peace and blessings be upon him) said, "I am not leaving behind me a more harmful trial for men than women." (Bukhari and Muslim)
(https://hadeethenc.com/en/browse/hadith/5830)

Narrated Abu Hurairah (May Allah have mercy on him): The Prophet (peace and blessings be upon him) said: "A woman is married for four things, i.e. her wealth, her family status, her beauty and her religion. So, you should marry the religious woman, (otherwise) you will be a loser." (Bukhari)

Anas ibn Malik (May Allah have mercy on him) reported: The Messenger of Allah (peace and blessings be upon him) said: "Whomsoever has been blessed with a pious wife from Allah, then Allah has certainly assisted him (to fulfill) half of his Deen. So, he should fear Allah in the remaining half." (Al Mu'jamul Awsat, Hadith: 976 and Mustadrak Hakim, vol.2, p.61. Declared authentic by Imam Hakim, https://hadithanswers.com/fulfilling-half-of-din-by-making-nikah)

Narrated Fatimah bint Qays: Her husband divorced her three times and the Messenger of Allah (peace and blessings be upon her) had not appointed her housing or maintenance. The Prophet said to her, "When your waiting period is over, come to me." Fatimah came to him and she was given a marriage proposal from Mu'awiyyah, Abu Jahm and Usamah ibn Zayd. The Prophet said, "As for Mu'awiyyah, he is poor and has no property. As for Abu Jahm, he is a man who often beats women. Rather, choose Usamah ibn Zayd." Fatimah indicated with her hand that she did not want Usamah. The Prophet said, "Obedience to Allah and his Messenger is better for you." Fatimah said, "I married him and I was envied." (Muslim)

Abdullah ibn 'Amr ibn al-'Ās (May Allah be pleased with him) reported: The Messenger (May Allah's peace and blessings be upon him) said: "This world is but an enjoyment and the best of its enjoyments is a righteous woman." (Muslim) (https://hadeethenc.com/en/browse/hadith/5794)

Thawban reported: The Prophet (peace and blessings be upon him) said, "The best wealth is a tongue that remembers Allah, a grateful heart and a believing wife to help one in his faith." (Tirmidhi)

Husband and wife, by entering into the relationship of marriage, secure each other's chastity, just as a garment hides the nakedness. The garment gives comfort to the body; so, does the husband find comfort in his wife's company and she in his. The garment is the grace, the beauty, the embellishment of the body, so too are wives to their husbands as their husbands are to them.

Choose Single Woman and Single Man

Allah, the Exalted, says:

"And marry those among you who are single (i.e. a man who has no wife and the woman who has no husband)…" (Qur'an, An-Nur 24:32)

Marry Virgin

Narrated Jabir bin 'Abdullah (May Allah be pleased with him): "When I got married, Allah's Messenger (peace and blessings be upon him) said to me, "What type of lady have you married?" I replied, "I have married a matron' He said, "Why, don't you have a liking for the virgins and for fondling them?" Jabir also said: Allah's Messenger (peace and blessings be upon him) said, "Why didn't you marry a young girl so that you might play with her and she with you?'" (Bukhari)

Narrated Aisha (May Allah be pleased with her): "I said, 'O Allah's Messenger! Suppose you landed in a valley where there is a tree of which something has been eaten and then you found trees of which nothing has been eaten, of which tree would you let your camel graze?" He said, "(I will let my camel graze) of the one of which nothing has been eaten before." (The sub-narrator added: 'Aisha meant that Allah's Messenger (peace and blessings be upon him) had not married a virgin besides herself). (Bukhari)

Poor Man is Better

Allah, the Exalted, says:

"If they be poor, Allah will enrich them out of His Bounty. And Allah is All-Sufficent for His creatures' needs, All-Knowing (about the state of the people)." (Qur'an, An-Nur 24:32)

Sahl ibn Sa'd As-Sa'idi (May Allah be pleased with him) reported that a man passed by the Prophet (May Allah's peace and blessings be upon him), so he said to a man who was sitting with him: "What do you say about this man?" He replied: "He is one of the noblest of people. By Allah, if he proposes marriage his proposal deserves to be accepted, and if he intercedes his intercession deserves to be accepted." The Messenger of Allah (May Allah's peace and blessings be upon him) remained silent. Then another man passed by. The Messenger of Allah (May Allah's peace and blessings be upon him) said: "What do you think about this man?" He replied: "O Messenger of Allah, this is one of the poor Muslims. If he proposes marriage, he does not deserve to get married, and if he intercedes his intercession does not deserve to be accepted, and if he speaks, he does not deserve to be listened to." The Messenger of Allah (peace and blessings be upon him) said: "This one (the second) is better than an earthful of the other (the first)." (Bukhari) (https://hadeethenc.com/en/browse/hadith/3880)

Ibn Abbas and 'Imran ibn al-Husayn (May Allah be pleased with them) reported that the Messenger of Allah (May Allah's peace and blessings be upon him) said: "I looked into Paradise and found that the majority of its people are the poor, and I looked into the Fire and found that the majority of its people are women." (Bukhari and Muslim) (https://hadeethenc.com/en/browse/hadith/3184)

The Benefits of Marriage are Many:

Protecting one's religion, helping one to adhere to it, protecting and taking care of women, producing righteous offspring and increasing the ranks of the Ummah.

Abu Hurairah (May Allah be pleased with him) reported: The Messenger of Allah (peace and blessings be upon him) said, "When a man dies, his deeds come to an end except for three things: Sadaqah Jariyah (ceaseless charity); a knowledge which is beneficial or a virtuous descendant who prays for him (for the deceased)." (Muslim)

209. Refusing Marriage Proposal

Abu Hatim Al-Muzani (May Allah have mercy on him) reported that Messenger of Allah (peace and blessings be upon him) said: "If someone approaches you (with a proposal) and his religion (piety) and character is pleasing to you, then get him married. If you do not do so, there will be trials (Fitnah) and chaos (fasad) on the earth…" (Tirmidhi)

210. Prohibited Marriage Proposals

1. One who Cannot Support a Wife Shouldn't Marry

   Abdullah ibn Masud (May Allah be pleased with him) reported: The Prophet (May Allah's peace and blessings be upon him) said: "O young men, those of you who can afford to should marry; it restrains the gaze and fortifies one's chastity. Those who cannot should fast; it controls the sexual desire." (Bukhari and Muslim) (https://hadeethenc.com/en/browse/hadith/5863)

2. Prohibition of Marriage Proposal Without Woman's Guardian Arrangement
3. Prohibition of Marriage Proposal or Arranging the Marriage of Another One in a State of Ihram
4. Prohibition of Marriage Proposal to Woman Already Engaged
5. Prohibition on a Woman Proposing to a Man who Has Proposed to Another Woman
6. Prohibition of Marriage Proposal by a Muslim Man to Non-Muslim Woman
7. Prohibition of Marriage Proposal to al-Maharim, the Relatives to whom Marriage is Forbidden
8. Prohibition of Marriage Proposal to Two Sisters at the Same Time
9. Prohibition of Marriage Proposal to a Woman whom Your Father Married
10. Prohibition of Marriage Proposal to a Woman if he is Married to her Paternal or Maternal Aunt at the Same Time
11. Prohibition of Marriage Proposal to a Woman Having a Foster Suckling Relationship
12. Prohibition of Secret Marriage Proposal
13. Prohibition of Shighar Marriage Proposal
14. Prohibition of Al-Mut'ah Marriage Proposal

15. Prohibition of Marriage Proposal to a Woman Already Married
16. Prohibition of Marriage Proposal to his Illegitimate Daughter
17. Prohibition of Marriage Proposal for Plural Marriage if he Cannot Treat Wives Equally
18. Prohibition of Same-Sex Marriage Proposal
19. Prohibition of "Paper" Marriage Proposal
20. Prohibition of the Marriage Proposal to the Orphan Girl under the Guardianship of her Guardian who Likes her Beauty and Wealth, and Wishes to (Marry her and) Curtails her Mahr
21. Prohibition of Marriage Proposals to a Divorced or Widowed Woman During her Iddah (the Waiting Period During which she is Not Allowed to Marry Again)
22. Prohibition of Marriage Proposal to a Woman who is Ungrateful and Displeased with Allah's Decree

211. Prohibition of Marriage Proposal or Arranging the Marriage of

Another One in the Estate of Ihram

Nubaih b. Wahb reported that 'Umar b. Ubaidullah intended to marry Talha b. 'Umar with the daughter of Shaiba b. Jubair; so, he sent a messenger to Aban b. Uthman to attend the marriage, and he was at that time the Amir of Hajj. Aban said: 'I heard 'Uthman b. 'Affan say that Allah's Messenger (peace and blessings be upon him) had stated: "A Muhrim must neither marry himself, nor arrange the marriage of another one, nor should he make the proposal of marriage."' (Muslim)

212. Prohibition of Marriage Proposal to Woman Already Engaged

Narrated Abu Hurairah (May Allah be pleased with him): The Prophet (peace and blessings be upon him) said: "A man should not propose marriage to a woman to whom his brother has already proposed and he should not outbid his brother. A man should not marry a woman if he is already married to her paternal aunt or maternal aunt. A woman should not ask for her sister to be divorced, so as to deprive her of what is rightfully hers and so that she may be married in her stead; rather she will have what Allah has decreed for her." (Bukhari and Muslim)

Narrated Ibn 'Umar (May Allah be pleased with him): "The Prophet (peace and blessings be upon him) already decreed that one should not try to cancel a bargain agreed upon between some other persons (by offering a bigger price). And a man should not ask for the hand of a girl who is already engaged to his Muslim brother, unless the first suitor gives her up or allows him to ask for her hand." (Bukhari)

Narrated Abu Hurairah (May Allah be pleased with him): The Prophet (peace and blessings be upon him) said, "Beware of suspicion (about others), as suspicion is the falsest talk, and do not spy upon each other, and do not listen to the evil talk of the people about others' affairs, and do not have enmity with one another, but be brothers. And none should ask for the hand of a girl who is already engaged to his (Muslim) brother, but one should wait till the first suitor marries her or leaves her." (Bukhari)

213. Prohibition on a Woman Proposing to a Man who Has Proposed to Another Woman

Narrated Abu Hurairah (May Allah be pleased with him): The Prophet (peace and blessings be upon him) said, "No town-dweller should sell for a Bedouin. Do not practice Najsh (i.e. Do not offer a high price for a thing which you do not want to buy, in order to deceive the people). No Muslim should offer more for a thing already bought by his Muslim brother, nor should he demand the hand of a girl already engaged to another Muslim. A Muslim woman shall not try to bring about the divorce of her sister (i.e. another Muslim woman) in order to take her place herself." (Bukhari)

Al-Haafiz (May Allah have mercy on him) said:

"This is quoted as evidence for the prohibition on a woman proposing to a man who has already proposed to another woman. This Hadith makes the ruling concerning men the same as the ruling concerning women with regard to proposing marriage. The scenario is: a woman proposes to a man, and he responds to that proposal, then another woman comes and encourages him to marry her, and tries to make him lose interest in the one who came before her, whom he has already agreed to marry. End quote." (Fath al-Baari 9/200) (229)

214. Prohibited Marriages

Ibn 'Abbas further said, "Seven types of marriages are unlawful because of blood relations, and seven because of marriage relations." Then Ibn 'Abbas recited the Verse: *"Forbidden for you (for marriages) are your mothers…" (4:23).* 'Abdullah bin Ja'far married the daughter and wife of 'Ali at the same time (they were step-daughter and mother). Ibn Sirin said, "There is no harm in that." But Al-Hasan Al-Basri disapproved of it at first, but then said that there was no harm in it. Al-Hasan bin Al-Hasan bin 'Ali married two of his cousins in one night. Ja'far bin Zaid disapproved of that because of it would bring hatred (between the two cousins), but it is not unlawful, as Allah said, *"Lawful to you are all others [beyond those (mentioned)]. (4:24).* Ibn 'Abbas said: "If somebody commits illegal sexual intercourse with his wife's sister, his wife does not become unlawful for him." And narrated Abu Ja'far, "If a person commits homosexuality with a boy, then the mother of that boy is unlawful for him to marry." Narrated Ibn 'Abbas, "If one commits illegal sexual intercourse with his mother in law, then his married relation to his wife does not become unlawful." Abu Nasr reported to have said that Ibn 'Abbas in the above case, regarded his marital relation to his wife unlawful, but Abu Nasr is not known well for hearing Hadith from Ibn 'Abbas. Imran bin Hussain, Jabir b. Zaid, Al-Hasan and some other Iraqi's, are reported to have judged that his marital relations to his wife would be unlawful. In the above case Abu Hurairah said, "The marital relation to one's wife does not become unlawful except if one as had sexual intercourse (with her mother)." Ibn Al-Musaiyab, 'Urwa, and Az-Zuhri allows such person to keep his wife. 'Ali said, "His marital relations to his wife does not become unlawful." (Bukhari)

1) Prohibition of Marriage Without Woman's Guardian Arrangement
2) Prohibition of Marriage Without Two Legally Acceptable Witnesses
3) Forced/Unconsented Marriage
4) Prohibition of Marriage Without Obligatory Mahr Paid
5) Prohibition of Dowry
6) Prohibition of Marriage Between Muslim Man and Non-Muslim Woman
7) Prohibition of Marriage Between Muslim Woman and Non-Muslim Man
8) Prohibition of Marriage to al-Maharim, the Relatives to whom Marriage is Forbidden
9) Prohibition of Marriage to Two Sisters at the Same Time
10) Prohibition of Marriage to a Woman whom Your Father Married
11) Prohibition of Marriage to a Woman if he is Married to her Paternal or Maternal Aunt at the Same Time
12) Prohibition of Marriage to a Woman Having a Foster Suckling Relationship
13) Prohibition of Secret Marriage
14) Prohibition of Shighar Marriage
15) Prohibition of Al-Mut'ah Marriage
16) Prohibition of Marriage to a Woman Already Married
17) Prohibition of Marriage to his Illegitimate Daughter
18) Prohibition of the Marriage to the Orphan Girl under the Guardianship of her Guardian who Likes her Beauty and Wealth and Wishes to (Marry her and) Curtails her Mahr
19) Prohibition of Marriage to a Divorced or Widowed Woman During her Iddah (the Waiting Period During which she is Not Allowed to Marry Again)
20) Prohibition of Marriage to a Woman who is Ungrateful and Displeased with Allah's Decree
21) Prohibition of Plural Marriage if he Cannot Treat Wives Equally
22) Prohibition of Same-Sex Marriage
23) Prohibition of "Paper" Marriage
24) Prohibition of Marriage between Human and Jinn

215. Prohibition of Marriage Without Woman's Guardian Arrangement

Narrated 'Urwa bin Az-Zubair: Aisha, the wife of the Prophet (peace and blessings be upon him), told him that there were four types of marriage during pre-Islamic period of Ignorance. One type was similar to that of the present day i.e. a man used to ask somebody else for the hand of a girl under his guardianship or for his daughter's hand, and give her Mahr and then marry her. The second type was that a man would say to his wife after she had become clean from her period. "Send for so-and-so and have sexual intercourse with him." Her husband would then keep away from her and would never sleep with her till she got pregnant from the other man with whom she was sleeping. When her pregnancy became evident, he husband would sleep with her if he wished. Her husband did so (i.e. let his wife sleep with some other man) so that he might have a child of noble breed. Such marriage was called as Al-Istibda'. Another type of marriage was that a group of less than ten men would assemble and enter upon a woman, and all of them would have sexual relation with her. If she became pregnant and delivered a child and some days had passed after delivery, she would sent for all of them and none of them would refuse to come, and when they all gathered before her, she would say to them, "You (all) know what you have done, and now I have given birth to a child. So, it is your child so-and-so!" naming whoever she liked, and her child would follow him and he could not refuse to take him. The fourth type of marriage was that many people would enter upon a lady and she would never refuse anyone who came to her. Those were the prostitutes who used to fix flags at their doors as sign, and he who would wish, could have sexual intercourse with them. If anyone of them got pregnant and delivered a child, then all those men would be gathered for her and they would call the Qa'if (persons skilled in recognizing the likeness of a child to his father) to them and would let the child follow the man (whom they recognized as his father) and she would let him adhere to him and be called his son. The man would not refuse all that. But when Muhammad (peace and blessings be upon him) was sent with the Truth, he abolished all the types of marriages observed in pre-Islamic period of Ignorance except the type of marriage the people recognize today." (Bukhari)

Narrated Aisha (May Allah be pleased with her): The Messenger of Allah (peace and blessings be upon him) said: "Whichever woman married without the permission of her Wali, her marriage is invalid, her marriage is invalid, her marriage is invalid. If he (the man) entered into her, then the Mahr is for her in lieu of what he enjoyed from her private part. If they disagree, then the Sultan is the Wali for one who has no Wali." (Tirmidhi)

Narrated Abu Musa: The Messenger of Allah (peace and blessings be upon him) said: "There is no marriage except with a guardian." (Ibn Majah)

216. Prohibition of Marriage Without Two Legally Acceptable Witnesses

The Prophet (peace and blessings of Allah be upon him) said: "There is no marriage except with a wali and two witnesses of good character." (al-Bayhaqi)
With regard to the witness, it is stipulated that he be male, an adult and of sound mind. The testimony of a child, woman or insane person is not valid.
It says in Sharh Muntaha'l-Iraadaat (2/648):

"The marriage contract cannot be done except with the witness of two males who are adults, of sound mind, able to speak and hear, Muslims – even if the wife is a dhimmi (Jew or Christian living under Muslim rule) – and of good character, even if it is only outwardly. End quote." (230)

217. Forced/Unconsented Marriage

Allah, the Exalted, says:

"O you who believe! You are forbidden to inherit women against their will…" (Qur'an, An-Nisa 4:19)

Narrated Abdullah ibn Abbas: "A virgin came to the Prophet (peace and blessings be upon him) and mentioned that her father had married her against her will, so the Prophet (peace and blessings be upon him) allowed her to exercise her choice." (Abu Dawud)

Khansa bint Khidam reported: "Her father gave her in marriage when she was a divorcee, but she disliked her marriage. She came to the Messenger of Allah (peace and blessings be upon him) and he annulled their marriage." (Bukhari)
Abdur Rahman bin Yazid Al-Ansari and Mujamma bin Yazid Al-Ansari said: "A man among them who was called Khidam arranged a marriage for his daughter, and she did not like the marriage arranged by her father. She went to the Messenger of Allah (peace and blessings be upon him) and told him about that, and he (peace and blessings be upon him) annulled the marriage arranged by her father. Then she married Abu Lubabah bin Abdul-Mundhir." (Ibn Majah)

Narrated Ibn Buraidah: His father said: "A girl came to the Prophet and said: 'My father married me to his brother's son so that he might raise his status thereby.' The Prophet (peace and blessings be upon him) gave her the choice, and she said: 'I approve of what my father did, but I wanted women to know that their fathers have no right to do that.'" (Ibn Majah)

Abu Hurairah (May Allah be pleased with him) reported that the Prophet (May Allah's peace and blessings be upon him) said: "A previously married woman should not be married until her verbal consent has been sought, and a virgin should not be married until her permission has been sought." They said: "O Messenger of Allah, what is her permission?" He said: "When she remains silent." (Bukhari and Muslim) (https://hadeethenc.com/en/browse/hadith/6088)

Marriage is one of a person's private affairs and it is impermissible for parents to force their daughter to marry someone she does not want to marry since that would be oppression and a transgression on the rights of others. In Islam women have complete freedom to accept or reject whoever comes to propose to them. Islamic marriages require acceptance of the groom, the bride and the consent of the custodian (wali) of the bride. The wali of the bride is normally a male relative of the bride, preferably her father. The consent of the woman is essential, and must be obtained, and any marriage which is forced is considered to be batil or void. (231, 232)

218. Prohibition of Marriage Without Obligatory Mahr Paid

Allah, the Exalted, says:

"And give to the women (whom you marry) their Mahr (obligatory bridal money given by the husband to his wife at the time of marriage) with a good heart, but if they, of their own good pleasure, remit any part of it to you, take it, and enjoy it without fear of any harm (as Allah has made it lawful)." (Qur'an, An-Nisa 4:4)
"(Lawful to you in marriage) are chaste women from the believers and chaste women from those who were given the Scripture (Jews and Christians) before your time, when you have given their due Mahr (bridal money given by the husband to his wife at the time of marriage), desiring chastity (i.e. taking them in legal wedlock) not committing illegal sexual intercourse, nor taking them as girlfriends." (Qur'an, Al-Ma'idah 5:5)

Narrated Sahl bin Sad As-Sa'idi: "A woman came to Allah's Apostle and said, "O Allah's Apostle! I have come to give you myself in marriage (without Mahr)." Allah's Apostle looked at her. He looked at her carefully and fixed his glance on her and then lowered his head. When the lady saw that he did not say anything, she sat down. A man from his companions got up and said, "O Allah's Apostle! If you are not in need of her, then marry her to me." The Prophet said, "Have you got anything to offer?" The man said, "No, by Allah, O Allah's Apostle!" The Prophet said (to him), "Go to your family and see if you have something." The man went and returned, saying, "No, by Allah, I have not found anything." Allah's Apostle said, "(Go again) and look for something, even if it is an iron ring." He went again and returned, saying, "No, by Allah, O Allah's Apostle! I could not find even an iron ring, but this is my Izar (waist sheet)." He had no rida. He added, "I give half of it to her." Allah's Apostle said, "What will she do with your Izar? If you wear it, she will be naked, and if she wears it, you will be naked." So, that man sat down for a long while and then got up (to depart). When Allah's Apostle saw him going, he ordered that he be called back. When he came, the Prophet said,

"How much of the Qur'an do you know?" He said, "I know such Surahs and such Surahs", counting them. The Prophet said, "Do you know them by heart?" He replied, "Yes." The Prophet (peace and blessings be upon him) said, "Go, I marry her to you for that much of the Qur'an which you have." (Bukhari)

Narrated Anas: 'Abdur Rahman bin 'Auf married a woman and gave her gold equal to the weight of a date stone (as Mahr). When the Prophet (peace and blessings be upon him) noticed the signs of cheerfulness of the marriage (on his face) and asked him about it, he said, "I have married a woman and gave (her) gold equal to a date stone in weight (as Mahr)." (Bukhari)

Narrated Sahl bin Sa`d: The Prophet (peace and blessings be upon him) said to a man: "Marry, even with (a Mahr equal to) an iron ring." (Bukhari)

Mahr is distinct from Dower in two ways:

1) Mahr is legally required for all Islamic marriages while Dower was optional.
2) Mahr is given at the time of marriage, while Dower is not paid until the death of the husband.

219. Prohibition of Dowry

Allah, the Exalted, ordered:

"And give to the women (whom you marry) their Mahr (obligatory bridal money given by the husband to his wife at the time of marriage) with a good heart..." (Qur'an, An-Nisa 4:4)

"Also (forbidden are) women already married, except those (captives and slaves) whom your right hands possess. Thus, has Allah ordained for you. All others are lawful, provided you seek (them in marriage) with Mahr (bridal money given by the husband to his wife at the time of marriage) from your property..." (Qur'an, An-Nisa 4:24)

Dowry is a demanded wedding gift (cash or valuables) from the bride's family to the groom's family. Dowry is an evil practice. The practice of Dowry transgresses Allah's command. Allah has made the Mahr obligatory for man to give to woman, and not vice versa. *(Qur'an, An-Nisa 4:4)*

220. Dowry Abuse

Allah, the Exalted, says:

"And when the news of (the birth of) a female (child) is brought to any of them, his face becomes dark, and he is filled with inward grief!" (Qur'an, An-Nahl 16:58)

"He hides himself from the people because of the evil of that whereof he has been informed. Shall he keep her with dishonor or bury her in the earth? Certainly, evil is their decision." (Qur'an, An-Nahl 16:59)

"Let there arise out of you a band of people inviting to all that is good, Enjoining what is right, and forbidding what is wrong: They are the ones to attain felicity." (Qur'an, Ali 'Imran 3:104)

Malik reported Allah's Messenger (May peace be upon him) as saying: "He, who brought up two girls properly till they grew up, he and I would come (together) (very closely) on the Day of Resurrection, and he interlaced his fingers (for explaining the point of nearness between him and that person)." (Muslim)

Aisha (May Allah be pleased with her) reported: "A woman, along with her two daughters, came to me asking (for charity). She found that I had nothing except one date, so I gave it to her. She divided it between her two daughters and ate nothing herself, then she got up and left. The Prophet (May Allah's peace and blessings be upon him) then came in, and I informed him about this and he remarked: "Whoever is tried by having daughters and he treats them kindly, they will be a screen for him from Hellfire." (Bukhari and Muslim. This is the wording of Al-Bukhari) (https://hadeethenc.com/en/browse/hadith/3358)

Dowry is a social evil which came into existence due to worldly greed. The cruelty to extract more and more dowry, unaffordable dowry results in mental and physical harassment and even suicide or murder of the bride. The practice of Dowry inevitably leads to discrimination against daughters and makes them vulnerable to various forms of violence. Many women remain unmarried due to Dowry. (233)

People rejoicing over the birth of a son and lamenting over the birth of daughter. Dowry leads to Dowry-related sex selective abortion, femicide or her parents may abandon or mistreat her.

The Qur'an and Sunnah emphasize the birth of daughters to be a great blessing and carry the message to value women. Islam ensures that boys and girls are treated equally and stresses fairness and kindness. It is so unfortunate to see people submitting themselves to the dictates and fitnah of culture rather than to the Will and Decree of Allah.

221. Dishonoring Woman

Allah, the Exalted, says:

"Whoever works righteousness, whether male or female, while he (or she) is a true believer (of Islamic Monotheism), verily, to him We will give a good life (in this world with respect, contentment and lawful provision), and We shall pay them certainly a reward in proportion to the best of what they used to do (i.e. Paradise in the Hereafter)." (Qur'an, An-Nahl 16:97)

"…And live with them honorably. If you dislike them, it may be that you dislike a thing and Allah brings through it a great deal of good." (Qur'an, An-Nisa 4:19)

"They are Libas [i.e. body cover or screen, or Sakan (i.e. you enjoy the pleasure of living with her - as in Verse 7:189) Tafsir At-Tabari] for you and you are the same for them." (Qur'an, Al-Baqarah 2:187)

Other Verses: *Al-Baqarah 2:228, Al-Ahzab 33:35, An-Nisa 4:1 and 4:129.*

Abu Hurairah (May Allah be pleased with him) reported: Messenger of Allah (peace and blessings be upon him) said: "Take my advice with regard to women: Act kindly towards women, for they were created from a rib, and the most crooked part of a rib is its uppermost. If you attempt to straighten it; you will break it, and if you leave it alone it will remain crooked; so, act kindly toward women." (Bukhari and Muslim)

'Abdullah bin Zam'ah (May Allah be pleased with him) reported that he heard the Prophet (peace and blessings be upon him) giving a speech when he mentioned the she-camel (of Prophet Salih) and the man who had killed her. Messenger of Allah (peace and blessings be upon him) said: *"When the most wicked man among them went forth (to kill the she-camel).' (91:12)* signifies that a distinguished, wicked and most powerful chief of the people jumped up to kill the she-camel." Then he (peace and blessings be upon him) made mention of women and said, "Some of you beat your wives as if they were slaves, and then have intercourse with them at the end of the day." Then he admonished them against laughing at another's passing of wind, saying, "Why does any of you laugh at another doing what he does himself." (Bukhari and Muslim)

The Prophet (May Allah's peace and blessings be upon him) said during his sermon: "Some of you would whip their wives as if they were slaves." This indicates harsh disciplining. The context of the Hadith indicates the improbability of these two being done by a rational person, i.e. that he would beat his wife severely and then have sexual intercourse with her the same day or night. This is because sexual intercourse normally requires a desire for companionship, love and affection, whereas the one who is whipped normally shuns the one who whipped him. So, the dispraise of this type of action was pointed out here. If beating is necessary, it should be a gentle beating that does not cause complete repulsion, so one should not exceed the proper limits in both beating and disciplining. Then, he warned them against laughing at the act of passing wind because it is against good manners and because it entails exposing other people. Out of criticism for such an attitude, he said: "Why should any of you laugh at another doing what he does himself?" This is because laughing is normally caused by something strange or astonishing that lead to smiling. If the smile gets stronger and is accompanied by a sound, it

will be considered laughter, and if it becomes even stronger than that, it will be called a guffaw. Since passing wind normally happens to all people, then what is the reason for laughing at the one who passes wind?
(https://hadeethenc.com/en/browse/hadith/3070)

Abu Hurairah (May Allah be pleased with him) reported: Messenger of Allah (peace and blessings be upon him) said, "A believer must not hate (his wife) believing woman; if he dislikes one of her characteristics, he will be pleased with another." (Muslim)

'Amr bin Al-Ahwas Al-Jushami (May Allah be pleased with him) reported that he had heard the Prophet (peace and blessings be upon him) saying on his Farewell Pilgrimage, after praising and glorifying Allah and admonishing people, "Treat women kindly, they are like captives in your hands; you do not owe anything else from them. In case they are guilty of open indecency, then do not share their beds and beat them lightly but if they return to obedience, do not have recourse to anything else against them. You have rights over your wives and they have their rights over you. Your right is that they shall not permit anyone you dislike to enter your home, and their right is that you should treat them well in the matter of food and clothing." (Tirmidhi)

Mu'awiyah bin Haidah (May Allah be pleased with him) reported: "I asked Messenger of Allah (peace and blessings be upon him): 'What right can any wife demand of her husband?' He replied, "You should give her food when you eat, clothe her when you clothe yourself, not strike her on the face, and do not revile her or separate from her except in the house." (Abu Dawud)

Abu Hurairah (May Allah be pleased with him) reported: The Messenger of Allah (peace and blessings be upon him) said, "The believers who show the most perfect faith are those who have the best behavior, and the best of you are those who are the best to their wives." (Tirmidhi)

Iyas bin 'Abdullah (May Allah be pleased with him) reported: The Messenger of Allah (peace and blessings be upon him) said, "Do not beat Allah's bondwomen." When 'Umar (May Allah be pleased with him) came to Messenger of Allah (peace and blessings be upon him) and complained saying: "The women have become very daring towards their husbands." He (peace and blessings be upon him) gave permission to beat them. Then many women went to the family of the Messenger of Allah (wives) complaining of their husbands, and he (the Prophet, peace and blessings be upon him) said, "Many women have gone round Muhammad's family complaining of their husbands. Those who do so, that is, those who take to beating their wives, are not the best among you." (Abu Dawud)

Commentary: This Hadith tells us that those who take to beating their wives are not perfect people. The decency of manners warrants that one must refrain from beating, as is evident from the conduct of the Prophet (peace and blessings be upon him) who neither resorted to beating with his own hand any of his wives nor slaves nor any other. He would avenge those who transgressed the limits of Allah. (234)

'Abdullah bin 'Amr bin Al-'as (May Allah be pleased with him) reported: The Messenger of Allah (peace and blessings be upon him) said, "The world is but a (quick passing) enjoyment; and the best enjoyment of the world is a pious and virtuous woman." (Muslim)

Aisha (May Allah be pleased with her) said: "The Messenger of Allah (peace and blessings of Allah be upon him) never struck a servant or a woman." (Abu Dawud)

Anas ibn Malik (May Allah have mercy on him) reported: The Messenger of Allah (peace and blessings be upon him) said: "Whomsoever has been blessed with a pious wife from Allah, then Allah has certainly assisted him (to fulfill) half of his Deen. So, he should fear Allah in the remaining half." (Al Mu'jamul Awsat)

Abu Shurayh Khuwaylid ibn 'Amr al-Khuzā'i and Abu Hurairah (May Allah be pleased with them) reported that the Messenger of Allah (May Allah's peace and blessings be upon him) said: "O Allah, I declare strictly inviolable the rights of the two weak ones: the orphan and the woman." (Ibn Majah, An-Nasa'i and Ahmad) (https://hadeethenc.com/en/browse/hadith/3468)

Jabir ibn Abdullah reported: The Messenger of Allah (peace and blessings be upon him) said, "Fear Allah regarding women. Verily, you have taken them as a trust from Allah, and intercourse has been made lawful by the Word of Allah. Your rights over them are that they do not let anyone in the house you dislike. If they do so, you may strike them without violence. Their rights over you are that you provide for them and clothe them in a reasonable manner." (Muslim)
Abu Hurairah (May Allah be pleased with him) reported that the Prophet (May Allah's peace and blessings be upon him) said: "The one who looks after the widow and the needy person is like the one who fights in the Cause of Allah." Abu Hurairah (May Allah be pleased with him) added: "I believe that he said: 'And like the one who constantly stands in (voluntary night) prayer and never slackens, and like the one who constantly fasts and never abandons fasting.'" (Bukhari and Muslim)
(https://hadeethenc.com/en/browse/hadith/3135)

Anas ibn Malik (May Allah be pleased with him) reported that the Prophet (May Allah's peace and blessings be upon him) said: "Whoever supports two girls till they grow up, he and I will come on the Day of Resurrection like this," joining his fingers. (Muslim)

Narrated 'Abdullah: "During some of the Ghazawat of the Prophet (peace be upon him) a woman was found killed. Allah's Messenger (peace and blessings be upon him) disapproved the killing of women and children." (Bukhari)

Narrated Thawban: "When the Verse concerning silver and gold was revealed, they said: 'What kind of wealth should we acquire?' Umar said: 'I will tell you about that.' So, he rode on his camel and caught up with the Prophet, and I followed him. He said: 'O Messenger of Allah what kind of wealth should we acquire?' He said: 'Let one of you acquire a thankful heart, a tongue that remembers Allah and a believing wife who will help him with regard to the Hereafter.'" (Ibn Majah)

Islam does not consider woman "an instrument of the Devil", but rather the Qur'an calls her Muhsana - a fortress against Satan because a good woman, by marrying a man, helps him keep to the path of rectitude in his life. It is for this reason that marriage was considered by the Prophet Muhammad (peace and blessings be upon him) as a most virtuous act. He said: "When a man marries, he has completed one half of his religion." He enjoined matrimony on Muslims by saying: "Marriage is part of my way and whoever keeps away from my way is not from me (i.e. is not my follower)." (232)

222. Prohibition of Marriage Between Muslim Man and Non-Muslim Woman

Allah, the Exalted, says:

"And do not marry Al-Mushrikat (idolatresses, etc.) till they believe (worship Allah Alone). And indeed, a slave woman who believes is better than a (free) Mushrikah (idolatress, etc.), even though she pleases you. And give not (your daughters) in marriage to Al-Mushrikun till they believe (in Allah Alone) and verily, a believing slave is better than a (free) Mushrik (idolater, etc.), even though he pleases you. Those (Al-Mushrikun) invite you to the Fire, but Allah invites (you) to Paradise and Forgiveness by His Leave, and makes His Ayat (proofs, evidences, verses, lessons, signs, revelations, etc.) clear to mankind that they may remember." (Qur'an, Al-Baqarah 2:221)

"...(Lawful to you in marriage) are chaste women from the believers and chaste women from those who were given the Scripture (Jews and Christians) before your time, when you have given their due Mahr (bridal money given by the husband to his wife at the time of marriage), desiring chastity (i.e. taking them in legal wedlock) not committing illegal sexual intercourse, nor taking them as girlfriends. And whosoever disbelieves in the Oneness of Allah and in all the other Articles of Faith [i.e. His (Allah's), Angels, His Holy Books, His Messengers, the Day of Resurrection and Al-Qadar (Divine Preordainments)], then fruitless is his work, and in the Hereafter, he will be among the losers." (Qur'an, Al-Ma'idah 5:5)

"The adulterer marries not but an adulteress or a Mushrikah and the adulteress none marries her except an adulterer or a Muskrik [and that means that the man who agrees to marry (have a sexual relation with) a Mushrikah (female polytheist, pagan or idolatress) or a prostitute, then surely, he is either an adulterer or a Mushrik (polytheist, pagan or idolater, etc.) And the woman who agrees to marry (have a sexual relation with) a Mushrik (polytheist, pagan or idolater) or an adulterer, then she is either a prostitute

or a Mushrikah (female polytheist, pagan or idolatress, etc.)]. Such a thing is forbidden to the believers (of Islamic Monotheism)." (Qur'an, An-Nur 24:3)
Other Verses: *Al-Mumtahanah 60:10, Al-Furqan 25:68-70, An-Nur 24:26)*

This Verse of the Prohibition of Marriage between Muslim Men and non-Muslim women was revealed with the connection to the story of Marthad Al-Ghanawi: https://www.youtube.com/watch?v=G9uJZJjjUog

Who are the Disbelievers?

The disbelief in Allah, His Messengers and transgression of Allah's Laws.

1. Polytheism
2. Idol Worshippers
3. Christians
4. Jews
5. Hypocrites
6. Atheists
7. Wrongdoers

Christians didn't follow Jesus' teaching.

The original Bible was sent by Allah to Jesus (Muslim man and Allah's Messenger) to call people to worship Allah, the Only One True God. But Christians deviated and worship Jesus, man, as an Idol.

Jews didn't follow Musa's teaching.

The original Torah was sent by Allah to Musa (Muslim man and Allah's Messenger) to call people to worship the Creator. But Jews worship Uzair, the human being, as an idol.
Narrated Nafi': "Whenever Ibn 'Umar was asked about marrying a Christian lady or a Jewess, he would say: "Allah has made it unlawful for the believers to marry ladies who ascribe partners in worship to Allah, and I do not know of a greater thing, as regards to ascribing partners in worship, etc. to Allah, than that a lady should say that Jesus is her Lord although he is just one of Allah's slave." (Bukhari)

Narrated Abu Burda's father: Allah's Apostle (peace and blessings be upon him) said, "Any man who has a slave girl whom he educates properly, teaches good manners, manumits and marries her, will get a double reward. And if any man of the people of the Scriptures believes in his own Prophet and then believes in me too, he will (also) get a double reward. And any slave who fulfills his duty to his master and to his Lord, will (also) get a double reward." (Bukhari)

Narrated Abu Hurairah: The Prophet (peace and blessings be upon him) said, "A woman is married for four things, i.e. her wealth, her family status, her beauty and her religion. So, you should marry the religious woman, (otherwise) you will be a loser." (Bukhari)

Narrated Abdullah bin 'Umar: Allah's Apostle (peace and blessings be upon him) said, "Evil omen is in the women, the house and the horse." (Bukhari)

Husband and wife should have the same religion.

Marriage (Nikah) is a contract between a Muslim man and a Muslim woman.

It is not permissible for a Muslim man or woman to marry a kafir, and the marriage is not valid, and intercourse with him is Zina (fornication, adultery).

No one can attain true life, happiness and peace of mind unless he believes in Allah as his Lord, Islam as his religion and Muhammad as his Prophet.

223. Prohibition of Marriage Between Muslim Woman and Non-Muslim Man

Allah, the Exalted, says:

"And give not (your daughters) in marriage to Al-Mushrikoon till they believe (in Allah Alone) and verily, a believing slave is better than a (free) Mushrik (idolater), even though he pleases you. Those (Al-Mushrikoon) invite you to the Fire, but Allah invites (you) to Paradise and forgiveness by His Leave, and makes His Ayat (proofs, evidences, verses, lessons, signs, revelations, etc.) clear to mankind that they may remember." (Qur'an, Al-Baqarah 2:221)

224. Prohibition of Marriage to al-Maharim, the Relatives to whom

Marriage is Forbidden

Allah, the Exalted, says:

"Forbidden to you (for marriage) are: your mothers, your daughters, your sisters, your father's sisters, your mother's sisters, your brother's daughters, your sister's daughters, your foster mother who gave you suck, your foster milk suckling sisters, your wives' mothers, your step daughters under your guardianship, born of your wives to whom you have gone in - but there is no sin on you if you have not gone in them (to marry their daughters), - the wives of your sons who (spring) from your own loins, and two sisters

in wedlock at the same time, except for what has already passed; verily, Allah is Oft-Forgiving, Most Merciful." *(Qur'an, An-Nisa 4:23)*

Samurah reported that the Messenger of Allah (May Allah's peace and blessings be upon him) said: "If anyone gets possession of a relative who is within the prohibited degrees, that person becomes free." (Ibn Majah, Tirmidhi, Abu Dawud and Ahmad) https://hadeethenc.com/en/browse/hadith/64706)

Ruling on marrying cousins

Allah, the Exalted, says:

"O Prophet (Muhammad SAW)! Verily, We have made lawful to you your wives, to whom you have paid their Mahr (bridal money given by the husband to his wife at the time of marriage), and those (captives or slaves) whom your right hand possesses - whom Allah has given to you, and the daughters of your 'Amm (paternal uncles) and the daughters of your 'Ammah (paternal aunts) and the daughters of your Khal (maternal uncles) and the daughters of your Khalah (maternal aunts)..." (Qur'an, Al-Ahzab 33:50)

Marriages between first cousins are allowed in Islam.

The Prophet (peace and blessings be upon him) married his daughter Fatima to Ali (May Allah be pleased with them) and he is the son of her father's uncle, as well as the marriage of the Prophet himself to Zainab bint Jahsh (May Allah be please with her) and she is his aunt's daughter (i.e. his cousin).

As for the fear of hereditary diseases, it is a good practice to have a blood test before marriage. While marriage between cousins is permissible, it is preferable to choose a marriage partner from outside one's family. (235, 236)

225. Prohibition of Marriage to Two Sisters at the Same Time

Allah, the Exalted, says:

"Forbidden to you (for marriage) are: your mothers, your daughters, your sisters, your father's sisters, your mother's sisters, your brother's daughters, your sister's daughters, your foster mother who gave you suck, your foster milk suckling sisters, your wives' mothers, your step daughters under your guardianship, born of your wives to whom you have gone in - but there is no sin on you if you have not gone in them (to marry their daughters), - the wives of your sons who (spring) from your own loins, and two sisters in wedlock at the same time, except for what has already passed; verily, Allah is Oft-Forgiving, Most Merciful." (Qur'an, An-Nisa 4:23)

Narrated Umm Habiba: "I said, 'O Allah's Messenger (peace and blessings be upon him)! Marry my sister, the daughter of Abu Sufyan." He said, "Do you like that?" I said, "Yes, for even now I am not your only wife; and the most beloved person to share the good with me is my sister." The Prophet (peace and blessings be upon him) said, "But that is not lawful for me (i.e. to be married to two sisters at a time.)" I said, "O Allah's Messenger (peace and blessings be upon him)! By Allah, we have heard that you want to marry Durrah, the daughter of Abu Salama." He said, "You mean the daughter of Umm Salama?" I said, "Yes." He said, "By Allah! Even if she were not my stepdaughter, she would not be lawful for me to marry, for she is my foster niece, for Thuwaiba has suckled me and Abu Salama; so, you should neither present your daughters, nor your sisters to me." (Bukhari)

Narrated Dailami: "I came to the Messenger of Allah, and I was married to two sisters whom I had married during the Ignorance period. He said: 'When you go back, divorce one of them.'" (Ibn Majah)

226. Prohibition of Marriage to a Woman whom Your Father Married

Allah, the Exalted, says:

"And marry not women whom your fathers married, except what has already passed; indeed, it was shameful and most hateful, and an evil way." (Qur'an, An-Nisa 4:22)

227. Prohibition of Marriage to a Woman if he is Married to her Paternal or Maternal Aunt at the Same Time

Narrated Abu Hurairah (May Allah be pleased with him): The Prophet (peace and blessings be upon him) said: "One may not combine in marriage a woman and her paternal aunt, or a woman and her maternal aunt." (Bukhari and Muslim) (https://hadeethenc.com/en/browse/hadith/6090)

228. Prohibition of Marriage to a Woman Having a Foster Suckling Relationship

Allah, the Exalted, says:

"Forbidden to you (for marriage) are: your mothers, your daughters, your sisters, your father's sisters, your mother's sisters, your brother's daughters, your sister's daughters, your foster mother who gave you suck, your foster milk suckling sisters…" (Qur'an, An-Nisa 4:23)

Narrated Abdullah bin Abi Mulaika from Uqba bin Al-Harith: Uqba married the daughter of Abu Ihab bin Aziz, and then a woman came and said, "I suckled Uqba and his wife." Uqba said to her, "I do not know that you have suckled me, and you did not inform me." He then sent someone to the house of Abu Ihab to enquire about that but they did not know that she had suckled their daughter. Then Uqba went to the Prophet (peace and blessings be upon him) in Madinah and asked him about it. The Prophet (peace and blessings be upon him) said to him, "How (can you keep your wife) after it has been said (that both of you were suckled by the same woman)?" So, he divorced her and she was married to another man." (Bukhari)

Narrated Ibn Abbas: The Prophet (peace and blessings be upon him) said about Hamza's daughter, "I am not legally permitted to marry her, as foster relations are treated like blood relations (in marital affairs). She is the daughter of my foster brother." (Bukhari)

Narrated Umm Habiba: "I said, 'O Allah's Messenger (peace and blessings be upon him)! Marry my sister, the daughter of Abu Sufyan.' He said, 'Do you like that?' I said, 'Yes, for even now I am not your only wife; and the most beloved person to share the good with me is my sister.' The Prophet (peace and blessings be upon him) said, 'But that is not lawful for me (i.e. to be married to two sisters at a time).' I said, 'O Allah's Messenger (peace and blessings be upon him)! By Allah, we have heard that you want to marry Durra, the daughter of Abu Salama.' He said, 'You mean the daughter of Umm Salama?' I said, 'Yes.' He said, 'By Allah! Even if she were not my stepdaughter, she would not be lawful for me to marry, for she is my foster niece, for Thuwaiba has suckled me and Abu Salama; so, you should neither present your daughters, nor your sisters to me.'" (Bukhari)

Narrated Aisha (May Allah be pleased with her): The Prophet Allah (peace and blessings be upon him) said: "Suckling once or twice does not make (marriage) unlawful." (Ibn Majah)

229. Prohibition of Secret Marriage

Allah, the Exalted, says:

"Marry them with the permission of their families and give them their due as is good, chaste women, neither fornicators nor secret mistresses." (Qur'an, An-Nisa 4:25)

Amir ibn 'Abdullah ibn Az-Zubayr reported from his father that the Prophet (May Allah's peace and blessings be upon him) said: "Announce marriages." (Ahmad) (https://hadeethenc.com/en/browse/hadith/58065)

Marrying secretly is not permissible for the following reasons: Firstly: the approval of her Guardian is one of the conditions of marriage being valid. Secondly: marriage must be witnessed or announced openly. A secret marriage that is not witnessed or announced openly is an invalid marriage. (237)

230. Prohibition of Shighar Marriage

Abdullah ibn 'Umar (May Allah be pleased with him) reported that the Messenger of Allah (May Allah's peace and blessings be upon him) prohibited Shighar marriage. Shighar marriage means that a man gives his daughter in marriage to another on condition that the other gives his daughter to him in marriage without any Mahr being paid by either." (Bukhari and Muslim) (https://hadeethenc.com/en/browse/hadith/5849)

231. Prohibition of Al-Mut'ah Marriage

Ali ibn Abi Talib (May Allah be pleased with him) reported that the Prophet (May Allah's peace and blessings be upon him) prohibited the fixed term marriage on the day of Khaybar and eating the flesh of domestic donkeys. (Bukhari and Muslim) (https://hadeethenc.com/en/browse/hadith/5922)

232. Prohibition of Marriage to a Woman Already Married

Allah, the Exalted, says:

"Also (forbidden are) women already married, except those (captives and slaves) whom your right hands possess. Thus, has Allah ordained for you." (Qur'an, An-Nisa 4:24)

233. Prohibition of Marriage to his Illegitimate Daughter

Allah, the Exalted, says:

"Forbidden to you (for marriage) are: your mothers, your daughters…" (Qur'an, An-Nisa 4:23)

Ibn Qudaamah (May Allah have mercy on him) said:

"It is haram for a man to marry his illegitimate daughter, or his illegitimate sister, or his (illegitimate) son's daughter, or his daughter's daughter, or his brother's daughter, or his sister who is illegitimate. This is the view of most of the fuqaha'." (End quote from Al-Mughni (7/485)

According to the majority of scholars, the rulings forbidding marriage still apply between the illegitimate child and his father and his father's relatives. (238)

234. Prohibition of the Marriage to the Orphan Girl under the Guardianship of her Guardian who Likes her Beauty and Wealth and Wishes to (Marry her and) Curtails her Mahr

Allah, the Exalted, says:

"And if you fear that you shall not be able to deal justly with the orphan girls, then marry (other) women of your choice, two or three, or four but if you fear that you shall not be able to deal justly (with them), then only one or (the captives and the slaves) that your right hands possess. That is nearer to prevent you from doing injustice." (Qur'an, An-Nisa 4:3)

"They ask your legal instruction concerning women, say: Allah instructs you about them, and about what is recited unto you in the Book concerning the orphan girls whom you give not the prescribed portions (as regards Mahr and inheritance) and yet whom you desire to marry, and (concerning) the children who are weak and oppressed, and that you stand firm for justice to orphans." (Qur'an, An-Nisa 4:127)

Narrated 'Urwa bin Az-Zubair that he asked Aisha regarding the Statement of Allah: *"If you fear that you shall not be able to deal justly with the orphans." (4:3)* She said, "O son of my sister! An orphan girl used to be under the care of a guardian with whom she shared property. Her guardian, being attracted by her wealth and beauty, would intend to marry her without giving her a just Mahr, i.e. the same Mahr as any other person might give her (in case he married her). So, such guardians were forbidden to do that unless they did justice to their female wards and gave them the highest Mahr their peers might get. They were ordered (by Allah), to marry women of their choice other than those orphan girls." Aisha added, "The people asked Allah's Apostle his instructions after the Revelation of this Divine Verse: *"They ask your legal instruction concerning the women..." (4:127)*. Aisha further said, "And the Statement of Allah: *'And yet whom you desire to marry...' (4:127)* So, Allah revealed to them that if the orphan girl had beauty and wealth, they desired to marry her and for her family status. They can only marry them if they give them their full Mahr. And if they had no desire to marry them because of their lack of wealth and beauty, they would leave them and marry other women. So, as they used to leave them, when they had no interest in them, they were forbidden to marry them when they had such interest, unless they treated them justly and gave them their full Mahr. Allah's Apostle (peace and blessings of Allah be upon him) said, 'If at all there is evil omen, it is in the horse, the woman and the house." Bukhari's Chapter: What evil omen of a lady is to be warded off. And the Statement of Allah: *"Truly, among your wives and your children, there are enemies for you (i.e. may stop you from the obedience of Allah)." (64:14)* (Bukhari)

235. Prohibition of Marriage to a Divorced or Widowed Woman During her Iddah (the Waiting Period During which she is Not Allowed to Marry Again)

Allah, the Exalted, says:

"There is no blame on you for subtly showing interest in ˹divorced or widowed˺ women or for hiding ˹the intention˺ in your hearts. Allah knows that you are considering them ˹for marriage˺. But do not make a secret commitment with them—you can only show interest in them appropriately. Do not commit to the bond of marriage until the waiting period expires. Know that Allah is aware of what is in your hearts, so beware of Him. And know that Allah is All-Forgiving, Most Forbearing." (Qur'an, Al-Baqarah 2:235)

Definition of Iddah Period

Iddah is the period of time that a woman that is in the process of officially being separated from her husband legislatively, in which she does not remarry. The Iddah period leaves open time for the husband and wife to reconcile and continue on with their marriage, as long as it is done before the period has ended.

What are the types of woman that has an Iddah Period?

1. The woman that her husband has passed away.
2. The woman that her husband is still alive.

What are the Iddah periods for these types of woman?

1. **The one whose husband has passed away:**

    1.1. If she is pregnant her Iddah period is until she delivers the child.
    1.2. If she is not pregnant her Iddah period is four months and ten days.

2. **The one whose husband is alive:**

   2.1. If she is pregnant her Iddah period is until she delivers the child.
   2.2. If she is not pregnant her Iddah period is;
         2.2.1. If she still has her menstrual cycle, three periods of purifying herself after her menses.
         2.2.2. If she no longer has menses, she must wait a period of three months.

There is no Iddah period if the divorce occurred before marriage was consummated. (239)

There are six categories of women as regards of Iddah. (240)

First, a pregnant woman: Her 'Iddah, whether she is a widow or divorced, expires upon delivery.

Allah, the Exalted, says:

"…And for those who are pregnant (whether they are divorced or their husbands are dead), their 'Iddah (prescribed period) is until they deliver (their burdens)…" (Qur'an, At-Talaq 65:4)

Subay'ah al-Aslamiyyah (May Allah be pleased with her) reported that she was married to Sa'd ibn Khawlah, who belonged to the tribe of 'Amir ibn Lu'ay. He was one of the Companions who participated in the battle of Badr. He died during the Farewell Hajj while Subay'ah was pregnant. Shortly after his death, she delivered her child. When her postnatal bleeding stopped, she beautified herself for prospective suitors. Abu As-Sanabil ibn Ba'kak (a man from the tribe of Banu 'Abd Ad-Dār) entered upon her and said: "Why are you thus adorned? Perhaps you wish to remarry? By Allah, you cannot remarry unless four months and ten days (of 'Iddah) have passed." Subay'ah said: "When he said that, I put on my clothes in the evening and I went to the Messenger of Allah (May Allah's peace and blessings be upon him). I asked him about that, and he gave me a Fatwa that remarrying had become lawful to me when I delivered my child, and he ordered me to marry if I so wished." Ibn Shihab said: "I do not find anything wrong with her marrying right after she gives birth, even if she is still bleeding (postpartum) except that her new husband should not approach her until she attains purity (when the bleeding stops)." (Bukhari and Muslim) (https://hadeethenc.com/en/browse/hadith/6046)

Second, a non-pregnant widow: Her 'Iddah is four months and ten days following her husband's death.

Allah, the Exalted, says:

"And those of you who die and leave wives behind them, they (the wives) shall wait (as regards their marriage) for four months and ten days…" (Qur'an, Al-Baqarah 2:234)

Third, a menstruating woman: Her 'Iddah is three menstrual periods.

Allah, the Exalted, says:

"And divorced women shall wait (as regards their marriage) for three menstrual periods…" (Qur'an, Al-Baqarah 2:228)

Fourth, a woman who does not menstruate, either because she is too young or too old: Her 'Iddah is three months.

Allah, the Exalted, says:

"And those of your women as have passed the age of monthly courses, for them the 'Iddah (prescribed period), if you have doubts (about their periods), is three months, and for those who have no courses [(i.e. they are still immature) their 'Iddah (prescribed period) is three months likewise, except in case of death]." (Qur'an, At-Talaq 65:4)

Fifth, a woman who no longer has menstrual periods for an unknown reason, her 'Iddah is one year.

Sixth, the wife of a lost man: Her 'Iddah is four months and ten days like a widow.

'Umar ibn al-Khattab (May Allah be pleased with him) said: "A woman whose husband is missing and whose whereabouts is unknown to her must wait for four years and then observe the 'Iddah (of a widow) for four months and ten days. After that, she is allowed to marry." (Malik) (No judgment by Sheikh Al-Albaani is available) (https://hadeethenc.com/en/browse/hadith/58170)

236. Prohibition of Marriage to a Woman who is Ungrateful and Displeased with Allah's Decree

Allah, the Exalted, says:

"Among His proofs is that He created for you spouses from among yourselves, in order to have tranquility and contentment with each other, and He placed in your hearts love and care towards your spouses. In this, there are sufficient proofs for people who think." (Qur'an, Ar-Rum 30:21)

Narrated Ibn Abbas: "…When he asked Ishmael's wife about him, she replied, 'He has gone in search of our livelihood.' Then he asked her about their way of living and their condition, and she replied, 'We are living in misery; we are living in hardship and destitution,' complaining to him. He said, 'When your husband returns, convey my salutation to him and tell him to change the threshold of the gate (of his house).' When Ishmael came, he seemed to have felt something unusual, so he asked his wife, 'Has anyone visited you?' She replied, 'Yes, an old man of so-and-so description came and asked me about you and I informed him, and he asked about our state of living, and I told him that we were living in a hardship and poverty.' On that Ishmael said, 'Did he advise you anything?' She replied, 'Yes, he told me to convey his salutation to you and to tell you to change the threshold of your gate.' Ishmael said, 'It was my father, and he has ordered me to divorce you. Go back to your family.' So, Ishmael divorced her and married another woman from amongst them (i.e. Jurhum). Then Abraham stayed away from them for a period as long as Allah wished and called on them again but did not find Ishmael. So, he came to Ishmael's wife and asked her about Ishmael. She said, 'He has gone in search of our livelihood.' Abraham asked her, 'How are you getting on?' asking her about their sustenance and living. She replied, 'We are prosperous and well-off (i.e. we have everything in abundance).' Then she thanked Allah. Abraham said, 'What kind of food do you eat?' She said. 'Meat.' He said, 'What do you drink?' She said, 'Water." He said, "O Allah! Bless their meat and water." The Prophet (peace and blessings be upon him) added, "At that time they did not have grain, and if they had grain, he would have also invoked Allah to bless it." The Prophet (peace and blessings be upon him) added, "If somebody has only these two things as his sustenance, his health and disposition will be badly affected, unless he lives in Makkah." The Prophet (peace and blessings be upon him) added," Then Abraham said Ishmael's wife, "When your husband comes, give my regards to him and tell him that he should keep firm the threshold of his gate.' When Ishmael came back, he asked his wife, 'Did anyone call on you?' She replied, 'Yes, a good-looking old man came to me,' so she praised him and added. 'He asked about you, and I informed him, and he asked about our livelihood and I told him that we were in a good condition.' Ishmael asked her, 'Did he give you any piece of advice?' She said, 'Yes, he told me to give his regards to you and ordered that you should keep firm the threshold of your gate.' On that Ishmael said, 'It was my father, and you are the threshold (of the gate). He has ordered me to keep you with me...'" (Bukhari)

This story teaches us a number of lessons, including the following:

1 - Gratitude to Allah is a cause of His blessing being increased, and ingratitude brings the opposite. This is clear from the fate of both women.

2 - It indicates how a woman should be: content and accepting whatever provision Allah grants her husband without being annoyed or displeased.

3 - One should be careful to choose a good wife who will help him with regard to the Hereafter. (241)

237. Prohibition of Plural Marriage if he Cannot Treat Wives Equally

Allah, the Exalted, says:

"And if you fear that you shall not be able to deal justly with the orphan girls, then marry (other) women of your choice, two or three, or four but if you fear that you shall not be able to deal justly (with them), then only one or (the captives and the slaves) that your right hands possess. That is nearer to prevent you from doing injustice." (Qur'an, An-Nisa 4:3)

"You will never be able to do perfect justice between wives even if it is your ardent desire, so do not incline too much to one of them (by giving her more of your time and provision) so as to leave the other hanging (i.e. neither divorced nor married). And if you do justice, and do all that is right and fear Allah by keeping away from all that is wrong, then Allah is Ever Oft-Forgiving, Most Merciful." (Qur'an, An-Nisa 4:129)

The Prophet Muhammad (peace and blessings be upon him) was married to one wife, Khadijah, until she died. He was a faithful husband to her for twenty-five years, and did not marry another woman, except after her death. Muhammad had one wife - from the age of 25 to 50.

He married his other wives thereafter for a social or political purpose; such that he wanted to honor the pious women, or wanted the loyalty of certain tribes so that Islam would spread amongst them. He was just and fair towards them all and did not differentiate between them. There are the conditions attached to Plural Marriage:

1 – **Justice and Fairness**

Allah, the Exalted, says:

"You will never be able to do perfect justice between wives even if it is your ardent desire." (Qur'an, An-Nisa 4:129)

Plural marriage is permitted when one is able to be fair and just and treat his wives equally in terms of spending, clothing, other material things, spending the bed. If a man is afraid that he will not be able to treat his wives justly, then it is forbidden for him to marry more than one.

2 – **The ability to spend on one's wives**

Allah, the Exalted, says:

"And let those who find not the financial means for marriage keep themselves chaste, until Allah enriches them of His Bounty." (Qur'an, An-Nur 24:33)

Having more wives, means having more children. He should provide for his wives and children, and educate his children.

The wisdom behind permitting plural marriage

1. Plural marriage helps to increase the numbers of the Ummah (Muslim community).

Wise people know that increasing the number of offspring will strengthen the Ummah and increase the number of workers in it, which will raise its economic standard in a proper manner.

Allah, All-Wise, Who has prescribed plural marriage, has guaranteed to provide provision for His slaves and has created on earth what is more than sufficient for them. Whatever shortfall exists is due to the injustice of administrations, governments and individuals, and due to bad management and sins.

2. Statistics show that the number of women is greater than the number of men; if each man were to marry just one woman, this would mean that some women would be left without a husband, which would have a harmful effect on her and on society. The harmful effect is that she would never find a husband to take care of her interests, to give her a place to live, to spend on her, to protect her from haram desires, and to give her children to bring her joy. This may lead to deviance and going astray, except for those on whom Allah has Mercy. With regard to the harmful effects on society, it is well known that this woman who is left without a husband may deviate from the Straight Path and follow the ways of promiscuity, so she may fall into the swamp of fornication and prostitution which leads to the spread of immorality and the emergence of fatal diseases such as AIDS and other contagious diseases for which there is no cure. It also leads to family breakdown and the birth of children whose identity is unknown, and who do not know who their fathers are. Those children do not find anyone to show compassion towards them or any mature man to raise them properly. When they go out into the world and find out the truth, that they are illegitimate, that is reflected in their behavior, and they become exposed to deviance, the means of their country's destruction, leaders of deviant gangs, as is the case in many nations in the world.

3. Men are exposed to incidents that may end their lives, for they work in dangerous professions. They are the soldiers who fight in battle, and more men may die than women. This is one of the things that raise the percentage of husbandless women, and the only solution to this problem is plural marriage.

4. There are some men who may have strong physical desires, for whom one wife is not enough. If the door is closed to such a man and he is told, you are not allowed more than one wife, this will cause great hardship to him, and his desire may find outlets in forbidden ways. In addition to that, a woman menstruates each month, and when she gives birth, she bleeds for thirty days (postpartum bleeding or nifaas in Arabic), at which time a man cannot have intercourse with his wife, because intercourse at the time of menstruation or nifaas is forbidden, and the harm that it causes has been proven medically.

5. A wife may be barren, or she may not meet her husband's needs, or he may be unable to have intercourse with her because she is sick. A husband may long to have children, which is a legitimate desire, and he may want to have a sex life within marriage, which is something permissible, and the only way is to marry another wife. It is only fair for the wife to agree to remain his wife and to allow him to marry another.

6. A woman may be one of the man's relatives and have no one to look after her, and she is unmarried or a widow whose husband has died, and the man may think that the best thing to do for her is to include her in his household as a wife along with his first wife, so that he will both keep her chaste and spend on her. This is better for her than leaving her alone and being content only to spend on her.

7. Plural marriage may strengthen the bonds between families, or between a leader and some of his people or group, and he may think that one of the ways of achieving this aim is to become related to them through marriage.

On the other hand, plural marriage can cause problems and negative consequences that may outweigh any benefits; in such cases, plural marriage is disallowed, as in the case where the husband is not able to treat all his wives fairly, and he is afraid of being unfair or unjust towards them, or other cases in which the negative consequences outweigh any benefits that may be sought. (242)

It is on this basis that the Prophet (peace and blessings of Allah be upon him) forbade Ali ibn Abi Talib to take another wife in addition to his daughter Fatima (May Allah be pleased with her), even though plural marriage was permissible in principle for him.

Narrated al-Miswar ibn Makhramah that Ali ibn Abi Talib proposed marriage to the daughter of Abu Jahl, when he was already married to Fatima, the daughter of the Messenger of Allah (peace and blessings of Allah be upon him). When Fatima heard about that, she went to the Prophet (peace and blessings of Allah be upon him) and said to him: "Your people are saying that you do not get angry for the sake of your daughters, and Ali is going to marry the daughter of Abu Jahl." Al-Miswar said: "The Prophet (peace and blessings of Allah be upon him) stood up and I heard him when he bore witness, then he said: "I gave a daughter of mine in marriage to Abu'l-'Aas ibn ar-Rabee'; when he spoke, he told me the truth and when he made me a promise, he fulfilled his promise. Fatima is a part of me, and whatever hurts her, hurts me. By Allah, the daughter of the Messenger of Allah and the daughter of the enemy of Allah will not be joined together as wives of one man." So, Ali abandoned that proposal." (Bukhari and Muslim)

238. Prohibition of Same-Sex Marriage

Allah, the Exalted, says:

"Verily, you practice your lusts on men instead of women. Nay, but you are a people transgressing beyond bounds (by committing great sins)." (Qur'an, Al-A'raf 7:81)

"And We rained down on them a rain (of stones). Then see what was the end of the Mujrimoon (criminals, polytheists and sinners)." (Qur'an, Al-A'raf 7:84)

Jabir (May Allah have mercy on him) reported that the Messenger of Allah (peace and blessings be upon him) said: "The greatest fear that I have for my Ummah, is (that they will engage in) the action of the people of Lut." (Tirmidhi)
Abdullah ibn Abbas (May Allah be pleased with him) reported that the Messenger of Allah (peace and blessings of Allah be upon him) said: "…Allah's Curse be upon those who do the action of the people of Lut." Nabi (peace and blessings of Allah be upon him) repeated this curse thrice!) (Ibn Hibban)
Narrated Ibn Abbas (May Allah be pleased with him): The Messenger of Allah (peace and blessings of Allah be upon him) said: "Whoever you find doing the action of the people of Lut, execute the one who does it and the one to whom it is done." (Tirmidhi, Abu Dawud and Ibn Majah)

The lesbian, gay, bisexual and transgender (LGBT) people go against the natural disposition (Fitrah) which Allah has created in mankind; whereby the male is inclined towards the female, and vice versa.

The spread of homosexuality has caused many diseases (AIDS, etc.). It also causes the breakup of the family and leads people to give up their work and study because they are preoccupied with these perversions. Allah did not test anyone with this Major sin before the people of Lut, and He punished them with a punishment that He did not send upon any other nation; He combined all kinds of punishment for them, such as destruction, turning their houses upside down, causing them to be swallowed up by the earth, sending stones down upon them from the sky, taking away their sight, punishing them and making their punishment ongoing. That was because of the greatness of the evil consequences of this crime which the earth can hardly bear if it is committed upon it, and the angels flee to the farthest reaches of heaven and earth if they witness it, lest the punishment be sent upon those who do it and they be stricken along with them. The earth cries out to its Lord, may He be Blessed and Exalted, and the mountains almost shift from their places. (243)

239. Prohibition of "Paper" Marriage

"Paper Marriage" is a marriage in which a man and a woman enter without any intention to be husband and wife into a contract in which they pretend to be husband and wife in front of the legal authorities.

If two persons are entering into any such contract to facilitate one or the other spouse to immigrate to any other country, or secure a Green Card, or citizenship, or acquire or inherit property, or adopt children, or get H1B visa, they may be fulfilling legal formalities but will be in fact, cheating the authorities without attracting any provisions of law.

Paper marriage may be validated in the sight of human law; however, it contradicts our Creator's Law.

The minimum conditions for the validity of marriage (nikah) are the following:

1. The Consent of the Guardian of the woman
2. Presence of Two Legal Witnesses and Announcement of marriage
3. Offering and Acceptance
4. Obligatory Mahr

Once the above conditions have been fulfilled, the marriage will be deemed as valid; but if these conditions are not fulfilled, then it will be considered as being null and void.

Major sins committed in "Paper Marriage" are:

1. Absence of Intention to marry and live together. Actions are judged by intention,
2. Absence of Guardian or Guardian acting Illegal way to arrange "Paper Marriage",
3. Absence of Two Legal Witnesses and Announcement of marriage,
4. False testimony,
5. Lying,
6. Consumption of Haram. "Paper Marriage" usually involves huge amount of money,
7. Cheating the legal authorities.

This process is going to be considered a huge negative factor on Judgment Day. (244)

240. Prohibition of Marriage between Human and Jinn

Allah, the Exalted, says:

"And Allah has made for you wives of your own kind..." (Qur'an, An-Nahl 16:72)

"And among His Signs is this, that He created for you wives from among yourselves, that you may find repose in them, and He has put between you affection and mercy. Verily, in that are indeed signs for a people who reflect." (Qur'an, Ar-Rum 30:21)

"O you assembly of Jinns and mankind! "Did not there come to you Messengers from amongst you, reciting unto you My Verses and warning you of the meeting of this Day of yours?" (Qur'an, Al-An'am 6:130)

Other Verse: *Al-A'raf 7:27.*

Aisha (May Allah be pleased with her) reported that the Prophet (May Allah's peace and blessings be upon him) said: "Angels were created from light, Jinn were created from a smokeless flame of fire, and Adam was created from what was described to you (in the Qur'an)." (Muslim) (https://hadeethenc.com/en/browse/hadith/8264)

Ibn Taymiyah (May Allah have mercy on him) said:

"The Jinn may take the form of animals like snakes, scorpions, camels, cows, goats, sheep, horses, mules, donkeys and birds. They may also assume the form of humans, as in the case where the Devil came to the Quraysh in the form of Suraqah ibn Malik when they wanted to set out to Badr. In reference to this incident, Allah, the Exalted, revealed the Verse: *(Qur'an, Al-Anfal 8:48)*. It is also narrated that Satan took the form of an old man from Najd when the leaders of Quraysh gathered in their assembly room to decide whether to kill the Prophet, imprison him or banish him." The Almighty said concerning this: *(Qur'an, Al-Anfal 8:30)*" (10)

He (May Allah have mercy on him) said:

"The occasional possession of man by the Jinn may be due to sensual desires on the part of the Jinn, capricious whims, or even love, just as it may be among humans. Jinns and humans may also have intercourse with each other and beget children."

"Without the possessed human's consent, it becomes a grave case of atrocity and oppression. In such cases, the Jinn should be addressed and informed that their acts are either abominable and prohibited, or vile and tyrannical, so that evidence may be brought against them on the Day of Judgement and they be made aware that they have broken the Laws of Allah and His Prophet whom He sent to both worlds; that of man and that of the Jinn."

He (May Allah have mercy on him) also said:

"Most legists have opposed marriage with the Jinn." (10)

Marriage between Jinn and human is impermissible, for they are of different types and characteristics. Jinn is unseen matter while human is seen matter.

Several of the issues will arise if marriage between human and Jinn is made permissible:

- Adultery will increase and then the pregnancy will be claimed to be from the Jinn realm.
- The purpose of marriage is to attain children and family life. To whom will the child be associated and how are they created?
- Interaction with Jinn isn't free from harm? Jinn are very jealous and just evil creatures; whereas Islam emphasizes maintaining and preserving a person's safety.
- It opens doors to more unresolvable issues and never-ending questions and problems. (245)

241. Prohibition of Islamic Concubinage

Allah, the Exalted, says:

"And those who guard their chastity (i.e. private parts, from illegal sexual acts) Except from their wives or (the slaves) that their right hands possess, for then, they are free from blame." (Qur'an, Al-Mu'minun 23:6)

"O Prophet (Muhammad, peace be upon him)! Verily, We have made lawful to you your wives, to whom you have paid their Mahr (bridal money given by the husband to his wife at the time of marriage), and those (captives or slaves) whom your right hand possesses - whom Allah has given to you…" (Qur'an, Al-Ahzab 33:50)

Other Verses: Al-Ma'arij 70:30, Al-Ahzab 33:52

Narrated Ali ibn Abu Talib: The last words which the Messenger of Allah (peace and blessings be upon him) spoke were: "Prayer, prayer; fear Allah about those whom your right hands possess." (Abu Dawud)
This Hadith was among the last Ahadith, but the Hadith of Aisha is the last of all. (See Fayd al-Qadeer by al-Manaawi, 5/250-251; https://islamqa.info/en/answers/45841)

Narrated Ibn 'Abbas: "All types of women were prohibited for the Messenger of Allah (peace be upon him) except for the believing women among those who emigrated. Allah said: *'It is not lawful for you (to marry other) women after this, nor to change them for other wives even though their beauty attracts you, except those whom your right hand possesses.'* (33:52) And Allah made your believing girls lawful *'And a believing woman if she offers herself to the Prophet.'* (33:50) and He made every woman of a religion other than Islam unlawful. Then He said: *'And whoever disbelieves in faith then fruitless is his work; and in the Hereafter he will be among the losers.'* (5:5) And He said: *'Verily We have made lawful to you your wives, to whom you have paid their Mahr, and those whom your right hands possess - whom Allah has given you'* up to His saying: *'A privilege to only you, not for the (rest of) the believers.'* (33:50) He made the other types of women forbidden." (Tirmidhi) (https://sunnah.com/tirmidhi:3215)

Narrated Anas: "The Prophet stayed between Khaibar and Al-Madinah for three days when he consummated his marriage to Safiyyah bint Huyayy, and I invited the Muslims to his Walimah, in which there was no bread or meat. He commanded that a leather cloth (be spread) and dates, cottage cheese and ghee were placed on it, and that was his Walimah. The Muslims said: '(Will she be) one of the Mothers of the Believers, or a female slave whom his right hand possesses?' They said: 'If he has a Hijab for her, then she will be one of the Mothers of the Believers and if she does not have a Hijab then she will be a female slave whom his right hand possesses.' When he rode on, he set aside a plate for her behind him and extended a Hijab between her and the people." (An-Nasa'i)

Narrated Ruwayfi' ibn Thaabit al-Ansaari: "I heard the Messenger of Allah (peace and blessings be upon him) say on the day of Hunayn: "It is not permissible for any man who

believes in Allah and the Last Day to irrigate the crop of another else – meaning to have intercourse with a woman who is pregnant. And it is not permissible for a man who believes in Allah and the Last Day to have intercourse with a captured woman until he has established that she is not pregnant. And it is not permissible for a man who believes in Allah and the Last Day to sell any booty until it has been shared out." (Abu Dawud)
Sheikh al-Shanqeeti (May Allah have mercy on him) said:

"When the Muslims take prisoners of war, they are given the right to enslave them by the Law of the Creator of all, and He is the All-Wise, All-Aware. If this right is established, then the slave becomes a Muslim after that, his right to be freed from slavery because of his Islam is superseded by the right of the mujaahid whose right to enslave him took effect before he was a Muslim. It is not just or fair to waive the former right because of a latter right, as is well known to all wise people. Yes, it is good for the owner to set him free if he becomes Muslim, and Islam enjoins that and encourages it, and opens the door to doing so in many ways – he is referring to the fact that Allah has decreed that when expiation takes the form of freeing a slave, the slave in question should be a Muslim. *"Glory be to the All-Wise, All-Aware: "And the Word of your Lord has been fulfilled in truth and in justice. None can change His Words. And He is the All-Hearer, the All-Knower." (Al-An'am 6:115)* (Adwa' al-Bayaan, 3/389) (246)

With regard to Muslims owning slaves, he should be very careful to establish that those who are bought or sold now are indeed slaves, because Islam has limited the sources of slaves which were many before Muhammad (peace and blessings be upon him), and has allowed only one source, which is kaafir prisoners of war, when the kuffaar are fighting the Muslims. There is no other way in which they may be enslaved except those who are captured as a result of fighting between kaffirs and Muslims or their children.

242. Wearing Engagement and Wedding Ring

Narrated Abu Hurairah (May Allah have mercy on him): "The Prophet (peace and blessings be upon him) forbade the wearing of a gold ring." (Bukhari)

The Prophet (peace and blessings be upon him) forbade gold for men. He saw a man wearing a ring of gold and he (peace and blessings be upon him) took it from his hand and said, "Would any one of you take a coal from the fire and hold it in his hand?" (Muslim)

Sheikh Saalih al-Fawzan (May Allah have mercy on him) said:

"Firstly, the wedding ring is not one of the customs of the Muslims. It is a custom that has come to the Muslims from the non-Muslims. Secondly, if it is believed that it generates love between the spouses, and that taking it off and not wearing it will have an effect on the marital relationship, then this is regarded as a form of Shirk and is a kind of jaahili belief. Laa hawla wa laa quwwata illa Billaah (there is no power and no strength except with Allah)." (From a Fatwa issued by Sheikh Saalih al-Fawzan) (247)

243. Refusing Wedding Invitation Without Valid Excuse

Narrated 'Abdullah bin 'Umar (May Allah be pleased with him): Allah's Messenger (peace and blessings be upon him) said, "If anyone of you is invited to a wedding banquet, he must go for it (accept the invitation)." (Bukhari)

Narrated Abu Hurairah (May Allah be pleased with him) used to say: "The worst food is the food of a wedding banquet to which only the rich are invited while the poor are left out. Anyone who does not answer the invitation has disobeyed Allah and His Messenger (May Allah's peace and blessings be upon him)." (Bukhari and Muslim) (https://hadeethenc.com/en/browse/hadith/58113)

244. Extravagance in Wedding Party and Honeymoon

Allah, the Exalted, says:

"And those, who, when they spend, are neither extravagant nor niggardly, but hold a medium (way) between those (extremes)." (Qur'an, Al-Furqan 25:67)

"...but waste not by extravagance, certainly He (Allah) likes not Al-Musrifun (those who waste by extravagance)." (Qur'an, Al-A'raf 7:31)

Other Verse: *At-Talaq 65:7.*

"The most blessed marriage is that which is affordable; the less the expenses are, the greater the blessings." (Sheikh Muhammad ibn Saalih al-'Uthaymeen, https://islamqa.info/en/answers/171265)

The "honeymoon" is a great waste of money. It involves other sins like singing, dancing, musical instruments, mixing between men and women, etc.

245. Husband's Rights Concerning his Wife

Allah, the Exalted, says:

"Men are the protectors and maintainers of women, because Allah has made one of them to excel the other, and because they spend (to support them) from their means. Therefore, the righteous women are devoutly obedient (to Allah and to their husbands), and guard in the husband's absence what Allah orders them to guard (e.g. their chastity and their husband's property)." (Qur'an, An-Nisa 4:34)

The Husband's Rights Over his Wife:

1. Obligation of Obedience to Husband in Doing Good Deeds

Ali reported: The Prophet (peace and blessings be upon him) said, "There is no obedience to anyone if it is disobedience to Allah. Verily, obedience is only in good conduct." (Bukhari and Muslim)
In another narration, The Prophet (peace and blessings be upon him) said, "There is no obedience to a created being if it is disobedience to Allah Almighty."

Abu Hurairah reported: The Messenger of Allah (peace and blessings be upon him) said, "If a woman prays her five prayers, fasts her month of Ramadan, guards her chastity, and obeys her husband, she will enter Paradise from any gate she wishes." (Ibn Ḥibban)

2. Making Herself Available to her Husband

Narrated Abu Hurairah (May Allah be pleased with him): The Messenger of Allah (peace and blessings be upon him) said, "When a man calls his wife to his bed, and she does not respond and he (the husband) spends the night angry with her, the angels curse her until morning." (Bukhari and Muslim)

Commentary: This Hadith makes it abundantly clear that obedience of the husband is compulsory on the wife. If, in the absence of any lawful reason, she refuses to obey the orders of her husband, she will be liable to the Wrath and Curse of Allah until she returns to obedience. This Hadith has a stern warning for those women who do not care for the displeasure of their husbands because of their bad temperament, stubbornness and habit of dominating their husbands. (248)

Abu 'Ali Talq bin 'Ali (May Allah be pleased with him) reported: The Messenger of Allah (peace and blessings be upon him) said, "When a man calls his wife to satisfy his desire, she must go to him even if she is occupied with the oven." (Tirmidhi and An-Nasa'i)

Umm Salamah (May Allah be pleased with her) reported: The Messenger of Allah (peace and blessings be upon him) said, "Any woman dies while her husband is pleased with her, she will enter Jannah." (Tirmidhi)

If a wife refuses to respond to her husband's request for intercourse, she has committed a Major sin, unless she has a valid excuse such as menses, obligatory fasting, sickness, etc. (249)

3. Not admitting anyone whom the husband dislikes

Narrated Abu Hurairah (May Allah be pleased with him): The Messenger of Allah (peace and blessings be upon him) said, "It is not lawful for a woman to observe (voluntary) fasting without the permission of her husband when he is at home; and she should not allow anyone to enter his house without his permission." (Bukhari and Muslim)

Sulaiman bin Amr bin Al-Ahwas said: "My father narrated to me that he will witness the farewell Hajj with the Messenger of Allah. So, he thanked and praised Allah, and he reminded and gave admonition. He mentioned a story in his narration and he (the Prophet) (peace and blessings be upon him) said: "And indeed, I order you to be good to the women, for they are but captives with you over whom you have no power than that, except if they come with manifest Fahishah (evil behavior). If they do that, then abandon their beds and beat them with a beating that is not harmful. And if they obey you then you have no cause against them. Indeed, you have rights over your women, and your women have rights over you. As for your rights over your women, then they must not allow anyone whom you dislike to treat on your bedding (furniture), nor to admit anyone in your home that you dislike." (Tirmidhi)

Narrated Jabir: The Prophet (peace and blessings of Allah be upon him) said: "Fear Allah concerning women! Verily you have taken them on the security of Allah, and intercourse with them has been made lawful unto you by Words of Allah. You too have right over them, and that they should not allow anyone to sit on your bed whom you do not like. But if they do that, you can chastise them but not severely. Their rights upon you are that you should provide them with food and clothing in a fitting manner. I have left among you the Book of Allah, and if you hold fast to it, you would never go astray. And you would be asked about me (on the Day of Resurrection)." (Muslim)

'Uqba b. 'Amir reported Allah's Messenger (peace and blessings be upon him) as saying: "Beware of getting, into the houses and meeting women (in seclusion). A person from the Ansar said: Allah's Messenger, what about husband's brother, whereupon he (peace be upon him) said: "Husband's brother is like death." (Muslim)

'Abdullah b. 'Amr. b. al-'As reported: "Some persons from Banu Hisham entered the house of Asma' daughter of 'Umais when Abu Bakr also entered (and she was at that time his wife). He (Abu Bakr) saw it and disapproved of it and he made a mention of that to Allah's Messenger (May peace and blessings be upon him) and said: 'I did not see but good only (in my wife).' Thereupon Allah's Messenger (May peace and blessings be upon him) said: 'Verily Allah has made her immune from all this.' Then Allah's Messenger (May peace and blessings be upon him) stood on the pulpit and said: 'After this day no man should enter the house of another person in his absence, but only when he is accompanied by one person or two persons.'" (Muslim)

4. Not Going out of the House Except with the Husband's Permission

One of the rights of the husband over his wife is that she should not go out of the house without his permission except going to the Mosque, to study, to work, to see relatives, buying necessary things. (250, 251)

5. Discipline

Allah, the Exalted, says:

"And live with them honorably. If you dislike them, it may be that you dislike a thing and Allah brings through it a great deal of good." (Qur'an, An-Nisa 4:19)

"O you who believe! Ward off yourselves and your families against a Fire (Hell) whose fuel is men and stones." (Qur'an, At-Tahrim 66:6)

Other Verses: *An-Nisa 4:34, Al-Ahzab 33:6.*

Abu Hurairah (May Allah be pleased with him) reported that the Messenger of Allah (May Allah's peace and blessings be upon him) said: "May Allah have mercy upon a man who wakes up at night and prays, and awakens his wife. If she refuses, he sprinkles water on her face. May Allah have mercy upon a woman who wakes up at night and prays, and awakens her husband. If he refuses, she sprinkles water on his face." (Ibn Majah, An-Nasa'i, Abu Dawud and Ahmad) (https://hadeethenc.com/en/browse/hadith/3717)

Iys ibn 'Abdullah ibn Abi Dhubāb (May Allah be pleased with him) reported that the Messenger of Allah (May Allah's peace and blessings be upon him) said: "Do not beat Allah's handmaidens." Later, 'Umar (May Allah be pleased with him) came to the Messenger of Allah (May Allah's peace and blessings be upon him) and said: "Women have become emboldened towards and disobedient to their husbands." So, he gave a license to beat them. Consequently, many women came around the families of the Messenger of Allah (May Allah's peace and blessings be upon him) complaining about their husbands. So, the Messenger of Allah (May Allah's peace and blessings be upon him) said: "Many women have gone around Muhammad's families complaining about their husbands. Those (husbands) are not the best of you." (Ibn Majah, Abu Dawud and Al-Darimi) (https://hadeethenc.com/en/browse/hadith/5821)

Beating (hitting) is subject to the condition that it should not be harsh or cause injury. Al-Hasan al-Basri said: "This means that it should not cause pain." 'Ata' said: "I said to Ibn 'Abbas, what is the kind of hitting that is not harsh?" He said, "Hitting with a siwaak and the like." (A siwaak is a small stick or twig used for cleaning the teeth) The purpose behind this is not to hurt or humiliate the woman, rather it is intended to make her realize that she has transgressed against her husband's rights, and that her husband has the right to set her straight and discipline her. (252)

There happened between his wives (May Allah be pleased with them) that which usually happens between co-wives, but nevertheless they would soon calm down and go back to their usual way of conduct based on faith, restraint, dignity and religious commitment. (253)

7. Kind Treatment

Allah' the Exalted, says:

"O you who believe! You are forbidden to inherit women against their will, and you should not treat them with harshness, that you may take away part of the Mahr you have given them, unless they commit open illegal sexual intercourse. And live with them honorably. If you dislike them, it may be that you dislike a thing and Allah brings through it a great deal of good." (Qur'an, An-Nisa 4:19)

Jabir Ibn Abdullah reported: The Messenger of Allah (peace and blessings be upon him) said: "Fear Allah regarding women. Verily, you have taken them as a trust from Allah." (Muslim)

Narrated Sulaiman bin Amr bin Ahwas: "My father told me that he was present at the Farewell Pilgrimage with the Messenger of Allah. He praised and glorified Allah, and reminded and exhorted (the people). Then he said: 'I enjoin good treatment of women, for they are prisoners with you, and you have no right to treat them otherwise, unless they commit clear indecency. If they do that, then forsake them in their beds and hit them, but without causing injury or leaving a mark. If they obey you, then do not seek means of annoyance against them. You have rights over your women and your women have rights over you. Your rights over your women are that they are not to allow anyone whom you dislike to tread on your bedding (furniture), nor allow anyone whom you dislike to enter your houses. And their right over you are that you should treat them kindly with regard to their clothing and food.'" (Ibn Majah)

Narrated Mu'adh bin Jabal (May Allah be pleased with him): The Prophet (peace and blessings be upon him) said, "Whenever a woman harms her husband in this world (that is without any due right), his wife among the Houris in Paradise says: ''Do not harm him! May Allah destroy you! He is but a passing guest with you, and he will soon leave you to join us.''" (Ibn Majah, Tirmidhi and Ahmad)
(https://hadeethenc.com/en/browse/hadith/5822)

8. Beautification

Narrated Jabir bin 'Abdullah (May Allah be pleased with him): "...When we were about to enter (Madinah), the Prophet (peace and blessings be upon him) said, "Wait so that you may enter (Madinah) at night so that the lady of unkempt hair may comb her hair and the one whose husband has been absent may shave her pubic region." (Bukhari)

Serving and running marital house as a favor and not as an obligation

Aisha (May Allah be pleased with her) was asked: "What did the Messenger of Allah (peace and blessings of Allah be upon him) do in his house?" She said: "He was a human being like any other; he would clean his garment, milk his sheep and serve himself." (Ahmad)

Narrated Al-Aswad bin Yazid (May Allah be pleased with him): "I asked Aisha "What did the Prophet (peace and blessings be upon him) use to do at home?" She said, "He used to work for his family, and when he heard the Adhan (Call for the prayer), he would go out." (Bukhari)

Acknowledge her efforts

The Prophet (peace and blessings be upon him) always appreciated even the littlest of things that his wives did for him, from cooking to taking care of the children. He never took his wives efforts for granted and showered her with respect and gratitude.

Help her with daily chores

Prophet Muhammad (peace and blessings be upon him) always supported his wives and helped them in household chores. He did his own work, and helped in cooking and cleaning of the house. Allah rewards the man who helps his wife in household chores.

246. Non-Fulfillment of Husband's Obligations

Husband's Obligations towards his Wife:

1. Mahr

Allah, the Exalted, says:

"And give to the women (whom you marry) their Mahr (obligatory bridal money given by the husband to his wife at the time of marriage) with a good heart..." (Qur'an, An-Nisa 4:4)

2. Husband is a Guardian of the family

Allah, the Exalted, says:

"Men are the protectors and maintainers of women, because Allah has made one of them to excel the other, and because they spend (to support them) from their means. Therefore, the righteous women are devoutly obedient (to Allah and to their husbands), and guard

in the husband's absence what Allah orders them to guard (e.g. their chastity, their husband's property, etc.). As to those women on whose part you see ill conduct, admonish them (first), (next) refuse to share their beds, (and last) beat them (lightly, if it is useful), but if they return to obedience, seek not against them means (of annoyance). Surely, Allah is Ever Most High, Most Great." (Qur'an, An-Nisa 4:34)

"...but the father of the child shall bear the cost of the mother's food and clothing on a reasonable basis." (Qur'an, Al-Baqarah 2:233)

"Let the rich man spend according to his means, and the man whose resources are restricted, let him spend according to what Allah has given him. Allah puts no burden on any person beyond what He has given him." (Qur'an, At-Talaq 65:7)

Other Verse: *Al-Baqarah 2:228.*

Narrated 'Abdullah bin 'Umar: The Prophet (peace and blessings be upon him) said, "Surely, everyone of you is a guardian and is responsible for his charges. The Imam (ruler) of the people is a guardian and is responsible for his subjects; a man is the guardian of his family (household) and responsible for his subjects; a woman is the guardian of her husband's home and of his children and is responsible for them; and the slave of a man is a guardian of his master's property and is responsible for it. Surely, everyone of you is a guardian and responsible for his charges." (Bukhari)

Narrated Sad: "…The Prophet (peace and blessings be upon him) said: "Whatever you spend will be considered a Sadaqah for you, even the mouthful of food you put in the mouth of your wife…" (Bukhari)

Narrated Aisha: "Hind bint 'Utbah, the wife of Abu Sufyan, entered upon the Messenger of Allah (peace and blessings of Allah be upon him) and said, 'O Messenger of Allah, Abu Sufyan is a stingy man who does not spend enough on me and my children, except for what I take from his wealth without his knowledge. Is there any sin on me for doing that?' The Messenger of Allah (peace and blessings of Allah be upon him) said, 'Take from his wealth on a reasonable basis, only what is sufficient for you and your children.'" (Bukhari and Muslim)

Narrated Jabir: The Messenger of Allah (peace and blessings be upon him) said in his Farewell Sermon: "Fear Allah concerning women! Verily you have taken them on the security of Allah, and intercourse with them has been made lawful unto you by Words of Allah. You too have rights over them, and that they should not allow anyone to sit on your bed (i.e. not let them into the house) whom you do not like. But if they do that, you can chastise them but not severely. Their rights upon you are that you should provide them with food and clothing in a fitting manner." (Muslim) (https://sunnah.com/muslim:1218a)

3. Accommodation

Allah, the Exalted, says:

"Lodge them (the divorced women) where you dwell, according to your means…" (Qur'an, At-Talaq 65:6)

One of the wife's rights is that her husband should provide her with accommodation. This may vary according to what the husband can afford.

It is not permissible for a husband to make anyone live with his wife whose presence will cause her harm such as his mother, father or children from another wife. If one of his parents needs him, and she will not be affected by his or her presence, then we advise the wife to fear Allah with regard to this one who is in need. She should realize that honouring her husband's parents is part of treating him kindly, and the wise husband should appreciate his wife's actions which will increase the bonds of love between them. (254)

The husband is financially in charge of all of them, provided no prejudice is caused to the wife from such accommodation.

The wife may not accommodate with her in the conjugal domicile her children from another man unless they have no other caretaker, they may be harmed from separation or by express, or implied agreement of the husband, provided he has the right to go back on his acceptance should he sustains a prejudice therefrom. The husband may not accommodate with his wife another wife of his unless she accepts provided, she can go back on this acceptance whenever it becomes detrimental to her. (255)

4. Taking Care of his Wife

Narrated Ibn 'Abbas: The Prophet (peace and blessings be upon him) said: "The best of you is the one who is best to his wife, and I am the best of you to my wives." (Ibn Majah)

Narrated Abu Hurairah: The Prophet (peace and blessings be upon him) said, "Whoever believes in Allah and the Last Day should not hurt (trouble) his neighbor. And I advise you to take care of the women, for they are created from a rib and the most crooked portion of the rib is its upper part; if you try to straighten it, it will break, and if you leave it, it will remain crooked, so I urge you to take care of the women." (Bukhari)

5. Loving for the sake of Allah

Allah, the Exalted, says:

"And among His Signs is this, that He created for you wives from among yourselves, that you may find repose in them, and He has put between you affection and mercy. Verily, in that are indeed signs for a people who reflect." (Qur'an, Ar-Rum 30:21)

Narrated Ibn Abbas (May Allah be pleased with him): The Messenger of Allah (peace and blessings be upon him) said: "There is nothing like marriage, for two who love one another." (Ibn Majah)

Abu Hurairah (May Allah be pleased with him) reported: The Messenger of Allah (May Allah's peace and blessings be upon him) said: "Allah the Almighty will say on the Day of Judgment: 'Where are those who loved each other for My Glory? Today, I will shelter them under My Shade the day when there is no shade but My Shade.'" (Muslim) (https://hadeethenc.com/en/browse/hadith/3369)

6. Respect his wife

The Qur'an implores men to treat women with kindness and respect even in times of disagreement. She works for you and your children's comfort and thus, value her efforts and respect her. She may become tired from housework and may become annoyed with the children. Others may upset her by their criticisms. Women, who experience hardship, need appeasing. Men must comfort them because they are their partners.

7. Kind Treatment

Allah, the Exalted, says:

"And verily, you (O Muhammad SAW) are on an exalted standard of character." (Qur'an, Al-Qalam 68:4)

Aisha, the wife of Allah's Apostle (peace and blessings be upon him), reported that Allah's Messenger (peace be upon him) said: "Aisha, Verily, Allah is Kind and He loves kindness and confers upon kindness which he does not confer upon severity and does not confer upon anything else besides it (kindness)." (Muslim)

Aisha (May Allah be pleased with her) reported: The Messenger of Allah (peace and blessings be upon him) said: "Verily, the most complete of believers in faith are those with the best character and who are most kind to their families." (Tirmidhī)

Abdullah Ibn Amr reported: The Messenger of Allah (peace and blessings be upon him) said: "Whoever would love to be delivered from Hellfire and admitted into Paradise, let him meet his end with faith in Allah and the Last Day, and let him treat people as he would love to be treated." (Muslim)

8. Non-infliction of bodily or moral prejudice to her

Allah, the Exalted, says:

"And live with them honorably. If you dislike them, it may be that you dislike a thing and Allah brings through it a great deal of good." (Qur'an, An-Nisa 4:19)

The Prophet (peace and blessings be upon him) said, "Fear Allah in regard to women. You were given them as a trust from Allah and by the Word of Allah they have become lawful for you." (Muslim)

Aisha (May Allah be pleased with her) reported: The Messenger of Allah (peace and blessings be upon him) said, "Overlook the faults of people of good mannerisms except the legal punishments." (Abu Dawud)

Abu Umamah al-Bahili (May Allah be pleased with him) reported: The Prophet (May Allah's peace and blessings be upon him) said: "I guarantee a house on the outskirts of Paradise for the one who refrains from arguing even if he is right, and a house in the middle of Paradise for the one who refrains from lying even if he is joking, and a house in the highest part of Paradise for the one who perfects his manners." (Abu Dawud) (https://hadeethenc.com/en/browse/hadith/5804)

9. Non-obstruction to complete her education

10. Non-opposition to visit her ascendants, descendants, brothers and sisters

Narrated Ali: "Fatima complained of what she suffered from the hand mill and from grinding, when she got the news that some slave girls of the booty had been brought to Allah's Messenger (peace and blessings be upon him). She went to him to ask for a maid-servant, but she could not find him, and told Aisha of her need. When the Prophet (peace and blessings be upon him) came, Aisha informed him of that. The Prophet (peace and blessings be upon him) came to our house when we had gone to our beds. (On seeing the Prophet) we were going to get up, but he said, 'Keep at your places,' I felt the coolness of the Prophet's feet on my chest. Then he said, "Shall I tell you a thing which is better than what you asked me for? When you go to your beds, say: 'Allahu Akbar (i.e. Allah is Greater)' for 34 times, and 'Al hamdu Lillah (i.e. all the praises are for Allah)' for 33 times, and Subhan Allah (i.e. Glorified be Allah) for 33 times. This is better for you than what you have requested." (Bukhari) (https://sunnah.com/bukhari:3113)

11. Non-interference with her personal properties

12. Protection

Allah, the Exalted, says:

"Men are protectors of women, because Allah has made some of them excel others and because they spend their wealth on them…" (Qur'an, An-Nisa 4: 34)

247. Wife's Rights Concerning his Husband

The Rights of the Wife:

The wife has financial rights over her husband, which are the Mahr, spending, accommodation, health expenses. And she has non-financial rights, such as fair division between co-wives, being treated in a good manner, and not being treated in a harmful way. The obligation upon women to obey the husband in the matters which do not contradict Allah's commands and prohibitions and take care of the matrimonial home and children. (232)

1. Mahr

Allah, the Exalted, says:

"And give to the women (whom you marry) their Mahr (obligatory bridal money given by the husband to his wife at the time of marriage) with a good heart." (Qur'an, An-Nisa 4:4)

2. Financial Maintenance

Allah, the Exalted, says:

"Men are the protectors and maintainers of women, because Allah has made one of them to excel the other, and because they spend (to support them) from their means." (Qur'an, An-Nisa 4:34)

"but the father of the child shall bear the cost of the mother's food and clothing on a reasonable basis." (Qur'an, Al-Baqarah 2:233)

"And they (women) have rights (over their husbands as regards living expenses) similar (to those of their husbands) over them (as regards obedience and respect) to what is reasonable" (Qur'an, Al-Baqarah 2:228)

Other Verse: At-Talaq 65:7.

Narrated Hakim bin Muawiyah, from his father: "A man asked the Prophet (peace and blessings be upon him): "What are the rights of the woman over her husband?" He said: "That he should feed her as he feeds himself and clothe her as he clothes himself; he should not strike her on the face nor disfigure her, and he should not abandon her except in the house (as a form of discipline)." (Ibn Majah)

Narrated Aisha (May Allah be pleased with her): "Hind bint 'Utbah, the wife of Abu Sufyan, entered upon the Messenger of Allah (peace and blessings be upon him) and said, 'O Messenger of Allah, Abu Sufyan is a stingy man who does not spend enough on me and my children, except for what I take from his wealth without his knowledge. Is there any sin on me for doing that?' The Messenger of Allah (peace and blessings be upon him) said, 'Take from his wealth on a reasonable basis, only what is sufficient for you and your children.'" (Bukhari and Muslim)

The wife has no financial responsibilities to the husband, her children or maintaining the household. Not even if she is rich or is working.

3. Accommodation

Allah, the Exalted, says:

"Lodge them (the divorced women) where you dwell, according to your means, and do not treat them in such a harmful way that they be obliged to leave…" (Qur'an, At-Talaq 65:6)

4. Non-Infliction of Bodily or Moral Prejudice to Wife

Allah, the Exalted, says:

"And live with them honorably. If you dislike them, it may be that you dislike a thing and Allah brings through it a great deal of good." (Qur'an, An-Nisa 4:19)

Narrated 'Ubaadah Ibn al-Saamit that the Messenger of Allah (peace and blessings be upon him) ruled,

"There should be no harming nor reciprocating harm." (Ibn Majah)

5. Wife Completes her Education without Husband's Obstruction

6. Wife visits her Ascendants, Descendants, Brothers and Sisters without Husband's Opposition

7. Wife Deals with her Personal Properties without Husband's Interference

8. Divorced or Widowed Woman Staying in the Marital House during her Waiting Period

Allah, the Exalted, says:

"O Prophet! When you divorce women, divorce them at their 'Iddah (prescribed periods) and count (accurately) their 'Iddah (periods). And fear Allah your Lord (O Muslims). And turn them not out of their (husband's) homes nor shall they (themselves) leave, except in case they are guilty of some open illegal sexual intercourse. And those are the set limits of Allah. And whosoever transgresses the set limits of Allah, then indeed he has wronged himself." (Qur'an, At-Talaq 65:1)

"Lodge them (the divorced women) where you dwell, according to your means, and do not treat them in such a harmful way that they be obliged to leave. And if they are pregnant, then spend on them till they deliver. Then if they give suck to the children for you, give them their due payment, and let each of you accept the advice of the other in a just way. But if you make difficulties for one another, then some other woman may give suck for him (the father of the child)." (Qur'an, At-Talaq 65:6)

"And those of you who die and leave behind wives should bequeath for their wives a year's maintenance and residence without turning them out, but if they (wives) leave, there is no sin on you for that which they do of themselves, provided it is honorable (e.g. lawful marriage). And Allah is All-Mighty, All-Wise." (Qur'an, Al-Baqarah 2:240)

9. Equitable Treatment Between Wives

Allah, the Exalted, says:

"The Prophet is closer to the believers than their own selves, and his wives are their (believers') mothers (as regards respect and marriage)." (Qur'an, Al-Ahzab 33:6)

Husband must provide them all with the same accommodation, living expenses and divide his time equally between the wives.

10. Kind Treatment

11. Love for the sake of Allah

12. Protection

13. Alimony

248. Non-Fulfillment of Wife's Obligations

<u>Wife's Obligations Towards her Husband:</u>

1. Obligation of Obedience to Husband in Doing Good Deeds

The Prophet (peace and blessings be upon him) said: "There is no obedience to a created being if it is disobedience to Allah Almighty." (Bukhari)

2. Making herself Available to her Husband

Abu Hurairah (Allah he pleased with him) reported Allah's Messenger (may, peace be upon him) as saying: "When a man invites his wife to his bed and she does not come, and he (the husband) spends the sight being with her, the angels curse her angry until morning." (Muslim)

3. Not Admitting Anyone in his House whom the Husband Dislikes

4. Not Going out of the House Except with the Husband's Permission

Allah, the Exalted, says:

"And stay in your houses, and do not display yourselves like that of the times of ignorance." (Qur'an, Al-Ahzab 33:33)

1) Husband shouldn't prevent his wife to pray in the Mosque and attend Islamic lectures,
2) Husband shouldn't oppose to wife to complete her education.
3) Wife doesn't need the husband's permission to go to toilet which is outside of the house.
4) Wife is permitted to visit her parents, her children if they live separately, sisters and brothers.
5) It is permissible for a woman to work or study so long as a number of conditions are met. (256)

Narrated Ibn 'Abbas: The Prophet (peace and blessings be upon him) said, "A woman should not travel except with a Dhu-Mahram (her husband or a man with whom that woman cannot marry at all according to the Islamic Jurisprudence), and no man may visit her except in the presence of a Dhu-Mahram." A man got up and said, "O Allah's Messenger! I intend to go to such and such an army and my wife wants to perform Hajj." The Prophet (peace and blessings be upon him) said (to him), "Go along with her (to Hajj)." (Bukhari)

Narrated 'Adi bin Hatim: "While I was in the city of the Prophet, a man came and complained to him (the Prophet) of destitution and poverty. Then another man came and complained of robbery (by highwaymen). The Prophet said, "Adi! Have you been to Al-Hira?" I said, "I haven't been to it, but I was informed about it." He said, "If you should live for a long time, you will certainly see that a lady in a Howdah traveling from Al-Hira will (safely reach Makkah and) perform the Tawaf of the Ka'bah, fearing none but Allah." (Bukhari)

If the wife leaves the marital house and then refuses to return without having an excuse, she is then considered recalcitrant, and is not entitled to financial support as of that date. (257)

5. Guarding Husband's Property and Honor

6. Kind Treatment

7. Love for the sake of Allah

8. Voluntary Fasting only with Husband's Permission

Narrated Abu Hurairah (May Allah be pleased with him): The Messenger of Allah (peace and blessings of Allah be upon him) said: "No woman should fast when her husband is present without his permission, and she should not allow anyone to enter his house when he is present without his permission." (Bukhari and Muslim)

10. Beautification for husband (within the Qur'an and Sunnah)

11. Guarding and Educating Children

12. Divorced or Widowed Woman Staying in the Marital House during the Waiting Period

Allah, the Exalted, says:

"O Prophet! When you divorce women, divorce them at their 'Iddah (prescribed periods) and count (accurately) their 'Iddah (periods). And fear Allah your Lord (O Muslims). And turn them not out of their (husband's) homes nor shall they (themselves) leave, except in case they are guilty of some open illegal sexual intercourse." (Qur'an, At-Talaq 65:1)

"And those of you who die and leave behind wives should bequeath for their wives a year's maintenance and residence without turning them out." (Qur'an, Al-Baqarah 2:240)

When the husband pronounces a revocable divorce, like the case when he divorces his non-pregnant wife once after the consummation of the marriage with no compensation conditioned, the wife has to remain at her husband's house. It is unlawful for her to leave the husband's house as long as the term of the 'Iddah has not expired yet. Likewise, it is unlawful for the husband to drive her out of the house until her 'Iddah expires unless a clear act of immorality has been committed. This is because a revocable divorced woman is still considered to be a wife. During the period of 'Iddah, the husband has the right to take her back in marriage, even if she does not agree, provided that this is done in the presence of two just witnesses. Neither a new marriage contract nor Mahr (mandatory gift to a bride from her groom) is required from the husband.

However, if the husband pronounces an irrevocable divorce, like the case when he divorces her prior to or after the consummation of the marriage while conditioning a compensation for the divorce, she becomes unlawful for him. He may take her back in marriage with a new marriage contract and a new Mahr provided that she gives her consent to remarry him. Pronouncement of irrevocable divorce makes it impermissible for the husband to sit in Khulwah (being alone with a member of the opposite sex) with his ex-wife or to see any part of her body which a non-Mahram (not a spouse or an unmarriageable relative) is not allowed to see. (258)

249. Disobedience to Husband

Allah, the Exalted, says:

"As to those women on whose part you see ill-conduct, admonish them (first), (next) refuse to share their beds, (and last) beat them (lightly, if it is useful); but if they return to obedience, seek not against them means (of annoyance). Surely, Allah is Ever Most High, Most Great." (Qur'an, An-Nisa 4:34)

Narrated Muadh bin Jabal: The Messenger of Allah (peace and blessings be upon him) said: "No woman annoys her husband but his wife among houris (of Paradise) says: 'Do not annoy him, may Allah destroy you, for he is just a temporary guest with you and soon he will leave you and join us.'" (Ibn Majah)

Narrated Abu Hurairah: Allah's Messenger (peace and blessings be upon him) said, "It is not lawful for a lady to fast (Nawafil) without the permission of her husband when he is at home; and she should not allow anyone to enter his house except with his permission; and if she spends of his wealth (on charitable purposes) without being ordered by him, he will get half of the reward." (Bukhari)

Narrated Ibn Abbas: The Messenger of Allah (peace and blessings be upon him) said: "There are three whose prayer do not rise more than a hand span above their heads: A man who leads people (in prayer) when they do not like him; a woman who has spent the night with her husband angry with her; and
two brothers who have severed contact with one another." (Ibn Majah)

Narrated Usama: The Prophet (peace and blessings be upon him) said, "I stood at the gate of Paradise and saw that the majority of the people who entered it were the poor, while the wealthy were stopped at the gate (for the accounts). But the companions of the Fire were ordered to be taken to the Fire. Then I stood at the gate of the Fire and saw that the majority of those who entered it were women." (Bukhari)

Happy homes are those which are built on mutual understanding and love and consolidated with affection and compassion between spouses. None of this can be achieved without the spouses doing the duties that are specific to them. The husband has to look for the causes of his wife's willful defiance and find out the ways in which he can treat her sickness and lead her to the way of guidance and salvation, so that she will be protected from the Punishment of Allah. These causes may include the husband! Yes, he may be one of the causes of her willful defiance, either because of sins that he is committing – as one of the salaf said: "I see the effect of my sins in my mount and my wife", in her bad attitude or refusal to obey him – or the husband may have a bad attitude towards his wife so her behavior is a reaction against the way he deals with her (https://hadeethenc.com/en/browse/hadith/5821)

If he knows that the reason for her willful defiance is something that he can remedy, then he should do that. If he cannot deal with her, then he should appoint someone else from among his/her family to undertake this mission. Someone else may have a stronger influence over her than him. If the wife is not praying, she is a kaafir woman and it is not permissible for him to be close to her or have intercourse with her. If she persists in this grave sin, the marriage contract with her will be rendered invalid. If she repents and prays, then praise be to Allah. (259)

250. Prohibition of Refusal by a Woman when her Husband Calls her to his Bed

Abu Hurairah (May Allah be pleased with him) said: The Messenger of Allah (peace and blessings be upon him) said, "If a man calls his wife to his bed and she refuses, and thus he spends the night angry with her, the angels continue cursing her till the morning." (Bukhari and Muslim)

Commentary: It is incumbent on every woman to respond to her husband's invitation to his bed for sexual intercourse. It would be a different matter if she has a lawful reason for it, such as observing an obligatory act of worship, like fasting during the month of Ramadan, illness, menses, etc... (260)

251. Ingratitude to Husband

Abu Sa'id al-Khudri (May Allah be pleased with him) reported: The Messenger of Allah (May Allah's peace and blessings be upon him) went out to the prayer grounds on Eid Al-Adha or 'Eid Al-Fitr and passed by the women. He said: "O womenfolk, give charity, for I have seen that you are from the majority of the inhabitants of Hellfire." They said: "Why is that, O Messenger of Allah?" He said: "You curse frequently and you are ungrateful to your husbands. I have not seen anyone deficient in intelligence and religion, yet a decisive and sensible man could be led and subdued by one of you." They said: "O Messenger of Allah, what is the deficiency in our religion and intelligence?" He said: "Isn't the testimony of two women equals to the testimony of one man?" They replied in the affirmative. He said: "That is the deficiency in her intelligence. Is it not true that a woman neither prays nor fasts during her menses?" They replied in the affirmative. He said: "That is the deficiency in her religion." (Bukhari and Muslim) (https://hadeethenc.com/en/browse/hadith/10011)

Ibn 'Abbas and 'Imran ibn al-Husayn (May Allah be pleased with both of them) reported that the Messenger of Allah (May Allah's peace and blessings be upon him) said: "I looked into Paradise and found that the majority of its people are the poor, and I looked into the Fire and found that the majority of its people are women." (Bukhari and Muslim) (https://hadeethenc.com/en/browse/hadith/3184)

252. Forcing Your Wife

Allah, the Exalted, says:

"O you who believe! You are forbidden to inherit women against their will, and you should not treat them with harshness, that you may take away part of the Mahr you have given them, unless they commit open illegal sexual intercourse. And live with them honorably. If you dislike them, it may be that you dislike a thing and Allah brings through it a great deal of good." (Qur'an, An-Nisa 4:19)

"As to those women on whose part you see ill-conduct, admonish them (first), (next) refuse to share their beds, (and last) beat them (lightly, if it is useful); but if they return to obedience, seek not against them means (of annoyance). Surely, Allah is Ever Most High, Most Great." (Qur'an, An-Nisa 4:34)

"And if a woman fears cruelty or desertion on her husband's part, there is no sin on them both if they make terms of peace between themselves; and making peace is better. And human inner-selves are swayed by greed. But if you do good and keep away from evil, verily, Allah is Ever Well-Acquainted with what you do." (Qur'an, An-Nisa 4:128)

Other Verse: Al-Baqarah 2:228.

The beating, forcing women, taking back the bridal gift are disapproved.

Aisha (May Allah be pleased with her) said: The Messenger of Allah (peace and blessings of Allah be upon him) never struck a servant or a woman." (Abu Dawud)

Abu Hurairah (May Allah be pleased with him) reported: The Messenger of Allah (peace and blessings be upon him) said, "The believers who show the most perfect Faith are those who have the best behaviour, and the best of you are those who are the best to their wives." (Tirmidhi)

Narrated Ja'far b Muhammad on the authority of his father: The Messenger of Allah (peace and blessings be upon him) said: "Fear Allah concerning women! Verily you have taken them on the security of Allah, and intercourse with them has been made lawful unto you by Words of Allah. You too have right over them, and that they should not allow anyone to sit on your bed whom you do not like. But if they do that, you can chastise them but not severely. Their rights upon you are that you should provide them with food and clothing in a fitting manner. I have left among you the Book of Allah, and if you hold fast to it, you would never go astray." (Muslim)

Aisha (May Allah be pleased with her) reported: "The Messenger of Allah (peace and blessings be upon him) never struck anything with his hand, neither a woman nor a servant, except when he was fighting in the Cause of Allah. He would never avenge himself concerning anything that was done to him except if the limits of Allah the Almighty were transgressed. Then (in that case) he would seek revenge for the sake of Allah the Almighty." (Muslim)

Narrated `Abdullah bin Zam`a: The Prophet (peace and blessings be upon him) said, "None of you should flog his wife as he flogs a slave and then have sexual intercourse with her in the last part of the day." (Bukhari)

253. Prohibition of Observing Silence from Dawn till Night

Qais bin Abu Hazim (May Allah be pleased with him) said: "Abu Bakr (May Allah be pleased with him) came upon a woman named Zainab from the Ahmas tribe and noticed that she was observing total silence. He said: "What has happened to her? Why does she not speak?" People informed him that she had sworn to remain silent. He then said to her: "You should speak, it is not permissible (to observe silence), for it is an act of the Days of Ignorance (Jahiliyyah)." (After hearing this) she started speaking." (Bukhari)

Commentary:
1. From the above narrations it becomes clear that one cannot be called an orphan when maturity is attained. The proof of maturity is night discharge and not any particular age. The age of maturity may differ in different countries according to the climate and individual body development. So, night discharge has been fixed as the condition and criterion or sign of maturity. Night discharge means ejaculation of semen during sleep.
2. During the pre-Islamic period, keeping quiet was also considered as a sort of worship or devotion to God. Islam does not allow such ascetic ceremonies and extravagance. So, such actions are forbidden. Further it has been stressed that instead of keeping quiet one should engage in good actions, such as enjoining good, forbidding evil, entertaining a guest, remembering Allah and glorifying Him. However, it is better to keep quiet rather than telling lies, indulging in indecent talk or backbiting. (261)

254. Disclosing Bedroom Secrets

Abu Sa'id Al-Khudri reported: Allah's Messenger (peace and blessings be upon him) said: "Verily, the most evil of people in front of Allah on the Day of Resurrection is a man who is intimate with his wife and then spreads her secrets." (Muslim)

It was reported from Asma bint Yazid that she was with the Prophet (peace and blessings of Allah be upon him) and men and women were sitting with him, and the Prophet (peace and blessings of Allah be upon him) said, "Would any man say what he did with his wife? Would any woman tell others what she did with her husband?" The people kept quiet and did not answer. I (Asma) said: "Yes, by Allah, O Messenger of Allah, they (women) do that, and they (men) do that." He said, "Do not do that. It is like a male Devil meeting a female Devil in the road and having intercourse with her whilst the people are watching." (Abu Dawud)

Sexual relations are among the important matters of life which Islam came to explain and to prescribe proper conduct and rulings which elevate it from the level of mere bestial pleasure and physical desire. Islam connects it to a righteous intention, supplications (Adhkar) and proper conduct which lift it up to the level of worship for which the Muslim will be rewarded. When engaging in intimate relations, have the sincere intention of doing this thing only for the sake of Allah. (262)

It was reported from Abu Dharr that the Messenger of Allah (peace and blessings of Allah be upon him) said: "In the sexual intercourse of any one of you there is reward (meaning, when he has intercourse with his wife)." They said, "O Messenger of Allah, when any one of us fulfils his desire, will he have a reward for that?" He (peace and blessings of Allah be upon him) said: "Do you not see that if he were to do it in a haram manner, he would be punished for that? So, if he does it in a halal manner, he will be rewarded. (Muslim)

255. Prohibition of Observing an Optional Saum (Fast) by a Woman Without the Permission of her Husband

Abu Hurairah (May Allah be pleased with him) said: The Messenger of Allah (peace and blessings be upon him) said, "It is not lawful for a woman to observe an optional Saum (fast) without the permission of her husband when he is at home. Nor should she allow anyone to enter his house without his permission." (Bukhari and Muslim)

Commentary: Fasting here signifies voluntary fasting. (263)

256. Prohibition of Describing the Charms of a Woman to a Man Without Valid Reason

Ibn Masud (May Allah be pleased with him) said: The Messenger of Allah (peace and blessings be upon him) said, "No woman should touch another woman's body and then describe the details of her figure to her husband in such a manner as if he was looking at her." (Bukhari)

Commentary: "Mubashirah" means "meeting of two bodies" and here it signifies that one should not see another person's body. Here, it is used in its literal as well as metaphorical sense. What it really means is that neither a woman should see the body of any other woman nor should she touch her own body with the body of some other woman, for if she does so, she will come to know the physical qualities of the other woman which she may disclose to her husband. Such disclosures may induce her husband to mischief and eventually ruin her own life. One is allowed, however, to disclose a woman's charms to a man who intends to marry her. (264)

257. Stoning of a Married Adulterer

'Abdullah b. 'Abbas reported that 'Umar b. Khattab sat on the pulpit of Allah's Messenger (peace and blessings be upon him) and said: "Verily, Allah sent Muhammad (peace and blessings be upon him) with Truth and He sent down the Book upon him, and the Verse of stoning was included in what was sent down to him. We recited it, retained it in our memory and understood it. Allah's Messenger (peace and blessings be upon him) awarded the punishment of stoning to death (to the married adulterer and adulteress) and, after him, we also awarded the punishment of stoning, I am afraid that with the lapse of time, the people (may forget it) and may say: 'We do not find the punishment of stoning in the Book of Allah, and thus go astray by abandoning this duty prescribed by Allah. Stoning is a duty laid down in Allah's Book for married men and women who commit adultery when proof is established, or there is a pregnancy, or a confession." (Muslim)

Narrated Abu Hurairah: "A man from Bani Aslam came to Allah's Apostle while he was in the Mosque and called (the Prophet) saying, "O Allah's Apostle! I have committed illegal sexual intercourse." On that the Prophet turned his face from him to the other side, whereupon the man moved to the side towards which the Prophet had turned his face, and said, "O Allah's Apostle! I have committed illegal sexual intercourse." The Prophet turned his face (from him) to the other side whereupon the man moved to the side towards which the Prophet had turned his face, and repeated his statement. The Prophet turned his face (from him) to the other side again. The man moved again (and repeated his statement) for the fourth time. So, when the man had given witness four times against himself, the Prophet called him and said, "Are you insane?" He replied, "No." The Prophet then said (to his companions), "Go and stone him to death." The man was a married one. Jabir bin 'Abdullah Al-Ansari said: 'I was one of those who stoned him. We stoned him at the Musalla (Eid praying place) in Madinah. When the stones hit him with their sharp edges, he fled, but we caught him at Al-Harra and stoned him till he died.'" (Bukhari)

258. Divorce is Mischief

Allah, the Exalted, says:

"They followed what the Shayateen (Devils) gave out (falsely of the magic) in the lifetime of Sulaiman (Solomon). Sulaiman did not disbelieve, but the Shayateen (Devils) disbelieved, teaching men magic and such things that came down at Babylon to the two angels, Harut and Marut, but neither of these two (angels) taught anyone (such things) till they had said, "We are only for trial, so disbelieve not (by learning this magic from us)." And from these (angels) people learn that by which they cause separation between man and his wife, but they could not thus harm anyone except by Allah's Leave. And they learn that which harms them and profits them not. And indeed, they knew that the buyers of it (magic) would have no share in the Hereafter. And how bad indeed was that for which they sold their own selves, if they but knew." (Qur'an, Al-Baqarah 2:102)

Jabir (May Allah be pleased with him) reported that the Messenger of Allah (May Allah's peace and blessings be upon him) said: "Satan places his throne upon water; he then sends his troops; the nearer to him in rank are those who are most skillful in creating mischief. One of them comes and says: 'I did such-and-such', to which Satan replies: 'You did nothing.' Then one among them comes and says: 'I did not leave so-and-so until I separated him from his wife.' Satan brings him near him and says: 'You did well.'" Al-A'mash said: "I think he said: 'He then embraces him.'" (Muslim) (https://hadeethenc.com/en/browse/hadith/10569)

Narrated Abdullah bin Umar (May Allah be pleased with him): The Messenger of Allah (peace and blessings be upon him) said: "The most hated of permissible things to Allah is divorce." (Ibn Majah)

"Divorce is a mischief. However, it is a measure that cannot be avoided for the welfare of the community, because it is the only remedy for another harm which may be more dangerous. The prohibition of divorce, whatever harm it may imply, is like the prohibition of surgery, because the surgeon is compelled to amputate some of the limbs of the patient's body. However, there is no danger whatsoever, in legislating for divorce (in accordance with the practice established by Islam) since it is not divorce that spoils married life and dissolves its sacred tie, but the misunderstanding that arises between the married couple and hinders the strengthening of this (union by marriage) and demolished it. Divorce alone puts an end to the hatred that may occur between the husband and his wife before it is aggravated and becomes an intolerable mischief to society." (Hasan Ibrahim Hasan, Islam, Religious, Political, Social and Economic Study, p.274) (Muslim)

Ibn 'Abbas (May Allah be pleased with him) reported: A man came to the Prophet (May Allah's peace and blessings be upon him) and said: "My wife does not object if anyone touches her." He said: "Divorce her." The man said: "I am afraid that I will miss her." The Prophet (May Allah's peace and blessings be upon him) said: "Then enjoy her." (An-Nasa'i and Abu Dawud) (https://hadeethenc.com/en/browse/hadith/58158)

Abu Darda (May Allah be pleased with him) reported: The Messenger of Allah (peace and blessings be upon him) said: "Shall I not tell you of what is better in degree than extra fasting, prayer and charity?" They said, "Of course!" The Prophet (peace and blessings be upon him) said: "Reconciliation between people. Verily, corrupted relations between people is the razor." (Tirmidhi)

259. Giving an Option to Divorce to Wife

Allah, the Exalted, says:

"But if you seek Allah and His Messenger and the Abode of the Hereafter, then surely Allah has prepared a great reward for those of you who do good." (Qur'an, Al-Ahzab 33:29)

Aisha (May Allah be pleased with her) reported: "When the Messenger of Allah (May peace and blessings be upon him) was commanded to give option to his wives, he started it from me saying: 'I am going to mention to you a matter which you should not (decide) in haste until you have consulted your parents.' She said that he already knew that my parents would never allow me to seek separation from him. She said: 'Then he said: 'Allah, the Exalted and Glorious, said: 'Prophet, say to thy wives: If you desire this world's life and its adornment, then come, I will give you a provision and allow you to depart a goodly departing; and if you desire Allah and His Messenger and the abode of the Hereafter, then Allah has prepared for the doers of good among you a great reward.' She is reported to have said: 'About what should I consult my parents, for I desire Allah and His Messenger and the abode of the Hereafter?' She (Aisha) said: 'Then all the wives of Allah's Messenger (May peace and blessings be upon him) did as I had done.'" (Muslim)

Narrated Aisha (May Allah be pleased with her): "Allah's Apostle gave us the option (to remain with him or to be divorced) and we selected Allah and His Apostle. So, giving us that option was not regarded as divorce." (Bukhari)

260. Divorce Not Following Allah's Law

Allah, the Exalted, says:

"O Prophet! `Instruct the believers: `When you intend to divorce women, then divorce them with concern for their waiting period, and count it accurately. And fear Allah, your Lord. Do not force them out of their homes, nor should they leave—unless they commit a blatant misconduct. These are the limits set by Allah. And whoever transgresses Allah's limits has truly wronged his own soul. You never know, perhaps Allah will bring about a change `of heart` later." (Qur'an, At-Talaq 65:1)

"Then when they have almost reached the end of their waiting period, either retain them honorably or separate from them honourably. And call two of your reliable men to witness either way—and let the witnesses bear true testimony for the sake of Allah. This is enjoined on whoever has faith in Allah and the Last Day. And whoever is mindful of Allah, He will make a way out for them, and provide for them from sources they could never imagine. And whoever puts their trust in Allah, then He Alone is sufficient for them. Certainly, Allah achieves His Will. Allah has already set a destiny for everything." (Qur'an, At-Talaq 65:2)

"Let them live where you live during their waiting period, according to your means. And do not harass them to make their stay unbearable. If they are pregnant, then maintain them until they deliver. And if they nurse your child, compensate them, and consult together courteously. But if you fail to reach an agreement, then another woman will nurse the child for the father." (Qur'an, At-Talaq 65:6)

Other Verse: Al-Baqarah 2:228.

Divorce Steps:

1. Evaluation and Reconciliation

Allah, the Exalted, says:

"And if a woman fears cruelty or desertion on her husband's part, there is no sin on them both if they make terms of peace between themselves; and making peace is better. And human inner-selves are swayed by greed. But if you do good and keep away from evil, verily, Allah is Ever Well-Acquainted with what you do." (Qur'an, An-Nisa 4:128)

2. Arbitration

Allah, the Exalted, says:

"If you fear a breach between them twain (the man and his wife), appoint (two) arbitrators, one from his family and the other from her's; if they both wish for peace, Allah will cause their reconciliation. Indeed, Allah is Ever All-Knower, Well-Acquainted with all things." (Qur'an, An-Nisa 4:35)

3. Filing the Divorce

4. Waiting Period (Iddah)

Iddah or Iddat (*period of waiting*) is the period a woman must observe after a divorce or after the death of her husband, during which she should not marry another man.

The waiting period is intended to give the couple an opportunity for reconciliation, and also a means to ensure that the wife is not pregnant. The wife retains all her rights during the waiting period.

The divorce becomes final when the waiting period expires. She is not permissible for him except with a new marriage contract.

For a menstruating woman, the Iddah is three menstrual periods.

Allah, the Exalted, says:

"And divorced women shall wait (as regards their marriage) for three menstrual periods…" (Qur'an, Al-Baqarah 2:228)

For non-menstruating women (post-menopause women and pre-menarche girls), the Iddah is three months.

Allah, the Exalted, says:

"And those of your women as have passed the age of monthly courses, for them the 'Iddah (prescribed period), if you have doubts (about their periods), is three months, and for those who have no courses [i.e. they are still immature] their 'Iddah (prescribed period) is three months likewise, except in case of death]…" (Qur'an, At-Talaq 65:4)

For pregnant (divorced or widowed) woman, the Iddah is until the birth.

Allah, the Exalted, says:

"…And for those who are pregnant (whether they are divorced or their husbands are dead), their 'Iddah (prescribed period) is until they deliver (their burdens), and whosoever fears Allah and keeps his duty to Him, He will make his matter easy for him." (Qur'an, At-Talaq 65:4)

For non-pregnant widowed woman, the Iddah is four lunar months and ten days.

Allah, the Exalted, says:

"And those of you who die and leave wives behind them, they (the wives) shall wait (as regards their marriage) for four months and ten days, then when they have fulfilled their term, there is no sin on you if they (the wives) dispose of themselves in a just and honorable manner (i.e. they can marry). And Allah is Well-Acquainted with what you do." (Qur'an, Al-Baqarah 2:234)

If a man takes an oath not to have sexual intercourse with his wife, which would lead to automatic divorce, is allowed a four-month period to break his oath.

Allah, the Exalted, says:

"Those who take an oath not to have sexual relation with their wives must wait four months, then if they return (change their idea in this period), verily, Allah is Oft-Forgiving, Most Merciful." (Qur'an, Al-Baqarah 2:226)

Atonement is essential for one who made his wife unlawful for himself without the intention to divorce.

5. Witnesses to Divorce

Allah, the Exalted, says:

"Then when they are about to attain their term appointed, either take them back in a good manner or part with them in a good manner. And take as witness two just persons from among you (Muslims)." (Qur'an, At-Talaq 65:2)

Narrated Mutarrif ibn Abdullah: "Imran ibn Husayn was asked about a person who divorces his wife, and then has intercourse with her, but he does not call any witness to her divorce nor to her restoration. He said: 'You divorced against the Sunnah and took her back against the Sunnah. Call someone to bear witness to her divorce, and to her return in marriage, and do not repeat it." (Abu Dawud)

6. Divorce Finalized

Allah, the Exalted, says:

"And when you have divorced women and they have fulfilled the term of their prescribed period, either take them back on reasonable basis or set them free on reasonable basis. But do not take them back to hurt them, and whoever does that, then he has wronged himself. And treat not the Verses (Laws) of Allah as a jest, but remember Allah's Favors on you (i.e. Islam), and that which He has sent down to you of the Book (i.e. the Qur'an) and Al-Hikmah (the Prophet's Sunnah - legal ways - Islamic jurisprudence, etc.) whereby He instructs you. And fear Allah, and know that Allah is All-Aware of everything." (Qur'an, Al-Baqarah 2:231)

The irrevocably divorced woman is not entitled to maintenance or accommodation, unless she is pregnant.

Narrated ash-Sha'bi: "I entered upon Fatimah bint Qays and asked her about the ruling of the Messenger of Allah (peace and blessings of Allah be upon him) concerning her. She said: 'My husband divorced me irrevocably, and I referred my dispute with him about maintenance and accommodation to the Messenger of Allah (peace and blessings of Allah be upon him). He did not grant me any accommodation or maintenance, and he told me to observe my 'iddah in the house of Ibn Umm Maktoom." (Muslim)

7. Child Custody

The husband must spend on his children, which includes accommodation, food, drink, clothing, school costs, medical care and all that they need. That should be worked out on a reasonable basis, paying attention to the husband's financial situation.

The wife does not have to pay anything towards the maintenance of the husband or children, even if the husband does not have a job. (265)

The Main Legal Categories are Talaq (repudiation), *khul'* (mutual divorce), judicial divorce and oaths. (266)

Talaq is considered in Islam to be a reprehensible means of divorce. The pronouncement of Talaq as forbidden or reprehensible unless it was motivated by a compelling cause such as impossibility of cohabitation due to irreconcilable conflict.

The initial declaration of Talaq is a revocable repudiation and sexual abstinence during the waiting period.

The Qur'an limited the number of repudiations (Talaq) to three, after which the man cannot take his wife back unless she first marries another man.

Allah, the Exalted, says:

"And if he has divorced her (the third time), then she is not lawful unto him thereafter until she has married another husband. Then, if the other husband divorces her, it is no sin on both of them that they reunite, provided they feel that they can keep the limits ordained by Allah. These are the limits of Allah, which He makes plain for the people who have knowledge." (Qur'an, Al-Baqarah 2:230)

Nafi' (May Allah have mercy on him) said: "When Ibn 'Umar was asked about person who had given three divorces, he said, "Would that you gave one or two divorces, for the Prophet (peace and blessings be upon him) ordered me to do so. If you give three divorces then she cannot be lawful for you until she has married another husband (and is divorced by him)." (Bukhari)

261. Condemnation of Divorce Without Compelling Reason

Narrated Thawban (May Allah have mercy on him): The Prophet (peace and blessings be upon him) said: "Any woman who asks her husband for a divorce without a compelling reason, the fragrance of Paradise will be forbidden to her." (Abu Dawud)

262. Divorce Before Consumption of the Marriage

Allah, the Exalted, says:

"O you who believe! When you marry believing women, and then divorce them before you have sexual intercourse with them, no 'Iddah [divorce prescribed period, see (V.65:4)] have you to count in respect of them. So, give them a present, and set them free i.e. divorce, in a handsome manner." (Qur'an, Al-Ahzab 33:49)

"There is no sin on you, if you divorce women while yet you have not touched (had sexual relation with) them, nor appointed unto them their Mahr (bridal money given by the husband to his wife at the time of marriage). But bestow on them (a suitable gift), the rich according to his means, and the poor according to his means, a gift of reasonable amount is a duty on the doers of good." (Qur'an, Al-Baqarah 2:236)

"And if you divorce them before you have touched (had a sexual relation with) them, and you have appointed unto them the Mahr (bridal money given by the husbands to his wife at the time of marriage), then pay half of that (Mahr), unless they (the women) agree to forego it, or he (the husband), in whose hands is the marriage tie, agrees to forego and give her full appointed Mahr. And to forego and give (her the full Mahr) is nearer to At-Taqwa (piety, righteousness, etc.). And do not forget liberality between yourselves. Truly, Allah is All-Seer of what you do." (Qur'an, Al-Baqarah 2:237)

263. Annulment of Marriage by Husband's Vow to Refrain from Intercourse (Ila)

Allah, the Exalted, says:

"Those who take an oath not to have sexual relation with their wives must wait for four months, then if they return (change their idea in this period), verily, Allah is Oft-Forgiving, Most Merciful. And if they decide upon divorce, then Allah is All-Hearer, All-Knower." (Qur'an, Al-Baqarah 2:226-227)

"Those among you who make their wives unlawful (Az-Zihar) to them by saying to them "You are like my mother's back." They cannot be their mothers. None can be their mothers except those who gave them birth. And verily, they utter an ill word and a lie. And verily, Allah is Oft-Pardoning, Oft-Forgiving." *(Qur'an, Al-Mujadilah 58:2)*

264. Atonement is Essential for the One who Made his Wife Unlawful for Himself Without the Intention to Divorce

Allah, the Exalted, says:

"And those who make unlawful to them (their wives) (by Az-Zihar) and wish to free themselves from what they uttered, (the penalty) in that case (is) the freeing of a slave before they touch each other. That is an admonition to you (so that you may not return to such an ill thing). And Allah is All-Aware of what you do." *(Qur'an, Al-Mujadilah 58:3)*

"And he who finds not (the money for freeing a slave) must fast two successive months before they both touch each other. And for him who is unable to do so, he should feed sixty of Miskin (poor). That is in order that you may have perfect faith in Allah and His Messenger. These are the limits set by Allah. And for disbelievers, there is a painful torment." *(Qur'an, Al-Mujadilah 58:4)*

Ibn Abbas (May Allah be pleased with him) reported: "When a man declares his wife unlawful for himself that is an oath which must be atoned, and he said: 'There is in the Messenger of Allah (May peace and blessings be upon him) a noble pattern for you.'" (Muslim)

Narrated Ibn 'Umar (May Allah be pleased with him) used to say concerning Ila: "If the period of Ila expires, then the husband has either to retain his wife in a handsome manner or to divorce her as Allah has ordered." (Bukhari)

Ibn 'Umar (May Allah be pleased with him) said: "When the period of four months has passed, the husband should be put in prison so that he divorces his wife, but the divorce does not occur unless the husband himself declares it." (Bukhari) (https://hadeethenc.com/en/browse/hadith/58151)

Ila is forbidden in Islam because it is a vow not to do something that is obligatory. It is in effect a vow not to have intercourse with one's wife, either never again or for a period that exceeds four months; or else it means vowing that if one's wife does not do a certain obligatory action, or does a certain haram action, he will not have intercourse with her. The fuqaha' also said that the one who does not have intercourse with his wife for more than four months without swearing an oath, in order to harm her and without having a valid excuse, also comes under the category of Ila. (267)

265. Ruling on Divorce at a Moment of Anger

Allah, the Exalted, says:

"Indeed, Allah has heard the statement of her (Khaulah bint Tha'labah) that disputes with you (O Muhammad SAW) concerning her husband (Aus bin AsSamit), and complains to Allah. And Allah hears the argument between you both. Verily, Allah is All-Hearer, All-Seer." (Qur'an, Al-Mujadilah 58:1)

Narrated Aisha (May Allah be pleased with her): The Prophet (peace and blessings be upon him) said:

"There is no divorce or emancipation in case of constraint or duress (ghalaq)." (Abu Dawud)

Anger may be of three types:

1 – When a person is angry and is no longer aware of what he is doing. This is likened to the insane, so divorce does not take place according to all scholars.

2 – Where a person is very angry but is still aware of what is going on, but his anger is so intense that it makes him say the words of divorce. In this case too, divorce does not take place according to the correct scholarly opinion.

3 – The ordinary type of anger which is not very intense. In this case, divorce takes place, according to all the scholars. (From Fataawa al-Talaaq, p.19-21, compiled by Dr. 'Abd-Allaah al-Tayyaar and Muhammad al-Moosa)

Ibn al-Qayyim wrote an essay on that entitled Ighaathat al-Lahfaan fi Hukm Talaq al-Ghadbaan, in which he said: "Anger is of three types…" (Mataalib Ooli al-Nuha, 5/323; see also, Zad Al-Ma'ad, 5/215) (268)

266. Divorce by One Strong Pronouncement of Divorce

Narrated Yahya related to me from Malik from Nafi that Abdullah ibn Umar said that statements like "I cut myself off from you" or "You are abandoned", were considered as three pronouncements of divorce. Malik said that any strong statements such as these or others were considered as three pronouncements of divorce for a woman whose marriage had been consummated. In the case of a woman whose marriage had not been consummated, the man was asked to make an oath on his Deen, as to whether he had intended one or three pronouncements of divorce. If he had intended one pronouncement, he was asked to make an oath by Allah to confirm it, and he became a suitor among other suitors, because a woman whose marriage had been consummated, required three pronouncements of divorce to make her inaccessible for the husband, whilst only one pronouncement was needed to make a woman whose marriage had not been consummated inaccessible. Malik added, "That is the best of what I have heard about the matter." (Malik Muwatta)

267. Pronouncements of Three Divorces

Allah, the Exalted, says:

"The divorce is twice, after that, either you retain her on reasonable terms or release her with kindness…" (Qur'an, Al-Baqarah 2:229)

"And if he has divorced her (the third time), then she is not lawful unto him thereafter until she has married another husband. Then, if the other husband divorces her, it is no sin on both of them that they reunite, provided they feel that they can keep the limits ordained by Allah. These are the limits of Allah, which He makes plain for the people who have knowledge." (Qur'an, Al-Baqarah 2:230)

"Divorce is of three kinds: the *Ahsan* or most laudable, the *Hasan* or laudable, and the *Bid'ah* or irregular.

Talaq Ahsan or the most laudable divorce is where the husband repudiates his wife by making one pronouncement within the term of Tahr (purity when the woman is not passing through the period of menses) during which he has not had sexual intercourse with her, and she is left to observe her 'Iddah.

Talaq Hasan or laudable divorce is where a husband repudiates an enjoyed wife by three sentences of divorce, in three Tuhrs.

Talaq Bid'ah or irregular divorce is where a husband repudiates his wife by three divorces at once.

According to the majority of the jurists, it is against the spirit of the Shariah, and, therefore, the man who follows this course in divorce is an offender in the eye of Islamic Law." (Muslim)

Giving Talaq (divorce) three times at once is Bid'ah, and goes against the Ayah:

"… When you divorce women, divorce them at their 'iddah (prescribed periods)…" (At-Talaq 65:1)

If a Muslim wants to divorce his wife, he should divorce her according to the Sunnah, which is to give one Talaq at a time when his wife is taahir (not menstruating) and he has not yet had intercourse with her following her period, or when it is clear that she is pregnant. According to the Shaafi'i madhhab and the majority of other madhhabs, giving three Talaqs at once counts as three separate Talaqs and is irrevocable, and the couple cannot remarry until the woman has been married to and divorced from another man. Other scholars say that three Talaqs given at once count as only one Talaq. And Allah knows best. (269)

Ibn 'Abbas (May Allah be pleased with him) reported that the (pronouncement) of three divorces during the lifetime of Allah's Messenger (peace be upon him) and that of Abu Bakr and two years of the caliphate of Umar (Allah be pleased with him) was treated as one. But Umar b. Khattab (Allah be pleased with him) said: "Verily the people have begun to hasten in the matter in which they are required to observe respite. So, if we had imposed this upon them, and he imposed it upon them." (Muslim)

Abu Sahba' said to Ibn 'Abbas (May Allah be pleased with them): "Do you know that three (divorces) were treated as one during the lifetime of Allah's Apostle (peace and blessing be upon him), and that of Abu Bakr, and during three (years) of the caliphate of Umar (Allah be pleased with them)?" Ibn Abbas (Allah be pleased with him) said: "Yes." (Muslim)

The fuqaha differed concerning the threefold divorce (Talaq). The correct view is that it counts as one divorce, whether it is uttered in a single phrase, such as saying "You are thrice divorced" or in repeated words such as saying, "You are divorced, you are divorced, you are divorced." This is the view favored by Sheikh al-Islam Ibn Taymiyah (May Allah have mercy on him) and was the view regarded as most correct by Sheikh al-Sa'di (May Allah have mercy on him) and Sheikh Ibn 'Uthaymeen (May Allah have mercy on him). (270)

Abdullah (b.'Umar) reported that he divorced a wife of his with the pronouncement of one divorce during the period of menstruation. Allah's Messenger (peace and blessings be upon him) commanded him to take her back and keep her until she was purified, and then she entered the period of menses in his house for the second time. And he should wait until she was purified of her menses. And then if he would decide to divorce her, he should do so when she was purified before having a sexual intercourse with her; for that was the 'Iddah which Allah had commanded for the divorce of women. Ibn Rumh in his narration made this addition: "When 'Abdullah was asked about it, he said to one of them: If you have divorced your wife with one pronouncement or two (then you can take her back), for Allah's Messenger (peace and blessings be upon him) commanded me to do it; but if you have divorced her with three pronouncements, then she is forbidden for you until she married another husband, and you disobeyed Allah in regard to the divorce of your wife what He had commanded you. (Muslim said: 'The word "one divorce" used by Laith is good') (Muslim)

268. Divorce Women at their Iddah (Prescribed Periods)

Allah, the Exalted, says:

"O Prophet (SAW)! When you divorce women, divorce them at their 'Iddah (prescribed periods), and count (accurately) their 'Iddah (periods). And fear Allah, your Lord (O Muslims), and turn them not out of their (husband's) homes, nor shall they (themselves) leave, except in case they are guilty of some open illegal sexual intercourse. And those are the set limits of Allah. And whosoever transgresses the set limits of Allah, then indeed he has wronged himself. You (the one who divorces his wife) know not, it may be that Allah will afterward bring some new thing to pass (i.e. to return her back to you if that was the first or second divorce)." (Qur'an, At-Talaq 65:1)

"Then when they are about to fulfil their term appointed, either take them back in a good manner or part with them in a good manner. And take for witness two just persons from among you (Muslims). And establish the witness for Allah. That will be an admonition given to him who believes in Allah and the Last Day. And whosoever fears Allah and keeps his duty to Him, He will make a way for him to get out (from every difficulty)." (Qur'an, At-Talaq 65:2)

"And those of your women as have passed the age of monthly courses, for them the 'Iddah (prescribed period), if you have doubts (about their periods), is three months, and for those who have no courses [(i.e. they are still immature) their 'Iddah (prescribed period) is three months likewise, except in case of death]. And for those who are pregnant (whether they are divorced or their husbands are dead), their 'Iddah (prescribed period) is until they deliver (their burdens), and whosoever fears Allah and keeps his duty to Him, He will make his matter easy for him." (Qur'an, At-Talaq 65:4)

Other Verses: *At-Talaq 65:5-6, 65:8-10.*

Narrated Abdullah ibn Abbas: "Abdu Yazid, the father of Rukanah and his brothers, divorced Umm Rukanah and married a woman of the tribe of Muzaynah. She went to the Prophet (peace and blessings be upon him) and said: 'He is of no use to me except that he is as useful to me as a hair; and she took a hair from her head. So, separate me from him.' The Prophet (peace and blessings be upon him) became furious. He called on Rukanah and his brothers. He then said to those who were sitting beside him: 'Do you see so-and-so who resembles Abdu Yazid in respect of so-and-so; and so-and-so who resembles him in respect of so-and-so?' They replied: 'Yes.' The Prophet (peace and blessings be upon him) said to Abdu Yazid: 'Divorce her.' Then he did so. He said: 'Take your wife, the mother of Rukanah and his brothers, back in marriage.' He said: 'I have divorced her by three pronouncements, Apostle of Allah.' He said: 'I know: take her back.' He then recited the Verse: *"O Prophet, when you divorce women, divorce them at their appointed periods." (At-Talaq 65:1)*

Abu Dawud said: The tradition narrated by Nafi' b. 'Ujair and 'Abd Allah b. Yazid b. Rukanah from his father on the authority of his grandfather reads: Rukanah divorced his wife absolutely (i.e. irrevocable divorce). The Prophet (peace be upon him) restored her to him. This version is sounder (than other versions), for they (i.e. these narrators) are the children of his man, and the members of the family are more aware of his case. Rukanah divorced his wife absolutely (i.e. three divorces in one pronouncement) and the Prophet (peace be upon him) made it a single divorce. (Abu Dawud) (https://sunnah.com/abudawud:2196)

269. Prohibition of Divorcing Woman During Menstruation

Allah, the Exalted, says:

"O Prophet (SAW)! When you divorce women, divorce them at their 'Iddah (prescribed periods), and count (accurately) their 'Iddah (periods). And fear Allah your Lord (O Muslims), and turn them not out of their (husband's) homes, nor shall they (themselves) leave, except in case they are guilty of some open illegal sexual intercourse. And those are the set limits of Allah. And whosoever transgresses the set limits of Allah, then indeed he has wronged himself. You (the one who divorces his wife) know not, it may be that Allah will afterward bring some new thing to pass (i.e. to return her back to you if that was the first or second divorce)." (Qur'an, At-Talaq 65:1)

Narrated 'Abdullah bin 'Umar that he had divorced his wife while she was menstruating during the lifetime of Allah's Messenger (peace and blessings be upon him). 'Umar bin Al-Khattab asked Allah's Messenger (peace and blessings be upon him) about that. Allah's Messenger (peace and blessings be upon him) said, "Order him (your son) to take her back and keep her till she is clean and then to wait till she gets her next period and becomes clean again, whereupon, if he wishes to keep her, he can do so, and if he wishes to divorce her, he can divorce her before having sexual intercourse with her; and that is the prescribed period which Allah has fixed for the women meant to be divorced." (Bukhari and Muslim)

270. Concealing What is in the Wombs

Allah, the Exalted, says:

"Divorced women remain in waiting for three periods, and it is not lawful for them to conceal what Allah has created in their wombs if they believe in Allah and the Last Day. And their husbands have more right to take them back in this (period) if they want reconciliation. And due to the wives is similar to what is expected of them, according to what is reasonable. But the men have a degree over them (in responsibility and authority). And Allah is Exalted in Might and Wise." (Qur'an, Al-Baqarah 2:228)

271. Taking Back Mahr

Allah, the Exalted, says:

"And it is not lawful for you (men) to take back (from your wives) any of your Mahr (bridal money given by the husband to his wife at the time of marriage) which you have given them, except when both parties fear that they would be unable to keep the limits ordained by Allah (e.g. to deal with each other on a fair basis). Then if you fear that they would not be able to keep the limits ordained by Allah, then there is no sin on either of them if she gives back (the Mahr or a part of it) for her Al-Khul' (divorce). These are the limits ordained by Allah, so do not transgress them. And whoever transgresses the limits ordained by Allah, then such are the Zalimun (wrong-doers, etc.)." (Qur'an, Al-Baqarah 2:229)

"…and you should not treat them with harshness, that you may take away part of the Mahr you have given them, unless they commit open illegal sexual intercourse…" (Qur'an, An-Nisa 4:19)

"But if you intend to replace a wife by another and you have given one of them a Cantar (of gold i.e. a great amount) as Mahr, take not the least bit of it back; would you take it wrongfully without a right and (with) a manifest sin?" (Qur'an, An-Nisa 4:20)

Other Verses: *An-Nisa 4:4 and 4:21.*

272. Khula' Divorce Initiated by the Wife

Allah, the Exalted, says:

"And it is not lawful for you (men) to take back (from your wives) any of your Mahr (bridal money given by the husband to his wife at the time of marriage) which you have given them, except when both parties fear that they would be unable to keep the limits ordained by Allah (e.g. to deal with each other on a fair basis). Then if you fear that they would not be able to keep the limits ordained by Allah, then there is no sin on either of them if she gives back (the Mahr or a part of it) for her Al-Khul' (divorce). These are the limits ordained by Allah, so do not transgress them. And whoever transgresses the limits ordained by Allah, then such are the Zalimun (wrongdoers, etc.)." (Qur'an, Al-Baqarah 2:229)

Khula' (Arabic: خلع) is the right of a woman to divorce from her husband by returning the Mahr.

Narrated Ibn Abbas: "The wife of Thabit bin Qais came to the Prophet (peace and blessings be upon him) and said, "O Allah's Messenger (peace and blessings be upon him)! I do not blame Thabit for defects in his character or his religion, but I, being a Muslim, dislike to behave in un-Islamic manner (if I remain with him)." On that Allah's Messenger (peace and blessings be upon him) said (to her), "Will you give back the garden which your husband has given you (as Mahr)?" She said, "Yes." Then the Prophet (peace and blessings be upon him) said to Thabit, "O Thabit! Accept your garden, and divorce her once." (Bukhari)

Narrated Abdullah ibn Amr ibn al-'As: The Prophet (peace and blessings be upon him) said: "There is no divorce except in what you possess; there is no possession, there is no sale transaction till you possess." (Abu Dawud)

273. Marriage Dissolution Not following the Law of Li'an in Husband's Accusation Against his Spouse or Denying Paternity

Allah, the Exalted, says:

"And those who accuse chaste women, and produce not four witnesses, flog them with eighty stripes, and reject their testimony forever, they indeed are the Fasiqun (liars, rebellious, disobedient to Allah)." (Qur'an, An-Nur 24:4)

"And for those who accuse their wives (of adultery), but have no witnesses except themselves, let the testimony of one of them be four testimonies (i.e. testifies four times) by Allah that he is one of those who speak the truth." (Qur'an, An-Nur 24:6)

"But it shall avert the punishment (of stoning to death) from her, if she bears witness four times by Allah, that he (her husband) is telling a lie." (Qur'an, An-Nur 24:8)

Other Verse: *An-Nur 24:9.*

The husband who accuses his wife of adultery or denies paternity of a child conceived by her and doesn't produce four witnesses, should be flogged with eighty stripes, and his testimony should be rejected forever, he is indeed the Fasiqun (liars, rebellious, disobedient to Allah). Then, the **Law of Li'an** should be applied.

The husband will be asked to testify four times with the wordings given in the Qur'an to the effect that he is honest, and the fifth time will say that if he was lying, then Allah's Curse be on him. If the husband hesitates from saying these words, then he should be arrested, and asked either to swear by saying these words five times or accept himself to be a liar. Until he accedes to one of the two alternatives, he should not be released. If he accepts himself to be a liar, then he should be awarded the punishment of false allegation of adultery, but in case he swears by repeating the required words five times, then the wife be asked to swear five times by uttering the words given in the Qur'an for this purpose. If she refuses to swear, then she should be put under arrest until such time that either she swears five times or accepts her guilt of adultery. The punishment for Zina should be carried out on her, and nothing can prevent the punishment except if she also swears the oath of condemnation (Li'an) and swears by Allah four times that he is one of those who lied, i.e. in what he is accusing her of; And the fifth; should be that the Wrath of Allah be upon her if he speaks the truth. This way they both have escaped the punishment in this world, but in the Hereafter, the one who has lied will suffer the punishment, as Allah knows best who is the liar. After the process of Li'an this couple will be forbidden to each other for ever. The husband should free the woman by divorcing her. If the husband does not divorce her, then the judge or the ruler can have them separated by His Decree, which will have the same force as divorce.

Allah, the Exalted, says:

"But it shall avert the punishment (of stoning to death) from her, if she bears witness four times by Allah, that he (her husband) is telling a lie. And the fifth (testimony) should be that the Wrath of Allah be upon her if he (her husband) speaks the truth." (Qur'an, An-Nur 24:8-9)

The Wrath of Allah is mentioned specially in the case of the woman, because usually a man would not go to the extent of exposing his wife and accusing her of Zina unless he is telling the truth and has good reason to do this, and she knows that what he is accusing her of is true. So, in her case the fifth testimony calls for the Wrath of Allah to be upon her, for the one upon whom is the Wrath of Allah, is the one who knows the truth yet deviates from it.

Allah, the Exalted, says:

"And had it not been for the Grace of Allah and His Mercy on you (He would have hastened the punishment upon you)! And that Allah is the One Who accepts repentance, the All-Wise." (Qur'an, An-Nur 24:10)

Ibn Abbas (May Allah be pleased with him) reported that Hilal ibn Umayyah went to the Prophet (May Allah's peace and blessings be upon him) and accused his wife of committing illegal sexual intercourse with Sharik ibn Sahma'. The Messenger of Allah (May Allah's peace and blessings be upon him) said: "Either you provide proof or you will receive the legal punishment on your back." Hilal said: "O Messenger of Allah, if one of us saw a man on top of his wife, should he go and look for witnesses?" The Prophet (May Allah's peace and blessings be upon him) kept saying: "Either you provide proof or you will receive the legal punishment on your back." Hilal then said: "By the One Who sent you with the Truth, I am truthful, and Allah will reveal to you what will save my back from the legal punishment." Then (the following) was revealed: *"And for those who accuse their wives..." (Qur'an, An-Nur 24:6)* He kept reciting until he reached: *"...if he was of the truthful." (Qur'an, An-Nur 24:9)* Then the Prophet (May Allah's peace and blessings be upon him) left and had her summoned. So, Hilal came and took an oath. So, the Prophet (May Allah's peace and blessings be upon him) was saying: "Allah knows that one of you is a liar, so will either of you repent?" Then the woman got up and took the oaths, and when she was about to take the fifth one, the people stopped her and said to her: "It will definitely bring about Allah's Curse upon you (if you are guilty)." So, she hesitated and recoiled so much that we thought that she would withdraw her denial. But she said: "I will not dishonor my family for the rest of their days." The Prophet (May Allah's peace and blessings be upon him) then said: "Watch her, if she delivers a child with eyes that appear to have kohl on them, big bottoms and fat shins, then it is Sharik ibn Sahma's child." (Later) she gave birth to a child fitting that description. So, the Prophet (May Allah's peace and blessings be upon him) said: "If it had not been settled in the Book of Allah, there would have been a matter between me and her." (Bukhari and Muslim) (This is the wording of Al-Bukhari) (https://hadeethenc.com/en/browse/hadith/58242)

Sa'id b Jubair reported: "I was asked about the invokers of Curses during the reign of Mus'ab (b. Zubair) whether they could separate (themselves by this process). He said: "I did not understand what to say.' So, I went to the house of Ibn 'Umar (Allah be pleased with him) in Makkah. I said to his servant: 'Seek permission for me.' He said that he (Ibn 'Umar) had been taking rest. He (Ibn 'Umar) heard my voice and said: 'Are you Ibn Jubair?' I said: 'Yes.' He said: 'Come in. By Allah, it must be some (great) need which has brought you here at this hour.' So, I got in and found him lying on a blanket reclining against a pillow stuffed with fibres of date-palm. I said: 'O Abu'Abd al-Rahman, should there be separation between the invokers of Curses?' He said: 'Hallowed be Allah, yes. The first one who asked about it was so and so.' He said: 'Messenger of Allah told me If one of us finds his wife committing adultery, what should he do? If he talks, that is something great, and if he keeps quiet that is also (something great) (which he cannot afford to do).' Allah's Prophet (peace be upon him) kept quiet (or some time). After some time, he (that very person) came to him (Allah's Messenger) and said: 'I have been involved in that very cage about which I had asked you. Allah, the Exalted and Majestic, then revealed (these) Verses of Surah An-Nur: *"Those who accuse their wives" (Verse 24:6)*, and he (the Holy Prophet) recited them to him and admonished him, and exhorted him, and informed him that the torment of the world is less painful than the torment of the Hereafter. He said: 'No, by Him Who sent you with Truth, I did not tell a lie against her.' He (the Holy Prophet) then called her (the wife of that person who had accused her) and admonished her, and exhorted her, and informed her that the torment of this world is less painful than the torment of the Hereafter. She said: 'No, by Him Who sent thee with Truth, he is a liar. (it was) the man who started the swearing of oath and he swore in the Name of Allah four times that he was among the truthful, and at the fifth turn he said, 'Let there be Curse of Allah upon him if he were among the liars.' Then the woman was called and she swore four times in the Name of Allah that he (her husband) was among the liars, and at the fifth time (she said), 'Let there be Curse upon her if he were among the truthful.' He (the Holy Prophet) then effected separation between the two." (Muslim)

Ibn Umar (May Allah be pleased with him) reported Allah's Messenger (peace and blessings be upon him) saying to the invokers of Curse:" Your account is with Allah. One of you must be a liar. You have now no right over this woman." He said: 'Messenger of Allah, what about my wealth (Mahr that I paid her at the time of marriage)?' He said: 'You have no claim to wealth. If you tell the truth, it (Mahr) is the recompense for your having had the right to intercourse with her, and if you tell a lie against her, it is still more remote from you than she is.' Zuhair said in his narration: 'Sufyan reported to us on the authority of 'Amr that he had heard Sa'id b Jubair saying: 'I heard Ibn Umar (May Allah be pleased with him) saying that Allah's Messenger (May peace be upon him) had said it.'" (Muslim)

Narrated Sahl bin Sa'd As-Sa'idi: 'Uwaimir Al-'Ajlani came to 'Asim bin 'Adi and said, "If a man found another man with his wife and killed him, would you sentence the husband to death (in Qisas) i.e. equality in punishment)?" "O 'Asim! Please ask Allah's Apostle about this matter on my behalf." 'Asim asked the Prophet but the Prophet disliked the question and disapproved of it. 'Asim returned and informed 'Uwaimir that the Prophet disliked that type of question. 'Uwaimir said, "By Allah, I will go (personally) to the Prophet." 'Uwaimir came to the Prophet when Allah had already revealed the Quranic Verses (in that respect), after 'Asim had left (the Prophet). So, the Prophet said to 'Uwaimir, "Allah has revealed Quranic Verses regarding you and your wife." The Prophet then called for them, and they came and carried out the order of Li'an. Then 'Uwaimir said, "O Allah's Apostle! Now if I kept her with me, I would be accused of telling a lie." So 'Uwaimir divorced her although the Prophet did not order him to do so. Later on, this practice of divorcing became the tradition of couples involved in a case of Li'an. The Prophet said (to the people). "Wait for her! If she delivers a red short (small) child like a Wahra (a short red animal), then I will be of the opinion that he ('Uwaimir) has told a lie but if she delivered a black big-eyed one with big buttocks, then I will be of the opinion that he has told the truth about her." 'Ultimately she gave birth to a child that proved the accusation. (Bukhari)

274. Divorce of Breastfeeding Woman

Sheikh Ibn 'Uthaymeen (May Allah have mercy on him) said:

"The words: "During a period of purity in which he has not had intercourse with her" exclude the case in which he divorces her during a period of purity in which he has had intercourse with her, because that is an innovated divorce, even if the period of purity lasted for a long time. If we assume that this man's wife became pure from nifaas (postpartum bleeding) and he had intercourse with her when she was still breastfeeding, and usually the woman who is breastfeeding does not menstruate until she has weaned her child, which is after approximately two years, then if he divorces her within those two years, it is an innovated divorce, because it has occurred during a period of purity in which he had intercourse with her. So, he should wait until her menses has come then she becomes pure. End quote." (Ash-Sharh al-Mumti' (13/37) (271)

275. Rights of Revocably and Irrevocably Divorced Women

If a woman has asked for divorce – when her husband has consummated the marriage with her – one of two scenarios must apply:

1 - First scenario.

Either she has asked for it because of the husband's shortcomings in fulfilling her rights or because of some attitude in him that annoys her and deprives her of her rights, or because he has fallen into sin, and other such reasons which make it permissible for her to ask for Talaq. The Shariah judge is the one who should evaluate them and decide whether they are valid reasons or not. If they are valid, then the husband must divorce her by Talaq in that case, and give her all her rights in full, which are:

1a. The full Mahr. The Messenger of Allah (peace and blessings be upon him) said: "If he has consummated the marriage with her, then the Mahr is hers because of his intimacy with her." (Tirmidhi)

1b. Reasonable maintenance, including food, drink, accommodation and clothing during the Iddah period in revocable divorce.

If the divorce is irrevocable, such as a third Talaq, then she is not entitled to maintenance or accommodation.

Fatima bint Qais reported that Abu 'Amr b. Hafs divorced her absolutely when he was away from home, and he sent his agent to her with some barley. She was displeased with him and when he said: "I swear by Allah that you have no claim on us." She went to Allah's Messenger (peace and blessings be upon him) and mentioned that to him. He said: "There is no maintenance due to you from him…" (Muslim)

1c. Payment for custody and breastfeeding.

Allah, the Exalted, says:

"The mothers shall give suck to their children for two whole years, (that is) for those (parents) who desire to complete the term of suckling, but the father of the child shall bear the cost of the mother's food and clothing on a reasonable basis. No person shall have a burden laid on him greater than he can bear." (Qur'an, Al-Baqarah 2:233)

1d. Maintenance for the children.

So, Allah has made it obligatory for the father of the child to spend on the mother who breastfeeds her child. This includes the woman who is pregnant or divorced; the father must pay for maintenance. (Tafsir al-Sa'di (p.105)

Sheikh Muhammad ibn Saalih al-'Uthaymeen (May Allah have mercy on him) said:

"The woman who is thrice-divorced is not entitled to maintenance from her husband for herself, but he should spend on her for the sake of the pregnancy. On that basis, whatever she needs of maintenance after the delivery. Allah, the Exalted, says: *"And if they are pregnant, then spend on them till they lay down their burden."* (Qur'an, At-Talaq 65:6) (Liqaa'aat al-Baab il-Maftooh (147/question no.8)

2 - The Second scenario.

The woman asks for divorce from the husband with no cause. In that case the husband may ask her to return the Mahr that he gave her, in return for divorcing her. This is what is called Khula'.

In this case the four rights mentioned above no longer remain, except payment for breastfeeding and custody, and maintenance of the child who is still being breastfed. (272)

276. Revocably Divorced Woman Should Stay in her Husband's House Until her Iddah is Over

Allah, the Exalted, says:

"...and turn them not out of their (husband's) homes nor shall they (themselves) leave, except in case they are guilty of some open illegal sexual intercourse. And those are the set limits of Allah. And whosoever transgresses the set limits of Allah, then indeed he has wronged himself..." (Qur'an, At-Talaq 65:1)

"...You (the one who divorces his wife) know not it may be that Allah will afterward bring some new thing to pass (i.e. to return her back to you if that was the first or second divorce)." (Qur'an, At-Talaq 65:1)

The woman who is revocably divorced should stay in her husband's house until her 'Iddah ends. (273)

277. The Iddah of Divorced Woman by Talaq

A. If the woman is divorced by Talaq before intercourse or intimacy with her and been alone, then she does not have to observe any Iddah at all.

B. But if he has been alone with her and had intercourse with her, then she has to observe the Iddah (waiting period) which takes one of the following forms:

1 – If she is pregnant then her Iddah lasts until the end of pregnancy.

Allah, the Exalted, says:

"And for those who are pregnant (whether they are divorced or their husbands are dead), their Iddah (prescribed period) is until they lay down their burden." (Qur'an, At-Talaq 65:4)

2 – If the woman is not pregnant and she menstruates, her Iddah is three menstrual cycles after the divorce, i.e. her period comes then she becomes pure, then her period comes again and she becomes pure, then her period comes again and she becomes pure. If he divorces his breastfeeding wife, then she remains in Iddah until she has had three menstrual cycles, so she may stay in this state for two years or more. Allah, the Exalted, says:

"And divorced women shall wait (as regards their marriage) for three menstrual periods." (Qur'an, Al-Baqarah 2:228)

3 – If a woman does not menstruate (very young or old (postmenopause), then her Iddah is three months. Allah, the Exalted, says:

"And those of your women as have passed the age of monthly courses, for them the 'Iddah (prescribed period), if you have doubt (about their periods), is three months; and for those who have no courses [(i.e. they are still immature) their 'Iddah (prescribed period) is three months likewise..." (Qur'an, At-Talaq 65:4)

4 – If a woman stopped menstruate (i.e. after hysterectomy...), her Iddah is three months.

5 – If her periods have ceased and she knows the cause, she should wait for the cause to cease and for her periods to return, then she should observe Iddah according to her menstrual cycle.

6 – If her periods have ceased and she does not know what caused that, then the scholars say that she should observe an Iddah of a full year, nine months for pregnancy and three months for Iddah. (274)

278. Prohibition to Marry a Woman Divorced by Three Pronouncements Until she is Married to Another Man and he has

a Sexual Intercourse with her and then he Abandons her and she Completes her Iddah

Allah, the Exalted, says:

"And if he has divorced her (the third time), then she is not lawful unto him thereafter until she has married another husband." (Qur'an, Al-Baqarah 2:230)

Narrated Aisha (May Allah be pleased with her): "Rifa'a Al-Qurazi divorced his wife irrevocably (i.e. that divorce was the final). Later on, 'Abdur-Rahman bin Az-Zubair married her after him. She came to the Prophet (peace and blessings be upon him) and said, "O Allah's Apostle! I was Rifa'a's wife and he divorced me thrice, and then I was married to 'Abdur-Rahman bin Az-Zubair, who, by Allah, has nothing with him except something like this fringe, O Allah's Apostle" showing a fringe she had taken from her covering sheet. Abu Bakr was sitting with the Prophet (peace and blessings be upon him) while Khalid Ibn Said bin Al-As was sitting at the gate of the room waiting for admission. Khalid started calling Abu Bakr, "O Abu Bakr! Why don't you reprove this lady from what she is openly saying before Allah's Apostle?" Allah's Apostle did nothing except smiling, and then said (to the lady), "Perhaps you want to go back to Rifa'a? No, (it is not possible), unless and until you enjoy the sexual relation with him ('AbdurRahman), and he enjoys the sexual relation with you." (Bukhari)

Narrated Aisha (May Allah be pleased with her): "A man divorced his wife thrice (by expressing his decision to divorce her thrice), then she married another man who also divorced her. The Prophet (peace and blessings be upon him) was asked if she could legally marry the first husband (or not). The Prophet (peace and blessings be upon him) replied, "No, she cannot marry the first husband unless the second husband consummates his marriage with her, just as the first husband had done." (Bukhari)

279. Prohibition of Tahleel Marriage

Allah, the Exalted, says:

"And if he has divorced her (the third time), then she is not lawful unto him thereafter until she has married another husband. Then, if the other husband divorces her, it is no sin on both of them that they reunite, provided they feel that they can keep the limits ordained by Allah. These are the limits of Allah, which He makes plain for the people who have knowledge." (Qur'an, Al-Baqarah 2:230)

'Ali (May Allah be pleased with him) reported: The Prophet (peace and blessings be upon him) said:

"May Allah curse the Muhallil and the Muhallal lahu." (Ibn Majah)

(https://hadeethenc.com/en/browse/hadith/58076)

Tahleel marriage takes several forms, including the following:

1. Where the husband who had issued the divorce, or the woman, or her guardian, hires a human "billy-goat", and stipulates that he must marry the divorced woman, consummate the marriage with her, then divorce her, and they give him a sum of money in return for that!

2. Where a man marries that divorced woman without making any agreement with anybody, but his aim is to make her permissible for the first husband, then he divorces her.

Tahleel marriage is unlawful, and those who do that deserve to be cursed. (275)

280. When Husband Disappears and the Wife Doesn't Know Where he is

Narrated Yahya from Malik from Yahya ibn Said from Said ibn al-Musayyab that Umar ibn al-Khattab said, "The woman who loses her husband and does not know where he is, waits for four years, then she does 'Iddah for four months, and then she is free to marry." Malik said, "If she marries after her 'Iddah is over, regardless of whether the new husband has consummated the marriage or not, her first husband has no means of access to her." Malik said, "That is what is done among us and if her husband reaches her before she has remarried, he is more entitled to her." Malik said that he had seen people disapproving of someone who said that one of the people (of knowledge) attributed to Umar ibn al-Khattab that he said, "Her first husband chooses when he comes either her bride-price or his wife." Malik said, "I have heard that Umar ibn al-Khattab, speaking about a woman whose husband divorced her while he was absent from her, and then he took her back and the news of his taking her back had not reached her, while the news of his divorcing her had, and so she had married again, said, 'Her first husband who divorced her has no means of access to her whether or not the new husband has consummated the marriage.'" Malik said, "This is what I like the best of what I heard about the missing man." (Malik Muwatta)

281. Alimony

1. Revocable Divorce

Allah, the Exalted, says:

"And for divorced women, maintenance (should be provided) on reasonable (scale). This is a duty on Al-Muttaqun (the pious - see V.2:2)." (Qur'an, Al-Baqarah 2:240)

"Let the rich man spend according to his means; and the man whose resources are restricted, let him spend according to what Allah has given him. Allah puts no burden on any person beyond what He has given him. Allah will grant after hardship, ease." (Qur'an, At-Talaq 65:7)

The woman (in first or second Talaq) must be given maintenance and accommodation during the Iddah, but when her Iddah ends, if she is not pregnant, she is not entitled to that.

Maintenance of children is a duty of the father whether he remains married to his wife or divorces her, and whether the wife is poor or rich. She is not obliged to spend on the children when their father is still alive. Maintenance of children includes providing accommodation, food, drink, clothing and education, and everything that they need, on a reasonable basis, depending on the husband's circumstances.

2. Irrevocable Divorce

An irrevocable divorce ends the marriage as soon as it has happened. (276)

The irrevocably divorced woman is not entitled to maintenance or accommodation, unless she is pregnant.

Fatima bint Qais (May Allah be pleased with her) reported that her husband divorced her with three pronouncements and Allah's Messenger (peace and blessings be upon him) made no provision for her lodging and maintenance allowance…" (Mulsim)

3. Breastfeeding Woman

Allah, the Exalted, says:

"Then if they give suck to the children for you, give them their due payment." (Qur'an, At-Talaq 65:6)

"The mothers shall give suck to their children for two whole years, (that is) for those (parents) who desire to complete the term of suckling, but the father of the child shall bear the cost of the mother's food and clothing on a reasonable basis." (Qur'an, Al-Baqarah 2:233)

Sheikh al-Islam Ibn Taymiyah (May Allah have mercy on him) said:

"As for payment for breastfeeding, she is entitled to that according to scholarly consensus, as Allah says:

"Then if they give suck to the children for you, give them their due payment." (At-Talaq 65:6)."
(End quote from al-Fataawa al-Kubra (3/347) (277)

4. Pregnant Woman

Allah, the Exalted, says:

"Lodge them (the divorced women) where you dwell, according to your means, and do not harm them so as to straighten them (that they be obliged to leave your house). And if they are pregnant, then spend on them till they lay down their burden." *(Qur'an, At-Talaq 65:6)*

Sheikh Ibn Baaz (May Allah have mercy on him) was asked whether a woman may be divorced by Talaq when she is pregnant. He said:

"...Rather the view of all the scholars is that a pregnant woman can be divorced by Talaq. There is consensus on this point among the scholars, and there is no dispute. Talaq according to the Sunnah means that a woman may be divorced in two cases:

1 - She may be divorced when she is pregnant; this is a Sunnah divorce and is not Bid'ah.

2 - "She should be taahir (pure, i.e. not menstruating) and her husband should not have touched her (i.e. had intercourse with her), i.e. she should have become taahir following menstruation or nifaas (post-natal bleeding) and before he has intercourse with her. Talaq in this case is in accordance with the Sunnah." (Fataawa al-Talaq by Sheikh Ibn Baaz, 1/45-46) (278)

5. Widowed woman

Allah, the Exalted, says:

"And those of you who die and leave behind wives should bequeath for their wives a year's maintenance and residence without turning them out, but if they (wives) leave, there is no sin on you for that which they do of themselves, provided it is honorable (e.g. lawful marriage). And Allah is All-Mighty, All-Wise. [The order of this Verse has been cancelled (abrogated) by Verse 4:12]." *(Qur'an, Al-Baqarah 2:240)*

6. Divorced before consummation of the marriage, whose Mahr had not been decided upon at the

time of the marriage contract.

Allah, the Exalted, says:

"There is no blame upon you if you divorce women you have not touched nor specified for them an obligation. But give them [a gift of] compensation - the wealthy according to his capability and the poor according to his capability - a provision according to what is acceptable, a duty upon the doers of good." (Qur'an, Al-Baqarah 2:236)

A gift of compensation to be given to a woman divorced before consummation of the marriage.

282. Woman Stipulating the Divorce of the Wife of the would-be-Husband

Narrated Abu Hurairah (May Allah have mercy on him): The Prophet (peace and blessings be upon him) said, "It is not lawful for a woman (at the time of wedding) to ask for the divorce of her sister (i.e. the other wife of her would-be husband) in order to have everything for herself, for she will take only what has been written for her." (Bukhari)

283. Prohibition of Inciting a Woman Against her Husband or a Slave Against his Master

Abu Hurairah (May Allah be pleased with him) reported that the Prophet (May Allah's peace and blessings be upon him) said: "Whoever incites a woman against her husband or a slave against his master is not one of us." (Abu Dawud) (https://hadeethenc.com/en/browse/hadith/8884)

284. Unlawful Sexual Intercourse - Zina

Allah, the Exalted, warned:

"And come not near to unlawful sex. Verily, it is a Fahishah (i.e. anything that transgresses its limits: a great sin) and an evil way that leads one to Hell unless Allah forgives him." (Qur'an, Al-Isra 17:32)

"The woman and the man guilty of illegal sexual intercourse, flog each of them with a hundred stripes. Let not pity withhold you in their case, in a punishment prescribed by

Allah, if you believe in Allah and the Last Day. And let a party of the believers witness their punishment. (This punishment is for unmarried persons guilty of the above crime but if married persons commit it, the punishment is to stone them to death, according to Allah's Law)." (Qur'an, An-Nur 24:2)

Abu Hurairah (May Allah be pleased with him) reported that the Prophet (May Allah's peace and blessings be upon him) said: "Hellfire is surrounded by lusts and Paradise is surrounded by adversities." (Bukhari and Muslim) (https://hadeethenc.com/en/browse/hadith/3702)

Narrated 'Uthman ibn Abi'l-'Aas al-Thaqafi: The Prophet (peace and blessings of Allah be upon him) said: "The gates of Heaven are opened halfway through the night and a Caller cries out: 'Is anyone supplicating so that he may be answered? Is anyone asking so that he might be given? Is anyone in distress, so that he might be granted relief?' And there will be no Muslim left who is supplicating but Allah will answer him, except for a zaaniyah who earns a living from committing Zina or an Extortionist." (Tabarani in al-Mu'jam al-Kabeer (9/59) and in al-Mu'jam al-Awsat (3/154). Al-Haythami said in Majma' al-Zawaa'id (10/156): Its men are the men of saheeh. Al-Albaani said in al-Silsilah al-Saheehah 91073): Its isnaad is Saheeh.

Zina is an Islamic legal term referring to unlawful sexual intercourse.

Islamic Law establishes two categories of legal sexual relationships: between husband and wife, and between a man and his concubine. All other sexual relationships are considered Zina including adultery, fornication, prostitution, rape, sodomy, homosexuality, incest and bestiality.

Pompeii, the symbol of the degeneration of the Roman Empire was involved in sexual perversity. Its end was similar to that of the people of Lut. The destruction of Pompeii came by means of the eruption of the volcano Vesuvius. The volcano Vesuvius is the symbol of Italy, primarily the city of Naples. Remaining silent for the last two millennia, Vesuvius is named the 'mount of warning'. The disaster that befell Sodom and Gomorrah is very similar to the disaster that destroyed Pompeii. The lava and ash of a huge volcanic eruption, that happened two millennia ago, caught the inhabitants of that city. The disaster happened so suddenly that everything in the town was caught in the middle of everyday life and remains today exactly as it was two millennia ago. It is as if the time had been frozen. The removal of Pompeii from the face of the earth by such a disaster was not purposeless. The historical records show that the city was exactly a center of dissipation and perversity. The city was marked by a rise in prostitution to such an extent that eventually the number of brothels was not known. Male organs in their original sizes were hung on the doors of brothels. Archeologists first excavated the city during Victorian times, shocked by the open sexual perversity of the people, a secret museum was formed to house some of the artifacts found. These included many phallic symbols, images of homosexuality and even bestiality. But the lava of Vesuvius wiped the whole city off the map in a single moment. Numerous petrified couples were found in the act of intercourse. The most interesting thing is that there were couples of the same sex and couples of young boys and young girls. The general expression on those faces was bewilderment. This aspect of the event shows that the disappearance of Pompeii was similar to the destructive events mentioned in the *Qur'an*, because the *Qur'an* particularly points to "sudden annihilation" while relating these events. For example, the "inhabitants of the city" described in *Surah Yasin* died all at once in a single moment.

Allah, the Exalted, says:

"It was no more than a single mighty blast, and behold! They were (like ashes) quenched and silent." (Qur'an, Yasin 36:29)

"For we sent against them a single mighty blast, and they became like the dry stubble used by one who pens cattle." (Qur'an, Al-Qamar 54:31)

Despite all these, things have not changed much where Pompeii once stood. The districts of Naples where debauchery prevails do not fall short of those licentious districts of Pompeii.

The island of Capri is a base where homosexuals and nudists rule. The island of Capri is represented as a "Homosexual Paradise" in tourist commercials. Not only in Italy, but in nearly all the world, a similar moral degeneration is at work and people insist on not learning from the awful experience of past peoples. (279)

285. Zina of the Eyes, Ears, Tongue, Hands, Feet and Heart

Allah, the Exalted, says:

"Tell the believing men to lower their gaze (from looking at forbidden things), and protect their private parts (from illegal sexual acts). That is purer for them. Verily, Allah is All-Aware of what they do." (Qur'an, An-Nur 24:30)

"Allah knows the fraud of the eyes, and all that the breasts conceal." (Qur'an, Ghafir 40:19)

Sheikh 'Abd al-'Azeez ibn Baaz (May Allah have mercy on him) said:

"In these two Verses, Allah commands the believing men and women to lower their gaze and guard their chastity, which is because of the serious nature of Zina and what it leads to of great corruption among the Muslims. Letting one's gaze wander freely is one of the causes of sickness in the heart and the occurrence of immoral actions, whereas lowering the gaze is one of the means of keeping oneself safe from that. Allah, the Exalted, says: *"Tell the believing men to lower their gaze (from looking at forbidden things), and protect their private parts (from illegal sexual acts). That is purer for them. Verily, Allah is All-Aware of what they do."* (Qur'an, An-Nur 24:30) Lowering one's gaze and guarding one's chastity is purer for the believer in this world and in the Hereafter, whereas letting one's gaze wander freely and not guarding one's chastity are among the greatest causes of doom and punishment in this world and in the Hereafter.

We ask Allah to keep us safe and sound. Allah tells us that He is All-Aware of what people do, and that nothing is hidden from Him. This is a warning to the believer against doing that which Allah has forbidden and turning away from that which Allah has prescribed for him, and it is a reminder to him that Allah sees him and knows all that he does, whether it is good or otherwise. Allah, the Exalted, says: *"Allah knows the fraud of the eyes, and all that the breasts conceal." (Qur'an, Ghafir 40:19)* End quote." (From al-Tabarruj wa Khataruhu) (280)

Abu Hurairah (May Allah have mercy on him) reported Allah's Messenger (peace and blessings of Allah be upon him) as saying, "Allah fixed the very portion of adultery which a man will indulge in. There would be no escape from it. The adultery of the eye is the lustful look and the adultery of the ears is listening to voluptuous (song or talk) and the adultery of the tongue is licentious speech and the adultery of the hand is the lustful grip (embrace) and the adultery of the feet is to walk (to the place) where he intends to commit adultery and the heart yearns, and desires which he may or may not put into effect." (Muslim)

Narrated Abu Musa (May Allah have mercy on him): The Prophet (peace and blessings of Allah be upon him) said: "Every eye commits adultery, and when the woman uses perfume and she passes by a gathering, then she is like this and that.'" Meaning an adulteress. (Tirmidhi)

Narrated Ibn Abbas (May Allah have mercy on him): "I did not see anything so resembling Minor sins as what Abu Hurairah said from the Prophet (peace and blessings be upon him), who said, 'Allah has written for the son of Adam his inevitable share of adultery whether he is aware of it or not: The adultery of the eye is the looking (at something which is sinful to look at), and the adultery of the tongue is to utter (what it is unlawful to utter), and the inner self wishes and longs for (adultery), and the private parts turn that into reality or refrain from submitting to the temptation.'" (Bukhari)

Abu Hurairah (May Allah be pleased with him) reported that the Prophet (May Allah's peace and blessings be upon him) said: "Whoever Allah saves from the evil of what is between his jaws and the evil of what is between his legs will enter Paradise." (Tirmidhi) (https://hadeethenc.com/en/browse/hadith/3477)

ShakI ibn Humayd (May Allah be pleased with him) reported: "I said: 'O Messenger of Allah, teach me a supplication." He said: "Say: O Allah, I seek refuge in You from the evil of my hearing, from the evil of my sight, from the evil of my tongue, from the evil of my heart, and from the evil of my semen (i.e. my lust)." (Tirmidhi, An-Nasa'i, Abu Dawud, Ahmad) (https://hadeethenc.com/en/browse/hadith/6163)

Looking at that which is forbidden is one of the arrows of the Shaytan, which leads a person to doom, even if he did not do it intentionally at first.

286. Prohibition of Incest

Incest is human sexual activity between family members or close relatives. This typically includes sexual activity between people in consanguinity (blood relations), and sometimes those related by affinity (marriage or stepfamily), adoption, clan or lineage. A common justification for prohibiting incest is avoiding inbreeding: a collection of genetic disorders suffered by the children of parents with a close genetic relationship. Such children are at greater risk for congenital disorders, death and developmental and physical disability.

Narrated Ibn'Abbas (May Allah have mercy on him) that the Messenger of Allah (peace and blessings be upon him) said: "Whoever has intercourse with a Mahram relative, kill him; and whoever has intercourse with an animal, kill him and kill the animal." (Ibn Majah)

Zina with a Mahram relative is a Major sin because it is severing the ties of kinship, and an act of aggression against those with whom we are enjoined to uphold ties of kinship.

Ibn al-Qayyim (May Allah have mercy on him) said concerning intercourse with one's mother, daughter or sister: "There is a totally natural repulsion towards that, and the Hadd punishment for that is one of the most severe of punishments according to one of the two opinions, which is execution in all cases, whether he was married or not…" (281)

287. Prescribed Punishment for Adultery and Fornication

Allah, the Exalted, says:

"And come not near to unlawful sex. Verily, it is a Fahishah (i.e. anything that transgresses its limits: a great sin, and an evil way that leads one to hell unless Allah Forgives him)." (Qur'an, Al-Isra 17:32)

"And those who invoke not any other ilaah (god) along with Allah, nor kill such person as Allah has forbidden, except for just cause, nor commit illegal sexual intercourse and whoever does this shall receive the punishment." (Qur'an, Al-Furqan 25:68)

"But there came after them an evil generation, who neglected prayers and followed the sexual desires, so they will meet perdition." (Qur'an, Maryam 19:59)

Other Verse: *An-Nur 24:2.*

Zina encompasses any sexual intercourse except that between husband and wife. It includes both extramarital sex and premarital sex, and is often translated as "fornication" in English. The degree of sin is worse and the punishment is multiplied if the woman is married, because that is a betrayal of her husband … Hence the punishment for an unmarried zaani is one hundred lashes during one year, and the punishment for a married zaani is stoning to death.

Fornication is a consensual sexual intercourse between two people not married to each other.

Adultery is when one of the partners to consensual sexual intercourse is a married person.

Abu Hurairah (May Allah be pleased with him) reported that the Prophet (May Allah's peace and blessings be upon him) said: "Verily, Allah the Almighty gets jealous. The jealousy of Allah the Almighty is when a person commits what Allah has made unlawful for him." (Bukhari and Muslim) (https://hadeethenc.com/en/browse/hadith/3354)

Narrated Ibn Masud (May Allah be pleased with him): "A man said: 'Allah's Messenger, which offense is the most grievous in Allah's Eye?" He replied: "That you associate a partner with Allah Who created you." He said: "What next?" He replied: "That you kill your child out of fear that he would join you in food." He said: "What next?" He replied: "That you commit adultery with your neighbor's wife." And the Almighty and Exalted Lord testified it: *"All those who call not unto another god along with Allah, and slay not any soul which Allah has forbidden, except in the cause of justice, nor commit fornication, and he who does this shall meet a requital of sin." (Qur'an 25:68)* (Muslim)

Narrated Abu Hurairah and Zaid bin Khalid Al-Juhani: "A Bedouin came to Allah's Apostle (peace and blessings be upon him) and said, "O Allah's apostle! I ask you by Allah to judge my case according to Allah's Laws." His opponent, who was more learned than he, said, "Yes, judge between us according to Allah's Laws, and allow me to speak." Allah's Apostle (peace and blessings be upon him) said, "Speak." He (i.e. the Bedouin or the other man) said, "My son was working as a labourer for this (man) and he committed illegal sexual intercourse with his wife. The people told me that it was obligatory that my son should be stoned to death, so in lieu of that I ransomed my son by paying one hundred sheep and a slave girl. Then I asked the religious scholars about it, and they informed me that my son must be lashed one hundred lashes and be exiled for one year, and the wife of this (man) must be stoned to death." Allah's Apostle (peace and blessings be upon him) said, "By Him in Whose Hands my soul is, I will judge between you according to Allah's Laws. The slave-girl and the sheep are to be returned to you, your son is to receive a hundred lashes and be exiled for one year. You, Unais, go to the wife of this (man) and if she confesses her guilt, stone her to death." Unais went to that woman next morning and she confessed. Allah's Apostle (peace and blessings be upon him) ordered that she be stoned to death. (Bukhari)

'Abdullah ibn 'Umar (May Allah be pleased with him) reported: "The Jews came to the Messenger of Allah (May Allah's peace and blessings be upon him) and informed him that a man and a woman from among them had committed unlawful sexual intercourse. The Messenger (May Allah's peace and blessings be upon him) asked them: "What do you find in the Torah about stoning?" They said: "We disclose their sin and flog them." 'Abdullah ibn Salam said: "You have lied! The Verse of stoning is there (in the Torah)." They fetched the Torah, spread it out, and one of them placed his hand over the Verse of stoning. He recited what was before it and what was after it. Thereupon, 'Abdullah ibn Salam told him to lift his hand. He lifted his hand and there was the Verse of stoning. They said: "He has spoken the truth, O Muhammad." So, the Messenger of Allah (May Allah's peace and blessings be upon him) ordered that they be stoned. 'Abdullah ibn 'Umar added: "I saw the man leaning over the woman to protect her from the stones." (Bukhari and Muslim) (https://hadeethenc.com/en/browse/hadith/2948)

'Ubada b. as-Samit reported: Allah's Messenger (peace and blessings be upon him) as saying: "Receive (teaching) from me, receive (teaching) from me. Allah has ordained a way for those (women). When an unmarried male commits adultery with an unmarried female (they should receive) one hundred lashes and banishment for one year. And in case of married male committing adultery with a married female, they shall receive one hundred lashes and be stoned to death." (Muslim)

'Imran ibn al-Husayn (May Allah be pleased with him) reported: A woman from the tribe of Juhaynah came to the Prophet (May Allah's peace and blessings be upon him) while she was pregnant from adultery, and she said to him: "O Messenger of Allah, I have committed a sin liable to the legal punishment, so execute the legal punishment on me." The Messenger of Allah called her guardian and said to him: "Treat her kindly and bring her to me after she delivers (her baby)." The man complied with the order, and the Prophet (May Allah's peace and blessings be upon him) commanded that the legal punishment be executed on her. Her clothes were secured around her and she was stoned to death. The Prophet then led the funeral prayer over her." (Muslim) (https://hadeethenc.com/en/browse/hadith/5649)

Narrated Ruwayfi' ibn Thaabit al-Ansaari: "I heard the Messenger of Allah (peace and blessings be upon him) say on the day of Hunayn: "It is not permissible for any man who believes in Allah and the Last Day to irrigate the crop of another else – meaning to have intercourse with a woman who is pregnant. And it is not permissible for a man who believes in Allah and the Last Day to have intercourse with a captured woman until he has established that she is not pregnant. And it is not permissible for a man who believes in Allah and the Last Day to sell any booty until it has been shared out." (Abu Dawud)

Narrated Anas: Allah's Apostle (peace and blessings be upon him) said, "From among the portents of the Hour are (the following): 1. Religious knowledge will be taken away (by the death of Religious learned men), 2. (Religious) ignorance will prevail, 3. Drinking of alcoholic drinks (will be very common), 4. There will be prevalence of open illegal sexual intercourse. (Bukhari)

Narrated Abdullah bin Umar: The Messenger of Allah (peace and blessings be upon him) turned to us and said: "O Muhajirun, there are five things with which you will be tested, and I seek refuge with Allah lest you live to see them: Immorality never appears among a people to such an extent that they commit it openly, but Plagues and Diseases that were never known among the predecessors will spread among them. They do not cheat in weights and measures but they will be stricken with famine, severe calamity and the oppression of their rulers. They do not withhold the Zakah of their wealth, but rain will be withheld from the sky, and were it not for the animals, no rain would fall on them. They do not break their covenant with Allah and His Messenger, but Allah will enable their enemies to overpower them and take some of what is in their hands. If their leaders do not rule according to the Book of Allah and seek all good from that which Allah has revealed, Allah will cause them to fight one another." (Ibn Majah)

Narrated Abu Hurairah (May Allah have mercy on him): The Messenger of Allah (peace and blessings be upon him) said, "There are three (types of) people whom Allah will neither speak to on the Day of Resurrection nor will He purify them (i.e. from their sins), nor will look upon them; and they will have a painful chastisement. These are: an old man who commits fornication; a king who is a great liar and a poor man who is proud." (Muslim)

Narrated Samura bin Jundab: "...They told me to proceed on; so, we proceeded on and passed by a hole like an oven; with a narrow top and wide bottom, and the fire was kindling underneath that hole. Whenever the fire-flame went up, the people were lifted up to such an extent that they about to get out of it, and whenever the fire got quieter, the people went down into it, and there were naked men and women in it... And those you saw in the hole (like oven) were adulterers (those men and women who commit illegal sexual intercourse)..." (Bukhari) (https://sunnah.com/bukhari:1386)

Narrated Abu Hurairah (May Allah have mercy on him): The Prophet (peace and blessings be upon him) said, "An adulterer, at the time he is committing illegal sexual intercourse is not a believer; and a person, at the time of drinking an alcoholic drink is not a believer; and a thief, at the time of stealing, is not a believer." Ibn Shihab said: 'Abdul Malik bin Abi Bakr bin 'Abdur-Rahman bin Al-Harith bin Hisham told me that Abu Bakr used to narrate that narration to him on the authority of Abu Hurairah. He used to add that Abu Bakr used to mention, besides the above cases, "And he who robs (takes illegally something by force) while the people are looking at him, is not a believer at the time he is robbing (taking)." (Bukhari)

Narrated Sahl bin Sa'd (May Allah have mercy on him): Allah's Messenger (peace and blessings be upon him) said, "Whoever can guarantee (the chastity of) what is between his two jaw-bones and what is between his two legs (i.e. his tongue and his private parts), I guarantee Paradise for him." (Bukhari)

288. Prohibition of Sodomy

Sodomy refers to anal or oral intercourse. "Sodomy is defined as any sexual act involving the sex organs of one person and the mouth or anus of another." (Court of Appeals, Georgia, US)

Sodomy has been referred to as a "crime against nature" by various courts and statutes. (282)

Prohibition of Oral Sex

Narrated Ali ibn Abu Talib: "Your mouths are the paths of the Qur'an, so perfume them with the tooth stick." (Ibn Majah)

There are some religious and medical objections regarding the Oral Sex. (283-285)

Firstly, such an act is contrary to honor and it is disgusting.

Secondly, some substances continually come out of sexual organs; and they are dirty fluids. In that case, a person will take in dirty substances into his/her mouth.

Thirdly, everybody knows that Islam gives great importance to human health. However, in this way, a person takes in a lot of microbes and puts himself/herself at risk.

The mouth was not created for sexual intercourse but for other purposes. Sexual intercourse through the mouth is contrary to the purpose of the creation of the mouth and to human nature; those people whose nature are not spoiled hate it. Oral sex is not a natural style of having sex and can cause feelings like hatred after a while and can affect the sexual happiness negatively.

Oral Sex and Mouth Cancer

Human papilloma virus (HPV) transmitted through sexual intercourse causes cervical, oral and anal cancers.

Oral Sex and Sexually Transmitted Diseases

Herpes, Gonorrhea, HIV, Syphilis, Chlamydia, Hepatitis B and C, HIV, etc.

Prohibition of Anal Sex

Narrated Abu Hurairah (May Allah have mercy on him): The Prophet (peace and blessings be upon him) said: "He who has intercourse with his wife through her anus is accursed." (Abu Dawud)

Ibn 'Abbas (May Allah have mercy on him) reported God's Messenger (peace and blessings be upon him) as saying, "God will not look at a man who has intercourse with a man or a woman through the anus." (Tirmidhi)

289. Lesbianism and Homosexuality

References to Lesbianism and Homosexuality in the Quran

Allah, the Exalted, says:

"*And (remember) Loot (Lot), when he said to his people: 'Do you commit the worst sin such as none preceding you has committed in the 'Alamin (mankind and Jinns)? 'Verily, you practice your lusts on men instead of women. Nay, but you are a people transgressing beyond bounds (by committing great sins).' And the answer of his people was only that they said: 'Drive them out of your town, these are indeed men who want to be pure (from sins)!' Then We saved him and his family, except his wife; she was of those who remained behind (in the torment). And We rained down on them a rain (of stones). Then see what was the end of the Mujrimoon (criminals, polytheists, sinners, etc.).*" (Qur'an, Al-A'raf 7:80-84)

"*Verily, by your life (O Muhammad), in their wild intoxication, they were wandering blindly. So As-Saihah (torment - awful cry) overtook them at the time of sunrise. And We turned (the towns of Sodom in Palestine) upside down and rained down on them stones of baked clay. Surely, in this are signs for those who see (or understand, or learn the lessons from the Signs of Allah). And verily, they (the cities) were right on the highroad (from Makkah to Syria, i.e. the place where the Dead Sea is now).*" (Qur'an, Al-Hijr 15:72-76)

"*And come not near to unlawful sex. Verily, it is a Fahishah (i.e. anything that transgresses its limits: a great sin), and an evil way (that leads one to Hell unless Allah Forgives him)."
(Qur'an, Al-Isra 17:32)*

Other Verses: *Al-Qamar 54:34, Al-'Ankabut 29:28, Al-Anbiya 21:74, An-Naml 27:54-58.*

<u>References to Lesbianism and Homosexuality in the Sunnah</u>

Ibn 'Abbas (May Allah have mercy on him) reported God's Messenger (peace and blessings be upon him) as saying, "God will not look at a man who has intercourse with a man or a woman through the anus." (Tirmidhi)

Narrated Jabir (May Allah have mercy on him): The Messenger of Allah (peace and blessings be upon him) said: "What I fear most from my Ummah is the behavior of the people of Lut." (Tirmidhi)

Ibn 'Abbas (May Allah have mercy on him) narrated that the Messenger of Allah (peace and blessings be upon him) said: "Whoever you find doing as the people of Lot did (i.e. homosexuality), kill the one who does it and the one to whom it is done, and if you find anyone having sexual intercourse with animal, kill him and kill the animal." (Ahmad and the four imams with a trustworthy chain of narrators)

Abdullah ibn 'Abbas (May Allah be pleased with him) reported that the Messenger of Allah (peace and blessings of Allah be upon him) said: "…Allah's Curse be upon those who do the action of the people of Lut." The Prophet (peace and blessings of Allah be upon him) repeated this curse thrice!) (Ibn Hibban)

The crime of Homosexuality is one of the greatest of crimes, the worst of sins and the most abhorrent of deeds, and Allah punished those who did it in a way that He did not punish other nations. It is indicative of violation of the Fitrah, total misguidance, weak intellect and lack of religious commitment, and it is a sign of doom and deprivation of the Mercy of Allah. (286)

290. Rape

The punishment for rape in Islam is same as the punishment for Zina, which is stoning if the perpetrator is married, and one hundred lashes and banishment for one year if he is not married. (287)

Some scholars also say that he is required to pay a Mahr to the woman.

Imam Malik (May Allah have mercy on him) said:

"In our view the man who rapes a woman, whether she is a virgin or not, if she is a free woman, he must pay a "Mahr" like that of her peers, and if she is a slave, he must pay whatever has been detracted from her value. The punishment is to be carried out on the rapist and there is no punishment for the woman who has been raped, whatever the case. End quote." (Malik Muwatta)

291. Prostitution

Allah, the Exalted, says:

"...And force not your maids to prostitution, if they desire chastity, in order that you may make a gain in the (perishable) goods of this worldly life..." (Qur'an, An-Nur 24:33)

"The adulterer marries not but an adulteress or a Mushrikah and the adulteress none marries her except an adulterer or a Muskrik [and that means that the man who agrees to marry (have a sexual relation with) a Mushrikah (female polytheist, pagan or idolatress) or a prostitute, then surely he is either an adulterer or a Mushrik (polytheist, pagan or idolater, etc.) And the woman who agrees to marry (have a sexual relation with) a Mushrik (polytheist, pagan or idolater) or an adulterer, then she is either a prostitute or a Mushrikah (female polytheist, pagan or idolatress, etc.)]. Such a thing is forbidden to the believers (of Islamic Monotheism)." (Qur'an, An-Nur 24:3)

Jabir (May Allah be pleased with him) reported: Abdullah ibn Ubayy would say to his servant girl, "Go earn us something from prostitution." Then, Allah Almighty revealed, *"Do not* compel your slave girls to prostitution if they desire chastity, seeking thereby the interests of worldly life. If someone compels them, Allah is Forgiving and Merciful to them after their compulsion." (24:33) (Muslim)

Narrated Abu Hurairah (May Allah be pleased with him): The Prophet (peace and blessings be upon him) prohibited the earnings of slave girls (through prostitution). (Bukhari)

Abu Masud (May Allah be pleased with him) reported: The Messenger of Allah (May Allah's peace and blessings be upon him) prohibited the price of a dog, the earning of a prostitute, and the money paid to a soothsayer." (Bukhari and Muslim) (https://hadeethenc.com/en/browse/hadith/6036)

292. Bestiality

Narrated Ibn Abbas (May Allah have mercy on him): The Messenger of Allah (peace and blessings be upon him) said: "Whoever has intercourse with a Mahram relative, kill him; and whoever has intercourse with an animal, kill him and kill the animal." (Ibn Majah)

Narrated Ibn 'Abbas (May Allah be pleased with him): The Messenger of Allah (peace and blessings be upon him) said: "Whomever you see having relations with an animal then kill him and kill animal." So, it was said to Ibn 'Abbas: "What is the case of the animal?" He said: "I did not hear anything from the Messenger of Allah (peace and blessings be upon him) about this, but I see that the Messenger of Allah (peace and blessings be upon him) disliked eating its meat or using it, due to the fact that such a (heinous) thing has been done with that animal." (Tirmidhi)

293. The Pimp and the One Who Permits His Wife to Fornicate

Allah, the Exalted, says:

"The adulterer marries not but an adulteress or a Mushrikah and the adulteress none marries her except an adulterer or a Muskrik [and that means that the man who agrees to marry (have a sexual relation with) a Mushrikah (female polytheist, pagan or idolatress) or a prostitute, then surely he is either an adulterer or a Mushrik (polytheist, pagan or idolater, etc.) And the woman who agrees to marry (have a sexual relation with) a Mushrik (polytheist, pagan or idolater) or an adulterer, then she is either a prostitute or a Mushrikah (female polytheist, pagan or idolatress, etc.)]. Such a thing is forbidden to the believers (of Islamic Monotheism)." (Qur'an, An-Nur 24:3)

Abdullah ibn Umar (May Allah be pleased with him) reported: The Messenger of Allah (peace and blessings be upon him) said, "Three persons will not be looked upon by Allah Almighty on the Day of Resurrection: one who disobeys his parents, a woman who imitates men, and a man who allows his women to fornicate…" (An-Nasa'i)

294. Masturbation

Allah, the Exalted, says:

"And those who guard their chastity (i.e. private parts, from illegal sexual acts). Except from their wives or (the captives and slaves) that their right hands possess, - for them, they are free from blame. But whoever seeks beyond that, then those are the transgressors." (Qur'an, Al-Mu'minun 23:5-7)

"But whoever seeks beyond that, then they are the transgressors." (Qur'an, Al-Ma'arij 70:31)

Abdullah ibn Masud (May Allah be pleased with him) said, "We were with the Prophet (peace and blessings be upon him) while we were young and had no wealth whatsoever. Allah's Messenger (peace and blessings be upon him) said, 'O young people! Whoever among you can marry, should marry, because it helps him lower his gaze and guard his modesty (i.e. his private parts from committing illegal sexual intercourse, etc.), and whoever is not able to marry, should fast, as fasting diminishes his sexual power.'" (Bukhari)

Masturbation (for both men and women) is haram (forbidden) in Islam. (288, 289)

295. Prohibition of Gazing at Women and Beardless Handsome Boys Except in Exigency

Allah, the Exalted, says:

"Tell the believing men to lower their gaze (from looking at forbidden things)." (Qur'an, An-Nur 24:30)

"Allah knows the fraud of the eyes, and all that the breasts conceal." (Qur'an, Ghafir 40:19)

Other Verses: *Al-Fajr 89:14, Al-Isra 17:36.*

Abu Hurairah (May Allah be pleased with him) said: The Prophet (peace and blessings be upon him) said, "Allah has written the very portion of Zina which a man will indulge in. There will be no escape from it. The Zina of the eye is the (lustful) look, the Zina of the ears is the listening (to voluptuous songs or talk), the Zina of the tongue is (the licentious) speech, the Zina of the hand is the (lustful) grip, the Zina of the feet is the walking (to the place where he intends to commit Zina), the heart yearns and desires and the private parts approve all that or disapprove it." (Bukhari and Muslim)

Abu Sa'id Al-Khudri (May Allah be pleased with him) said: The Prophet (peace and blessings be upon him) said, "Avoid sitting on roadsides." His Companions said: "O Messenger of Allah (peace and blessings be upon him), there is no other alternative but to sit there to talk." Thereupon the Messenger of Allah (peace and blessings be upon him) said, "If you have to sit at all, then fulfill the rights of the road." They asked: "What are their rights?" Thereupon he said, "Lowering the gaze (so that you may not stare at wrong things); refraining from doing some harm to others, responding to greeting (i.e. saying 'Wa'alaikumus-salam' to one another) and commanding the good and forbidding the evil." (Bukhari and Muslim)

Jarir bin 'Abdullah (May Allah be pleased with him) said: "I asked the Messenger of Allah (peace and blessings be upon him) about (the Islamic ruling on) accidental glance (i.e. at a woman one is not Islamically allowed to look at) and he ordered me to turn my eyes away." (Muslim)

Abu Sa'id Al-Khudri (May Allah be pleased with him) said: The Messenger of Allah (peace and blessings be upon him) said, "A man must not look at a man's private parts nor must a woman look at a woman's private parts; Neither should two men lie naked under one cover, nor should two women lie naked under the same cover." (Muslim)

Commentary: This Hadith tells us how Islam has closed all doors of immodesty and obscenity... (290)

296. Looking at Non-Mahram

Allah, the Exalted, says:

"Tell the believing men to lower their gaze (from looking at forbidden things) and protect their private parts (from illegal sexual acts, etc.). That is purer for them. Verily, Allah is All-Aware of what they do." (Qur'an, An-Nur 24:30)

"And tell the believing women to lower their gaze (from looking at forbidden things) and protect their private parts (from illegal sexual acts, etc.) and not to show off their adornment except only that which is apparent (like palms of hands or one eye or both eyes for necessity to see the way, or outer dress like veil, gloves, head-cover, apron, etc.), and

to draw their veils all over Juyubihinna (i.e. their bodies, faces, necks and bosoms, etc.) and not to reveal their adornment except to their husbands, their fathers, their husband's fathers, their sons, their husband's sons, their brothers or their brother's sons, or their sister's sons, or their (Muslim) women (i.e. their sisters in Islam), or the (female) slaves whom their right hands possess, or old male servants who lack vigour, or small children who have no sense of the shame of sex." (Qur'an, An-Nur 24:31)

Jarir b. 'Abdullah reported: "I asked Allah's Messenger (peace and blessings of Allah be upon him) about the sudden glance (that is cast) on the face (of a non-Mahram). He commanded me that I should turn away my eyes." (Muslim)

Commenting on this Hadith, al-Mubaarakpoori said: "Accidental means that his gaze fell on a non-Mahram woman unintentionally. He commanded me to turn my gaze away means that he was not to look a second time, because the first glance was not by choice and would be forgiven, but any further glances would be counted as sin, and he should heed the Words of Allah): *"Tell the believing men to lower their gaze (from looking at forbidden things)."* (An-Nur 24:30) (291)

Buraydah reported: The Messenger of Allah (peace and blessings be upon him) said, "Do not follow one glance at a woman with another. Verily, you have the first one and not the second." (Tirmidhi)

297. Looking at the Sexual Organs of the Same or the Opposite Sex

The Great Virtue of Lowering Gaze

Allah, the Exalted, says:

"Tell the believing men to lower their gaze (from looking at forbidden things) and protect their private parts (from illegal sexual acts, etc.). That is purer for them. Verily, Allah is All-Aware of what they do." (Qur'an, An-Nur 24:30)

"Allah knows the fraud of the eyes, and all that the hearts conceal." (Qur'an, Ghafir 40:190)

Abu Sa'id (May Allah be pleased with him) reported that the Messenger of Allah (May Allah's peace and blessings be upon him) said: "A man must not look at another man's 'Awrah, nor must a woman look at another woman's 'Awrah; neither should two men lie undressed and touch under one cover, nor should two women lie undressed and touch under one cover." (Muslim)

(https://hadeethenc.com/en/browse/hadith/8904)

Jabir b. 'Abdullah (May Allah be pleased with him) reported: "The Messenger of Allah (peace and blessings be upon him) was carrying along with them (his people) stones for the Ka'bah and there was a waist wrapper around him. His uncle, Abbas, said to him: '0 son of my brother! if you take off the lower garment and place it on the shoulders underneath the stones, it would be better. He (the Holy Prophet) took it off and placed it on his shoulder and fell down unconscious. He (the narrator) said: 'Never was he seen naked after that day.'" (Muslim)

Narrated Abu Hurairah (May Allah be pleased with him): Allah's Messenger (peace and blessings be upon him) said, "(The Prophet) Moses was a shy person and used to cover his body completely because of his extensive shyness. One of the children of Israel hurt him by saying, 'He covers his body in this way only because of some defect in his skin, either leprosy or scrotal hernia, or he has some other defect.' Allah wished to clear Moses of what they said about him, so one day while Moses was in seclusion, he took off his clothes and put them on a stone and started taking a bath. When he had finished the bath, he moved towards his clothes so as to take them, but the stone took his clothes and fled; Moses picked up his stick and ran after the stone saying, 'O stone! Give me my garment!' Till he reached a group of Bani Israel who saw him naked then, and found him the best of what Allah had created, and Allah cleared him of what they had accused him of. The stone stopped there and Moses took and put his garment on and started hitting the stone with his stick. By Allah, the stone still has some traces of the hitting, three, four or five marks. This was what Allah refers to in His Saying: *"O you who believe! Be you not like those who annoyed Moses, but Allah proved his innocence of that which they alleged, And he was honorable In Allah's Sight." (33.69)* (Bukhari)

Ibn Taymiyah (May Allah have mercy on him) said:

"Just as lowering the gaze includes not looking at the 'awrahs of other people and other haram things, it also includes refraining from looking into people's houses. A man's house conceals his body just as his garments conceal him." (Majmoo' al-Fataawa (15/379) (292)

The lowering one's gaze from (seeing) the prohibited things necessarily leads to three benefits that carry tremendous value and are of great significance.

The First: experiencing the delight and sweetness of faith.

This delight and sweetness are far greater and more desirable that which might have been attained from the object that one lowered his gaze from for the sake of Allah. Indeed, "... whosoever leaves something for the sake of Allah then Allah, the Mighty and Magnificent, will replace it with something better than it." (Ahmad, al-Marwazi, An-Nasa'i)

The soul is a temptress and loves to look at beautiful forms and the eye is the guide of the heart. The heart commissions its guide to go and look to see what is there and when the eye informs it of a beautiful image it shudders out of love and desire for it. Frequently such interrelations tire and wear down both the heart and the eye as is said: When you sent your eye as a guide. For your heart one day, the object of sight fatigued you. For you saw one over whom you had no power. Neither a portion or in totality, instead you had to be patient. Therefore, when the sight is prevented from looking and investigating the heart finds relief from having to go through the arduous task of (vainly) seeking and desiring. Whosoever lets his sight roam free will find that he is in a perpetual state of loss and anguish for sight gives birth to love (*mahabbah*) the starting point of which is the heart being devoted and dependent upon that which it beholds. This then intensifies to become fervent longing (*sababah*) whereby the heart becomes totally dependent and devoted to the (object of its desire). Then this further intensifies and becomes infatuation (*gharamah*) which clings to the heart like the one seeking repayment of a debt clings firmly to the one who has to pay the debt. Then this intensifies and becomes passionate love (*ishk*) and this is a love that transgresses all bounds. Then this further intensifies and becomes crazed passion (*shaghafa*) and this a love that encompasses every tiny part of the heart. Then this intensifies and becomes worshipful love (*tatayyuma*). *Tatayyum* means worship and it is said: *tayyamallah* i.e. he worshipped Allah. Hence the heart begins to worship that which is not correct for it to worship and the reason behind all of this was an illegal glance. The heart is now bound in chains whereas before it used to be the master, it is now imprisoned whereas before it was free. It has been oppressed by the eye and it complains to it upon which the eye replies: 'I am your guide and messenger and it was you who sent me in the first place!' All that has been mentioned applies to the heart that has relinquished the love of Allah and being sincere to Him for indeed the heart must have an object of love that it devotes itself to. Therefore, when the heart does not love Allah Alone and does not take Him as its God then it must worship something else.

Allah said concerning Yusuf as-Siddiq:

"Thus (did We order) so that We might turn away from him all evil and indecent actions for he was one of Our sincere servants." *(Qur'an, Yusuf 12:24)*

It was because the wife of al-Aziz was a polytheist that (the passionate love) entered her heart despite her being married. It was because Yusuf (May Allah have mercy on him) was sincere to Allah that he was saved from it despite his being a young man, unmarried and a servant.

The Second: the illumination of the heart, clear perception and penetrating insight.

Ibn Shuja' al-Kirmani said, "Whosoever builds his outward form upon following the Sunnah, his internal form upon perpetual contemplation and awareness of Allah, he restrains his soul from following desires, he lowers his gaze from the forbidden things and he always eats the lawful things then his perception and insight shall never be wrong."

Allah mentioned the people of Lut and what they were afflicted with and then He went on to say:

"Indeed, in this are signs for the Mutawassimin." *(Qur'an, Al-Hijr 15:75)*

The Mutwassimin are those who have clear perception and penetrating insight, those who are secure from looking at the unlawful and performing indecent acts.

Allah said after mentioning the Verse concerning lowering the gaze:

"Allah is the Light of the heavens and the earth." (Qur'an, An-Nur 24:35)

The reason behind this is that the reward is of the same type as the action. So, whosoever lowers his gaze from the unlawful for the sake of Allah, the Mighty and Magnificent, He will replace it with something better than it of the same type. So just as the servant restrained the light of his eye from falling upon the unlawful, Allah blesses the light of his sight and heart thereby making him perceive what he would not have seen and understood had he not lowered his gaze. This is a matter that the person can physically sense in himself for the heart is like a mirror and the base desires are like rust upon it. When the mirror is polished and cleaned of the rust then it will reflect the realities (*haqa'iq*) as they actually are. However, if it remains rusty then it will not reflect properly and therefore its knowledge and speech will arise from conjecture and doubt.

The Third: the heart becoming strong, firm and courageous.

Allah will give it the might of aid for its strength just as He gave it the might of clear proofs for its light. Hence the heart shall combine both of these factors and as a result, Shaytan shall flee from it. It is mentioned in the narration, "Whosoever opposes his base desires, the Shaytan shall flee in terror from his shade." This is not established as a *Hadith* of the Prophet (peace be upon him). This is why the one who follows his base desires shall find in himself the ignominy of the soul, its being weak, feeble and contemptible. Indeed, Allah places nobilty for the one who obeys Him and disgrace for the one who disobeys Him:

"So do not lose heart nor fall into despair; for you must gain mastery if you are true in faith." (Qur'an, Ali 'Imran 3:139)

"Whosoever desires honour, power and glory then to Allah belong all honour, power and glory [and one can get honour, power and glory only by obeying and worshipping Allah (Alone)]." (Qur'an, Fatir 35:10)

Meaning that whosoever seeks after disobedience and sin then Allah, the Mighty and Magnificent, will humiliate the one who disobeys Him.

Some of the salaf said, "The people seek nobility and power at the door of the Kings and they will not find it except through the obedience of Allah."

This is because the one who obeys Allah has taken Allah as his friend and Protector, and Allah will never humiliate the one who takes his Lord as friend and patron. (293)

Lowering gaze is also reducing the chance of receiving or projecting the Evil Eye, the poisonous arrow (Satan), with the glances which can cause catastrophic consequences.

298. Prohibition of Meeting a Non-Mahram Woman in Seclusion

Allah, the Exalted, says:

"And when you ask (his wives) for something, ask them from behind a partition. That is purer for your hearts and their hearts." (Qur'an, Al-Ahzab 33:53)

"O you who believe! Follow not the footsteps of Shaitan (Satan). And whosoever follows the footsteps of Shaitan (Satan), then, verily he commands Al-Fahsha' [i.e. to commit indecency (illegal sexual intercourse, etc.)], and Al-Munkar [disbelief and polytheism (i.e. to do evil and wicked deeds; to speak or to do what is forbidden in Islam, etc.)]." (Qur'an, An-Nur 24:21)

'Uqbah bin 'Amir (May Allah be pleased with him) said: The Messenger of Allah (peace and blessings be upon him) said, "Avoid (entering a place) in which are women (uncovered or simply to mix with them in seclusion)." A man from the Ansar said, "Tell me about the brother of a woman's husband." He replied, "The brother of a woman's husband is death." (Bukhari and Muslim)

Ibn Abbas (May Allah be pleased with him) said: The Messenger of Allah (peace and blessings be upon him) said, "No one of you should meet a woman in privacy unless she is accompanied by a Mahram (i.e. a relative within the prohibited degrees)." (Bukhari and Muslim)

Commentary: This Hadith strictly prohibits Muslims from meeting a non-Mahram woman in seclusion without her Mahram, in order to avoid the temptation to commit sin of adultery and fornication. (294)

Buraidah (May Allah be pleased with him) said: The Messenger of Allah (peace and blessings be upon him) said, "The sanctity of the wives of Mujahidun (i.e. those who strive hard and fight in the way of Allah) for those who remain at home (i.e. those who do not go to the battlefield to fight Jihad) is like the sanctity of their own mothers. Anyone who remains behind to look after the family of a Mujahid and betrays his trust, will be made to stand on the Day of Resurrection before the Mujahid who will take away from his meritorious deeds whatever he likes till he is satisfied." The Messenger of Allah (peace and blessings be upon him) turned toward us and said, "Now, what do you think (i.e. will he leave anything with him)?" (Muslim)

Prohibition to sit with a strange lady in privacy or to enter her house when she is alone.

Jabir reported Allah's Messenger (peace and blessings be upon him) as saying: "Behold, no person should spend the night with a married woman, but only in case he is married to her or he is her Mahram." (Muslim)

299. Prohibition of Shaking Hands with Non-Mahram Women

Narrated Ma'qil ibn Yassaar: The Messenger of Allah (peace and blessings be upon him) said: "For one of you to be stabbed in the head with an iron needle is better for him than that he should touch a woman who is not permissible for him." (Tabarani)

Muhammad bin Munkadir said that he heard Umaimah bint Ruqaiqah say: "I came to the Prophet (peace be upon him) with some other women, to offer our pledge to him. He said to us: '(I accept your pledge) with regard to what you are able to do. But I do not shake hands with women.'" (Ibn Majah)

Narrated Aisha, the wife of the Prophet (peace and blessings of Allah be upon him): "When the believing women migrated to the Messenger of Allah (peace and blessings of Allah be upon him), they would be tested in accordance with the Words of Allah: *"O Prophet! When believing women come to you to give you the Bai'a (pledge), that they will not associate anything in worship with Allah, that they will not steal, that they will not commit illegal sexual intercourse, that they will not kill their children, that they will not utter slander, intentionally forging falsehood (i.e. by making illegal children belonging to their husbands), and that they will not disobey you in any Ma'ruf (Islamic Monotheism and all that which Islam ordains) then accept their Bai'a (pledge), and ask Allah to forgive them, Verily, Allah is Oft-Forgiving, Most Merciful."* (Qur'an, Al-Mumtahanah 60:12) Aisha said: 'Whoever among the believing women agreed to that, had passed the test, and when the women agreed to that, the Messenger of Allah (peace and blessings of Allah be upon him) said to them: 'Go, for you have given your oath of allegiance.' No, by Allah, the hand of the Messenger of Allah (peace and blessings of Allah be upon him) never touched the hand of any woman, rather they would give their oath of allegiance with words only.' And Aisha said: 'By Allah, the Messenger of Allah (peace and blessings of Allah be upon him) only took the oath of allegiance from the women in the manner prescribed by Allah, and the hand of the Messenger of Allah (peace and blessings of Allah be upon him) never touched the hand of any woman. When he had taken their oath of allegiance he would say, 'I have accepted your oath of allegiance verbally.'" (Bukhari)

There is no doubt that for a man to touch a non-Mahram woman is one of the causes of Fitnah (turmoil, temptation), provocation of desire and committing haram deeds.

300. Meeting and Mixing of Men and Women

Narrated Abdullah (May Allah have mercy on him): The Prophet (peace and blessings be upon him) said: "The woman is Awrah, so when she goes out, the Shaitan seeks to tempt her." (Tirmidhi)

The meeting together, mixing and intermingling of men and women in one place, the crowding of them together, and the revealing and exposing of women to men are prohibited by Almighty Allah. These acts are prohibited because they are among the causes for Fitnah (temptation or trial which implies evil consequences), the arousing of desires, and the committing of indecency and wrongdoing. (295)

A look has the same effect on the heart as a poisonous arrow (Evil Eye) has on its victim. If it does not kill him, it will wound him. It is like a spark of fire in dried grass; if it does not burn all of it; it will still burn some of it.

Allah, the Exalted, says:

"And when you ask (his wives) for anything you want, ask them from behind a screen, that is purer for your hearts and for their hearts." (Qur'an, Al-Ahzab 33:53)

In explaining this Verse, Ibn Kathir (May Allah have mercy on him) said:

"Meaning, as I forbade you to enter their rooms, I forbid you to look at them at all. If one wants to take something from them, one should do so without looking at them. If one wants to ask a woman for something, the same has to be done from behind a screen." (295)

301. Correspondence Between the Sexes

Allah, the Exalted, said:

"O wives of the Prophet! You are not like any other women. If you keep your duty (to Allah), then be not soft in speech, lest he in whose heart is a disease (of hypocrisy, or evil desire for adultery) should be moved with desire, but speak in an honourable manner." (Qur'an, Al-Ahzab 33:32)

To protect lineages and honour, Allah has forbidden Zina (illicit sexual relationships) and has forbidden the means that may lead to that, such as a man being alone with a woman who is not his Mahram, sinful looking, travelling without a Mahram, a woman going out of her house wearing perfume and makeup, and clothed yet naked. Another of these means is a man talking with a woman and her speaking softly to him and tempting him and provoking his desire, making him fall into her trap, whether that is when they meet in the street or talk on the phone, or correspond in writing, etc.

Allah forbade the wives of His Messenger (peace and blessings of Allah be upon him) – who were pure women – to display themselves like that of the times of Ignorance (Jaahiliyyah) or to speak in soft tones lest those in whose hearts was a disease be moved with desire, and He commanded them to speak in an honourable manner. (296)

302. Dating and Romance Scam

Allah, the Exalted, warned:

"O ye who believe! Follow not Satan's footsteps: if any will follow the footsteps of Satan, he will (but) command what is indecent and wrong." (Qur'an, An-Nur 24:21)

Ibn 'Umar (May Allah have mercy on him) narrated: 'Umar delivered a Khutbah to us at Al-Jabiyah. He said: "O you people! Indeed, I have stood among you as the Messenger of Allah (peace and blessings be upon him) stood among us, and he said: "I order you (to stick) to) my Companions, then those who come after them, then those who come after them. Then will spread a man will take an oath when no oath was sought from him, and a witness will testify when his lying testimony was not sought. Behold!

A man is not alone with a woman but the third of them is Shaytan. Adhere to the Jama'ah, beware of separation, for indeed Shaitan is with one, and he is further away from two. Whoever wants the best place in Paradise, then let him stick to the Jama'ah. Whoever rejoices with his good deeds and grieves over his evil deeds, then that is the believer among you." (Tirmidhi)

Dating and romance scams through dating websites or social media with fake profiles designed to lure you in, such as military personnel, professional working abroad, businessman, claiming to be from the western country. As the number of the single women has been increasing, desperate to find their partners, they spend time chatting online, then going out for meeting with possibly sexual adventure. Once the scammers have gained their trust, they will ask for money, gifts or offer the incredible fruitful investment, steal the identity, credit card details, money. The person may pretend to love but in reality, bears enmity and malice for her/him in her/his heart, for example, to get her/his money through love intrigue. Deception through dating with fake love, relationship and along with possible other problems like sexually transmitted diseases.

Islam dictates strict rules: it forbids all forms of "dating" and isolating oneself with a member of the opposite sex, as well indiscriminate mingling and mixing. (297)

Allah, the Exalted, says:

"And if the people of the towns had believed and had the Taqwa (piety), certainly, We should have opened for them blessings from the heaven and the earth." (Qur'an, Al-A'raf 7:96)

A good life is the fruit of faith and righteous deeds.

Allah, the Exalted, says:

"Whoever works righteousness — whether male or female — while he (or she) is a true believer (of Islamic Monotheism) verily, to him We will give a good life (in this world with respect, contentment and lawful provision), and We shall pay them certainly a reward in proportion to the best of what they used to do (i.e. Paradise in the Hereafter)." (Qur'an, An-Nahl 16:97)

303. Revealing one's Nudity

Allah, the Exalted, says:

"and to draw their veils all over Juyubihinna (i.e. their bodies, faces, necks and bosoms, etc.)…" (Qur'an, An-Nur 24:31)

"O Children of Adam! We have bestowed raiment upon you to cover yourselves (screen your private parts, etc.) and as an adornment, and the raiment of righteousness, that is better. Such are among the Ayat (proofs, evidences, verses, lessons, signs, revelations, etc.) of Allah, that they may remember (i.e. leave falsehood and follow Truth)." (Qur'an, Al-A'raf 7:26)

Yahya related to me from Malik from Muslim ibn Abi Maryam from Abu Salih that Abu Hurairah said, "Women who are naked even though they are wearing clothes, go astray and make others go astray, and they will not enter the Garden and they will not find its scent, and its scent is experienced from as far as the distance traveled in five hundred years." (Malik Muwaṭṭa)

Mu'awiyah ibn Haydah reported: "I said, "O Messenger of Allah, when should we cover our *Awrah* (parts of the body that need to be covered in front of others) and when may we uncover it?" He said, "Protect (cover) your *Awrah* from everyone except your wife and those whom your right hand possesses." I said, "O Messenger of Allah, what about when one of us is alone?" He said, "Allah is more deserving than the people that you should be modest before Him." (Tirmidhi)

Jabir b. 'Abdullah reported: "The Messenger of Allah (peace and blessings be upon him) was carrying along with them (his people) stones for the Ka'bah and there was a waist wrapper around him. His uncle, Abbas, said to him: 'O son of my brother! if you take off the lower garment and place it on the shoulders underneath the stones, it would be better. He (the Holy Prophet) took it off and placed it on his shoulder and fell down unconscious. He (the narrator) said: 'Never was he seen naked after that day.'" (Muslim)

On the authority of Abu Dharr al-Ghifaree (May Allah be pleased with him) from the Prophet (peace and blessings of Allah be upon him) from his Lord, that He said: "…O My servants, all of you are astray except those whom I have guided, so seek guidance from Me and I shall guide you. O My servants, all of you are hungry except those whom I have fed, so seek food from Me and I shall feed you. O My servants, all of you are naked except those whom I have clothed, so seek clothing from Me and I shall clothe you. O My servants, you commit sins by day and by night, and I forgive all sins, so seek forgiveness from Me and I shall forgive you….O My servants, it is but your deeds that I account for you, and then recompense you for. So, he who finds good, let him praise Allah, and he who finds other than that, let him blame no one but himself." (Muslim) (https://sunnah.com/nawawi 40:24)

304. Touching the Body of a Stranger

Narrated Ma'qil ibn Yassaar: The Messenger of Allah (peace and blessings of Allah be upon him) said: "For one of you to be stabbed in the head with an iron needle is better for him than that he should touch a woman who is not permissible for him." (Tabarani)

Narrated Aisha, the wife of the Prophet (peace and blessings be upon him). She said: "When the believing women migrated (to Madinah) and came to the Messenger of Allah (peace be upon him), they would be tested in accordance with the following Words of Allah the Almighty and Exalted: "O Prophet, when believing women come to thee to take the oath of fealty to thee that they will not associate in worshiping anything with God, that they will not steal. that, they will not commit adultery… to the end of the Verse (*60:12*). Whoso from the believing women accepted these conditions and agreed to abide by them were considered to have offered themselves for swearing fealty. When they had (formally) their declared resolve to do so, the Messenger of Allah (may peace be upon him) would say to them: You may go. I have confirmed your faith. By God, the hand of the Messenger of Allah (peace be upon him) never touched the hand of a woman. He would take the oath of fealty from them by oral declaration. By God, the Messenger of Allah (peace be upon him) never took any vow from women except that which God had ordered him to take, and his palm never touched the palm of a woman. When he had taken their vow, he would tell them that he had taken the oath from them orally." (Muslim)

305. Accusation of Immorality Without Proof

Allah, the Exalted, says:

"Verily, those who accuse chaste women, who never even think of anything touching their chastity and are good believers - are cursed in this life and in the Hereafter, and for them will be a great torment." (Qur'an, An-Nur 24:23)

"And those who accuse chaste women and produce not four witnesses, flog them with eighty stripes, and reject their testimony forever. They, indeed, are the Fasiqun (liars, rebellious, disobedient to Allah)." (Qur'an, An-Nur 24:4)

Narrated Abu Hurairah (May Allah have mercy on him): The Prophet (peace and blessings be upon him) said, "Avoid the seven great destructive sins." The people enquire, "O Allah's Apostle! What are they?" He said, "To join others in worship along with Allah, to practice sorcery, to kill the life which Allah has forbidden except for a just cause (according to Islamic Law), to eat up Riba (usury), to eat up an orphan's wealth, to show one's back to the enemy and fleeing from the battlefield at the time of fighting, and to accuse chaste women, who never even think of anything touching chastity and are good believers." (Bukhari)

The wisdom behind the Hadd punishment for slander:

1. It prevents accusations of immorality.
2. It protects people's honor from being transgressed and protects their reputations from being tarnished.
3. It prevents enmity and grudges; wars may break out because of slurs against people's honor.
4. It prevents such things becoming part of public opinion and protects people from having to hear them
5. It prevents the spread of rumours among the believers, because when there are a lot of accusations and such talk becomes common and is easily spoken of, the foolish become bold enough to commit such actions. (298)

The story of the accusation of adultery levied against Aisha (May Allah be pleased with her), the wife of the Prophet Muhammad (peace and blessings be upon him), also known as the Event of Ifk. Muhammad (peace and blessings be upon him) came to speak directly with Aisha about the rumors. He was still sitting in her house when he announced that he had received a Revelation from God confirming Aisha's innocence. (299)

Allah, the Exalted, said:

"Allah forbids you from it (slander) and warns you not to repeat the like of it forever, if you are believers." (Qur'an, An-Nur 24:17)

Aisha (May Allah be pleased with her) reported: "When my vindication was revealed, the Prophet (May Allah's peace and blessings be upon him) got up onto the pulpit, mentioned what happened, and recited (the Verses of the Qur'an that had been revealed). When he came down from the pulpit, he ordered that the two men and the woman (who made the false accusation) be given their prescribed punishment (eighty lashes)." (Ibn Majah) (https://hadeethenc.com/en/browse/hadith/58241)

Slandering Aisha implies insulting the Prophet (peace and blessings be upon him) because Allah, the Exalted, says:

"Bad statements are for bad people (or bad women for bad men) and bad people for bad statements (or bad men for bad women)..." (Qur'an, An-Nur 24:26)

306. Accusation of Pedophilia Against Prophet Muhammad

Allah, the Exalted, says:

"And those of your women as have passed the age of monthly courses, for them the 'Iddah (prescribed period), if you have doubts (about their periods), is three months, and for those who have no courses [(i.e. they are still immature) their 'Iddah (prescribed period) is three months likewise, except in case of death]." (Qur'an, At-Talaq 65:4)

"And verily, you (O Muhammad SAW) are on an exalted standard of character." (Qur'an, Al-Qalam 68:4)

Narrated Aisha (May Allah be pleased with her): Allah's Apostle (peace and blessings be upon him) said to me, "You have been shown to me twice in my dreams. A man was carrying you in a silken cloth and said to me, 'This is your wife.' I uncovered it; and behold, it was you. I said to myself, 'If this dream is from Allah, He will cause it to come true.'" (Bukhari)

Aisha (May Allah be pleased with her) said: "The Prophet (peace and blessings of Allah be upon him) married me when I was six years old. Then we came to Madinah and stayed in Bani al-Haarith ibn Khazraj. I fell ill and my hair started to fall out (due to the illness; then it grew back thick again). My mother Umm Roomaan came to me whilst I was on a swing and my friends were with me. She shouted for me and I came to her, not knowing what she wanted. She took me by the hand and led me to the door of the house. I was out of breath and we waited until I had calmed down, then she took some water and wiped my face and head, then took me inside. There were some women of the Ansar in the house, and they said: "'Alaa al-khayri wa'l-baraka wa 'ala khayri taa'ir (blessings, best wishes, etc.)." My mother handed me over to them and they tidied me up, then suddenly the Messenger of Allah (peace and blessings of Allah be upon him) was there. It was mid-morning, and they handed me over to him. At that time, I was nine years old." (Bukhari)

'Urwah said: "Khadeejah died three years before the Prophet (peace and blessings of Allah be upon him) migrated to Madinah. He stayed alone for two years or thereabouts, then he married Aisha when she was six years old, and consummated the marriage when she was nine years old." (Bukhari)

The marriage of the Prophet Muhammad (peace and blessings be upon him) with Aisha (May Allah be pleased with her) was indeed a Divine Decree.

Puberty in Islam starts with getting the first period (menstruation). From the age of puberty, the marriage is allowed.

Marriage in Islam is not simply about sex. Marriage is a spiritual agreement based upon *"love and mercy."*

Allah, the Exalted, says:

"And among His Signs is this, that He created for you wives from among yourselves, that you may find repose in them, and He has put between you affection and mercy. Verily, in that are indeed signs for a people who reflect." (Qur'an, Ar-Rum 30:21)

Ratifying a marriage contract does not necessitate sex. There is no evidence whatsoever that the Prophet had sex with Aisha before puberty. In light of this, it cannot be said that there is any evidence at all that the Prophet committed pedophilia. (300)

Being young and the closest to the Holy Prophet, Aisha had an important role in early Islamic history, both during Muhammad's life and after his death. In Sunni tradition, Aisha is portrayed as scholarly and inquisitive. She contributed to the spread of Muhammad's message and served the Muslim community for 44 years after his death. She is known for narrating 2,210 Ahadith. That's was Allah's Plan.

This unjust accusation of the Prophet of pedophilia includes many Major sins: Disbelieving in Destiny (Qadar), Speaking without knowledge, Slander, Defamation, Skepticism, Making Fun, etc.

307. Prohibition of Sexual Intercourse During Menstruation and Post-Natal Bleeding

Allah, the Exalted, says:

"They ask you concerning menstruation. Say: that is an Adha (a harmful thing for a husband to have a sexual intercourse with his wife while she is having her menses), therefore keep away from women during menses and go not unto them till they have purified (from menses and have taken a bath). And when they have purified themselves, then go in unto them as Allah has ordained for you (go in unto them in any manner as long as it is in their vagina). Truly, Allah loves those who turn unto Him in repentance and loves those who purify themselves (by taking a bath, and cleaning and washing thoroughly their private parts, bodies, for their prayers, etc.)." (Qur'an, Al-Baqarah 2:222)

Ibn 'Abbas said: "If one has intercourse in the beginning of the menses, (one should give) one dinar; in case one has intercourse towards the end of the menses, then half a dinar (should be given)." (Abu Dawud)

Ibn 'Abbas (May Allah's peace and blessings be upon him) reported: The Prophet (May Allah's peace and blessings be upon him) said concerning a man who engages in sexual intercourse with his wife during her menses: "Let him give one dinar or half a dinar in charity." (Ibn Majah, An-Nasa'i, Abu Dawud, Ahmad, Al-Darimi) (https://hadeethenc.com/en/browse/hadith/10012)

308. Not Performing Ghusl after Menstruation and Post-Natal Bleeding

Allah, the Exalted, says:

"And when they have purified themselves, then come to them from where Allah has ordained for you." (Qur'an, Al-Baqarah 2:222)

309. Praying and Fasting while Menstruating

Narrated 'Aisha (May Allah be pleased with her): The Prophet (peace and blessings of Allah be upon him) said to me, "Give up the prayer when your menses begin, and when it has finished, wash the blood off your body (take a bath) and start praying." (Bukhari)

Narrated Abu Sa'id Al-Khudri: "Once Allah's Messenger (peace and blessings of Allah be upon him) went out to the Musalla (to offer the prayer) of EId-al-Adha or Al-Fitr prayer. Then he passed by the women and said, "O women! Give alms, as I have seen that the majority of the dwellers of Hellfire were you (women)." They asked, "Why is it so, O Allah's Messenger?" He replied, "You curse frequently and are ungrateful to your husbands. I have not seen anyone more deficient in intelligence and religion than you. A cautious sensible man could be led astray by some of you." The women asked, "O Allah's Messenger! What is deficient in our intelligence and religion?" He said, "Is not the evidence of two women equal to the witness of one man?" They replied in the affirmative. He (peace and blessings of Allah be upon him) said, "This is the deficiency in her intelligence. Isn't it true that a woman can neither pray nor fast during her menses?" The women replied in the affirmative. He said, "This is the deficiency in her religion." (Bukhari)

Narrated Mu'adha: "A woman asked Aisha, "Should I offer the prayers that which I did not offer because of menses?" Aisha said, "Are you from the Huraura' (a town in Iraq)? We were with the Prophet (peace and blessings of Allah be upon him) and used to get our periods but he never ordered us to offer them (the Prayers missed during menses)." Aisha perhaps said, "We did not offer them." (Muslim)

310. Not Performing Ghusl After Sexual Intercourse or Seminal Emission

Ghusl is obligatory when:

1. Emission of semen even if it is not through intercourse.

Abu Sa'id al-Khudri (May Allah be pleased with him) reported: "The Apostle of Allah (peace and blessings be upon him) observed: "Bathing is obligatory in case of seminal emission." (Muslim)

Abu Sa'id al-Khudri (May Allah be pleased with him) said: The Prophet (peace and blessings of Allah be upon him) said: "Water is for water (i.e. Ghusl must be done when semen is emitted)." (Muslim)

2. When male and female come in close contact, Ghusl becomes compulsory.

Narrated Abu Hurairah (May Allah be pleased with him): The Prophet (peace and blessings of Allah be upon him) said: "When a man sits between the four parts of woman and has intercourse with her, then Ghusl is obligatory." (Bukhari and Muslim added: "Even if he does not ejaculate.")

Aisha (May Allah have mercy on her) reported: "When Allah's Messenger (peace and blessings be upon him) bathed because of sexual intercourse, he first washed his hands, he then poured water with his right hand on his left hand and washed his private parts. He then performed ablution as is done for prayer. He then took some water and put his fingers and moved them through the roots of his hair. And when he found that these had been properly moistened, then poured three handfuls on his head and then poured water over his body and subsequently washed his feet." (Muslim)

Narrated Abu Hurairah (May Allah be pleased with him): The Apostle of Allah (peace and blessings be upon him) said: "When a man has sexual intercourse, bathing becomes obligatory (both for the male and the female). In the Hadith of Matar the words are: Even if there is no orgasm. Zuhair has narrated it with a minor alteration of words." (Muslim)

Abu Sa'id al-Khudri (May Allah be pleased with him) reported: The Messenger of Allah (peace and blessings be upon him) said: "When anyone amongst you has sexual intercourse with his wife and then he intends to repeat it, he should perform ablution." (Muslim)

311. Not Performing Ghusl for a Woman After Experiencing Orgasm in Dream

Umm Salamah (May Allah be pleased with her) reported: Umm Sulaym, the wife of Abu Talhah, came to the Messenger of Allah (May Allah's peace and blessings be upon him) and said: "O Messenger of Allah, verily, Allah does not feel shy of the truth. If a woman had a wet dream, would it be obligatory on her to take a ritual bath (Ghusl)?" He replied: "Yes, if she sees vaginal fluid." (Bukhari and Muslim) (https://hadeethenc.com/en/browse/hadith/3351)

Anas b. Malik reported: "Umm Sulaim who was the grandmother of Ishaq came to the Messenger of Allah (May peace and blessings be upon him) in the presence of Aisha and said to him: 'Messenger of Allah, in case or woman sees what a man sees in dream and she experiences in dream what a man experiences (i.e. experiences orgasm)?' Upon this Aisha remarked: 'O Umm Sulaim, you brought humiliation to women; may your right hand be covered with dust. He (the Holy Prophet) said to Aisha: 'Let your hand be covered with dust', and (addressing Umm Sulaim) said: 'Well, O Umm Sulaim, she should take a bath if she sees that (i.e. she experiences orgasm in dream).'" (Muslim)

Ibn 'Abbas said: "Water is for water' is only about the wet dream." (Tirmidhi)

312. Pornography

Allah, the Exalted, warns:

"O you who believe! Follow not the footsteps of Shaitan (Satan). And whosoever follows the footsteps of Shaitan (Satan), then, verily he commands Al-Fahisha' [i.e. to commit indecency (illegal sexual intercourse, etc.)]…" (Qur'an, An-Nur 24:21)

"Tell the believing men to lower their gaze (from looking at forbidden things) and protect their private parts (from illegal sexual acts, etc.). That is purer for them. Verily, Allah is All-Aware of what they do." (Qur'an, An-Nur 24:30)

"Verily, the hearing, and the sight, and the heart of each of those ones will be questioned (by Allah)." (Qur'an, Al-Isra 17:36)

Other Verses: *An-Nur 24:31, Al-Isra 17:32, Al-Jathiyah 45:23, Ali 'Imran 3:14, Ghafir 40:19, Al-An'am 6:128.*

Sahl ibn Sa'd (May Allah be pleased with him) reported that the Prophet (May Allah's peace and blessings be upon him) said: "Whoever guarantees for me to safeguard what is between his jaws and what is between his legs, I shall guarantee Paradise for him." (Bukhari)

'Abdullah ibn Masud (May Allah be pleased with him) reported: The Prophet (May Allah's peace and blessings be upon him) said: "O young men, those of you who can support a wife should marry; for it eyes from casting (evil glances). and preserves one from immorality; but those who cannot, should fast; it controls the sexual desire." (Bukhari and Muslim) (https://hadeethenc.com/en/browse/hadith/5863)

Abu Hurairah (May Allah be pleased with him) reported Allah's Messenger (peace and blessings be upon him) as saying: "Allah fixed the very portion of adultery which a man will indulge in. There would be no escape from it. The adultery of the eye is the lustful look and the adultery of the ears is listening to voluptuous (song or talk) and the adultery of the tongue is licentious speech and the adultery of the hand is the lustful grip (embrace) and the adultery of the feet is to walk (to the place) where he intends to commit adultery and the heart years and desires which he may or may not put into effect." (Muslim)

Pornography is one of signs of the Jinn (Demonic) Possession. Satan will approach you by tempting you first into Minor sins, leading you step by step into the commission of bigger evils. Looking upon that which is forbidden is a classic tactic of Satan; one that sets you on a path that will lead you to commit a more serious evil. When one continues to look at that which is forbidden, one can get hooked and addicted to these illicit images. Satan can lay a firm grip on his victim, to the point that the individual will not be able to control him or herself.

Dangers of Pornography:

Amongst the harms of watching pornographic images or videos are its negative effects and ultimate destroyer of one's Iman (faith), heart and spirituality. Porn consumption weakens one's connection with God, weakening one's prayers. The eyes are the most direct path to the heart. The act of seeing that which is prohibited violates and corrupts the soul. Do not stand amongst those who are enslaved by their desires, as the one who is controlled by his whims and desires is indeed a prisoner.

Effects of not lowering your gaze: beneficial knowledge deprivation, removal of Allah's blessings, support, protection, provision, capabilities of accomplishing certain acts of worship, physical weakness, anxiety, hardening of the heart, lowering one's self-esteem or confidence, shame, morals and even motivation. Watching pornographic images and videos increases the risk of loneliness and depression, and deplete valuable time that can be spent on more beneficial things.

Pornography can wreck many negative effects on one's marriage, mind, eyes, organs and reproductive system. Pornography can lead to sexual dysfunctions, such as erectile dysfunction or delayed ejaculation. Watching pornography has devastating effects on the brain and will have one constantly checking out the people around them with a lustful gaze and intent.

Pornography Addiction:

Pornography Addiction involves the Evil Jinn. Pornography addiction leads to other sins and destructive outcomes, and punishment in the Hereafter.

How to Stop Watching Pornography:

Allah, the Exalted, says:

"Till, when they reach it (Hellfire), their hearing (ears) and their eyes, and their skins will testify against them as to what they used to do." (Qur'an, Fussilat 41:20)

Other Verses: Hud 11:114, Al-'Ankabut 29:45.

Pray to God to seek forgiveness, help and guidance. Fear the Judgment Day when everyone will be held accountable for the actions. One's own body parts will testify against him, for using them to disobey the Creator.

God the Almighty connects the respectful lowering of one's gaze with the protecting of one's private parts. He mentions the gaze first, as what the eyes view influences the heart. When one lowers their gaze, they are in obedience to God's command. Lowering one's gaze purifies the eyes and the soul and illuminates the heart. It increases one's wisdom, steadfastness, courage and quality of intuition. The one that lowers gaze will feel the sweetness and pleasure of his or her Iman (faith) in their heart. (301)

313. Distributing Massage Parlour Cards

Distribution of massage service cards with lewd images of undressed women by throwing cards on the roadside or sticking them on vehicles, by internet is a Major sin.

314. Public Massage and Bathhouse

Abu Said (May Allah be pleased with him) reported: The Messenger of Allah (May Allah's peace and blessings be upon him) said: "A man must not look at another man's 'Awrah, nor must a woman look at another woman's 'Awrah; neither should two men lie undressed and touch under one cover, nor should two women lie undressed and touch under one cover." (Muslim)

(https://hadeethenc.com/en/browse/hadith/8904)

Narrated Aisha (May Allah be pleased with her): "The Prophet (peace and blessings be upon him) forbade men and women to enter bathhouses, then he allowed men to enter them wearing a waist wrap, but he did not make the same allowance for women." (Ibn Majah)

Al-Qasim bin Abil-Qasim as-Saba'i narrated from a preacher who was addressing the troops in al-Qustanteeniyyah, that he heard him narrate that Umar bin al-Khattab (May Allah be pleased with him, said: "O people, I heard the Messenger of Allah (peace and blessings be upon him) say: 'Whoever believes in Allah and the Last Day, let him not sit at passed a table where alcohol is being around; Whoever believes in Allah and the Last Day, let him not enter a bathhouse unless he is wearing a waist wrapper; and whoever (among women) believes in Allah and the Last Day, let her not enter bathhouses (at all).'" (Ahmad)

Narrated Yala: "The Messenger of Allah (peace and blessings be upon him) saw a man performing Ghusl in an open place, so he ascended the Minbar and praised and glorified Allah, then he said; 'Allah, the Mighty and Sublime, is Forbearing, Modest and Concealing, and He loves modesty and concealment. When any one of you performs Ghusl, let him conceal himself.'" (An-Nasa'i)

Narrated Abu Malih Al-Hudhail that some women from the people of Hims asked permission to enter upon Aisha. She (May Allah be pleased with her) said: "Perhaps you are among those (women) who enter bathhouses? I heard the Messenger of Allah (peace and blessings be upon him) say: 'Any woman who takes off her clothes anywhere but in her husband's house, has torn the screen between her and Allah.'" (Ibn Majah)

Narrated Bahz bin Hakim: "My father narrated to me from my grandfather, who said: 'I said: "O Messenger of Allah! Regarding our 'Awrah, what of it must we cover and what of it may we leave?" He said: "Protect your 'Awrah except from your wife or what your right hand possesses."' He said: "What about a man with another man?" He said: "If you are able to not let anyone see it, then do so." I said: "What about a man when he is alone?" He said: "Allah is most deserving of being shy from Him." (Tirmidhi)

Looking at 'Awrahs and touching and massaging parts of the body may provoke desire and lead to temptation and evil.

The massage is a kind of pleasure which can be done at home by one's wife or using machines.

315. Night, Strip, Sex Clubs

Night, Strip, Sex clubs involve multiple Major sins: alcohol, smoking, mixing and intermingling of men and women, music, dance, singing, looking at non-mahram, touching, forbidden dress, Zina of eyes, ears, hand, feet, etc.

316. Begging

Allah, the Exalted, says:

"And in their properties, there was the right of the beggar, and the Mahrum (the poor who does not ask the others)." (Qur'an, Adh-Dhariyat 51:19)

"For the beggar who asks, and for the unlucky who has lost his property and wealth, (and his means of living has been straitened)." (Qur'an, Al-Ma'arij 70:25)

"…And whosoever fears Allah and keeps his duty to Him, He will make a way for him to get out (from every difficulty). And He will provide him from (sources) he never could imagine. And whosoever puts his trust in Allah, then He will suffice him. Verily, Allah will accomplish his purpose. Indeed, Allah has set a measure for all things." (Qur'an, At-Talaq 65:2-3)

Other Verses: Hud 11:6, Al-Baqarah 2:177 and 2:273, Adh-Dhariyat 51:56-57, Ad-Duha 93:10.

Narrated Abu Hurairah: The Prophet (peace and blessings be upon him) said, "Richness is not the abundance of wealth, rather it is self-sufficiency." (Bukhari and Muslim)

'Abdullah bin 'Amr bin Al-As (May Allah be pleased with him) reported: The Messenger of Allah (peace and blessings be upon him) said, "Successful is the one who has entered the fold of Islam and is provided with sustenance which is sufficient for his needs, and Allah makes him content with what He has bestowed upon him." (Muslim)

Hakim bin Hizam (May Allah be pleased with him) reported: "I begged Messenger of Allah (peace and blessings be upon him) and he gave me; I begged him again and he gave me. I begged him again and he gave me and said, "O Hakim, wealth is pleasant and sweet. He who acquires it with self-contentment, it becomes a source of blessing for him; but it is not blessed for him who seeks it out of greed. He is like one who goes on eating but his hunger is not satisfied. The upper hand is better than the lower one." I said to him, "O Messenger of Allah, by Him Who sent you with the Truth, I will not, after you, ask anyone for anything till I leave this world." So, Abu Bakr (May Allah be pleased with him) would summon Hakim

(May Allah be pleased with him) to give his rations, but he would refuse. Then 'Umar (May Allah be pleased with him) would call him but he would decline to accept anything. So 'Umar (May Allah be pleased with him) said addressing Muslims: "O Muslims, I ask you to bear testimony that I offer Hakim his share of the booty that Allah has assigned for him but he refuses my offer." Thus, Hakim did not accept anything from anyone after the death of Messenger of Allah (peace and blessings be upon him), till he died. (Bukhari and Muslim)

Hakim bin Hizam (May Allah be pleased with him) reported: The Prophet (peace and blessings be upon him) said, "The upper hand is better than the lower one; and begin (charity) with those who are under your care; and the best charity is (the one which is given) out of surplus; and he who wishes to abstain from begging will be protected by Allah; and he who seeks self-sufficiency will be made self-sufficient by Allah." (Bukhari)

Abu Sufyan (May Allah be pleased with him) reported: The Messenger of Allah (peace and blessings be upon him) said, "Do not be importunate in begging. By Allah! If one of you asks me for something and I give it to him unwillingly, there is no blessing in what I give him." (Muslim)

'Auf bin Malik Al-Ashja'i (May Allah be pleased with him) reported: "Seven, eight or nine people, including myself, were with Messenger of Allah (peace be upon him) on an occasion when he (peace be upon him) remarked, "Would you pledge allegiance to Messenger of Allah?" As we had taken oath of allegiance shortly before, we said, "We have already done so, O Messenger of Allah." He again asked, "Would you not pledge allegiance to Messenger of Allah?" So, we stretched out our hands and said, "We have already made our pledge with you, O Messenger of Allah, on what should we make a pledge with you?" He said, "To worship Allah and not to associate anything with Him, to perform the five (daily) Salat and to obey." Then he added in a low tone, "And not to ask people for anything." Thereafter, I noticed that some of these people who were present did not ask anyone to pick up even the whip for them if it fell from their hands. (Muslim)

Abdullah ibn Umar reported: The Prophet (peace and blessings be upon him) said, "A man continues to beg people until he will come on the Day of Resurrection without any flesh on his face." (Bukhari and Muslim)

Narrated Ibn Umar: "I heard Allah's Apostle (peace and blessings be upon him) while he was on the pulpit speaking about charity, to abstain from asking others for some financial help and about begging others, saying, "The upper hand is better than the lower hand. The upper hand is that of the giver and the lower (hand) is that of the beggar." (Bukhari)

Abu Hurairah (May Allah be pleased with him) reported: The Messenger of Allah (peace and blessings be upon him) said, "He who begs to increase his riches is in fact asking only for a live coal. It is up to him to decrease it or increase it." (Muslim)

Samurah bin Jundub (May Allah be pleased with him) reported: The Messenger of Allah (peace be upon him) said, "Begging is a cut that a person inflicts upon his face; except for asking a ruler, or under the stress of circumstances from which there is no escape." (Tirmidhi)

Ibn Masud (May Allah be pleased with him) reported that the Prophet (May Allah's peace and blessings be upon him) said: "He who is inflicted with poverty and seeks relief from people, he will not be relieved; whereas he who seeks relief from Allah, he will be given sustenance from Allah sooner or later." (Tirmidhi and Abu Dawud)

Thawban, the client of the Messenger of Allah (May peace and blessings be upon him), reported him as saying: "If anyone guarantees me that he will not beg from people, I will guarantee him Paradise." Thawban said: "I (will not beg). He never asked anyone for anything." (Sunan Abi Dawud)

Abu Hurairah (May Allah be pleased with him) reported: The Messenger of Allah (May Allah's peace and blessings be upon him) said: "The needy is not the one who can be turned away with a date-fruit or two, or a morsel or two. But the needy is the one who abstains from begging." (Bukhari and Muslim)

Commentary: The professional beggars and the truly needy have clearly been identified here. The point is that we should try to find out deserving people and spend on them. Because, despite being needy, they do not wear a professional look nor do they approach anybody to receive alms. In no way will it be counted as charity if we satisfy ourselves by giving a few coins to a professional beggar whom we come across on the road. (302)

Narrated Abu Sa'id al-Khudri (May Allah be pleased with him) that some people from among the Ansaar asked the Messenger of Allah (peace and blessings of Allah be upon him) and he gave them, then they asked him and he gave them, then they asked him and he gave them, until what he had was exhausted. He said: "Whatever I have of good I will never withhold from you, but whoever refrains from asking (of people), Allah will make him content; whoever seeks to be independent of means, Allah will make him independent; and whoever strives to be patient, Allah will bestow patience upon him, and no one is ever given anything better and more abundant than patience." (Bukhari and Muslim)

Narrated Al-Mughira bin Shuba: The Prophet (peace and blessings be upon him) said, "Allah has forbidden for you to be undutiful to your mothers, to bury your daughters alive, do not to pay the rights of the others (e.g. charity, etc.) and to beg of men (begging). And Allah has hated for you Qil and Qal (useless talk or that you talk too much about others), to ask too many questions (in disputed religious matters) and to waste the wealth (by extravagance with lack of wisdom and thinking)." (Bukhari)

Here are more of Prohibition of Begging

1. Benefiting from Begging

Many people misunderstood the meaning of begging, take it as one way to collect money. They even make begging as a fixed job. To assure others, they pretend to be sick and wear torn clothes. This act of lie is not allowed, as Allah, the Exalted, says:

"In their hearts is a disease (of doubt and hypocrisy) and Allah has increased their disease. A painful torment is theirs because they used to tell lies." (Qur'an, Al-Baqarah 2:10)

2. Begging is Not asking for help. If a Muslim thinks that begging is similar with asking for a help, it's completely wrong. It called help when the benefits can be felt by others as well. This one example is when the Prophet (peace be upon him) asked help to make a pulpit.

3. Begging makes someone depend on others for living. It's not the right act since one can only depend on Allah and himself in any condition.

4. Don't make begging as a habit or even a job since all you will get from begging is endless laziness by getting money without having to work hard. Islam is a religion who value work hard more than anything.

5. Our Creator prohibited to live on the wealth of other people. Working on your own even when you don't make much is better.

6. Begging brings inconvenience to others. For an instance, begging from someone who doesn't have money, who lost job or begging on the traffic lights. People who are travelling and some of them are probably in a rush may feel disturbed by the beggars.

7. Begging could become a big sin when someone has an ill intention behind it. Such as enriching himself.

The above warnings are for those who are able to earn a livelihood, and thereby have no excuse for begging.

However, when we are approached by beggars, we should not reproach them. Either donate something or speak what is good, or politely excuse yourself. (303)

Encouraging working

Allah, the Exalted, says:

"Then when the (Jumu'ah) Salat (prayer) is finished, you may disperse through the land, and seek the Bounty of Allah (by working, etc.), and remember Allah much, that you may be successful." (Qur'an, Al-Jumu'ah 62:10)

Zubair bin 'Awwam (May Allah be pleased with him) reported: The Messenger of Allah (peace and blessings be upon him) said, "It is far better for you to take your rope, go to the mountain (cut some firewood), carry it on your back, and sell it and thereby save your face than begging from people whether they give you or refuse." (Bukhari)

Abu Hurairah (May Allah be pleased with him) reported: The Messenger of Allah (peace and blessings be upon him) said, "It is better for anyone of you to carry a bundle of wood on his back and sell it than to beg of someone whether he gives him or refuses." (Bukhari and Muslim)

Abu Hurairah (May Allah be pleased with him) reported: The Prophet (peace be upon him) said, "(Prophet) Dawud (peace be upon him) ate only out of that which he earned through his manual work." (Bukhari)

Commentary: Labor and manual work make the living of a man good, laudable and excellent. The Prophets also earned their living with their own work. Upon such earnings we get the blessing of Allah. (304)

Abu Hurairah (May Allah be pleased with him) reported: Messenger of Allah (peace be upon him) said, "(Prophet) Zakariyya (peace be upon him) was a carpenter." (Bukhari)

Begging is allowed in certain circumstances

Qabisah bin Al-Mukhariq (May Allah be pleased with him) reported: "I stood as surety for a debt and came to Messenger of Allah (peace and blessings be upon him) to seek his help in discharging it. Messenger of Allah (peace and blessings be upon him) said, "Wait till we receive charity and I shall give you out of it." He (peace and blessings be upon him) added, "O Qabisah, begging is not lawful except for three people. One who has incurred debt (for assuming guarantee), for him begging is permissible till the guarantee is discharged and he should then refrain; a person whose property has been destroyed by a calamity is allowed to beg till he attains self-sufficiency; a person who meets with dire necessity (due to hunger) provided that three men of understanding from his people affirm the genuineness (of his poverty), for him begging is lawful till he attains means of his subsistence. Other than these, O Qabisah, anything received through begging is unlawful, its recipient devours it unlawfully." (Muslim)

Commentary: This Hadith explicitly tells us about the three types of men who are allowed to beg of others. (302)

317. About Begging in the Name of Allah

Jabir (May Allah be pleased with him) said: The Messenger of Allah (peace and blessings be upon him) said, "No one should ask in the Face of Allah for anything except Jannah." (Abu Dawud)

Ibn 'Umar (May Allah be pleased with him) said: The Messenger of Allah (peace and blessings be upon him) said, "Grant shelter to him who begs for it in the Name of Allah, give to him who begs in the Name of Allah, accept the invitation of him who invites you, and requite him who does a favor to you, but if you are unable to requite him, go on praying for him till you are sure that you have requited him adequately." (Abu Dawud and An-Nasa'i)

Commentary: The following points are clear from this Hadith:

First, supplicating for safety and asking in the Name of Allah is endorsed.

Second, if a person begs in the Name of Allah, he should not be turned down. He must be given something to honor the Name of Allah. However, if one is sure that the petitioner is a professional beggar and does not stand in need of what he is begging, then it is better to turn him down in order to discourage the evil of begging in the society. (305)

318. Greediness

Allah, the Exalted, says:

"But he who is greedy miser and thinks himself self-sufficient. And gives the lie to Al-Husna; We will make smooth for him the path for evil; And what will his wealth benefit him when he goes down (in destruction)." (Qur'an, Al-Layl 92:8-11)

"And do not let those who greedily withhold Allah's bounties think it is good for them—in fact, it is bad for them! They will be leashed´ by their necks` on the Day of Judgment with whatever ´wealth` they used to withhold. And Allah is the ´sole´ inheritor of the heavens and the earth. And Allah is All-Aware of what you do." (Qur'an, Ali 'Imran 3:180)

Other Verses: Al-Baqarah 2:268, At-Tawbah 9:34-35.

Hakim ibn Hizam (May Allah be pleased with him) reported: "I asked the Messenger of Allah (May Allah's peace and blessings be upon him) for some money and he gave me. Then I asked him again and he gave me. Then I asked him again and he gave me, and then he said: "O Hakim, this money is like a sweet fresh fruit; whoever takes it without greediness, he is blessed in it, and whoever takes it with greediness, he is not blessed in it, and he is like a person who eats but is never satisfied; and the giving hand is better than the receiving hand.'" Hakim added: "I said: 'O Messenger of Allah, by the One Who sent you with the truth, I shall never accept anything from anyone after you until I leave this world.'" Then Abu Bakr (May Allah be pleased with him) (during his caliphate) would call Hakim to give him his share from the war booty and he would refuse to take anything. Then 'Umar (May Allah be pleased with him) (during his caliphate) called him to give him his share but he refused. Upon that, 'Umar said: "O Muslims, I would like you to bear witness that I offer Hakim his share from this booty that Allah entitled him to, and he refuses to take it." Thus, Hakim never took anything from anybody after the Prophet (May Allah's peace and blessings be upon him) till he died." (Bukhari and Muslim)

Narrated Anas bin Malik (May Allah have mercy on him): Allah's Messenger (peace and blessings be upon him) said, "If Adam's son had a valley full of gold, he would like to have two valleys, for nothing fills his mouth except dust. And Allah forgives him who repents to Him." (Bukhari)

319. Not Spending of Good for Parents, Kindred, Orphans, Poor and Wayfarers

Allah, the Exalted, says:

"They ask you (O Muhammad SAW) what they should spend. Say: Whatever you spend of good must be for parents and kindred, and orphans, and Al-Masakin (the poor), and the wayfarers, and whatever you do of good deeds, truly, Allah knows it well." (Qur'an, Al-Baqarah 2:215)

"And give the relative his right, and (also) the poor, and the traveler…" (Qur'an, Al-Isra 17:26)

"Worship Allah and join none with Him in worship, and do good to parents, kinsfolk, orphans, Al-Masakin (the poor), the neighbour who is near of kin, the neighbour who is a stranger, the companion by your side, the wayfarer (you meet), and those (slaves) whom your right hands possess. Verily, Allah does not like such as are proud and boastful." (Qur'an, An-Nisa 4:36)

Other Verses: Al-Insan 76:8, Al-Fajr 89:17, Al-Isra 17:28, Al-Baqarah 2:177.

In order for it to be obligatory to spend on fathers and grandfathers, they should be poor and the child should be rich, because the Prophet (peace and blessings of Allah be upon him) said: "Start with yourself and give charity to yourself. If there is anything left over, then (give) to your family. If there is anything left over from your family, then (give) to your relatives." (Muslim)

Narrated Abu Hurairah (May Allah be pleased with him): The Messenger of Allah (peace and blessings be upon him) said: "The best house among the Muslims is a house in which there is an orphan who is treated well. And the worst house among the Muslims is a house in which there is an orphan who is treated badly." (Ibn Majah)

Narrated Abu Hurairah (May Allah be pleased with him): Allah's Messenger (peace and blessings be upon him) said, "The one who looks after and works for a widow and for a poor person is like a warrior fighting for Allah's Cause." (The narrator Al-Qa'nabi is not sure whether he also said "Like the one who prays all the night without slackness and fasts continuously and never breaks his fast.") (Bukhari)

Jabir ibn 'Abdullah (May Allah be pleased with him) reported: "We were with Messenger of Allah (May Allah's peace and blessings be upon him) shortly after dawn when there came to him some people clad in woolen rags, or covered with sleeveless blankets; and with swords hanging down from their necks. Most of them, rather all of them, belonged to the Mudar tribe. The Prophet's face changed when he saw them starving. Then he went into his house and came out; then he commanded Bilal to proclaim the Adhan. So, he proclaimed the Adhan and recited Iqamah and the Prophet led the prayer. Then he delivered a sermon saying: "O mankind, fear your Lord, who created you from one soul and created from it its mate and dispersed from both of them many men and women. And fear Allah, through whom you ask one another, and the wombs. Indeed, Allah is ever, over you, an Observer." (Surah An-Nisa 4:1) He also recited a Verse at the end of Surah Al-Hashr: "O you who believe, fear Allah and keep your duty to Him. And let everyone look what he has sent forth for the tomorrow." Thereafter, every man gave in charity dinar, dirham, clothes, measure-full of wheat and measure-full of dates till he said: "Give in charity be it half a date." Then a man from the Ansar came with a bag which was difficult for him to hold in his hand. Thereafter, the people came successively with charity till I saw two heaps of food and clothes. I noticed that the Messenger's face was glowing like that of the bright moon or glittering gold. Then he said: "Whosoever introduces a good practice in Islam, there is for him its reward and the reward of those who act upon it after him without anything being diminished from their rewards. And whosoever introduces an evil practice in Islam will shoulder its sin and the sins of all those who will act upon it, without diminishing in any way their burden." (Muslim)

Narrated Abu 'Amir or Abu Malik Al-Ash'ari that he heard the Prophet (peace and blessings be upon him) saying, "From among my followers there will be some people who will consider illegal sexual intercourse, the wearing of silk, the drinking of alcoholic drinks and the use of musical instruments, as lawful, be some people who will stay near the side of a mountain and in the evening their shepherd will come to them with their sheep and ask them for something, but they will say to him, 'Return to us tomorrow.' Allah will destroy them during the night and will let the mountain fall on them, and He will transform the rest of them into monkeys and pigs and they will remain so till the Day of Resurrection." (Bukhari)

320. Not Giving in Charity

Allah, the Exalted, says:

"(Charity is) for Fuqara (the poor), who in Allah's Cause are restricted (from travel), and cannot move about in the land (for trade or work). The one who knows them not, thinks that they are rich because of their modesty. You may know them by their mark, they do not beg of people at all. And whatever you spend in good, surely Allah knows it well." (Qur'an, Al-Baqarah 2:273)

"The example of those who spend their wealth in the way of God is like a seed (of grain) which grows seven spikes; in each spike is a hundred grains. And God multiplies (His reward) for whom He wills. And God is all-Encompassing and Knowing." (Qur'an, Al-Baqarah 2:261)

"Those who spend their wealth in the Cause of Allah, and do not follow up their gifts with reminders of their generosity or with injury, their reward is with their Lord. On them shall be no fear, nor shall they grieve." (Qur'an, Al-Baqarah 2:262)

Other Verses: *At-Tawbah 9:79.*

Narrated Ibn Abbas (May Allah be pleased with him): Allah's Apostle (peace and blessings be upon him) was the most generous of all the people, and he used to reach the peak in generosity in the month of Ramadan when Gabriel met him. Gabriel used to meet him every night of Ramadan to teach him the Qur'an. Allah's Apostle was the most generous person, even more generous than the strong uncontrollable wind (in readiness and haste to do charitable deeds). (Bukhari)

Narrated Sad (May Allah be pleased with him): "I became seriously ill at Makkah and the Prophet came to visit me. I said, "O Allah's Apostle! I shall leave behind me a good fortune, but my heir is my only daughter; shall I bequeath two third of my property to be spent in charity and leave one third (for my heir)?" He said, "No." I said, "Shall I bequeath half and leave half?" He said, "No." I said, "Shall I bequeath one third and leave two thirds?" He said, "One third is alright, though even one third is too much." Then he placed his hand on his forehead and passed it over my face and abdomen and said, "O Allah! Cure Sad and complete his emigration." I feel as if I have been feeling the coldness of his hand on my liver ever since." (Bukhari)

Narrated Asma (May Allah be pleased with her): Allah's Apostle (peace and blessings be upon him) said,

"Give (in charity) and do not give reluctantly lest Allah should give you in a limited amount; and do not withhold your money lest Allah should withhold it from you." (Bukhari)

Narrated Abu Hurairah (May Allah be pleased with him): The Prophet (peace and blessings be upon him) owed somebody a camel of a certain age. When he came to demand it back, the Prophet (peace and blessings be upon him) said (to some people), "Give him (his due)." When the people searched for a camel of that age, they found none, but found a camel one year older. The Prophet (peace and blessings be upon him) said, "Give (it to) him." On that, the man remarked, "You have given me my right in full. May Allah give you in full." The Prophet (peace and blessings be upon him) said, "The best amongst you is the one who pays the rights of others generously." (Bukhari)

Narrated Abu Hurairah (May Allah be pleased with him): A man asked the Prophet (peace and blessings be upon him), "O Allah's Apostle (peace and blessings be upon him)! What kind of charity is the best?" He replied. "To give in charity when you are healthy and greedy hoping to be wealthy and afraid of becoming poor. Don't delay giving in charity till the time when you are on the death bed when you say, 'Give so much to so-and-so and so much to so-and so,' and at that time the property is not yours but it belongs to so-and-so (i.e. your inheritors)." (Bukhari)

Narrated Abu Hurairah (May Allah be pleased with him): "Whenever a meal was brought to Allah's Apostle (peace and blessings be upon him), he would ask whether it was a gift or Sadaqah (something given in charity). If he was told that it was Sadaqah, he would tell his companions to eat it, but if it was a gift, he would hurry to share it with them." (Bukhari)

Narrated Abu Dhar (May Allah be pleased with him): "I asked the Prophet (peace and blessings be upon him), "What is the best deed?" He replied, "To believe in Allah and to fight for His Cause." I then asked, "What is the best kind of manumission (of slaves)?" He replied, "The manumission of the most expensive slave and the most beloved by his master." I said, "If I cannot afford to do that?" He said, "Help the weak or do good for a person who cannot work for himself." I said, "If I cannot do that?" He said, "Refrain from harming others for this will be regarded as a charitable deed for your own good." (Bukhari)

Narrated 'Adi ibn Hatim (May Allah be pleased with him): The Messenger of Allah (peace and blessings be upon him) said: "Guard yourself from the Hellfire even with half of a date in charity. If he cannot find it, then with a kind word." (Bukhari)

Abu Hurairah (May Allah be pleased with him) reported: The Messenger of Allah (peace and blessings be upon him) said: "Charity does not decrease wealth, no one forgives another but that Allah increases his honor, and no one humbles himself for the sake of Allah but that Allah raises his status." (Muslim)

Narrated Jabir bin Abdullah (May Allah be pleased with him): The Messenger of Allah (peace and blessings be upon him) said: "Every good is charity. Indeed, among the good is to meet your brother with a smiling face, and to pour what is left in your bucket into the vessel of your brother." (Tirmidhi)

Narrated Abu Hurairah (May Allah be pleased with him): The Prophet (peace and blessings be upon him) said, "A man felt very thirsty while he was on the way, there he came across a well. He went down the well, quenched his thirst and came out. Meanwhile he saw a dog panting and licking mud because of excessive thirst. He said to himself, "This dog is suffering from thirst as I did." So, he went down the well again and filled his shoe with water and watered it. Allah thanked him for that deed and forgave him. The people said, "O Allah's Messenger! Is there a reward for us in serving the animals?" He (peace and blessings be upon him) replied: "Yes, there is a reward for serving any animate (living being)." (Bukhari)

Narrated Abu 'Amir or Abu Malik Al-Ash'ari that he heard the Prophet (peace and blessings be upon him) saying, "From among my followers there will be some people who will consider illegal sexual intercourse, the wearing of silk, the drinking of alcoholic drinks and the use of musical instruments, as lawful, be some people who will stay near the side of a mountain and in the evening their shepherd will come to them with their sheep and ask them for something, but they will say to him, 'Return to us tomorrow.' Allah will destroy them during the night and will let the mountain fall on them, and He will transform the rest of them into monkeys and pigs and they will remain so till the Day of Resurrection." (Bukhari)

Abu Hurairah (May Allah be pleased with him) reported that the Prophet (May Allah's peace and blessings be upon him) said: "Hasten to good deeds before being overtaken by tribulations that are like parts of the dark night. A man would be a believer in the morning and turn to a disbeliever in the evening, or he would be a believer in the evening and turn to a disbeliever in the morning. He sells his religion for a worldly gain." (Muslim) (https://hadeethenc.com/en/browse/hadith/3138)

321. Taking Advantages of Other People for their Own Benefit

Allah, the Exalted, says:

"O you who believe! Do your duty to Allah and fear Him. Seek the means of approach to Him, and strive hard in His Cause as much as you can. So that you may be successful." (Qur'an, Al-Ma'idah 5:35)

"Whoever works righteousness - whether male or female - while he (or she) is a true believer (of Islamic Monotheism) verily, to him We will give a good life (in this world with respect, contentment and lawful provision), and We shall pay them certainly a reward in proportion to the best of what they used to do (i.e. Paradise in the Hereafter." (Qur'an, An-Nahl 16:97)

"and whatsoever you spend of anything (in Allah's Cause), He will replace it. And He is the Best of providers." (Qur'an, Saba 34:39)

Narrated Abu Hurairah (May Allah have mercy on him): The Messenger of Allah (peace and blessings of Allah be upon him) said: "Allah says: 'O son of Adam, spend and I will spend on you.'" (Bukhari and Muslim)

Narrated Anas bin Malik (May Allah have mercy on him): The Prophet (peace and blessings be upon him) said, "Make things easy for the people, and do not make it difficult for them, and make them calm (with glad tidings) and do not repulse (them)." (Bukhari)

Some people are constantly asking you to do favors for them, taking advantage of your kindness, of your property, etc. And they may waste your time, energy and money if they return back your property with damages. They only reach out when they need help.

So, you should think what is your priority, think about possible negative consequences for you (sins) or negative emotions, wasting precious time for unnecessary things instead of remembering Allah. Your property maybe used for sinful things. (306, 307)

1. Learn to say "No" when possibly you think you may commit sins answering to a requested favor.
2. Prefer to help really poor or needy people to have Allah's rewards.
3. Adhere to commands and prohibitions in the Qur'an and Sunnah.
4. Maintain your self-respect, so that people have to think twice before asking your help.
5. Strive for higher standards of righteous actions, keep distance from all unnecessary burdens, time-wasters and obstacles that come between you and the Pleasure of Allah.

322. Undesirability of Giving a Gift and then Ask Back for it

Narrated Ibn 'Abbas (May Allah be pleased with him): The Messenger of Allah (peace and blessings be upon him) said, "The one who takes back the gift he has given to someone is like one who eats his vomit." In another wording: "The one who takes back the charity that he gave is like a dog that vomits then eats its vomit." (Bukhari and Muslim) (https://hadeethenc.com/en/browse/hadith/6074)

'Umar bin Al-Khattab (May Allah be pleased with him) reported: "I donated a horse for Jihad. The man who had the horse neglected it, so I wanted to buy it back, thinking that he would sell it for a cheap price. I asked the Prophet about this, and he said: "Do not buy it back and do not take back your charity, even if he gives it to you for one dirham, for the one who takes back his gift is like the one who takes back his vomit." (Bukhari and Muslim) (https://hadeethenc.com/en/browse/hadith/6073)

Commentary: We learn from this Hadith that even to purchase something which one has already given in charity is not legal. (308)

323. Looking Down Upon the Gift

Narrated Abu Hurairah (May Allah have mercy on him): The Prophet (peace and blessings be upon him) said, "O Muslim women! None of you should look down upon the gift sent by her she-neighbour even if it were the trotters of the sheep (fleshless part of legs)." (Bukhari)

324. Not Rewarding People for the Gift or Favor

Narrated Aisha (May Allah be pleased with her): The Messenger of Allah (peace and blessings of Allah be upon him) used to accept gifts and used to give something in return." (Bukhari)

Jabir ibn 'Abdillah (May Allah have mercy on him) reported that the Messenger of Allah (peace and blessings be upon him) said: "Whomsoever is gifted something, and is able to reciprocate, should do so. Whoever is unable to do so, then he should (at least) praise (or supplicate for the person who gave the gift), for the one who praises has shown gratitude and whoever conceals (and refrains from praising) has certainly been ungrateful." (Tirmidhi and Abu Dawud)

Narrated Abdullah ibn Umar (May Allah be pleased with him): The Prophet (peace and blessings be upon him) said: "If anyone seeks protection in Allah's Name, grant him protection; if anyone begs in Allah's Name, give him something; if anyone gives you an invitation, accept it; and if anyone does you a kindness, recompense him; but if you have not the means to do so, pray for him until you feel that you have compensated him." (Abu Dawud)

Usama bin Zaid (May Allah be pleased with him) reported: The Messenger of Allah (peace and blessings of Allah be upon him) said: "He who is favored by another and says to his benefactor: 'Jazak-Allah khairan (May Allah reward you well), indeed praised (the benefactor) satisfactorily." (Tirmidhi)

325. Prohibition of Miserliness

Allah, the Exalted, says:

"But as for he who withholds and considers himself free of need. And denies the best (reward), We will ease him toward difficulty. And what will his wealth avail him when he falls?" (Qur'an, Al-Layl 92:8-11)

"So, fear Allah as much as you are able and listen and obey, and spend (in the way of Allah); it is better for yourselves. And whoever is protected from the stinginess of his soul - it is those who will be the successful." (Qur'an, At-Taghabun 64:16)

"Thus, will Allah show them their deeds to be intense regret to them and they shall not come forth from the fire." (Qur'an, Al-Baqarah 2:167)

Other Verses: Al-Furqan 25:67, At-Talaq 65:7, Al-Hashr 59:9, Al-Insan 76:8.

Jabir bin 'Abdullah (May Allah be pleased with him) reported: The Messenger of Allah (peace be upon him) said, "… beware of stinginess, as it ruined those who were before you…" (Muslim)

(https://hadeethenc.com/en/browse/hadith/5787)

Narrated Abu Hurairah (May Allah be pleased with him): The Prophet (peace and blessings be upon him) said: "Every day two angels come down from Heaven and one of them says, 'O Allah! Compensate every person who spends in Your Cause, and the other (angel) says, 'O Allah! Destroy every miser.'" (Bukhari)

326. Prohibition of Consumption of Unlawful Food and Income

Allah, the Exalted, says:

"O mankind, eat from whatever is on earth (that is) lawful and good and do not follow the footsteps of Satan. Indeed, he is to you a clear enemy." (Qur'an, Al-Baqarah 2:168)

"He has forbidden you only the Maytatah (dead animals) and blood, and the flesh of swine, and that which is slaughtered as a sacrifice for others than Allah (or has been slaughtered for idols, etc., on which Allah's Name has not been mentioned while slaughtering)." (Qur'an, Al-Baqarah 2:173)

"And eat up not one another's property unjustly (in any illegal way e.g. stealing, robbing, deceiving, etc.) nor give bribery to the rulers (judges before presenting your cases) that you may knowingly eat up a part of the property of others sinfully." (Qur'an, Al-Baqarah 2:188)

Other Verses: Al-Baqarah 2:219 and 275, Ali 'Imran 3:130, An-Nisa 4:29, Al-Ma'idah 5:3 and 62-63,

Al-Mu'minun 23:51.

Pursuit of lawful means of Livelihood.

Ibn 'Abbas (May Allah be pleased with him) reported, "Once, when I recited the Verses of the Qur'an, *'O you people! Eat of what is on earth, lawful and good.' (2:168)* in the presence of the Prophet (peace and blessings be upon him) Sa'd b. Abi Waqqas got up and said, 'O Messenger of Allah! Ask Allah to make me one whose supplication is heard.' At this the Prophet (peace and blessings be upon him) said, 'O Sa'd, consume lawful things and your supplications will be heard, and by Him in Whose hands is the soul of Muhammad, when a man puts into his stomach a morsel of what is forbidden, his prayers are not accepted for forty days, and a servant of Allah whose body is nourished by usury or by what is forbidden becomes more deserving of the Hellfire." (Al-Hafiz b. Marduwiyah) (Fiqh-us-Sunnah, vol.4: Supplications)

Abu Hurairah (May Allah be pleased with him) reported: The Prophet (May Allah's peace and blessings be upon him) said: "Indeed, Allah is Good and accepts only what is good. And Allah commanded the believers as He commanded the Messengers. He says: *"O (you) Messengers! Eat of the Taiyibat [all kinds of Halal (legal) foods which Allah has made legal (meat of slaughtered eatable animals, milk products, fats, vegetables, fruits, etc.], and do righteous deeds. Verily! I am Well-Acquainted with what you do." (Qur'an, Al-Mu'minun 23:51).* And Allah the Almighty also said: *"O you who believe! Eat of the lawful things that We have provided you with." (Qur'an, Al-Baqarah 2:172).* He (the Prophet) then mentioned a person who travels for so long that his hair is disheveled and covered with dust. He lifts his hand toward the sky (saying): 'O Lord, O Lord,' but his food is unlawful, his drinks are unlawful and his clothing is unlawful, and he has been nourished by the unlawful. So, how can his supplication be accepted?" (Muslim) (https://hadeethenc.com/en/browse/hadith/4316)

Narrated Anas Ibn Malik (May Allah be pleased with him): "The Messenger of Allah (peace and blessings be upon him) cursed ten with regard to wine: the one who squeezes (the grapes etc.), the one who asks for it to be squeezed, the one who drinks it, the one who carries it, the one to whom it is carried, the one who pours it, the one who sells it and consumes its price, the one who buys it and the one for whom it is bought." (Tirmidhi)

Narrated Abu Hurairah (May Allah be pleased with him): The Prophet (peace and blessings be upon him) said, "A time will come when one will not care how one gains one's money, legally or illegally." (Bukhari)

Narrated Ibn 'Umar(May Allah be pleased with him): Allah's Messenger (peace and blessings be upon him) forbade the eating of donkey-meat." (Bukhari)

Abu Hurairah (May Allah be pleased with him) reported God's Messenger as saying, "Eating any fanged beast of prey is prohibited." (Muslim)

Ibn 'Abbas (May Allah be pleased with him) reported: "Allah's Messenger (peace and blessings be upon him) prohibited the eating of all fanged beasts of prey, and all the birds having talons." (Muslim)

Narrated Jabir bin Abdullah (May Allah be pleased with him): "I heard Allah's Apostle, in the year of the Conquest of Makkah, saying, 'Allah and His Apostle made illegal the trade of alcohol, dead animals, pigs and idols.' The people asked, "O Allah's Apostle! What about the fat of dead animals, for it was used for greasing the boats and the hides; and people use it for lights?' He said, 'No, it is illegal.' Allah's Apostle further said, 'May Allah curse the Jews, for Allah made the fat (of animals) illegal for them, yet they melted the fat and sold it, and ate its price.'" (Bukhari)

Narrated Jabir (May Allah be pleased with him): "The Messenger of Allah (peace be upon him) forbade eating cats and he forbade their price." (Ibn Majah)

Narrated AbdurRahman ibn Shibl (May Allah be pleased with him): "The Messenger of Allah (peace and blessings be upon him) forbade to eat the flesh of lizard." (Abu Dawud)

Narrated Ibn 'Umar (May Allah be pleased with him): "Who eats crows? The Messenger of Allah (peace and blessings be upon him) called them vermin, By Allah, they are not from among the good and permissible things." (Ibn Majah)

Narrated Aisha (May Allah be pleased with her): The Prophet (peace and blessings be upon him) said: "Snakes are vermin, scorpions are vermin, mice are vermin and crows are vermin." (Ibn Majah)

'Adi b. Hatim (May Allah be pleased with him) reported: "I asked Allah's Messenger (peace and blessings be upon him) saying: 'We are a people who hunt with these (trained) dogs, then (what should we do)?' Thereupon he (the Holy Prophet) said: 'When you set of your trained dogs having recited the Name of Allah, then eat what these (hounds) have caught for you, even if it (the game) is killed, provided (the hunting dog) has not eaten (any part of the game). If it has eaten (the game), then you don't eat it as I fear that it might have caught for its own self. And do not eat it if other dogs have joined your trained dogs." (Muslim)

Narrated Adi bin Hatim (May Allah be pleased with him): "I asked the Prophet about the game killed by a Mi'rad (i.e. a sharp-edged piece of wood or a piece of wood provided with a sharp piece of iron used for hunting)." He (peace and blessings be upon him) said, "If the game is killed with its sharp edge, eat of it, but if it is killed with its shaft, with a hit by its broad side then the game is unlawful to eat for it has been beaten to death." I asked him about the game killed by a trained hound. He said, "If the hound catches the game for you, eat of it, for killing the game by the hound, is like its slaughtering. But if you see with your hound or hounds another dog, and you are afraid that it might have shared in hunting the game with your hound and killed it, then you should not eat of it, because you have mentioned Allah's Name on (sending) your hound only, but you have not mentioned it on some other hound." (Bukhari)

Mus'ab b. Sa'd (May Allah be pleased with him) reported: Abdullah son of Umar came to Ibn 'Amir in order to inquire after his health as he was ailing. He said: "Ibn 'Umar, Why don't you pray to Allah for me?" He said: "I heard of Allah's Messenger (May peace and blessings be upon him) say: "Neither the prayer is accepted without purification nor is charity accepted out of the ill-gotten (wealth), and thou wert the (governor) of Basra." (Muslim)

Narrated Abdul Malik (May Allah be pleased with him): The Prophet (peace and blessings be upon him) said: "Allah does not accept charity from goods acquired by embezzlement as He does not accept prayer without purification." (Abu Dawud)

Narrated Ka'b bin Ujrah (May Allah be pleased with him): The Messenger of Allah (peace and blessings be upon him) said to me: "…There is no flesh raised that sprouts from the unlawful except that the Fire is more appropriate for it." (Tirmidhi)

Narrated Miqdam bin Ma'dikarib (Ar-Zubaidi) (May Allah be pleased with him): The Messenger of Allah (peace and blessings be upon him) said: "No man earns anything better than that which he earns with his own hands, and what a man spends on himself, his wife, his child and his servant, then it is charity." (Ibn Majah)

Narrated Abu Hurairah (May Allah be pleased with him): The Prophet (peace and blessings be upon him) prohibited the earnings of slave girls (through prostitution)." (Bukhari)

Haram money should be returned back to the owners or you must seek their pardon. If the original owners have died, then you must return the item to their heirs or seek their pardon. If the owners of the haram item are unknown (interest money or money obtained through gambling), then you must give away the amount in charity without the intention of receiving rewards.

Also, a deal or sale during Friday's prayers is unlawful action.

Narrated Ibn 'Umar (May Allah have mercy on him): Allah's Messenger (peace and blessings be upon him) said, "A believer eats in one intestine (is satisfied with a little food), and a kafir (unbeliever) or a hypocrite eats in seven intestines (eats too much)." (Bukhari)

Ibn Taymiyah (May Allah have mercy on him) said:

"Allah forbade like blood, animals which died of themselves, died from strangulation, goring, falling or butting, animals partly eaten by wild animals and animals slaughtered in names other than that of Allah. And even the best of them [i.e. the Prophet (peace and blessings be upon him) used to dislike things which were not forbidden by Allah. For example, lizard (Dabb) meat was disliked by the Prophet who on one occasion said: "It is not to be found in the land of my people so I find it distasteful." However, he added, "Certainly, it is not haram. On another occasion it was eaten at the table at which he was eating and he said, "I do not eat it and I do not forbid it."

The majority of scholars hold that the good things which Allah has made permissible are whatever will benefit the religious practice of one who eats it and filth is that which will harm his religious practice. Justice forms the basis of Divine religion which Allah the Almighty sent

His Messengers to establish. Consequently, Allah forbade foods which produce aggression, ruthlessness and ferocity. He forbade all fanged predatory animals because they are aggressive and ruthless since the eater is similar to what he eats. Hence, if human flesh is produced from the meat of predatory carnivores, there develops in man the instinctual predatory characteristics of violent aggressiveness and ferocity.

Pork produces in man the most filthy habits and characteristics, as the pig feeds on a wider range of substances than any other animal and it is not repulsed by anything. Similarly, blood contains and conveys the powerful forces of sexual desire and anger which spring from the soul. If one is nourished from it, his desires and anger will soon become abnormal. Consequently, only flowing blood has been forbidden, while small amounts like what remains in the blood vessels are allowable since they are harmless. Aisha (May Allah be pleased with her) mentioned that they used to put meat in the pot and see traces of blood in it. As a result, the majority of scholars excused small amounts of blood on the body or clothes if it was not flowing." (10)

Pig is awfully filthy, lives and eats dirty things including his own feces and urine. Pig is shameless, immoral and does not honor its own females and invites other males to the group sexual activity. Consumption of pork, therefore, leads to moral degradation, anger and spiritual bankruptcy. Pork meat causes many diseases. The Qur'an prohibits eating the flesh of swine, because it is a SIN and an IMPIETY (Rijss). The word Rijss has been explained as meaning "filthy" and "dirty" as mentioned in the *Qur'an 9:95-96, 7:70, 10:100, 22:30* and *33:33*. (309)

The studies emphasizing the links between digestion, mood, behavior, health and even the way of thinking; brain-gut connection, communications between the big brain and the brain in our gut.

Scientists call this little brain the *Enteric Nervous System* (ENS). And it's not so little. The ENS is two thin layers of more than 100 million nerve cells lining the gastrointestinal tract from esophagus to rectum.

The ENS may trigger big emotional shifts experienced by people coping with irritable bowel syndrome (IBS) and functional bowel problems such as constipation, diarrhea, bloating, pain and stomach upset. (310)

The Gut-Brain-Axis is a bidirectional signaling pathway between the gastrointestinal (GI) tract and the brain. The hundreds of trillions of microorganisms populating the gastrointestinal tract are thought to modulate this connection, and have far reaching effects on the immune system, central and autonomic nervous systems and GI functioning. These interactions diagnostic and statistical manual of mental disorders have also been linked to various psychiatric illnesses such as depression, anxiety, substance abuse, autism spectrum disorder and eating disorders. It is hypothesized that techniques aimed at strengthening and repopulating the gut microbiome, such as Fecal Microbiota Transplant (FMT), may be useful in the prevention and treatment of psychiatric illnesses. (311)

The theory that the trillions of microbes living in the human gut are in constant communication with the brain affecting the way a person feels has been strengthened thanks to the increasing prevalence of faecal transplants.

Anecdotal evidence that recipients of a faecal transplant - a procedure to restore the gut microbiota - mimick the mood and other characteristics of their donor.

Associate Professor Patrick Charles from the Department of Infectious Diseases at Austin Health says they have heard of some "very interesting" things from faecal transplant recipients, including stories about patients experiencing fluctuations in mood. "There have even been reports that patients with no prior history of depression have become depressed after receiving a transplant from someone with depression", he said. "There have also been cases where dramatic body changes have occurred - both rapid weight gain and weight loss, each time aligned to the donor."

A faecal microbiota transplant, known as an FMT, is a procedure which replaces the 'gut bacteria' in an unhealthy individual with those of someone who is healthy. Essentially, it involves taking 'healthy' poo from a donor and using it to create a liquid preparation that is then transplanted into the patient, normally via a colonoscopy. It is becoming increasingly popular for the treatment of multiple conditions including chronic fatigue, irritable bowel syndrome, Parkinson's and autism. Typically, it is performed to treat someone with Clostridium Difficile infections when antibiotics fail. Despite more research being needed, Ass Prof Charles says that its only now that scientists are beginning to recognize and understand the influence of the microbiome on both the mind and body. "We're still really only just scratching the surface of what impacts microbiomes have on health and disease but as DNA sequencing techniques advance so will our understanding of their role," he said. (312)

The study by De Palma has shown that fecal material from humans with irritable bowel syndrome (IBS) with diarrhea (IBS-D) invoked physical changes in the intestinal environment and in behavior. In the De Palma study, stool was collected from five healthy controls (HCs) and eight IBS-D patients. Patients with IBS were diagnosed using the Rome-III criteria and Bristol stool form scale (≥ 6), with more than three bowel movements per day and symptoms for at least 2 years. Of the IBS-D patients, four were characterized as having anxiety by the Hospital Anxiety and Depression Scale (HADS) (HADS score, 11–14) and four IBS-D patients did not have anxiety (HADS score, 5–7). Eight- to 10-week-old germ-free National Institutes of Health (NIH) Swiss mice were gavaged with stool from either HCs or IBS-D patients with or without anxiety. The authors found that mice colonized with microbiota originating from IBS-D patients with anxiety spent longer amounts of time in the dark compartment during the light-preference test than mice colonized by HCs and IBS-D patients without anxiety, as well as longer latency in stepping off an elevated platform in the step-down test, indicating these mice had an altered behaviour when colonized with the microbiota of IBS-D patients with anxiety. Faster transit time was observed in mice colonized by the microbiota of IBS-D patients than HCs. Gut barrier function was impaired in mice colonized by IBS-D patients' microbiota and the authors found that there was increased ion transport in IBS-D colonized mouse colonic tissue (but not jejunal tissue) compared to HCs. An increase in CD3+ T lymphocytes was observed in the IBS-D with anxiety mice compared to IBS-D without anxiety and HC mice. A total of 22 genes involved in inflammatory pathways were found to be upregulated in IBS-D mice. They found that humans with IBS-D had a higher relative abundance of the genus *Blautia* and humans with anxiety had higher relative abundances of the genera *Blautia, Coprococcus, Streptococcus*, and the species *Clostridium butyricum* and *Eggerthella lenta*. Mice colonized by IBS patients had higher relative abundances of the genera *Oscillospira, Bacteroides*, and the species *Clostridium citronia* and mice with anxiety had higher relative abundances of the genus *Oscillospira* and the species *Bacteroides fragilis, Akkermansia muciniphila, Shewanella algae*, and *Blautia producta*.

Past research from these authors demonstrated antibiotics administered to mice altered their behaviour and this was the basis for their hypothesis that an altered microbiota could contribute to the psychiatric conditions commonly observed in IBS patients. (313)

My commentary:

Majority of diseases are caused by the Evil Jinn because of sins. The Jinn eat the feces, that's way they live in the toilets. Medications excite the Evil Jinn and excited Jinn spread more diseases. The anaerobic atmosphere is suitable for the Jinn (being composed from Carbon Dioxide, Positive Ions). They cannot tolerate Negative Ions, alkalinity. And Allah knows the best.

An unhealthy gut triggers changes in normal breast tissue that helps breast cancer spread to other parts of the body, new research from UVA Cancer Center reveals. The gut microbiome – the collection of microbes that naturally live inside us – can be disrupted by poor diet, long-term antibiotic use, obesity or other factors. When this happens, the ailing microbiome reprograms important immune cells in healthy breast tissue, called mast cells, to facilitate cancer's spread. (314)

My commentary:

Cancer is a Jinn Possession disease and in majority cases because of sins.

Acidosis causes an imbalance in the body's pH. If the kidneys and lungs are unable to get rid of excess acid, it can cause serious health problems. If a disease or health condition is causing acidosis, treating the condition can help lower acidity in the body. Different types and possible causes of Acidosis were discussed in the article 'What to know about Acidosis." (315)

Most fruits and vegetables, soybeans, tofu, nuts, seeds are alkaline-promoting foods. Raw fruit and vegetables are the best.

Dairy, eggs, meat, most grains, refined sugar, processed foods, like canned and packaged snacks and convenience foods, fall on the acid side. Alcohol, carbonated drinks and caffeine are acidic. (316, 317)

Drug and chemical-induced metabolic acidosis. The most common drugs and chemicals that induce the anion gap type of acidosis are biguanides, alcohols, polyhydric sugars, salicylates, cyanide and carbon monoxide. Normal anion gap acidosis is caused by carbonic anhydrase inhibitors, hydrochloride salts of amino acids, toluene, amphotericin, spironolactone and non-steroidal anti-inflammatory drugs. (318)

327. Slaughtering for Other than Allah

Allah, the Exalted, says:

"Say: Verily my prayer, my sacrifice, my living and my dying are for Allah, the Lord of the worlds. He has no partner. And of this I have been commanded, and I am the first of the Muslims." (Qur'an, Al-An'am 6:162-163)

"Therefore, turn in prayer to your Lord and sacrifice (to Him only)." (Qur'an, Al-Kawthar 108:2)

Ali bin Abi Talib (May Allah be pleased with him) said: "Allah's Messenger (May the peace and blessing of Allah be upon him) informed me about four Judgments (of Allah): 1) Allah's Curse is upon the one who slaughters (devoting his sacrifice) to anything other than Allah; 2) Allah's Curse is upon the one who curses his own parents; 3) Allah's Curse is upon the one who shelters a heretic (who has brought a *Bid'ah* in religion); 4) Allah's Curse is upon the one who alters the landmarks (who changes boundary lines)." (Muslim)

Narrated Tariq bin Shihab that Allah's Messenger (peace and blessing of Allah be upon him) said: "A man entered Paradise because of a fly, and a man entered Hellfire because of a fly." They (the Companions) asked, "How was that possible O Messenger of Allah?" He said, "Two men passed by the people who had an idol by which they would not allow anyone to pass without making sacrifice to it. They ordered one man to make a sacrifice. He said, 'I have nothing to present as an offering.' The people told him, 'Sacrifice something, even if it be a fly.' So, he presented a fly (to their idol). They opened the way for him, and thus he entered the Hellfire. They said to the other man, 'Sacrifice something.' He said, 'I will never sacrifice anything to any other than Allah, Most Majestic and Glorious.' So, they struck his throat and killed him and he, therefore, entered Paradise." (Ahmad)

Narrated 'Abdullah: "Allah's Messenger (peace and blessings be upon him) said that he met Zaid bin 'Amr Nufail at a place near Baldah and this had happened before Allah's Messenger (peace and blessings be upon him) received the Divine Inspiration. Allah's Messenger (peace and blessings be upon him) presented a dish of meat (that had been offered to him by the pagans) to Zaid bin 'Amr, but Zaid refused to eat of it and then said (to the pagans), "I do not eat of what you slaughter on your stone altars (Ansa's) nor do I eat except that on which Allah's Name has been mentioned on slaughtering." (Bukhari)

328. Non-Islamic Slaughtering of Animal

Allah, the Exalted, says:

"It is neither their meat nor their blood that reaches Allah, but it is piety from you that reaches Him. Thus, have We made them subject to you that you may magnify Allah for His Guidance to you. And give glad tidings (O Muhammad SAW) to the Muhsinun (doers of good)." (Qur'an, Al-Hajj 22:37)

"Forbidden to you (for food) are: Al-Maitah (the dead animals - cattle - beast not slaughtered), blood, the flesh of swine, and that on which Allah's Name has not been mentioned while slaughtering (that which has been slaughtered as a sacrifice for others than Allah, or has been slaughtered for idols) and that which has been killed by strangling, or by a violent blow, or by a headlong fall, or by the goring of horns — and that which has been (partly) eaten by a wild animal — unless you are able to slaughter it (before its death)." (Qur'an, Al-Ma'idah 5:3)

"So, eat of that (meat) on which Allah's Name has been pronounced (while slaughtering the animal), if you are believers in His Ayat (proofs, evidences, verses, lessons, signs, revelations, etc.). And why should you not eat of that (meat) on which Allah's Name has been pronounced (at the time of slaughtering the animal), while He has explained to you in detail what is forbidden to you, except under compulsion of necessity? And surely, many do lead (mankind) astray by their own desires through lack of knowledge. Certainly, your Lord knows best the transgressors." (Qur'an, Al-An'am 6:118-119)

Other Verse: Al-An'am 6:121.

The sacrifice in Islam is nothing else than a natural expression of homage and gratitude to the Creator. It is only piety of heart, nobility of soul and righteousness of conduct, that is acceptable to Him. It is essentially symbolic, an external symbol of dedication, devotion to Allah. Tafsir Ibn Kathir stresses this point: "The man who offers sacrifice should keep this fact uppermost in his mind that the most important motive behind this is the willing submission to Allah." (vol.VI, p.183)

The Holy Qur'an makes a pointed reference to the fact that this sacrifice of animals is commemorative of Abraham's offer of his son's life at the Command of Allah, who was substituted by a ram, and it has been perpetuated by Islam. It is narrated that once the Companions of the Holy Prophet (May peace be upon him) asked him about the sacrifice. He replied: "This is commemorative Sunnah of your father Abraham" (vide Ibn Kathir, vol. III, p.221). (Muslim, Kitab Al-Adahi (Book of Sacrifices)

Age of the animal to be slaughtered

Jabir reported Allah's Messenger (peace and blessings be upon him) as saying: "Sacrifice only a grown-up animal, unless it is difficult for you, in which case sacrifice a ram (of even less than a year, but more than six months' age)." (Muslim)

It says in Fataawa al-Lajnah al-Daa'imah (11/377):

"The Shariah evidence indicates that a sheep that has reached the age of six months may count as a sacrifice, as may a goat that has reached the age of one year, a cow that has reached the age of two years, and a camel that has reached the age of five years. Anything younger than that does not count as a hadiy or udhiyah. This is what the Qur'an refers to when it says (interpretation of the meaning): "sacrifice a Hady (animal, i.e. a sheep, a cow or a camel) such as you can afford." (Qur'an, A-Baqarah 2:196), because the texts of the Qur'an and Sunnah explain one another." End quote. (319)

It is forbidden to sacrifice the animal for anyone besides Allah and curse upon one who does it.

Abu Tufail reported: "Ali was asked whether Allah's Messenger (peace and blessings be upon him) had showed special favor (by disclosing to him) a thing (which he kept secret from others). Thereupon he said: Allah's Messenger (peace and blessings be upon him) singled us not for (disclosing to us) anything (secret) which he did not make public, (but those few things) which lie in the sheath of my sword. He drew out the written document contained in it and on that (it was mentioned): Allah cursed him who sacrificed for anyone else besides Allah, and Allah cursed him who stole the signposts (demarcating the boundary lines of the land), and Allah cursed him who cursed his father, and Allah cursed him who accommodated an innovator (in religion)." (Muslim)

329. Do Not Mentioning the Name of Allah Before Eating and Drinking

Allah, the Exalted, says:

"And do not eat of that upon which the Name of Allah has not been mentioned, for indeed, it is grave disobedience. And indeed, do the Devils inspire their allies (among men) to dispute with you. And if you were to obey them, indeed, you would be associates (of others with Him)." (Qur'an, Al-An'am 6:121)

'Umar ibn Abu Salamah (May Allah be pleased with him) reported: "I was a young boy under the care of the Messenger of Allah (May Allah's peace and blessings be upon him) and my hand used to wander all over the platter (of food). The Messenger of Allah (May Allah's peace and blessings be upon him) said to me: "O boy, mention Allah's Name, eat with your right hand, and eat from what is nearer to you." Since then, I have been eating that way." (Bukhari and Muslim) (https://hadeethenc.com/en/browse/hadith/58120)

Ibn Umar narrated that the Messenger of Allah (peace and blessings be upon him) said: "When one of you eats, he should eat with his right hand, and when he drinks, he should drink with his right hand, for the Devil eats and drinks with his left hand." (Muslim)

Jabir (May Allah be pleased with him) reported: "I heard Messenger of Allah (peace and blessings be upon him) saying, "If a person mentions the Name of Allah upon entering his house or eating, Satan says, addressing his followers: 'You will find nowhere to spend the night and no dinner.' But if he enters without mentioning the Name of Allah, Satan says (to his followers); 'You have found (a place) to spend the night in, and if he does not mention the Name of Allah at the time of eating, Satan says: 'You have found (a place) to spend the night in as well as food.'" (Muslim)

330. Prohibition of Using Utensils Made of Gold and Silver

Umm Salamah (May Allah be pleased with her) said: The Messenger of Allah (peace and blessings be upon him) said, "Whosoever drinks in utensils of silver, in fact, kindles in his belly the fire of Hell." (Bukhari and Muslim)

Hudhaifah (May Allah be pleased with him) reported: The Prophet (peace and blessings be upon him) prohibited us from wearing silk or Dibaj and from drinking out of gold and silver vessels and said, "These are meant for them (non-Muslims) in this world and for you in the Hereafter." (Bukhari and Muslim)

Anas bin Sirin (May Allah be pleased with him) said: "I was with Anas bin Malik (May Allah be pleased with him) in the company of some Magians when Faludhaj (a sweet made of flour and honey) was brought in a silver utensil, and Anas did not take it. The man was told to change the utensil. So, he changed the utensil and when he brought it to Anas, he took it." (Al-Baihaqi)

Islam encourages simplicity and piety in eating, drinking, dress and living; and forbids luxury and ease that creates resemblance and likeness with the disbelievers. It includes also gold or silver-plated utensils, cutlery, etc. (320)

331. Throwing Leftover Food

Allah, the Exalted, says:

"Indeed, the wasteful are brothers of the Devils, and ever has Satan been to his Lord ungrateful." *(Qur'an, Al-Isra 17:27)*

"O children of Adam, take your adornment at every Masjid, and eat and drink, but not excessive. Indeed, He likes not those who commit excess." *(Qur'an, Al-A'raf 7:31)*

Narrated Anas (May Allah be pleased with him): "When the Messenger of Allah (peace and blessings be upon him) finished eating his food, he would lick his three fingers (i.e. the forefinger, the middle finger and the thumb). He (peace and blessings be upon him) said, "If anyone of you drops a morsel, he should remove anything harmful from it and then eat it. He should not leave it for Shaitan." He commanded us to clean out the dish saying, "You do not know in what portion of your food the blessing lies." (Muslim)

Commentary: This Hadith also stresses humbleness, simplicity and regard for the blessings of Allah… (321)

Al-Miqdam ibn Ma'di Karib (May Allah be pleased with him) reported: "I heard the Messenger of Allah (May Allah's peace and blessings be upon him) say: "The son of Adam does not fill any vessel worse than his stomach. It is enough for the son of Adam to eat a few mouthfuls to straighten his back, but if he must (fill his stomach), then one third for his food, one third for his drink and one third for his breath." (Ibn Majah) (https://hadeethenc.com/en/browse/hadith/4723)

'Abdullah ibn 'Amr ibn al-'As (May Allah be pleased with him) reported that the Prophet (May Allah's peace and blessings be upon him) said: "Eat, drink, give charity and wear clothes without extravagance or pride." (Ibn Majah) (https://hadeethenc.com/en/browse/hadith/5363)

Narrated Abu Hurairah (May Allah be pleased with him): Allah's Messenger (peace and blessings be upon him) said, "The food for two persons is sufficient for three and the food of three persons is sufficient for four persons." (Bukhari)

Throwing the leftover food means throwing Allah's money. We will be asked about it on Judgment Day. The remaining food can be frozen or given to the neighbours, poor, needy people or to the animals and birds.

332. Gluttony

Allah, the Exalted, says:

"and eat and drink but waste not by extravagance, certainly He (Allah) likes not Al-Musrifoon (those who waste by extravagance)." *(Qur'an, Al-A'raf 7:31)*

Salman (May Allah be pleased with him) reported: The Messenger of Allah, peace and blessings be upon him, said, "Verily, the people who ate to their fill the most in this world will be the hungriest on the Day of Resurrection." (Ibn Majah)

Narrated Nafi' (May Allah be pleased with him): "Ibn 'Umar never used to take his meal unless a poor man was called to eat with him. One day I brought a poor man to eat with him, the man ate too much, whereupon Ibn 'Umar said, "O Nafi'! Don't let this man enter my house, for I heard the Prophet (peace and blessings be upon him) saying, "A believer eats in one intestine (is satisfied with a little food), and a kafir (unbeliever) eats in seven intestines (eats much food)." (Bukhari)

Ibn 'Umar (May Allah be pleased with him) said: A man burped in the presence of the Prophet (blessings and peace of Allah be upon him) and he said: "Keep your burps away from us, for the one who eats his fill the most in this world will be hungry for the longest time on the Day of Resurrection." (Tirmidhi)

Burping results from eating too much, and eating too much is regarded as blameworthy according to Islamic teaching. (322)

Overeating is bad for the body, for his spiritual health and wellbeing. (323)

333. Prohibition of Criticizing Food

Abu Hurairah (May Allah be pleased with him) reported: "The Messenger of Allah (peace and blessings be upon him) never found fault with food. If he had inclination to eating it, he would eat, and if he disliked it, he would leave it." (Bukhari and Muslim)

Jabir (May Allah be pleased with him) reported: "The Prophet (peace and blessings be upon him) asked for sauce and was told that there was nothing except vinegar. He asked for it and began to eat from it saying, "How excellent is vinegar when eaten as sauce! How excellent is vinegar when eaten as Udm!" (Muslim)

Commentary: This Hadith speaks about the simplicity and humility of Messenger of Allah (peace and blessings be upon him) with regard to food. As he abstained from a luxurious lifestyle, he hardly craved for delicious food. No mention of dainties, he would readily eat whatever was available to him. (324)

334. Prohibition of Eating Two Date-Fruits Simultaneously

Jabalah bin Suhaim (May Allah be pleased with him) reported: "We were with 'Abdullah bin Az-Zubair (May Allah be pleased with them) in a time of famine, then we were provided with dates. (Once) when we were eating, 'Abdullah bin 'Umar (May Allah be pleased with him) passed by us and said: "Do not eat two dates together, for Messenger of Allah (peace and blessings be upon him) prohibited it, unless one seeks permission from his brother (partner)." (Bukhari and Muslim)

Commentary: The person, unconcerned about others around him, will fill his own plate with food. Such a greed of eating is against the Prophet's teaching and guidance which inspire us to have a due regard for others, share food, care about others first. (325)

335. Prohibition of Selling and Buying Unripe Fruit

Anas ibn Malik (May Allah be pleased with him) reported that the Messenger of Allah (May Allah's peace and blessings be upon him) forbade the sale of fruits until they are ripe. They said: "What is meant by ripe?" He said: "When they become red." He added: "What if Allah prevents the fruits, how could one of you consider his brother's money lawful for himself?" (Bukhari and Muslim) (https://hadeethenc.com/en/browse/hadith/5851)

Jabir ibn 'Abdullah (May Allah be pleased with him) reported that the Prophet (May Allah's peace and blessings be upon him) forbade the sales called Mukhabarah, Muhaqalah, Muzabanah and the selling of fruits until they are fit for eating. He also forbade the selling of fruits but for money, except in the case of 'Araya." (Bukhari and Muslim) (https://hadeethenc.com/en/browse/hadith/5917)

Narrated Ibn 'Umar (May Allah be pleased with him) that the Prophet (peace and blessings of Allah be upon him) forbade selling fruits before their condition is known, and he forbade both the seller and the buyer." (Bukhari and Muslim)

Fruits are often destroyed before their condition is known.

336. Alcohol and Intoxicants

Allah, the Exalted, says:

"They ask you about wine and gambling. Say, "In them is great sin and (yet, some) benefit for people. But their sin is greater than their benefit." (Qur'an, Al-Baqarah 2:219)

"O you who believe! Intoxicants (all kinds of alcoholic drinks), gambling, Al-Ansab and Al-Azlam (arrows for seeking luck or decision) are an abomination of Shaitan's (Satan) handiwork. So, avoid (strictly all) that (abomination) in order that you may be successful. Shaitan (Satan) wants only to excite enmity and hatred between you with intoxicants (alcoholic drinks) and gambling, and hinder you from the remembrance of Allah and from As-Salat (the prayer). So, will you not then abstain?" (Qur'an, Al-Ma'idah 5:90-91)

"Bad statements are for bad people (or bad women for bad men) and bad people for bad statements (or bad men for bad women). Good statements are for good people (or good women for good men) and good people for good statements (or good men for good women), such (good people) are innocent of (each and every) bad statement which they say, for them is Forgiveness, and Rizqun Karim (generous provision i.e. Paradise)." (Qur'an, An-Nur 24:26)

Narrated Aisha (May Allah be pleased with her): "When the last Verses of Surah Al-Baqarah were revealed, the Prophet went out (of his house to the Mosque) and said, "The trade of alcohol has become illegal." (Bukhari)

Aisha (May Allah be pleased with her) reported that the Messenger of Allah (May Allah's peace and blessings be upon him) was asked about mead, and he said: "Every drink that intoxicates is unlawful." (Bukhari and Muslim) (https://hadeethenc.com/en/browse/hadith/2952)

Narrated Anas (May Allah be pleased with him): Allah's Apostle (peace and blessings be upon him) said, "From among the portents of the Hour are (the following): 1. Religious knowledge will be taken away (by the death of Religious learned men), 2. (Religious) ignorance will prevail, 3. Drinking of Alcoholic drinks (will be very common), 4. There will be prevalence of open illegal sexual intercourse. (Bukhari)

Narrated Abu Hurairah (May Allah be pleased with him): The Messenger of Allah (peace and blessings be upon him) said: "The one who is addicted to wine is like one who worships idols." (Ibn Majah)

Narrated Abu Darda (May Allah be pleased with him): "My close friend (peace and blessings be upon him) advised me: "Do not associate anything with Allah, even if you are cut and burned. Do not neglect any prescribed prayer deliberately, for whoever neglects it deliberately no longer has the Protection of Allah. And do not drink wine, for it is the key to all evil." (Ibn Majah)

Narrated Ibn Umar (May Allah be pleased with him): The Messenger of Allah (peace and blessings of Allah be upon him) said: "Wine is cursed from ten angles: The wine itself, the one who squeezes (the grapes, etc.), the one for whom it is squeezed, the one who sells it, the one who buys it, the one who carries it, the one to whom it is carried, the one who consumes its price, the one who drinks it and the one who pours it." (Ibn Majah)

Jabir ibn 'Abdullah (May Allah be pleased with him) reported that he heard the Messenger of Allah (May Allah's peace and blessings be upon him) in the year of the Conquest, when he was in Makkah, say: "Indeed, Allah and His Messenger have forbidden selling alcohol, dead animals, swine and idols." It was said: "O Messenger of Allah, what about the fat of the dead animals that is used for coating boats and as hides, and people use it for lighting purposes?" He said: "No, it is forbidden." Then the Messenger (May Allah's peace and blessings be upon him) said: "May Allah destroy the Jews. Indeed, Allah had forbidden fat to them, but they melted it and then sold it and consumed its price." (Bukhari and Muslim) (https://hadeethenc.com/en/browse/hadith/4556)

The Mother of All Sins

Al-Harith (May Allah be pleased with him) reported: Uthman (May Allah be pleased with him) said, "Stay away from wine, for it is the mother of wickedness. By Allah, faith and addiction to wine cannot be combined but that one of them will eventually expel the other." (An-Nasa'i)

Narrated Abu Bakr bin 'Abdur-Rahman bin Al-Harith that his father said: "I heard 'Uthman (May Allah be pleased with him) say: 'Avoid Khamr for it is the mother of all evils. There was a man among those who came before you who was a devoted worshipper. An immoral woman fell in love with him. She sent her slave girl to him, saying: 'We are calling you to bear witness.' So, he set out with her slave girl, and every time he entered a door, she locked it behind him, until he reached a beautiful woman who has with her a boy and a vessel of wine. She said: 'By Allah, I did not call you to bear witness, rather I called you to have intercourse with me or to drink a cup of this wine, or to kill this boy.' He said: 'Pour me a cup of this wine.' So, she poured him a cup. He said: 'Give me more.' And soon he had intercourse with her and killed the boy. So, avoid Khamr, for by Allah faith and addiction to Khamr cannot coexist, but one of them will soon expel the other." (An-Nasa'i)

337. Prescribed Punishment for Drinking Alcohol

Abu Hurairah (May Allah be pleased with him) reported that a man who drank wine was brought to the Prophet (May Allah's peace and blessings be upon him), who said: "Beat him." Abu Hurairah added: "So some of us beat him with our hands, some with their sandals and some with their garments (by twisting it like a lash). Then, when the man left, someone said: "May Allah disgrace you!" Upon that, the Prophet (May Allah's peace and blessings be upon him) said: "Do not say this! Do not help the Devil to overpower him." (Bukhari) (https://hadeethenc.com/en/browse/hadith/3262)

Anas ibn Malik (May Allah be pleased with him) reported: A man who had drunk alcohol was brought to the Prophet (May Allah's peace and blessings be upon him), who hit him with a palm stalk with about forty lashes." (Bukhari and Muslim) (https://hadeethenc.com/en/browse/hadith/2946)

'Abdullah ibn 'Umar (May Allah be pleased with him) reported that the Messenger of Allah (May Allah's peace and blessings be upon him) said: ''Every intoxicant is alcohol, and every intoxicant is prohibited. He who drinks alcohol in this world and dies while he is addicted to it, not having repented, will not drink it in the Hereafter.'' (Muslim) (https://hadeethenc.com/en/browse/hadith/58259)

Abu Musa al-Ash'ari (May Allah be pleased with him) reported that the Messenger of Allah (peace be upon him) said: "Three will not enter Paradise: the habitual drinker of alcohol, the one who severs the ties of kinship and the one who believes in sorcery." (Ibn Hibban and Ahmad) (https://hadeethenc.com/en/browse/hadith/5951)

Narrated 'Abdullah bin' Amr (May Allah be pleased with him): The Messenger of Allah (peace be upon him) said: "Whoever drinks wine and gets drunk, his prayer will not be accepted for forty days, and if he dies, he will enter Hell, but if he repents, Allah will accept his repentance. If he drinks wine again and gets drunk, his prayer will not be accepted for forty days, and if he dies, he will enter Hell, but if he repents, Allah will accept his repentance. If he drinks wine again and gets drunk, his prayer will not be accepted for forty days, and if he dies, he will enter Hell, but if he repents Allah will accept his repentance. But if he does it again, then Allah will most certainly make him drink of the mire of the puss or sweat on the Day of Resurrection." They said: "O Messenger of Allah, what is the mire of the pus or sweat? He said: "The drippings of the people of Hell." (Ibn Majah)

338. Blowing and Breathing into the Vessel

Abu Sa'id al-Khudri (May Allah be pleased with him) reported that the Prophet (May Allah's peace and blessings be upon him) prohibited blowing in one's drink. A man said: "Sometimes, I see a speck in the vessel. What should I do then?" He replied: "Spill it." Then the man said: "My thirst is not quenched with one draught." He said: "Then remove the cup from your mouth (in between three gulps, and take a breath)." (Tirmidhi, Ahmad, Malik and Al-Darimi) (https://hadeethenc.com/en/browse/hadith/5453)

Narrated Abu Qatada (May Allah be pleased with him): Allah's Messenger (peace and blessings be upon him) said, "When you drink (water), do not breathe in the vessel; and when you urinate, do not touch your penis with your right hand. And when you cleanse yourself after defecation, do not use your right hand." (Bukhari)

339. Prohibited Drinking Directly from the Mouth of a Waterskin

Abu Hurairah and Ibn 'Abbas (May Allah be pleased with them) reported: The Messenger of Allah (May Allah's peace and blessings be upon him) prohibited drinking directly from the mouth of a waterskin." (Bukhari and Muslim) (https://hadeethenc.com/en/browse/hadith/5451)

340. Undesirability of Drinking While Standing

Abu Hurairah (May Allah be pleased with him) reported that the Prophet (May Allah's peace and blessings be upon him) said: "None of you should drink while standing, and whoever forgets, then let him induce vomit." (Muslim with its two versions) (https://hadeethenc.com/en/browse/hadith/5450)

Narrated Ibn Masud (May Allah be pleased with him): "I brought water to the Messenger of Allah (peace and blessings of Allah be upon him) from Zamzam and he drank whilst standing." (Bukhari and Muslim)

Al-Nawawi (May Allah have mercy on him) said:

"There is no contradiction in these Ahadith, Praise be to Allah, and none of them are da'eef (weak). Rather they are all Saheeh. The correct view is that the forbidding mentioned in them is to be understood as meaning that it is disliked…" (326)

341. Declining the Invitation to a Meal Without Valid Reason

Abu Hurairah (May Allah be pleased with him) reported: The Messenger of Allah (peace and blessings be upon him)) said, "Every Muslim has five rights over another Muslim (i.e. he has to perform five duties for another Muslim): to return the greetings, to visit the sick, to accompany funeral processions, to accept an invitation, to respond to the sneezer (i.e. to say: 'Yarhamuk-Allah (May Allah bestow His Mercy on you)' when the sneezer praises Allah)." (Bukhari and Muslim)

Narrated Nafi` (May Allah be pleased with him): 'Abdullah bin `Umar said, "Allah's Messenger (peace and blessings be upon him) said, 'Accept the marriage invitation if you are invited to it.' Ibn `Umar used to accept the invitation whether to a wedding banquet or to any other party, even when he was fasting.'" (Bukhari)

Abu Hurairah (May Allah be pleased with him) reported that the Messenger of Allah (May Allah's peace and blessings be upon him) said: "No people leave a gathering in which they did not remember Allah the Almighty, except that it will be as if they are leaving the carcass of a donkey, and it will be a cause of regret for them." (Abu Dawud) (https://hadeethenc.com/en/browse/hadith/3910)

The scholars divided the invitations which the Muslim is commanded to accept into two categories:

1) Invitation to a wedding party (waleemah). The majority of scholars said that it is obligatory to accept such an invitation, unless there is a legitimate Shariah reason.

Narrated Abu Hurairah (May Allah be pleased with him): "The worst food is that of a wedding banquet to which only the rich are invited while the poor are not invited. And he who refuses an invitation (to a banquet) disobeys Allah and His Apostle." (Bukhari)

2) Invitation to various kinds of gatherings other than wedding feasts. The majority of scholars say that accepting these invitations is mustahabb (recommended)…

But the scholars have stipulated conditions for accepting an invitation; if these conditions are not met then it is not obligatory or mustahabb to accept the invitation, rather it may be haram to attend.

These conditions were summed up by Sheikh Muhammad ibn 'Uthaymeen, who said:

1-There should be nothing objectionable (munkar) in the place where the party, etc., is to be held. If there is something objectionable and it is possible to remove it, then it is obligatory to attend for two reasons: to accept the invitation and to change the objectionable thing. If it is not possible to remove it then it is haram to attend.

2-The person who invited him should not be someone whom it is obligatory or Sunnah to forsake (such as one who openly commits immoral actions or sin, where forsaking him may be of benefit in bringing about his repentance).

3-The person who invited him should be a Muslim. If he is not, then it is not obligatory to accept the invitation, because the Prophet (peace and blessings of Allah be upon him) said: "The rights of a Muslim over his fellow Muslim are five…"

4-The food offered should be halal (lawful).

5-Accepting the invitation should not lead to ignoring a more important duty; if that is the case then it is haram to accept the invitation.

6- It should not cause any trouble to the person who is invited. For example, if he needs to travel or to leave his family who need him there, and so on. (al-Qawl al-Mufeed, 3/111).

Some scholars added:

7- If the host issued a general invitation, saying that everyone is welcome, then it is not obligatory to accept the invitation. (327)

342. Dishonoring the Guest

Allah, the Exalted, says:

"Has the story reached you, of the honored guests [three angels; Jibreel (Gabriel) along with another two] of Ibrahim (Abraham)? When they came in to him and said: 'Salam (peace be upon you),' He answered: 'Salam (peace be upon you)', and said: 'You are a people unknown to me.' Then he turned to his household and brought out a roasted calf (as the property of Ibrahim (Abraham) was mainly cows). And placed it before them, (saying): 'Will you not eat?'" (Qur'an, Adh-Dhariyat 51:24-27)

"And his (Lut's) people came rushing towards him, and since aforetime they used to commit crimes (sodomy), he said: 'O my people! Here are my daughters (i.e. the women of the nation), they are purer for you (if you marry them lawfully). So, fear Allah and disgrace me not with regard to my guests! Is there not among you a single right-minded man?'" (Qur'an, Hud 11:78)

Abu Hurairah (May Allah be pleased with him) reported: The Prophet (peace and blessings be upon him) said, "He who believes in Allah and the Last Day, let him show hospitality to his guest; and he who believes in Allah and the Last Day, let him maintain good relation with kins; and he who believes in Allah and the Last Day, let him speak good or remain silent." (Bukhari and Muslim)

Abu Shurayh Khuwaylid ibn 'Amr al-Khuza'i (May Allah be pleased with him) reported that the Prophet (May Allah's peace and blessings be upon him) said: "Whoever believes in Allah and the Last Day let him honor his guest with his due reward." They said: "O Messenger of Allah, what is his due reward?" He said: "A day and a night (of excellent accommodation), and hospitality is for three days, and whatever is beyond that is charity offered to him." In another version: "It is not lawful for a guest to stay (for long) at the home of his brother to the point that he causes him to sin." They said: "O Messenger of Allah, how does he cause him to sin?" He said: "He overstays with him till he has nothing to serve to him." (Bukhari and Muslim with its two versions) (https://hadeethenc.com/en/browse/hadith/3042)

Commentary: This Hadith throws light on something more of the etiquette and scope of hospitality. A guest ought to be given the best entertainment on the first day and night. For the next two days, hospitality should be moderate. On the fourth day, the guest should leave for his destination. Yet if he chooses to stay, hospitality will be in the sense of charity. (328)

Abu Hurairah (May Allah be pleased with him) reported that the Prophet (May Allah's peace and blessings be upon him) said: "Whoever believes in Allah and the Last Day, let him say good words or remain silent. Whoever believes in Allah and the Last Day, let him be generous to his neighbor. Whoever believes in Allah and the Last Day, let him be hospitable to his guest." (Bukhari and Muslim)

(https://hadeethenc.com/en/browse/hadith/5437)

343. Remaining in the Invited Home Unnecessarily After a Meal

Allah, the Exalted, says:

"Believers, do not enter the houses of the Prophet for a meal without permission. if you are invited, you may enter, but be punctual (so that you will not be waiting while the meal is being prepared). When you have finished eating, leave his home. Do not sit around chatting among yourselves. This will annoy the Prophet but he will feel embarrassed to tell you. God does not feel embarrassed to tell you the truth. When you want to ask something from the wives of the Prophet, ask them from behind the curtain. This would be more proper for you and for them. You are not supposed to trouble the Prophet or to ever marry his wives after his death, for this would be a grave offense in the sight of God." (Qur'an, Al-Ahzab 33:53)

Narrated Anas bin Malik (May Allah be pleased with him): "Then he called the men in batches of ten to eat of it, and he said to them, "Mention the Name of Allah, and each man should eat of the dish the nearest to him." When all of them had finished their meals, some of them left and a few remained there talking, over which I felt unhappy. Then the Prophet (peace be upon him) went out towards the dwelling places (of his wives) and I too, went out after him and told him that those people had left. Then he returned and entered his dwelling place and let the curtains fall while I was in (his) dwelling place, and he was reciting the Verses: 'O you who believe! Enter not the Prophet's house leave until is given you for a meal, (and then) not (as early as) to what for its preparation. But when you are invited, enter, and when you have taken your meals, disperse without sitting for a talk. Verily such (behavior) annoys the Prophet; and he would be shy of (asking) you (to go), but Allah is not shy of (telling you) the Truth.' (33-53) Abu Uthman said: Anas said, "I served the Prophet for ten years." (Bukhari)

344. Uninvited Guests

Abu Masud Al-Badri (May Allah be pleased with him) reported: "A man prepared some food especially for the Prophet (peace and blessings be upon him) and invited him along with four others. But a man accompanied him. Having arrived at the door, Messenger of Allah (peace and blessings be upon him) said to the host, "This person has followed us. You may allow him, if you like, and if you like, he will return." He said: "O Messenger of Allah, I allow him too." (Bukhari and Muslim)

Commentary: It will be considered an expression of bad manners if somebody participates in a feast as an uninvited, parasitic guest. Yet, he stands a chance in case he is allowed by the host… (329)

345. Abomination of Selecting Friday, Single Day, for Fasting

Narrated Abu Hurairah (May Allah be pleased with him): "I heard the Messenger of Allah (peace and blessings be upon him) as saying: "None of you should observe fast on Friday except that he should observe fast either one day before it or one day after it." (Bukhari and Muslim)

Narrated Juwairiyah bint Al-Harith (May Allah be pleased with her): The Prophet (peace and blessings be upon him) visited her on a Friday and she was observing fast. He (peace and blessings be upon him) asked, "Did you observe fast yesterday?" She said, "No." He asked, "Do you intend to observe fast tomorrow?" She said, "No." He (peace and blessings be upon him) said, "In that case, give up your fast today." (Bukhari)

Narrated Abu Hurairah (May Allah be pleased with him): The Prophet (peace and blessings be upon him) said, "Do not choose the Friday night among all other nights for standing in (Tahajjud) prayer, and do not choose Friday among all other days for Saum (fasting) except that one you have accustomed to." (Muslim)

Commentary: It is undesirable to fix Jumu'ah for voluntary fast. One can, however, observe fasting if Friday occurs in his routine of fasts, i.e. if one observes fast on alternate days and Jumu'ah occurs on the day when he observes fast, or if one observes the fast of the Day of 'Arafah, or the Day of 'Ashura', and Friday occurs on that day, or if Friday occurs during the Ayyam Al-Beid, or Friday occurs when one is observing fasts of Nadhr (fasts one has vowed for). (330)

346. Fasting on Saturday, Single Day

Narrated As-Samma' sister of Abdullah ibn Busr: The Prophet (peace and blessings be upon him) said: "Do not fast on Saturday except what has been made obligatory on you, and if one of you can get nothing but a grape skin or a piece of wood from a tree, he should chew it." (Tirmidhi and Abu Dawud;

Tirmidhi said: "This is a hasan Hadith. What is makrooh in this case is for a man to single out Saturday for fasting, because the Jews venerate Saturday. End quote.) (331)

Fasting on Saturday is permissible when:

1. Coupled with fasting the day before or after.

2. It coincides with other fasting like the fasting of Ashura or Shawwal.

3. Coinciding with the fasting of the Prophet Dawud on every alternate day

347. Prohibition of Extending Fast Beyond One Day

Abu Hurairah and Aisha (May Allah be pleased with them) said: "The Prophet (peace and blessings be upon him) prohibited observing continuous voluntary fasts beyond one day." (Bukhari and Muslim)

Ibn 'Umar (May Allah be pleased with him) said: "The Messenger of Allah (peace and blessings be upon him) prohibited observing continuous fasts beyond one day. The Companions submitted: "But you do it." He replied, "I am not like you. I am given to eat and to drink (from Allah)." (Bukhari and Muslim)

Commentary:

1. Through this Hadith we learn that in certain matters the Prophet (peace and blessings be upon him) had some specific injunctions which were obligatory for him but not for his Ummah. Such things were permissible for him but not for his followers. All these things are called his special distinctions. It is not permissible for Muslims to follow such practices. One of these things is Saum Al-Wisal, which means to observe fast for several days at a stretch without taking any food. Since Allah had granted him special power and patience, he could observe fast continuously for days. As his followers are not endowed with that energy and patience, they are not permitted to do so.

2. "I am not like you" does not mean that "I am not a man like you," because such an interpretation goes against a categorical statement of the Qur'an to the effect that "I am a man like you". What the statement "I am not like you" really means is "you do not possess that special power which has been granted to me."

3. "I am given to eat and to drink" signifies that Allah the Almighty provides him with the strength and energy which he can derive from food and drink without necessarily having them. (332)

348. Fasting on Eid Al-Fitr, Eid Al-Adha and Three Days of Tashreeq

Narrated Abu Ubaid (May Allah be pleased with him): "I was present for Eid with Umar bin Khattab. He started with the prayer before the sermon, and said: 'The Messenger of Allah (peace and blessings of Allah be upon him) forbade fasting on these two days, the Day of Fitr and the Day of Adha. As for the Day of Fitr, it is the day when you break your fast, and on the Day of Adha you eat the meat of your sacrifices.'" (Ibn Majah)

Narrated Bishr bin Suhaim (May Allah be pleased with him): The Messenger of Allah (peace and blessings of Allah be upon him) delivered a sermon on the days of Tashreeq (11th, 12th, and 13th of Dhul-Hijjah) and said: "No one will enter Paradise but a Muslim soul, and these days are the days of eating and drinking." (Ibn Majah)

Narrated Aisha and Ibn Umar (May Allah be pleased with them): "Nobody was allowed to fast on the days of Tashreeq except those who could not afford the Hadi (Sacrifice)." (Bukhari)

Narrated Qazaa Maula (freed slave of) Ziyad: "I heard Abu Said Al-khudri narrating four things from the Prophet and I appreciated them very much. He said, conveying the words of the Prophet. 1) "A woman should not go on a two-day journey except with her husband or a Dhi-Mahram, 2) No fasting is permissible on two days: Eid-al-Fitr and Eid-al-Adha, 3) No prayer after two prayers, i.e. after the Fajr prayer till the sun rises and after the 'Asr prayer till the sun sets, 4) Do not prepare yourself for a journey except to three Mosques, i.e. Al-Masjid Al-Haram, the Mosque of Aqsa (Jerusalem) and my Mosque." (Bukhari)

349. Relieving Oneself Facing Qiblah or Turning Back Towards

Salman (May Allah be pleased with him) reported that it was said to him: "Your Prophet taught you everything, even how to relieve yourself." Salman replied: "Yes, he did. He prohibited us from facing the Qiblah when defecating or urinating and from using the right hand, using less than three stones, and using dung and bones in Istinja.'" (Muslim) (https://hadeethenc.com/en/browse/hadith/10048)

350. Prohibition of Relieving Nature on the Paths

Allah, the Exalted, says:

"And those who annoy believing men and women undeservedly, they bear (on themselves) the crime of slander and plain sin." (33:58)

Narrated Abu Hurairah (May Allah be pleased with him): The Messenger of Allah (peace and blessings be upon him) said, "Avoid two habits which provoke cursing." The Companions said: "What are those things which provoke cursing?" He said, "Relieving on the thoroughfares or under the shades where people take shelter and rest." (Muslim)

Commentary: We learn from this Hadith that a Muslim must avoid all such things which cause inconvenience to other Muslims... (333)

Public pathways and shaded areas are two areas, where people would be offended from excrement and filth. The same curse would apply to those who leave filth behind for the next person. The curse has two meanings: people are cursed by the one who has to deal with the dirt they left behind and they are cursed by Allah for their careless and disgusting habits.

351. Not Concealing One's' Private Part while Bathing or Relieving Oneself

'Abdullah b. Ja'far (May Allah be pleased with him) reported: "The Messenger of Allah (peace and blessings be upon him) one day made me mount behind him and he confided to me something secret which I would not disclose to anybody; and the Messenger of Allah (peace and blessings be upon him) liked the concealment provided by a lofty place or cluster of dates (while answering the call of nature), Ibn Asma' said in his narration: 'It implied an enclosure of the date-trees.'" (Muslim)

Narrated Jabir ibn Abdullah (May Allah be pleased with him): "When the Prophet (peace and blessings be upon him) felt the need of relieving himself, he went far off where no one could see him." (Abu Dawud)

Ali bin Abi Talid (May Allah be pleased with him) narrated: The Messenger of Allah said: "The screen between the eyes of the Jinn and nakedness of the children of Adam when one of you enters the area of relieving oneself is saying: 'Bismillah.'" (Tirmidhi)

Ya'la ibn Umayyah (May Allah be pleased with him) reported that the Messenger of Allah (May Allah's peace and blessings be upon him) saw a man bathing in an open area without a lower garment. So, he mounted the pulpit, praised and extolled Allah, and said: "Verily, Allah, Glorified and Exalted, is characterized by modesty and concealment, and He loves modesty and concealment. Therefore, when any of you bathes, let him conceal himself." (An-Nasa'i) (https://hadeethenc.com/en/browse/hadith/8292)

352. Greeting, Speaking and Eating in the Toilet

Narrated Jabir bin 'Abdullah (May Allah be pleased with him): "A man passed by the Prophet while he was urinating, and greeted him by the Salam. The Messenger of Allah said to him: "If you see me in this situation, do not greet me with the Salam, for if you do that, I will not respond to you." (Ibn Majah)

The Islamic greeting is Asalam Alaykum (peace be upon you). "Asalam" is one of the Names of Allah. One should not greet a person who is answering the call of nature or return a greeting whilst one is answering the call of nature, out of respect to Allah by not mentioning His Name in a dirty place. The majority of scholars said that it is makrooh (disliked) to speak in the restroom unnecessarily.

Sheikh Ibn 'Uthaymeen (May Allah have mercy on him) was asked about the ruling on eating and drinking in the bathroom. He replied: "The bathroom is a place for relieving oneself only and one should not stay there longer than is necessary. Eating or doing other things there requires staying there for a length of time that is not appropriate." (End quote from Majmoo' al-Fataawa, 11/110) (334)

353. Prohibition of Using the Right Hand for Cleaning After Toilet Without Valid Reason

Allah, the Exalted, says:

"Then as for him who will be given his Record in his right hand will say: 'Take, read my Record!'" (Qur'an, Al-Haqqah 69:19)

"So those on the right hand (i.e. those who will be given their Records in their right hands), Who will be those on the right hand? (As a respect for them, because they will enter Paradise). And those on the left hand (i.e. those who will be given their Record in their left hands), Who will be those on the left hand? (As a disgrace for them, because they will enter Hell)." *(Qur'an, Al-Waqi'ah 56:8-9)*

Aisha (May Allah be pleased with her) reported: "The Messenger of Allah (peace and blessings be upon him) was used to using his right hand for performing Wudu and for eating his food whereas he was used to using his left hand in his toilet and for other similar purposes." (Abu Dawud)

Commentary: The Messenger of Allah (peace and blessings be upon him) used to use his left hand in washing his private parts and cleaning his nose and similar things. (335)

Hafsah (May Allah be pleased with her) reported: "The Messenger of Allah (peace and blessings be upon him) used to use his right hand for eating, drinking and wearing his clothes and used to use his left hand for other purposes." (Abu Dawud)

Abu Qatadah (May Allah be pleased with him) said: The Prophet (peace and blessings be upon him) said, "Do not touch your private parts with your right hand while urinating, nor for washing or cleaning (your private parts); and do not breathe into the drinking vessel from which you drink." (Bukhari and Muslim)

Commentary: Muslims are required to take food and do other such things with their right hand. They have been ordained to do all the other essential but not much liked acts with their left hand. (336)

354. Not Cleaning Oneself from All Traces of Urine

Narrated Ibn Abbas (May Allah have mercy on him): "Once the Prophet (peace and blessings be upon him), while passing through one of the graveyards of Madinah or Makkah, heard the voices of two persons who were being tortured in their graves. The Prophet (peace and blessings be upon him) said, "These two persons are being tortured not for a Major sin (to avoid)." The Prophet then added, "Yes! (they are being tortured for a Major sin). Indeed, one of them never saved himself from being soiled with his urine while the other used to go about with calumnies (to make enmity between friends). The Prophet (peace and blessings be upon him) then asked for a green leaf of a date-palm tree, broke it into two pieces and put one on each grave. On being asked why he had done so, he replied, "I hope that their torture might be lessened, till these get dried." (Bukhari)

Narrated Aisha (May Allah have mercy on her): The Messenger of Allah (peace and blessings be upon him) said: "Ten are the acts according to Fitrah: clipping the moustache, letting the beard grow, using the tooth stick, snuffing water in the nose, cutting the nails, washing the finger joints, plucking the hair under the armpits, shaving the pubes and cleaning one's private parts with water. The narrator said: 'I have forgotten the tenth, but it may have been rinsing the mouth.'" (Muslim)

355. Urinating in a Hole

Narrated Abdullah ibn Sarjis (May Allah be pleased with him): "The Prophet (peace and blessings be upon him) prohibited to urinate in a hole." (Abu Dawud)

Narrated Qatadah from Abdullah bin Sarjis: The Prophet of Allah (peace and blessings be upon him) said: "None of you should urinate into a burrow in the ground." They said to Qatadah: "Why is it disliked to urinate into a burrow in the ground?" He said: "It is said that these are dwelling places of the Jinns." (An-Nasa'i)

356. Prohibition of Urinating into Stagnant Water

Jabir (May Allah be pleased with him) said: The Messenger of Allah (peace and blessings be upon him) forbade urinating into stagnant water." (Muslim)

Commentary: "Stagnant water" means water which is not flowing, like the water in a pond or a tank. When urination is prohibited at such places, defecating would be more sternly prohibited… (337)

357. Uncleanliness

Allah, the Exalted, says:

"*Truly, Allah loves those who turn to Him constantly and He loves those who keep themselves pure and clean.*" *(Qur'an, Al-Baqarah 2:222)*

"*…Verily, the Mosque whose foundation was laid from the first day on piety is more worthy that you stand therein (to pray). In it are men who love to clean and to purify themselves. And Allah loves those who make themselves clean and pure (i.e. who clean their private parts with dust (i.e. to be considered as soap) and water from urine and stools, after answering the call of nature].*" *(Qur'an, At-Tawbah 9:108)*

Narrated Abu Sufyan (May Allah be pleased with him) said: "Abu Ayyub Al-Ansari, Jabir bin 'Abdullah, and Anas bin Malik told me that when this Verse: *"In it (the Mosque) are men who love to clean and to purify themselves. And Allah loves those who make themselves clean and pure." (Qur'an, At-Tawbah 9:108)* was revealed, the Messenger of Allah (peace and blessings be upon him) said: 'O Ansar! Allah has praised you for your cleanliness. What is the nature of your cleanliness?' They said: 'We perform ablution for prayer and we take a bath to cleanse ourselves of impurity due to sexual activity, and we clean ourselves with water (after urinating).' He said: 'This is what it is. So, adhere to it.'" (Ibn Majah)

Narrated Abu Musa al-Ashari (May Allah be pleased with him): The Messenger of Allah (peace and blessings be upon him) said: "Cleanliness is half of Faith and al-Hamdu Liliah (Praise be to Allah) fills the scale, and Subhan Allah (Glory be to Allah) and al-Hamdu Liliah (Praise be to Allah) fill up what is between the heavens and the earth, and prayer is a light, and charity is proof (of one's faith) and endurance is a brightness and the Holy Qur'an is a proof on your behalf or against you. All men go out early in the morning and sell themselves, thereby setting themselves free or destroying themselves." (Muslim)

358. Prohibition of Magic - Sorcery - Witchcraft

Allah, the Exalted, says:

"And verily, there were men among mankind who took shelter with the masculine among the Jinns, but they (Jinns) increased them (mankind) in sin and disbelief." (Qur'an, Al-Jinn 72:6)

"He [Musa (Moses)] said: "Throw you (first)." So, when they threw, they bewitched the eyes of the people, and struck terror into them, and they displayed a great magic." (Qur'an, Al-A'raf 7:116)

"Sulaiman (Solomon) did not disbelieve, but the Shayateen (Devils) disbelieved, teaching men magic." (Qur'an, Al-Baqarah 2:102)

Other Verses: *Ash-Shu'ara 26:221-222, Taha 20:69, Al-An'am 6:59.*

Narrated Abu Hurairah (May Allah be pleased with him): The Prophet (peace and blessings be upon him) said, "Avoid the seven destructive things." It was asked (by those present): "What are they, O Messenger of Allah?" He replied, "Associating anyone or anything with Allah in worship; practicing sorcery, killing of someone without a just cause whom Allah has forbidden, devouring the property of an orphan, eating of usury, fleeing from the battlefield and slandering chaste women who never even think of anything touching chastity and are good believers." (Bukhari and Muslim)

Commentary: The teaching, learning and practicing of Magic are all unlawful. (338)

Malik (May Allah be pleased with him) related to me that he heard that Umar ibn al-Khattab wanted to go to Iraq, and Kabal-Ahbar said to him, "Do not go there, amir al-muminin. There is nine-tenths of sorcery there and it is the place of the rebellious Jinns and the disease which the doctors are unable to cure." (Malik Muwatta)

Aisha (May Allah be pleased with her) reported: "A man from the Banu Zurayq, whose name was Labid ibn al-A'sam, performed Magic on the Messenger of Allah (May Allah's peace and blessings be upon him) and he began to imagine that he had done something that he had not. One day, while he was with me, he supplicated to Allah the Almighty, and he supplicated for a prolonged period and then said: 'O Aisha, do you know that Allah has told me regarding the matter I asked Him about? Two men came to me, one of them sat near my head and the other sat near my feet. One of them asked his companion: "What is wrong with this man?" The other replied: "He is under a Magic spell." The first one asked: "Who performed Magic on him?" The other replied: "Labid ibn al-A'sam." The first one asked: "What did he do it with?" The other replied: "With a comb and the hair stuck in it, and the skin of a male date palm pollen." The first one asked: "Where is it?" The other replied: "In the well of Dharwan." The Messenger of Allah (May Allah's peace and blessings be upon him) went with some of his Companions to the well. He returned to me and said: 'O Aisha, by Allah, the water in that well was (red) like a Henna leaf infusion, and the date palms were like the heads of Devils.' I said: 'O Messenger of Allah, should you take (those things) out (of the pollen skin)?' He said: 'No. Allah has healed me, and I was afraid that I would spread evil among the people.' He then ordered the well be filled with earth, and it was filled with earth." (Bukhari and Muslim) (https://hadeethenc.com/en/browse/hadith/10570)

Narrated Abu Hurairah (May Allah be pleased with him): "The Messenger of Allah (peace and blessings be upon him) said: 'Whoever ties a knot and blows on it, he has practiced Magic; and whoever practices Magic, he has committed Shirk; and whoever hangs up something (as an amulet) will be entrusted to it.'" (An-Nasa'i)

Safiyya (May Allah be pleased with her) reported from some of the wives of Allah's Apostle (peace be upon him): Allah's Apostle (peace and blessings be upon him) having said: "He who visits a diviner ('Arraf) and asks him about anything, his prayers extending to forty nights will not be accepted." (Muslim)

Narrated Zainab (May Allah be pleased with her): "There was an old woman who used to enter upon us and perform Ruqyah from Erysipelas: contagious disease which causes fever and leaves a red coloration of the skin. We had a bed with long legs, and when 'Abdullah entered he would clear his throat and make noise. He entered one day and when she heard his voice, she veiled herself from him. He came and sat beside me and touched me, and he found a sting. He said: 'What is this?' I said: 'An amulet against Erysipelas.' He pulled it, broke it and threw it away, and said: 'The family of 'Abdullah has no need of polytheism.' I heard the Messenger of Allah (peace and blessings be upon him) say: "Ruqyah (i.e. which consist of the names of idols and Devils, etc.), amulets and Tiwalah (charms) are polytheism.'" I said: 'I went out one day and so-and-so looked at me, and my eye began to water on the nearest side him. When I recited Ruqyah for it, it stopped, but if I did not recite Ruqyah it watered again.' He said: 'That is Satan, if you obey him, he leaves you alone but if you disobey him, he pokes you with his finger in your eye. But if you do what the Messenger of Allah (peace be upon him) used to do, that will be better for you and more effective in healing. Sprinkle water in your eye and say: 'Adhibil-bas Rabban-nas, washfi Antash-Shafi, la shifa'a illa shafi'uka, shafi'an la yughadiru saqaman (Take away the pain, O Lord of mankind, and grant healing, for You are the Healer, and there is no healing but Your Healing that leaves no trace of sickness).'" (Ibn Majah)

Malik related to me from Zayd ibn Aslam that Abdullah ibn Umar said, "Two men from the east stood up and spoke, and people were amazed at their eloquence. The Messenger of Allah (peace and blessings be upon him) said, 'Some eloquence is sorcery,' or he said, 'Part of eloquence is sorcery.'" (Malik Muwatta)

Bajalah ibn 'Abadah (May Allah be pleased with him) reported that 'Umar ibn al-Khattab (May Allah be pleased with him) wrote: "Kill every sorcerer and sorceress." Bajalah said: "So we killed three sorceresses." Ibn 'Umar (May Allah be pleased with him) said: "A maid-servant of Hafsah (the Prophet's wife) bewitched her and admitted practicing sorcery. So Hafsah ordered 'Abdur-Rahman ibn Zayd to kill her." Also, Abu 'Uthman An-Nahdi said: "Al-Walid had a magician who used to perform shows before him. He once slaughtered a man, cutting off his head, and we were astonished. Then he returned the head to its proper place, so Jundub al-Azdi came and killed him." (Bayhaqi) (https://hadeethenc.com/en/browse/hadith/5946)

Taweez, Amulets, Talismans for Good Luck Charms or to Ward off the Evil Eye is an act of Idolatry (Shirk)

Ruwaifi' b. Thabit told that God's Messenger said to him, "You may live for a long time after I am gone, Ruwaifi', so tell people that if anyone ties his beard or wears round his neck a string to ward off the Evil Eye, or cleanses himself with animal dung or bone, Muhammad has nothing to do with him." (Abu Dawud)

Abu Bashir al-Ansari (May Allah be pleased with him) reported: "He was with the Messenger of Allah (May Allah's peace and blessings be upon him) on one of his journeys, so he sent a messenger ordering: 'There should not remain any necklace of bowstring or any other kind of necklace around the necks of camels without being cut." (Bukhari and Muslim) (https://hadeethenc.com/en/browse/hadith/6761)

'Uqbah ibn 'Amir reported: The Messenger of Allah (peace and blessings be upon him) received a group of men and he accepted the pledge of nine of them, while he refrained from one. They said, "O Messenger of Allah, you accepted the pledge of nine men and left this one out?" The Prophet said, "Verily, there is an amulet upon him." The man took it in his hand and cut it, then the Prophet accepted his pledge and he said, "Whoever hangs an amulet around his neck has committed an act of idolatry." (Ahmad)

Narrated 'Imran bin Husain: The Prophet (peace and blessings be upon him) saw a man with a brass ring on his hand. He said: "What is this ring?" He said: "It is for Wahinah." He said: "Take it off, for it will only increase you in weakness." (Ibn Majah)

Jabir told that when the Prophet (peace and blessings be upon him) was asked about a charm for one who is possessed (*nushra*)*, he replied, "It pertains to the work of the Devil." (Abu Dawud)

* *Nushra* comes from a root meaning to disperse and is said to be used meaning a charm for one who is possessed because it disperses the trouble.

'Isa b. Hamza told that he went to visit 'Abdallah b. 'Ukaim* who was suffering from Erysipelas and asked why he did not attach an amulet. He replied, "We seek refuge in God from that. God's Messenger said that if anyone hangs anything on himself, he will be left to it."** (Abu Dawud)

* *Mirqat*, iv, 510 wrongly gives Hukaim. Cf. Tahdhib, v, 323 f. ** If anyone puts his trust in a charm instead of seeking God's help, His help will be withheld from him.

Sorcery (Witchcraft, Black Magic or Sihr in Arabic) can only be performed with the aid of Devils (the Unseen world of Jinn) whose help is attained under one condition: the sorcerer must carry out, under Satan's request, shameful and haram acts which are strictly forbidden by Islam and actions that are Shirk and kufr and in return the Evil Jinn will obey the sorcerer and help him mislead and harm people. It is real and there are kinds of witchcraft that may affect people psychologically and physically, so that they become sick or even die, or cause infertility, miscarriage or divorce. Its effects happen by the Will of Allah.

The beneficial knowledge about Black Magic were described by Ibn Taymiyah, Abdul-'Azeez Ibn Baaz, Wahid Ibn Adbessalam, Muhammad Tim Humble, etc. (10, 339-341)

Another form of fortune telling is the practice of predicting information about a person's life. Sometimes called "reading" or "spiritual consultation", fortune teller gives the client advice and predictions which are said to have come from spirits or in visions.

Alectromancy: by observation of a rooster pecking at grain.
Astrology: by the movements of celestial bodies.
Astromancy: by the stars.
Augury: by the flight of birds.
Bazi or four pillars: by hour, day, month, and year of birth.
Bibliomancy: by books; frequently, but not always, religious texts.
Cartomancy: by playing cards, tarot cards, or oracle cards.
Ceromancy: by patterns in melting or dripping wax.
Chiromancy: by the shape of the hands and lines in the palms.
Chronomancy: by determination of lucky and unlucky days.
Clairvoyance: by spiritual vision or inner sight.

Cleromancy: by casting of lots, or casting bones or stones.
Cold reading: by using visual and aural clues.
Crystallomancy: by crystal ball also called scrying.
Extispicy: by the entrails of animals.
Face reading: by means of variations in face and head shape.
Feng shui: by earthen harmony.
Gastromancy: by stomach-based ventriloquism (historically).
Geomancy: by markings in the ground, sand, earth, or soil.
Haruspicy: by the livers of sacrificed animals.
Horary astrology: the astrology of the time the question was asked.
Hydromancy: by water.
I Ching divination: by yarrow stalks or coins and the I Ching.
Kau cim by means of numbered bamboo sticks shaken from a tube.
Lithomancy: by stones or gems.
Molybdomancy: by molten metal after dumped in cold water
Naeviology: by moles, scars, or other bodily marks
Necromancy: by the dead, or by spirits or souls of the dead.
Nephomancy: by shapes of clouds.
Numerology: by numbers.
Oneiromancy: by dreams.
Onomancy: by names.
Palmistry: by lines and mounds on the hand.
Parrot astrology: by parakeets picking up fortune cards
Paper fortune teller: origami used in fortune-telling games.
Pendulum reading: by the movements of a suspended object.
Pyromancy: by gazing into fire.
Rhabdomancy: divination by rods.
Runecasting or Runic divination: by runes.
Scrying: by looking at or into reflective objects.
Spirit board: by planchette or talking board.
Taromancy: by a form of cartomancy using tarot cards.
Tasseography or tasseomancy: by tea leaves or coffee grounds. (342)

Counteracting Magic with Magic - It is an Act of Devil

Jabir (May Allah be pleased with him) reported that when the Messenger of Allah (May Allah's peace and blessings be upon him) was asked about the 'Nushrah' (counteracting Magic with Magic), he said: "It is an act of the Devil." (Abu Dawud and Ahmad) (https://hadeethenc.com/en/browse/hadith/3402)

Narrated 'Abdullah bin 'Amr bin Al-As (May Allah be pleased with him): "This Verse: *'Verily We have sent you (O Muhammad) as a witness, as a bringer of glad tidings and as a warner.' (48.8)* which is in the Qur'an, appears in the Torah thus: 'Verily We have sent you (O Muhammad) as a witness, as a bringer of glad tidings and as a warner, and as a protector for the illiterates (i.e. the Arabs.) You are My slave and My Apostle, and I have named you Al-Mutawakkil (one who depends upon Allah). You are neither hard-hearted nor of fierce character, nor one who shouts in the markets. You do not return evil for evil, but excuse and forgive. Allah will not take you unto Him till He guides through you a crocked (curved) nation on the Right Path by causing them to say: "None has the right to be worshipped but Allah." With such a statement He will cause to open blind eyes, deaf ears and hardened hearts.'" (Bukhari)

Ibn Taymiyah (May Allah have mercy on him) in his book - Ibn Taymiyah's Essay on Jinn (Demons) - described the way how the sorcery is done, the contract between the fortune teller and Jinn, the mystery of the Unseen world of Jinn. (10)

"If a man's soul goes bad, his nature will then desire what is harmful and he will take pleasure in corruption and love it dearly. As a result, the character, health and wealth of such a man will also become corrupted and destroyed. Satan is himself vile, so if one seeks to gain his favor through the things which he loves, like incantations, oaths, books on spiritualism and Magic, disbelief and idolatry, etc., he will fulfil some of the person's desires. Sacrilegious acts are like a bribe to Satan. It is similar to the case wherein a man may give another money to kill someone he wishes killed or to help him in performing some obscene act. Consequently, much of these amulets have Qur'anic Verses written in impurities like blood, etc., or some Qur'anic Words written backwards, or other things which please the Devil may be written or spoken over them. When that which pleases the Devil is written or spoken by men, he may help them attain some of their desires, like removing large quantities of water from some place, or carrying them in the air to other places, or bringing them wealth stolen from the treacherous and those who do not mention Allah's Name on their wealth, etc.

The deviant ascetics and heretics devoted to prayer who experience illuminations and visions, usually retreat to locations frequented by the Devils in which Salah has been prohibited. They choose such places because the Devils visit them there and communicate with them in the same way that they communicate with Magicians and Fortune tellers. The Jinn also enter idols, speak to those who worship the idols and fulfil some of their needs. They often help star worshippers when they perform acts of worship which the Jinn consider suitable, like singing praises to idols representing the sun, moon and the planets, dressing the idols in luxurious garments, and burning incense in their presence, etc. The Devils may appear to these servants of theirs in forms which humans mistakenly identify as heavenly spirits and the Devils may fulfil some of their requests by killing some of their enemies, making others sick, attracting someone whom they desire, or bringing them some wealth. However, the harm they receive from such service is often many times greater than the benefit.

Many of those who utilize the Jinn in these ways claim that Prophet Sulayman (May Allah have mercy on him) used the Jinn in the same manner for the same purpose. More than one of the early scholars have mentioned that when Sulayman died, the Devils wrote books on Magic filled with acts of disbelief and put them under his chair. When the books were discovered, the Devils then claimed that Sulayman used to use the Jinn by these methods. As a result, some Christians and Jews have falsely discredited Prophet Sulayman. Others claimed that if Magic were not permissible, Sulayman would not have practiced it. Both groups went astray, one by debasing Prophet Sulayman and the other by practicing Magic. Consequently, Almighty Allah revealed the following Verse:

"They followed what the Shayateen (Devils) gave out (falsely of the Magic) in the lifetime of Sulaiman (Solomon). Sulaiman did not disbelieve, but the Shayateen (Devils) disbelieved, teaching men Magic and such things that came down at Babylon to the two angels, Harut and Marut, but neither of these two (angels) taught anyone (such things) till they had said, "We are only for trial, so disbelieve not (by learning this Magic from us)." And from these (angels) people learn that by which they cause separation between man and his wife, but they could not thus harm anyone except by Allah's Leave. And they learn that which harms them and profits them not. And indeed, they knew that the buyers of it (Magic) would have no share in the Hereafter. And how bad indeed was that for which they sold their own selves, if they but knew." *(Qur'an, Al-Baqarah 2:102)*

Jinn Transformation from Invisible to Physical Forms

The Jinn may take the form of animals like snakes, scorpions, camels, cows, goats, sheep, horses, mules, donkeys and birds. They may also assume the form of humans, as in the case where the Devil came to the Quraysh in the form of Suraqah ibn Malik when they wanted to set out to Badr. In reference to this incident, Allah, the Exalted, revealed the Verse:

"And (remember) when Shaitan (Satan) made their (evil) deeds seem fair to them and said, "No one of mankind can overcome you this Day (of the battle of Badr) and verily, I am your neighbour (for each and every help)." But when the two forces came in sight of each other, he ran away and said "Verily, I have nothing to do with you. Verily! I see what you see not. Verily! I fear Allah for Allah is Severe in punishment." *(Qur'an, Al-Anfal 8:48)*

It is also narrated that Satan took the form of an old man from Najd when the leaders of Quraysh gathered in their assembly room to decide whether to kill the Prophet, imprison him or banish him." (10)

359. Prohibition of Consultation with Soothsayers

Allah, the Exalted, says:

"And with Him are the keys of the Ghaib (all that is hidden), none knows them but He. And He knows whatever there is in (or on) the earth and in the sea; not a leaf falls, but he knows it. There is not a grain in the darkness of the earth nor anything fresh or dry, but is written in a Clear Record." *(Qur'an, Al-An'am 6:59)*

"Say (O Muhammad SAW): "I possess no power of benefit or hurt to myself except as Allah wills. If I had the knowledge of the Ghaib (unseen), I should have secured for myself an abundance of wealth, and no evil should have touched me. I am but a warner, and a bringer of glad tidings unto people who believe." *(Qur'an, Al-A'raf 7:188)*

Aisha (May Allah be pleased with her) said: "Some people asked the Messenger of Allah (peace and blessings be upon him) about soothsayers. He (peace and blessings be upon him) said, "They are of no account." Upon this they said to him, "O Messenger of Allah! But they sometimes make true predictions." Thereupon the Messenger of Allah (peace be upon him) said, "That is a word to truth which is a Jinn snatches (from the angels) and whispers into the ears of his friend (the soothsayers) who will then mix more than a hundred lies with it." (Bukhari and Muslim)

Narrated Safiyyah, daughter of Abu 'Ubaid, on the authority of some of the wives of the Prophet (peace and blessings be upon him) who said, "He who goes to one who claims to tell about matters of the Unseen and believes in him, his Salah (prayers) will not be accepted for forty days." (Muslim)

Commentary: We learn from this Hadith that visiting soothsayers and astrologers for the purpose of knowing from them what lies hidden in the future is such a great offense that he who does it, loses all merits of his forty days Salah… (343)

Qabisah bin Al-Mukhariq (May Allah be pleased with him) said: "I heard the Messenger of Allah (peace and blessings be upon him) saying, "The practice of 'Iyafah, the interpretation of omens from the flight of birds, the practice of divination by drawing lines on the ground and taking evil omens are all practices of Al-Jibt (the idol, the diviner or sorcerer)." (Abu Dawud)

Mu'awiyah bin Al-Hakam (May Allah be pleased with him) reported: "I said: 'O Messenger of Allah, I have recently emerged from ignorance, and Allah has favored me with Islam. There are still some men among us who visit the soothsayers to consult them (on matters relating to the future).' He (peace be upon him) replied, 'Do not visit them.' I said: 'There are some men who are guided by omens.' He replied, 'These are the ideas which come up in their minds but you should not be influenced by them (i.e. these things) should not prevent them from pursuing their works.' I said: 'There are some men who practice divination by drawing lines on the ground.' The Messenger of Allah (peace be upon him) replied, 'There was a Prophet who drew lines."

'Imran Ibn Husayn and Ibn 'Abbas (May Allah be pleased with them) reported that the Prophet (May Allah's peace and blessings be upon him) said: "He is not one of us who seeks omens or has omens interpreted for him, or who practices soothsaying or has it done for him. And whoever goes to a soothsayer and believes in what he says has disbelieved in what was revealed to Muhammad (May Allah's peace and blessings be upon him)." (Al-Bazzar and Tabarani) (https://hadeethenc.com/en/browse/hadith/5981)

Narrated Abu Hurairah (May Allah be pleased with him): "The Messenger of Allah said: 'Whoever has intercourse with a menstruating woman, or with a woman in her rear, or who goes to a fortune teller and believes what he says, he has disbelieved in that which was revealed to Muhammad.'" (Ibn Majah)

Nobody knows tomorrow (Unseen) except Allah

Narrated Masruq (May Allah be pleased with him): "I said to Aisha, "O Mother! Did Prophet Muhammad see his Lord?" Aisha said, "What you have said makes my hair stand on end! Know that if somebody tells you one of the following three things, he is a liar: Whoever tells you that Muhammad saw his Lord, is a liar." Then Aisha recited the Verse: *'No vision can grasp Him, but His grasp is over all vision. He is the Most Courteous Well-Acquainted with all things.' (6:103) 'It is not fitting for a human being that Allah should speak to him except by inspiration or from behind a veil.' (42:51)* Aisha further said, "And whoever tells you that the Prophet knows what is going to happen tomorrow, is a liar." She then recited: *'No soul can know what it will earn tomorrow.' (31:34)* She added: "And whoever tells you that he concealed (some of Allah's orders), is a liar." Then she recited: *'O Apostle! Proclaim (the Message) which has been sent down to you from your Lord.' (5:67)* Aisha added. "But the Prophet (peace and blessings be upon him) saw Gabriel in his true form twice." (Bukhari)

360. Forbiddance of Believing in Ill Omens

Allah, the Exalted, says:

"No afflictions strike in the earth nor befalls you except According to what was written prior." (Qur'an, Hadid 57:22)

"And if Allah touches you with hurt, there is none who can remove it but He; and if He intends any good for you, there is no one who can repel His Favor . . ." (Qur'an, Yunus 10:107)

Narrated Anas (May Allah be pleased with him): The Messenger of Allah (peace and blessings be upon him) said, "Not the transmission of disease of one person to another and no evil omen, but I am pleased with good omens." He was asked: "What is good omen?" He replied, "A good word." (Bukhari and Muslim)

Narrated Ibn 'Umar (May Allah be pleased with him): The Messenger of Allah (peace and blessings be upon him) said, "There is no infection and no evil omen; but if there is anything (that may be a source of trouble) then it could be a house, a horse and a woman." (Bukhari and Muslim)

Buraidah (May Allah be pleased with him) said: "The Prophet never took ill omens." (Abu Dawud)

Narrated 'Urwah bin' Amir (May Allah be pleased with him): "When talking of omens was mentioned in the presence of the Messenger of Allah (peace and blessings be upon him), he said, "The best type of omen is the good omen." He (peace and blessings be upon him) added, "A Muslim should not refrain from anything because of an omen." He (peace and blessings be upon him) told them, "When any of you sees anything which he dislikes, he should say:

'Allahuma la ya'ti bil-hasanati illa Anta, wa la yadfa'us-sayyi'ati illa Anta, wa la hawla wa la quwwata illa Bika (O Allah! You Alone bring good things; You Alone avert evil things, and there is no might or power but in You).'" (Abu Dawud)

Commentary:
Muslim should pray to Allah for granting him the power and ability to abstain from evils. (344)

Abdullah ibn Masud reported that the Prophet (peace and blessings be upon him) said, "Paying attention to the bad omen (tayyara) is association (Shirk). It has nothing to do with us. Allah will remove it by reliance on Him." (Al-Adab Al-Mufrad, Bukhari)

Islam invalidated these practices as they corrode the foundation of Tawheed al- ibaadah, by directing the form of worship known as Trust (Tawakkul) to other than Allah; and Tawheed Al Asma was sifath, by attributing to man the power to predict the coming of good and evil, and the ability to avoid Allah's destiny. The knowledge of the future belongs to Allah Alone. Therefore, the Prophet (peace and blessings be upon him) denounces the very idea of bad omen, describing it as a form of associating partners with Allah. (10)

361. Believing in Horoscope and Astrology

Allah, the Exalted, says:

"Say: 'None in the heavens and the earth knows the Ghayb (Unseen) except Allah...'" (Qur'an, An-Naml 27:65)

"And with Him are the keys of the Ghaib (all that is hidden), none knows them but He. And He knows whatever there is in (or on) the earth and in the sea; not a leaf falls, but he knows it. There is not a grain in the darkness of the earth nor anything fresh or dry, but is written in a Clear Record." (Qur'an, Al-An'am 6:59)

"Say (O Muhammad SAW): "I possess no power of benefit or hurt to myself except as Allah wills. If I had the knowledge of the Ghaib (unseen), I should have secured for myself an abundance of wealth, and no evil should have touched me. I am but a warner, and a bringer of glad tidings unto people who believe." (Qur'an, Al-A'raf 7:188)

Narrated Abdullah ibn Abbas (May Allah have mercy on him): The Prophet (peace and blessings be upon him) said: "If anyone acquires any knowledge of astrology, he acquires a branch of Magic (Sihr) which he gets more as long as he continues to do so." (Abu Dawud)

Commentary: In this Hadith, astrology has been regarded as a part of Magic. In Islam the learning of Magic has been held equivalent to infidelity. Thus, it is evident that in Islam, astrology and soothsaying are highly dangerous, and learning them is a great sin. (343)

Since the Unseen is known only to Allah, the Prophet (May Allah's peace and blessings be upon him) forbade all attempts to figure it out. Astrology is thus forbidden, as it is an attempt to use celestial conditions to predict terrestrial events. (https://hadeethenc.com/en/browse/hadith/5989)

Qutadah said: "Allah created these stars for three purposes: to adorn the heavens, to stone the Devils and as signs by which to navigate. Whoever seeks anything else in them is mistaken and does not benefit from them, and he is wasting his time and effort in seeking something of which he has no knowledge." (Bukhari, Baab fi'l-Nujoom 2/240)

Astrology, horoscope, superstition and fortune telling are all actions of jaahiliyyah (period of Ignorance) which Islam came to show as false and to explain that they are Shirk, because they involve depending on something other than Allah, and believing that benefit and harm come from something other than Him, and believing the words of fortune tellers and soothsayers who falsely claim to have knowledge of the Unseen in order to cheat people of their money and change their beliefs. (345)

Astrology, horoscope, superstition and fortune telling are all the work of Satan.

362. Prohibition of Attributing Rain to the Stars

Narrated Zaid bin Khalid (May Allah be pleased with him): The Messenger of Allah (peace and blessings be upon him) led the Fajr prayer at Al-Hudaibiyyah after a rainfall during the night. At the conclusion of prayer, he turned towards the people and said, "Do you know what your Rubb has said?" They replied: 'Allah and His Messenger know better.' Upon this he remarked, 'He has said: Some of My slaves have entered the morning as My believers and some as unbelievers. He who said: 'We have had a rainfall due to the Grace and Mercy of Allah, believes in Me and disbelieves in the stars', and he who said: 'We have had a rainfall due to the rising of such and such star, disbelieves in Me and affirms his faith in the stars.'" (Bukhari and Muslim)

Commentary:
People of the period of Ignorance used to ascribe the rain which occurred at the appearance or setting of some star, to that star and would thus accept it as the real cause of it. In this Hadith, such ascription has been regarded as Kufr and Shirk. (346)

363. Prohibition of Wearing String and Thread

Allah, the Exalted, says:

"And most of them believe not in Allah except that they attribute partners unto Him (i.e. they are Mushrikun - polytheists - see Verse 6:121)." (Qur'an, Yusuf 12:106)

"Say: "I seek refuge with (Allah) the Lord of the daybreak, From the evil of what He has created; And from the evil of the darkening (night) as it comes with its darkness; (or the moon as it sets or goes away). And from the evil of the witchcrafts when they blow in the knots, And from the evil of the envier when he envies." (Qur'an, Al-Falaq)

Zainab, the wife of 'Abdallah b. Masud, told that 'Abdallah saw a thread on her neck and asked what it was. When she told him that it was a thread over which a spell had been recited for her, he took it, cut it up and said, "You, family of 'Abdallah, are independent of polytheism. I have heard God's Messenger say that spells, charms and love-spells are polytheism." She replied, "Why do you speak like this? My eye was discharging and I kept going to so and so, the Jew, and when he applied a spell to it, it calmed down." 'Abdallah said, "That was just the work of the Devil who was pricking it with his hand, and when a spell was uttered, he desisted. All you need to do is to say as God's Messenger (peace and blessings be upon him) did, 'Remove the harm, O Lord of men, and heal. Thou art the Healer. There is no remedy but Thine which leaves no disease behind." (Abu Dawud)

Ruwaifi' b. Thabit told that God's Messenger said to him, "You may live for a long time after I am gone, Ruwaifi', so tell people that if anyone ties his beard or wears round his neck a string to ward off the Evil Eye, or cleanses himself with animal dung or bone, Muhammad has nothing to do with him." (Abu Dawud)

'Imran ibn Husayn (May Allah be pleased with him) reported that the Prophet (May Allah's peace and blessings be upon him) saw a man wearing a brass ring on his hand and said: "What is that?" The man said: "It is for a weakening ailment." He said: "Take it off, for it will only increase your weakness. If you die with it on, you will never succeed." (Ibn Majah) (https://hadeethenc.com/en/browse/hadith/6362)

Wearing a thin scarlet wool thread or crimson string (Hebrew: khutt hasheni) as a type of talisman is a Jewish folk custom as a way to ward off misfortune brought about by the Evil Eye. The tradition is popularly thought to be associated with Kabbalah and religious forms of Judaism. (347, 348)

Red strings around the wrist are common in many folk beliefs; for example, the *kalava* is a Hindu version.

String and thread worn with the intention of warding off the Evil Eye, problem, sickness, bad luck or to bring good luck and the like, they are all Shirk and involve the Evil Jinn. It works as Taweez.

364. Prohibition of Wearing the Evil Eye Jewelry

Allah, the Exalted, says:

"Say: "I seek refuge with (Allah) the Lord of the daybreak, From the evil of what He has created, And from the evil of the darkening (night) as it comes with its darkness; (or the moon as it sets or goes away), And from the evil of the witchcrafts when they blow in the knots, And from the evil of the envier when he envies." (Qur'an, Al-Falaq 113:1-5)

"Say: "I seek refuge with (Allah) the Lord of mankind, the King of mankind, The Ilah (God) of mankind, From the evil of the whisperer (Devil who whispers evil in the hearts of men) who withdraws (from his whispering in one's heart after one remembers Allah), Who whispers in the breasts of mankind, of Jinn and men." (Qur'an, An-Nas 114:1-6)

The Evil Eye jewelry, which people think that it wards off the Evil Eye and harm, is a Shirk. (349, 350)

Abu Abbas Abdullah bin Abbas (May Allah be pleased with him) who said: "One day I was behind the Prophet (peace and blessings of Allah be upon him) (riding on the same mount) and he said, "O young man, I shall teach you some words (of advice): Be mindful of Allah and Allah will protect you. Be mindful of Allah and you will find Him in front of you. If you ask, then ask Allah (Alone); and if you seek help, then seek help from Allah (Alone). And know that if the nation were to gather together to benefit you with anything, they would not benefit you except with what Allah had already prescribed for you. And if they were to gather together to harm you with anything, they would not harm you except with what Allah had already prescribed against you. The pens have been lifted and the pages have dried." (Tirmidhi)

365. Belief in Superstitions

Abu Hurairah (May Allah be pleased with him) reported: The Prophet (May Allah's peace and blessings be upon him) said: "(There is) no 'Adwa (no contagious disease is conveyed without Allah's permission), nor is there any bad omen (from birds), nor is there any Hamah, nor is there any bad omen in the month of Safar, and one should run away from the leper as one runs away from a lion." (Bukhari)

Sheikh Muhammad Saalih al-Munajjid gave a beautiful explainataion of this Hadith: https://islamqa.info/en/answers/13930

Some people regard black cat crossing one's path as a bad luck or unlucky number such as 13, or lucky day such as Friday 13 for lottery; or auspicious date, certain day and time good for the business contract, marriage or the birth, etc. Superstitions through crossing fingers, knocking on the wood for protection… Superstitions are Shirk, the belief that something other than Allah has the power.

Abu Musa (May Allah be pleased with him) reported: The Messenger of Allah (peace and blessings be upon him) said to me, "Shall I not guide you to a treasure from the treasures of Jannah?" I said: "Yes, O Messenger of Allah!" Thereupon he (peace be upon him) said, "(Recite) 'La hawla wa la quwwata illa billah' (There is no power and no strength except with Allah)." (Bukhari and Muslim)

No one brings about good save Allah, and no one wards off evil save Him.

366. Seeking Decision Through Divining Arrows

Allah, the Exalted, says:

"and (prohibited is) that you seek decision through divining arrows. That is grave disobedience." (Qur'an, Al-Ma'idah 5:3)

"and divining arrows (for seeking luck or decision) are but defilement from the work of Satan, so avoid it that you may be successful." (Qur'an, Al-Ma'idah 5:90)

367. Playing Games of Chance Without Betting

Allah, the Exalted, says:

"O you who believe! Intoxicants (all kinds of alcoholic drinks), gambling, Al-Ansab (stone altars for sacrifices to idols etc.) and Al-Azlam (arrows for seeking luck or decision) are an abomination of Shaitan's (Satan) handiwork. So, avoid (strictly all) that (abomination) in order that you may be successful. Shaitan (Satan) wants only to excite enmity and hatred between you with intoxicants (alcoholic drinks) and gambling, and hinder you from the remembrance of Allah and from As-Salat (the prayer). So, will you not then abstain?" (Qur'an, Al-Ma'idah 5:90-91)

Buraida (May Allah be pleased with him) reported: The Prophet (peace and blessings be upon him) as saying, "He who plays backgammon is as though he had dipped his hand in a pig's flesh and blood." (Muslim)

Yahya related to me from Malik from Musa ibn Maysara from Said ibn Abi Hind from Abu Musa al-Ashari that the Messenger of Allah (peace and blessings be upon him) said, "Whoever plays games of dice has disobeyed Allah and His Messenger." (Malik Muwatta)

Abdullah ibn Masud (May Allah be pleased with him) said, "Beware of these two marked cubes. They should be forcibly prohibited. They are part of gambling." (Bukhari)

Alqama ibn Abi 'Alqama reported from his mother that Aisha (May Allah be pleased with her) heard that some people living in a room in her house had a backgammon game. She sent to them, saying, "If you do not remove it, I will evict you from my house." He censured them for playing that." (Bukhari, Al-Adab Al-Mufrad)

Games, with or without betting, that rely on luck, conjecture and guessing are regarded as haram by a number of fuqaha', by analogy with dice games. Playing with dice is completely based on conjecture and guessing, and is very foolish and silly. Games of chance is when there is a chance to win a prize but have no control over the outcome: lotteries, sports betting, casino games such as roulette and poker: all prohibited. (351)

368. Prohibition of Envy

Allah, the Exalted, says:

"Or do they envy people for what Allah has given them of His bounty? But we had already given the family of Abraham the Scripture and wisdom and conferred upon them a great kingdom." (Qur'an, An-Nisa 4:54)

"Truly, the religion with Allah is Islam. Those who were given the Scripture (Jews and Christians) did not differ except, out of mutual jealousy, after knowledge had come to them. And whoever disbelieves in the Ayat (proofs, evidences, verses, signs, revelations, etc.) of Allah, then surely, Allah is Swift in calling to account." (Qur'an, Ali 'Imran 3:19)

"And those who, before them, had homes (in Al-Madinah) and had adopted the Faith, love those who emigrate to them, and have no jealousy in their breasts for that which they have been given (from the booty of Bani An-Nadir), and give them (emigrants) preference over themselves, even though they were in need of that. And whosoever is saved from his own covetousness, such are they who will be the successful." (Qur'an, Al-Hashr 59:9)

Other Verses: *An-Nahl 16:71, Al-Falaq 113:1-5.*

Abu Hurairah (May Allah be pleased with him) said: The Prophet (peace and blessings be upon him) said, "Beware of envy because envy consumes (destroys) the virtues just as the fire consumes the firewood", or he said "grass." (Abu Dawud)

Commentary: Envy is one of the Major sins which are bound to destroy virtues as fast as the fire burns the wood and dry grass to ashes. (352)

Yahya related to me from Malik that Muhammad ibn Abi Umama ibn Sahl ibn Hunayf heard his father say, "My father, Sahl ibn Hunayf did a Ghusl at al-Kharrar. He removed the jubbah he had on while Amir ibn Rabia was watching, and Sahl was a man with beautiful white skin. Amir said to him, 'I have never seen anything like what I have seen today, not even the skin of a virgin.' Sahl fell ill on the spot, and his condition grew worse. Somebody went to the Messenger of Allah (peace and blessings be upon him) and told him that Sahl was ill, and could not go with him. He (peace and blessings be upon him) came to him, and Sahl told him what had happened with Amir. The Messenger of Allah (peace and blessings be upon him) said, "Why does one of you kill his brother? Did you not say, 'May Allah bless you (Tabarak Allah).' The Evil Eye is true. Do Wudu from it." Amir did Wudu from it and Sahl went with the Messenger of Allah (peace and blessings be upon him) and there was nothing wrong with him." (Malik Muwatta)

Ibn 'Abbas (May Allah be pleased with him) reported Allah's Messenger (peace and blessings be upon him) as saying: "The influence of an Evil Eye is a fact; If anything would precede the destiny it would be the influence of an Evil Eye, and when you are asked to take bath (as a cure) from the influence of an Evil Eye, you should take bath." (Muslim)

Narrated Aisha (May Allah be pleased with her): "The Prophet (peace and blessings be upon him) ordered me or somebody else to do Ruqyah (if there was danger) from an Evil Eye." (Bukhari)

Narrated Ibn Masud (May Allah be pleased with him): "I heard the Prophet (peace and blessings be upon him) saying, "There is no envy except in two: a person whom Allah has given wealth and he spends it in the right way, and a person whom Allah has given wisdom (i.e. religious knowledge) and he gives his decisions accordingly and teaches it to the others." (Bukhari)

Abu Dharr (May Allah be pleased with him) reported: The Messenger of Allah (peace and blessings be upon him) said, "Verily, the Evil Eye might attach itself to a man by permission of Allah, until he climbs a tall mountain and then throws himself off it." (Aḥmad)

Jabir (May Allah be pleased with him) reported: The Messenger of Allah (peace and blessings be upon him) said, "A great many from my nation who die, after the Judgment, Decree and Providence of Allah, die by the Evil Eye." (Abu Dawud)

Sahl ibn Hunayf (May Allah be pleased with him) reported: The Messenger of Allah (peace and blessings be upon him) said, "If one of you sees something from his brother, or in himself, or in his wealth which impresses him, then supplicate for him to be blessed in it. Verily, the Evil Eye of envy is real." (Aḥmad)

Ibn Abbas (May Allah be pleased with him) reported: The Prophet (peace and blessings be upon him) would seek refuge for his grandsons Hasan and Husayn, saying, "Verily, your forefather would seek refuge for Ishmael and Isaac. I seek refuge in the perfect Words of Allah from every Devil and scourge and every harmful Eye." (Bukhari)

Narrated 'Ubaid bin Rifa'ah Az-Zuraqi: Asma said: "O Messenger of Allah! The children of Ja'far have been afflicted by the Evil Eye, shall I recite Ruqyah for them?' He said: 'Yes, for if anything were to overtake the Divine Decree it would be the Evil Eye.'" (Ibn Majah)

Abu Sa'id Al-Khudri (May Allah be pleased with him) reported: "Jibreel (Gabriel) came to the Prophet (peace and blessings be upon) and said: "O Muhammad! Do you feel sick?" He (peace and blessings be upon him) said, "Yes." Jibreel supplicated thus (i.e. he performed Ruqyah): "Bismillahi arqika, min kulli shay'in yu'dhika, min sharri kulli nafsin aw 'ayni hasidi, Allahu yashfika, bismillahi arqika. (With the Name of Allah, I recite over you (to cleanse you) from all that troubles you and from every harmful mischief and from the Evil of the Eye of an envier. Allah will cure you and with the Name of Allah, I recite over you)." (Muslim) (https://hadeethenc.com/en/browse/hadith/5650)

369. Amulets to Ward off the Evil Eye and Hasad (Envy)

Narrated Abdullah ibn Masud (May Allah be pleased with him): "The Prophet of Allah (peace and blessings of Allah be upon him) disliked ten things: "Yellow colouring, meaning khalooq (a perfume made from saffron), dyeing grey hair, trailing the lower garment, wearing a gold ring, throwing dice, a woman adorning herself before people who are not her mahrams, using spells (Ruqyah) except with the Mu'awwidhatan, wearing amulets, coitus interruptus and having intercourse with a woman who is breastfeeding a child; but he did not declare them to be prohibited." (An-Nasa'i and Abu Dawud; classed as da'eef (weak) by al-Albaani)

Narrated 'Uqbah ibn 'Aamir (May Allah be pleased with him): "I heard the Messenger of Allah (peace and blessings of Allah be upon him) say: "Whoever wears an amulet, may Allah not fulfil his need, and whoever wears a seashell, may Allah not give him peace." (Ahmad)

Narrated 'Uqbah ibn 'Aamir al-Juhani that a group came to the Messenger of Allah (peace and blessings of Allah be upon him) [to swear their allegiance (bay'ah) to him]. He accepted the bay'ah of nine of them but not of one of them. They said, "O Messenger of Allah, you accepted the bay'ah of nine but not of this one." He said, "He is wearing an amulet." The man put his hand (in his shirt) and took it off, then he (the Prophet (peace and blessings of Allah be upon him) accepted his bay'ah. He said, 'Whoever wears an amulet has committed Shirk." (Ahmad)

Amulets are worn on the necks of children or adults, or are hung up in houses or cars, in order to ward off evil (Evil Eye) or to bring some benefits – are Shirk.

Amulets contain spells (Ruqyah) using the names of Shayateen (Devils) and others, and hanging them up, and even being attached to those Shayateen, seeking refuge in them, slaughtering animals for them, asking them to ward off harm and bring benefits – actions which are pure Shirk.

Narrated 'Eesa ibn Hamzah (May Allah be pleased with him): "I entered upon Abdullah ibn 'Akeem and his face was red due to high fever. I said, 'Why don't you hang up an amulet?' He said, 'We seek refuge with Allah from that.' The Messenger of Allah (peace and blessings of Allah be upon him) said: "Whoever hangs up anything will be entrusted to its care…'" (Abu Dawud)

Sheikh Haafiz Hukami said:

"…they make amulets for seeking refuge, on which they write an Ayah or Surah or the phrase "Bismillaah ir-Rahmaan ir-Raheem (In the Name of Allah, the most Gracious, the Most Merciful), then underneath it they put some Devilish mumbo-jumbo, the meaning of which no one knows except one who has read their books. Or they divert the hearts of the common folk from putting their trust in Allah and make them dependent on the things that they have written, and most of them frighten the people, before anything even happens to them. One of them will come to the person whom he wants to trick out of his money, knowing that the person is relying on him and trusts him, and he says: "Such and such is going to happen to your family or your wealth, or to you," Or he says, "You have a qareen (constant companion) from among the Jinn," or the like, and he describes things to him and tells him things about himself that the Shaytan whispers to him, to make him think that he has true insight and that he cares about him and wants to bring him some benefit. When the heart of the ignorant fool is filled with fear of what has been described to him, he turns away from his Lord and turns to this charlatan with all his heart and soul; he puts his trust in him and relies on him instead of Allah, and says to him, "What is the way out from the things that you have described? What are the means of warding them off?" It is as if he (the charlatan) has control over benefit and harm, at which point his hopes are raised and he becomes more greedy, wondering how much he will be able to take. So, he tells him, "If you give me such and such, I will write an amulet for that which will be this long and this wide" – he describes it and speaks to him in a nice manner. Then he hangs up this amulet to protect him from such and such diseases. Do you think, after all that we have mentioned, that this belief is a form of Minor Shirk? No way; it means that one is taking as one's god someone other than Allah, putting one's trust in someone other than Him, turning to someone other than Him, relying on the deeds of created beings and trying to divert people from their religion. Can the Shaytan do any of these tricks except with the help of his Devilish brethren among mankind?

"Say: 'Who can guard and protect you in the night or in the day from the (punishment of the) Most Gracious (Allah)?' Nay, but they turn away from the remembrance of their Lord." *(Qur'an, Al-Anbya 21:42)*

Then along with the Devilish mumbo-jumbo, he writes on the amulet something from the Qur'an, and hangs it up when he is not taahir (in a state of purity), when he is in a state of minor or major impurity, and he never shows any respect towards it or keeps it away from other things. By Allah, none of the enemies of Allah have treated His Book with as much contempt as these heretics who claim to be Muslims. By Allah, the Qur'an was revealed to be recited and followed, for its commandments to be obeyed and its prohibitions heeded, for its information to be believed and its limits to be adhered to, for its parables and stories to serve as lessons, and for it to be believed in.

"… the whole of it (clear and unclear Verses) are from our Lord…" (Qur'an, Ali 'Imran 3:7)

But these people have ignored all of that and cast it behind their backs; they have merely memorized a few Words in order to earn their living from them, like any other means of earning a living that enables them to do haram things, not things which are permitted. If a king or a governor wrote a letter to his subordinate, telling him to do so such and such and not to do such and such, commanding the people in your city to do such and such and forbidding them to do such and such, etc., and he took that letter and did not read it or think about its instructions, and he did not convey that to those to whom he was commanded to convey it, but instead he took it and hung it around his neck or his arm, and did not pay any attention at all to what was in it, the king would punish him severely for that. So how about that which was revealed from the Compeller of the heavens and the earth, Who has the highest description in the heavens and on earth, to Whom is all Praise in the beginning and at the end, to Whom all things return, so worship Him and put your trust in Him, He is sufficient for me, there is no god but He, in Him I put my trust and He is the Lord of the Mighty Throne. And if they (amulets) contain anything but the two revelations (i.e. Qur'an and Saheeh Sunnah) then this is Shirk without a doubt, and is more akin to the azlaam (arrows used during the jaahiliyyah for seeking luck or help in decision making) in being far-removed from the characteristics of Islam. If they (amulets) contain anything other than the two revelations and instead contain mumbo-jumbo from the Jews or worshippers of the temple, stars or angels, or those who use the services of the Jinn, etc., or they are made of pearls, strings, iron rings, etc., then this is Shirk, i.e. hanging them up or wearing them is Shirk, beyond a doubt, because they are not among the permissible means or known forms of treating disease. It is simply a belief that they will ward off such and such a problem or pain because of their so-called special features. This is like the belief of idol-worshippers concerning their idols, and they are like the azlaam (arrows) which the people of the jaahiliyyah used to take everywhere with them and consult whenever they had to make a decision. These were three arrows, on the first of which was written 'Do', on the second 'Do not do' and on the third 'Try again.' If the person picked out the one which said 'Do', he would go ahead and do that thing; if it said, 'Do not do', he would not do it, and if it said, 'Try again,' he would consult them again. Instead of this, Allah – to Whom be Praise – has given us something better, which is the prayer of Istikharah… (Ma'aarij al-Qubool, 2/510-512) (353)

370. Saying "Ma Shaa Allah" to Prevent the Evil Eye is a Bid'ah

There is no authentic Hadith that telling "Ma shaa Allah" will prevent the Evil Eye. The correct action according to the Sunnah is for the individual to pray for blessing (barakah) when he sees something that he likes and fears that the may affect its owner.

The Messenger of Allah (peace and blessings of Allah be upon him) said: "If one of you sees something in himself or his wealth, or his brother that he likes, let him pray for blessing (barakah) for it, for the Evil Eye is real." (Ibn as-Sunni in 'Amal al-Yawm wa'l-Laylah, p.168, al-Hakim)

Narrated Abu Umamah ibn Sahl ibn Hunayf: "Amir ibn Rabi'ah passed by Sahl ibn Hunayf when he was doing ghusl and said: 'I have never seen such beautiful skin, not even the skin of young women in seclusion.' Straightaway, he (Sahl) fell to the ground. He was brought to the Prophet (peace and blessings of Allah be upon him) and it was said to him: 'Help Sahl, for he has had a fit (seizure).' He said: 'Whom do you accuse with regard to him?' They said: 'Amir ibn Rabi'ah.' He said: 'Why would any one of you kill his brother? If he sees something in his brother that he likes, then let him pray for blessing (barakah) for him.' Then he called for water, and he told 'Amir to do Wudu, so he washed his face and his arms up to the elbows, his knees and inside his lower garment, then he told him to pour the water over him." (Ibn Majah, Ahmad and Malik)

Narrated Abu Ya'la in his Musnad, as is mentioned in al-Matalib al-'Aliyah (10/348) and Tafsir Ibn Kathir (5/158), from Anas ibn Malik (May Allah be pleased with him): The Messenger of Allah (peace and blessings of Allah be upon him) said: "Allah, may He be Glorified and Exalted, never bestows any blessing – such as family, wealth or a child – upon a person and he says "Ma shaa Allah la quwwata illa Billah," but he will never see any troubles in it except death." And he used to recite this Verse: *"And why did you, when you entered your garden, not say, 'What Allah willed (has occurred); there is no power except in Allah."* (Al-Kahf 18:39)

But the Hadith mentioned is da'eef (weak). It was narrated from 'Abd al-Malik ibn Zarah, whose Hadith is da'eef. See: *al-Asma wa's-Sifat* by al-Bayhaqi, annotated by 'Abdullah al-Hashidi (1/417).

He should say to ward off his own Evil Eye against his own wealth, family or beauty:

If a person sees something that he likes in his own wealth, and he says, "Ma shaa Allah la quwwata illa Billah", it is still valid and he acknowledges that the source of this blessing is Allah, the Most Powerful, and he is powerless and it will avoid him to ascribe partner to Allah. Allah knows the best.

He can also say: Allahumma Barik - May Allah bless. (354)

He should say to ward off his own Evil Eye against someone's wealth, family and beauty:

Tabarak Allahu 'alayka - May Allah bless it for you (for man).
Tabarak Allahu 'alayki - May Allah bless it for you (for woman).
Allahumma barik lahu - May Allah bless him.
Allahumma barik laha - May Allah bless her.
Allahumma barik lahum - May Allah bless them.

Sheikh Ibn 'Uthaymeen (May Allah have mercy on him) said:

"The best, if someone fears that he may have affected someone else with the Evil Eye because he liked or admired him, is for him to say: 'Tabarak Allahu 'alayka (May Allah bless it for you', because the Prophet (peace and blessings of Allah be upon him) said to the man who affected his brother with the Evil Eye: "Why did you not pray for blessing for him?" With regard to saying "Ma shaa Allah la quwwata illa Billah," this should be said by the one who admires his own wealth or property, as the owner of the garden said to his companion: "And why did you, when you entered your garden, not say, 'What Allah willed (has occurred); there is no power except in Allah." (Qur'an, Al-Kahf 18:39) (355)

371. Belief in Reincarnation

What is Reincarnation?

Reincarnation or the transmigration of souls is that when the body dies, the soul moves to another body, where it will be happy or miserable as a result of its previous actions, and thus it moves from one body to another. (356, 357)

Ruling on Reincarnation

This is one of the falsest of false beliefs, and one of the worst forms of disbelief in Allah, His Books and His Messengers. For belief in the Hereafter, the Reckoning, Paradise and Hell is among the things that are well known in the teachings of the Messengers and in the Words of the Books which were revealed to them. Belief in Reincarnation is tantamount to disbelief in all of that. (358)

The Resurrection is stated clearly in the Book of Allah and the Sunnah of His Messenger.

<u>Resurrection in the Quran</u>

Allah, the Exalted, says:

"Everyone shall taste death. Then unto Us you shall be returned." (Qur'an, Al-'Ankabut 29:57)

"To Him is the return of all of you. The Promise of Allah is true. It is He Who begins the creation and then will repeat it, that He may reward with justice those who believed and did deeds of righteousness. But those who disbelieved will have a drink of boiling fluids and painful torment because they used to disbelieve." (Qur'an, Yunus 10:4)

"The Day We shall gather the Muttaqoon (the pious) unto the Most Gracious (Allah), like a delegation (presented before a king for honor). And We shall drive the Mujrimoon (polytheists, sinners, criminals, disbelievers in the Oneness of Allah) to Hell, in a thirsty state (like a thirsty herd driven down to water)." (Qur'an, Maryam 19:85-86)

Other Verses: Maryam 19:94-95, An-Nisa 4:87, At-Taghabun 64:7, Al-Jathiyah 45:26.

Resurrection in the Sunnah

Narrated Ibn Abbas (May Allah have mercy on him): Allah's Messenger (peace and blessings be upon him) delivered a sermon and said, "O people! You will be gathered before Allah barefooted, naked and not circumcised." Then (quoting Qur'an) he said: *"As We began the first creation, We shall repeat it. A promise We have undertaken: Truly We shall do it." (21:104)* The Prophet (peace and blessings of Allah be upon him) then said, "The first of the human beings to be dressed on the Day of Resurrection, will be Abraham. Lo! Some men from my followers will be brought and then (the angels) will drive them to the left side (Hellfire). I will say. 'O my Lord! (They are) my companions!' Then a reply will come (from Almighty), 'You do not know what they did after you.' I will say as the pious slave (the Prophet Jesus) said: *"And I was a witness over them while I dwelt amongst them. When You took me up. You were the Watcher over them and You are a Witness to all things." (5:117)* Then it will be said, "These people have continued to be apostates since you left them." (Bukhari)

Narrated Abu Hurairah (May Allah have mercy on him): The Messenger of Allah (peace and blessings of Allah be upon him) said: "There is no part of man that will not disintegrate, apart from a single bone at the base of the coccyx, from which he will be recreated on the Day of Resurrection." (Ibn Majah)

Narrated Anas bin Malik (May Allah have mercy on him): The Messenger of Allah (peace and blessings be upon him) said: "I will come to the gate of Paradise on the Day of Resurrection and would seek its opening, and the keeper would say: 'Who art thou?' I would say: 'Muhammad'. He would then say: 'It is for thee that I have been ordered, and not to open it for anyone before thee.'" (Muslim)

Does the Soul Move to Another Body?

The Islamic teachings concerning torment or blessing in the grave and the questioning of the two angels clearly prove that the soul of man does not move to another body, rather the soul and body experience torment or blessing, until the Judgment Day, then on Judgment Day and in Hereafter, eternal Paradise (blessing) or eternal Hellfire (torment).

The belief that the body will perish and will not be restored to experience blessing or punishment is a means that leads man to indulge in desires, wrongdoing and evil. This is what the Satan wants for those who follow this corrupt belief, in addition to pushing them further into kufr when he makes them believe in this false idea. (359)

372. Prohibition of Suspicion

Allah, the Exalted, says:

"O you, who believe! Avoid much suspicions, indeed some suspicions are sins." (Qur'an, Al-Hujurat 49:12)

Narrated Abu Hurairah (May Allah have mercy on him): The Prophet (peace and blessings be upon him) said, "Beware of suspicion, for suspicion is the worst of false tales; and do not look for the others' faults and do not spy, and do not be jealous of one another, and do not desert (cut) your relation with) one another, and do not hate one another; and O Allah's worshipers! Be brothers (as Allah has ordered you)." (Bukhari)

373. Prohibition of Spying on Muslims and to be Inquisitive about Others

Allah, the Exalted, says:

"…And spy not…" (Qur'an, Al-Hujurat 49:12)

"And those who annoy believing men and women undeservedly, bear on themselves the crime of slander and plain sin." (Qur'an, Al-Ahzab 33:58)

"O you who believe! Enter not houses other than your own, until you have asked permission…" (Qur'an, An-Nur 24:27)

Abu Hurairah (May Allah be pleased with him) said: The Messenger of Allah (peace and blessings be upon him) said, "Beware of suspicion, for suspicion is the worst of false tales. Do not look for other's faults. Do not spy one another, and do not practice Najsh (means to offer a high price for something in order to allure another customer who is interested in the thing). Do not be jealous of one another and do not nurse enmity against one another. Do not sever ties with one another. Become the slaves of Allah, and be brothers to one another as He commanded. A Muslim is the brother of a Muslim. He should neither oppress him nor humiliate him. The piety is here! The piety is here!" While saying so he pointed towards his chest. "It is enough evil for a Muslim to look down upon his Muslim brother. All things of a Muslim are inviolable for his brother in Faith: his blood, his wealth and his honor. Verily, Allah does not look to your bodies nor to your faces but He looks to your hearts and your deeds." (Muslim)

Muawiyah (May Allah be pleased with him) said: I heard the Messenger of Allah (peace and blessings be upon him) saying, "If you find faults with Muslims, you will corrupt them." (Abu Dawud)

Commentary: If a Muslim looks for the defects of another and hunts for his weaknesses, other Muslims will also adopt the same attitude towards him, and this situation will create dissension and conflict in society. This also will make them fall prey to sins and make them persistent in committing them. For this reason, spying and finding faults with Muslims has been prohibited by Shariah. (360)

Narrated Abu Hurairah (May Allah have mercy on him): The Prophet (peace and blessings be upon him) said, "Beware of suspicion, for suspicion is the worst of false tales; and do not look for the others' faults and do not spy, and do not be jealous of one another, and do not desert (cut) your relation with) one another, and do not hate one another; and O Allah's worshipers! Be brothers (as Allah has ordered you)." (Bukhari)

Narrated Ibn 'Abbas (May Allah have mercy on him): The Prophet (peace and blessings be upon him) said: "Whoever claims to have seen a dream which he did not see, will be ordered to make a knot between two barley grains which he will not be able to do; and if somebody listens to the talk of some people who do not like him (to listen) or they run away from him, then molten lead will be poured into his ears on the Day of Resurrection; and whoever makes a picture, will be punished on the Day of Resurrection and will be ordered to put a soul in that picture, which he will not be able to do." (Bukhari)

Abu Barza Al-Aslami (May Allah be pleased with him) narrated that the Prophet (peace and blessings be upon him) said: "O community of people, who believed by their tongue, and belief did not enter their hearts, do not back-bite Muslims, and do not search for their faults, for if anyone searches for their faults, Allah will search for his fault, and if Allah searches for the fault of anyone, He disgraces him in his house." (Abu Dawud)

Salamah ibn al-Akwa' (May Allah be pleased with him) said: "A spy from among the polytheists came to the Prophet (May Allah's peace and blessings be upon him) while he was on a journey. The spy stayed with the Prophet's Companions (May Allah be pleased with them) and talked to them, and then he left. Thereupon, the Prophet (May Allah's peace and blessings be upon him) said: 'Go in pursuit of him and kill him.' I killed him, and the Prophet (May Allah's peace and blessings be upon him) gave me his belongings (as an extra share)." (Muslim)

374. Spying in Order to Catch the Faults of Others

Allah, the Exalted, says:

"Allah does not like that the evil should be uttered in public except by him who has been wronged. And Allah is Ever All-Hearer, All-Knower." (Qur'an, An-Nisa 4:148)

"Avoid much suspicion; indeed, some suspicions are sins. And spy not…" (Qur'an, Al-Hujurat 49:12)

"And desire not corruption in the land. Indeed, Allah does not like corrupters." (Qur'an, Al-Qasas 28:77)

Abu Said al-Khudri reported: The Messenger of Allah (peace and blessings be upon him) said: "I have not been commanded to pierce through the hearts of people, nor to split their bellies (insides)." (Muslim) (https://sunnah.com/muslim:1064b)

Spying on the employees, on the wife or husband, and be suspicious about them, will corrupt them and make them lose trust, as the Prophet (peace and blessings of Allah be upon him) said: "If you seek out people's faults you will corrupt them or almost corrupt them." (Abu Dawud)

Abdullah ibn Amr reported: The Messenger of Allah (peace and blessings be upon him) said, "Whoever is silent has been saved." (Tirmidhi)

Spying is a path to hatred and an instigator of vengeance. Spying is a manifestation of ill faith. Spying leads to a corrupt life, making it rife with doubts and fears. It is a way for amicable ties to be broken, relations to become void, dear ones having enmity against each other and brothers splitting up.

375. Spying on Phones

Allah, the Exalted, says:

"O you who believe! Avoid much suspicions, indeed some suspicions are sins. And spy not…" (Qur'an, Al-Hujurat 49:12)

Abdullah ibn Amr (May Allah be pleased with him) reported: The Messenger of Allah (peace and blessings be upon him) said, "Whoever would love to be delivered from Hellfire and admitted into Paradise, let him meet his end with faith in Allah and the Last Day, and let him treat people as he would love to be treated." (Muslim)

Narrated Abu Hurairah (May Allah be pleased with him: The Prophet (peace and blessings of Allah be upon him) said, "Beware of suspicion, for suspicion is the worst of false tales; and do not look for the others' faults and do not spy, and do not be jealous of one another, and do not desert (cut your relation with) one another, and do not hate one another; and O Allah's worshipers! Be brothers (as Allah has ordered you)." (Bukhari)

Prohibition of spying in all its forms and in all situations is clear from the Qur'an and Ahadith. Therefore, the basic rule is to deal with people with trust and do not go towards the investigations and monitoring their private matters and circumstances without legal justification. A person being of suspicious nature and accusing others of various things and interpreting things in the strange ways doesn't justify for him to compromise privacy of other people, therefore, perpetrating two evils: holding evils suspicions and also having bad conduct, including spying on others. (361)

Spying or checking on somebody else's mobile phone without permission is committing a forbidden act. It happens when there is a lack of trust and confidence, suspicion which can only lead to a troubled life.

Violation of privacy of individuals, checking a person's phone without permission, disclosing or spreading information stored on a victim's mobile phone, obtaining a confidential number, code or password used to access any electronic site without permission can invite both imprisonment and fine.

Eavesdropping, recording conversations without the knowledge of the person, installing tracking devices on the phone, installing tracking devices on a vehicle are acts that can be punished for privacy violation if they are committed without the consent and knowledge of the other person whose privacy is being breached. These violations are criminal actions and penalties of both fines and imprisonment can be imposed. (362)

376. Prohibition of Obscenity

Ibn Masud (May Allah be pleased with him) said: The Messenger of Allah (peace and blessings be upon him) said, "A true believer does not taunt or curse, or abuse, or talk indecently." (Tirmidhi)

Anas (May Allah be pleased with him) said: The Messenger of Allah (peace and blessings be upon him) said, "Indecency does not leave anything untainted and decency does not leave anything ungraced and embellished." (Tirmidhi)

Commentary: This Hadith induces us to abandon indecency and adopt decency. (363)

Narrated Abu Ad-Dardh: The Messenger of Allah (peace and blessings be upon him) said: "Nothing is heavier on the believer's scale on the Day of Judgment than good character. For indeed Allah, Most High, is angered by the shameless obscene person." (Tirmidhi)

Abu 'Abdullah al-Jadali (May Allah be pleased with him reported: "I asked Aisha (May Allah be pleased with her) about the moral character of the Messenger of Allah (May Allah's peace and blessings be upon him) and she said: "He was not unseemly or obscene in his speech, nor was he loud-voiced in the markets, nor did he return evil for evil, but he would forgive and pardon." (Tirmidhi)

(https://hadeethenc.com/en/browse/hadith/10974)

377. Abomination of Self-Condemnation

Narrated Aisha (May Allah be pleased with her): The Prophet (peace and blessings be upon him) said,

"None of you should say: 'My soul has become evil.' He should say: 'My soul is in bad shape.'" (Bukhari and Muslim)

Commentary:
Imam Al-Khattabi says that this is a guidance for speaking in a proper manner. One should always use a decent word and abstain from impolite language. (364)

378. Prohibition of Maligning

Allah, the Exalted, says:

"And those who annoy believing men and women undeservedly, bear on themselves the crime of slander and plain sin." (Qur'an, Al-Ahzab 33:58)

'Abdullah bin 'Amr bin Al-'As (May Allah be pleased with him) reported: The Messenger of Allah (peace and blessings be upon him) said, "A (true) Muslim is one from whose tongue and hand the Muslims are safe; and a Muhajir (Emigrant) is he who leaves the deeds which Allah has prohibited." (Bukhari and Muslim)

Narrated 'Abdullah bin 'Amr bin Al-'As (May Allah be pleased with him): The Messenger of Allah (peace and blessings be upon him) said, "He who desires to be rescued from the Fire of

Hell and to enter Jannah, should die in a state of complete belief in Allah and the Last Day, and should do unto others what he wishes to be done unto him." (Muslim)

Commentary: It stresses steadfastness in Faith and virtuous deeds because the time of death is not known to anyone. Since one can die at any moment, one should never be unmindful of the obligations of Faith and good deeds so that he embraces death in a state of perfect Faith. This Hadith has the same meanings which are contained in the Verse 102 of the Surah Ali 'Imran exhorting the Muslims thus: *"And die not except in a state of Islam [(as Muslim) with complete submission to Allah]." (3:102)* (365)

379. Prohibition of Nursing Rancor and Enmity

Allah, the Exalted, says:

"The believers are nothing else than brothers (in Islamic religion)." (Qur'an, Al-Hujurat 49:10)

"... humble towards the believers, stern towards the disbelievers ..." (Qur'an, Al-Ma'dah 5:54)

"Muhammad (peace and blessings be upon him) is the Messenger of Allah, and those who are with him are severe against disbelievers, and merciful among themselves." (Qur'an, Al-Fath 48:29)

Anas bin Malik (May Allah be pleased with him) said: The Prophet (peace and blessings be upon him) said, "Do not harbour grudge against one another, nor jealousy, nor enmity; and do not show your backs to one another; and become as fellow brothers and slaves of Allah. It is not lawful for a Muslim to avoid speaking with his brother beyond three days." (Bukhari and Muslim)

Abu Hurairah (May Allah be pleased with him) said: The Messenger of Allah (peace and blessings be upon him) said, "The gates of Jannah are opened on Mondays and Thursdays, and then every slave of Allah is granted forgiveness if he does not associate anything with Allah in worship. But the person in whose heart there is rancour against his Muslim brother, they will not be pardoned and with regard to them it will be said twice: 'Hold both of them until they are reconciled with each other.'" (Muslim)

Commentary: We learn from this Hadith that mutual enmity, grudge and malice are bound to deprive a man from Jannah in the Hereafter. (366)

380. Prohibition of Two Holding Secret Counsel to the Exclusion of the Third in a Gathering of Three People

Allah, the Exalted, says:

"O you who believe! When you hold secret counsel, do it not for sin and wrong and disobedience to the Messenger, but do it for righteousness and self-restraint; and fear Allah, to Whom you shall be brought back." (Qur'an, Al-Mujadila 58:9)

"Secret counsels (conspiracies) are only from Shaitan (Satan), in order that he may cause grief to the believers. But he cannot harm them in the least, except as Allah permits, and in Allah let the believers put their trust." (Qur'an, Al-Mujadilah 58:10)

Ibn 'Umar (May Allah be pleased with him) said: The Messenger of Allah (peace and blessings be upon him) said, "In the presence of three people, two should not hold secret counsel, to the exclusion of the third." (Bukhari and Muslim)

Abu Dawud, Abu Salih related: "I asked Ibn 'Umar: "What if there are four people." He said, "There is no harm in that."

'Abdullah bin Dinar related: "Ibn 'Umar and I were together in Khalid bin 'Uqbah's house which was situated in the market place. A man came to consult Ibn 'Umar. None besides me was present. Ibn 'Umar called another man in and we became four and said to me and the man he had called: 'Move away a bit because I have heard the Messenger of Allah (peace and blessings be upon him) saying, "The two people should not hold secret counsel together excluding the third."' (https://sunnah.com/riyadussalihin:1598)

Ibn Masud (May Allah be pleased with him) said: The Messenger of Allah (peace and blessings be upon him) said, "When three of you are together, two of you must not converse privately ignoring the third till the number increases, lest the third should be grieved." (Bukhari and Muslim)

Commentary: This Hadith tells us that holding private counsel has been prohibited for the reason that it hurts the feelings of the Muslim who is ignored; and to hurt the feelings of a Muslim is a great sin indeed. Allah says: *"And those who annoy believing men and women undeservedly, bear on themselves the crime of slander and plain sin." (33:58)* Whispering of the two is permissible when all the three mix up in a crowd. Then the two can speak to each other in confidence. (367)

381. Prohibition of Rejoicing Over Another's Trouble

Allah, the Exalted, says:

"The believers are but brothers, so make settlement between your brothers. And fear Allah that you may receive mercy." (Qur'an, Al-Hujurat 49:10)

"Verily, those who like that (the crime of) illegal sexual intercourse should be propagated among those who believe, they will have a painful torment in this world and in the Hereafter." (Qur'an, An-Nur 24:19)

Wathilah bin Al-Asqa' (May Allah be pleased with him) said: The Messenger of Allah (peace and blessings be upon him) said, "Do not express pleasure at the misfortune of a (Muslim) brother lest Allah should bestow mercy upon him and make you suffer from a misfortune." (Tirmidhi)

Commentary: A true believer is one who feels unhappy to see Muslims suffering and rejoices on the happiness of his other fellows in Faith. It is contrary to the conduct of a true believer to rejoice over the trouble of another Muslim as this attitude is very much disliked by Allah. There is every possibility that Allah may punish such a person in this world and relieve the one who is in trouble. (368)

Abu Hurairah (May Allah be pleased with him) reported that the Prophet (peace and blessings be upon him) said: "If one sees an afflicted person and says, 'Praise and thanks be to Allah Who has saved me from what He has afflicted you with, and has honored me over many of His creatures,' he will be saved from that affliction." (Tirmidhi)

382. Prohibition of Cruelty

Allah, the Exalted, says:

"And do good to parents, kinsfolk, orphans, Al-Masakin (the poor), the neighbour who is near of kin, the neighbour who is a stranger, the companion by your side, the wayfarer (you meet), and those (slaves) whom your right hands possess. Verily, Allah does not like such as are proud and boastful." (Qur'an, An-Nisa 4:36)

Ibn 'Umar (May Allah be pleased with him) said: The Messenger of Allah (peace and blessings be upon him) said, "A woman was punished in Hell because of a cat which she had confined until it died. She did not give it to eat or to drink when it was confined, nor did she free it so that it might eat the vermin of the earth." (Bukhari and Muslim)

Ibn 'Umar (May Allah be pleased with him) reported: "I happened to pass by some lads of the Quraish who had tied a bird at which they have been shooting arrows. Every arrow that they missed came into the possession of the owner of the bird. No sooner had they seen Ibn 'Umar, they dispersed. Thereupon, Ibn 'Umar said: "Who has done this? May Allah curse him who has done so. Verily, the Messenger of Allah (peace and blessings be upon him) has cursed anyone who makes a live thing the target (of one's marksmanship)." (Bukhari and Muslim)

Anas (May Allah be pleased with him) said: "The Messenger of Allah (peace and blessings be upon him) forbade animals being tied (as targets)." (Bukhari and Muslim)

Abu Ali Suwaid bin Muqarrin (May Allah be pleased with him) said: "I was the seventh child of Banu Muqarrin and we had only one slave girl. When the youngest of us once happened to slap her (on the face) the Messenger of Allah (peace and blessings be upon him) ordered us to set her free." (Muslim)

Abu Masud Al-Badri (May Allah be pleased with him) said: "I was beating my slave with a whip when I heard a voice behind me which said: "Abu Masud! Bear in mind..." I did not recognize the voice for the intense anger I was in. Abu Masud added, "As he came near me, I found that he was the Messenger of Allah (peace and blessings be upon him) who was saying, "Abu Masud! Bear in mind that Allah has more dominance upon you than you have upon your slave." Then I said: "I will never beat any slave in future."

Commentary:

1. This Hadith has a stern warning for those who punish their slaves and servants without reason or far more than what they deserve.

2. This Hadith also gives a hint of the aura of awe and majesty that characterized the person of the Prophet (peace and blessings be upon him). (369)

Ibn 'Umar (May Allah be pleased with him) reported: The Prophet (peace and blessings be upon him) said, "The expiation for beating or slapping a slave on the face for something he has not done is to set him free." (Muslim)

Narrated Hisham bin Hakim bin Hizam (May Allah be pleased with him) happened to pass by some (non-Arab) farmers of Syria who had been made to stand in the sun, and olive oil was poured on their heads. He said: "What is the matter?" He was told that they had been detained for the non-payment of Jizyah. (Another narration says that they were being tortured for not having paid Al-Kharaj). Thereupon Hisham said: "I bear testimony to the fact that I heard the Messenger of Allah (peace and blessings be upon him) saying, 'Allah will torment those who torment people in the world.'" Then he proceeded towards their Amir and reported this Hadith to him. The Amir then issued orders for their release. (Muslim)

Ibn Abbas (May Allah be pleased with him) said: "The Messenger of Allah (peace and blessings be upon him) saw an ass which had been branded on the face. He disapproved of it. Upon this Ibn 'Abbas (May Allah be pleased with him) said, "By Allah, I shall not brand (the animal) but on a part at a distance from the face." Ibn 'Abbas (May Allah be pleased with him) then commanded branding on the hips; he was the first person to brand the animals on hips." (Muslim)

Ibn Abbas (May Allah be pleased with him) said: "An ass with a brand on the face happened to pass before the Prophet (peace and blessings be upon him). Thereupon he said, "May Allah curse the one who has branded it (on the face)." (Muslim)

383. Throwing Stones

Abdullah ibn Mughaffal (May Allah be pleased with him) reported: The Messenger of Allah (peace and blessings be upon him) forbade throwing stones and said: "It does not kill the quarry or harm the enemy. Instead, it can gouge out an eye or break a tooth." (Bukhari and Muslim)
(https://hadeethenc.com/en/browse/hadith/3080)

384. Killing a Human Being

Allah, the Exalted, says:

"And do not kill anyone which Allah has forbidden except for a just cause. And whoever is killed (intentionally with hostility and oppression, and not by mistake), We have given his heir the authority [to demand Qisas, Law of Equality in punishment or to forgive, or to take Diya (blood money)]. But let him not exceed limits in the matter of taking life (i.e. he should not kill except the killer only). Verily, he is helped (by the Islamic Law)."
(Qur'an, Al-Isra 17:33)

"Because of that We ordained for the Children of Israel that if anyone killed a person not in retaliation of murder, or (and) to spread mischief in the land - it would be as if he killed all mankind, and if anyone saved a life, it would be as if he saved the life of all mankind. And indeed, there came to them Our Messengers with clear proofs, evidences and signs, even then after that many of them continued to exceed the limits (e.g. by doing oppression unjustly and exceeding beyond the limits set by Allah by committing the Major sins) in the land!" (Qur'an, Al-Ma'idah 5:32)

Other Verse: *Ali 'Imran 3:145.*

385. Answering to Evil by the Greater Evil

Allah, the Exalted, says:

"O you who believe! Take care of your own selves. If you follow the (Right) Guidance [and enjoin what is right (Islamic Monotheism and all that Islam orders one to do) and forbid what is wrong (polytheism, disbelief and all that Islam has forbidden)] no hurt can come to you from those who are in error." (Qur'an, Al-Ma'idah 5:105)

"Let there arise out of you a group of people inviting to all that is good (Islam), enjoining Al-Ma'ruf (i.e. Islamic Monotheism and all that Islam orders one to do) and forbidding Al-Munkar (polytheism and disbelief and all that Islam has forbidden). And it is they who are the successful." (Qur'an, Ali 'Imran 3:104)

"The recompense for an evil is an evil like thereof, but whoever forgives and makes reconciliation, his reward is due from Allah. Verily, He likes not the Zalimun (oppressors, polytheists and wrongdoers, etc.)." (Qur'an, Ash-Shuraa 42:40)

Narrated Abu Sa`id Al-Khudri (May Allah be pleased with him): "I heard the Messenger of Allah (peace and blessings be upon him) say, "Whosoever of you sees an evil, let him change it with his hand; and if he is not able to do so, then (let him change it) with his tongue; and if he is not able to do so, then with his heart - and that is the weakest of faith." (Muslim)

Narrated Qais (May Allah have mercy on him): Abu Bakr stood up and praised and glorified Allah, then he said: "O people, you recite this Verse: "*O you who believe! Take care of your own selves. If you follow the (Right) Guidance and enjoin what is right (Islamic Monotheism and all that Islam orders one to do) and forbid what is wrong (polytheism, disbelief and all that Islam has forbidden) no hurt can come to you from those who are in error." (Al-Ma'idah 5:105)* We heard the Messenger of Allah (peace and blessings be upon him) say: `If the people see evil and do not change it, soon Allah will send His punishment upon them all." (Ahmad)

It is not permitted to remove an evil by means of a greater evil; evil must be warded off by that which will remove it or reduce it. (370)

All people are obliged to enjoin what is good and forbid what is evil. But it is essential that it is done with wisdom, kindness and gentleness, because Allah sent Moosa and Haroon to Pharaoh and said:

"And speak to him mildly, perhaps he may accept admonition or fear (Allah)." (Qur'an, Taha 20:44)

Sheikh Muhammad ibn Saalih al-'Uthaymeen (May Allah have mercy on him) said:

"The first condition is that he should know the Islamic ruling concerning that which he is enjoining or forbidding, so he should only enjoin that which he knows that Shariah enjoins, and he should only forbid that which he knows Shariah forbids, and he should not rely on his taste or customs with regard to that.

The second condition is that he should know the situation of the person addressed: is he one who should be enjoined or forbidden, or not? If he sees a person who he is not sure whether he is accountable or not, he should not enjoin anything upon him until he finds out.

The third condition is that he should know about the person who appears to be accountable: has he done the action he wants to enjoin or not? If he sees someone enter the Mosque and sit down, and he is not sure whether he did the two Rak'ahs or not, he should not denounce him or tell him to do them, rather he should find out more.

The fourth condition is that he should be able to enjoin what is good and forbid what is bad, without bringing harm upon himself. If it will bring harm upon him, then he does not have to do it, but if he is patient and does it, that is better, because all duties are subject to the condition that one be able to do them.

The fifth condition is that enjoining what is good and forbidding what is evil should not result in any evil greater than keeping quiet. If that will result then he does not have to do it, rather it is not permissible for him to enjoin what is good and forbid what is evil." (Sheikh al-'Uthaymeen, Majmoo' Fataawa (8/652-654)

When Muslim sees evil being committed, then not advising the one who is doing it means that he is sinning if there is no one else to advise the evildoer except him. But if there is someone else who undertakes to advise the evildoer, then it becomes a communal obligation and he is not sinning if someone else fulfils the duty of Shariah.

Sheikh Ibn Baaz (May Allah have mercy on him) said:

"It is not permissible to keep quiet about that to avoid upsetting the husband, brother or anyone else. But it should be done with good manners and kind words, not with violence and harshness, paying attention to suitable times. Some people may not be open to advice at some times, but at other times they may be willing to accept it. The believing man and woman pay attention to the appropriate times for denouncing evil and enjoining good, and they should not despair and think that the one who does not accept it today will not accept it tomorrow. The believing man should not despair and the believing woman should not despair, rather they should carry on denouncing evil and enjoining what is good with sincerity towards Allah and His slaves, and thinking positively of Allah and hoping for the reward that is with Allah." (Fataawa al-Sheikh Ibn Baaz (4/50) (371)

386. Spreading and Exposing his Own Sins

'Abdullah ibn 'Umar (May Allah be pleased with him) reported that the Prophet (May Allah's peace and blessings be upon him) stood up after stoning Al-Aslami and said: "Avoid these filthy practices which Allah has prohibited. The one who commits any of these deeds should conceal himself with Allah's veil (he should not speak about them) and repent to Allah, for if anyone exposes his hidden sins (to us), we shall inflict the punishment prescribed by Allah the Almighty on him." (Al-Bayhaqi and Al-Hakim) (https://hadeethenc.com/en/browse/hadith/58240)

387. Spreading and Exposing Someone's Sins

Allah, the Exalted, says:

"Verily, those who love that the evil and indecent actions of those who believe should be propagated (and spread), they will have a painful torment in this world and in the Hereafter. And Allah knows and you know not. And had it not been for the Grace of Allah and His Mercy on you, (Allah would have hastened the punishment on you) and that Allah is full of kindness, Most Merciful." (Qur'an, An-Nur 24:19-20)

"And said, 'Ask Forgiveness of your Lord. Indeed, He is ever a Perpetual Forgiver. He will send (rain from) the sky upon you in (continuing) showers. And give you increase in wealth and children and provide for you gardens and provide for you rivers." (Qur'an, Nuh 71:10-12)

Abu Hurairah (May Allah be pleased with him) reported that the Prophet (May Allah's peace and blessings be upon him) said: "There is no servant who conceals the faults of another servant in this worldly life, except that Allah will conceal his faults on the Day of Resurrection." (Muslim) (https://hadeethenc.com/en/browse/hadith/3777)

Ibn Qudamah Al-Maqdisy (May Allah have mercy on him) in his famous book Kitabut Tawwabin said:

"It was narrated that in the days that Musa (May Allah have mercy on him) wandered with Bani Israel in the desert an intense drought befell them. Together, they raised their hands towards the heavens praying for the blessed rain to come. Then, to the astonishment of Musa (May Allah have mercy on him) and all those watching, the few scattered clouds that were in the sky vanished, the heat poured down, and the drought intensified. It was revealed to Musa that there was a sinner amongst the tribe of Bani Israel whom had disobeyed Allah, the Exalted, for more than forty years of his life. "Let him separate himself from the congregation," Allah, the Exalted, told Musa (May Allah have mercy on him). "Only then shall I shower you all with rain." Musa (May Allah have mercy on him) then called out to the throngs of humanity, "There is a person amongst us who has disobeyed Allah for forty years. Let him separate himself from the congregation and only then shall we be rescued from the drought." That man, waited, looking left and right, hoping that someone else would step forward, but no one did. Sweat poured forth from his brow and he knew that he was the one. The man knew that if he stayed amongst the congregation, all would die of thirst and that if he stepped forward, he would be humiliated for all eternity. He raised his hands with a sincerity he had never known before, with a humility he had never tasted, and as tears poured down on both cheeks, he said: "O Allah, have mercy on me! O Allah, hide my sins! O Allah, forgive me!" As Musa (May Allah have mercy on him) and the people of Bani Israel waited for the sinner to step forward, the clouds hugged the sky and the rain poured. Musa (May Allah have mercy on him) asked Allah: "O Allah, You blessed us with rain even though the sinner did not come forward." And Allah, the Exalted, replied, "O Musa, it is for the repentance of that very person that I blessed all of Bani Israel with water." Musa (May Allah have mercy on him) wanted to know who this blessed man was, asked, "Show him to me, O Allah!" Allah, the Exalted, replied, "O Musa, I hid his sins for forty years, do you think that after his repentance I shall expose him?" (372, 373)

388. Throwing a Fault or a Sin on to Someone Innocent

Allah, the Exalted, says:

"And whoever earns a fault or a sin and then throws it on to someone innocent, he has indeed burdened himself with falsehood and a manifest sin." (Qur'an, An-Nisa 4:112)

389. Committing Evil Deeds Openly and Blatantly

Abu Hurairah (May Allah be pleased with him) reported: The Messenger of Allah (peace and blessings be upon him) said, "Everyone from my nation will be forgiven except those who sin in public. Among them is a man who commits an evil deed in the night that Allah has hidden for him, then in the morning he says: 'O people, I have committed this sin!' His Lord had hidden it during the night but in the morning, he reveals what Allah has hidden." (Bukhari and Muslim)

390. Not Denouncing or Advising the Sinner Committing Evil Deeds

Openly and Blatantly

Narrated Abu Sa`id al-Khudri (May Allah be pleased with him): "I heard the Messenger of Allah (peace and blessings be upon him) say, "Whosoever of you sees an evil, let him change it with his hand; and if he is not able to do so, then (let him change it) with his tongue; and if he is not able to do so, then with his heart - and that is the weakest of faith." (Muslim)

Narrated Qais (May Allah have mercy on him): "Abu Bakr stood up and praised and glorified Allah, then he said: 'O people, you recite this Verse: *"O you who believe! Take care of your own selves. If you follow the (right) guidance (and enjoin what is right (Islamic Monotheism and all that Islam orders one to do) and forbid what is wrong (polytheism, disbelief and all that Islam has forbidden) no hurt can come to you from those who are in error." (Al-Ma'idah 5:105)* We heard the Messenger of Allah (peace and blessings be upon him) say: 'If the people see evil and do not change it, soon Allah will send His punishment upon them all.'" (Ahmad)

Narrated Abu Hurairah (May Allah be pleased with him): "A man who had drunk alcohol was brought to the Prophet (peace and blessings of Allah be upon him), and he said: "Beat him." Abu Hurairah said: "Some of us beat him with their hands, some beat him with their sandals and some beat him with their garments. When they had finished, one of the people said: 'May Allah disgrace you.' The Prophet (peace and blessings of Allah be upon him) said: "Do not say such things; do not help the Shaytan against him." (Bukhari)

The Muslim should sincerely advise his Muslim brother and love good for him. If he falls into sin, he should not help the Shaytan against him or pray against him, or despise him; rather he should advise him sincerely, rebuke him and hate his action; he should ask Allah to guide him, and enable him to repent. But if this sinner commits a sin openly and blatantly, then this is blameworthy and reprehensible; and he should be hated for the sake of Allah commensurate with his sin. All possible measures should be taken to stop him and protect the people from his evil, even if that is by means of shunning him, because he is persisting in sin and boasting about it, and people are no longer safe from his evil. (374)

391. Accusing Innocent Person

Allah, the Exalted, says:

"And whoever earns a fault or a sin and then throws it on to someone innocent, he has indeed burdened himself with falsehood and a manifest sin." (Qur'an, An-Nisa 4:112)

"Bad statements are for bad people (or bad women for bad men) and bad people for bad statements (or bad men for bad women). Good statements are for good people (or

good women for good men) and good people for good statements (or good men for good women), such (good people) are innocent of (each and every) bad statement which they say, for them is Forgiveness and Rizqun Karim (generous provision i.e. Paradise)."
(Qur'an, An-Nur 24:26)

Narrated Abu Dhar that he heard the Prophet (peace and blessings be upon him) saying, "If somebody accuses another of Fusuq (by calling him 'Fasiq' i.e. a wicked person) or accuses him of Kufr, such an accusation will revert to him (i.e. the accuser) if his companion (the accused) is innocent." (Bukhari)

Narrated 'Ubada bin As-Samit who took part in the battle of Badr and was a Naqib (a person heading a group of six persons), on the night of Al-'Aqaba pledge: "Allah's Apostle said while a group of his companions were around him, "Swear allegiance to me for:

1. Not to join anything in worship along with Allah.
2. Not to steal.
3. Not to commit illegal sexual intercourse.
4. Not to kill your children.
5. Not to accuse an innocent person (to spread such an accusation among people).
6. Not to be disobedient (when ordered) to do good deed."

The Prophet (peace and blessings be upon him) added: "Whoever among you fulfills his pledge will be rewarded by Allah. And whoever indulges in any one of them (except the ascription of partners to Allah) and gets the punishment in this world, that punishment will be an expiation for that sin. And if one indulges in any of them, and Allah conceals his sin, it is up to Him to forgive or punish him (in the Hereafter)." 'Ubada bin As-Samit added: "So we swore allegiance for these." (points to Allah's Apostle) (Bukhari).

The story of the accusation of adultery levied against Aisha (May Allah be pleased with her), the wife of the Prophet Muhammad (peace and blessings be upon him), also known as the Event of Ifk, can be traced to *Surah An-Nur* of the Qur'an. As the story goes, Aisha left her *howdah* in order to search for a missing necklace. Aisha's accusers were subjected to punishments of 80 lashes. (375)

Allah would not have made Aisha (May Allah be pleased with her) the wife of His Messenger (peace and blessings be upon him) unless she had been good, because he (peace and blessings be upon him) was the best of mankind. Had she been evil, she would not have been a suitable partner according to Allah' Laws and Decree.

392. Condemning Instead of Advising

Allah, the Exalted, says:

"Verily, those who love that the evil and indecent actions of those who believe should be propagated (and spread), they will have a painful torment in this world and in the Hereafter. And Allah knows and you know not. And had it not been for the grace of Allah and His mercy on you, (Allah would have hastened the punishment on you) and that Allah is full of kindness, Most Merciful." (Qur'an, An-Nur 24:19-20)

"The believers, men and women, are Auliya' (helpers, supporters, friends, protectors) of one another." (Qur'an, At-Tawbah 9:71)

Jundub ibn Abdullah (May Allah be pleased with him) reported: The Messenger of Allah (May Allah's peace and blessings be upon him) said: "A man said: 'By Allah, Allah will not forgive so-and-so.' Thereupon, Allah said: 'Who is that who swears that I will not forgive so-and-so? Indeed, I have forgiven him and rendered worthless your deeds.'" In a similar Hadith reported by Abu Hurairah: ''The sayer was a worshiper.'' Abu Hurairah said: ''He said a word that ruined his life and Hereafter.'' (Muslim) (https://hadeethenc.com/en/browse/hadith/3415)

Abu Hurairah (May Allah be pleased with him) reported: The Messenger of Allah (May Allah's peace and blessings be upon him) said: "If a man says: 'People are ruined, he himself will be the most ruined among them all." (Muslim) (https://hadeethenc.com/en/browse/hadith/8877)

Ibn al-Qayyim (May Allah have mercy on him) said:

"It may be that what he meant is that your criticizing your brother for his sin is an even greater sin than his, because it means that you feel pride in your obedience and you are praising yourself for that, and claiming to be free from sin, whereas your brother has fallen into sin. But it may be that his feeling humble because of his sin and what has happened to him, such as his feeling humble and submissive, thinking less of himself, ridding himself of pious pretensions, arrogance and self-admiration, standing before Allah with his head bowed, his gaze lowered and his heart broken – it may be that all of that is better for him than your feeling proud of your obedience, thinking that you are doing much good, believing that by doing so you are important, and reminding Allah and mankind of that. How close this sinner is to the Mercy of Allah, and how close this conceited one is to the Wrath of Allah! A sin that leads to humility is more beloved to Him than an act of obedience which fills a person with conceit. If you sleep all night then wake up feeling regret (for not having prayed Qiyaam al-Layl), that may be better for you than if you were to pray all night and wake up in the morning filled with self-admiration. For the deeds of the one who admires himself are not accepted. Perhaps your laughing whilst admitting to shortcomings is better than your weeping with piety but being filled with conceit. The groaning of the sinners is more beloved to Allah than the tasbeeh of the conceited. It may be that by means of this sin, Allah has caused him to drink the medicine that will cure a fatal disease which you also have, but you do not realize it. Allah has reason for what He does to both those who are obedient and those who sin, which are known to no-one except Him, and which no one recognizes except those who have insight, and then only within the limits of human understanding; beyond that there are reasons which are not even known to the honorable scribes (i.e. the recording angels). The Prophet said: "If the slave woman of any one of you commits adultery, let him carry out the punishment on her and not criticize." And Yusuf (peace be upon him) said: *"No reproach on you this day." (Yusuf 12:92)* For the scale is in the Hand of Allah, and the ruling is His. The point is to carry out the punishment (prescribed by Allah) and not to shame and criticize. No one feels safe from what has been decreed for them and from the power of His Decree except those who are ignorant of Allah. Allah said to the one who had more knowledge of Him than anyone else and was closer to Him: *"And had We not made you stand firm, you would nearly have inclined to them a little." (Al-Isra 17:74)* And Yusuf said: *"Unless You turn away their plot from me, I will feel inclined towards them and be one (of those who commit sin and deserve blame or those who do deeds) of the ignorant." (Yusuf 12:33)* One of the ways in which the Messenger of Allah used to swear was "No, by the One Who turns hearts." And he said, "There is no heart which is not between two of the Fingers of the Most Merciful. If He wills, He guides it aright and if He wills, He sends it astray." Then he said, "O Allah, the One Who turns hearts over, make our hearts steadfast in adhering to Your religion. O Allah, musrif al-Quloob, sirf our hearts to obey You." (Madaarij al-Saalikeen, 1/177, 178) (376)

393. Claiming Yourselves to be Pure

Allah, the Exalted, says:

"Those who avoid great sins (see the Qur'an, Verses: 6:152-153) and Al-Fawahish (illegal sexual intercourse, etc.) except the small faults, verily, your Lord is of vast forgiveness. He knows you well when He created you from the earth (Adam), and when you were fetuses in your mothers' wombs. So, ascribe not purity to yourselves. He knows best him who fears Allah and keep his duty to Him [i.e. those who are Al-Muttaqun (pious - see V.2:2)]." (Qur'an, An-Najm 53:32)

394. Prohibition of Taking Ar-Riba (The Usury)

Allah, the Exalted, says:

"Those who consume interest cannot stand (on the Day of Resurrection) except as one stands who is being beaten by Satan into insanity. That is because they say, "Trade is (just) like interest." But Allah has permitted trade and has forbidden interest. So, whoever has received an admonition from his Lord and desists may have what is past, and his affair rests with Allah. But whoever returns to (dealing in interest or usury) - those are the companions of the Fire; they will abide eternally therein. Allah will destroy Riba (usury) and will give increase for Sadaqat (deeds of charity, alms, etc.) And Allah

likes not the disbelievers, sinners. Truly those who believe and do deeds of righteousness, and perform As-Salat (Iqamat-as-Salat), and give Zakat, they will have their reward with their Lord. On them shall be no fear, nor shall they grieve. O you who believe! Be afraid of Allah and give up what remains (due to you) from Riba (usury) (from now onward), if you are (really) believers. And if you do not do it, then take a notice of war from Allah and His Messenger but if you repent, you shall have your capital sums. Deal not unjustly (by asking more than your capital sums), and you shall not be dealt with unjustly (by receiving less than your capital sums)." (Qur'an, Al-Baqarah 2:275-279)

"O believers! Do not consume interest, multiplying it many times over. And be mindful of Allah, so you may prosper." (Qur'an, Ali 'Imran 3:130)

"Whatever you pay as interest so that it may increase (li yarbu) the wealth of people does not increase (fa la yarbu) in the sight of Allah." (Qur'an, Ar-Rum 30:39)

Abdullah bin Masud (May Allah be pleased with him) reported: The Messenger of Allah (peace and blessings be upon him) cursed the one who accepts Ar-Riba (the usury) and the one who pays it." (Muslim)

Commentary: Both the parties, that is the one who charges interest and the one who pays it, are equally guilty in the matter of usury (or Riba)… (377)

Narrated Aun bin Abi Juhaifa (May Allah be pleased with him): "I saw my father buying a slave whose profession was cupping, and ordered that his instruments (of cupping) be broken. I asked him the reason for doing so. He replied, "Allah's Apostle (peace and blessings be upon him) prohibited taking money for blood, the price of a dog and the earnings of a slave girl by prostitution; he cursed her who tattoos and her who gets tattooed, the eater of Riba (usury), and the maker of pictures." (Bukhari)

Narrated Aisha (May Allah be pleased with her): "When the Verses of Surah "Al-Baqarah"' about the usury Riba were revealed, the Prophet went to the Mosque and recited them in front of the people and then banned the trade of alcohol." (Bukhari)

Narrated Abu Hurairah (May Allah be pleased with him): The Prophet (peace and blessings be upon him) said, "Avoid the seven great destructive sins." The people enquire, "O Allah's Apostle (peace and blessings be upon him)! What are they? "He said, "To join others in worship along with Allah, to practice sorcery, to kill the life which Allah has forbidden except for a just cause (according to Islamic Law), to eat up Riba (usury), to eat up an orphan's wealth, to show one's back to the enemy and fleeing from the battlefield at the time of fighting, and to accuse chaste women who never even think of anything touching chastity and are good believers." (Bukhari)

Narrated Abu Said Al-Khudri (May Allah be pleased with him): "Once Bilal brought Barni (i.e. a kind of dates) to the Prophet (peace and blessings be upon him) and the Prophet (peace and blessings be upon him) asked him, "From where have you brought these?" Bilal replied, "I had some inferior type of dates and exchanged two Sas of it for one Sa of Barni dates in order to give it to the Prophet (peace and blessings be upon him) to eat." Thereupon the Prophet (peace and blessings be upon him) said, "Beware! Beware! This is definitely Riba (usury)! This is definitely Riba (Usury)! Don't do so, but if you want to buy (a superior kind of dates) sell the inferior dates for money and then buy the superior kind of dates with that money." (Bukhari)

Narrated Ibn Shihab (May Allah be pleased with him): Malik bin Aus said, "I was in need of change for one-hundred dinars. Talha bin Ubaid-Ullah called me and we discussed the matter, and he agreed to change (my dinars). He took the gold pieces in his hands and fidgeted with them, and then said, "Wait till my storekeeper comes from the forest." Umar was listening to that and said, "By Allah! You should not separate from Talha till you get the money from him, for Allah's Apostle (peace and blessings be upon him) said, 'The selling of gold for gold is Riba (usury) except if the exchange is from hand to hand and equal in amount, and similarly, the selling of wheat for wheat is Riba (usury) unless it is from hand to hand and equal in amount, and the selling of barley for barley is usury unless it is from hand to hand and equal in amount, and dates for dates is usury unless it is from hand to hand and equal in amount" (Bukhari)

Narrated Ibn Abu Aufa (May Allah be pleased with him): "A man displayed some goods in the market and took a false oath that he had been offered so much for them though he was not offered that amount. Then the following Divine Verse was revealed: *"Verily! Those who purchase a little gain at the cost of Allah's covenant and their oaths . . . Will get painful punishment." (Qur'an, Ali 'Imran 3:77)*

Ibn Abu Aufa added, "Such person as described above is a treacherous Riba eater (i.e. eater of usury). (Bukhari)

395. Mortgage

Allah, the Exalted, says:

"Those who eat Riba (usury) will not stand (on the Day of Resurrection) except like the standing of a person beaten by Shaytan (Satan) leading him to insanity. That is because they say: "Trading is only like Riba (usury)," whereas Allah has permitted trading and forbidden Riba (usury). So, whosoever receives an admonition from his Lord and stops eating Riba (usury) shall not be punished for the past; his case is for Allah (to judge); but whoever returns (to Riba (usury)), such are the dwellers of the Fire - they will abide therein." (Qur'an, Al-Baqarah 2:275)

A mortgage is a haram Riba-based transaction that is based on a loan with interest in which the owner of the money takes as collateral the property for the purchase of which the borrower is taking out the loan, until the debt has been paid off along with the interest (Riba). (378)

396. Credit Card as Riba

Allah, the Exalted, says:

"Those who eat Riba (usury) will not stand (on the Day of Resurrection) except like the standing of a person beaten by Shaytan (Satan) leading him to insanity…" (Qur'an, Al-Baqarah 2:275)

The credit card is a new kind of Riba-based transaction and of consuming people's wealth unlawfully, making them fall into sin and contaminating their earnings and dealings.

Sheikh Ibn 'Uthaymeen (May Allah have mercy on him) was asked about this and he said:

"The answer is that a contract of this type is not permissible, because it involves Riba which is the price of the card, and it also means committing to pay interest if payment is delayed." (379)

397. Stock Market

Allah, the Exalted, says:

"O you who believe! Fear Allah and give up what remains (due to you) from Riba (from now onward) if you are (really) believers. And if you do not do it, then take a notice of war from Allah and His Messenger but if you repent, you shall have your capital sums. Deal not unjustly (by asking more than your capital sums), and you shall not be dealt with unjustly (by receiving less than your capital sums)." (Qur'an, A-Baqarah 2:278-279)

"Those who eat Riba (usury) will not stand (on the Day of Resurrection) except like the standing of a person beaten by Shaytan (Satan) leading him to insanity…" (Qur'an, Al-Baqarah 2:275)

Ruling on dealing in Stocks:

Dealing in stocks is haram according to Shariah, because it is a loan in return for agreed-upon interest, and this is Riba (usury) which Allah has forbidden and warned against.

The difference between shares and stocks:

A share represents a stake in a company, meaning that the shareholder is a partner, whereas a stock represents a debt owed by the company, meaning that the stockholder is a lender. Based on this, the shareholder only earns profits when the company makes a profit, whereas the stockholder earns guaranteed annual interest whether the company makes a profit or not.

Also based on this, if the company makes a loss, the shareholder has to bear some part of the loss, depending on the amount of shares he has, because he is a partner and owner of part of the company, so he must bear some part of the loss. The stockholder, on the other hand, does not bear any of the company's losses because he is not a partner in the company, rather he is simply a lender, who lends money in return for benefits agreed upon whether the company makes a profit or makes losses. (380)

398. Money Exchange

Narrated Abu Al-Minhal (May Allah be pleased with him): "I used to practice money exchange, and I asked Zaid bin Arqam about it, and he narrated what the Prophet said in the following: Abu Al-Minhal said, "I asked Al-Bara bin Azib and Zaid bin Arqam about practicing money exchange. They replied, 'We were traders in the time of Allah's Apostle and I asked Allah's Apostle about money exchange. He replied, 'If it is from hand to hand, there is no harm in it; otherwise, it is not permissible.'" (Bukhari)

Narrated Abu Salih Az-Zaiyat (May Allah be pleased with him): "I heard Abu Sa'id Al-Khudri saying, "The selling of a dinar for a dinar, and a dirham for a dirham is permissible." I said to him, "Ibn 'Abbas does not say the same." Abu Sa'id replied, "I asked Ibn 'Abbas whether he had heard it from the Prophet (peace and blessings of Allah be upon him) or seen it in the Holy Book. Ibn 'Abbas replied, "I do not claim that, and you know Allah's Messenger (peace and blessings of Allah be upon him) better than I, but Usama informed me that the Prophet had said, 'There is no Riba (in money exchange) except when it is not done from hand to hand (i.e. when there is delay in payment).'" (Bukhari)

Narrated 'Ubaadah ibn as-Saamit (May Allah be pleased with him): The Messenger of Allah (peace and blessings of Allah be upon him) said: "Gold for gold, silver for silver, wheat for wheat, barley for barley, dates for dates, salt for salt, like for like, same for same, hand to hand. But if these commodities differ, then sell as you like, as long as it is hand to hand." (Muslim)

If the money cannot be transferred directly to final destination (i.e. your family), and you have to use a middleman. If the money will reach this middleman in riyals or dollars, then he will exchange it himself for liras and then transfer it to your family through the transfer office, this process is not permissible, because there is no hand-to-hand exchange between you and this person. (381, 382)

Scholars who specialize in contemporary financial dealings have pointed out that selling currencies via the internet is not a transaction in which hand-to-hand exchange can take place, so it is haram according to Shariah.

Moreover, there is another reason for forbidding the transaction asked about here, which is that the company gives investors profits of between 8 and 12% on a weekly basis, and this renders the investment contract invalid, because what is required in the case of an investment contract is that profits should be distributed by percentage among the partners, so each partner should get a specific share of the profits, such as one half or one quarter and so on; taking a fixed percentage based on the capital invested is not permissible.

To sum up:

Selling currencies via this method is not permissible for two reasons:

1-Selling currencies via the internet is not a transaction in which hand-to-hand exchange can take place.

2-The investment contract stipulates that the profits should be shared among the partners as a percentage, and it is not permissible for that percentage to be calculated only on the basis of the capital invested.

We should point out that it is not permissible to borrow from these middlemen or agents in what is called the "margin system", which is where you required to deposit part of the value of the loan you give them with them so that they can deal on the stock exchange – and especially with currencies – and these agents make deals worth many times more than what you gave them, and any losses will be deducted from the money you have deposited with them.

You should know that dealing with the margin system is haram according to Shariah and it is not permissible for anyone to deal with it. Many people – even non-Muslims – have warned against it because of the bad effects it has on financial dealings in the stock exchange. One of the main causes of the collapse of the New York Stock Exchange on "Black Monday" was dealings with the margin system, because of commands to sell that were programmed into brokers' computers, telling them to sell in the event that prices dropped to a certain level. When the prices actually fell, the commands to sell were triggered automatically, which led to an unprecedented flooding of the market when there was no demand, and this is what led to the collapse. (383)

399. Bitcoin and Cryptocurrency

An-Nu'man bin Bashir (May Allah be pleased with him) reported: The Messenger of Allah (peace and blessings be upon him) said, "What is lawful is clear and what is unlawful is clear, but between them are certain doubtful things which many people do not know. So, he who guards against doubtful things keeps his religion and his honor blameless. But he who falls into doubtful things falls into that which is unlawful, just as a shepherd who grazes his cattle in the vicinity of a pasture declared prohibited (by the king); he is likely to stray into the pasture. Mind you, every king has a protected pasture and Allah's involved limits is that which He has declared unlawful. Verily, there is a piece of flesh in the body, if it is healthy, the whole body is healthy, and if it is corrupt, the whole body is corrupt. Verily, it is the heart." (Bukhari and Muslim)

Any investment involving interest and ambiguity is prohibited. (383, 384)

400. Prohibition of Devouring the Property of an Orphan

Allah, the Exalted, says:

"Do not handle the property of the orphans except with a good reason until they become mature and strong. Maintain equality in your dealings by the means of measurement and balance. No soul is responsible for what is beyond its ability. Be just in your words, even if the party involved is one of your relatives and keep your promise with God. Thus, does your Lord guide you so that you may take heed." (Qur'an, Al-An'am 6:152)

"Give orphans their wealth when they reach maturity, and do not exchange your worthless possessions for their valuables, nor cheat them by mixing their wealth with your own. For this would indeed be a great sin." (Qur'an, An-Nisa 4:2)

"Verily, those who unjustly eat up the property of orphans, they eat up only fire into their bellies, and they will be burnt in the blazing fire!" (Qur'an, An-Nisa 4:10)

Other Verses: *An-Nisa 4:5-6, Al Fajr 89:17, Al-Baqarah 2:220.*

Abu Hurairah (May Allah be pleased with him) said: The Prophet (peace and blessings be upon him) said, "Keep away from the seven fatalities." It was asked: "What are they, O Messenger of Allah?" He (peace be upon him) replied, "Associating anything with Allah in worship (i.e. committing an act of Shirk), sorcery, killing of one whom Allah has declared inviolable without a just cause, devouring the property of an orphan, the eating of usury (Riba), fleeing from the battlefield and accusing chaste believing women, who never even think of anything touching their chastity." (Bukhari and Muslim)

Commentary: All the sins mentioned in the Hadith are Major sins but Shirk is the greatest of all… (385)

Narrated Nafi (May Allah be pleased with him): "Ibn Umar never refused to be appointed as a guardian." The most beloved thing to Ibn Sirin concerning an orphan's wealth was that the orphan's advisors and guardians would assemble to decide what is best for him. When Tawus was asked about the something concerning an orphan's affairs, he would recite: '…*And Allah knows him who means mischief from him who means good…*' *(2:220)* Ata said concerning some orphans, "The guardian is to provide for the young and the old orphans according to their needs from their shares." (Bukhari)

Narrated Abu Hurairah (May Allah be pleased with him): The Messenger of Allah (peace and blessings be upon him) said: "The best house among the Muslims is a house in which there is an orphan who is treated well. And the worst house among the Muslims is a house in which there is an orphan who is treated badly." (Ibn Majah)

Narrated Abu Dharr (May Allah be pleased with him): The Messenger of Allah (peace and blessings be upon him) said: "Abu Dharr, I find that thou art weak and I like for thee what I like for myself. Do not rule over (even) two persons and do not manage the property of an orphan." (Muslim)

401. Taking People's Property Unjustly

Allah, the Exalted, says:

"And eat up not one another's property unjustly (in any illegal way, e.g. stealing, robbing, deceiving), nor give bribery to the rulers (judges before presenting your cases) that you may knowingly eat up a part of the property of others sinfully." (Qur'an, Al-Baqarah 2:188)

"O you who have believed, do not consume one another's wealth unjustly but only (in lawful) business by mutual consent." (Qur'an, An-Nisa 4:29)

Narrated Abu Wail: Abdullah bin Masud said, "Whoever takes a (false) oath in order to grab some property (unjustly), Allah will be angry with him when he will meet Him. Allah confirmed that through His Divine Revelation: *"Verily! Those who purchase a little gain at the cost of Allah's covenant and their oaths . . . they will have a painful punishment." (3:77)* Al-Ashath bin Qais came to us and asked, 'What is Abu Abdur-Rahman (i.e. Abdullah) telling you? 'We told him what he was narrating to us. He said, 'He was telling the Truth; this Divine Verse was revealed in connection with me. There was a dispute between me and another man about something and the case was filed before Allah's Apostle (peace and blessings be upon him) who said, 'Produce your two witnesses or else the defendant is to take an oath.' 'I said, the defendant will surely take a (false) oath caring for nothing.' The Prophet (peace and blessings be upon him) said, 'Whoever takes a false oath in order to grab other's property, then Allah will be angry with him when he will meet Him.' Then Allah revealed its confirmation. Al-Ashath then recited the above Divine Verse." (3:77) (Bukhari)

Narrated Abu Salama that there was a dispute between him and some people (about a piece of land). When he told Aisha about it, she said, "O Abu Salama! Avoid taking the land unjustly, for the Prophet (peace and blessings be upon him) said, 'Whoever usurps even one span of the land of somebody, his neck will be encircled with it down the seven earths.'" (Bukhari)

The property that is seized by force, false oath or action, may be a real estate or it may be moveable goods, any wealth, any things which belong to someone else. The one who has seized anything unlawfully must repent to Allah and return the seized property to its owner and ask him for forgiveness. If the seized property is still there, it should be returned as it is, and if it is not there, then he must replace it. Wrongful seizure of property is not restricted only to taking it by force; it may also include taking it by way of false dispute, false oaths, etc. The matter is serious and the reckoning will be severe. The one who has seized anything unlawfully must repent to Allah and return the seized property to its owner and ask him for forgiveness. The Prophet (peace and blessings of Allah be upon him) said: "Whoever has done any wrong to his brother, let him seek his forgiveness today, before there will be no dinar and no dirham (i.e. the Day of Resurrection), when if he has any hasanat (good deeds), some of his hasanat will be taken and given to the one who was wronged, and if he does not have any hasanat, some of the sayi'aat (bad deeds) of the one who was wronged will be taken and thrown onto him, and he will be thrown into Hell," or as he (peace and blessings of Allah be upon him) said it. If the seized property is still there, it should be returned as it is, and if it is not there, then he must replace it. Similarly, he is obliged to return the seized property along with any increase, whether it is connected to it or separate, because that is the growth of the seized property, so it also belongs to the original owner. If the one who seized the property has built anything or planted crops on the seized land, he has to remove the buildings or crops if the owner asks him to, because the Prophet (peace and blessings of Allah be upon him) said, "The sweat of the evildoer counts for nothing." (Tirmidhi)

If that has caused any damage to the land, he is to be penalized for that damage. He also has to erase any traces of building or planting that remain, so that the land may be given back to its owner in good condition. He also has to pay rent covering the period from the time when he seized the land to the time when he gave it back - i.e. the rent for a similar piece of land – because he unlawfully prevented its owner from benefiting from it during this time. (386, 387)

402. Illegally Using Someone's Property

Allah, the Exalted, says:

"And eat up not one another's property unjustly (in any illegal way, e.g. stealing, robbing, deceiving)." (Qur'an, Al-Baqarah 2:188)

Narrated `Ikrima: Ibn `Abbas said: Allah's Messenger (peace and blessings be upon him) delivered a sermon on the Day of Nahr and said, "…No doubt! Your blood, your properties and your honor are sacred to one another…" (Bukhari) (https://sunnah.com/bukhari:5550)

Narrated Said bin Zaid (May Allah be pleased with him): Allah's Apostle (peace and blessings be upon him) said, "Whoever usurps the land of somebody unjustly, his neck will be encircled with it down the seven earths (on the Day of Resurrection)." (Bukhari)

In Islam one cannot use anything belonging to the other without the permission of the owner.

If tenant doesn't pay rent and refuses to leave, then they are usurping the property and are sinning.

You can pray against him – for the prayer of the oppressed is answered - or you can leave their case to Allah to take your rights from them for you. (388)

The ex-worker may continue to live illegally in the company's apartment after his resignation.

The squatters may deliberately enter and occupy the property with no legal claim to the property (no title, right or lease).

Using other people's property wrongfully, no matter how small it may be (can be a needle), is one of the most heinous sins in Islam.

Narrated Ibn 'Umar (May Allah be pleased with him): The Prophet (peace and blessings be upon him) said, "Oppression will be a darkness on the Day of Resurrection." (Bukhari)

403. Consuming One Another's Wealth

Allah, the Exalted, says:

"And do not consume one another's wealth." (Qur'an, Al-Baqarah 2:188)

"O you who have believed, do not consume one another's wealth unjustly." (Qur'an, An-Nisa 4:29)

404. Carelessness in Guarding the Trust

Allah, the Exalted, says:

"Truly, We did offer al-Amanah (the trust or moral responsibility, or honesty and all the duties which Allah has ordained) to the heavens and the earth, and the mountains, but they declined to bear it and were afraid of it (i.e. afraid of Allah's Torment). But man bore it. Verily, he was unjust (to himself) and ignorant (of its results)." (Qur'an, Al-Ahzab 33:72)

"Those who are faithfully true to their Amanat (all the duties which Allah has ordained, honesty, moral responsibility and trusts etc.) and to their covenants." (Qur'an, Al-Mu'minun 23:8)

"O you who believe! Betray not Allah and His Messenger, nor betray knowingly your Amanat (things entrusted to you, and all the duties which Allah has ordained for you)." (Qur'an, Al-Anfal 8:27)

Other Verse: An-Nisa 4:58.

There are four well-known scenarios with regard to Amanah or Trust:

1. Financial rights

Financial rights that are established by contracts and covenants, such as items left with a person for safekeeping, hiring and rentals, and so on; and those concerning found items and what people pick up of the lost property of others, where there is no contract.

2. Positions of responsibility, whether social, public or private

One should carry out such positions of trust and responsibility on a basis of truth and justice. A position of rulership is a trust, a judicial position is a trust, a management position is a trust, responsibility for a family is a trust, and the same applies to all positions of responsibility.

Narrated Abu Hurairah (May Allah be pleased with him): The Messenger of Allah (peace and blessings of Allah be upon him) said: "When honesty is lost, then wait for the Hour." It was asked, "How will honesty be lost, O Allah's Messenger?" He said, "When authority is given to those who do not deserve it, then wait for the Hour." (Bukhari)

Abu Dharr (May Allah be pleased with him) reported: "I said: 'O Messenger of Allah, will you not appoint me to (an official position)?" He patted me on my shoulder with his hand and said: "O Abu Dharr, you are weak and it is a trust. It will be a cause of disgrace and remorse on the Day of Resurrection, except for the one who takes it up with a full sense of responsibility and fulfills what is entrusted to him." (Muslim) (https://hadeethenc.com/en/browse/hadith/3467)

3. Marriage

Jabir ibn Abdullah (May Allah be pleased with him) reported: The Messenger of Allah (peace and blessings be upon him) said, "Fear Allah regarding women. Verily, you have taken them as a trust from Allah, and intercourse has been made lawful by the Word of Allah..." (Muslim)

4. Keeping people's secrets

Narrated Abu Sa'id al-Khudri (May Allah have mercy on him): The Messenger of Allah (peace and blessings of Allah be upon him) said: "One of the most evil people before Allah on the Day of Resurrection will be a man who is intimate with his wife and she is intimate with him, then he broadcasts her secrets." (Muslim)

Narrated Jabir ibn 'Abdullah (May Allah be pleased with him): The Messenger of Allah (peace and blessings of Allah be upon him) said: "When a man tells something and then departs, it is a trust (which should not be disclosed by the one who heard it)." (Abu Dawud)

When a man was to set out on a journey, Abdullah ibn 'Umar (May Allah be pleased with him) would say to him: "Draw near to me so that I may bid you farewell as the Messenger of Allah (May Allah's peace and blessings be upon him) used to bid us farewell. He would say: 'I entrust Allah with your religion, your trusts and your last deeds.'" Abdullah ibn Yazīd al-Khatmi (May Allah be pleased with him) reported that the Messenger of Allah (May Allah's peace and blessings be upon him) would bid farewell to the departing army by saying: "I entrust Allah with your religion, your trusts and your last deeds." (Ibn Majah) (https://hadeethenc.com/en/browse/hadith/3058)

The individual is obliged to take care of, uphold and fulfil of the rights of others. Neglecting or betrayal of trusts are Major sin. Betrayal of trusts is one of the signs of hypocrisy. (389)

405. Taking More than Your Allotment

Al-Hasan narrated from Abu Hurairah (May Allah be pleased with them) that the Messenger of Allah (peace and blessings be upon him) said: "Who will take these statements from me, so that he may act upon them or teach one who will act upon them?" So, Abu Hurairah said: "I said: 'I shall, O Messenger of Allah!' So he (peace and blessings be upon him) took my hand and enumerated five (things), he said: "Be on guard against the forbidden and you shall be the most worshiping among the people, be satisfied with what Allah has allotted for you and you shall be the richest of the people, be kind to your neighbor and you shall be a believer, love for the people what you love for yourself and you shall be a Muslim. And do not laugh too much, for indeed increased laughter kills the heart." (Tirmidhi)

Umm Salamah (May Allah be pleased with her) told on the Prophet's authority about two men, who brought a dispute before him about inheritances, but had no proof beyond their claim. He (peace and blessings be upon him) said, "If I give a decision in favor of one respecting what is rightly his brother's I am allotting him only a portion of Hell." Thereupon both the men said, "Messenger of God, this right of mine may go to my brother," but he replied, "No; rather go and divide it up, aiming at what is right, then draw lots, and let each of you consider the other to have what is legitimately his." In a version he said, "I judge between you only by my opinion regarding matters about which no Revelation has been sent down to me." (Abu Dawud)

Narrated Anas bin Malik (May Allah be pleased with him): "Some people used to allot some date palm trees to the Prophet (peace and blessings be upon him) as gift till he conquered Banu Quraiza and Bani An-Nadir, where upon he started returning their date palms to them." (Bukhari)

Narrated Ibn 'Umar (May Allah have mercy on him): "On the Day of Khaibar, the Messenger of Allah (peace and blessings be upon him) allotted two shares for a horse, and one share (from the war booty) for the fighter." (Bukhari)

Allah allotted men and women different rights and cultural expectations. Hadith Saheeh Bukhari states that a man is expected to be the "guardian of (his) family," whereas a woman is expected to be the "guardian of her husband's home and his children."

406. Prohibition of Seeking out a Position of Authority

Abu Hurairah (May Allah be pleased with him) reported: The Prophet (May Allah's peace and blessings be upon him) said: "You will eagerly seek out a position of authority, but it will be a source of regret on the Day of Judgment. How excellent is the wet nurse, and how evil is the weaning one." (Bukhari) (https://hadeethenc.com/en/browse/hadith/64681)

Abu Musa al-Ash'ari (May Allah be pleased with him) reported: "I and two of my paternal cousins entered upon the Prophet (May Allah's peace and blessings be upon him). One of them said: "O Messenger of Allah, appoint us rulers over some of what Allah the Almighty has entrusted you with." The other said the same. The Prophet (May Allah's peace and blessings be upon him) said: "By Allah! We do not entrust this post to anyone who seeks it or is keen to attain it.'" (Bukhari and Muslim)

(https://hadeethenc.com/en/browse/hadith/3517)

Narrated 'Abd al-Rahman b. Samura: "The Messenger of Allah (peace be upon him) said to me: "Abd al-Rahman, do not ask for a position of authority, for if you are granted this position as a result of your asking for it, you will be left alone (without God's help to discharge the responsibilities attendant thereon); and if you are granted it without making any request for it, you will be helped (by God in the discharge of your duties). (Muslim)

407. The Leader Who Misleads his Followers, the Tyrant and the Oppressor

Allah, the Exalted, says:

"The cause is only against the ones who wrong the people and tyrannize upon the earth without right. Those will have a painful punishment." (Qur'an, Ash-Shuraa 42:42)

Hisham ibn Hakim ibn Hizam (May Allah be pleased with him) reported that while in the Levant he passed by some Nabataean peasants who had been made to stand in the sun with oil poured on their heads. He asked, "What is this?" He was told, "They are being punished on account of the land tax." In another narration, "They have been imprisoned on account of the Jizyah." So, Hisham said: "I testify that I heard the Messenger of Allah (May Allah's peace and blessings be upon him) saying: 'Verily, Allah tortures those who torture people in this world.'" He then went to the ruler and spoke with him, and the ruler ordered their release." (Muslim) (https://hadeethenc.com/en/browse/hadith/8888)

Abu Dharr (May Allah be pleased with him) reported: The Messenger of Allah (peace and blessings be upon him) said, "Allah Almighty said: 'O My servants, I have forbidden injustice for Myself and I have forbidden it among you, so do not oppress one another…'" (Muslim)

Abu Sa'id Al-Khudri (May Allah be pleased with him) reported: The Prophet (peace and blessings be upon him) said, "The best type of Jihad (striving in the way of Allah) is speaking a true word in the presence of a tyrant ruler." (Abu Dawud and Tirmidhi)

The tyrant ruler is accountable not only for his oppressive deeds but he incurs the intense Wrath of Allah because of his ingratitude and denial of Allah's blessings.

408. The Unjust Ruler

Allah, the Exalted, says:

"And if you judge, judge between them with justice. Indeed, Allah loves those who act justly." (Qur'an, Al-Ma'idah 5:42)

"Verily, Allah enjoins Al-'Adl (justice) and Al-Ihsan (performing duties in a perfect manner)." (Qur'an, An-Nahl 16:90)

"And be equitable. Verily! Allah loves those who are the equitable." (Qur'an, Al-Hujurat 49:9)

Other Verse: *An-Nisa 4:59.*

Narrated Abu Hurairah (May Allah be pleased with him): The Prophet (peace and blessings be upon him) said, "Seven are (the people) whom Allah will give protection with His Shade on the Day when there will be no shade except His Shade (i.e. on the Day of Resurrection), and they are: a just ruler, a youth who grew up with the worship of Allah, a person whose heart is attached to the Mosque, two people who love and meet each other and depart from each other for the sake of Allah, a man whom a beautiful and high-ranking woman seduces (for illicit relation) but he rejects this offer by saying: "I fear Allah", a person who gives a charity and conceals it to such an extent that the left hand might not know what the right has given, and a person who remembers Allah in solitude and his eyes well up." (Bukhari and Muslim)

Narrated 'Abdullah bin 'Amr bin Al-'As (May Allah be pleased with him): The Messenger of Allah (peace and blessings be upon him) said, "The just will be seated upon pulpits of light. Those who are fair with regards to their judgment and their family, and those who are under them." (Muslim)

Commentary: The Hadith throws light on the excellence of justice and the high rank of those who do justice. (390)

Narrated 'Auf bin Malik (May Allah be pleased with him): The Messenger of Allah (peace and blessings be upon him) said, "The best of your rulers are those whom you love and who love you, and those who supplicate Allah in your favor and you supplicate Allah in their favor. The worst of your rulers are those whom you hate and who hate you; and whom you curse and who curse you." It was asked (by those who were present): "Should not we oppose them?" He said, "No, as long as they establish Salat; as long as they establish Salat in your midst." (Muslim)

'Iyad ibn Himar (May Allah be pleased with him) reported that the Prophet (May Allah's peace and blessings be upon him) said: "The people of Paradise are three: a ruler who is just and successful; a man who is compassionate and soft-hearted toward every relative and Muslim; and a man with dependents who is chaste and abstains from begging." (Muslim) (https://hadeethenc.com/en/browse/hadith/5324)

409. Obligation of Obedience to the Ruler in what is Lawful and

Prohibition of Obeying him in what is Unlawful

Allah, the Exalted, says:

"O you who believe! Obey Allah and obey the Messenger (Muhammad, peace be upon him), and those of you (Muslims) who are in authority." (Qur'an, An-Nisa 4:59)

Ibn 'Umar (May Allah be pleased with him) reported: The Prophet (peace and blessings be upon him) said, "It is obligatory upon a Muslim to listen (to the ruler) and obey whether he likes it or not, except when he is ordered to do a sinful thing; in such case, there is no obligation to listen or to obey." (Bukhari and Muslim)

Ibn 'Umar (May Allah be pleased with him) reported: "Whenever we took a pledge of allegiance to Messenger of Allah (peace and blessings be upon him) to hear and obey, he (peace and blessings be upon him) would say to us, "As far as you are capable of." (Bukhari and Muslim)

Ibn 'Umar (May Allah be pleased with him) reported: The Messenger of Allah (peace and blessings be upon him) said, "One who withdraws his hand from obedience (to the Amir), will find no argument (in his defense) when he stands before Allah on the Day of Resurrection; and one who dies without having sworn allegiance, will die the death of one belonging to the Days of Ignorance." (Muslim)

Anas (May Allah be pleased with him) reported: The Messenger of Allah (peace and blessings be upon him) said, "Hear and obey even if an Abyssinian slave whose head is like a raisin is placed in authority over you." (Bukhari)

Abu Hurairah (May Allah be pleased with him) reported: The Messenger of Allah (peace and blessings be upon him) said, "It is obligatory upon you to listen and obey the orders of the ruler in prosperity and adversity, whether you are willing or unwilling, or when someone is given undue preference to you." (Muslim)

Abdullah bin 'Amr (May Allah be pleased with him) reported: "We accompanied Messenger of Allah (peace and blessings be upon him) on a journey. We halted at a place to take a rest. Some of us began to set right their tents, others began to graze their animals, while others were engaged in competing with one another in archery when an announcer of Messenger of Allah (peace and blessings be upon him) announced that people should gather for Salat. We gathered around the Messenger of Allah and he (peace and blessings be upon him) addressed us, saying, "Every Prophet before me was under obligation to guide his followers to what he knew was good for them and to warn the evil thing which he knew. As for this Ummah, it will have sound state and in its early stage of existence; but the last phase of its existence, will be faced with trials and with things you do not recognize. There will be tremendous trials, one after the other, and to each the believer will say, 'That is it'. Whenever a trial arrives the believer will say: 'This is going to bring about my destruction.' When this pass, another calamity will approach and he will say: 'This surely is going to be my end.' Whosoever wishes to be removed from the Fire (Hell) and admitted to Jannah should die with faith in Allah and the Last Day; and he should treat others as he wishes to be treated. He who swears allegiance to an imam, he should give him the pledge in ratification and the sincerity of his heart. He should obey him to the best of his capacity. If another man comes forward as a claimant (when one has already been installed), behead the second." (Muslim)

Narrated Wa'il bin Hujr (May Allah be pleased with him): "Salamah bin Yazid Al-Ju'f (May Allah be pleased with him) asked Messenger of Allah (peace and blessings be upon him): 'O Prophet of Allah! Tell us, what you command us to do if there arises over us rulers who demand of us what is due to them and refuse us what is due to us.' Messenger of Allah (peace and blessings be upon him) turned away from him, but he repeated the same question. Thereupon Messenger of Allah (peace and blessings be upon him) said, 'Listen to them and obey them. They are responsible for their obligations and you are accountable for yours." (Muslim)

Commentary:
This Hadith means that both the ruler and the ruled have their own respective obligations. (391)

Narrated Abdullah bin Masud (May Allah be pleased with him): The Messenger of Allah (peace and blessings be upon him) said, "There will be discrimination after my death and there will be other matters that you will disapprove." He was asked: "O Messenger of Allah! What do you command us to do when we are encountered with such happenings?" He answered, "Give what is due from you and supplicate to Allah for your rights." (Bukhari and Muslim)

Narrated Abu Hurairah (May Allah be pleased with him): The Messenger of Allah (peace and blessings be upon him) said, "Whosoever obeys me, obeys Allah; and he who disobeys me, disobeys Allah; and whosoever obeys the Amir (leader), in fact, obeys me; and he who disobeys the Amir, in fact, disobeys me." (Bukhari and Muslim)

Narrated Ibn Abbas (May Allah be pleased with him): The Messenger of Allah (peace and blessings be upon him) said, "If a person notices in his ruler what he dislikes, he should show patience because he who departs from the (Muslim) community a cubit, dies like those who died in the Days of Ignorance." (Bukhari and Muslim)

Narrated Abu Bakrah (May Allah be pleased with him): "I heard Messenger of Allah (peace and blessings be upon him) saying, "He who insults the rulers, Allah will insult him." (Tirmidhi)

410. Fighting the Ruler, Rebelling Against Him Even if He Oppresses

Allah, the Exalted, says:

"And do not kill yourselves (nor kill one another). Surely, Allah is Most Merciful to you." (Qur'an, An-Nisa 4:29)

"O you who believe! Obey Allah and obey the Messenger (Muhammad SAW), and those of you (Muslims) who are in authority. (And) if you differ in anything amongst yourselves, refer it to Allah and His Messenger (SAW), if you believe in Allah and in the Last Day. That is better and more suitable for final determination." (Qur'an, An-Nisa 4:59)

Narrated Junida b. Abu Umayya: "We called upon 'Ubada b. Samit who was ill and said to him: 'May God give you health I Narrate to us a tradition which God may prove beneficial (to us) and which you have heard from the Messenger of Allah (May Allah's peace and blessings be upon him). He said: 'The Messenger of Allah (May Allah's peace and blessings be upon him) called us and we took the oath of allegiance to him. Among the injunctions he made binding upon us was: 'Listening and obedience (to the Amir) in our pleasure and displeasure, in our adversity and prosperity, even when somebody is given preference over us, and without disputing the delegation of powers to a man duly invested with them (Obedience shall be accorded to him in all circumstances) except when you have clear signs of his disbelief in (or disobedience to) God-signs that could be used as a conscientious justification (for non-compliance with his orders)." (Muslim)

Abu Hurairah (May Allah be pleased with him) reported that the Messenger of Allah (May Allah's peace and blessings be upon him) said: "Whoever gives up obedience and separates from the Muslim community and then dies, has died a death like that of the pre-Islamic era of Ignorance. Whoever fights under the banner of a blind, unguided cause, getting flared up for his people's pride, calling to fight for the sake of his people's pride or in support of his people's pride, or personal inclination, and, therefore, is killed, his killing is like that of the pre-Islamic era of Ignorance. Whoever breaks his allegiance to my Ummah, killing the righteous and the wicked of them, paying no heed to the believers among them, and not fulfilling a covenant with those with whom he has made covenants, he does not belong to me and I do not belong to him." (Muslim) (https://hadeethenc.com/en/browse/hadith/58218)

Narrated 'Abd al-Rahman b. Abd Rabb al-Ka'ba (May Allah have mercy on him): "…He (peace and blessings be upon him) said: 'It was the duty of every Prophet that has gone before me to guide his followers to what he knew was good for them and warn them against what he knew was bad for them; but this Ummah of yours has its days of peace and (security) in the beginning of its career, and in the last phase of its existence it will be afflicted with trials and with things disagreeable to you. (In this phase of the Ummah), there will be tremendous trials one after the other, each making the previous one dwindles into insignificance. When they would be afflicted with a trial, the believer would say: 'This is going to bring about my destruction. When at (the trial) is over, they would be afflicted with another trial, and the believer would say:' This surely is going to be my end. Whoever wishes to be delivered from the Fire and enter the Garden should die with Faith in Allah and the Last Day and should treat the people as he wishes to be treated by them. He who swears allegiance to a Caliph should give him the pledge of his hand and the sincerity of his heart (i.e. submit to him both outwardly as well as inwardly). He should obey him to the best of his capacity. If another man comes forward (as a claimant to Caliphate), disputing his authority, they (the Muslims) should behead the latter. The narrator says: 'I came close to him ('Abdullah b. 'Amr b. Al-'As) and said to him: 'Can you say on oath that you heard it from the Messenger of Allah (peace be upon him)?' He pointed with his hands to his ears and his heart and said: 'My ears heard it and my mind retained it.' I said to him: 'This cousin of yours, Mu'awiya, orders us to unjustly consume our wealth among ourselves and to kill one another, while Allah says: *"O ye who believe, do not consume your wealth among yourselves unjustly, unless it be trade based on mutual agreement, and do not kill yourselves. Verily, God is Merciful to you." (4:29)* The narrator says that (hearing this) Abdullah b. 'Amr b. Al-'As kept quiet for a while and then said: 'Obey him in so far as he is obedient to God; and disobey him in matters involving disobedience to God." (Muslim)

Narrated through a different chain of transmitters, on the authority of Hudhaifa b. al-Yaman: "Messenger of Allah, no doubt, we had an evil time (i.e. the days of Jahiliyya or Ignorance) and God brought us a good time (i.e. Islamic period) through which we are now living. Will there be a bad time after this good time? He (the Holy Prophet) said: 'Yes.' I said: 'Will there be a good time after this bad time?' He said: 'Yes.' I said: 'Will there be a bad time after good time?' He said: 'Yes.' I said: 'How?' Whereupon he said: 'There will be leaders who will not be led by my guidance and who will not adopt my ways. There will be among them men who will have the hearts of Devils in the bodies of human beings.' I said: 'What should I do, Messenger of Allah, if I (happen) to live in that time?' He replied: 'You will listen to the Amir and carry out his orders; even if your back is flogged and your wealth is snatched, you should listen and obey." (Muslim)

Narrated 'Auf b. Malik (May Allah have mercy on him): The Messenger of Allah (peace and blessings be upon him): "The best of your rulers are those whom you love and who love you, who invoke God's blessings upon you and you invoke His blessings upon them. And the worst of your rulers are those whom you hate and who hate you, and whom you curse and who curse you. It was asked (by those present): Shouldn't we overthrow them with the help of the sword? He said: No, as long as they establish prayer among you. If you then find anything detestable in them. You should hate their administration, but do not withdraw yourselves from their obedience." (Muslim)

Narrated Alqama b. Wai'l al-Hadrami who learnt the tradition from his father. The latter said: "Salama b. Yazid al-ju'afi asked the Messenger of Allah (peace and blessings be upon him): "Prophet of Allah, what do you think if we have rulers who rule over us and demand that we discharge our obligations towards them, but they (themselves) do not discharge their own responsibilities towards us? What do you order us to do?' The Messenger of Allah (peace be upon him) avoided giving any answer. Salama asked him again. He (again) avoided giving any answer. Then he asked again - it was the second time or the third time - when Ash'ath b. Qais (finding that the Holy Prophet was unnecessarily being pressed for answer) pulled him aside and said: 'Listen to them and obey them, for on them shall he their burden and on you shall be your burden." (Muslim)

Warding off evil by means of a greater evil is not permitted according to the scholarly consensus (ijmaa') of the Muslims. (392)

Abdullah b. Zaid (May Allah be pleased with him) reported: The Prophet (peace and blessings be upon him) said, "…And you would soon find after me preferences (over you in getting material benefits). So, you should show patience till you meet me at the Haud (Kawthar)." (Muslim)

411. Strike

Allah, the Exalted, says:

"O you who believe! Fulfil (your) obligations…" (Qur'an, Al-Ma'idah 5:1)

"Seek not mischief in the land, for Allah loves not those who do mischief." (Qur'an, Al-Qasas 28:77)

Striking is a breach of the contract between the worker and his employer, and Allah calls on us in His Book to honour and uphold the contracts that one person may take upon himself towards another person. So, the worker has to do all the work that he agreed to do in a manner that pleases Allah.

Strikes are often accompanied by trouble, discord and violence which is unacceptable in Islam because of the Fiqhi principle that warding off evil takes priority over achieving benefits. There are a number of other means which can be resorted to in order to achieve one's goals, and which may be more effective than striking. A wise man would not leave any legitimate avenue unexplored. (393)

As for stopping work because one has not been paid, this is permissible, because in this case the employer is in breach of contract, so the worker has the right to stop work until he gets paid. The Prophet (peace and blessings of Allah be upon him) said: "Give the hired worker his wages before his sweat dries." (Ibn Majah).

412. Betraying the Leader

Allah, the Exalted, says:

"If you (have reason to) fear from a people betrayal, throw (their treaty) back to them, (putting you) on equal terms. Indeed, Allah does not like traitors." (Qur'an, Al-Anfal 8:58)

Narrated Ibn 'Umar (May Allah be pleased with him): Allah's Messenger (peace and blessings be upon him) said, "A flag will be fixed on the Day of Resurrection for every betrayer, and it will be announced (publicly in front of everybody), 'This is the betrayal (perfidy) so-and-so, the son of sound- so." (Bukhari)

Narrated Abu Hurairah (May Allah be pleased with him): Allah's Messenger (peace be upon him) said, "Whoever obeys me, obeys Allah, and whoever disobeys me, disobeys Allah, and whoever obeys the ruler, obeys me, and whoever disobeys him, disobeys me." (Bukhari)

413. Betrayal of Trust and Cheating Others

Allah, the Exalted, says:

"And argue not on behalf of those who deceive themselves. Verily, Allah does not like anyone who is a betrayer of his trust and indulges in crime." (Qur'an, An-Nisa 4:107)

"Verily! Allah commands that you should render back the trusts to those, to whom they are due; and that when you judge between men, you judge with justice. Verily, how excellent is the teaching which He (Allah) gives you! Truly, Allah is Ever All-Hearer, All-Seer." (Qur'an, An-Nisa 4:58)

Narrated Yahya related to me from Malik from Yahya ibn Said that he had heard that Abdullah ibn Abbas said, "Stealing from the spoils does not appear in a people but that terror is cast into their hearts. Fornication does not spread in a people but that there is much death among them. A people do not lessen the measure and weight but that provision is cut off from them. A people do not judge without right but that blood spreads among them. A people do not betray the pledge but that Allah gives their enemies power over them." (Malik Muwatta)

414. Acceptance of Gifts on the Part of State Officer is Forbidden

Narrated Abu Humaid as-Sa'idi (May Allah have mercy on him): The Messenger of Allah (peace and blessings be upon him) appointed a man from the Asad tribe who was called Ibn Lutbiyya in charge of Sadaqah (i.e. authorized hign to receive Sadaqah from the people on behalf of the State. When he returned (with the collections), he said: "This is for you and (this is mine as), it was presented to me as a gift." The narrator said: "The Messenger of Allah (peace and blessings be upon him) stood on the pulpit and praised God and extolled Him. Then he said: "What about a State official whom I give an assignment and who (comes and) says: 'This is for you and this has been presented to me as a gift?' Why didn't he remain in the house of his father or the house of his mother so that he could observe whether gifts were presented to him or not. By the Being in Whose Hand is the life of Muhammad, any one of you will not take anything from it but will bring it on the Day of Judgment, carrying on his neck a camel that will be growling or a cow that will be bellowing, or an ewe that will be bleating." Then he raised his hands so that we could see the whiteness of his armpits. Then he said twice: "O God, I have conveyed (Thy Commandments)." (Muslim)

415. Legislation Not Following Allah's Laws

Allah, the Exalted, says:

"And whosoever does not judge by what Allah has revealed (then) such (people) are the Fasiqoon (the rebellious i.e. disobedient (of a lesser degree) to Allah." (Qur'an, Al-Ma'idah 4:47)

"O you who believe! Stand out firmly for justice, as witnesses to Allah, even though it be against yourselves or your parents, or your kin, be he rich or poor, Allah is a Better Protector to both (than you). So, follow not the lusts (of your hearts), lest you may avoid justice, and if you distort your witness or refuse to give it, verily, Allah is Ever Well Acquainted with what you do." (Qur'an, An-Nisa 4:135)

"They have no Wali (Helper, Disposer of affairs, Protector, etc.) other than Him, and He makes none to share in His Decision and His Rule." (Qur'an, Al-Kahf 18:26)

Other Verses: *An-Nisa 4:60, Yusuf 12:40.*

Man-made legislation contradicts the Laws of Allah, permitting what is forbidden. Giving the legislators the right to do that, so they have the right to permit whatever they want and to forbid whatever they want; whatever the majority agrees upon by voting (without reference to the Qur'an and Sunnah). This is the ultimate kufr (disbelief).

416. Usurping the Rights of Others or Non-Fulfillment of Rights

Usurping Rights of Others:

1) The Right to Life

Allah, the Exalted, says:

"Whosoever kills a human being without (any reason like) man slaughter, or corruption on earth, it is as though he had killed all mankind." (Qur'an, Al-Ma'idah 5:32)

The right to life is conferred by the Qur'an even on one's enemy during war as Muslims are forbidden from using force except in self-defense.

Abu Bakr (May Allah be pleased with him) said: "Delivering the sermon during the Farewell Pilgrimage on the day of Sacrifice at Mina, the Messenger of Allah (peace and blessings be upon him) said, 'Verily your blood, your property and your honor are as sacred and inviolable as the sanctity of this day of yours, in this month of yours and in this town of yours. Verily! I have conveyed this message to you.'" (Bukhari and Muslim)

2) The Right to Live in Dignity

Life is a Divine bestowal on humanity that should be secured and defended by all means. It is the individual and universal duty of Muslims, according to the Qur'an, to protect the human merits and virtues of others. The Qur'an forbids the taking of life without due process of the Law, and it also obligates Muslims to provide for those who cannot provide for themselves. Also protected by the Qur'an are the elderly, parents, women, children, orphans, animals, trees, etc.

3) The Right to Justice

Allah, the Exalted, says:

"Verily! Allah commands that you should render back the trusts to those, to whom they are due; and that when you judge between men, you judge with justice. Verily, how excellent is the teaching which He (Allah) gives you! Truly, Allah is Ever All-Hearer, All-Seer." (Qur'an, An-Nisa 4:58)

4) The Right to Equal Protection of the Law

Allah, the Exalted, says:

"O you who believe! Stand out firmly for justice, as witnesses to Allah, even though it be against yourselves or your parents, or your kin, be he rich or poor, Allah is a Better Protector to both (than you). So, follow not the lusts (of your hearts), lest you may avoid justice, and if you distort your witness or refuse to give it, verily, Allah is Ever Well-Acquainted with what you do." (Qur'an, An-Nisa 4:135)

"Verily, Allah enjoins Al-Adl (i.e. justice and worshipping none but Allah Alone - Islamic Monotheism) and Al-Ihsan [i.e. to be patient in performing your duties to Allah, totally for Allah's sake and in accordance with the Sunnah (legal ways) of the Prophet SAW in a perfect manner], and giving (help) to kith and kin (i.e. all that Allah has ordered you to give them e.g. wealth, visiting, looking after them or any other kind of help, etc.); and forbids Al-Fahisha (i.e. all evil deeds, e.g. illegal sexual acts, disobedience of parents, polytheism, to tell lies, to give false witness, to kill a life without right, etc.), and Al-Munkar (i.e. all that is prohibited by Islamic Law: polytheism of every kind, disbelief and every kind of evil deeds, etc.), and Al-Baghy (i.e. all kinds of oppression), He admonishes you, that you may take heed." (Qur'an, An-Nahl 16:90)

5) The Right of Choice

Allah, the Exalted, says:

"And say: "The truth is from your Lord." Then whosoever wills, let him believe, and whosoever wills, let him disbelieve. Verily, We have prepared for the Zalimun (polytheists and wrongdoers, etc.), a Fire whose walls will be surrounding them (disbelievers in the Oneness of Allah). And if they ask for help (relief, water, etc.), they will be granted water like boiling oil, that will scald their faces. Terrible the drink, and an evil Murtafaqa (dwelling, resting place, etc.)!" (Qur'an, Al-Kahf 18:29)

"There is no compulsion in religion. Verily, the Right Path has become distinct from the wrong path. Whoever disbelieves in Taghut and believes in Allah, then he has grasped the most trustworthy handhold that will never break. And Allah is All-Hearer, All-Knower." (Qur'an, Al-Baqarah 2:256)

6) The Right of Free Expression within the Glorious Qur'an and Sunnah

Allah, the Exalted, says:

"Not a word does he (or she) utter but there is a watcher by him ready (to record it)." (Qur'an, Qaf 50:18)

Narrated Abu Hurairah (May Allah be pleased with him): The Messenger of Allah (peace and blessings be upon him) said: "Whoever believes in Allah and the Last Day, let him speak good or else keep silent." (Bukhari and Muslim)

7) The Right to Privacy

Allah, the Exalted, says:

"O you who believe! Avoid much suspicions, indeed some suspicions are sins. And spy not, neither backbite one another. Would one of you like to eat the flesh of his dead brother? You would hate it (so hate backbiting). And fear Allah. Verily, Allah is the One Who accepts repentance, Most Merciful." (Qur'an, Al-Hujurat 49:12)

"Do not enter any houses except your own homes unless you are sure of their occupants' consent." (Qur'an, An-Nur 24:27)

Narrated Abu Hurairah (May Allah be pleased with him): The Messenger of Allah (May Allah's peace and blessings be upon him) said: "If a man - or someone - peeped at you without your permission and you threw a pebble at him that gouged out his eye, you would not be at fault." (Bukhari and Muslim)
(https://hadeethenc.com/en/browse/hadith/2989)

8) The Right to Own and Protect Property

Allah, the Exalted, says:

"O you who believe! Eat not up your property among yourselves unjustly except it be a trade amongst you, by mutual consent. And do not kill yourselves (nor kill one another). Surely, Allah is Most Merciful to you." (Qur'an, An-Nisa 4:29)

"Surely, those who unjustly devour the property of the orphans do nothing but devour Fire into their bellies, and soon they shall enter a blazing Hell." (Qur'an, An-Nisa 4:10)

9) The Right to Basic Necessities of Life

Allah, the Exalted, says:

"And in their properties, there was the right of the beggar and the Mahrum (the poor who does not ask the others)." (Qur'an, Adh-Dhariyat 51:19)

"Verily, you have (a promise from Us that you will never be hungry therein nor naked. And you (will) suffer not from thirst therein nor from the sun's heat." (Qur'an, Taha 20:118-119)

"The father of the child shall bear the cost of the mother's food and clothing on a reasonable basis." (Qur'an, Al-Baqarah 2:233)

Four basic needs arise from the Qur'an: water, food, clothes and shelter from heat and cold (a home). (394)

In the Holy Qur'an, the 'basic necessaries' have been declared as the right of the poor and needy as a share in the wealth of the rich. The rich do not give any share of their own wealth in the form of Zakat but give back only what belongs to the poor. Thus, it is incumbent on the wealthy Muslims to help out the poor and the needy irrespective of the fact whether they ask for assistance or not, it is their duty to reach them and give all the help that they can extend.

417. Not Enjoining Good and Forbidding Evil

Allah, the Exalted, says:

"Let there arise out of you a group of people inviting to all that is good (Islam), enjoining Al-Ma'ruf (i.e. Islamic Monotheism and all that Islam orders one to do) and forbidding Al-Munkar (polytheism and disbelief, and all that Islam has forbidden). And it is they who are the successful." (Qur'an, Ali 'Imran 3:104)

"(The believers whose lives Allah has purchased are) those who repent to Allah (from polytheism and hypocrisy, etc.), who worship Him, who praise Him, who fast (or go out in Allah's Cause), who bow down (in prayer), who prostrate themselves (in prayer), who enjoin (people) for Al-Ma'ruf (i.e. Islamic Monotheism and all what Islam has ordained) and forbid (people) from Al-Munkar (i.e. disbelief, polytheism of all kinds and all that Islam has forbidden), and who observe the limits set by Allah (do all that Allah has ordained and abstain from all kinds of sins and evil deeds which Allah has forbidden). And give glad tidings to the believers." (Qur'an, At-Tawbah 9:112)

"O my son! Aqim As-Salat (perform As-Salat), enjoin (people) for Al-Ma'ruf (Islamic Monotheism and all that is good) and forbid (people) from Al-Munkar (i.e. disbelief in the Oneness of Allah, polytheism of all kinds and all that is evil and bad), and bear with patience whatever befall you. Verily! These are some of the important commandments ordered by Allah with no exemption." (Qur'an, Luqman 31:17)

Other Verses: Ali 'Imran 3:110, At-Tawbah 9:71, Al-Ma'idah 5:105.

Abu Sa`id al-Khudri (May Allah be pleased with him) said: "I heard the Messenger of Allah (peace and blessings be upon him) say, "Whosoever of you sees an evil, let him change it with his hand; and if he is not able to do so, then (let him change it) with his tongue; and if he is not able to do so, then with his heart - and that is the weakest of faith." (Muslim)

Abu Sufyan Sakhr ibn Harb (May Allah be pleased with him) reported: Heraclius said: "What does the Prophet (peace and blessings be upon him) enjoin you to do?" I said: "He tells us to worship Allah Alone, not to associate anything with Him and to give up all that our ancestors said. He also commands us to perform prayers, adhere to truthfulness, be chaste and maintain ties of kinship." (Bukhari and Muslim)

(https://hadeethenc.com/en/browse/hadith/3154)

An-Nu'man ibn Bashir (May Allah be pleased with him) reported that the Prophet (May Allah's peace and blessings be upon him) say: "The example of the one who abides by the limits prescribed by Allah and the one who transgresses them is like the example of a people who boarded a ship after casting lots. Some of them were in its lower deck and others were in its upper deck. When those in the lower deck needed water, they had to go up and pass by those above them. So, they said: 'If we could make a hole in our share of the ship, so that we would not bother those above us.' If those in the upper deck leave them do as they wish, they will all perish, but if they stop them, they will all survive." (Bukhari)

(https://hadeethenc.com/en/browse/hadith/3341)

Narrated 'Ubaidullah bin Jarir that his father said: The Messenger of Allah (peace and blessings be upon him) said: "There is no people among whom sins are committed when they are stronger and of a higher status (i.e. they have the power and ability to stop the sinners) and they do not change them, but Allah will send His punishment upon them all." (Ibn Majah)

Abu Bakr (May Allah be pleased with him) said: "O people, you recite this Verse: *"O you who believe, upon you is responsibility for yourselves. Those who have gone astray will not harm you when you have been guided." (Qur'an, Al-Ma'idah 5:105)*, but I have heard Messenger of Allah (May Allah's peace and blessings be upon him) say: 'When people see an oppressor but do not prevent him committing sin, it is likely that Allah will punish them all.'" (Ibn Majah, Tirmidhi, An-Nasa'i, Abu Dawud and Ahmad) (https://hadeethenc.com/en/browse/hadith/3470)

Abu Hurairah (May Allah be pleased with him) reported that the Prophet (May Allah's peace and blessings be upon him) said: "'Do you know who is the bankrupt?" They said: "The bankrupt among us is the one who has neither money nor property." He said: "The bankrupt in my Ummah is the one who will come on the Day of Judgment with prayer, fasting and Zakat, but since he hurled abuse at others, accused others of committing adultery without evidence, unlawfully consumed the wealth of others, and shed the blood of others and beat others, his good deeds will be credited to the accounts of others (who suffered at his hands), and if his good deeds fall short to clear his account, others' sins will be cast on him and he will then be thrown in the Fire." (Muslim) (https://hadeethenc.com/en/browse/hadith/6454)

Narrated Umm Habiba, the wife of the Prophet, that the Prophet (peace and blessings be upon him) said: "The words of the son of Adam count against him, not for him, except what is good and forbidding what is evil, and remembering Allah." (Ibn Majah)

Before forbidding evil there are the conditions to follow:

- he should know the Islamic ruling concerning that which he is enjoining or forbidding,

- he is accountable or not,

- forbid what is bad, without bringing harm upon himself,

- forbidding what is evil should not result in any evil greater. (395)

Allah, the Exalted, says:

"And speak to him mildly, perhaps he may accept admonition or fear (Allah)." (Qur'an, Taha 20:44)

"Invite (mankind, O Muhammad) to the way of your Lord (i.e. Islam) with wisdom (i.e. with the Divine Revelation and the Qur'an) and fair preaching, and argue with them in a way that is better. Truly, your Lord knows best who has gone astray from His Path, and He is the Best Aware of those who are guided." (Qur'an, An-Nahl 16:125)

418. Chastisement for One who Enjoins Good and Forbids Evil but Acts Otherwise

Allah, the Exalted, says:

"Enjoin you Al-Birr (piety and righteousness and every act of obedience to Allah) on the people and you forget (to practice it) yourselves, while you recite the Scripture [the Taurat (Torah)]! Have you then no sense?" (Qur'an, Al-Baqarah 2:44)

"(Shu'aib said:) I wish not, in contradiction to you, to do that which I forbid you." (Qur'an, Hud 11:88)

Usamah ibn Zayd ibn Harithah (May Allah be pleased with him) reported that the Messenger of Allah (May Allah's peace and blessings be upon him) said: "A man will be brought on the Day of Resurrection and thrown into the Fire, and his intestines will slip out and he will go around by them like a donkey goes around a millstone. The dwellers of Hell will gather around him and say: 'So-and-so, what is the matter with you? Did you not use to command us to do right and forbid us from doing wrong?' He will reply: 'Yes, I commanded you to do right but I did not do it myself, and I forbade you from doing wrong but I did it myself.'" (Bukhari and Muslim) (https://hadeethenc.com/en/browse/hadith/3345)

419. Extortion

Narrated 'Uthman ibn Abi'l-'Aas al-Thaqafi: The Prophet (peace and blessings of Allah be upon him) said: "The gates of Heaven are opened halfway through the night and a Caller cries out: 'Is anyone supplicating so that he may be answered? Is anyone asking so that he might be given? Is anyone in distress, so that he might be granted relief?' And there will be no Muslim left who is supplicating but Allah will answer him, except for a zaaniyah who earns a living from committing Zina or an Extortionist." (Tabarani in al-Mu'jam al-Kabeer (9/59) and in al-Mu'jam al-Awsat (3/154). Al-Haythami said in Majma' al-Zawaa'id (10/156): Its men are the men of Saheeh. Al-Albaani said in al-Silsilah al-Saheehah 91073): Its isnaad is Saheeh.

Extortion occurs when someone attempts to obtain money or property by threatening to commit violence or even to kill, accusing the victim of a crime or of some other disgraceful conduct, expose a secret, by intimidation, pressure or revealing private or damaging information about the victim.

The type of property someone tries to obtain when using extortion encompasses almost anything that has value. However, the property doesn't need to be actual physical property and can be property that does not have a dollar value. It is also not necessary for the accused to actually deprive the victim of property, as attempting to extort property is also a crime.

Punishment for Extortion in this world: fines, restitution, incarceration, probation. Severe torment in the Hereafter.

420. Prohibition of Following the Manners of Satan and Disbelievers

Allah, the Exalted, says:

"His power is only over those who obey and follow him (Satan) and those who join partners with Him (Allah, i.e. those who are Mushrikoon, i.e. polytheists)." (Qur'an, An-Nahl 16:98)

"(Their allies deceived them) like Shaitan (Satan), when he says to man: "Disbelieve in Allah." But when (man) disbelieves in Allah, Shaitan (Satan) says: "I am free of you, I fear Allah, the Lord of the 'Alamin (mankind, Jinns and all that exists)!" (Qur'an, Al-Hashr 59:16)

Ibn 'Umar (May Allah be pleased with him) reported that the Messenger of Allah (May Allah's peace and blessings be upon him) said: "If anyone of you eats, let him eat with his right hand, and if he drinks, let him drink with his right hand, for indeed the Devil eats with his left hand and drinks with his left hand."
(Muslim) (https://hadeethenc.com/en/browse/hadith/58122)

Narrated Abu Hurairah (May Allah be pleased with him) said: "I heard the Messenger of Allah (peace and blessings be upon him) as saying: 'Jews and Christians do not dye (their grey hair), so do the opposite of what they do." (Bukhari and Muslim)

Commentary: We learn from this Hadith that the Prophet (peace and blessings be upon him) has advised the Muslims to dye the hair of their head and beard with yellow or red colour. (396)

421. Condemnation of Pride and Self-Conceit

Allah, the Exalted, says:

"...and he was proud, and he was one of the unbelievers." (Qur'an, Al-Baqarah 2:34)

"Your Ilah (God) is One Ilah (God Allah, none has the right to be worshipped but He). But for those who believe not in the Hereafter, their hearts deny (the faith in the Oneness of Allah), and they are proud." (Qur'an, An-Nahl 16:22)

"That home of the Hereafter (i.e. Jannah), We shall assign to those who rebel not against the truth with pride and tyranny in the land nor do mischief by committing crimes. And the good end is for the Muttaqun (the pious and righteous persons)." (Qur'an, Al-Qasas 28:83)

Other Verses: *Al-Isra 17:37, Luqman 31:18, Al-Qasas 28:76-78.*

Narrated Haritha bin Wahab (May Allah be pleased with him): Messenger of Allah (peace and blessings be upon him) said, "May I not inform you about the denizens of Hellfire?" They said: "Yes." And he said: "Every haughty, fat and proud (person)." (Muslim)

Commentary: Flouting at Divine rules, niggardliness (to keep from spending in the way of Allah) and haughtiness are condemnable habits, and those who indulge in them will be pushed into Hell. (397)

Narrated Abu Hurairah (May Allah be pleased with him): The Messenger of Allah (peace and blessings be upon him) said, "On the Day of Resurrection, Allah will not look at him who trails his lower garment out of pride." (Bukhari and Muslim)

Narrated Abu Hurairah (May Allah have mercy on him): The Messenger of Allah (peace and blessings be upon him) said, "There are three (types of) people to whom Allah will not speak on the Day of Resurrection, nor will He purify them, nor look at them, and they will have a painful punishment. These are: an aged man who commits Zina (illicit sexual act), a ruler who lies and a proud poor person." (Muslim)

Narrated Jabir ibn Atik (May Allah be pleased with him): The Prophet (peace and blessings be upon him) said: "There is jealousy which Allah loves and jealousy which Allah hates. That which Allah loves is jealousy regarding a matter of doubt, and that which Allah hates is jealousy regarding something which is not doubtful. There is pride which Allah hates and pride which Allah loves. That which Allah loves is a man's pride when fighting and when giving Sadaqah and that which Allah hates is the pride shown by oppression. The narrator Musa said: "by boasting." (Abu Dawud)

Narrated Abu Hurairah (May Allah be pleased with him): Allah's Apostle (peace and blessings be upon him) said, "The main source of disbelief is in the east. Pride and arrogance are characteristics of the owners of horses and camels, and those Bedouins who are busy with their camels and pay no attention to Religion; while modesty and gentleness are the characteristics of the owners of sheep." (Bukhari)

422. Prohibition of Arrogance, Vanity and Haughtiness

Allah, the Exalted, says:

"Thus, does Allah set a seal over the heart of every proud, haughty one." (Qur'an, Ghafir 40:35)

"He refused and was arrogant and became a disbeliever." (Qur'an, Al-Baqarah 2:34)

"(Allah) said: "What prevented you (O Iblees) that you did not prostrate, when I commanded you?" Iblees said: "I am better than him (Adam), You created me from fire, and him You created from clay." Qur'an, Al-A'raf 7:12)

Other Verses: Al-A'raf 7:27 and 7:146, Az-Zumar 39:72, Luqman 31:18, Al-Baqarah 2:206.

Narrated Abu Hurairah (May Allah be pleased with him): The Messenger of Allah (peace and blessings be upon him) said, "While a man was walking, dressed in clothes admiring himself, his hair combed, walking haughtily when Allah caused the earth to swallow him. Now he will continue to go down in it (as a punishment) until the Day of Resurrection." (Muslim)

Narrated Salamah bin Al-Akwa' (May Allah be pleased with him): The Messenger of Allah (peace and blessings be upon him) said, "Man continues to display haughtiness and arrogance until he is recorded among the arrogant and will be therefore afflicted with what afflicts them." (Tirmidhi)

Commentary: The Hadith says that a man who has even an iota of pride in his heart will be barred from entering Jannah. (397)

Narrated Abdullah bin Masud: The Messenger of Allah (peace and blessings be upon him) observed:

"None shall enter the Fire (of Hell) who has in his heart the weight of a mustard seed of Iman and none shall enter Paradise who has in his heart the weight of a mustard seed of pride." (Muslim)

Narrated Thawban (the freed slave of the Messenger of Allah (peace and blessings be upon him): The Messenger of Allah (peace and blessings be upon him) said: "Anyone whose soul leaves his body and he is free of three things, will enter Paradise: arrogance, stealing from the spoils of war and debt." (Ibn Majah)

Narrated Abdullah bin Umar: "The Messenger of Allah (peace and blessings be upon him) said: 'Whoever wears a garment of pride and vanity in this world, Allah will clothe him in a garment of humiliation on the Day of Resurrection, then set it ablaze.'" (Ibn Majah)

Narrated 'Iyad bin Himar (May Allah be pleased with him): The Messenger of Allah (peace and blessings be upon him) said, "Verily, Allah has revealed to me that you should adopt humility. So, that no one may wrong another and no one may be disdainful and haughty towards another." (Muslim)

Narrated Abu Hurairah (May Allah be pleased with him): The Messenger of Allah (peace and blessings be upon him) said, "When a person says: 'People have been ruined, he is the one to be ruined the most.'" (Muslim)

Commentary: This Hadith prohibits a Muslim from saying the statement in the Hadith or something similar to it out of arrogance and pride. (398)

Salamah bin Al-Akwa' (May Allah be pleased with him) reported: "A man ate with his left hand in the presence of the Messenger of Allah (May Allah's peace and blessings be upon him), whereupon he said: "Eat with your right hand." The man said: "I cannot do that." Thereupon, he said: "May you not be able to do that." It was only arrogance that prevented the man from doing it, and consequently he could not raise it (his right hand) up to his mouth afterwards." (Muslim) (https://hadeethenc.com/en/browse/hadith/3372)

Abu Sa'id al-Khudri (May Allah be pleased with him) reported that the Prophet (May Allah's peace and blessings be upon him) said: "Paradise and Hell debated. Hell said: 'The tyrants and the arrogant are in me.' Paradise said: 'The weak and the poor are in me.' So, Allah judged between them and said to Paradise: 'You are My Mercy. I show Mercy through you to whom I will.' And He said to Hell: 'You are My Punishment, I punish through you whom I will. And I guarantee to fill both of you completely.'" (Muslim) (https://hadeethenc.com/en/browse/hadith/3261)

Narrated Jabir (May Allah be pleased with him): The Messenger of Allah (peace and blessings be upon him) said, "The dearest and nearest among you to me on the Day of Resurrection will be one who is the best of you in manners; and the most abhorrent among you to me and the farthest of you from me will be the pompous, the garrulous and Al-Mutafaihiqun." The Companions asked him: "O Messenger of Allah! We know about the pompous and the garrulous, but we do not know who Al-Mutafaihiqun are." He replied: "The arrogant people." (Tirmidhi)

When God created Adam and ordered the angels to bow down, Iblees, being a Jinn created from fire, refused, and disobeyed God, considering himself better than man, leading to his downfall. Iblees was expelled from Paradise because of his pride and arrogance, and it was a matter of few minutes but with tremendous consequences, all his good deeds, worshipping Allah for thousands of years, were cancelled.

Man should be aware of his weakness and helpless, and whatever strength he has developed is given by Allah, the Exalted. Besides his strength and power are limited, Allah has made him susceptible to hunger, thirst and sleep. He is needful of clothing, dwelling and other requirements without which he would perish. He is prone to diseases, calamities and disasters, over which he has no control.

Misguided by Satan, man is prone to dispute, arrogance and pride. And he is attracted towards the things in which there is destruction for him and dislikes the things which are beneficial to him. Apart from this, he is in constant dread of losing something which is dear and precious to him, like wealth or children, or his physical powers.

The proud person loses all awareness of the reality that he is an insignificant creature, whose very existence and all that he possesses is only because of Allah's Favor on him. He regards himself as someone very special, in full control of his life, which no other power can influence.

Islam considers it the worst sin since through arrogance all other sins are committed.

423. Prohibition of Oppression

The Oppressor

Allah, the Exalted, says:

"The way (of blame) is only against those who oppress men and wrongly rebel in the earth without justification; for such there will be a painful torment." (Qur'an, Ash-Shuraa 42:42)

"Verily, Allah enjoins Al-Adl (i.e. justice and worshipping none but Allah Alone - Islamic Monotheism) and Al-Ihsan [i.e. to be patient in performing your duties to Allah, totally for Allah's sake and in accordance with the Sunnah (legal ways) of the Prophet SAW in a perfect manner], and giving (help) to kith and kin (i.e. all that Allah has ordered you to give them e.g. wealth, visiting, looking after them or any other kind of help, etc.); and forbids Al-Fahisha (i.e. all evil deeds, e.g. illegal sexual acts, disobedience of parents, polytheism, to tell lies, to give false witness, to kill a life without right, etc.), and Al-Munkar (i.e. all that is prohibited by Islamic Law: polytheism of every kind, disbelief and every kind of evil deeds, etc.), and Al-Baghy (i.e. all kinds of oppression), He admonishes you, that you may take heed." (Qur'an, An-Nahl 16:90)

Anas ibn Malik (May Allah be pleased with him) reported that the Prophet (May Allah's peace and blessings be upon him) said: "Support your brother whether he is an oppressor or oppressed." A man said: "O Messenger of Allah, I should support him if he is oppressed, but how should I support him if he is an oppressor?" The Prophet (May Allah's peace and blessings be upon him) said: "Support him by preventing him from practicing oppression." (Bukhari) (https://hadeethenc.com/en/browse/hadith/4236)

Narrated Abu Dharr al-Ghifari (May Allah be pleased with him): The Prophet (peace and blessings of Allah be upon him) related from his Lord, the Exalted, Who said: "O My servants, I have forbidden oppression for Myself and have made it forbidden amongst you, so do not oppress one another..." (Muslim)

Narrated Abu Hurairah (May Allah be pleased with him): Allah's Apostle (peace and blessings be upon him) said, "Whoever has oppressed another person concerning his reputation or anything else, he should beg him to forgive him before the Day of Resurrection when there will be no money (to compensate for wrong deeds), but if he has good deeds, those good deeds will be taken from him according to his oppression which he has done, and if he has no good deeds, the sins of the oppressed person will be loaded on him." (Bukhari)

Narrated Ibn Umar (May Allah be pleased with him): The Prophet (peace and blessings be upon him) said, "Az-Zulm (Oppression) will be a darkness on the Day of Resurrection." (Bukhari)

Jabir ibn 'Abdullah (May Allah be pleased with him) reported: The Messenger of Allah (May Allah's peace and blessings be upon him) said: "Beware of oppression, for oppression will be layers of darkness on the Day of Resurrection; and beware of stinginess, as it ruined those who were before you. It incited them to shed their blood and regard the unlawful as lawful." (Muslim)
(https://hadeethenc.com/en/browse/hadith/5787)

Az-Zubayr ibn 'Adiyy reported: "We went to Anas ibn Malik (May Allah be pleased with them) and complained to him about the oppression we were suffering at the hands of Al-Hajjaj. So, Anas said: "Be patient, for no time will come but will be followed by a worse one until you meet your Lord. I heard it from your Prophet (May Allah's peace and blessings be upon him)." (Bukhari)
(https://hadeethenc.com/en/browse/hadith/4953)

Abu Kabshah 'Amr ibn Sa'd (May Allah be pleased with him) reported that the Messenger of Allah (May Allah's peace and blessings be upon him) said: "I swear by Allah for three things which I am going to tell you about. Remember them well: The wealth of a man will not diminish by charity, Allah augments the honor of a man who endures an oppression patiently; and he who opens a gate of begging, Allah opens a gate of poverty (or he said a word similar to it)." He also said: "Remember well what I am going to tell you: The world is for four kinds of people. 1) One upon whom Allah has bestowed wealth and knowledge and so he fears his Lord in respect to them, maintains the ties of kinship and acknowledges the rights of Allah on him; this type will have the best position. 2) One upon whom Allah has conferred knowledge but no wealth, and he is sincere in his intention and says: 'Had I possessed wealth, I would have acted like so-and-so.' He will be treated according to his intention, and his reward is the same as that of the other. 3) One whom Allah has given wealth but no knowledge and he squanders his wealth ignorantly, does not fear Allah in respect to it, does not discharge the obligations of kinship and does not acknowledge the rights of Allah. Such a person will be in the worst position. 4) One upon whom Allah has bestowed neither wealth nor knowledge and he says: 'Had I possessed wealth, I would have acted like so-and-so (i.e. he would squander his wealth).' He will be treated according to his intention, and both will have equal sin." (Tirmidhi) (https://hadeethenc.com/en/browse/hadith/5833)

Ibn Masud (May Allah be pleased with him) reported that the Prophet (May Allah's peace and blessings be upon him) said: "There will see after me selfishness and other matters that you will disapprove of." They asked: "What do you order us to do then, O Messenger of Allah?" He said: "Fulfill your duty (to the rulers) and ask Allah for your rights." (Bukhari) (https://hadeethenc.com/en/browse/hadith/3156)

Umm Salamah (Hind bint Abi Umayyah Hudhayfah) (May Allah be pleased with her) reported that the Prophet (May Allah's peace and blessings be upon him) said: "There shall be rulers in charge of you, and you will approve and disapprove. So, anyone who hates shall be absolved, and anyone who denies shall be safe, except for those who approve and comply." They said: ''O Messenger of Allah, shall we not fight them?" He replied: "No, so long as they establish prayer among you." (Muslim)
(https://hadeethenc.com/en/browse/hadith/3481)

Not Preventing Oppression

Allah, the Exalted, says:

"And do not incline to those who are unjust, lest the fire touch you, and you have no guardians besides Allah, then you shall not be helped." (Qur'an, Hud 11:113)

"...and do not help one another in sin and oppression; and be careful of (your duty to) Allah; surely Allah is severe in requiting evil." (Qur'an, Al-Ma'idah 5:2)

Hudhaifah bin Al-Yaman narrated that the Prophet (peace and blessings be upon him) said: "By the One in Whose Hand is my soul! Either you command good and forbid evil, or Allah will soon send upon you a punishment from Him, then you will call upon Him, but He will not respond to you." (Tirmidhi)

Not Helping the Oppressed

Allah, the Exalted, says:

"if they seek your help in religion, it is your duty to help them…" (Qur'an, Al-Anfal 8:72)

Narrated Ibn Abbas (May Allah be pleased with him): The Prophet (peace and blessings be upon him) sent Muadh to Yemen and said, "Be afraid, from the curse of the oppressed as there is no screen between his invocation and Allah." (Bukhari)

Narrated Abu Hurairah (May Allah be pleased with him): The Messenger of Allah (peace and blessings be upon him) said: "The supplications of three persons are never turned away: a fasting person until he breaks his fast, a just ruler and the supplication of the oppressed which is raised by Allah above the clouds, the gates of heaven are opened for it, and the Lord says: 'By My Might, I will help you in due time.'" (Tirmidhi)

Abu Hurairah (May Allah be pleased with him) reported: The Prophet (May Allah's peace and blessings be upon him) said: "There are three supplications that will undoubtedly be answered: the supplication of the oppressed, the supplication of the traveler and the supplication of a parent against his child." (Ibn Majah) (https://hadeethenc.com/en/browse/hadith/5909)

When the Oppressed One Becomes an Oppressor

Aisha (May Allah be pleased with her) reported: A man came and sat in front of the Messenger of Allah (May Allah's peace and blessings be upon him) and said: "O Messenger of Allah, I have two slaves who lie to me, deceive me and disobey me, and I scold them and hit them. So, what is my case concerning them?" He said: "The extent to which they betrayed you, disobeyed you and lied to you will be measured against how much you punish them. If your punishing them is equal to their sins, the two will be the same, nothing for you and nothing against you. If your punishing them is above their sins, some of your rewards will be taken from you and given to them." The man left, and began weeping and crying aloud. The Messenger of Allah (May Allah's peace and blessings be upon him) said: "You should read what Allah says in His Book: *"We will place the scales of justice on the Day of Resurrection, and no soul will be wronged in the least. Even if a deed is the weight of a mustard seed, We will bring it forth. Sufficient are We as Reckoners." (Surah Al-Anbya 21:47)* Thereupon, the man said: "By Allah, O Messenger of Allah, I see nothing better for myself and them than parting with them. Bear witness that they are all free." (Tirmidhi) (https://hadeethenc.com/en/browse/hadith/65065)

Abu Hurairah (May Allah be pleased with him) reported that the Messenger of Allah (May Allah's peace and blessings be upon him) said: "When two people insult each other, the one who started will be the sinner until the oppressed exceeds the limits (in retorting)." (Muslim) (https://hadeethenc.com/en/browse/hadith/8878)

Praising an Oppressor

Abu Musa al-Ash'ari (May Allah be pleased with him) reported: The Prophet (May Allah's peace and blessings be upon him) heard a man praising another and exaggerating in his praise, whereupon he said: 'You have ruined - or cut - the man's back." (Bukhari and Muslim)

(https://hadeethenc.com/en/browse/hadith/5734)

424. Unlawfulness of Oppression and Restoring Others Rights

Allah, the Exalted, says:

"There will be no friend, nor an intercessor for the Zalimun (polytheists and the wrongdoers) who could be given heed to." (Qur'an, Ghafir 40:18)

"And for the Zalimun (wrongdoers, polytheists and disbelievers in the Oneness of Allah) there is no helper." (Qur'an, Al-Hajj 22:71)

Jabir bin 'Abdullah (May Allah be pleased with him) reported: The Messenger of Allah (peace and blessings be upon him) said, "Beware of injustice, for oppression will be darkness on the Day of Resurrection; and beware of stinginess because it doomed those who were before you. It incited them to shed blood and treat the unlawful as lawful." (Muslim)

Abu Hurairah (May Allah be pleased with him) reported: The Messenger of Allah (peace and blessings be upon him) said, "On the Resurrection Day, the rights will be paid to those to whom they are due so much so that a hornless sheep will be retaliated for by punishing the horned sheep which broke its horns." (Muslim)

Aisha (May Allah be pleased with her) reported: The Messenger of Allah (peace and blessings be upon him) said, "Whoever usurps unlawfully even a hand span of land a collar measuring seven times (this) land will be placed around his neck on the Day of Resurrection." (Bukhari and Muslim)

Commentary: This Hadith tells us that even a minor injustice to anybody in this world can cause great trouble on the Day of Resurrection. (399)

Abu Musa (May Allah be pleased with him) reported: The Messenger of Allah (peace and blessings be upon him) said, "Verily, Allah gives respite to the oppressor. But when He seizes him, He does not let him escape." Then he (peace and blessings be upon him) recited, *"Such is the Seizure of your Rubb when He seizes the (population of) towns while they are doing wrong. Verily, His Seizure is painful (and) severe."* (11:102) (Bukhari and Muslim)

Mu'adh (May Allah be pleased with him) reported: The Messenger of Allah (peace and blessings be upon him) sent me (as a governor of Yemen) and instructed me thus: "You will go to the people of the Book. First call them to testify that 'there is no true god except Allah, that I am (Muhammad) the Messenger of Allah.' If they obey you, tell them that Allah has enjoined upon them five Salat (prayers) during the day and night; and if they obey you, inform them that Allah has made Zakat obligatory upon them; that it should be collected from their rich and distributed among their poor; and if they obey you refrain from picking up (as a share of Zakat) the best of their wealth. Beware of the supplication of the oppressed, for there is no barrier between it and Allah." (Bukhari and Muslim)

Abu Humaid bin Sa'd As-Sa'idi (May Allah be pleased with him) reported: "The Prophet (peace and blessings be upon him) employed a man from the tribe of Al-Azd named Ibn Lutbiyyah as collector of Zakat. When the employee returned (with the collections) he said: "(O Prophet! This is for you and this is mine because it was presented to me as gift." Messenger of Allah (peace and blessings be upon him) rose to the pulpit and praised Allah and extolled Him. Then he said, "I employ a man to do a job and he comes and says: 'This is for you and this has been presented to me as gift'? Why did he not remain in the house of his father or the house of his mother and see whether gifts will be given to him or not? By Allah in Whose Hand is the life of Muhammad, if any one of you took anything wrongfully, he will bring it on the Day of Resurrection, carrying it on (his back), I will not recognize anyone of you on the Day of Resurrection with a grunting camel or a bellowing cow, or a bleating ewe." Then he raised his hands till we could see the whiteness of his armpits. Then he said thrice, ''O Allah! have I conveyed (Your Commandments).'' (Bukhari and Muslim)

Abu Hurairah (May Allah be pleased with him) reported: The Prophet (peace and blessings be upon him) said, "He who has done a wrong affecting his brother's honor or anything else, let him ask his forgiveness today before the time (i.e. the Day of Resurrection) when he will have neither a dinar nor a dirham. If he has done some good deeds, a portion equal to his wrong doings will be subtracted from them; but if he has no good deeds, he will be burdened with the evil deeds of the one he had wronged in the same proportion." (Bukhari)

'Abdullah bin 'Amr bin Al-'as (May Allah be pleased with him) reported: The Prophet (peace and blessings be upon him) said, "A Muslim is the one from whose tongue and hands the Muslims are safe; and a Muhajir (Emigrant) is the one who refrains from what Allah has forbidden." (Bukhari and Muslim)

'Abdullah bin 'Amr bin Al-'as (May Allah be pleased with him) reported: "A man named Kirkirah, who was in charge of the personal effects of Messenger of Allah (peace and blessings be upon him), passed away and the Prophet (peace and blessings be upon him) said, "He is in the (Hell) Fire." Some people went to his house looking for its cause and found there a cloak that he had stolen.'" (Bukhari)

Abu Bakrah (May Allah be pleased with him) reported: The Prophet (peace and blessings be upon him) said, "…Your blood, your property and your honor are inviolable to you all like the inviolability of this day of yours, in this city of yours and in this month of yours. You will soon meet your Rubb and He will ask you about your deeds. So do not turn to disbelief after me by striking the necks of one another…" (Bukhari and Muslim) (https://sunnah.com/bukhari:5550)

Abu Umamah (May Allah be pleased with him) reported: The Messenger of Allah (peace and blessings be upon him) said, "Allah decrees the (Hell) Fire and debars Jannah for the one who usurps the rights of a believer by taking a false oath." One man asked: "O Messenger of Allah! Even if it should be for an insignificant thing?" He said, "Even if it be a stick of the Arak tree (i.e. the tree from which Miswak sticks are taken)." (Muslim)

'Adi bin 'Umairah (May Allah be pleased with him) reported: The Messenger of Allah (peace and blessings be upon him) said, "Whosoever among you is appointed by us to a position and he conceals from us even a needle or less, it will amount to misappropriation and he will be called upon to restore it on the Day of Resurrection." 'Adi bin 'Umairah added: "A black man from the Ansar stood up - I can see him still - and said: "O Messenger of Allah, take back from me your assignment." He (the Prophet (peace and blessings be upon him) said, "What has happened to you?" The man replied: "I have heard you saying such and such." He (peace and blessings be upon him) said, "I say that even now: Whosoever from you is appointed by us to a position, he should render an account of everything, big or small, and whatever he is given therefrom, he should take and he should desist from taking what is unlawful." (Muslim)

'Umar bin Al-Khattab (May Allah be pleased with him) reported: "On the day (of the battle) of Khaibar, some Companions of the Prophet (peace and blessings be upon him) came and remarked: "So-and-so is a martyr and so-and-so is a martyr". When they came to a man about whom they said: "So-and-so is a martyr," the Prophet (peace and blessings be upon him) declared, "No. I have seen him in Hell for a mantle (or cloak) which he has stolen." (Muslim)

Abu Qatadah Al-Harith bin Rib'i (May Allah be pleased with him) reported: The Messenger of Allah (peace and blessings be upon him) said, "Faith in Allah and striving in His Cause (Jihad) are the deeds of highest merit." A man stood up and said: "O Messenger of Allah! Tell me if I am killed in the Cause of Allah, will all my sins be forgiven?" He (peace and blessings be upon him) replied, "Yes, if you are killed in the Cause of Allah while you are patient, hopeful of your reward and marching forward not retreating." Then the Prophet (peace and blessings be upon him) said to him, "Repeat what you have said." The man said: "Tell me if I am killed in the Cause of Allah, will all my sins be remitted?" He replied, "Yes, if you are martyred while you are patient, hopeful of your reward and march forward without retreating, unless, if you owe any debt, that will not be remitted. Angel Jibreel told me that." (Muslim)

Abu Hurairah (May Allah be pleased with him) reported: The Messenger of Allah (peace and blessings be upon him) said, "Do you know who is the bankrupt?" They said: "The bankrupt among us is one who has neither money with him nor any property." He said, "The real bankrupt of my Ummah would be he who would come on the Day of Resurrection with Salat, Saum and Sadaqah (charity), but he will find himself bankrupt on that Day as he will have exhausted the good deeds because he reviled others, brought calumny against others, unlawfully devoured the wealth of others, shed the blood of others and beat others; so his good deeds would be credited to the account of those who suffered at his hand. If his good deeds fall short to clear the account, their sins would be entered in his account and he would be thrown in the (Hell) Fire." (Muslim)

Ibn 'Umar (May Allah be pleased with him) reported: The Messenger of Allah (peace and blessings be upon him) said, "A believer continues to guard his faith (and thus hopes for Allah's Mercy) so long as he does not shed blood unjustly." (Bukhari)

Khaulah bint 'Thamir (May Allah be pleased with her) reported: The Messenger of Allah (peace and blessings be upon him) said, "Many people misappropriate (acquire wrongfully)

Allah's Property (meaning Muslims' property). These people will be cast in Hell on the Day of Resurrection." (Bukhari)

425. Terrorism, Extremism

Allah, the Exalted, says:

"And desire not corruption in the land. Indeed, Allah does not like corrupters." (Qur'an, Al-Qasas 28:77)

"And do not kill yourselves (nor kill one another). Surely, Allah is the Most Merciful." (Qur'an, An-Nisa 4:29)

"O you, who have believed, do not follow the footsteps of Satan. And whoever follows the footsteps of Satan - indeed, he enjoins immorality and wrongdoing." (Qur'an, An-Nur 24:21)

Other Verses: *Al-Ma'idah 5:32-33, An-Naba 78:30, All-Jumu'ah 62:5.*

Abdullah ibn Masud (May Allah be pleased with him) reported: The Prophet (May Allah's peace and blessings be upon him) said: "Ruined are the extremists!" He said it thrice." (Muslim)

There is a severe punishment for one who terrorizes and frightens people, such as gangs of bandits, who spread mischief and corruption on earth. Allah has prescribed the severest punishments for them, so as to ward off their evil and protect people's lives, honor and wealth.

"False propaganda accuses Muslims in the terroristic acts.
But use your logic and just try to think deeply and justly:
Who started the First World War? Not Muslims?
Who started the Second World War? Not Muslims?
Who killed about 20 million of Aborigines in Australia? Not Muslims?
Who sent the nuclear bombs in Hiroshima and Nagasaki? Not Muslims?
Who killed more than 50 million of Indians in South America? Not Muslims?
Who took about 180 million of African people as slaves and 88% of them died and were thrown in Atlantic Ocean? Not Muslims?
No! Not Muslims!
First of all, you have to define Terrorism properly...
If a non-Muslim does something bad... It is a crime. But if Muslim commits the same... he is a terrorist...So, first remove this double standard... Then come to the point!
I am proud to be a Muslim! Are you?" (from German man reverted to Islam (reverted is more appropriate than converted as the souls of all people were created Muslims)

In this deluded world, the Jinn Possession is widespread because of humanity's sins. In case of the complete Jinn Possession, the free will of the human is replaced by the free will of Satan and Satan does only evil actions.

The monsters behind the terroristic attacks on innocent human beings do not represent any faith or community. They only represent extremism and terrorism. The same applies to those extremists that kill innocent worshippers in the Mosque.

426. Humble before a Disbeliever, Transgressor, Arrogant People

Allah, the Exalted, says:

"Indeed, Allah does not guide the defiantly disobedient people." (Qur'an, Al-Munafiqun 63:6)

"And to Allah belongs (all) honor and to His Messenger, and to the believers, but the hypocrites do not know." (Qur'an, Al-Munafiqun 63:8)

Thawban (May Allah be pleased with him) reported that the Prophet (May Allah's peace and blessings be upon him) said: "Make frequent prostration to Allah, for every prostration that you make for Allah, He will raise your position a degree and will remit one of your sins." (Muslim)

(https://hadeethenc.com/en/browse/hadith/3732)

Sa'd ibn Abi Waqqas (May Allah be pleased with him) reported that the Prophet (May Allah's peace and blessings be upon him) that he said: "Allah loves the one who is pious, content and restraint (humble)." (Muslim) (https://hadeethenc.com/en/browse/hadith/5340)

'Iyad ibn Himar (May Allah be pleased with him) reported that the Prophet (May Allah's peace and blessings be upon him) said: "Verily, Allah, the Exalted, revealed to me that you must be humble, so that no one oppresses another or boasts of oneself before another." (Muslim)
(https://hadeethenc.com/en/browse/hadith/5497)

427. Prohibition of Conferring a Title of Honor upon a Sinner, a Hypocrite and the Like

Narrated Buraidah (May Allah be pleased with him): The Messenger of Allah (peace and blessings be upon him) said, "Do not address a hypocrite with the title of chief (or similar titles of respect), for even if he deserves this title you will invite Allah's Wrath by using it for him." (Abu Dawud)

Commentary: A sinner does not deserve any respect. His respect amounts to inviting the Wrath of Allah. Hypocrites, innovators in religion, disbelievers, polytheists, atheists, heretics and those who disobey Allah and His Prophet (peace and blessings be upon him) fall in this category, and none of them deserve any respect… (400)

428. Saying "You are our Master"

Buraidah (May Allah be pleased with him) reported that the Messenger (May Allah's peace and blessings be upon him) said: "Do not call a hypocrite a master, for if he is a master, you will have angered your Almighty Lord." (An-Nasa'i) (https://hadeethenc.com/en/browse/hadith/8962)

'Abdullah ibn Ash-Shikhir (May Allah be pleased with him) reported: "I set out with the delegation of Banu 'Āmir to meet the Messenger of Allah (May Allah's peace and blessings be upon him). We said (to him): "You are our master." He said: "The Master is Allah, Blessed and Exalted." We said: "How about the best of us in excellence and the greatest of us in authority." He said: "Say what you like, but do not let the Devil play you." (Abu Dawud and Ahmad) (https://hadeethenc.com/en/browse/hadith/3389)

429. To Honor a Wealthy and Powerful Person for his Wealth and Power

Allah, the Exalted, says:

"And do not stretch your eyes after that with which We have provided different classes of them, (of) the splendor of this world's life, that We may thereby try them…" (Qur'an, Taha 20:131)

430. To Point a Sharp Object at Someone

The Prophet (peace and blessings be upon him) said: "Whoever points a piece of iron at his brother, the angels curse him." (Tirmidhi)

To point anything sharp, like fork, knife, scissor, etc. One cannot terrify a Muslim, not even trying to come behind and scare him or wear a mask and jump at him. Sometimes a person doesn't know, why there is no barakah in his life and this is good to account himself and look at his sins.

431. Prohibition of Pointing with a Weapon at Another Brother in Faith

Narrated Abu Hurairah (May Allah be pleased with him) said: The Messenger of Allah (peace and blessings be upon him) said, "None of you should point at his brother with a weapon because he does not know that Satan may make it lose from his hand and, as a result, he may fall into a pit of Hellfire (by accidentally killing him)." (Bukhari and Muslim)

Commentary:
"Silah" is that weapon which is used in war for attack and defense, i.e. sword, gun, pistol, lance, etc. To point any such weapon towards a Muslim or Dhimmi, even to frighten him, is forbidden. (401)

Narrated Jabir (May Allah be pleased with him) said: "The Messenger of Allah (peace and blessings be upon him) prohibited from presenting a drawn sword to another." (Abu Dawud and Tirmidhi)

432. Prohibition of Chastisement with Fire

Abu Hurairah (May Allah be pleased with him) said: The Messenger of Allah (peace and blessings be upon him) sent us on an expedition and said to us, "If you find so-and-so (he named two persons belonging to the Quraish) commit them to the fire." When we were on the verge of departure, he said to us, "I ordered you to burn so-and-so, but it is Allah Alone Who punishes with the fire. So, if you find them put them to death." (Bukhari)

Ibn Masud (May Allah be pleased with him) reported: "We were with the Messenger of Allah (peace and blessings be upon him) in a journey when he drew apart (to relieve nature). In his absence, we saw a red bird which had two young ones with it. We caught them and the red mother bird came, beating the earth with its wings. In the meantime, the Prophet (peace and blessings be upon him) returned and said, "Who has put this bird to distress on account of its young? Return them to her." He (peace and blessings be upon him) also noticed a mound of ants which we had burnt up. He asked, "Who has set fire to this?" We replied: "We have done so." He (peace and blessings be upon him) said, "None can chastise with fire except the Rubb of the Fire." (Abu Dawud)

Commentary:
1. To catch nestlings of a bird and torment them or to burn the holes of insects along with their inmates is forbidden. One can, however, burn their vacant holes.
2. If somebody has burnt a person to death, it is not permissible to kill him in return by burning. If the heirs of the victim want to kill him in the same way under Al-Qisas (the Law of equality in punishment) they can do so; otherwise he can be put to the sword. (402)

'Ikrimah reported that 'Ali (May Allah be pleased with him) burned some people and this news reached Ibn 'Abbas, who said: "Had I been in his place, I would not have burned them, as the Prophet (May Allah's peace and blessings be upon him) said: 'Do not punish (anybody) with Allah's Punishment.' No doubt, I would have killed them, for the Prophet (May Allah's peace and blessings be upon him) said: 'If a Muslim changes his religion, kill him.'" (Bukhari) (https://hadeethenc.com/en/browse/hadith/58227)

433. Prohibition of Leaving the Fire Burning

Narrated Ibn 'Umar (May Allah be pleased with him): The Prophet (peace and blessings be upon him) said, "Do not keep the fire burning in your homes when you go to bed." (Bukhari and Muslim)

Narrated Abu Musa Al-Ash'ari (May Allah be pleased with him) said: "A house in Al-Madinah was burnt with its occupants inside it one night. When this was reported to the Messenger of Allah (peace and blessings be upon him), he said, "Fire is your enemy. So, put it out before going to bed." (Bukhari and Muslim)

Narrated Jabir (May Allah be pleased with him) said: The Messenger of Allah (peace and blessings be upon him) said, "Cover up the (kitchen) containers (i.e. pots, pans, etc.), tie up the mouth of the water-skin, lock up the doors and extinguish the lamps, because Satan can neither untie the waterskin nor open the door nor uncover the containers. If one can cover the cooking pot even by placing a piece of wood across it, and pronounce the Name of Allah on it, let him do it. A mouse can sometimes cause a house to burn along its dwellers." (Muslim)

Commentary:

The Ahadith mentioned above stress the fact that one must put out the fire before going to bed, no matter whether this fire is in the form of a lamp, a fireplace or a heater. Experience shows that leaving the fire alive sometime proves very dangerous... (403)

434. Prohibition of Putting Oneself to Undue Hardship

Allah, the Exalted, says:

"Say (O Muhammad SAW): 'No wage do I ask of you for this (the Qur'an), nor am I one of the Mutakallifun (those who pretend and fabricate things which do not exist).'" (Qur'an, Sad 38:86)

'Umar (May Allah be pleased with him) said: "We have been forbidden to go into excess." (Bukhari)

Commentary: Affectation and artificiality are also different forms of formality which some people exercise in their speech, dress and manners. To make unusual effort in hospitality and preparation of several dishes for meals also come in the category of formality which is greatly disliked... (404)

Masruq (May Allah be pleased with him) said: "We visited 'Abdullah bin Masud (May Allah be pleased with him) and he said to us: 'O people! He who has the knowledge of any matter may convey it to the others. And he who has no knowledge, thereof, should say: "Allahu a'lam (Allah knows better)."' It is a part and parcel of knowledge that a man who has no knowledge of a matter should say: "Allah knows better." Allah Almighty said to His Prophet (peace and blessings be upon him): *"Say (O Muhammad SAW): 'No wage do I ask of you for this (the Qur'an), nor am I one of the Mutakallifun (those who pretend and fabricate things which do not exist).'" (Qur'an, Sad 38:86)* (Bukhari)

435. Democracy, Telling "Rules of People"

Allah, the Exalted, says:

"So, the judgment is only with Allah, the Most High, the Most Great!" (Qur'an, Ghafir 40:12)

"The decision is only for Allah, He declares the Truth, and He is the Best of judges." (Qur'an, Al-An'am 6:57)

"...O my son, do not associate (anything) with Allah. Indeed, association (with Him) is great injustice." (Qur'an, Luqman 31:13)

Other Verse: *Yusuf 12:40.*

Democracy is a system giving the power of legislation to people, it is ascribing partner to Allah. In these systems, legislation has been promulgated allowing abortion, same-sex marriage, usurious interest (Riba), alcohol, etc.

In non-Muslim countries, the legislation has been implying "no intervention of religion into political matters." Human beings are unaware of what is best for them. Hence, in societies that are ruled by people in terms of legislation and laws, the unlawful things by Allah became lawful creating only corruption, immorality, deception and disintegration of the society and none is protected.

It says in Mawsoo'ah al-Adyaan wa'l-Madhaahib al-Mu'aasirah (2/1066):

"Undoubtedly democratic systems are one of the modern forms of Shirk in terms of obedience and submission or in legislation as it disregards the Authority of the Creator, Glorified and Exalted, and His absolute right of Legislation." (405)

436. Electoral Fraud

Allah, the Exalted, says:

"The decision is only for Allah." (Qur'an, An-An'am 6:57)

"You do not worship besides Him but only names which you have named (forged) - you and your fathers - for which Allah has sent down no authority. The command (or the judgement) is for none but Allah. He has commanded that you worship none but Him (i.e. His Monotheism); that is the True) Straight Religion, but most men know not." (Qur'an, Yousuf 12:40)

It says in Mawsoo'at al-Adyaan wa'l-Madhaahib al-Mu'aasirah (2/1066, 1067):

"Undoubtedly the democratic system is one of the modern forms of Shirk, in terms of obedience and submission or legislation, as it denies the sovereignty of the Creator and His absolute right to issue Laws…" (405)

Narrated 'Abd al-Rahman b. Samura (May Allah be pleased with him): The Messenger of Allah (peace and blessings be upon him) said to me: "Abd al-Rahman, do not ask for a position of authority, for if you are granted this position as a result of your asking for it, you will be left alone (without God's help to discharge the responsibilities attendant thereon); and if you are granted it without making any request for it, you will be helped (by God in the discharge of your duties)." (Muslim)

Abu Bakrah (May Allah be pleased with him) reported: "During the days (of the battle) of Al-Jamal (the Camel), Allah benefited me with a word that I had heard from the Messenger of Allah (May Allah's peace and blessings be upon him) after I had been about to join the Companions of the Camel and fight along with them. When the Messenger of Allah (May Allah's peace and blessings be upon him) was informed that the Persians had crowned the daughter of Khosrow as their ruler, he said: "A people who appointed a woman to be in charge of their affairs will never succeed." (Bukhari) (https://hadeethenc.com/en/browse/hadith/64687)

437. Discrimination

Allah, the Exalted, says:

"O mankind! We have created you from a male and a female and made you into nations and tribes, that you may know one another. Verily, the most honorable of you with Allah is that (believer) who has At-Taqwa (i.e. he is one of the Muttaqoon (the pious). Verily, Allah is All-Knowing, All-Aware." (Qur'an, Al-Hujurat 49:13)

"Whoever works righteousness - whether male or female - while he (or she) is a true believer (of Islamic Monotheism) verily, to him We will give a good life (in this world with respect, contentment and lawful provision), and We shall pay them certainly a reward in proportion to the best of what they used to do (i.e. Paradise in the Hereafter)." (Qur'an, An-Nahl 16:97)

"(Allah) said: "What prevented you (O Iblees) that you did not prostrate, when I commanded you?" Iblis said: "I am better than him (Adam)…" (Qur'an, Al-A'raf 7:12)

Other Verse: An-Nisa 4:94.

Narrated Abu Nadrah (May Allah be pleased with him): Someone who heard the Khutbah of the Messenger of Allah (peace and blessings of Allah be upon him) on the second of the days of at-Tashreeq told me that he said: "O people, verily your Lord is One and your father is one. Verily there is no superiority of an Arab over a non-Arab or of a non-Arab over an Arab, or of a red man over a black man, or of a black man over a red man, except in terms of Taqwa. Have I conveyed the message?" They said: "The Messenger of Allah (peace and blessings of Allah be upon him) has conveyed the message." (Ahmad)

Narrated Ibn 'Umar (May Allah be pleased with him): The Prophet (peace and blessings be upon him) addressed the people at the conquest of Makkah and said, "O Mankind! Indeed, Allah has taken away from you the arrogance of Jahiliyyah and its pride in forefathers. People are of two types: righteous and pious, who are dear to Allah, and doomed evildoers, who are insignificant before Allah. People are the descendants of Adam, and Allah created Adam from dust." (Tirmidhi)

Safiyyah (May Allah be pleased with her), the wife of the Prophet (peace and blessings be upon him), came to know that Hafsah (May Allah be pleased with her) had said about her that she is the daughter of a Jew. When the Prophet (peace and blessings be upon him) met her, she was weeping. So, he asked, 'Why are you weeping?' She replied, 'Hafsah said that I am the daughter of a Jew.' Nabi (peace and blessings be upon him) said: 'You are the daughter of a Prophet Harun (peace be upon him), and your uncle was a Prophet as well, Musa (peace be upon him), and you are the wife of a Prophet, so what is she boasting about?' Then Nabi (peace and blessings be upon him) told Hafsah, 'O Hafsah! Fear Allah!' (Tirmidhi)

Abu Hurairah (May Allah have mercy on him) reported that Prophet (peace and blessings be upon him) said: "Verily, Allah does not look at your appearance or wealth, but rather He looks at your hearts and actions." (Muslim)

Abdullah ibn 'Abbassaid (May Allah be pleased with him): "I don't think anyone who practices on the Verse (quoted below) will say, 'I am more noble than you are.' None is more noble than another person except by Taqwa." *"O Mankind! We created you from a single pair of a male and a female and made you into nations and tribes so that you may get to know each other. Surely, the noblest among you in sight of Allah is the most righteous. Allah is All-Knowledgeable, All-Aware (Surah Al-Hujurat 49:13).*" (Bukhari, Al Adab Al Mufrad)

A dark-skinned person once came to Sa'id ibn Al Musayyab (May Allah have mercy on him) asking for something. Sa'id (May Allah have mercy on him) told him, 'You being dark skinned, should not be a cause of grief/distress, for certainly three dark skinned men/African men were among the best of people; Bilal (May Allah have mercy on him), Mihja', the freed slave of 'Umar (May Allah have mercy on them) and Luqman Al Hakim." (Tafsir Tabari; Jami'ul Bayan and Tafsir Ibn Kathir, Surah Luqman 31:12) (https://hadithanswers.com/hadiths-on-racism)

Narrated 'Uqbah ibn 'Amir (May Allah have mercy on him): The Prophet (peace and blessings be upon him) said: "No one is better than anyone else except by religion or good deeds. It is enough (to regard a person) evil if he is profane, vulgar, greedy or cowardly." (Ahmad and Bayhaqi) (https://hadithanswers.com/no-one-is-better-than-anyone-else-except-through-religion-or-good-deeds)

438. Freedom

Allah, the Exalted, says:

"Namely, that no bearer of burdens can bear the burden of another. That man can have nothing but what he strives for." (Qur'an, An-Najm 53:38-39)

"And We have fastened every man's deeds to his neck, and on the Day of Resurrection, We shall bring out for him a book which he will find wide open. (It will be said to him): "Read your book. You yourself are sufficient as a reckoner against you this Day." (Qur'an, Al-Isra 17:13-14)

"And shown him the two ways (good and evil)?" (Qur'an, Al-Balad 90:10)

Other Verses: *Az-Zumar 39:6, At-Tariq 86:5, Al-Qiyamah 75:14.*

Freedom of Belief

Allah, the Exalted, says:

"There shall be no compulsion in (acceptance of) the religion. The Right Path has become distinct from the wrong path. So, whoever disbelieves false deities, evil and believes in Allah has grasped the most trustworthy handhold with no break in it. And Allah is Hearing and Knowing." (Qur'an, Al-Baqarah 2:256)

"It is He Who has sent His Messenger (Muhammad SAW) with guidance and the religion of Truth (Islam), to make it superior over all religions even though the Mushrikun (polytheists, pagans, idolaters, disbelievers in the Oneness of Allah) hate (it)." (Qur'an, At-Tawbah 9:33)

"And say, "The Truth is from your Lord, so whoever wills - let him believe; and whoever wills - let him disbelieve." Indeed, We have prepared for the wrongdoers a fire whose walls will surround them. And if they call for relief, they will be relieved with water like murky oil, which scalds (their) faces. Wretched is the drink, and evil is the resting place." (Qur'an, Al-Kahf 18:29)

Other Verses: *Al-Ma'idah 5:48, Al-An'am 6:107, Ash-Shuraa 42:48, Az-Zumar 39:7.*

The freedom of belief created more than 4200 religions/beliefs while Allah is the Only One True God.

If it was to God's Will, the idea of recompense or punishment on Judgment Day would be meaningless.

Allah, the Owner of the Universe, has chosen Islam for all people from the creation of the first man.

Any other religions/beliefs by free will because the parents are disbelievers or because you reject the Oneness of Allah or transgress His Laws (Qur'an and Sunnah - is the result of misguidance by Satan.

<u>Freedom of Actions</u>

"What does 'freedom' mean?

Does the eagle want to swim in the sea,
Restricted by the sky?

Does the fish want to dance on the wind,
Not enough river to explore?

Yet the sky is freedom for the bird
but death for the fish,

The sea is wide for the fish
but will engulf the bird.

We ask for freedom but freedom to do what?
We can only express our nature as it was created.

The prayer mat of the earth is freedom,
freedom from slavery to other than the One,
Who offers a shoreless ocean of love to swim in
and a horizon that extends to the next life,
Yet we chose the prison and call it freedom." (Anonymous)

Belief in al-Qadar (the Divine Will and Decree) is one of the pillars of Faith. We have no choice of the day when and where a person will be born or die, male or female, the colour of the skin, eyes, the shape, etc. All of these are matters over which people have no control.

Allah, the Exalted, says:

"Verily, We have created all things with Qadar (Divine Preordainments of all things before their creation as written in the Book of Decrees Al-Lawh Al-Mahfuz)." (Qur'an, Al-Qamar 54:49)

All the deeds of mankind are written with Allah, because Allah has prior knowledge of them. This does not mean that Allah compels people to do what they do, rather they have freedom of choice but it is a subject to Allah's Will.

Allah, the Exalted, says:

"And you do not will except that Allah wills. Indeed, Allah is ever Knowing and Wise." (Qur'an, Al-Insan 76:30)

"Verily, We showed him the way, whether he be grateful or ungrateful." (Qur'an, Al-Insan 76:3)

Some actions are the subject of choice, such as whether to believe or disbelieve, or worldly matters such as choosing what to eat or drink, how to dress, etc.

But their actions are not compelled by Allah, for Allah does not force His slaves to do anything.

Imam Ibn Abi'l-'Izz al-Hanafi said concerning a similar matter:

"If it is said, how can Allah will something that He is not pleased with and does not like? How can He will it and create it? How can His Will be reconciled with His hatred for it?

It should be said (in response) that this is the question which has caused divisions among the people and has caused them to follow different paths and opinions.

It should be noted that what is willed may be of two types: that which is willed or wanted for itself, and that which is willed or wanted for something else.

That which is willed or wanted for itself is that which is wanted and loved for what it is and for the goodness it contains. So, it comes under the heading of aims and goals. That which is willed or wanted for something else may not be what is wanted, but it serves a purpose; it may not serve any purpose in and of itself, even though it may be a means to attain that which he wants and is aiming for. So, it may be something that is disliked in and of itself, but he may seek it because it serves a purpose and helps him reach what he wants. So, in this case he will have two opposing feelings, his dislike (of the means) and his desire (for the end). There is no contradiction, as these feelings are related to different things. This is like unpleasant medicine which the one who takes it knows will cure him, or like cutting off a wasted limb when he knows that will save the rest of his body, or travelling a difficult route when he knows that it will bring him to what he wants and loves. The wise man would rather accept the disliked thing on the basis that he is likely to get good results even though the ultimate end may not be quite certain. So how about Allah, from Whom nothing is hidden? He may dislike something but it may not be against His Will for it to exist, because it may be a means to an end, and it may be a means to something that Allah likes. For example, Allah created Iblees, who is the cause of the corruption of religions, deeds, beliefs and human wills; but nevertheless, he is a means to a lot of things that Allah likes, which result from the creation of Iblees. For these things to exist is dearer to Allah than if they did not exist at all." (Sharh al-'Aqeedah al-Tahhaawiyyah, 252-253) (406)

Freedom to Form Opinion/Decision

Allah, the Exalted says:

"Verily, those who conceal what Allah has sent down of the Book, and purchase a small gain therewith (of worldly things), they eat into their bellies nothing but Fire. Allah will not speak to them on the Day of Resurrection, nor purify them, and theirs will be a painful torment." (Qur'an, Al-Baqarah 2:174)

"Those who conceal the clear Signs We have sent down, and the Guidance, after We have made it clear for the People in the Book, - on them shall be God's Curse, and the curse of those entitled to curse." (Qur'an, Al-Baqarah 2:159)

"O you who believe! If a rebellious evil person comes to you with a news, verify it, lest you harm people in ignorance, and afterwards you become regretful to what you have done." (Qur'an, Al-Hujurat 49:6)

Those who don't have enough knowledge or data, or experience about a particular issue cannot form an educated opinion or beneficial decision.

Islam is very much assertive on the decision-making because faults and mistakes are very costly in the life of individuals and the community.

Freedom of Expression

See the next Sin.

Freedom of the Relationships

Allah, the Exalted, says:

"Shaitan (Satan) threatens you with poverty and orders you to commit Fahisha (evil deeds, illegal sexual intercourse, sins etc.); whereas Allah promises you Forgiveness from Himself and Bounty, and Allah is All-Sufficient for His creatures' needs, All-Knower." (Qur'an, Al-Baqarah 2:268)

Freedom of the relationships is the cause of multiples sins: immorality, adultery and fornication, homosexuality, prostitution, deception, abortion, etc. If the sexual drive is uncontrolled, man behaves worse than an animal.

God's commands and prohibitions are clear in the Qur'an and Sunnah regarding the husband and wife rights and duties, the rules of marriage, divorce, family life, Mahram and non-Mahram relations, prohibition of Zina, etc.

Freedom of the Food

Allah, the Exalted, says:

"Eat not (O believers) of that (meat) on which Allah's Name has not been pronounced (at the time of the slaughtering of the animal), for sure it is Fisq (a sin and disobedience of Allah). And certainly, the Shayatin (Devils) do inspire their friends (from mankind) to dispute with you, and if you obey them [by making Al-Maytatah (a dead animal) legal by eating it], then you would indeed be Mushrikun (polytheists) [because they (Devils and their friends) made lawful to you to eat that which Allah has made unlawful to eat and you obeyed them by considering it lawful to eat, and by doing so you worshipped them, and to worship others besides Allah is polytheism]." (Qur'an, Al-An'am 6:121)

"O (you) Messengers! Eat of the Taiyibat [all kinds of Halal (legal) foods which Allah has made legal (meat of slaughtered eatable animals, milk products, fats, vegetables, fruits, etc.], and do righteous deeds. Verily! I am Well-Acquainted with what you do." (Qur'an, Al-Mu'minun 23:51)

THE EATER IS SIMILAR TO WHAT HE EATS

Narrated Abu Hurairah (May Allah have mercy on him): The Messenger of Allah (peace and blessings be upon him) said, "Allah the Almighty is Good and accepts only that which is good. And verily Allah has commanded the believers to do that which He has commanded the Messengers. So, the Almighty has said: *"O (you) Messengers! Eat of the tayyibat [all kinds of halal (legal) foods], and perform righteous deeds." (23:51)* and the Almighty has said: *"O you who believe! Eat of the lawful things that We have provided you." (2:172)* Then he (peace and blessings be upon him) mentioned (the case) of a man who, having journeyed far, is disheveled and dusty, and who spreads out his hands to the sky saying "O Lord! O Lord!" while his food is haram (unlawful), his drink is haram, his clothing is haram, and he has been nourished with haram, so how can (his supplication) be answered?" (Muslim)

Eating what is lawful and good, according the Qur'an and Sunnah, helps one to be pious, do righteous deeds, have good manners and behavior, be healthy. If you eat good, you do good and you are healthy.

Eating what is unlawful and bad according the Qur'an and Sunnah, causes one to be unrighteous, do bad deeds, have bad manners and behavior, causes diseases, depression, anxiety, aggression, arrogance, immorality, laziness, etc.

Narrated Abdullah bin 'Amr (May Allah be pleased with him): The Messenger of Allah (peace and blessings be upon him) said: "Whoever drinks wine and gets drunk, his prayer will not be accepted for forty days, and if he dies, he will enter Hell, but if he repents, Allah will accept his repentance. If he drinks wine again and gets drunk, his prayer will not be accepted for forty days, and if he dies, he will enter Hell, but if he repents, Allah will accept his repentance. If he drinks wine again and gets drunk, his prayer will not be accepted for forty days, and if he dies, he will enter Hell, but if he repents Allah will accept his repentance. But if he does it again, then Allah will most certainly make him drink of the mire of the puss or sweat on the Day of Resurrection." They said: "O Messenger of Allah, what is the mire of the pus or sweat?" He said: "The drippings of the people of Hell." (Ibn Majah)

Jabir (May Allah be pleased with him) reported Allah's Messenger (peace and blessings be upon him) as saying, "Flesh which has grown out of what is unlawful will not enter Paradise*, but Hell is more suitable for all flesh which has grown out of what is unlawful." (Ahmad, Darimi, and Baihaqi, in *Shu'ab al-Iman*, transmitted it) *The reference here is to people who live on an unlawful source of income. (https://sunnah.com/mishkat:2772)

Miqdam bin Ma'dikarib (May Allah be pleased with him) said: "I heard the Messenger of Allah (peace and blessings be upon him) saying: 'The human does not fill any container that is worse than his stomach. It is sufficient for the son of Adam to eat what will support his back. If this is not possible, then a third for food, a third for drink and a third for his breath." (Tirmidhi)

Narrated Ibn 'Umar (May Allah be pleased with him): Allah's Messenger (peace and blessings be upon him) said, "A believer eats in one intestine (is satisfied with a little food), and a kafir (unbeliever) or a hypocrite eats in seven intestines (eats too much)." (Bukhari)

For more details, refer to the sin: Prohibition of Consumption of Unlawful Food and Income.

Freedom of the Dress

Allah, the Exalted, says:

"And tell the believing women to lower their gaze (from looking at forbidden things), and protect their private parts (from illegal sexual acts) and not to show off their adornment except only that which is apparent (like both eyes for necessity to see the way, or outer palms of hands, or one eye or dress like veil, gloves, headcover, apron), and to draw their veils all over Juyubihinna (i.e. their bodies, faces, necks and bosoms) and not to reveal their adornment except to their husbands, or their fathers, or their husband's fathers, or their sons, or their husband's sons, or their brothers or their brother's sons, or their sister's sons, or their (Muslim) women (i.e. their sisters in Islam), or the (female) slaves whom their right hands possess, or old male servants who lack vigour, or small children who have no sense of feminine sex. And let them not stamp their feet so as to reveal what they hide of their adornment. And all of you beg Allah to forgive you all, O believers, that you may be successful." (Qur'an, An-Nur 24:31)

Abu Hurairah (May Allah be pleased with him) reported that the Prophet (May Allah's peace and blessings be upon him) said: "While a man was walking, dressed in fine clothes and admiring himself, with his hair well-combed and he was walking haughtily, suddenly Allah caused the earth to swallow him, and he continues to sink therein until the Day of Judgment." (Bukhari and Muslim) (https://hadeethenc.com/en/browse/hadith/5905)

Abu Hurairah (May Allah be pleased with him) reported Allah's Messenger (peace and blessings be upon him) having said this: "Two are the types of the denizens of Hell whom I did not see: people having flogs like the tails of the ox with them and they would be beating people, and the women who would be dressed but appear to be naked, who would be inclined (to evil) and make their husbands incline towards it. Their heads would be like the humps of the bukht camel inclined to one side. They will not enter Paradise and they would not smell its odour whereas its odour would be smelt from such and such distance." (Muslim)

Abu Dharr al-Ghifari (May Allah be pleased with him) reported that the Prophet (May Allah's peace and blessings be upon him) said that Allah the Almighty said: "…O My slaves, all of you are naked except those whom I clothe, so ask Me for clothes and I shall clothe you…" (Muslim)

God ordered women to cover entire body, prohibited women imitating men in dress and manners and vice versa, etc.

Conclusion:
Freedom is only by submitting to our Creator's Will and Decree, to be Allah's slave.

Those who are not with Allah, are the slaves of Satan. Satan incites people to commit immorality, mischief, corruption, transgress Allah's Laws and brings people to the Hellfire.

439. Freedom of Expression

Allah, the Exalted, says:

"Not a word does he (or she) utter, but there is a watcher by him ready (to record it)." (Qur'an, Qaf 50:18)

"Invite (mankind, O Muhammad SAW) to the Way of your Lord (i.e. Islam) with wisdom (i.e. with the Divine Inspiration and the Qur'an) and fair preaching, and argue with them in a way that is better. Truly, your Lord knows best who has gone astray from His Path, and He is the Best Aware of those who are guided." (Qur'an, An-Nahl 16:152)

THE TONGUE IS THE MOST DANGEROUS ORGAN

Ibn Masud (May Allah be pleased with him) said: The Messenger of Allah (peace and blessings be upon him) said, "None of my Companions should convey to me anything regarding another because I desire to meet every one of you with a clean heart." (Abu Dawud and Tirmidhi)

Sufyan bin 'Abdullah (May Allah be pleased with him) reported: "I asked: 'O Messenger of Allah! Tell me, of something to which I may remain steadfast.'" He (peace and blessings be upon him) said, "Say: My Rubb is Allah and then remain steadfast." Then I said: "O Messenger of Allah! What do you fear most about me?" He took hold of his own tongue and said: "This." (Tirmidhi)

Abu Sa'id al-Khudri (May Allah be pleased with him) reported that the Prophet (May Allah's peace and blessings be upon him) said: "When the son of Adam gets up in the morning, all of his body organs humble themselves before the tongue and say: 'Fear Allah concerning us! For indeed, we are only as you are (our condition depends upon yours); if you are upright, we shall be upright, and if you are crooked, we shall be crooked.'" (Tirmidhi) (https://hadeethenc.com/en/browse/hadith/3579)

Abu Hurairah (May Allah be pleased with him) reported: The Prophet (peace and blessings of Allah be upon him) said, "He who believes in Allah and the Last Day must either speak good or remain silent." (Muslim)

Narrated Umm Habiba (May Allah be pleased with her): The Prophet (peace and blessings of Allah be upon him) said: "The words of the son of Adam count against him, not for him, except what is good and forbidding what is evil, and remembering Allah." (Ibn Majah)

Narrated Malik (May Allah be pleased with him): Malik related to me that he heard that Isa ibn Maryam used to say, "Do not speak much without the mention of Allah for you will harden your hearts. A hard heart is far from Allah, but you do not know. Do not look at the wrong actions of people as if you were lords. Look at your wrong actions as if you were slaves. Some people are afflicted by wrong action and some people are protected from it. Be merciful to the people of affliction and praise Allah for His Protection." (Malik Muwatta)

Narrated Muadh bin Jabal (May Allah be pleased with him): "I said: 'O Messenger of Allah, tell me of an act which will take me into Paradise and will keep me away from Hellfire.' He (peace and blessings be upon him) said: 'You have asked me about a major matter, yet it is easy for him for whom Allah Almighty makes it easy. You should worship Allah, associating nothing with Him, you should perform the prayers, you should pay the zakat, you should fast in Ramadan, and you should make the pilgrimage to the House.' Then he (peace and blessings be upon him) said: 'Shall I not show you the gates of goodness? Fasting [which] is a shield, charity (which) extinguishes sin as water extinguishes fire; and the praying of a man in the depth of night.' Then he recited: *'Who forsake their beds to cry unto their Lord in fear and hope, and spend of that We have bestowed on them. No soul knoweth what is kept hid for them of joy, as a reward for what they used to do." (As-Sajdah 32:16)* Then he said: 'Shall I not tell you of the peak of the matter, its pillar and its topmost part?' I said: 'Yes, O Messenger of Allah.'

He said: 'The peak of the matter is Islam; the pillar is prayer; and its topmost part is Jihad.' Then he said: 'Shall I not tell you of the controlling of all that?' I said: 'Yes, O Messenger of Allah', and he took hold of his tongue and said: 'Restrain this.' I said: 'O Prophet of Allah, will what we say be held against us?' He said: 'May your mother be bereaved of you, Muadh! Is there anything that topples people on their faces – or he said on their noses into Hellfire other than the jests of their tongues?'" (Tirmidhi)

Abu Hurairah (May Allah be pleased with him) reported that the Messenger of Allah (May Allah's peace and blessings be upon him) said: "If people sit in a session where they neither remember Allah nor invoke blessings upon the Prophet (May Allah's peace and blessings be upon him) that will be for them a cause of grief on the Day of Judgment." (Tirmidhi) (https://hadeethenc.com/en/browse/hadith/5511)

Abu Hurairah (May Allah be pleased with him) reported: The Prophet (peace and blessings be upon him) said, "A man utters a word pleasing to Allah without considering it of any significance for which Allah exalts his ranks (in Jannah); another one speaks a word displeasing to Allah without considering it of any importance, and for this reason he will sink down into Hell." (Bukhari)

Abu Hurairah (May Allah be pleased with him) reported: "A person utters a word thoughtlessly (i.e. without thinking about its being good or not) and, as a result of this, he will fall down into the Fire of Hell deeper than the distance between the east and the west." (Bukhari and Muslim)

Hudhaifah (May Allah be pleased with him) said: The Messenger of Allah (peace and blessings be upon him) said, "The person who goes about with calumnies will never enter Jannah." (Bukhari and Muslim)

Narrated Ibn Abbas (May Allah be pleased with him): The Prophet (peace and blessings be upon him) once passed by two graves, and those two persons (in the graves) were being tortured. He said, "They are being tortured not for a great thing (to avoid). One of them never saved himself from being soiled with his urine, while the other went about committing slander (to make enmity between friends). He then took a green leaf of a date-palm tree, split it into two pieces and fixed one on each grave. The people said, "O Allah's Messenger (peace and blessings be upon him)! Why have you done so?" He replied, "I hope that their punishment may be lessened till they (the leaf) become dry." (Bukhari)

Abu Musa Al-Ash'ari (May Allah be pleased with him) reported: "I asked the Messenger of Allah (peace and blessings be upon him): "Who is the most excellent among the Muslims?" He said, "One from whose tongue and hands the other Muslims are secure." (Bukhari and Muslim)

Sahl bin Sa'd (May Allah be pleased with him) reported: The Messenger of Allah (peace and blessings be upon him) said, "Whosoever gives me a guarantee to safeguard what is between his jaws and what is between his legs, I shall guarantee him Jannah." (Bukhari)

Ibn 'Umar (May Allah be pleased with him) reported: The Messenger of Allah (peace and blessings be upon him) said, "Do not indulge in excessive talk except when remembering Allah. Excessive talking without the Remembrance of Allah hardens the heart, and those who are the farthest from Allah are those whose hearts are hard." (Tirmidhi)

Anas (May Allah be pleased with him) said: The Messenger of Allah (peace and blessings be upon him) said, "During the Mi'raj (the Night of Ascension), I saw a group of people who were scratching their chests and faces with their copper nails. I asked, 'Who are these people, O Jibreel?' Jibreel replied: 'These are the people who ate flesh of others (by backbiting) and trampled people's honor.'" (Abu Dawud)

Uqbah bin' Amir (May Allah be pleased with him) said: "I asked the Messenger of Allah (peace and blessings be upon him), 'How can salvation be achieved?' He replied, 'Control your tongue, keep to your house and weep over your sins.'" (Tirmidhi)

Abu 'Abdur-Rahman Bilal bin Al-Harith Al-Muzani (May Allah be pleased with him) reported: The Messenger of Allah (peace and blessings be upon him) said, "A man speaks a good word without knowing its worth, Allah records for him His Good Pleasure till the day he will meet Him; and a man utters an evil word without realizing its importance, Allah records for him His displeasure till the day he will meet Him." (Malik and Tirmidhi)

440. Prohibition of Making Fun and Mockery

Allah, the Exalted, says:

"That shall be their recompense, Hell; because they disbelieved and took My Ayat (proofs, evidences, verses, lessons, signs, revelations, etc.) and My Messengers by way of jest and mockery." (Qur'an, Al-Kahf 18:106)

"And already were Messengers ridiculed before you, but those who mocked them were enveloped by that which they used to ridicule." (Qur'an, Al-An'am 6:10)

"Beautified is the life of this world for those who disbelieve, and they mock at those who believe. But those who obey Allah's Orders and keep away from what He has forbidden, will be above them on the Day of Resurrection. And Allah gives (of His Bounty, Blessings, Favors and Honors on the Day of Resurrection) to whom He wills without limit." (Qur'an, Al-Baqarah 2:212)

Other Verses: *Al-Mutaffifin 83:29-32, At-Tawbah 9:64-66, Al-Kahf 18:56, An-Nisa 4:140.*

Aisha (May Allah be pleased with her) said, "A man suffering from an affliction passed by some women and they laughed together, mocking him, and so one of them got that same affliction." (Bukhari in Al-Adab Al-Mufrad)

Mu'awiyah ibn Haydah (May Allah be pleased with him) reported that the Prophet (May Allah's peace and blessings be upon him) said: "Woe to him who speaks and tells lies so as to make people laugh thereby. Woe to him! Woe to him!" (Tirmidhi) (https://hadeethenc.com/en/browse/hadith/5519)

Aisha (May Allah be pleased with her) said: "I said to the Prophet (peace and blessings be upon him): "Such and such thing of Safiyyah (May Allah be pleased with her) is sufficient for you." (She means to say that she was a woman with a short stature). He said, "You have indeed uttered a word which would pollute the sea if it were mixed in it." She further said: "I imitated a person before him" and he said, "I do not like that I should imitate someone even (if I am paid) in return such and such." (Abu Dawud and Tirmidhi)

441. Prohibition of Excessive Laughing

Allah, the Exalted, says:

"And that it is He (Allah) Who makes (whom He wills) laugh, and makes (whom He wills) weep." (Qur'an, An-Najm 53:43)

Abu Hurairah reported that the Prophet (peace and blessings be upon him) said, "Laugh little. Much laughter kills the heart." (Bukhari in Al-Adab Al-Mufrad)

Anas (May Allah be pleased with him) reported: The Messenger of Allah (May Allah's peace and blessings be upon him) gave us a speech the like of which I never heard before. He said: "Paradise and Hellfire were presented to me, and I have never seen good and evil like what I saw today. If you knew what I know, you will rarely laugh and you will cry abundantly."

In another narration: "The Messenger of Allah was told of something about his Companions. So, he gave a speech, in which he said: "Paradise and Hell were presented to me, and I have never seen good and evil like what I saw today. If you knew what I know, you will rarely laugh and you will cry abundantly." The Companions had never had a harder day. They covered their heads, crying and sobbing." (Bukhari and Muslim) (https://hadeethenc.com/en/browse/hadith/4814)

Anas ibn Malik (May Allah be pleased with him) reported: The Messenger of Allah, peace and blessings be upon him, said to the angel Gabriel, "Why do I never see the angel Michael laughing?" Gabriel said, "Michael has not laughed since the creation of the Hellfire." (Aḥmad)

Narrated Abu Dharr (May Allah be pleased with him): The Messenger of Allah (peace and blessings be upon him) said, "I see what you do not see and I hear what you do not hear; heaven has squeaked, and it has right to do so. By Him, in Whose Hand my soul is, there is not a space of four fingers in which there is not an angel who is prostrating his forehead before Allah, the Exalted. By Allah, if you knew what I know, you would laugh little, weep much, and you would not enjoy women in beds, but would go out to the open space beseeching Allah." (Tirmidhi)

Aisha (May Allah be pleased with her) reported: "I never saw the Messenger of Allah (May Allah's peace and blessings be upon him) laugh so heartily that his palate could be seen; rather, he would only smile." (Bukhari and Muslim) (https://hadeethenc.com/en/browse/hadith/3060)

Excessive laughing indicates that one is careless and forgetful of the Hereafter.

Excessive Laughing can also cause life-threatening conditions e.g. rupture of brain aneurysm. Laughing too hard may prevent adequate breathing or cause a person to stop breathing, depriving their body of oxygen.

Uncontrollable laughing can be one of the signs of the Jinn Possession. Gelastic seizures often associated with uncontrollable laughing or giggling while awake or asleep. The person having the seizure may appear to laugh, smile or smirk. Some diseases are accompanied by episodes of sudden uncontrollable, exaggerated and inappropriate laughing or crying (for example, Pseudobulbar affect). Spontaneous Manic laughter is commonly part of Bipolar disorder (Jinn Possession).

Jabir (May Allah be pleased with him) reported that the Messenger of Allah (peace and blessings be upon him) said, "Every act of kindness is Sadaqah. Part of kindness is that you offer your brother a cheerful face and you pour some of your bucket into his water vessel."

442. Skepticism

Skepticism is by no means synonymous with atheism. It is, rather, the admission that one cannot convincingly demonstrate a Truth claim with certainty, and Islam's scholars, like their counterparts elsewhere, acknowledged such impasses, only to be inspired to find new ways to resolve the conundrums they faced. (407)

According to the Qur'anic epistemology elaborated by Ibn Taymiyah and his student Ibn Qayyim al-Jawzīyah, a person's faith in God is fully justified and meaningfully grounded without need for logical deductive argumentation. It is instead justified because it is the only meaningful outlook that emerges naturally from a person's *Fiṭrah* (innate disposition) - just like belief in the existence of good and evil, causality, numbers, truth, existence itself, and so on. To deny a core pillar of one's *Fiṭrah* leaves a person without a coherent system of interpreting existence in a meaningful way and, if taken to its logical conclusion, one's beliefs dissolve into endless doubt as in *safsaṭah* - a term used in the Islamic tradition to designate radical (Pyrrhonian) skepticism. (408)

443. Abusive Language

Allah, the Exalted, says:

"And do not abuse those whom they call upon besides Allah, lest exceeding the limits they should abuse Allah out of ignorance." (Qur'an, Al-An'am 6:108)

"And incite (to senselessness) whoever you can among them with your voice and assault them with your horses and foot soldiers and become a partner in their wealth and their children and promise them." But Satan does not promise them except delusion." (Qur'an, Al-Isra 17:64)

Narrated Abu Hurairah (May Allah be pleased with him): The Prophet (peace and blessings be upon him) said: "The gravest sin is going to lengths in talking unjustly against a Muslim's honor, and it is a Major sin to abuse twice for abusing once." (Abu Dawud)

Narrated 'Abdullah (May Allah be pleased with him): Allah's Messenger peace and blessings be upon him) said, "Abusing a Muslim is Fusuq (i.e. an evildoing), and killing him is Kufr (disbelief)." (Bukhari)

Ibn Masud (May Allah be pleased with him) reported: The Messenger of Allah (peace and blessings be upon him) said, "A true believer is not involved in taunting or frequently cursing (others), or in indecency, or abusing." (Tirmidhi)

444. Calling Others with Bad Names

Allah, the Exalted, says:

"... nor insult one another by nicknames. How bad is it, to insult one's brother after having faith [i.e. to call your Muslim brother (a faithful believer) as: "O sinner" or "O wicked", etc.]. And whosoever does not repent, then such are indeed Zalimun (wrongdoers, etc.)." (Qur'an, Al-Hujurat 49:11)

445. Listening to the People's Private Conversations

Narrated Ibn Abbas (May Allah be pleased with him): The Prophet (peace and blessings be upon him) said: "Whoever claims to have seen a dream which he did not see, will be ordered to make a knot between two barley grains which he will not be able to do; and if somebody listens to the talk of some people who do not like him (to listen) or they run away from him, then molten lead will be poured into his ears on the Day of Resurrection; and whoever makes a picture, will be punished on the Day of Resurrection and will be ordered to put a soul in that picture, which he will not be able to do." (Bukhari)

446. Disclosing Secret

Abu Sa'id al-Khudri (May Allah be pleased with him) reported that the Prophet (May Allah's peace and blessings be upon him) said: "Among the most wicked people in the sight of Allah on the Day of Judgment is the man who has sexual intercourse with a woman and then divulges her secret." (Muslim) (https://hadeethenc.com/en/browse/hadith/3328)

447. Reading the Other's Letter

Allah, the Exalted, says:

"O you who believe! Avoid much suspicion; indeed, some suspicions are sins. And spy not." *(Qur'an, Al-Hujurat 49:12)*

"But verily, over you (are appointed angels in charge of mankind) to watch you, Kiraman (honorable) Katibin writing down (your deeds), They know all that you do." *(Qur'an, Al-Infitar 82:10-12)*

Neither parents or husband, or wife, or anyone else have the right to read your letters, emails, messages, watch over someone or inspect their personal belongings because that comes under the heading of suspicion and spying, which Allah, the Most High, has forbidden. It may involve others sins: backbiting, gossip, disclosing secret, etc., unless speaking of it will bring some benefit to a Muslim or ward off some harm.

448. Prohibition of Calumny

Allah, the Exalted, says:

"A slanderer, going about with calumnies." (Qur'an, Al-Qalam 68:11)

"Not a word does he (or she) utter, but there is a watcher by him ready (to record it)." (Qur'an, Qaf 50:18)

"Allah does not love the public utterance of hurtful speech unless (it be) by one to whom injustice has been done." (Qur'an, An-Nisa 4:148)

Other Verse: An-Nur 24:19.

Narrated Hudhaifah (May Allah be pleased with him): The Messenger of Allah (peace and blessings be upon him) said, "The person who goes about with calumnies will never enter Jannah." (Bukhari and Muslim)

Narrated Ibn Abbas (May Allah be pleased with him): The Prophet (peace and blessings be upon him) once passed by two graves, and those two persons (in the graves) were being tortured. He said, "They are being tortured not for a great thing (to avoid). One of them never saved himself from being soiled with his urine, while the other went about committing slander (to make enmity between friends). He then took a green leaf of a date-palm tree, split it into two pieces and fixed one on each grave. The people said, "O Allah's Messenger (peace and blessings be upon him)! Why have you done so?" He replied, "I hope that their punishment may be lessened till they (the leaf) become dry." (Bukhari)

The Prophet (May Allah's peace and blessings be upon him) told his Companions so as to warn Muslim community. The dwellers of these two graves were being tormented for sins which they could have easily avoided. One of them would not keep urine off his clothes when he urinated. Therefore, his clothes and his body would be spoiled. The other person used to spread malicious gossip. He would spread slander among people and thus create enmity and resentment, especially among friends and relatives. He would go about people and tell this person what another person had said, and then he would go and tell that person what this person had said, so he would bring about feuds and animosity between them. Meanwhile, Islam preaches love and affection, rather than disputes and broken relations among the people. However, the Prophet (May Allah's peace and blessings be upon him) felt compassion for the dwellers of the two graves. So, he took a green stalk from a palm tree, split it in two halves and inserted one on each grave. The Companions asked the Prophet (May Allah's peace and blessings be upon him) why he did such a strange thing. He said: "Perhaps Allah will decrease their torment because of my intercession for them for as long as these stalks stay moist (green)." This act was exclusive for the Prophet (May Allah's peace and blessings be upon him). (https://hadeethenc.com/en/browse/hadith/3010)

Commentary:
1. "La yastatiru min baulihi" has another meaning, namely: "he does not pass urine in privacy but does it shamelessly in the presence of other people." Obviously, shamelessness is also a sin. Talebearing, carelessness in saving oneself from splash of urine drops, and lack of observance of privacy are sins which are liable to punishment.
2. The Hadith also proves punishment in the grave. (409)

Ibn Masud (May Allah be pleased with him) said: The Prophet (peace and blessings be upon him) said, "Shall I tell you what 'Al-'Adhu' (falsehood and slandering) is? It is calumny which is committed among the people." (Muslim)

449. Prohibition of Carrying Tales of the Officers

Allah, the Exalted, says:

"... Do not help one another in sin and transgression." (Qur'an, Al-Ma'idah 5:2)

"And those who break asunder the covenant of Allah after its confirmation and cut asunder that which Allah has ordered to be joined and make mischief in the land; (as for) those, upon them shall be curse and they shall have the evil (issue) of the abode." (Qur'an, Ar-Ra'd 13:25)

"If an evildoer comes to you with a report, look carefully into it." (Qur'an, Al-Hujurat 49:6)

Ibn Masud (May Allah be pleased with him) said: The Messenger of Allah (peace and blessings be upon him) said, "None of my Companions should convey to me anything regarding another because I desire to meet every one of you with a clean heart." (Abu Dawud and Tirmidhi)

Commentary: 'Should not convey to me anything harmful' here signifies anything undesirable or which is for the person concerned... (410)

450. Arguing, Picking Apart Another's Words and Quarreling

Allah, the Exalted, says:

"But man is ever more quarrelsome than anything." (Qur'an, Al-Kahf 18:54)

"And of mankind there is he whose speech may please you (O Muhammad SAW), in this worldly life, and he calls Allah to witness as to that which is in his heart, yet he is the most quarrelsome of the opponents." (Qur'an, Al-Baqarah 2:204)

"And when he turns away (from you "O Muhammad SAW "), his effort in the land is to make mischief therein and to destroy the crops and the cattle, and Allah likes not mischief." (Qur'an, Al-Baqarah 2:205)

Other Verse: Al-Ghafir 40:4.

Narrated Aisha (May Allah be pleased with her): The Prophet (peace and blessings be upon him) said, "The most hated person in the sight of Allah is the most quarrelsome person of the opponents." (Bukhari)

451. Prohibition of Backbiting and Slander

Allah, the Exalted, says:

"O you who have believed, avoid much (negative) assumption. Indeed, some assumption is sin. And do not spy or backbite each other. Would one of you like to eat the flesh of his brother when dead? You would detest it. And fear Allah; indeed, Allah is Accepting of repentance and Merciful." (Qur'an, Al-Hujurat 49:12)

"Woe to every slanderer and backbiter." (Qur'an, Al-Humaza 104:1)

"Nay! Verily, he will be thrown into the crushing Fire." (Qur'an, Al-Humaza 104:4)

Other Verses: Al-Hujurat 49:11, An-Nur 24:16 and 24:19, Al-Isra 17:36 and 17:53, Qaf 50:18.

Abu Hurairah (May Allah be pleased with him) said: The Messenger of Allah (peace and blessings be upon him) said, "Do you know what is backbiting?" The Companions said: "Allah and His Messenger know better." Thereupon he said, "Backbiting is talking about your (Muslim) brother in a manner which he dislikes." It was said to him: "What if my (Muslim) brother is as I say." He said, "If he is actually as you say, then that is backbiting; but if that is not in him, that is slandering." (Muslim)

Anas (May Allah be pleased with him) said: The Messenger of Allah (peace and blessings be upon him) said, "During the Mi'raj (the Night of Ascension), I saw a group of people who were scratching their chests and faces with their copper nails. Jibreel replied: 'These are the people who ate flesh of others (by backbiting) and trampled people's honor." (Abu Dawud)

Commentary: "These are the people who ate flesh of others" is a metaphor for backbiting. "To trample people's honor" is akin to harming their goodwill and honor. The punishment for these things mentioned in Hadith makes their seriousness obvious. (411)

Narrated Abu Hurairah (May Allah be pleased with him): Allah's Messenger (peace and blessings be upon him) said, "Whoever has wronged his brother, should ask for his pardon (before his death), as (in the Hereafter) there will be neither a Dinar nor a Dirham. Before some of his good deeds are taken and paid to his brother, or if he has done no good deeds, some of the bad deeds of his brother are taken to be loaded on him (in the Hereafter)." (Bukhari)

Ibn Masud (May Allah be pleased with him) said: The Messenger of Allah (peace and blessings be upon him) said, "None of my Companions should convey to me anything regarding another because I desire to meet every one of you with a clean heart." (Abu Dawud and Tirmidhi)

Expiation for backbiting, slander and gossip

Everyone who does any kind of Backbiting, Slander or Malicious Gossip has to repent and pray for forgiveness, and that is between him and Allah. If he knows that any of his words reached the person about whom he was speaking, then he should go to him and ask him to forgive him. But if he does not know, then he should not tell him; rather he should pray for forgiveness for him and make Du'a (supplication) for him, and speak well of him in his absence just as he spoke against him. Similarly, if he knows that telling him will provoke more enmity, then it is sufficient to make Du'a for him, speak well of him and pray for forgiveness for him. (412)

452. Prohibition of Listening to Backbiting and Slander

Allah, the Exalted, says:

"And when they hear Al-Laghw (dirty, false, evil vain talk), they withdraw from it…" (Qur'an, Al-Qasas 28:55)

"And those who turn away from Al-Laghw (dirty, false, evil vain talk, falsehood and all that Allah has forbidden)." (Qur'an, Al-Mu'minun 23:3)

"And why did you not, when you heard it, say? "It is not right for us to speak of this. Glory be to You, O Allah! This is a great lie." (Qur'an, An-Nur 24:16)

Other Verses: *Al-Isra 17:36, Al-An'am 6:68.*

Abu Darda' (May Allah be pleased with him) said: "The Prophet (peace and blessings be upon him) said, 'He who defends the honor of his (Muslim) brother, Allah will secure his face against the Fire on the Day of Resurrection.'" (Tirmidhi)

'Itban bin Malik (May Allah be pleased with him) said in his long Hadith cited in the Chapter entitled 'Hope' reported: "When the Prophet (peace and blessings be upon him) stood up to offer As-Salat (the prayer) he asked, "Where is Malik bin Ad-Dukhshum?" A man replied: "He is a hypocrite. He does not love Allah and His Messenger." The Prophet (peace and blessings be upon him) said, "Do not say that. Do you not know that he said: 'La ilaha illallah (there is no true god except Allah)', seeking His Pleasure. Allah has made the Fire of Hell unlawful for him who affirms that none has the right to be worshipped but Allah." (Bukhari and Muslim)

Ka'b bin Malik (May Allah be pleased with him) said in his long story about his repentance: "The Prophet (peace and blessings be upon him) was sitting among the people in Tabuk. He (peace and blessings be upon him) said, "What happened to Ka'b bin Malik?" A person from the tribe of Banu Salamah said: "O Messenger of Allah! the embellishment of his cloak and an appreciation of his sides have allured him, and he was thus detained." Mu'adh bin Jabal (May Allah be pleased with him) said: "Woe be upon you! You have passed indecent remarks. O Messenger of Allah! by Allah, we know nothing about him but good." The Messenger of Allah (peace and blessings be upon him) remained silent." (Bukhari and Muslim)

Commentary:

This Hadith has already been mentioned in detail in the Chapter on Repentance. Here it is repeated to show how important it is to defend a Muslim when someone accuses him in his absence. In the presence of the Prophet (peace and blessings be upon him) a person expressed misgivings about Ka'b bin Malik that his obsession (for fine dress) had prevented him from coming to the battlefield. Mu'adh immediately defended him saying that there was no justification for such misgivings. The Prophet's silence endorsed the stand taken by Mu'adh (May Allah be pleased with him). This goes to prove that if a Muslim brother or sister is disgraced in his or her absence in a gathering, then it is incumbent on others to defend his or her honor. (413)

452a. Some Cases where it is Permissible to Backbite

Backbiting is permissible only for valid reasons approved by Shariah. These reasons are as follows:

1- It is permissible for an oppressed person to speak before the judge or someone in a similar position of authority to help him or her establish his or her rights by telling him 'so-and-so wronged me and has done such and such to me', etc.

2- It is permissible to seek somebody's assistance in forbidding evil and helping someone change his or her immoral conduct. One can say to the person who can offer such assistance, 'so-and-so does such and such evil deeds. Can you exhort him?', etc. This is permissible as long as one intends to forbid evil. If, however, one intends something else apart from this, then this act becomes unlawful.

3- One who seeks legal verdict on a certain matter may point out the defaults of another person or relate something else. One in this case can say to the Mufti (religious scholar who issues verdicts): "My father or brother (for example) treated me unjustly. Can I get my right established?", etc. This is permissible to say only if you need be, but it is better to say 'What do you think of someone who did such and such?' This does not mean, however, that naming the person in question is not legal.

4- One who criticizes those who openly commit acts of disobedience, such as drinking wine, gambling, engaging in immoral habits, fornication, hypocrisy and making mischief.

5- It is permissible to call into question the narrators of Hadith and witnesses in the court when the need arises. It is also right to mention the bad qualities of somebody for marriage purposes in case an advice is sought. Also, if one has noticed that a "seeker of knowledge" frequently goes to the gatherings of an innovator in religion and one fears that this "seeker of knowledge" may be affected by this so-called scholar, then he must in this case give counsel to the "seeker of knowledge" by telling him about the "innovator", etc.

6- It is such permissible to use names such as "Al-a'mash" which means 'the blear-eyed' to talk about people who are known by names for the sake of identification and not for disparaging people and underestimating them. To identify them without resorting to such names is however better.

Aisha (May Allah be pleased with her) said: "A man sought permission for an audience with the Prophet (peace and blessings be upon him). He said, "Give him permission but he is a bad member of his tribe." (Bukhari and Muslim)

Fatima bint Qais (May Allah be pleased with her) said: "I came to the Prophet (peace and blessings be upon him) and said to him: 'Muawiyah and Abul-Jahm sent me a proposal of marriage.' The Messenger of Allah (peace and blessings be upon him) said, 'Muawiyah is destitute and he has no property, and Abul-Jahm is very hard on women.'" (Bukhari and Muslim)

Zaid bin Al-Arqam (May Allah be pleased with him) said: "We set out on a journey along with the Messenger of Allah (peace and blessings be upon him) and we faced many hardships. 'Abdullah bin Ubaiy (the chief of the hypocrites at Al-Madinah) said to his friends: "Do not spend on those who are with the Messenger of Allah (peace and blessings be upon him) until they desert him." He also said: "If we return to Al-Madinah, the more honorable (meaning himself, i.e. Abdullah bin Ubaiy) will drive out therefrom the meaner (meaning Messenger of Allah, peace be upon him)." I went to the Messenger of Allah (peace be upon him) and informed him about that and he sent someone to 'Abdullah bin Ubaiy. He asked him whether he had said that or not. Abdullah took an oath that he had not done anything of that sort and said that it was Zaid who carried a false tale to the Messenger of Allah (peace be upon him).

Zaid said: "I was so much perturbed because of this until this Verse was revealed verifying my statement: *"When the hypocrites come to you (O Muhammad, peace and blessings be upon him), they say: 'We bear witness that you are indeed the Messenger of Allah.' Allah knows that you are indeed His Messenger, and Allah bears witness that the hypocrites are liars indeed." (63:1)* Then the Messenger of Allah (peace and blessings be upon him) called the hypocrites in order to seek forgiveness for them from Allah, but they turned away their heads." (Bukhari and Muslim)

Aisha (May Allah be pleased with her) said: "Hind, the wife of Abu Sufyan, said to the Prophet (peace and blessings be upon him): 'Abu Sufyan is a niggardly man and does not give me and my children adequate provisions for maintenance unless I take something from his possession without his knowledge.' The Prophet (peace and blessings be upon him) said to her, "Take from his possessions on a reasonable basis that much which may suffice for you and your children." (Bukhari and Muslim)

Commentary: Hind was the mother of Mu'awiyah (May Allah be pleased with him). Along with her husband, Abu Sufyan, she embraced Islam in the year of conquest of Makkah.

We learn from this Hadith that:

1. In order to know religious injunctions, husband and wife can mention each other's shortcomings before a Mufti (a religious scholar who is in a position to issue verdicts on religious matters).

2. If a husband does not give his wife enough money to cover the domestic expenses, then it is permissible for his wife to take some of his money without his permission, provided the amount thus taken is for essential expenses not for superfluous matters. (414)

453. Ascertainment of What One Hears and Narrates

Allah, the Exalted, says:

"O you who believe! If a Faasiq (liar - evil person) comes to you with any news, verify it, lest you should harm people in ignorance, and afterwards you become regretful for what you have done." (Qur'an, Al-Hujurat 49:6)

Narrated Abu Hurairah (May Allah be pleased with him): The Prophet (peace and blessings be upon him) said, "It is enough for a man to prove himself a liar when he goes on narrating whatever he hears." (Muslim)

Narrated Samurah (May Allah be pleased with him): The Messenger of Allah (peace and blessings be upon him) said, "He who relates from me something which he deems false is one of the liars." (Muslim)

Narrated Asma (May Allah be pleased with her): "A woman came to the Messenger of Allah (peace and blessings be upon him) and said: "I have a co-wife. Is there any harm for me if I give her the false impression of getting something from my husband which he has not in fact given me?" The Messenger of Allah (peace and blessings be upon him) said, "The one who creates a false impression of receiving what one has not been given is like one who wears two garments of falsehood." (Bukhari and Muslim)

Commentary: Some people disguise themselves as pious to create a false impression of their piety; some put up the appearance of scholars to establish their scholarship; and some take to highly expensive clothes to give the impression of being rich. Since these things are fabricated and false, they constitute great sins. One should live as one really is. Similarly, the second wife should not invent false stories to give wrong impression of herself to the other wife. Nor should make false claims of greater love and attention of the husband only to incite the jealousy of the other one while the real position is far from that. In fact, even if this is so, she should not expose the weakness of the husband so that the feelings of his other wife are not injured. (415)

454. Useless Talk or Talk too Much About Others

Allah, the Exalted, says:

"No Laghw (dirty, false, evil vain talk) will they hear therein, nor any sinful speech (like backbiting, etc.)." (Qur'an, Al-Waqi'ah 56:25)

"And those who turn away from Al-Laghw (dirty, false, evil vain talk, falsehood and all that Allah has forbidden)." (Qur'an, Al-Mu'minun 23:3)

The Laghw (unnecessary, useless and idle speech and actions) kills heart.

Narrated Al-Mughira bin Shuba (May Allah be pleased with him): The Prophet (peace and blessings be upon him) said, "Allah has forbidden for you: 1) to be undutiful to your mothers, 2) to bury your daughters alive, 3) do not to pay the rights of the others (e.g. charity, etc.) and 4) to beg of men (begging). And Allah has hated for you: 1) Qil and Qal (useless talk or that you talk too much about others), 2) to ask too many questions (in disputed religious matters) and 3) to waste the wealth (by extravagance with lack of wisdom and thinking)." (Bukhari)

Ibn 'Umar (May Allah be pleased with him) reported: The Messenger of Allah (peace and blessings of Allah be upon him) said, "Do not indulge in excessive talk except when remembering Allah. Excessive talking without the Remembrance of Allah hardens the heart; and those who are the farthest from Allah are those whose hearts are hard." (Tirmidhi)

455. Anger

Allah, the Exalted, says:

"Those who spend (in Allah's Cause - deeds of charity, alms, etc.) in prosperity and in adversity, who repress anger, and who pardon men; verily, Allah loves Al-Muhsinun (the good doers)." (Qur'an, Ali 'Imran 3:134)

"Those who have believed and whose hearts are assured by the remembrance of Allah. Unquestionably, by the remembrance of Allah hearts are assured." (Qur'an, Ar-Ra'd 13:28)

Sulayman ibn Surad (May Allah be pleased with him) reported: "While I was sitting with the Prophet (May Allah's peace and blessings be upon him), two men began to insult each other, and the face of one of them turned red and the veins of his neck got swollen. The Messenger of Allah (May Allah's peace and blessings be upon him) said: "I know a word that if he said, his rage would go away. If he said, 'I seek refuge with Allah from the accursed Devil', his rage would subside." So, they said to him: "The Prophet (May Allah's peace and blessings be upon him) tells you to seek refuge with Allah from the accursed Devil." (Bukhari and Muslim) (https://hadeethenc.com/en/browse/hadith/3578)

Narrated Abu Hurairah (May Allah be pleased with him): "A man said to the Prophet (peace and blessings be upon him): "Advise me!" The Prophet (peace and blessings be upon him) said, "Do not become angry and furious." The man asked (the same) again and again, and the Prophet (peace and blessings be upon him) said in each case, "Do not become angry and furious." (Bukhari)

Narrated Abu Hurairah (May Allah be pleased with him): Allah's Messenger (peace and blessings be upon him) said, "The strong is not the one who overcomes the people by his strength, but the strong is the one who controls himself while in anger." (Bukhari)

Narrated Atiyyah as-Sa'di (May Allah be pleased with him): AbuWa'il al-Qass said: "We entered upon Urwah ibn Muhammad ibn as-Sa'di. A man spoke to him and made him angry. So, he stood and performed ablution; he then returned and performed ablution, and said: 'My father told me on the authority of my grandfather Atiyyah who reported the Apostle of Allah (peace and blessings be upon him) as saying: 'Anger comes from the Devil, the Devil was created of fire, and fire is extinguished only with water; so, when one of you becomes angry, he should perform ablution.'" (Abu Dawud)

Narrated Abu Dharr (May Allah be pleased with him): The Apostle of Allah (peace and blessings be upon him) said to us: "When one of you becomes angry while standing, he should sit down. If the anger leaves him, well and good; otherwise he should lie down." (Abu Dawud)

Narrated Abdullah bin Amr (May Allah be pleased with him): The Prophet (peace and blessings be upon him) said: "The Lord's Pleasure is in the parent's pleasure, and the Lord's Anger is in the parent's anger." (Tirmidhi)

Muʿadh ibn Anas (May Allah be pleased with him) reported that the Prophet (May Allah's peace and blessings be upon him) said: "Whoever suppresses his rage while being able to vent it, Allah, Glorified and Exalted, will call him before the entire creation on the Day of Judgment so that he can choose whomever of the houris he wishes to have." (Ibn Majah) (https://hadeethenc.com/en/browse/hadith/3287)

Abu Hurairah (May Allah be pleased with him) reported: The Messenger of Allah (peace and blessings be upon him) said, "When a man calls his wife to his bed, and she does not respond, and he (the husband) spends the night angry with her, the angels curse her until morning." (Bukhari and Muslim)

Narrated Samurah ibn Jundub (May Allah be pleased with him): The Prophet (peace and blessings be upon him) said: "Do not invoke Allah's Curse, Allah's Anger or Hell." (Abu Dawud)

When a person does not restrain his anger, he insults, curses, swears and hits. Anger is a door to all kinds of evils. Shaytan enters easily into human body in the state of anger.

Narrated Abu Hurairah (May Allah be pleased with him): The Prophet (peace and blessings be upon him) said, "Allah, the Exalted, becomes angry, and His Anger becomes provoked when a person does what Allah has declared unlawful." (Bukhari and Muslim)

Narrated Abu Hurairah (May Allah be pleased with him) that Aisha (May Allah be pleased with her) said:

"I noticed the Prophet (peace and blessings be upon him) was not there one night, so I started looking for him with my hand. My hand touched his feet and they were held upright, and he (peace and blessings be upon him) was prostrating saying: 'I seek refuge in Your Pleasure from Your Anger, in Your Forgiveness from Your Punishment, and I seek refuge in You from You. I cannot praise You enough, You are as You have praised Yourself.'" (An-Nasa'i)

Narrated Abu Ad-Dardh (May Allah be pleased with him): The Messenger of Allah (peace and blessings of Allah be upon him) said: "Nothing is heavier on the believer's scale on the Day of Judgment than good character. For indeed Allah, Most High, is angered by the shameless obscene person." (Tirmidhi)

Narrated Abu Hurairah (May Allah be pleased with him): Allah's Apostle (peace and blessings be upon him) said, "When Allah completed the creation, He wrote in His Book which is with Him on His Throne, "My Mercy overpowers My Anger." (Bukhari)

456. Harming and Insulting Others

Allah, the Exalted, warns:

"O you who believe! Let not a group scoff at another group, it may be that the latter are better than the former; nor let (some) women scoff at other women, it may be that the latter are better than the former, nor defame one another, nor insult one another by nicknames. How bad is it, to insult one's brother after having faith [i.e. to call your Muslim brother (a faithful believer) as: "O sinner" or "O wicked", etc.]. And whosoever does not repent, then such are indeed Zalimun (wrongdoers, etc.)." (Qur'an, Al-Hujurat 49:11)

"And tell My servants to say that which is best. Indeed, Satan induces (dissension) among them. Indeed, Satan is ever, to mankind, a clear enemy." (Qur'an, Al-Isra 17:53)

Abu Sa'id al-Khudri (May Allah be pleased with him) reported that the Prophet (May Allah's peace and blessings be upon him) said: ''There should be neither harm nor reciprocating harm." (Ibn Majah)

(https://hadeethenc.com/en/browse/hadith/4711)

Narrated 'Abdullah (May Allah be pleased with him): The Messenger of Allah (peace and blessings be upon him) said: "The believer does not insult the honor of others, nor curse, nor commit Fahisha, nor is he foul." (Tirmidhi)

Narrated 'Abdullah bin 'Amr (May Allah be pleased with him): The Prophet (peace and blessings be upon him) said, "A Muslim is the one who avoids harming Muslims with his tongue and hands. And a Muhajir (emigrant) is the one who gives up (abandons) all what Allah has forbidden." (Bukhari)

Ibn Masud (May Allah be pleased with him) reported that the Prophet (May Allah's peace and blessings be upon him) said: "There is nothing heavier on the scale than good manners. Indeed, Allah detests the one who is indecent and foulmouthed." Abu Ad-Darda (May Allah be pleased with him) reported that the Prophet (May Allah's peace and blessings be upon him) said: "A believer is neither a slanderer or an invoker of curse, nor is he indecent or foulmouthed." (Tirmidhi) (https://hadeethenc.com/en/browse/hadith/5371)

457. Prohibition of Cursing one Particular Man or Animal

Narrated Abu Zaid Thabit bin Ad-Dahhak Al-Ansari (May Allah be pleased with him) (he is one of those who gave their pledge of allegiance to the Messenger of Allah (peace and blessings be upon him) under the Tree): The Messenger of Allah (peace and blessings be upon him) said, "He who swears by a religion other than that of Islam, is like what he has professed. He who kills himself with something, will be tormented with it on the Day of Resurrection. A person is not bound to fulfill a vow about something which he does not possess. Cursing a believer is like murdering him." (Bukhari and Muslim)

Narrated Abud-Darda' (May Allah be pleased with him): The Messenger of Allah (peace and blessings be upon him) said, "Those who frequently resort to cursing (people) would neither be accepted as witnesses nor as intercessors on the Day of Resurrection." (Muslim)

Samurah bin Jundub (May Allah be pleased with him): The Messenger of Allah (peace and blessings be upon him) said, "Do not curse one another, invoking Curse of Allah or Wrath of Allah, or the fire of Hell." (Abu Dawud and Tirmidhi)

Ibn Masud (May Allah be pleased with him): The Messenger of Allah (peace and blessings be upon him) said, "A true believer is not involved in taunting or frequently cursing (others), or in indecency, or abusing." (Tirmidhi)

Narrated Abud-Darda' (May Allah be pleased with him): The Messenger of Allah (peace and blessings be upon him) said, "When a person curses somebody or something, the curse ascends to heaven and the gates of heaven are closed against it. Then it descends to earth and its gates are closed against it. and its gates get closed. Then it turns right and left and when it finds no exit it returns to what was cursed if it deserves to be cursed; otherwise, it rebounds to the one who uttered it." (Abu Dawud)

(https://hadeethenc.com/en/browse/hadith/6986)

Narrated 'Imran bin Husain (May Allah be pleased with him) said: "We were with the Messenger of Allah (peace and blessings be upon him) on a journey and there was a woman from the Ansar riding a she-camel. She abused and invoked curse upon it. The Messenger of Allah (peace be upon him) heard it and said, "Off load the she-camel and set it free because it has been cursed." (Muslim)

Narrated Abu Barzah Nadlah bin 'Ubaid Al-Aslami (May Allah be pleased with him): "A young woman was riding a she-camel on which there was the luggage of people. Suddenly she saw the Prophet (peace be upon him). The pass of the mountain became narrow for her people (because of fear). The young woman said to the she-camel: "Go ahead." When it did not move, she said, "O Allah! Curse it." The Prophet (peace be upon him) said, "The she-camel that has been cursed should not accompany us." (Muslim)

Commentary: This Hadith proves that it is not legal to associate with people who are given to sins and heresies in religion because they have been cursed. When one is not permitted to keep an animal which has been cursed, how can one possibly keep company with people who commit acts as a result of which they have been cursed. (416)

457a. Justification of Cursing the Wrongdoers Without Specifying One of Them

Narrated Abu Barzah Nadlah bin 'Ubaid Al-Aslami (May Allah be pleased with him): "A young woman was riding a she-camel on which there was the luggage of people. Suddenly she saw the Prophet (peace and blessings be upon him). The pass of the mountain became narrow for her people (because of fear). The young woman said to the she-camel: "Go ahead." When it did not move, she said, "O Allah! Curse it." The Prophet (peace and blessings be upon him) said, "The she-camel that has been cursed should not accompany us." (Muslim)

Commentary: Some people have taken this Hadith to mean that the she-camel cursed by the young woman was abandoned there and it was neither used for transport nor conveyance, as was the practice in the pre-Islamic period with she-camels which were let loose for free pasture for the polytheists' false gods, and nothing was allowed to be carried on them. Such she-camels were called as "As-Sa'ibah" There is no justification for such interpretation because the she-camel was not set absolutely free like As-Sa'ibah. All that was done was that because of the curse, it was considered unworthy of the entourage company of the Prophet (peace and blessings be upon him). Except for this bar, it was valid for all other purposes. Thus, this Hadith proves that it is not permissible to associate with people who are given to sins and heresies in religion because they have been cursed. When one is not permitted to keep an animal which has been cursed, how can one possibly keep company with people who commit acts as a result of which they have been cursed. (417)

458. Prohibition of Invoking the Curse or Wrath of Allah

Allah, the Exalted, says,

"And were Allah to hasten for mankind the evil (they invoke for themselves and for their children, while in a state of anger) as He hastens for them the good (they invoke) then they would have been ruined. So, We leave those who expect not their Meeting with Us, in their trespasses, wandering blindly in distraction." (Qur'an, Yunus 10:11)

"And if you punish (your enemy, O you believers in the Oneness of Allah), then punish them with the like of that with which you were afflicted. But if you endure patiently, verily, it is better for As-Sabirin (the patient ones, etc.)." (Qur'an, An-Nahl 16:126)

"Then He showed him what is wrong for him and what is right for him…" (Qur'an, Ash-Shams 91:8)

Abu Ad-Darda (May Allah be pleased with him) reported that the Prophet (May Allah's peace and blessings be upon him) said: "When a person curses something, the curse ascends to heaven and the gates of Heaven are closed against it. Then it descends to earth and its gates are closed against it. Then it turns right and left and when it finds no exit it returns to what was cursed if it deserves to be cursed; otherwise, it rebounds to the one who uttered it." (Abu Dawud)

Jabir ibn Abdullah (May Allah be pleased with him) reported: The Messenger of Allah (peace and blessings be upon him) said, "Do not supplicate against yourselves, do not supplicate against your children, and do not supplicate against your wealth, lest it coincide with a time in which Allah is asked and He gives and your supplication is answered." (Muslim)

Narrated Abu Sa'id al-Khudri (May Allah be pleased with him) said: The Messenger of Allah (peace and blessings of Allah be upon him) came out on Eid Al-Adha or Eid Al-Fitr to the prayer place, and he went to the women and said: "O women, give in charity, for I have seen that you are the majority of the people of Hell." They said: "Why, O Messenger of Allah?" He replied: "You curse frequently and are ungrateful to your husbands. I have not seen anyone more deficient in intelligence and religion than you. A keen sensible man could be led astray by some of you." The women asked, "O Allah's Messenger (peace be upon him)! What is deficient in our intelligence and religion?" He said, "Is not the evidence of two women equal to the witness of one man?" They replied in the affirmative. He said, "This is the deficiency in her intelligence, isn't." (Bukhari and Muslim)

Narrated Abu Hurairah (May Allah be pleased with him): It was said to Allah's Messenger (peace and blessings of Allah be upon him): "Invoke curse upon the polytheists", whereupon, he said: "I have not been sent as the invoker of curse, but I have been sent as mercy." (Muslim)

However, in cases of oppression, whether by men or Jinns, it becomes allowable based on the Prophet's own practice in this case.

Narrated Abu ad-Darda (May Allah have mercy on him): The Prophet (peace and blessings be upon him) said thrice to a Devil who wanted to break his Salah, "I seek refuge in Allah from you! I curse you by Allah's perfect Curse!" (Muslim)

The use of a curse in this case is similar to a curse used to repel the oppressive and sinful disbelievers among mankind. The Prophet also cursed a tribe in Najd when a group of forty Qur'anic reciters whom he had sent to teach them at their request were ambushed and massacred in the 4th year after the migration. (Bukhari (Arabic-English), vol.2, p.61-62, Hadith no. 116; Saheeh Muslim (English Trans.), vol.1, p.329-331, Hadith no. 1433 and The Life of Muhammad, p. 433- 434) (10)

459. Ignorance

Allah, the Exalted, says:

"Keep to forgiveness (O Muhammad) and enjoin kindness, and turn away from the ignorant." (Qur'an, Al-A'raf 7:199)

"Allah accepts only the repentance of those who do evil in ignorance and foolishness, and repent soon afterwards." (Qur'an, An-Nisa 4:17)

"Shaytan wants only to incite enmity and hatred between you with intoxicants (alcoholic drinks) and gambling, and hinder you from the remembrance of Allah and from as-Salah (the prayer). So, will you not then abstain?" (Qur'an, Al-Ma'idah 5:91)

Other Verses: Al-An'am 6:19, An-Nahl 16:125.

Abdullah ibn 'Amr ibn al-'As (May Allah be pleased with him) reported that the Prophet (May Allah's peace and blessings be upon him) said: "Convey (my teachings) to the people even one Verse, and narrate from the Children of Israel (which have been taught to you), and there is no sin in that. And whoever intentionally tells a lie against me, let him assume his seat in Hellfire." (Bukhari)
(https://hadeethenc.com/en/browse/hadith/3686)

Abu 'Abdur-Rahman Abdullah ibn Masud (May Allah be pleased with him) said: "It is as though I am looking at Allah's Messenger as he tells the story of one of the Prophets (peace be upon them) as his people struck him and caused him to bleed, and he wiped the blood from his face, saying: 'Allah, forgive my people for they do not know.'" (Bukhari and Muslim)

(https://hadeethenc.com/en/browse/hadith/3594)

Jabir (May Allah be pleased with him) reported: "We set out on a journey. One of our people was hit by a stone that injured his head. He then had a wet dream. He asked his fellow travelers: "Do you find a concession for me to perform Tayammum?" They said: "We do not find any concession for you since water is available to you." He, thus, took a bath and died (as a result). When we came to the Prophet (May Allah's peace and blessings be upon him) the incident was reported to him. He said: "They killed him, may Allah kill them! Why had they not asked when they did not know? The cure for ignorance is inquiry. It would have been enough for him to perform Tayammum and to press – or bind – a cloth over his wound then wipe with wet hands over it and wash the rest of his body." (Abu Dawud)

(https://hadeethenc.com/en/browse/hadith/10019)

Ignorance is the absence of knowledge - is a source of everything contrary to Islam (Deen) as knowledge.

Ignorance is the reason for sin and it incites sin and leads to it. The cure for ignorance is to question and to learn.

Jabir (May Allah have mercy on him) reported: The Messenger of Allah (peace and blessings be upon him) said, "Verily, the only cure for ignorance is to ask questions." (Abu Dawud)

Ibn al-Qayyim (May Allah have mercy on him) said in his Ash-Shaafiyatul-Kaafiyah:

"Ignorance is a fatal malady and its cure is in two things in agreement: A text from the Qur'an or from the Sunnah, and a physician possessing knowledge of the Deen."

Qatadah (May Allah have mercy on him) said: "The companions of the Messenger of Allah (peace and blessings be upon him) agreed that everything by which Allah is disobeyed is ignorance." (418)

The Prophet (peace and blessings of Allah be upon him) sent his Companions as teachers and conveyors of glad tidings and warnings. If leaving the people in ignorance was acceptable, the Messengers would not have been sent, the Books would not have been sent down and the callers would not have been charged with their duty. (419)

No one should imagine that leaving the ignorant in their ignorance is permissible. No rational person would say this, let alone any scholar. The fact that Allah may excuse the ignorant person whose ignorance is not the result of negligence does not mean that the scholar should refrain from doing what he has been commanded to do of conveying and explaining.

Allah, the Exalted, says:

"(And remember) when Allah took a covenant from those who were given the Scripture (Jews and Christians) to make it (the news of the coming of Prophet Muhammad, peace and blessings be upon him) and the religious knowledge) known and clear to mankind, and not to hide it." (Qur'an, Ali 'Imran 3:187)

"They know only the outside appearance of the life of the world (i.e. the matters of their livelihood, like irrigating or sowing, or reaping), and they are heedless of the Hereafter." (Qur'an, Ar-Rum 30:7)

"When it is said to them: "Follow what Allah has sent down." They say: "Nay! We shall follow what we found our fathers following." (Would they do that!) Even though their fathers did not understand anything nor were they guided?" (Qur'an, Al-Baqarah 2:170)

It should be noted that if the ignorant person finds someone who can teach him, but he falls short and is negligent, then he is sinning because he has not learnt what he was required to learn and he is not excused, whether the matter has to do with belief, acts of worship or interactions with others. Hence Allah criticized the heedless people who know about their worldly matters but are ignorant of their religion.

460. Seeing Oneself as Superior to Others in Any Way

Allah, the Exalted, says:

"I am greater than you in wealth and mightier in (numbers of) men. And he entered his garden while he was unjust to himself. He said, "I do not think that this will perish - ever. And I do not think the Hour will occur." (Qur'an, Al-Kahf 18:34-36)

"Wealth and children are the adornment of the life of this world. But the good righteous deeds (five compulsory prayers, deeds of Allah's obedience, good and nice talk, remembrance of Allah with glorification, praises and thanks, etc.), that last, are better with your Lord for rewards and better in respect of hope." (Qur'an, Al-Kahf 18:46)

"(Allah) said: "What prevented you (O Iblees) that you did not prostrate, when I commanded you?" Iblees said: "I am better than him (Adam), You created me from fire, and him You created from clay." (Qur'an, Al-A'raf 7:12)

Other Verses: *Taha 20:131, Al-Hujurat 49:13, An-Nisa 4:1.*

Ibn 'Umar (May Allah be pleased with him) reported: The Messenger of Allah (May Allah's peace and blessings be upon him) delivered a speech on the day of the Conquest of Makkah. He said: "O people, verily Allah has removed the arrogance of the Jahiliyyah from you and their boastfulness about their ancestry. So, now there are two types of people: a righteous, pious and honorable person in the sight of Allah, and a wicked, miserable and insignificant person in the sight of Allah. People are the children of Adam, and Allah created Adam from dust. Allah says: *"O mankind, We have created you from a male and a female, and made you into nations and tribes so that you may recognize one another. Indeed, the most noble of you before Allah is the most righteous among you. Indeed, Allah is All-Knowing, All-Aware." (Surah Al-Hujurat 49:13).* (Tirmidhi) (https://hadeethenc.com/en/browse/hadith/65074)

The Messenger of Allah (peace and blessings be upon him) mentioned in a sermon he delivered during the days of Hajj: "O People! Certainly, your Rabb is One, your father is one. An Arab has no virtue over a Non-Arab, nor does a Non-Arab have virtue over an Arab, a red skinned person is not more virtuous than a dark-skinned person nor is a dark-skinned person more virtuous than a red skinned person except through Taqwa." (Ahmad) (https://hadithanswers.com/virtue-is-based-on-taqwa-and-not-ethnicity)

Safiyyah (May Allah be pleased with her), the wife of the Prophet (peace and blessings be upon him) came to know that Hafsah (May Allah be pleased with her) had said about her that she is the daughter of a Jew. When the Prophet (peace and blessings be upon him) met her, she was weeping. So, he asked, "Why are you weeping?" She replied, "Hafsah said that I am the daughter of a Jew." The Prophet (peace and blessings be upon him) said: "You are the daughter of a Prophet (Harun, peace be upon him), and your uncle was a Prophet as well (Musa, peace be upon him] and you are the wife of a Prophet, so what is she boasting about?" Then the Prophet (peace and blessings be upon him) told Hafsah, "O Hafsah! Fear Allah!" (Tirmidhi)

Narrated Abu Hurairah (May Allah have mercy on him): The Prophet (peace and blessings be upon him) said: "Verily, Allah does not look at your appearance or wealth, but rather He looks at your hearts and actions." (Muslim)

Narrated 'Uthman (May Allah have mercy on him): The Prophet (peace and blessings be upon him) said, "The best among you (Muslims) are those who learn the Qur'an and teach it." (Bukhari)

461. Disputes and the Virtue of Reconciling Between Two Disputing Parties

Allah, the Exalted, says:

"And obey Allah and His Messenger, and do not dispute (with one another) lest you lose courage and your strength departs, and be patient. Surely, Allah is with those who are As-Sabirun (the patient)." (Qur'an, Al-Anfal 8:46)

"And hold fast, all of you together, to the Rope of Allah (i.e. this Qur'an), and be not divided among yourselves, and remember Allah's Favour on you, for you were enemies one to another but He joined your hearts together, so that, by His Grace, you became brethren (in Islamic Faith), and you were on the brink of a pit of Fire, and He saved you from it. Thus, Allah makes His Ayat (proofs, evidences, verses, lessons, signs, revelations, etc.) clear to you, that you may be guided." (Qur'an, Ali 'Imran 3:103)

Narrated Umm Kulthum bint 'Uqba (May Allah have mercy on her) that she heard Allah's Messenger (peace and blessings of Allah be upon him) saying, "He who makes peace between the people by inventing good information or saying good things, is not a liar." (Bukhari)

Narrated Sahl bin Sad (May Allah have mercy on him): Once the people of Quba fought with each other till they threw stones on each other. When Allah's Apostle (peace and blessings be upon him) was informed about it, he said, "Let us go to bring about a reconciliation between them." (Bukhari)

Narrated Abu Hurairah (May Allah be pleased with him): The Prophet (peace and blessings of Allah be upon him) said: "The gates of Paradise are opened on Monday and Thursday, and everyone who does not associate anything with Allah is forgiven, except a man who has had an argument with his brother. It is said: 'Wait for these two until they reconcile, wait for these two until they reconcile, wait for these two until they reconcile." (Muslim)

Abu Khirash Hadrad al-Aslami (May Allah be pleased with him) reported that the Prophet (May Allah's peace and blessings be upon him) said: "Whoever forsakes his brother for a year is like shedding his blood." (Abu Dawud) (https://hadeethenc.com/en/browse/hadith/8885)

Narrated Abu Darda' (May Allah have mercy on him): The Prophet (peace and blessings be upon him) said, "Shall I not tell you something that is better than the status of (voluntary) fasting, prayer and charity?" They said: 'Yes.' He said: 'Reconciling in a case of discord, for the evil of discord is the shaver.' At-Tirmidhi said: 'It was narrated that the Prophet (peace and blessings of Allah be upon him) said: 'It is the shaver, and I do not say that it shaves hair, but that it shaves (i.e. destroys) religious commitment.'" (Abu Dawud and Tirmidhi)

462. Debt

Allah, the Exalted, says:

"O you who believe! When you contract a debt for a fixed period, write it down. Let a scribe write it down in justice between you. Let not the scribe refuse to write as Allah has taught him, so let him write. Let him (the debtor) who incurs the liability dictate, and he must fear Allah, his Lord, and diminish not anything of what he owes. But if the debtor is of poor understanding or weak, or is unable himself to dictate, then let his guardian dictate in justice. And get two witnesses out of your own men. And if there are not two men (available), then a man and two women, such as you agree for witnesses, so that if one of them (two women) errs, the other can remind her. And the witnesses should not refuse when they are called on (for evidence). You should not become weary to write it (your contract), whether it be small or big, for its fixed term, that is more just with Allah; more solid as evidence, and more convenient to prevent doubts among yourselves, save when it is a present trade which you carry out on the spot among yourselves, then there is no sin on you if you do not write it down. But take witnesses whenever you make a commercial contract. Let neither scribe nor witness suffer any harm, but if you do (such harm), it would be wickedness in you. So be afraid of Allah; and Allah teaches you. And Allah is the All-Knower of each and everything." (Qur'an, Al-Baqarah 2:282)

"If the debtor is in a difficulty, grant him time till it is easy for him to repay. But if you remit it by way of charity, that is best for you if you only knew." (Qur'an, Al-Baqarah 2:280)

Narrated Samurah (May Allah have mercy on him): The Messenger of Allah (peace and blessings be upon him) addressed us and said: "...Your companion has been detained (from entering Paradise) on account of his debt. Then I saw him that he paid off all his debt on his behalf, and there remained no one to demand from him anything." (Abu Dawud)

Hudhayfah (May Allah have mercy on him) reported: The Messenger of Allah (peace and blessings be upon him) said: "There was a man in the past who was about to die. The Angel asked him: 'Have you ever did any good?' He replied: 'I am unaware of such.' He was told to think again after which he said: 'I don't know of anything (good that I did) besides the fact that I would be lenient when dealing with people; I would give time to the one who could still afford and waive (the debt of) the one who couldn't afford it.' Allah, the Exalted, admitted this person to Jannah." (Bukhari)

Abdullah ibn 'Umar (May Allah have mercy on him) related that the Prophet (peace and blessings be upon him) was asked, "O Messenger of Allah, which of the people are most beloved to Allah, and which deeds are most beloved to Allah?" The Messenger of Allah (peace and blessings be upon him) said: "The people most beloved to Allah are those who are most beneficial to the people; and the most beloved deed to Allah is to make a Muslim happy or remove one of his troubles, or to fulfill his debt, or to satiate his hunger. Walking to fulfill a need of my Muslim brother is more beloved to me than sitting in i'tikaf in a Masjid for two months. Whomsoever averts his anger, Allah will conceal his faults and whomsoever suppresses his anger while he is able to vent it, Allah will fill his heart with happiness. Whoever walks with his brother to fulfill his need and fulfills it for him, then Allah the Almighty will make his footing firm (on the bridge) on the Day when the footings are shaken. Evil character spoils one's deeds just as vinegar spoils honey." (Imam Abu Bakr Ibn Abid Dunya (May Allah have mercy on him) has recorded this narration. (Qada-ul Hawaij, Hadith: 36) (https://hadithanswers.com/a-hadith-encouraging-fulfilling-the-needs-of-a-muslim)

Abu Musa Al Ash'ari (May Allah have mercy on him) reported that the Messenger of Allah (peace and blessings be upon him) said: "Among the greatest of sins in Allah's sight which a man commits, after the Major sins which Allah has prohibited, is that a man should die while in debt, without making any (arrangement) for it to be paid off." (Ahmad)

Abu Hurairah (May Allah have mercy on him) reported that the Messenger of Allah (peace and blessings be upon him) said: "A Believer's soul is suspended as long as he has a debt." (Ahmad)

Abu Hurairah (May Allah be pleased with him) reported that the Messenger of Allah (May Allah's peace and blessings be upon him) mentioned that a man from the Children of Israel asked another to lend him one thousand dinars. The man asked him to bring witnesses. The former replied: "Allah is sufficient as witness." The second said: "Bring me a surety." The former replied: "Allah is sufficient as surety." The man said: "You are right", and lent him the money for a certain period. The first man went across the sea. When he finished his job, he searched for a conveyance so that he might reach the other in time for the repayment of the debt, but he could not find any. So, he took a piece of wood and made a hole in it, inserted one thousand dinars and a letter to the lender in it, and then firmly closed (i.e. sealed) the hole. He took the piece of wood to the sea and said: "O Allah, You know well that I took a loan of one thousand dinars from so-and-so. He demanded a surety from me, but I told him that Allah's guarantee was sufficient, and he accepted Your guarantee. He then asked for a witness, and I told him that Allah was sufficient as witness, and he accepted You as Witness. No doubt, I tried hard to find a conveyance so that I could give him his money, but I could not find any, so I hand over this money to You." Saying that, he threw the piece of wood into the sea till it went out far into it, and then he went away. Meanwhile, he started searching for a conveyance in order to reach the creditor's country. One day, the lender came out to see whether a ship had arrived bringing his money, when all of a sudden, he saw the piece of wood in which his money had been deposited. He took it home to use it for fire. When he sawed it, he found his money and the letter inside it. Shortly after that, the debtor came, bringing one thousand dinars to him, and he said: "By Allah, I had been trying hard to find a boat so that I could send you your money, but I failed to find one before the one I have come by." The lender asked: "Have you sent something to me?" The debtor replied: "I told you I could not find a boat other than the one I have come by." The lender said: "Allah has delivered the money which you sent in the piece of wood on your behalf. So, you may keep your one thousand dinars and depart while being guided on the Straight Path." (Bukhari)

Abu Qatadah (May Allah have mercy on him) once demanded payment from his debtor who then disappeared. Abu Qatadah (May Allah have mercy on him) located him and (the debtor) said:

"I am unable to pay." After taking an oath from him that he is unable to pay, Abu Qatadah (May Allah have mercy on him) said, "I heard the Messenger of Allah (peace and blessings be upon him) say:

'Whomsoever wishes that Allah save him from the torments of the Day of Qiyamah, should grant respite to the insolvent or waive off the debt.'" (Muslim)

Anas ibn Malik (May Allah be pleased with him) reported: The Messenger of Allah (May Allah's peace and blessings be upon him) used to say: "O Allah, I seek refuge with You from incapacity, laziness, cowardice, senility and miserliness. And I seek refuge with You from the torment of the grave. And I seek refuge with You from the trials of life and death." Another narration adds: "... and from the burden of heavy debt and the tyranny of men." (Bukhari) (https://hadeethenc.com/en/browse/hadith/5914)

Ali (May Allah be pleased with him) reported that a slave who had made a contract with his master to pay for his freedom, came to him and said: "I am unable to fulfill my obligation (of paying for my freedom to my master), so help me." Ali (May Allah be pleased with him) said to him: "Shall I not teach you some words which the Messenger of Allah (May Allah's peace and blessings be upon him) taught me (it will surely prove so useful), that if you have a debt as large as a mountain, Allah will surely pay it on your behalf? Say: *'Allahummak fini bi halalika an haramik wa aghnini bi fadhlika amman siwak.'* O Allah! Let the halal things you provide suffice me from haram, and by Your Grace, keep me independent from all besides You." (Tirmidhi) (https://hadeethenc.com/en/browse/hadith/5884)

Narrated Aisha (May Allah be pleased with her), the wife of the Prophet: Allah's Messenger (peace and blessings be upon him) used to invoke Allah in the prayer saying "Allahumma inni a'udhu bika min 'adhabi l-qabr, wa a'udhu bika min fitnati l-masihi d-dajjal, wa a 'udhu bika min fitnati l-mahya wa fitnati l-mamat. Allahumma inni a'udhu bika mina l-ma'thami wa l-maghram. (O Allah, I seek refuge with You from the punishment of the grave, from the afflictions of the imposter- Messiah, and from the afflictions of life and death. O Allah, I seek refuge with you from sins and from debt). Somebody said to him, "Why do you so frequently seek refuge with Allah from being in debt?" The Prophet (peace and blessings of Allah be upon him) replied, "A person in debt tells lies whenever he speaks, and breaks promises whenever he makes (them)." (Bukhari)

Anas ibn Malik (May Allah have mercy on him) reported that the Messenger of Allah (peace and blessings be upon him) told Mu'adh (May Allah have mercy on him), "Should I not teach you a Du'a which if you recite, your debts will be cleared even if they equal to mount Uhud?" The Du'a is:

"Allahumma Malikal Mulk, Tu-til mulka man tasha u watanzi'ul mulka mimman tasha u, wa tu'izzu man tasha u, watudhillu man tasha u, biyadikal khayru innaka 'ala kulli shay in Qadir Rahmanad Dunya wal Akhirati tu'tihima man tasha u wa tamna'u minhuma man tasha u irhamni rahmatan tughni ni biha 'an Rahmati man siwak." O Allah! Possessor of the kingdom, You give the kingdom to whom You will, and You take the kingdom from whom You will. You grant honor to whom You will and disgrace whom You will. In Your Hand is all good. Verily, You are able to do all things. (O Most Merciful of this world and the Hereafter, You grant them to whomsoever You wish and You deprive whomsoever You wish. Shower upon me such mercy, which will make me independent from the mercy of those besides You)." (Al Mu'jamus Saghir, Hadith: 558. Also see: Al Mu'jamul Kabir, vol.20, Hadith: 323)

Abu Hurairah (May Allah be pleased with him) reported: A man came to the Prophet (May Allah's peace and blessings be upon him) demanding repayment of a loan in such a rude manner that vexed the Companions and they were about to harm him, but the Messenger of Allah (May Allah's peace and blessings be upon him) said: "Leave him, for he who has a right is entitled to demand it. Give him a camel of the same age as his." They said: "O Messenger of Allah, we found none but older than his." He said: "Give it to him, for the best among you are those who settle their debts in the best manner." (Bukhari and Muslim) (https://hadeethenc.com/en/browse/hadith/3628)

'Abdullah ibn 'Amr ibn al-'As (May Allah be pleased with him) reported that the Prophet (May Allah's peace and blessings be upon him) said: "Allah forgives everything for the martyr except the debt." (Muslim) (https://hadeethenc.com/en/browse/hadith/3589)

Narrated Salama bin Al-Akwa (May Allah be pleased with her): "Once, we were sitting in the company of the Prophet (peace and blessings be upon him), a dead body was brought. The

Prophet (peace and blessings be upon him) was requested to lead the funeral salat (prayer) for the deceased. He (peace and blessings be upon him) said, "Is he in debt?" The people replied in the negative. He (peace and blessings be upon him) said, "Has he left any wealth?" They said, "No." So, he (peace and blessings be upon him) led his funeral prayer. Another dead person was brought and the people said, "O Allah's Messenger! Lead his funeral salat (prayer)." The Prophet (peace and blessings be upon him) said, "Is he in debt?" They said, "Yes." He (peace and blessings be upon him) said, "Has he left any wealth?" They said, "Three Dinar." So, he (peace and blessings be upon him) led the funeral prayer. Then a third dead person was brought and the people said (to the Prophet), "Please lead his funeral prayer." He (peace and blessings be upon him) said, "Has he left any wealth?" They said, "No." He (peace and blessings be upon him) asked, "Is he in debt?" They said, "Yes! He has to pay three Dinar." He (peace and blessings be upon him) refused to offer funeral salat (prayer) and said, "Then offer salat for your (dead) companion." Abu Qatada said, "O Allah's Messenger! Lead his funeral prayer, and I will pay his debt." So, he (peace and blessings be upon him) led the salat (prayer)." (Bukhari)

The same applies to an item that is sold but not delivered. The seller is obliged to deliver the goods to the buyer on time.

463. Prohibition of Procrastinating by a Rich Person to Fulfill his Obligation

Allah, the Exalted, says:

"Verily, Allah commands that you should render back the trusts to those, to whom they are due." (Qur'an, An-Nisa 4:58)

"Then if one of you entrust the other, let the one who is entrusted discharge his trust (faithfully)." (Qur'an, Al-Baqarah 2:283)

Abu Hurairah (May Allah be pleased with him) said: The Messenger of Allah (peace and blessings be upon him) said, "It is an act of oppression on the part of a person to procrastinate in fulfilling his obligation; if the repayment of a debt due to any of you is undertaken by a rich person, you should agree to the substitution." (Bukhari and Muslim)

Commentary:
1. Evasion or procrastination in the payment of debt, when a person is in a position to make its payment immediately, is prohibited.
2. If for the settlement of dispute, a rich man is entrusted to the lender for recovery of his debt, the lender should accept this decision. Thus, this Hadith induces one for an amicable way of settling disputes. (420)

Narrated Abu Hurairah (May Allah have mercy on him): Allah's Apostle (peace and blessings be upon him) said, "Procrastination (delay) in repaying debts by a wealthy person is injustice." (Bukhari)

464. Borrowing the Item with No Intention of Return or Without Taking Care

Allah, the Exalted, says:

"Verily, Allah commands that you should render back the trusts to those, to whom they are due." *(Qur'an, An-Nisa 4:58)*

Narrated Abu Hurairah (May Allah have mercy on him): The Prophet (peace and blessings be upon him) said: "Whoever takes people's money with the intention of repaying it, Allah will help him to repay it; whoever takes people's money with the intention of wasting it, Allah will destroy him." (Bukhari)

Narrated Anas bin Malik (May Allah be pleased with him): "I heard the Messenger of Allah (peace and blessings be upon him) say: 'Borrowed items are to be returned and an animal borrowed for milking is to be returned.'" (Ibn Majah)

Narrated Ya'la bin Umaiya (May Allah have mercy on him): Allah's Messenger (peace and blessings be upon him) said to me, "When my messengers come to you, give them thirty coats of armor." I asked, "O Allah's Messenger, is it a loan with a guarantee (of its return), or a borrowed object that must be returned?" He replied, "No, it is a borrowed object that must be returned." (Ahmad, Abu Dawud and An-Nasa'i)

Malik related to me from Humayd ibn Qays al-Makki that Mujahid said, "Abdullah ibn Umar borrowed some dirhams from a man, then he discharged his debt with dirhams better than them. The man said, 'Abu Abdar-Rahman. These are better than the dirhams which I lent you.' Abdullah ibn Umar said, 'I know that. But I am happy with myself about that.'" Malik said, "There is no harm in a person who has borrowed gold, silver, food or animals, taking to the person who lent it, something better than what he lent, when that is not a stipulation between them nor a custom. If that is by a stipulation or promise, or custom, then it is disapproved, and there is no good in it." He said, "That is because the Messenger of Allah (May Allah's peace and blessings be upon him) discharged his debt with a good camel in its seventh year in place of a young camel which he borrowed, and Abdullah ibn Umar borrowed some dirhams, and repaid them with better ones. If that is from the goodness of the borrower, and it is not by a stipulation, promise or custom, it is halal and there is no harm in it." (Malik Muwatta)

Narrated Ibn 'Umar (May Allah be pleased with him): "There was a Makhzumi woman who used to borrow things, saying that her neighbors needed them, then she would deny that she had borrowed them, so the Messenger of Allah ordered that her hand be cut off." (An-Nasa'i)

The borrower is responsible, has to take care of the loaned item until he has given it back to its owner in the same condition. He should not expose the item to the risk of destruction because it is a trust and because the owner has done him a favor.

465. Public Nuisance

Allah, the Exalted, says:

"And be moderate in your pace and lower your voice; indeed, the most disagreeable of sounds is the voice of donkeys." (Qur'an, Luqman 31:19)

"And of mankind is he who purchases idle talk (i.e. music, singing, etc.) to mislead (men) from the Path of Allah without knowledge, and takes it (the Path of Allah, the Verses of the Qur'an) by way of mockery. For such there will be a humiliating torment (in the Hellfire)." (Qur'an, Luqman 31:6)

"And those who annoy believing men and women undeservedly, bear on themselves the crime of slander and plain sin." (Qur'an, Al-Ahzab 33:58)

Narrated Anas bin Malik (May Allah have mercy on him): The Prophet (peace and blessings be upon him) said, "Make things easy for people, and do not make it difficult for them…" (Bukhari)

Annoying people by playing or running music, or speaking loudly, smoking, causes greater nuisance, discomfort. Music is prohibited, music is the instrument of Satan. Smoking is prohibited, the smoker burns Allah's money and his body which belongs to Allah. Smoker destroys his health and life. Smoking is harmful also to people around and to environment. Oxygen is the most important element. Without Oxygen we die within 4-6 minutes. Smoking causes many diseases. On Judgment Day, Allah, the Bestower, will ask for what we spent His money and how we preserved our bodies and health which belong to Him.

Public nuisance may interfere with public health (e.g. keeping of diseased animals).

Public safety nuisances include shooting fireworks in the streets, storing explosives, practicing medicine without a license or harboring a vicious dog.

Houses of prostitution, bars, night clubs, gaming houses and unlicensed prizefights are public moral nuisances.

Obstructing a highway or creating a condition to make travel unsafe or highly disagreeable are

examples of nuisances threatening the public convenience. Protesters blocking train and airport services causing commuter chaos, etc.

Closing the city's largest and busiest road for many hours for the world's largest sportive activities, like Run or Ride, may cause great inconvenience for the pregnant women to reach the hospital in case of premature rupture of membranes, bleeding or delivery, or in case of other medical emergencies, like heart attack or stroke. Those who work, should wake up earlier to take other roads which would be overcrowded to reach their job's place.

New Year celebration is a sinful noisy innovation, where the majority people forget the Creator, heedless of the Judgment Day. Whole world celebrates the innovated day with massive fireworks, public nuisance, wasting Allah's money for unlawful things (alcohol, music, dance, decorations, gifts, costumes, extravagance, etc.), the public transportation working extra night time, etc. The noisy fireworks are harmful for the environment and may hit the Jinn with possible Jinn Possession by vengeance.

God didn't create a month of 31 days!

466. Prohibition of Giving False Testimony

Allah, the Exalted, says:

"And shun lying speech (false statements)." (Qur'an, Al-Hajj 22:30)

"Not a word does he (or she) utter, but there is a watcher by him ready (to record it)." (Qur'an, Qaf 50:18)

"Verily, your Rubb is Ever Watchful (over them)." (Qur'an, Al-Fajr 89:14)

Other Verses: Al-Furqan 25:72, An-Nisa 4:135.

Abu Bakrah (May Allah be pleased with him) reported: The Prophet (May Allah's peace and blessings be upon him) said: "Shall I inform you of the gravest of the Major sins?" He repeated these three times, and then said: "Associating partners with Allah, mistreatment of parents." He was reclining, and then sat up and said: "And indeed the false statement and the false testimony." He kept repeating this so many times that we wished he should be quiet." (Bukhari and Muslim) (https://hadeethenc.com/en/browse/hadith/2941)

ShakI ibn Humayd (May Allah be pleased with him) reported: "I said: 'O Messenger of Allah, teach me a supplication.'" He said: "Say: O Allah, I seek refuge in You from the evil of my hearing, from the evil of my sight, from the evil of my tongue, from the evil of my heart, and from the evil of my semen (i.e. my lust)." (Tirmidhi) (https://hadeethenc.com/en/browse/hadith/6163)

467. Concealing Evidence

Allah, the Exalted, says:

"...and do not conceal testimony and whoever conceals it, his heart is surely sinful; and Allah knows what you do." (Qur'an, Al-Baqarah 2:283)

"O you who have believed, be persistently standing firm in justice, witnesses for Allah, even if it be against yourselves or parents and relatives. Whether one is rich or poor, Allah is worthier of both. So, follow not (personal) inclination, lest you not be just. And if you distort (your testimony) or refuse (to give it), then indeed Allah is ever, with what you do, Acquainted." (Qur'an, An-Nisa 4:135)

"...and the witnesses should not refuse when they are summoned." (Qur'an, Al-Baqarah 2:282)

Other Verse: *Ali 'Imran 3:161.*

Narrated Abu Sa'id Al-Khudri (May Allah have mercy on him): "The Messenger of Allah said: 'Whoever conceals knowledge which Allah has made beneficial for mankind's affairs of religion, Allah will bridle him with reins of Fire on the Day of Resurrection." (Ibn Majah)

Hakim b. Hizam (May Allah have mercy on him) reported God's Messenger as saying, "Both parties in a business transaction have a right to annul it so long as they have not separated; and if they tell the truth and make everything clear they will be blessed in their transaction, but if they conceal anything and lie, the blessing on their transaction will be blotted out." (Bukhari and Muslim.)

'Adi b. 'Amira (May Allah have mercy on him) reported God's Messenger as saying, "If I appoint any of you to deal with a matter and he conceals from me a needle and what is above that, it is dishonesty, and he will bring it on the Day of Resurrection." * (Muslim) *Qur'an 3:161*

468. Prohibition of Swearing in the Name of Anyone or Anything Besides Allah

Ibn 'Umar (May Allah be pleased with him) said: The Prophet (peace and blessings be upon him) said,

"Allah has prohibited you from taking an oath by your fathers. He who must take an oath, may do so by swearing in the Name of Allah or he should remain silent." (Bukhari and Muslim)

'Abdur-Rahman bin Samurah (May Allah be pleased with him) said: The Messenger of Allah (peace and blessings be upon him) said, "Swear neither by the name of Taghut (i.e. false deities, false leaders, etc.) nor by your fathers." (Muslim)

Ibn 'Umar (May Allah be pleased with him) said: "I heard a man saying: 'No, by the Ka'bah.' I admonished him: 'Do not swear by anything besides Allah, for I heard the Messenger of Allah (peace and blessings be upon him) saying, 'He who swears by anyone or anything other than Allah, has indeed committed an act of Kufr or Shirk.'" (Tirmidhi)

Some 'Ulama' are of the opinion that the words of the Prophet (peace and blessings be upon him) that "He who swears by anyone or anything other than Allah has indeed committed an act of Kufr or Shirk," are in the nature of extreme admonition. And in fact, it is not Shirk. The same applies to the saying of the Prophet (peace and blessings be upon him), who said, "showing off is Shirk."

Commentary: Imam An-Nawawi has regarded the saying "showing off is Shirk" as Hadith is not narrated in these words. It is, however, true that what the Prophet (peace and blessings be upon him) has stated about the evil and sinfulness of showing off implies that it is also a (Minor) Shirk. For instance, he stated that "He who kept fast or offered Salat for mere show, has indeed committed Shirk." In any case, to take oath of anyone other than Allah is strictly forbidden. It is, therefore, necessary to abstain from swearing by other than Allah. Unfortunately, such oaths are very common and people do not realize that they are prohibited and unlawful. (421)

469. Illegality of Swearing Falsely

Allah, the Exalted, says:

"Verily, those who purchase a small gain at the cost of Allah's Covenant and their oaths, they shall have no portion in the Hereafter. Neither will Allah speak to them nor look at them on the Day of Resurrection nor will He purify them, and they shall have a painful torment." (Qur'an, Ali 'Imran 3:77)

Ibn Masud (May Allah be pleased with him) said: The Prophet (peace and blessings be upon him) said,

"If anyone undertakes to take a false oath to appropriate the wealth of a Muslim, he will meet Allah while He is angry with him." It was revealed: *"Verily, those who purchase a small gain at the cost of Allah's Covenant and their oaths, they shall have no portion in the Hereafter. Neither will Allah speak to them nor look at them on the Day of Resurrection nor will He purify them, and they shall have a painful torment." (3:77)* (Bukhari and Muslim) (https://hadeethenc.com/en/browse/hadith/2996)

Abu Umamah Iyas bin Tha'labah Al-Harithi (May Allah be pleased with him) said: The Messenger of Allah (peace and blessings be upon him) said, "He who misappropriates the right of a Muslim by taking a false oath, Allah will condemn him to the Fire of Hell and will forbid Jannah for him." A person asked: "O Messenger of Allah, even if it is something insignificant?" He replied, "Yes, even if it is the twig of the Arak tree." (Muslim)

'Abdullah bin' Amr bin Al-As (May Allah be pleased with him) said: The Prophet (peace and blessings be upon him) said, "Of the Major sins are: Associating anything in worship with Allah, disobedience to the parents, killing without justification and taking a false oath (intentionally)." (Bukhari)

Narrated Thabit bin Ad-Dahhak: The Prophet (peace and blessings be upon him) said, "Whoever intentionally swears falsely by a religion other than Islam, then he is what he has said (e.g. if he says, 'If such a thing is not true then I am a Jew" he is really a Jew). And whoever commits suicide with a piece of iron will be punished with the same piece of iron in the Hellfire." Narrated Jundab the Prophet (peace be upon him) said, "A man was inflicted with wounds and he committed suicide, and so Allah said: My slave has caused death on himself hurriedly, so I forbid Paradise for him." (Bukhari)

470. Cheating on Exams No Matter what the Motives

Narrated Abu Hurairah (May Allah have mercy on him): The Prophet (peace ad blessings be upon him) said, "He who deceives is not of me (is not my follower)." (Muslim)

Aisha (May Allah be pleased with her) reported: The Messenger of Allah (peace and blessings be upon him) said, "Whoever seeks Allah's Pleasure by the people's wrath, Allah will suffice him from the people. And who ever seeks the people's pleasure by Allah's Wrath, Allah will entrust him to the people." (Tirmidhi)

Sheikh Ibn 'Uthaymeen (May Allah have mercy on him) said:

"Cheating in exams is forbidden; in fact, it is a Major sin, especially since this cheating will lead to a number of things in the future, it will affect the person's salary and position, and other things that are needed in order to succeed." (End quote. Fataawa Noor 'ala ad-Darb, 24/2) (422)

471. Smoking

Allah, the Exalted, says:

"...do not throw (yourselves) with your (own) hands into destruction..." (Qur'an, Al-Baqarah 2:195)

Ibn Masud (May Allah have mercy on him) reported: The Prophet (peace and blessings be upon him) said, "The son of Adam will not be dismissed from his Lord on the Day of Resurrection until he is questioned about five issues: his life and how he lived it, his youth and how he used it, his wealth and how he earned it and he spent it, and how he acted on his knowledge." (Tirmidhi)

Our body and soul belong to Allah. Health is one of countless Allah's blessings. Allah ordered to preserve health.

Smoking is a Major sin. Sins summon other sins.

1. Wasting (burning) Allah's money.
2. Not preserving health as commanded by our Creator. Lack of Oxygen because of Smoking increases acidity in the body. Smoking causes many diseases. Then, the sinner will spend Allah's money for the doctors, hospital, poisonous drugs, unnecessary surgeries; for medicine which doesn't follow the Glorious Qur'an and Prophetic Medicine, which means, the modern medicine cannot cure.
3. Harming people around Including pregnant women.
4. Harming other Allah's creations: cats, dogs, birds, trees, flowers…
5. Environment pollution.
6. Not enjoining good and forbidding evil.
7. Consumption of Haram.

The sins include all people from Tobacco factories, transportation, storage, sales, consumers.

472. Gambling

Allah, the Exalted, warns:

"O you who believe! Intoxicants (all kinds of alcoholic drinks) and gambling, and Al-Ansab (stone altars for sacrifices to idols, etc.), and Al-Azlaam (arrows for seeking luck or decision) are an abomination of Shaytan's (Satan's) handiwork. So, avoid (strictly all) that (abomination) in order that you may be successful." (Qur'an, Al-Ma'idah 5:90)

473. Theft

Allah, the Exalted, says:

"And (as for) the male thief and the female thief, cut off (from the wrist joint) their (right) hands as a recompense for that which they committed, a punishment by way of example from Allah. And Allah is All-Powerful, All-Wise." (Qur'an, Al-Ma'idah 5:38)

Narrated Abu Hurairah (May Allah be pleased with him): The Messenger of Allah (peace and blessings be upon him) observed: "The fornicator who fornicates is not a believer so long as he commits it, and no thief who steals is a believer as long as he commits theft, and no drunkard who drinks wine is a believer as long as he drinks it. Abdul-Malik b. Abi Bakr narrated this on the authority of Abu Bakr b. Abdur-Rahman b. Harith and then said: Abu Hurairah made this addition: "No plunderer who plunders a valuable thing that attracts the attention of people is a believer so long as he commits this act." (Muslim)

Aisha (May Allah be pleased with her) reported: "The Quraish were much worried about the case of a Makhzumi woman who had committed theft and wondered who should intercede for her with Messenger of Allah (peace and blessings be upon him) (so that she would not get punished for her crime). Some said Usama bin Zaid (May Allah be pleased with him) was his beloved and so he may dare do so. So, Usama (May Allah be pleased with him) spoke to him about that matter and the Prophet (peace and blessings be upon him) said to him, "Do you intercede when one of the legal punishments ordained by Allah has been violated?" Then he got up and addressed the people saying, "The people before you were ruined because when a noble person amongst them committed theft, they would leave him, but if a weak person amongst them committed theft, they would execute the legal punishment on him. By Allah, were Fatima, the daughter of Muhammad, to commit the theft, I would have cut off her hand." (Bukhari and Muslim)

Narrated Urwa bin Az-Zubair (May Allah be pleased with him): "A woman committed theft in the Ghazwa of the Conquest (of Makkah) and she was taken to the Prophet (peace and blessings be upon him) who ordered her hand to be cut off. Aisha said, "Her repentance was perfect and she was married (later) and used to come to me (after that) and I would present her needs to Allah's Apostle (peace and blessings be upon him)." (Bukhari)

Narrated Anas (May Allah be pleased with him): "The climate of Madinah did not suit some people, so the Prophet (peace be upon him) ordered them to follow his shepherd, i.e. his camels, and drink their milk and urine (as a medicine). So, they followed the shepherd that is the camels and drank their milk and urine till their bodies became healthy. Then they killed the shepherd and drove away the camels. When the news reached the Prophet (peace and blessings be upon him) he sent some people in their pursuit. When they were brought, he cut their hands and feet and their eyes were branded with heated pieces of iron." (Bukhari)

Aisha (May Allah be pleased with her) reported that the Prophet (May Allah's peace and blessings be upon him) said: "The hand of a thief is to be cut off for a quarter of a dinar or more." (Bukhari and Muslim) (https://hadeethenc.com/en/browse/hadith/2964)

Abu Hurairah (May Allah be pleased with him) reported that the Prophet (May Allah's peace and blessings be upon him) said: "May Allah curse the thief who steals an egg and his hand is cut off for that, and he steals a rope and his hand is cut off for that." (Bukhari and Muslim)

(https://hadeethenc.com/en/browse/hadith/58245)

'Abdullah ibn 'Amr ibn al-'As (May Allah be pleased with him) reported that the Messenger of Allah (May Allah's peace and blessings be upon him) was asked about fruit on the tree. He said: "Whatever a needy person eats without putting any in his pocket (and taking it away), there is no penalty on him. But whoever takes something away, he must pay a fine of twice its value and receive punishment. Whoever steals something after it has been stored properly, and its value amounts to the price of a shield, his hand must be cut off." (Ibn Majah) (https://hadeethenc.com/en/browse/hadith/58251)

474. Prohibition of Recession Regarding Prescribed Punishment for the Theft and Other (Crimes) in Case of Important Persons

Aisha (May Allah be pleased with her) reported that the Quraish had been anxious about the Makhzumi woman who had committed theft, and said: "Who will speak to Allah's Messenger (May peace be upon him) about her?" They said: "Who dare it, but Usama, the loved one of Allah's Messenger (May peace be upon him)?" So, Usama spoke to him. Thereupon, Allah's Messenger (peace be upon him) said: "Do you intercede regarding one of the punishments prescribed by Allah?" He then stood up and addressed (people) saying: "O people, those who have gone before you were destroyed, because if anyone of high rank committed theft amongst them, they spared him; and it anyone of low rank committed theft, they inflicted the prescribed punishment upon him. By Allah, if Fatima, daughter of Muhammad, were to steal, I would have her hand cut off. In the Hadith transmitted on the authority of Ibn Rumh (the words are): "Verily those before you perished." (Muslim)

475. Highwaymen Who Menace the Road

Allah, the Exalted, warns:

"Indeed, the penalty for those who wage war against Allah and His Messenger and strive upon earth (to cause) corruption is none but that they be killed or crucified, or that their hands and feet be cut off from opposite sides, or that they be exiled from the land. That is for them a disgrace in this world; and for them in the Hereafter is a great punishment." (Qur'an, Al-Ma'idah 5:33)

"The recompense for an evil is an evil like thereof." (Qur'an, Ash-Shuraa 42:40)

Hiraabah (Aggression) means ambushing people and threatening them with weapons and so on, killing them, terrorizing them and seizing their property by force and openly. Wealth is mentioned specifically because this is what usually happens, but the ruling applies also to people who terrorize others for the purposes of rape or sodomy. (423)

476. Stopping Others in the Street and Taking their Money

Allah, the Exalted, warns:

"Indeed, the penalty for those who wage war against Allah and His Messenger and strive upon earth (to cause) corruption is none but that they be killed or crucified, or that their hands and feet be cut off from opposite sides, or that they be exiled from the land. That is for them a disgrace in this world; and for them in the Hereafter is a great punishment." (Qur'an, Al-Ma'idah 5:33)

477. Prohibition of the Treachery and Breaking One's Covenant

Allah, the Exalted, says:

"O you who believe! Fulfill (your) obligations." (Qur'an, Al-Ma'idah 5:1)

"And fulfill (every) covenant. Verily! The covenant will be questioned about." (Qur'an, Al-Isra 17:34)

"Who break the covenant of Allah after its confirmation and cut as under what Allah has ordered to be joined, (that is mutual relationships), and make mischief in the land; these it is that are the losers." (Qur'an, Al-Baqarah 2:27)

Other Verse: Al-Ma'idah 5:89.

Ibn Masud, Ibn Umar and Anas (May Allah be pleased with them) said: The Prophet (peace and blessings be upon him) said, "For every one who breaks his covenant, there will be a (huge) flag on the Day of Resurrection and it will be said: 'This flag proclaims a breach of covenant by so-and-so.'" (Bukhari and Muslim)

Abu Sa'id Al-Khudri (May Allah be pleased with him) said: The Prophet (peace and blessings be upon him) said, "Everyone who breaks a covenant will have a flag by his buttocks on the Day of Resurrection. It will be raised higher according to the nature of his breach. Behold, there will be no greater a sin with respect to breaking the covenant than that of a ruler who breaks his covenant with the Muslim masses." (Muslim)

Abu Hurairah (May Allah be pleased with him) reported: The Prophet (peace and blessings be upon him) said, "Allah, the Exalted, says: 'I will contend on the Day of Resurrection against three (types of) people: One who makes a covenant in My Name and then breaks it; one who sells a free man as a slave and devours his price; and one who hires a workman and having taken full work from him, does not pay him his wages." (Bukhari)

Commentary: This Hadith highlights the importance of fulfillment of promise, the prohibition of the sale of a free person, and the payment of due wages to the laborers. (424)

477a. Desirability of Expiating the Oath Taken by a Person who Afterwards

Breaks it for a Better Alternative

'Abdur-Rahman bin Samurah (May Allah be pleased with him) said: The Messenger of Allah (peace and blessings be upon him) said to me, "When you take an oath and consider something else to be better than it, make expiation for your oath and choose the better alternative." (Bukhari and Muslim)

Abu Musa (May Allah be pleased with him) said: The Messenger of Allah (peace and blessings be upon him) said, "Verily, I swear by Allah, if Allah wills, I shall not swear to do something but that if I consider something else to be better than it, then I shall make expiation for my oath and adopt the thing that is better." (Bukhari and Muslim)

Abu Hurairah (May Allah be pleased with him) said: The Messenger of Allah (peace and blessings be upon him) said, "Persistence in respect of his oath about his family is more sinful with Allah than the payment of its expiation prescribed by Allah." (Bukhari and Muslim)

Commentary:
1. "Ahl" means wife, children and other members of one's family. For example, if a man takes an oath regarding some matter relating to his wife, although the act he has forbidden himself is better for him, it will be sinful to stick to the oath. Far less than this sin would be the breaking of the oath to normalize his relation with his wife and children. The essence of all these Ahadith is that if one comes to realize that, after taking an oath, his oath was wrong, then he must break the oath and do what he had vowed not to do. There are different forms of breaking the oaths. For instance, if one has taken an oath that he will drink alcohol, it will be obligatory for him to break his oath. Or if one takes an oath to not to do a thing which is desirable, or taken an oath to do something which is not desirable, then it will be desirable to break the oath. Similarly, if one takes an oath to not to do something permissible then the act of breaking the oath will also come in the category of permissible.
2. The expiation of an oath is necessary. This can be done by means of feeding ten poor persons, or by providing clothes to a similar number of persons, or by setting a slave free. If one does not have the capacity to do any of the three acts, then he should observe fast for three days.
3. If, in spite of realizing that the act one has vowed not to do is better, one still sticks to his oath, he would be then more sinful.
4. The teachings and practices of the Prophet (peace and blessings be upon him) tell us that to adopt the better course is preferable to sticking to the oath. (425)

477b. Expiation of Oaths

Allah, the Exalted, says:

"Allah will not punish you for what is unintentional in your oaths, but He will punish you for your deliberate oaths; for its expiation (a deliberate oath) feed ten Masakin (poor persons), on a scale of the average of that with which you feed your own families, or clothe them, or manumit a slave. But whosoever cannot afford (that), then he should observe fast for three days. That is the expiation for the oaths when you have sworn. And protect your oaths (i.e. do not swear much)." (Qur'an, Al-Ma'idah 5:89)

Aisha (May Allah be pleased with her) reported: "The Ayah: *"Allah will not punish you for what is unintentional in your oaths ..."* was revealed in respect of those persons who are in the habit of repeating: 'No, by Allah'; and 'Yes, by Allah.'" (Bukhari)

Commentary:
1. From the previous as well as present chapter we learn that there are three kinds of oaths:
   1.1. First, false oath (Al-Yamin Al-Ghamus).

- 1.2. Second, absurd (Laghw) oath, which is neither sinful nor is there any expiation for its violation.
- 1.3. Third, Al-Mu'aqqadah. It is an oath which one takes wholeheartedly for doing or not doing anything. It is liable for expiation if one violates it. Its expiation is mentioned in this Hadith.
2. What will be the quantity of the average food that is to be served to the ten people by way of expiation? We do not find any elaboration of this in any Hadith. Some 'Ulama' have stated that it means meals of the day and night. Some scholars have taken support of a Hadith and suggested that it should be one Mudd (about half kilogram) per head because this is the quantity which the Prophet (peace and blessings be upon him) prescribed as expiation for sexual intercourse with one's wife during fasting. The expiation prescribed by him was 15 Sa' dates which were to be divided among sixty poor fellows. Since one Sa' consists of four Mudd, the quantity of food, without curry, for ten persons would be six kilograms. (Ibn Kathir). This means that it would be six kilograms of flour or rice, or dates, etc. Thus, even if ten poor persons are served with an average meal, it would be a substantial quantity. Allah Alone knows what is correct. (426)

The following is a very basic explanation of promises, oaths and vows, just to appreciate the difference between them: https://seekersguidance.org/answers/hanafi-fiqh/what-is-the-difference-between-a-promise-an-oath-and-a-vow.

478. Abomination of Swearing in Transaction

Abu Hurairah (May Allah be pleased with him) said: "I heard the Messenger of Allah (peace and blessings be upon him) saying, 'Swearing produces a ready sale for a commodity, but blots out the blessing.'" (Bukhari and Muslim)

Abu Qatadah (May Allah be pleased with him) said: "I heard the Messenger of Allah (peace and blessings be upon him) saying, 'Beware of excessive swearing in sale, because it may promote trade but this practice will eliminate the blessing.'" (Muslim)

Commentary: This Hadith also mentions the same thing which has been stated in the preceding Hadith. It has food for thought that when oath robs the deal of its blessing, even if one's oath is perfectly true, how great a sin those commit who take false oaths to sell their goods! May Allah save us from committing this sin. (427)

479. Collecting Taxes

Allah, the Exalted, says:

"O you who believe! Eat not up your property among yourselves unjustly except it be a trade amongst you, by mutual consent." (Qur'an, An-Nisa 4:29)

"Zakah expenditures are only for the poor and for the needy, and for those employed to collect (Zakah), and for bringing hearts together (for Islam), and for freeing captives (or slaves), and for those in debt, and for the Cause of Allah, and for the (stranded) traveler - an obligation (imposed) by Allah. And Allah is Knowing and Wise." (Qur'an, At-Tawbah 9:60)

Ibn 'Abbas (May Allah have mercy on him) narrated: The Messenger of Allah (peace and blessings be upon him) said (the following) to Mu'adh ibn Jabal (May Allah have mercy on him) when he sent him to Yemen: 'Certainly, you are proceeding to a people that are Ahlul Kitab. When you come to them then invite them to bear witness that there is none worthy of worship besides Allah and that Muhammad (peace and blessings be upon him) is the Messenger of Allah. If they (accept and) obey you regarding that, then inform them that Allah the Almighty has made five prayers incumbent upon them, every day and night. If they obey you regarding that, then inform them that Allah the Almighty has ordained upon them charity (i.e. Zakah) to be taken from their wealthy and given to their poor. If they obey you regarding that, then be wary of the valuables of their wealth. And fear the Du'a (supplication) of the oppressed, for indeed there is no barrier between him and Allah." (Bukhari)

Abu Humayd As-Sa'idi (May Allah be pleased with him) reported: The Prophet (May Allah's peace and blessings be upon him) employed a man from the tribe of Azd, named Ibn al-Lutbiyyah, as a collector of Zakah. When he returned, he said: "This is for you, and this was given to me as a gift." Thereupon, the Messenger of Allah (May Allah's peace and blessings be upon him) ascended the pulpit, and after praising Allah and extolling Him, he said: "I employ a man from amongst you to do a job, as part of the authority in which Allah has put me, and he comes and says: 'This is for you and this was given to me as a gift.' Why did he not remain in his father's or mother's house and see whether gifts would be given to him, if he is telling the truth? By Allah! If anyone of you takes anything wrongfully, he will certainly meet Allah the Almighty carrying it on the Day of Judgment. I will not recognize anyone of you who will meet Allah while carrying a grunting camel, a bellowing cow, or a bleating ewe.'" Then, he raised his hands till we could see the whiteness of his armpits and said: "O Allah, have I not conveyed (Your message)?" (Bukhari and Muslim)

'Amr ibn 'Awf al-Ansari (May Allah be pleased with him) reported that the Messenger of Allah (May Allah's peace and blessings be upon him) sent Abu 'Ubaydah ibn al-Jarrāh to Bahrain to collect the Jizyah (yearly tax), and he returned from Bahrain with money. The Ansar heard the news of Abu 'Ubaydah's return and they gathered for the Fajr prayer with the Messenger of Allah (May Allah's peace and blessings be upon him). After he had prayed and left, the Ansar presented themselves before him. When he saw them, he smiled and said: "I believe you heard that Abu 'Ubaydah has returned from Bahrain with something." They replied: "Yes, O Messenger of Allah." The Prophet (May Allah's peace and blessings be upon him) said: "Rejoice, and hope for that which will please you. By Allah, it is not poverty that I fear for you. What I fear for you is that the world expands (with lots of wealth) for you just as it did for the people before you. Then you will compete as they competed, then it will destroy you just as it destroyed them." (Bukhari and Muslim)

Narrated Uqbah ibn Amir: "I heard the Messenger of Allah (peace and blessings be upon him) as saying: 'One who wrongfully takes an extra tax (sahib maks) will not enter Paradise.'" (Abu Dawud)

The basic principle is that it is prohibited to impose taxes, because they come under the heading of makoos (levies) that are haram. However, there is a concession allowing the imposition of taxes in exceptional circumstances, when the state needs that, on condition that it should be just and equitable, and that the taxes should be spent on valid purposes.

In al-Mawsoo'ah al-Fiqhiyyah (8/247) it says that one of the sources of income for the bayt al-maal (treasury) is:

"Taxes that are taken from the people to be spent on their interests, whether that is for Jihad or other purposes. They are not to be imposed on the people except in the case that there are not sufficient funds in the treasury to cover that, and that it is only done in the case of necessity. Otherwise, it is an illegitimate source of income. End quote."

If the taxes are of the prohibited type, it is prescribed to avoid them, so long as that will not result in greater harm, whether this is in a Muslim country or otherwise. (428)

Taxes come under the heading of man-made systems and are not prescribed by Allah. The tax collector is one of the closest supporters of the oppressors. Rather, he may be of the oppressors. He takes what is not lawful to him and gives it to those who do not deserve it.

480. Injustice

Allah, the Exalted, says:

"and whoever shall incline therein to wrong unjustly, We will make him taste of a painful chastisement." (Qur'an, Al-Hajj 22:25)

"Verily, Allah enjoins Al-Adl (i.e. justice and worshipping none but Allah Alone - Islamic Monotheism) and Al-Ihsan [i.e. to be patient in performing your duties to Allah, totally for Allah's sake and in accordance with the Sunnah (legal ways) of the Prophet SAW in a perfect manner], and giving (help) to kith and kin (i.e. all that Allah has ordered you to give them, e.g. wealth, visiting, looking after them or any other kind of help, etc.); and forbids Al-Fahisha' (i.e. all evil deeds, e.g. illegal sexual acts, disobedience of parents, polytheism, to tell lies, to give false witness, to kill a life without right, etc.), and Al-Munkar (i.e. all that is prohibited by Islamic Law: polytheism of every kind,

disbelief and every kind of evil deeds, etc.), and Al-Baghy (i.e. all kinds of oppression), He admonishes you, that you may take heed." (Qur'an, An-Nahl 16:90)

Abdullah ibn Amr (May Allah have mercy on him) reported: The Messenger of Allah (peace and blessings be upon him) said: "Verily, those who were just will be in the presence of Allah upon pulpits of light, near the Right Hand of the Merciful, the Exalted, and both of His Sides are honorable. They are those who practiced justice in their judgments and with their families and in all that they did." (Muslim)

Abu Hurairah (May Allah have mercy on him) reported: The Messenger of Allah (peace and blessings be upon him) said: "Whoever has oppressed another person concerning his reputation/honor or anything else should seek to be absolved by him before (the Day when) there will be neither dinar nor dirham. If he (the oppressor) has right actions, they will be taken from him to balance the injustice he did, and if he does not have any good actions, the bad deeds of (the oppressed) will be loaded onto him." (Bukhari)

Ibn 'Umar (May Allah be pleased with him) reported: The Prophet (May Allah's peace and blessings be upon him) said: "Injustice will be excessive darkness on the Day of Judgment." Jabir (May Allah be pleased with him) reported: "The Prophet (May Allah's peace and blessings be upon him) said: 'Fear injustice, for indeed, injustice will be excessive darkness on the Day of Judgment. And fear miserliness, for it destroyed those who were before you.'" (Muslim) (https://hadeethenc.com/en/browse/hadith/5328)

Narrated Ibn Umar (May Allah be pleased with him): The Messenger of Allah (peace and blessings be upon him) said, "Whoever takes the wrongdoer's side in a dispute or supports wrongdoing, he will remain subject to the Wrath of Allah until he gives it up." (Ibn Majah)

Anas ibn Malik (May Allah be pleased with him) reported that people said: "O Messenger of Allah, the prices have shot up, so fix the prices for us." The Messenger of Allah (May Allah's peace and blessings be upon him) said: "Indeed, Allah is the One Who fixes prices, the Withholder, the Extender and the Provider. Indeed, I wish to meet Allah while none of you will have any claim against me for an injustice regarding blood or property." (Ibn Majah) (https://hadeethenc.com/en/browse/hadith/8290)

481. Dishonest Judge

Allah, the Exalted, says:

"O you who believe! Stand out firmly for justice, as witnesses to Allah, even though it be against yourselves, or your parents, or your kin, be he rich or poor, Allah is a Better Protector to both (than you). So, follow not the lusts (of your hearts), lest you may

avoid justice, and if you distort your witness or refuse to give it, verily, Allah is Ever Well-Acquainted with what you do." (Qur'an, An-Nisa 4:135)

"No Prophet could ever act dishonestly. If any person acts dishonestly, he shall, on the Day of Judgment, restore what he misappropriated, then shall every soul receive its due whatever it earned." (Qur'an, Al-Baqarah 2:161)

"He it is Who sent among the unlettered ones a Messenger (Muhammad SAW) from among themselves, reciting to them His Verses, purifying them (from the filth of disbelief and polytheism), and teaching them the Book (this Qur'an, Islamic Laws and Islamic jurisprudence) and Al-Hikmah (As-Sunnah: legal ways, orders, acts of worship, etc. of Prophet Muhammad SAW). And verily, they had been before in manifest error." (Qur'an, Al-Jumu'ah 62:2)

Ali (May Allah have mercy on him) said, "The Prophet (peace and blessings be upon him) told me: "When two people come to you for a judgment, do not pass any ruling for the first person until you hear the other person's case. You will then know how to pass a ruling." (TirmidhI)

Narrated Buraidah ibn al-Hasib: The Prophet (peace and blessings be upon him) said: "Judges are of three types, one of whom will go to Paradise and two to Hell. The one who will go to Paradise is a man who knows what is right and gives judgment accordingly; but a man who knows what is right and acts tyrannically in his judgment will go to Hell; and a man who gives judgment for people when he is ignorant, will go to Hell." (Abu Dawud)

Abdullah ibn Amr reported: The Messenger of Allah (peace and blessings be upon him) said, "Verily, those who were just will be in the presence of Allah upon pulpits of light, near the right Hand of the Merciful, the Exalted, and both of His Sides are honorable. They are those who practiced justice in their judgments, with their families, and in all that they did." (Muslim)

Abu Hurairah (May Allah be pleased with him) reported: The Messenger of Allah (May Allah's peace and blessings be upon him) cursed the one who gives a bribe and the one who receives a bribe to influence a Judgment. (Tirmidhi) (https://hadeethenc.com/en/browse/hadith/64689)

'Amr ibn al-'As (May Allah be pleased with him) reported: The Messenger of Allah (May Allah's peace and blessings be upon him) said: "If a judge issues a ruling, having tried his best to decide correctly, and his ruling is right, he will have a double reward, but if he issues a ruling, having tried his best to decide correctly, and his ruling is wrong, he will have a single reward." (Bukhari and Muslim)

(https://hadeethenc.com/en/browse/hadith/64682)

Narrated Abu Hurairah (May Allah be pleased with him): The Prophet (peace and blessings be upon him) said: "He who has been appointed a judge has been killed without a knife." (Abu Dawud)

Narrated 'Abdullah bin Abu Awfa (May Allah be pleased with him): The Messenger of Allah (peace and blessing be upon him) said: "Allah is with the judge so long as he is not unjust, but if he rules unjustly, He entrusts him to himself." (Ibn Majah)

482. Ruling on Financial Penalties

The majority of scholars, including the four imams, said that imposing financial penalties is not permitted. Some of them responded to the cases in which it was reported that the punishment took the form of imposing a financial penalty by saying that this had been abrogated, and that it had been prescribed at the beginning of Islam but was later abrogated. They gave as the reason for not allowing punishment by seizing money the fact that this kind of punishment could be a means for unjust rulers to seize people's wealth unlawfully.

But Sheikh al-Islam Ibn Taymiyah and his student Ibn al-Qayyim suggested that it is permissible to punish a person by imposing a financial penalty if the authorities think that this will serve the purpose and deter wrongdoers and put a stop to evil, because Ta'zeer (punishments to be decided in cases where no specific punishment has been prescribed) is a broad category ranging from verbal rebuke to execution, if evil cannot be stopped in any other way. Imposing financial penalties is one form of Ta'zeer punishment which may serve as a deterrent to aggressors.

The two Sheikhs refuted the claim that this had been abrogated, and they denied that in strong terms. They quoted as evidence the reports of numerous cases in which financial penalties played a part.

The Sheikh said: "Those who claim that this was abrogated do not have any Shariah evidence, either from the Qur'an or the Sunnah. It is permissible according to the principles set out by Ahmad, because there was no dispute among his companions concerning the fact that financial penalties were not abrogated in totality.

Among the evidence that Ta'zeer may take the form of a financial penalty are the following:

The Prophet (peace and blessings of Allah be upon him) allowed seizing the property of one who hunted in the sanctuary of Madinah for the one who found it.

He commanded that the amphorae and vessels for wine should be smashed.

He commanded 'Abd-Allaah ibn 'Umar to burn the two garments which were dyed with safflower.

He increased the penalty for one who stole something that was not secured.

He destroyed the Mosque built by the hypocrites by way of harm (masjid al-diraar).

He denied the murderer the right to inherit or to be a beneficiary of a will.

Sheikh al-Islam said: "Financial penalties are of three kinds:

1 – Destruction. This means the destruction of evil items, such as breaking and burning idols, breaking musical instruments, smashing wine vessels, burning down taverns in which wine is sold, destroying books of heresy and atheism, and promiscuous movies, and three-dimensional pictures, and so on.

2 – Changing, such as destroyed forged money and curtains on which there are images, and making them into cushions and so on.

3 – Confiscation. Such as confiscating stolen dates or adulterated saffron and giving it in charity. Such things should be confiscated and given in charity, or their price should be given in charity. (429)

483. Prohibition to Judge while Judge Being in a State of Anger

Abdur-Rahman ibn Abu Bakrah reported: "My father wrote, or I wrote on his behalf, to his son 'Ubaydullāh ibn Abu Bakrah, a judge in Sijistan, saying: "Do not judge between two people while being in a state of anger, for indeed I heard the Messenger of Allah (May Allah's peace and blessings be upon him) say: 'Let no one judge between two people while being angry.'" Another narration reads: "Let no judge pass judgment between two people while being angry." (Bukhari and Muslim)
(https://hadeethenc.com/en/browse/hadith/2988)

484. Doubtful Matters

An-Nu'man ibn Bashir (May Allah be pleased with him) reported that he heard the Prophet (May Allah's peace and blessings be upon him) say: "Verily, the lawful is clear and the unlawful is clear, and between them are doubtful matters which many people do not know. Whoever avoids doubtful matters clears his liability regarding his religion and his honor, and whoever falls into doubtful matters will fall into the unlawful, just like the shepherd who grazes his animals in the vicinity of a pasture declared prohibited (by the king) and is, thus, likely to let them graze in a prohibited area (and be punished for that). Verily, every king has a protected area and the protected area of Allah is His prohibitions. Verily, in the body there is a piece of flesh which if upright then the entire body will be upright, and if it is diseased (corrupted), then the entire body is diseased (corrupted). Verily, it is the heart." (Bukhari and Muslim)

(https://hadeethenc.com/en/browse/hadith/4314)

Al-Hasan bin Ali (May Allah have mercy on him) said: "I remember that the Messenger of Allah (peace and blessings be upon him) said: 'Leave what makes you in doubt for what does not make you in doubt. The truth brings tranquility while falsehood sows doubt." (Tirmidhi)

An-Nawwas bin Sam'an (May Allah be pleased with him) reported: The Prophet (peace and blessings be upon him) said, "Piety is good manner, and sin is that which creates doubt and you do not like people to know of it." (Muslim)

Zirr bin Jubaish reported from Ali (May Allah be pleased with them) that he said: "We were still in doubt concerning the torment of the grave, until *'the mutual rivalry diverts you'* was revealed.'" (Tirmidhi)

Abu Hurairah (May Allah be pleased with him) reported: The Messenger of Allah (peace and blessings be upon him) said, "Satan will come to one of you and he will say, 'Who created this and that?' until he says to him, 'Who created your Lord?' When it comes to this, let him seek refuge in Allah and stop such thoughts." In another narration, the Prophet said, "Let him say: I have faith in Allah." (Bukhari and Muslim) (https://www.abuaminaelias.com/dailyhadithonline/2012/09/12/satan-devil-comes-doubts)

485. Bribery

Allah, the Exalted, says:

"And do not consume one another's wealth unjustly or send it (in bribery) to the rulers in order that (they might aid) you (to) consume a portion of the wealth of the people in sin, while you know (it is unlawful)." (Qur'an, Al-Baqarah 2:188)

Abu Hurairah (May Allah be pleased with him) reported: "The Messenger of Allah (May Allah's peace and blessings be upon him) cursed the one who gives a bribe and the one who receives a bribe to influence a Judgment." (Tirmidhi) (https://hadeethenc.com/en/browse/hadith/64689)

'Amr b. al-'As (May Allah be pleased with him) told that he heard God's Messenger say, "Fornication will not appear among any people without their being punished by famine, and bribery will not appear among any people without their being punished by terror." (Ahmad)

Regarding the intercession of someone who can help him to get a job, it says in Fataawa al-Lajnah al-Daa'imah (25/389):

"If the intercession of someone who can help him to get a job will result in one who is more qualified and has more right to it, due to greater knowledge of the field and more ability to do the job correctly, being deprived of the job, then such intercession is haram, because it is wronging one who is more deserving of the job, and it is wronging the bosses too, by depriving them of the work of one who is more qualified and of his services and help. It is also a transgression against the ummah because it deprives them of one who can take care of this aspect of their affairs in the best manner. In addition to that it generates resentment and suspicion and corrupts society. But if this intercession will not result in any violation of people's rights, then it is permissible and even encouraged in Shariah, and the intercessor will be rewarded for it, in shaa Allah. It is proven that the Prophet (peace and blessings of Allah be upon him) said: "Intercede, and you will be rewarded, and Allah will decree what He wills through the lips of His Messenger." (Bukhari) End quote."

With regard to giving money to this intercessor, this is subject to further discussion:

1 – If this intercessor is the one who is responsible for selection of employees, or he can exercise his influence and authority in that, then giving money to him is a bribe and is haram. The Messenger of Allah (peace and blessings of Allah be upon him) cursed the one who gives a bribe and the one who takes it, and the one who mediates between them.

Narrated Abu Humayd al-Sa'idi (May Allah be pleased with him): The Messenger of Allah (peace and blessings of Allah be upon him) appointed an agent (to collect the Zakah). The agent came when he had finished his work and said: "O Messenger of Allah, this is for you, and this was given to me." He said to him: "Why don't you sit in the house of your father and mother and see whether you are given anything or not?" Then the Messenger of Allah (peace and blessings of Allah be upon him) stood up that evening after the prayer and bore witness and praised Allah as He deserves to be praised, then he said: "What is the matter with an agent whom we appoint, and he comes to us and says, 'This is for you and this was given to me'? Why doesn't he sit in the house of his father and mother and see if he is given anything or not? …" (Bukhari and Muslim)

2 – If you are qualified for this job, and paying the bribe will not result in the transgression of anyone's rights, or depriving anyone who is your equal or more qualified than you, and you will be deprived of your rights if you do not pay this bribe, then it is permissible for you to pay it in this case, in order to attain your rights, although it is haram for the one who takes it.

This applies whether the money is given to the one who is in charge of that or to someone else who takes the money in return for interceding on your behalf with the one who is in charge.

Ibn Hazm (May Allah have mercy on him) said in al-Muhalla (8/118):

"Bribes are not permitted, i.e. that which a person gives so that he will judge falsely in his favour, or appoint him to a position of authority, or wrong someone for him. This is a sin on the part of the one who gives it and the one who takes it.

As for one who is deprived of his rights and gives a bribe so as to ward off wrong from himself, this is permissible for the one who gives it but the one who takes it is sinning. End quote."

Sheikh Ibn 'Uthaymeen (May Allah have mercy on him) said:

"As for the bribe which will help a man to attain his rights, such as if he cannot attain his rights except by giving this money, this is haram for the one who takes it but it is not haram for the giver, because the giver is only giving it in order to attain his rights, but the taker who accepts this bribe is the sinner, because he is taking what he is not entitled to." (End quote from Fataawa Islamiyyah (4/302) (430)

486. Make People Pay in Order to Pass Through, though it is Not a Rule from the Authority

Allah, the Exalted, warns:

"The cause is only against the ones who wrong the people and tyrannize upon the earth without right. Those will have a painful punishment." (Qur'an, Ash-Shuraa 42:42)

He will not let pass someone unless he is given money, and he is doing this unlawfully on his own; it can include bribery.

Ibn Taymiyah (May Allah have mercy on him) said:

"If he gives him a gift so that he will refrain from wronging him or so that he will give him his rights, this gift is haram for the one who takes it, but it is permissible for the giver to give it to him, as the Prophet (peace and blessings of Allah be upon him) said: "I give a gift to one of them…" (End quote from al-Fataawa al-Kubra (4/174)

He (May Allah have mercy on him) also said:

"The scholars said that it is permissible to give a bribe to an official so as to ward off mistreatment, not to make him withhold a right, but his taking the bribe is haram…" (Majmoo' al-Fataawa (20/252)

He also said:

"The scholars said: The one who gives a gift to the one who is in authority so that he will do something for him that is not permissible, it is haram for both the one who gives it and the one who takes it. This is the kind of bribe of which the Prophet (peace and blessings of Allah be upon him) said: "Allah has cursed the one who gives a bribe and the one who takes it."

But if he gives him a gift so that he will refrain from wronging him or so that he will give him a right that is his due, then this gift is haram for the one who takes it but it is permissible for the giver to give it to him. The Prophet (peace and blessings of Allah be upon him) used to say: "I give one of them something and he goes out with it under his arm, but it is fire." It was said: O Messenger of Allah, why do you give to them? He said: "They insist on asking me, and Allah insists that I should not be stingy." (Majmoo' al-Fataawa 31/278)

Conclusion:
It is permissible to give a bribe and it is haram for the official who takes it, but there are two conditions:

1-You should be giving it in order to take your rights or to ward off harm from yourself. But if you are giving it in order to take something to which you are not entitled, then it is haram and is a Major sin.

2-There should be no other means of obtaining your rights or warding off harm from yourself except this bribe. (431)

487. Prohibition of Show-Off

Allah, the Exalted, says:

"O you who believe! Do not render in vain your Sadaqah (charity) by reminders of your generosity or by injury, like him who spends his wealth to be seen of men." (Qur'an, Al-Baqarah 2:264)

"So, woe unto those performers of Salat (prayers) (hypocrites), Who delay their Salat (prayer) from their stated fixed times, Those who do good deeds only to be seen (of men), And refuse Al-Ma'un (small kindnesses e.g. salt, sugar, water, etc.)." (Qur'an, Al-Ma'un 107:4-7)

"Verily, the hypocrites seek to deceive Allah, but it is He Who deceives them. And when they stand up for As-Salat (the prayer), they stand with laziness and to be seen of men, and they do not remember Allah but little." (Qur'an, An-Nisa 4:142)

Other Verses: *Az-Zumar 39:47, An-Nisa 4:88.*

Abu Hurairah (May Allah be pleased with him) said: "I heard the Messenger of Allah (peace and blessings be upon him) saying, "The first to be judged on the Day of Resurrection will be a man who had died as a martyr. He will be brought forward. Allah will remind him of the favors He had bestowed upon him and the man will acknowledge them. Then He will ask him: 'What did you do to express gratitude for it?' The man will reply: 'I fought for Your Cause till I was martyred.' Allah will say: 'You have lied. You fought so that people might call you courageous; and they have done so.' Command will then be issued about him and he will be dragged on his face and thrown into Hell. Next a man who had acquired and imparted knowledge and read the Qur'an will be brought forward, Allah will remind him of the favors He had bestowed upon him and the man will acknowledge them. Then He will ask him: 'What did you do to express gratitude for it?' The man will reply: 'I acquired knowledge and taught it, and read the Qur'an for Your sake.' Allah will say to him: 'You have lied. You acquired knowledge so that people might call you a learned (man), and you read the Qur'an so that they might call you a reciter, and they have done so.' Command will then be issued about him, and he will be dragged on his face and thrown into Hell. Next a man whom Allah had made affluent and to whom Allah had given plenty of wealth, will be brought forward, Allah will remind him of the favors He had bestowed upon him and the man will acknowledge them. He will ask him: 'What did you do to express gratitude for it?' The man will reply: 'I did not neglect any of the ways you liked wealth to be spend liberally for Your sake'. Allah will say to him: 'You have lied. You did it so that people might call you generous, and they have done so.' Command will then be issued about him and he will be dragged on his face and thrown into Hell." (Muslim)

Jundub (May Allah be pleased with him) said: The Prophet (peace and blessings be upon him) said,

"He who so acts to show off, Allah will disgrace him on the Day of Resurrection, and he who does good deeds so that people may hold him in high esteem, Allah will expose his hidden evil intentions before the people on the Day of Resurrection." (Bukhari and Muslim)

Abu Hurairah (May Allah be pleased with him) said: The Messenger of Allah (peace and blessings be upon him) said, "A person who acquires (religious) knowledge, which is (normally) acquired to gain the Pleasure of Allah, (for the sole reason) to secure worldly comforts will not even smell the fragrance of Jannah on the Day of Resurrection (i.e. will not enter Jannah)." (Abu Dawud)

Commentary: It is an act of great virtue to acquire religious knowledge provided it is attained for the Pleasure of Allah. If one acquires it for worldly gains, he will be in fact committing a grave sin for which he will not even smell the fragrance of Jannah, that is to say in the first instance because after suffering the punishment for it in Hell, he will be sent to Jannah when Allah will so desire it. (432)

487a. Things Not to be Considered as Showing Off

Narrated Abu Dharr (May Allah be pleased with him): The Messenger of Allah (peace and blessings be upon him) was asked: "Tell us about a person who does some good deed and people praise him, will this be considered as showing off?" He replied, "This is the glad tidings which a believer receives (in this life)." (Muslim)

Commentary: We learn from this Hadith that if a person does a virtuous act to please Allah (i.e. not with the intention to show off) and people praise him for it, then there is nothing wrong with it. In fact, such praise is the glad tidings which he receives in this world. Expression of such good opinion about him by the public is akin to a declaration that Allah is pleased with him. Sincere admiration and praise of someone by the public is not a disqualification. It is, in fact, an evidence of his virtuous conduct and its recognition by Allah. (433)

488. Prohibition of Recounting of Favors

Allah, the Exalted, says:

"O you who believe! Do not render in vain your Sadaqah (charity) by reminders of your generosity or by injury, like him who spends his wealth to be seen of men, and he does not believe in Allah, nor in the Last Day. His likeness is the likeness of a smooth rock on which is a little dust; on it falls heavy rain which leaves it bare. They are not able to do anything with what they have earned. And Allah does not guide the disbelieving people."
(Qur'an, Al-Baqarah 2:264)

"Those who spend their wealth in the Cause of Allah, and do not follow up their gifts with reminders of their generosity or with injury." (Qur'an, Al-Baqarah 2:262)

Abu Dharr (May Allah be pleased with him) said: The Prophet (peace and blessings be upon him) observed: "There are three (types of) people to whom Allah will neither speak on the Day of Resurrection nor look at them, nor purify them, and they will have a painful chastisement." The Messenger of Allah (peace and blessings be upon him) repeated it three times. Abu Dharr (May Allah be pleased with him) remarked: "They are ruined. Who are they, O Messenger of Allah?" Upon this, the Messenger of Allah (peace and blessings be upon him) said, "One who lets down his lower garments (below his ankles) out of arrogance, one who boasts of his favors done to another; and who sells his goods by taking a false oath." (Muslim)

Commentary: The Hadith makes it evident that it is forbidden for a man to let his lower-body garment go beyond his ankles out of arrogance. The Hadith also makes it clear that it is forbidden to take a false oath with a view to sell one's goods. Messenger of Allah (peace and blessings be upon him) also said in a Hadith reported by Al-Bukhari: "Taking a false oath" helps one sell one's goods well but takes away Allah's blessings from it." (434)

489. Not Returning a Favor (Kindness) to the One Who Did you a Favor

Allah, the Exalted, says:

"Is there any reward for good other than good?" (Qur'an, Ar-Rahman 55:60)

Narrated Jabir ibn Abdullah (May Allah have mercy on him): The Prophet (peace and blessings be upon him) said, "Whoever is treated well, let him repay them. If he cannot find repayment, let him praise them for that is thanking them. If he conceals it, he was been ungrateful to them. Whoever adorns himself with what he has not been given, it is as if he wears a garment of lies." (Al-Adab Al-Mufrad)

Abdullah Ibn Umar (May Allah be pleased with him) reported: The Messenger of Allah (peace and blessings be upon him) said, "If anyone seeks protection in the Name of Allah, grant him protection; if anyone begs in the Name of Allah, give him something; if anyone gives you an invitation, accept it; and if anyone does something good for you, reciprocate him. If you do not have anything to reciprocate, supplicate for him until he sees that you have repaid him." (Abu Dawud)

Usama bin Zaid (May Allah be pleased with him) reported: The Messenger of Allah (peace and blessings be upon him) said, "He who is favored by another and says to his benefactor: 'Jazak Allah khairan (May Allah reward you well (with goodness), indeed praised (the benefactor) satisfactorily." (Tirmidhi)

Reciprocating kindness means choosing that which will make the one who did you a favor feel happy, just as he made you feel happy.

If you are not able to reciprocate with a gift or helping with some task, or offering some service, etc., then at least you can say Du'a for him, and this Du'a may be a means of bringing him happiness in this world and in the Hereafter. (435)

490. Stinging to "Jazak Allah"

The meaning of just the Arabic word Jazak Allah is "May Allah reward you", this itself is incomplete, as you can say may God reward you with bad or evil.

Usama bin Zaid (May Allah be pleased with him) reported: The Messenger of Allah (peace and blessings be upon him) said, "Whoever says 'Jazaka Allahu khayran' to the one who has done good to him, has certainly extolled him in praise." (Tirmidhi, Ibn Hibban)

We were unable to locate a narration that has 'jazakAllah' only. (https://hadithanswers.com/saying-jazakallahukhaira)

491. Answering to "Jazak Allah Khayran" by "Wa 'antum fa-jazākumu-llahu khayran"

Sheikh Moulana Muhammad Abasoomar said: "I haven't come across any response in the Hadith. Some people say: *'Amin* (O Allah accept)' and others says: *'Wa iyyak* (same to you)'. Both make sense and will not be wrong, although they are not proven from the Hadith. One should not consider these responses as Sunnah though.

Note: Some people cite a narration in Sahih Ibn Hibban; Al Ihsan, Hadith: 7279 in which the words: "Wa antum fa jazakumullahu khayran appear." According to the writer, this is a misinterpretation.

The reason for this is that when the Sahabi (May Allah have mercy on them) told Nabi (peace and blessings be upon him) "Jazak Allahu khayran", Nabi (peace and blessings be upon him) replied: "Wa antum fa jazakumullahu khayran" (rather, you deserve to be told; Jazakumullahu khayran) and he went on praising the good qualities of the Ansar.

In actual fact Nabi (peace and blessings be upon him) was saying to them (in this case) I should be telling you "Jazak Allahu khayr", instead of you telling me.

This explains why Nabi (peace and blessings be upon him) gave that particular reply. It doesn't mean that: "Wa antum fa jazakumullahu khayran" is a standard reply to such a Du'a. Rather when the situation is like the above, then this could be said in reply. (https://hadithanswers.com/the-reply-to-jazakallahukhairan)

492. Ingratitude

Allah, the Exalted, says:

"O you who believe (in the Oneness of Allah — Islamic Monotheism)! Eat of the lawful things that We have provided you with, and be grateful to Allah, if it is indeed, He Whom you worship." (Qur'an, Al-Baqarah 2:172)

"And if you would count the favors of Allah, never could you be able to count them. Truly, Allah is Oft-Forgiving, Most Merciful." (Qur'an, An-Nahl 16:18)

"And whatever of blessings and good things you have, it is from Allah." (Qur'an, An-Nahl 16:53)

Other Verses: Ibrahim 14:34, Al-Isra 17:111, Yunus 10:10, Al-A`raf 7:10, Adh-Dhariyat 51:58, Fatir 35:3, Ash-Shuraa 42:12, Al-'Ankabut 29:60, Az-Zumar 39:7, Ar-Rahman 55:10-14, Saba 34:17, Luqman 31:46, Al-Ma'idah 5:6.

Abu Hurairah (May Allah be pleased with him) reported: "On the Night of Al-Isra (the Night of Ascension) the Prophet (peace and blessings of Allah be upon him) was presented with two drinking vessels: one full of wine and the other one full of milk. He looked at them. Then he took the vessel which was full of milk. Thereupon Jibreel (Gabriel) said: "Al-hamdu lillah (praise be to Allah) Who has guided you to that, which is in accord with Fitrah (i.e. Islamic Monotheism, pure nature of Islam). Had you selected wine, your people would have gone astray." (Muslim)

Abu Hurairah (May Allah be pleased with him) reported: The Messenger of Allah (peace and blessings of Allah be upon him) said, "Any matter of importance which is not begun with Al-hamdu lillah (praise be to Allah) remains defective." (Abu Dawud)

Abu Musa Al-Ash'ari (May Allah be pleased with him) reported: The Messenger of Allah (peace and blessings of Allah be upon him) said, "When a slave's child dies, Allah, the Most High, asks His angels, 'Have you taken out the life of the child of My slave?' They reply in the affirmative. He then asks, 'Have you taken the fruit of his heart?' They reply in the affirmative. Thereupon he asks, 'What has My slave said?' They say: 'He has praised You and said: 'Inna lillahi wa inna ilaihi raji'un' (We belong to Allah and to Him we shall be returned). Allah says: 'Build a house for My slave in Jannah and name it as Bait-ul-Hamd (the House of Praise).'" (Tirmidhi)

Anas bin Malik (May Allah be pleased with him) reported: The Messenger of Allah (peace and blessings of Allah be upon him) said, "Allah is pleased with His slave who says: 'Al-hamdu lillah (praise be to Allah)' when he takes a morsel of food and drinks a draught of water." (Muslim)

Commentary: "Aklah" means to take a meal at one time, whether in the morning, the evening or at any other time. Similarly, "Sharba" means to drink water at any time. What the Hadith means is that to praise Allah on eating and drinking every time is a source of Allah's Pleasure, no matter whether the quantity one consumes is small or large. (436)

Abu Hurairah (May Allah be pleased with him) reported: The Prophet (May Allah's peace and blessings be upon him) say: ''There were three (men) from the Children of Israel: a leper, a bald-headed, and a blind…" (https://hadeethenc.com/en/browse/hadith/5926) Hadith was mentioned before.

Narrated Ibn Abbas (May Allah be pleased with him): The Prophet (peace and blessings be upon him) said: "I was shown the Hellfire and that the majority of its dwellers were women who were ungrateful." It was asked, "Do they disbelieve in Allah?" (or are they ungrateful to Allah?) He replied, "They are ungrateful to their husbands and are ungrateful for the favors and the good (charitable deeds) done to them. If you have always been good (benevolent) to one of them and then she sees something in you (not of her liking), she will say, 'I have never received any good from you." (Bukhari)

Narrated Abu Hurairah (May Allah be pleased with him): The Messenger of Allah (peace and blessings be upon him) said: "Look at those who are beneath you and do not look at those who are above you, for it is more suitable that you should not consider as less the blessing of Allah." (Ibn Majah)

Narrated Abu Bakrah (May Allah be pleased with him): "When the Prophet (peace and blessings of Allah be upon him) heard any news that made him glad, he would fall down prostrating to Allah, may He be Exalted." (Abu Dawud)

Gratitude towards Allah

The one who is most deserving of thanks and praise from people is Allah, may He be Glorified and Exalted, because of the great favors and blessings that He has bestowed upon His slaves.

Allah, the Exalted, says:

"Therefore, remember Me (by praying, glorifying). I will remember you, and be grateful to Me (for My countless favors on you) and never be ungrateful to Me." (Qur'an, Al-Baqarah 2:152)

The greatest ones who thanked Allah

The greatest ones, who obeyed this command and gave thanks to their Lord until they deserved to be described as shakir and shakur (thankful), are the Prophets and Messengers (peace and blessings of Allah be upon them).

Allah, the Exalted, says:

"Verily, Ibrahim was an Ummah (a leader having all the good righteous qualities) or a nation, obedient to Allah, Hanif (i.e. to worship none but Allah), and he was not one of those who were Al-Mushrikun (polytheists, idolaters, disbelievers in the Oneness of Allah, and those who joined partners with Allah). (He was) thankful for His (Allah's) Favors. He (Allah) chose him (as an intimate friend) and guided him to a Straight Path (Islamic Monotheism - neither Judaism nor Christianity)." (Qur'an, An-Nahl 16:120-121)

"O offspring of those whom We carried (in the ship) with Nuh (Noah)! Verily, he was a grateful slave." (Qur'an, Al-Isra 17:3)

Asking Allah to give thanks to Him

Narrated Mu'adh ibn Jabal (May Allah be pleased with him): The Messenger of Allah (peace and blessings of Allah be upon him) took his hand and said: "O Mu'adh, by Allah I love you, by Allah I love you." Then he said, "I advise you, O Mu'adh, do not fail following every prayer to say: 'O Allah help me to remember You, thank You and worship You properly.'" (Abu Dawud and An-Nasa'i)

Gratitude for Allah's blessings is a cause of them being increased.

Allah, the Exalted, says:

"And (remember) when your Lord proclaimed: 'If you give thanks (by accepting faith and worshipping none but Allah), I will give you more (of My blessings); but if you are thankless (i.e. disbelievers), verily, My punishment is indeed severe'." (Qur'an, Ibrahim 14:7)

Aisha (May Allah be pleased with her) said: When the Messenger of Allah (peace and blessings of Allah be upon him) prayed, he would stand for so long that his feet became swollen. Aisha said: "O Messenger of Allah, are you doing this when Allah has forgiven your past and future sins?" He said: "O 'Aisha, should I not be a thankful slave?" (Bukhari and Muslim)

Narrated Abu Hurairah (May Allah be pleased with him): The Prophet (peace and blessings of Allah be upon him) said: "He who does not thank the people is not thankful to Allah." (Abu Dawud)

Remember that gratitude for blessings is a blessing which needs to be given thanks for, so that one will continue to enjoy the blessings of his Lord, thanking his Lord for those blessings and praising Him for helping him to be among those who give thanks. (437)

Narrated Abu Dharr Al-Ghafari (May Allah be pleased with him) from the Prophet (peace and blessings of Allah be upon him) from his Lord, that He said: "…O My servants, it is but your deeds that I account for you, and then recompense you for. So, he who finds good, let him praise Allah, and he who finds other than that, let him blame no one but himself." (Muslim)

Abu Hurairah (May Allah be pleased with him) reported: The Messenger of Allah (peace and blessings be upon him) said, "Verily, the first thing a servant will be asked about on the Day of Resurrection will be his blessings. It will be said to him: Have We not given you health in your body and nourished you with cool water to drink?" (Timidhi)

Jabir (May Allah be pleased with him) reported: "My father owed some dates to a Jew, but he was killed on the day of Uhud and he left behind two gardens. The dates owed to the Jew would take up everything in the two gardens. The Prophet (peace and blessings be upon him) said, "Will you take half this year and half the next year?" But the Jew refused. The Prophet said, "Call me when it is time to pick the dates." So, I called him and he arrived accompanied by Abu Bakr. The dates were weighed and picked from the lowest parts of the tree, and the Prophet was praying for blessings until we paid off everything that we owed him from the smaller of the two gardens, as calculated by 'Ammar. Then, I brought them some fresh dates and water and they ate and drank, and the Prophet said, *"This is part of the blessings about which you will be asked." (102:8)* (An-Nasa'i)

493. Preoccupation with What Does Not Concern Him

Allah, the Exalted, says:

"There is no good in most of their secret talks save (in) him who orders Sadaqah (charity in Allah's Cause) or Ma'ruf (Islamic Monotheism and all the good and righteous deeds which Allah has ordained), or conciliation between mankind, and he who does this, seeking the good Pleasure of Allah, We shall give him a great reward." (Qur'an, An-Nisa 4:114)

Narrated Abu Hurairah (May Allah have mercy on him): The Messenger of Allah (peace and blessings be upon him) said: "Part of the perfection of one's Islam is his leaving that which does not concern him." (Tirmidhi)

494. Prohibition of Vowing

Ibn 'Umar (May Allah be pleased with him) reported that the Prophet (May Allah's peace and blessings be upon him) forbade vowing and said: "Indeed, a vow does not bring any good; rather it is only a means to extract something from the miser." (Bukhari and Muslim) (https://hadeethenc.com/en/browse/hadith/2960)

'Uqbah ibn 'Amir (May Allah be pleased with him) reported that the Messenger of Allah (May Allah's peace and blessings be upon him) said: "The expiation for a vow is the same as the expiation for an oath." (Muslim) (https://hadeethenc.com/en/browse/hadith/64675)

Thabit ibn Ad-Dahhak (May Allah be pleased with him) reported: "I gave an oath of allegiance to the Messenger of Allah (May Allah's peace and blessings be upon him) under the tree. Then, the Messenger (May Allah's peace and blessings be upon him) said: "If anyone swears by a religion other than Islam falsely and intentionally, he is as he has said. If anyone kills himself with something, he will be punished with it on the Day of Judgment. A man cannot make a vow on something that he does not possess." Another narration reads: "Cursing a believer is like killing him." A third narration stipulates: "If anyone makes a false claim to an increase of something, Allah, the Exalted and Glorified, will only give him a decrease." (Bukhari and Muslim) (https://hadeethenc.com/en/browse/hadith/2995)

495. Breaking Promise

Allah, the Exalted, says:

"and fulfill the promise, surely (every) promise shall be questioned about." (Qur'an, Al-Isra 17:34)

"...and be faithful to (your) covenant with Me, I will fulfill (My) covenant with you." (Qur'an, Al-Baqarah 2:40)

"And of them are some who made a covenant with Allah (saying): 'If He bestowed on us of His Bounty, we will verily, give Sadaqah (Zakah and voluntary charity in Allah's Cause) and will be certainly among those who are righteous.'" (Qur'an, At-Tawbah 9:75)

Other Verses: Al-Mu'minun 23:8, Al-An'am 6:152, Al-Ma'idah 5:89.

Narrated Abu Hurairah (May Allah be pleased with him): The Prophet (peace and blessings be upon him) said, "The signs of a hypocrite are three: Whenever he speaks, he tells a lie; whenever he is entrusted, he proves dishonest; whenever he promises he breaks his promise." (Bukhari)

'Abdullah said, "Lying is not correct, neither in seriousness nor in jest. None of you should promise his child something and then not give it to him." (Al-Adab Al-Mufrad)

Dawud said, "Be like a merciful father towards the orphan. Know that you will reap as you sow. How ugly poverty is after wealth! More than that: how ugly is misguidance after guidance! When you make a promise to your friend, fulfil your promise. If you do not, it will bring about enmity between you and him. Seek refuge in Allah from a companion who, when you mention something to him, does not help you and who does not remind you when you forget." (Al-Adab Al-Mufrad)

496. Prohibition of Drawing Portraits

Allah, the Creator and Fashioner, says:

"He it is Who shapes you in the wombs as He wills." (Qur'an, Ali 'Imran 3:6)

"And surely, We created you (your father Adam) and then gave you shape (the noble shape of a human being); then We told the angels, 'Prostrate yourselves to Adam.'" (Qur'an, Al-A'raf 7:11)

"O man! What has made you careless about your Lord, the Most Generous? Who created you, fashioned you perfectly, and gave you due proportion? In whatever form He willed, He put you together." (Qur'an, Al-Infitar 82:6-8)

Ibn 'Umar (May Allah be pleased with him) said: The Messenger of Allah (peace and blessings be upon him) said, "Those who draw pictures will be punished on the Day of Resurrection; and it will be said to them: 'Breathe soul into what you have created.'" (Bukhari and Muslim)

Ibn 'Abbas (May Allah be pleased with him) said: "I heard the Messenger of Allah (peace and blessings be upon him) saying, 'Every painter will go to Hell, and for every portrait he has made, there will be appointed one who will chastise him in the Hell.' Ibn 'Abbas said: 'If you have to do it, draw pictures of trees and other inanimate things.'" (Bukhari and Muslim)

Ibn 'Abbas (May Allah be pleased with him) said: "I heard the Messenger of Allah (peace and blessings be upon him) saying, 'Whosoever makes a picture, will be punished on the Day of Resurrection, and will be asked to infuse soul therein, which he will not be able to do.'" (Bukhari and Muslim)

Ibn Masud (May Allah be pleased with him) said: "I heard the Messenger of Allah (peace and blessings be upon him) saying, 'Those who will receive the most severe punishment from Allah on the Day of Resurrection will be painters (of living objects).'" (Bukhari and Muslim)

Abu Hurairah (May Allah be pleased with him) said: The Messenger of Allah (peace and blessings be upon him) said, "The Almighty Allah said: 'Who is more an oppressor than him who goes to create like My creation? Let him make an ant or a grain of corn, or a grain of barley.'" (Bukhari and Muslim)

Abu Talhah (May Allah be pleased with him) said: The Messenger of Allah (peace and blessings be upon him) said, "The angels do not enter a house in which there is a dog or a portrait." (Bukhari and Muslim)

Ibn 'Umar (May Allah be pleased with him) said: "Jibreel (Gabriel) promised to visit the Messenger of Allah (peace and blessings be upon him) but delayed and this grieved him very much. When he came out of his house, Jibreel met him. The Messenger of Allah (peace and blessings be upon him) asked him about the reason of delay, and he replied: 'We do not enter a house in which there is a dog or a portrait.'" (Bukhari)

Aisha (May Allah be pleased with her) said: "Jibreel (Gabriel) (peace and blessings be upon him) made a promise with the Messenger of Allah (peace and blessings be upon him) to come at a definite hour; that hour came but he did not visit him. There was a staff in the hand of the Messenger of Allah (peace and blessings be upon him). He threw it from his hand and said, 'Never does Allah back out of His Promise, nor do His messengers.' Then he noticed a puppy under his bed and said, 'O Aisha, when did this dog enter?' She said: 'By Allah, I don't know.' He then commanded that it should be turned out. No sooner than had they expelled it, Jibreel came and the Messenger of Allah (peace and blessings be upon him) said to him, 'You promised to visit me. I waited for you but you did not come.' Whereupon he said: 'The dog kept me from coming. We do not enter a house in which there is a dog or a picture.'" (Muslim)

Abul-Haiyaj Haiyan bin Husain said: Ali bin Abu Talib (May Allah be pleased with him) said to me: "Shall I not send you to do a task that the Messenger of Allah (peace and blessings be upon him) had assigned to me? Spare no portrait unwiped out, and leave not a high grave unlevelled." (Muslim)

Commentary: Drawing pictures and raising graves over the height of a span are forbidden and their removal is the responsibility of Muslim rulers. An Islamic state neither allows pictures, nor does it permit permanent structures over graves, nor graves over a span's height.

"Leave not a high grave unlevelled" does not mean levelling them to the ground. What it really means is that these should be reduced to the permissible height. (438)

Narrated Aisha (May Allah be pleased with her): "I purchased a cushion with pictures on it. The Prophet (peace and blessings be upon him) came and stood at the door but did not enter. I said (to him), "I repent to Allah for what (the guilt) I have done." He said, "What is this cushion?" I said, "It is for you to sit on and recline on." He said, "The makers of these pictures will be punished on the Day of Resurrection and it will be said to them, 'Make alive what you have created.' Moreover, the angels do not enter a house where there are pictures." (Bukhari)

Narrated Aisha (May Allah be pleased with her): The Prophet (peace and blessings be upon him) entered upon me while there was a curtain having pictures (of animals) in the house. His face got red with anger, and then he got hold of the curtain and tore it into pieces. The Prophet (peace and blessings be upon him) said, "Such people as paint these pictures will receive the severest punishment on the Day of Resurrection." (Bukhari)

Narrated Aisha (May Allah be pleased with her): "Umm Habiba and Umm Salama mentioned about a church they had seen in Ethiopia in which there were pictures. They told the Prophet about it, on which he (peace and blessings of Allah be upon him) said, "If any religious man dies amongst those people, they would build a place of worship at his grave and make these pictures in it. They will be the worst creature in the sight of Allah on the Day of Resurrection." (Bukhari)

Narrated Abu Juhaifa (May Allah be pleased with him): "I saw my father buying a slave whose profession was cupping, and ordered that his instruments (of cupping) be broken. I asked him the reason for doing so. He replied, "Allah's Apostle forbade taking the price of blood, the price of a dog and the earnings of a prostitute, and cursed the one who took or gave (Riba) usury, and the lady who tattooed others or got herself tattooed, and the picture-maker." (Bukhari)

Narrated Ali ibn Abu Talib (May Allah be pleased with him): The Prophet (peace and blessings of Allah be upon him) said: "Angels do not enter the house where there is a picture or a dog, or a person who is sexually defiled." (Abu Dawud)

497. Photography

Allah, the Exalted, says:

"So, fear Allah as much as you are able and listen and obey, and spend (in the way of Allah); it is better for your selves. And whoever is protected from the stinginess of his soul - it is those who will be the successful." (Qur'an, At-Taghabun 64:16)

Aisha (May Allah be pleased with her) reported that the Messenger of Allah (May Allah's peace and blessings be upon him) said: "The people who will receive the severest punishment on the Day of Resurrection will be those who try to emulate Allah's creation." (Bukhari and Muslim)

(https://hadeethenc.com/en/browse/hadith/5931)

Ibn 'Umar (May Allah be pleased with him) reported that the Messenger of Allah (May Allah's peace and blessings be upon him) said: "Verily, those who make these images will be tortured on the Day of Resurrection. It will be said to them: 'Bring to life what you have created.'" (Bukhari and Muslim)

Photography (tasweer) means the taking of pictures of living, animate moving beings, like people, animals, birds, etc. The ruling is that it is forbidden on the basis of a number of reports. (439)

Sorcery can be done on photography. Pictures may attract the Evil Eye by admiration or envy.

498. Prohibition of Bewailing the Deceased or When Afflicted with Adversity

Narrated Umar bin Al-Khattab (May Allah be pleased with him): The Prophet (peace and blessings be upon him) said, "The deceased is tortured in his grave for bewailing over him." (Bukhari and Muslim)

Narrated Ibn Masud (May Allah be pleased with him): The Messenger of Allah (peace and blessings be upon him) said, "He who (on befalling a calamity) slaps his cheeks, tears his clothes and follows the ways and traditions of the days of Ignorance is none of us." (Bukhari and Muslim)

Narrated Abu Burdah (May Allah be pleased with him): "(My father) Abu Musa got seriously ill and lost his consciousness. His head was in the lap of a woman of the family and she began to wail. When Abu Musa recovered his consciousness, he said: "I am innocent of those from whom Messenger of Allah (peace and blessings be upon him) is innocent. Verily, the Messenger of Allah (peace and blessings be upon him) declared himself free of (the responsibility) for a woman who wails, shaves her head and tears up her clothes." (Bukhari and Muslim)

Narrated Al-Mughirah bin Shu'bah (May Allah be pleased with him): "I heard the Messenger of Allah (peace and blessings be upon him) saying, "He who allows (others) to wail over his death, will be punished for it on the Day of Resurrection." (Bukhari and Muslim)

Narrated Umm 'Atiyyah (May Allah be pleased with her): "At the time of giving the pledge of allegiance, the Messenger of Allah (peace and blessings be upon him) took from us an oath that we would not wail." (Bukhari and Muslim)

Narrated An-Nu'man bin Bashir (May Allah be pleased with him): "When 'Abdullah bin Rawahah (May Allah be pleased with him) became unconscious, his sister began to weep and shout: "Alas! For the mountain among men. Alas! for such and such (mentioning his virtuous qualities)." When he recovered his consciousness, he said: "I was asked (disapprovingly, by the angels) about everything you said concerning me whether I am as you said." (Bukhari)

Narrated Ibn 'Umar (May Allah be pleased with him): The Messenger of Allah (peace and blessings be upon him) visited Sa'd bin 'Ubadah during his illness. He was accompanied by 'Abdur-Rahman bin 'Auf, Sa'd bin Abu Waqqas and 'Abdullah bin Masud (May Allah be pleased with them). When they entered his house, they found him unconscious. The Messenger of Allah asked, "Has he died?" They replied: "No, O Messenger of Allah." Hearing this the Messenger of Allah (peace and blessings be upon him) began to weep. When his Companions saw this, they also began to weep too. He said, "Listen attentively: Allah does not punish for the shedding of tears or the grief of the heart, but takes to task or show mercy because of the utterances of this (and he pointed to his tongue)." (Bukhari and Muslim)

Narrated Abu Malik Al-Ash'ari (May Allah be pleased with him): The Messenger of Allah (peace and blessings be upon him) said, "If the wailing woman does not repent before she dies, she will be made to stand on the Day of Resurrection wearing a garment of pitch and a garment of scabies (Allah knows the nature thereof)." (Muslim)

Narrated Asid bin Abu Usaid (May Allah be pleased with him): "A woman who had taken a pledge of allegiance at the hand of the Messenger of Allah (peace and blessings be upon him) said: "Among the matters in respect of which we gave the Messenger of Allah (peace and blessings be upon him) the pledge not to disobey him in any Ma'ruf [i.e. all that Islam ordains (V:60:12)] was that we should not slap our faces, bewail, tear our clothes up and tear out our hair (in grief)." (Abu Dawud)

Narrated Abu Hurairah (May Allah be pleased with him): The Messenger of Allah (peace and blessings be upon him) said, "Two things are signs of disbelief on the part of those who indulge in them: slandering one's lineage and wailing over the dead." (Muslim)

Commentary: Both the evils pointed out here are those sins which invite Allah's Wrath and will certainly take one out of the fold of Islam if one considers them lawful. Hence a person who practices them, revives the evils of the infidels. (440)

Narrated Anas bin Malik (May Allah be pleased with him): The Prophet passed by a woman who was weeping beside a grave. He told her to fear Allah and be patient. She said to him, "Go away, for you have not been afflicted with a calamity like mine." And she did not recognize him. Then she was informed that he was the Prophet (peace and blessings be upon him). So, she went to the house of the Prophet (peace and blessings be upon him) and there she did not find any guard. Then she said to him, "I did not recognize you." He said, "Verily, the patience is at the first stroke of a calamity." (Bukhari)

499. Praying at the Grave, in the Graveyard

Allah, the Exalted, says:

"Worship Allah and join none with Him (in worship)." (Qur'an, An-Nisa 4:36)

"Verily, Allah forgives not (the sin of) setting up partners (in worship) with Him, but He forgives whom He wills, sins other than that, and whoever sets up partners in worship with Allah, has indeed strayed far away." (Qur'an, An-Nisa 4:116)

Praying at graves is of two types:

The first type is praying to the occupant of the grave. This is Major Shirk which puts a person beyond the pale of Islam, because prayer is an act of worship, and it is not permissible to do any act of worship to anyone other than Allah.

The second type is praying to Allah in the graveyard. This covers a number of issues:

1 – Praying the Funeral (Janaazah) prayer at the graveside, which is permissible.

Narrated Abu Hurairah that a black man or a black woman used to clean the Mosque, and he (or she) died. The Prophet (peace and blessings of Allah be upon him) asked about him and they said, "He died." He said, "Why did you not tell me? Show me to his grave (or her grave)." So, he went to the grave and offered the funeral prayer." (Bukhari and Muslim)

2 – Praying in the graveyard - apart from the funeral (janaazah) prayer - this prayer is invalid and does not count, whether it is an obligatory prayer or a naafil prayer.

Abu Sa'id al-Khudri (May Allah be pleased with him) reported that the Prophet (May Allah's peace and blessings be upon him) said: "All of the earth is a Mosque (prayer place) except the graveyard and the bathroom." (Ibn Majah) (https://hadeethenc.com/en/browse/hadith/10645)

Aisha (May Allah be pleased with her) reported: "As the Messenger of Allah (May Allah's peace and blessings be upon him) was about to breathe his last, he kept drawing his sheet upon his face, and when he felt uneasy, he would uncover his face and say in that very state: "May the Curse of Allah be upon the Jews and the Christians, for they took the graves of their prophets as places of worship - He wanted to warn against what they did." If it were not for that, his grave would be made prominent; yet, he feared it might be taken as a place of worship." (Bukhari and Muslim)

(https://hadeethenc.com/en/browse/hadith/3330)

Sheikh Abdul Aziz Ibn Baaz (May Allah have mercy on him) said:

"Praying in the graveyard - apart from the funeral (Janazah) prayer - is invalid and does not count, whether it is an obligatory prayer or a nafil prayer." (Fataawa al-Lajnah al-Daa'imah 8/392) (441)

500. Prohibition of Facing the Graves During Prayer

Marthad al-Ghanawi (May Allah be pleased with him) reported: The Prophet (May Allah's peace and blessings be upon him) said: "Do not pray facing graves and do not sit on them." (Muslim)

Explanation

The Prophet (May Allah's peace and blessings be upon him) forbade praying towards graves in such a way that the person praying is facing in the direction of a grave and he forbade sitting on them. This also includes debasing them by putting one's feet on them or relieving oneself on them. All these things are unlawful.

Imam An-Nawawi said:

"Our companions (the scholars) said that it is Makruh (undesirable) to plaster the grave; while sitting, leaning against it or resting on it is haram (forbidden)." (442)

501. Congregational Du'a after Funeral Prayer

Narrated Uthman ibn Affan (May Allah be pleased with him): Whenever the Prophet (peace be upon him) became free from burying the dead, he used to stay at him (i.e. his grave) and say: "Seek forgiveness for your brother and beg steadfastness for him, for he will be questioned now." (Abu Dawud)

Abu Hurairah (May Allah be pleased with him) reported: The Messenger of Allah (peace and blessings be upon him) said, "When the human being dies, his deeds end except for three: ongoing charity, beneficial knowledge or a righteous child who prays for him." (Muslim)

Congregational Du'a after the burial, if it happens occasionally and does not become a regular practice, or if one of them offers Du'a and the others say Ameen, is regarded as permissible by some of the scholars. But if they always do it this way every time there is a funeral or they visit the deceased, or they single out a specific time to gather, or they recite Du'as in unison, then this is a kind of Bid'ah (innovation). (443)

502. Prohibition of Mourning Beyond Three Days (for Women)

Zainab bint Abu Salamah (May Allah be pleased with her) said: "I went to Umm Habiba (May Allah be pleased with her), the wife of the Prophet (peace and blessings be upon him), when her father Abu Sufyan bin Harb (May Allah be pleased with him) died. Umm Habiba (May Allah be pleased with her) sent for a yellow coloured perfume or something else like it, and she applied it to a slave girl and then rubbed it on her own cheeks and said: "By Allah, I have no need for perfume, I heard the Messenger of Allah (peace and blessings be upon him) saying from the pulpit, 'It is not permissible for a woman who believes in Allah and the Last Day to mourn for the dead beyond three days, except for the death of her husband; in which case the period of mourning is of four months and ten days.' Zainab said: 'I then visited Zainab, daughter of Jahsh (May Allah be pleased with her) when her brother died; she sent for perfume and applied it and then said: "Beware! By Allah, I don't feel any need of perfume but I heard the Messenger of Allah (peace and blessings be upon him) saying from the pulpit, 'It is not permissible for a woman who believes in Allah and the Last Day to mourn the dead beyond three days except in case of her husband (for whom the period is) four months and ten days.'" (Bukhari and Muslim)

Commentary: The period of mourning the husband's death is four months and ten days while ordinarily it is three days only (for others). The reasons behind mourning the dead husband is: Firstly, the purification of womb. Secondly, it is a mark of respect for the relation and love between husband and wife. The scent which was used in the two incidents reported in this Hadith occurred after the stipulated period of mourning in ordinary cases - that is three days. After the expiry of the mourning period, the woman is allowed to resume her routine. (444)

503. Prohibition of Sitting on the Graves

Narrated Abu Hurairah (May Allah be pleased with him): The Messenger of Allah (peace and blessings be upon him) said, "It is much better for one of you to sit on a live coal, which will burn his clothes and get to his skin than to sit on a grave." (Muslim)

Commentary:
To sit on the grave is strictly prohibited. Ibn Hajar Al-Haithami and others, however, regard this act to be only Makruh (undesirable) and maintain that the warning contained in the Hadith is for those people who sit on them for urinating or defecating. The Hadith also elucidates the fact that graves should be respected and that glorifying the people in them by plastering them or building over them is not permissible. (445)

504. Prohibition of Plastering and Building over the Graves

Narrated Jabir (May Allah be pleased with him): "The Messenger of Allah (peace and blessings be upon him) forbade that the graves should be plastered (made into permanent structures), used as sitting places (for the people) or building over them." (Muslim)

Commentary:

1. The construction of permanent graves is sheer extravagance because they do not benefit the dead. This act is 'disliked' and reaches the level of prohibition when graves are ornamented and embellished.

2. Sitting on the graves is a disliked act, as has been made clear in the previous Hadith.

3. It is such a respect for the dead which inclines people to Shirk. Construction of dome etc., over the graves have also the same effect. (446)

Narrated Abu'l-Hayaaj al-Asadi said: "Ali ibn Abi Taalib said to me: 'Shall I not send you on the same mission as the Messenger of Allah (peace and blessings of Allah be upon him) sent me? Do not leave any statue without erasing it, and do not leave any raised grave without leveling it." (Muslim)

505. Touching Graves and Looking for Help from the Occupants

Allah, the Exalted, says:

"And who is more astray than one who calls on (invokes) besides Allah, such as will not answer him till the Day of Resurrection, and who are (even) unaware of their calls (invocations) to them? And when mankind is gathered (on the Day of Resurrection), they (false deities) will become their enemies and will deny their worshipping." (Qur'an, Al-Ahqaf 46:5-6)

"And (remember) when Allah will say (on the Day of Resurrection): "O 'Eesa (Jesus), son of Maryam (Mary)! Did you say unto men: 'Worship me and my mother as two gods besides Allah?'" He will say: "Glory be to You! It was not for me to say what I had no right (to say)." (Qur'an, Al-Ma'idah 5:116)

"They (Jews and Christians) took their rabbis and their monks to be their lords besides Allah (by obeying them in things which they made lawful or unlawful according to their own desires without being ordered by Allah), and (they also took as their Lord) Messiah, son of Maryam (Mary), while they (Jews and Christians) were commanded [in the Tawrat (Torah) and the Injeel (Gospel)] to worship none but One Ilaah (God - Allah) Laa ilaaha illa Huwa (none has the right to be worshipped but He). Praise and Glory be to Him (far above is He) from having the partners they associate (with Him)." (Qur'an, At-Tawbah 9:31)

Aisha (May Allah be pleased with her) reported that, during his terminal illness, the Messenger of Allah (May Allah's peace and blessings be upon him) said: "May Allah curse the Jews and the Christians, they took the graves of their prophets as places of worship." She added: "Had it not been for that, his grave would have been made prominent, but it was feared that it might be taken as a place of worship." (Bukhari and Muslim) (https://hadeethenc.com/en/browse/hadith/5379)

With regard to the 'Urs which is held every year: if this involves some kinds of acts of worship or if the people who attend think that this will bring them closer to Allah, or if it involves acts of disobedience and sin, then it is not permissible to attend it or take part in it. Even if it is free of all these matters, you should still not attend it, because adopting an occasion as an "Eid" or festival (a regular annual event) other than the Eids prescribed in Islam is Bid'ah (reprehensible innovation) and is forbidden. The belief of those present, that the soul of the "wali" attends this 'Urs is an innovated and forbidden belief.

Ibn Taymiyah (May Allah have mercy on him) said:

"To explain further: if what the person wants is something that none is able to do except Allah - such as asking for healing from sickness, for people or animals, or for his debts to be paid off in some manner that he does not specify, or for his family to be safe and sound, or to be protected from calamity in this world or the next, or for help against his enemy, or for his heart to be guided, or for his sins to be forgiven, or for him to be admitted to Paradise or saved from Hell, or for help to learn knowledge and the Qur'an, or for his heart to be reformed, his attitude to be made good, his soul to be purified and so on - all of these are things which it is not permissible to seek from anyone other than Allah. It is not permissible to say to an angel or a Prophet, or a sheikh, whether he is alive or dead, "forgive my sin" or "help me against my enemy", or "heal my sick loved one", or "protect my family or my livestock" and the like. Whoever asks any created being - no matter who he is - for any of these things, is a mushrik who associates others with his Lord. He is like the mushrikeen who worship angels, Prophets and statues which they have created in their image, and his prayer is like the prayers of the Christians to the Messiah and his mother…(Majmoo' al-Fataawa, 27/67-68)

And he (Ibn Taymiyah) said:

"Whoever comes to the grave of a Prophet or a righteous man, or what he believes to be the grave of a Prophet or a righteous man although it is not, and asks him for something and seeks his help, one of the three following scenarios applies: he is asking him for something that he needs, such as to cure his sick animals or to pay off his debt, or to take revenge on his enemy or to protect him, his family and his livestock, and other things which no one can do except Allah. This is obvious Shirk and he must be told to repent. If he repents, all well and good, otherwise he must be executed. If he says, 'I am asking him because he is closer to Allah, so that he can intercede for me with regard to these matters, because I am seeking Allah's help through his virtue, just as people seek the ruler's help through those who are close to him - this is also like the actions of the mushrikeen and Christians, who claim that they take their priests and monks as intercessors and ask them to intercede for them with their requests.

Allah, the Exalted, says:

"We worship them only that they may bring us near to Allah." (Qur'an, Az-Zumar 39:3)

"You (mankind) have none, besides Him, as a Wali (protector or helper) or an intercessor. Will you not then remember (or receive admonition)?" (Qur'an, As-Sajdah 32:4)

"Who is he that can intercede with Him except with His Permission?" (Qur'an, Al-Baqarah 2:255)

Other Verse: *Az-Zumar 39:43-44, Al-Baqarah 2:186.*

The difference between Him and His creation is clear: people usually ask some of their leading figures who are in positions of honor to intercede for them with their leaders, so that intercessor asks the leader and he meets the person's request because he hopes to gain something thereby, or because he is afraid of him, or because he is too shy to refuse, or because he is being friendly towards him, etc. But no one intercedes with Allah, may He be Glorified, until He gives permission to the intercessor. He only does what He wills, and the intercession of the intercessor is only made by His permission. The entire matter rests with Him. The idea of many misguided people, that this person is closer to Allah than I am, and I am far away from Allah and cannot call upon Him except through this mediation etc., all of these ideas are ideas of Shirk.

In al-Saheeh it was reported that when they were on a journey, they were saying Takbeer ("Allahu Akbar") in loud voices, and the Prophet (peace and blessings of Allah be upon him) said: "O people, take it easy! You are not calling upon One Who is deaf or absent; you are calling upon One Who is All-Hearing and Ever Near. The One upon Whom you are calling is closer to any one of you than the neck of his camel."

Allah has commanded all people to pray to Him and call on Him, and He has commanded them all to say:

"You (Alone) we worship, and You (Alone) we ask for help (for each and everything)." (Qur'an, Al-Fatihah 1:5)

Moreover, it may be said to this mushrik: "If you call upon this person, that means you think that he knows more about your situation, is more able to grant you what you ask for and is more merciful towards you. This is ignorance, misguidance and kufr. If you know that Allah has more knowledge and is more able and more Merciful, then why do you fail to ask Him, and instead turn to others? Have you not heard what al-Bukhari and others narrated from Jabir (May Allah be pleased with him), who said: the Messenger of Allah (peace and blessings of Allah be upon him) used to teach us to pray Istikhara and make Du'a seeking guidance from Allah) in all our affairs, just as he taught us the Surahs of the Qur'an.

Even if you know that this person is closer to Allah than you and of a higher status than you, this may be true, but what you are implying is wrong. Even if he is indeed closer to Allah and of a higher status, that only means that Allah will reward him and give him more than you. It does not mean that if you call on him, Allah will answer your prayer more than He would do if you called upon Him yourself. If you are deserving of being punished and of having your supplication rejected, for example, because your Du'a is offered in an improper manner, then no Prophet or righteous person will help you to do something that Allah dislikes and is angry with. Even if that is not the case, then you should ask from Allah because Allah is the Most Merciful." (Majmoo' al-Fataawa, 27/72-75) (447)

506. Prohibition of Abusing the Deceased Without a Valid Legal Reason

Allah, the Exalted, says:

"Every soul will taste death, and you will only be given your (full) compensation on the Day of Resurrection. So, he who is drawn away from the Fire and admitted to Paradise has attained (his desire). And what is the life of this world except the enjoyment of delusion." (Qur'an, Ali 'Imran 3:185)

"Not for you (O Muhammad, but for Allah) is the decision; whether He turns in mercy to (pardons) them or punishes them; verily, they are the Zalimoon (polytheists, disobedient and wrongdoers)." (Qur'an, Ali 'Imran 3:128)

Narrated Aisha (May Allah be pleased with her): The Prophet (peace and blessings of Allah be upon him) said, "Don't abuse the dead, because they have attained that which they had forwarded (i.e. their deeds, good or bad)." (Bukhari)

Commentary: We should not censure or condemn the deceased because they have reached their end and they are receiving in the Hereafter return for whatever deeds they did in their life. There is no harm, however, in abusing the disbelievers who died in a state of Kufr. (448)

507. Prohibition of Disclosing the Physical Defects of the Deceased

Narrated Abu Rafi' Aslam, the freed slave of the Messenger of Allah (May Allah be pleased with him):

The Messenger of Allah (peace and blessings be upon him) said, "He who washes a dead body and conceals what he notices of physical defects, he will be forgiven forty times." (Al-Hakim)

Commentary: If during washing a man's dead body, the washer has noticed some physical defect or some sort of deformation in it, he should avoid disclosing it to others so that a bad name may not come to the departed soul… (449)

508. Not Performing Funeral Prayer for the Muslim Believer

Narrated Abu Hurairah (May Allah be pleased with him): "A black person, a male or a female, used to clean the Mosque and then died. The Prophet (peace and blessings be upon him) did not know about it. One day the Prophet (peace and blessings be upon him) remembered him and said, "What happened to that person?" The people replied, "O Allah's Apostle! He died." He (peace and blessings be upon him) said, "Why did you not inform me?" They said, "His story was so and so (i.e. regarded him as insignificant)." He (peace and blessings be upon him) said, "Show me his grave." He then went to his grave and offered the funeral prayer." (Bukhari)

Narrated Salama bin Al-Akwa (May Allah be pleased with him): "Once, we were sitting in the company of the Prophet (peace and blessings be upon him), a dead body was brought. The Prophet (peace and blessings be upon him) was requested to lead the funeral salat (prayer) for the deceased. He (peace and blessings be upon him) said, "Is he in debt?" The people replied in the negative. He (peace and blessings be upon him) said, "Has he left any wealth?" They said, "No." So, he (peace and blessings be upon him) led his funeral prayer. Another dead person was brought and the people said, "O Allah's Messenger! Lead his funeral salat (prayer)." The Prophet (peace and blessings be upon him) said, "Is he in debt?" They said, "Yes." He (peace and blessings be upon him) said, "Has he left any wealth?" They said, "Three Dinar." So, he (peace and blessings be upon him) led the funeral prayer. Then a third dead person was brought and the people said (to the Prophet), "Please lead his funeral prayer." He (peace and blessings be upon him) said, "Has he left any wealth?" They said, "No." He (peace and blessings be upon him) asked, "Is he in debt?" They said, ("Yes! He has to pay) three Dinar." He (peace and blessings be upon him) (refused to offer funeral salat (prayer) and) said, "Then offer salat for your (dead) companion." Abu Qatada said, "O Allah's Messenger! Lead his funeral prayer, and I will pay his debt." So, he (peace and blessings be upon him) led the salat (prayer)." (Bukhari)

Narrated Abu Hurairah (May Allah be pleased with him): Allah's Apostle (peace and blessings be upon him) said, "(A believer) who accompanies the funeral procession of a Muslim out of sincere faith and hoping to attain Allah's reward and remains with it till the funeral prayer is offered and the burial ceremonies are over, he will return with a reward of two Qirats. Each Qirat is like the size of the (Mount) Uhud. He who offers the funeral prayer only and returns before the burial, will return with the reward of one Qirat only." (Bukhari)

Narrated Umm-Atiya al-Ansariya (May Allah be pleased with her): Allah's Apostle (peace and blessings be upon him) came to us when his daughter died and said, "Wash her thrice or five times or more, if you see it necessary, with water and Sidr and then apply camphor or some camphor at the end; and when you finish, notify me." So, when we finished it, we informed him and he gave us his waist-sheet and told us to shroud the dead body in it." (Bukhari)

Narrated Samura bin Jundab (May Allah be pleased with him): "The Prophet (peace and blessings be upon him) offered the funeral prayer for the dead body of a woman who died of (during) delivery (i.e. child birth) and he stood by the middle of her body." (Bukhari)

Narrated Abu Hurairah (May Allah be pleased with him): The Prophet (peace and blessings be upon him) said, "Hurry up with the dead body for if it was righteous, you are forwarding it to welfare; and if it was otherwise, then you are putting off an evil thing down your necks." (Bukhari)

509. Burying the Dead at Three Forbidden Times

'Uqbah ibn 'Amir al-Juhani (May Allah be pleased with him) reported: "The Messenger of Allah (peace and blessings be upon him) used to forbid us from praying or burying our deceased ones at three times: when the sun begins to rise until it is fully risen; when the sun is at its highest point in the sky at noon until it passes its zenith and when the sun starts setting until it fully sets." (Muslim) (https://hadeethenc.com/en/browse/hadith/10604)

510. Mourning on the 3rd, 10th, 40th and on the Yearly Death Anniversary of the Deceased

Waiting for three days, then offering Du'a for the deceased for a period of ten days or twenty, or thirty, or forty days, on the grounds that his body goes through a number of stages of trials during this period, is an act that is contrary to the Sunnah and is a claim that is devoid of any evidence; it is a fabricated innovation (Bid'ah).

Sunnah is to offer Du'a for the deceased at the grave immediately after his burial. Moreover, offering Du'a for the Muslim dead in general and some in particular is something that is recommended, without specifying any particular period or time.

The idea that the head of the deceased explodes in the first three days, and his stomach explodes after ten days, and his entire body explodes after forty days, is a false notion and a fabricated claim for which there is no evidence. Perhaps this idea is the basis for the innovations surrounding the fortieth day after death, when tents are set up, and people come to offer condolences, and the reciter recites the Qur'an. The scholars have stated that these acts are innovations (Bid'ah).

Ibn 'Uthaymeen (May Allah have mercy on him) was asked:

"What is the ruling on observing the fortieth day after death, during which Qur'an is recited and people gather to offer condolences?" He replied:

"This is one of the innovations that are practiced by some people. When forty days have passed since the death, they organize a condolence gathering in which people gather at the house of the deceased, and they read Qur'an and illuminate in the place. In fact, this comes under the heading of renewing grief, which is prohibited." (End quote from Fataawa Noor 'ala ad-Darb (9/2)

The forty-day commemoration is a pharaonic custom.

Ibn 'Uthaymeen (May Allah have mercy on him) was asked:

"When seven days have passed since the death, the women of the bereaved family go to him in the graveyard, and they start to weep again. When fifteen days have passed, they repeat the same action, and again when forty days have passed, they mourn for him for a year or more, and they do not let children play or be happy. Is this permissible or not?" He replied:

"This action is not permissible, because for women to visit graveyards, if the woman goes out of her house for this purpose, then she is cursed – Allah forbid. The same applies to morning for a whole year; it is a reprehensible act that is not permissible." (End quote from Fataawa Noor 'ala ad-Darb (9/2)

By the same token, if the three-day period mentioned is also something that people do, whereby they set up tents for receiving condolences for their loss for three days, during which they recite Qur'an and receive condolences, this is also an innovation. (450)

511. Women Wearing Black Clothes at Times of Calamity and Death

Sheikh Ibn 'Uthaymeen (May Allah have mercy on him) was asked:

"What is the ruling on women attending funerals? And on wearing black clothes?" He replied: "It is haram for women to attend funerals because they have little patience and because it exposes them to fitnah and mixing with men. With regard to wearing black clothes at times of calamity, this is an innovation." (Majmoo' Fataawa Ibn 'Uthaymeen, 17/329)

He was also asked (17/410):

"What is the ruling on singling out certain kinds of clothes for offering condolences such as women wearing black?" He replied:

"Singling out a certain type of clothes for offering condolences is an innovation as far as we know, and it may stem from a person's being displeased with the Decree of Allah. Although some people think there is nothing wrong with it, the salaf did not do this and as it is to some extent an expression of displeasure with the Decree of Allah, undoubtedly, it is better not to do it, because if a person does that, he may be closer to sin than not." (451)

512. Prohibition of Funeral Prayer for the Disbeliever

Narrated Jabir (May Allah have mercy on him): "The leader of the hypocrites in Al-Madinah died, and left instructions that The Prophet (peace and blessings of Allah be upon him) should offer the funeral prayer for him and shroud him in his shirt. He offered the funeral prayer for him and shrouded him in his shirt, and stood by his grave. Then Allah revealed the Words: *'And never pray (the funeral prayer) for any of them (hypocrites) who dies, nor stand at his grave."* (Qur'an, 9:84) (Ibn Majah)

Narrated Anas bin Malik (May Allah have mercy on him): Allah's Apostle (peace and blessings be upon him) said, "When (Allah's) slave is put in his grave and his companions return, and he even hears their footsteps, two angels come to him and make him sit and ask, 'What did you use to say about this man (i.e. Muhammad)?' The faithful believer will say, 'I testify that he is Allah's slave and His Apostle.' Then they will say to him, 'Look at your place in the Hellfire; Allah has given you a place in Paradise instead of it.' So, he will see both his places." (Qatada said, "We were informed that his grave would be made spacious." Then Qatada went back to the narration of Anas who said, whereas a hypocrite or a non-believer will be asked, "What did you use to say about this man." He will reply, "I do not know; but I used to say what the people used to say." So, they will say to him, "Neither did you know nor did you take the guidance (by reciting the Qur'an)." Then he will be hit with iron hammers once, that he will send such a cry as everything near to him will hear, except Jinns and human beings. (Bukhari)

513. Abomination of Longing for Death

Narrated Abu Hurairah (May Allah be pleased with him): The Messenger of Allah (peace and blessings be upon him) said, "None of you should wish for death. If he is righteous, perhaps he may add to his good works, and if he is a sinner, possibly he may repent (in case he is given a longer life)." (Bukhari)

Narrated Abu Hurairah (May Allah be pleased with him): The Messenger of Allah (peace and blessings be upon him) said, "Let none of you wish for death, nor he ask for it before it comes to him, because when he dies, his actions will be terminated; certainly, the age of a true believer does not add but good." (Muslim)

Narrated Anas bin Malik (May Allah be pleased with him): The Messenger of Allah (peace and blessings be upon him) said, "Let none of you wish for death on account of an affliction that befalls him. If he has no alternative, let him pray: 'Allahumma ahyine ma kanatil-hayatu khairan li, wa tawaffani idha kanatil-wafatu khairan li (O Allah! Give my life so long as the life is good for me, and take away my life if death is good for me).'" (Bukhari and Muslim)

Commentary: Here, too, a believer has been prevented from wishing for death. Because it betrays that he is far from agreeing to what Allah wills or has ordained. If at all his wishing becomes intense and indispensable under the pressure of circumstances, he should pray in the Prophetic words mentioned in the Hadith above. (452)

In the Prophet's statement "None of you should wish for death", the prohibition here indicates unlawfulness, because in wishing for death there is a kind of displeasure with the Decree of Allah, and the believer must be patient when a calamity befalls him. When he is patient during hardships, he will achieve two important things:

1. Expiation of sins - because no worry, grief or annoyance befalls a person except that Allah expiates his sins for it - even the prick of a thorn expiates his sins;
2. If he succeeds in anticipating reward from Allah, and is patient for the sake of Allah, then he will be rewarded. Regarding his wish for death, this is an indication of lack of patience and content with what Allah, Exalted and Glorified, has decreed.

The Messenger of Allah (May Allah's peace and blessings be upon him) explained that if he is of the doers of good, he will increase in good deeds while still alive, since the believer may still increase in good deeds as long as he is living, even if he is afflicted with a calamity. On the other hand, if he is an evildoer who committed sins, he may give up his evil ways, i.e. seek the Pleasure and Pardon of Allah, so then he will die after having repented of his sins. So do not wish for death, because the matter in its entirety is decreed. So, one should be patient and anticipate reward from Allah, because nothing lasts forever. In the Hadith, there is also an indication that the meaning behind the prohibition of wishing for death is that death is the end of deeds. Life is the time of performing deeds, and deeds achieve an increase in reward, and even if there was nothing except continuous monotheism, then indeed it is the most virtuous of deeds. This is not refuted by claiming that apostasy is possible after having faith, because that is rare, and after the heart mixes with the purity of true faith, no one can reject it – taking into consideration that this may happen, but it is rare. Whoever is predestined to have a bad end, it must happen, whether his lifespan is long or short. So, it does a person no good in hastening it by wishing for death. In the Hadith there is also a sign of glad tidings for the doer of good because of His Benevolence; and a warning to the evildoer for his evil deeds. It is as if it is saying: "Whoever is a doer of good should avoid wishing for death in order to continue to do good and increase in it; and whoever is an evildoer should avoid wishing for death in order to desist from his evil deeds and not die upon it, putting himself in danger." (https://hadeethenc.com/en/browse/hadith/5652)

Narrated Qais bin Abu Hazim (May Allah be pleased with him): "I went to visit Khabbab bin Aratt (May Allah be pleased with him) during his illness. He had been cauterized in seven places. He said: 'Our companions who have died have left (this world) without having enjoyed the pleasures of the world (in order to get a great full reward in the Hereafter) while we have amassed wealth exceeding our needs for which there is no place to keep except in the earth. Had Messenger of Allah (peace and blessings be upon him) not prohibited us from longing for death, I would have prayed for it." Then we visited him again and he was building a wall. He said: "There is a reward in store for a Muslim in respect of everything on which he spends except for something he places in the earth (i.e. something exceeding our needs or essentials)." (Bukhari and Muslim)

514. Suicide

Allah, the Exalted, says:

"....and do not kill ourselves; surely Allah is Merciful to you. And whoever does this aggressively and unjustly, We will soon cast him into Fire; and this is easy for Allah." (Qur'an, An-Nisa 4:29-30)

Narrated Thabit bin Dahhak (May Allah be pleased with him): The Prophet (peace and blessings be upon him) said, "Whoever intentionally swears falsely by a religion other than Islam, then he is what he has said (e.g. if he says, 'If such thing is not true then I am a Jew,' he is really a Jew). And whoever commits suicide with piece of iron will be punished with the same piece of iron in the Hellfire." Narrated Jundab: The Prophet said, "A man was inflicted with wounds and he committed suicide, and so Allah said: "My slave has caused death on himself hurriedly, so I forbid Paradise for him." (Bukhari)

Narrated Abu Hurairah (May Allah be pleased with him): The Prophet (peace and blessings be upon him) said, "Whoever purposely throws himself from a mountain and kills himself, will be in the Hellfire falling down into it and abide therein perpetually forever; and whoever drinks poison and kills himself with it, he will be carrying his poison in his hand and drinking it in the Hellfire wherein he will abide eternally forever; and whoever kills himself with an iron weapon, will be carrying that weapon in his hand and stabbing his abdomen with it in the Hellfire wherein he will abide eternally forever." (Bukhari)

Jundub ibn 'Abdullah al-Bajali (May Allah be pleased with him) reported that the Prophet (May Allah's peace and blessings be upon him) said: "Among those who were before you, there was a man who was injured. He was impatient, so he took a knife and made a cut in his hand and bled to death. Allah, the Exalted, said: 'My servant hastened to bring about his demise; I have forbidden Paradise to him.'"

(Bukhari and Muslim) (https://hadeethenc.com/en/browse/hadith/2981)

515. Asking Forgiveness for the Disbelievers Alive and Dead

Allah, the Exalted, says:

"And Nuh (Noah) called upon his Lord and said, "O my Lord! Verily, my son is of my family! And certainly, Your Promise is true, and You are the Most Just of the judges." (Qur'an, Hud 11:45)

"He said: "O Nuh (Noah)! Surely, he is not of your family; verily, his work is unrighteous, so ask not of Me that of which you have no knowledge! I admonish you, lest you be one of the ignorants." (Qur'an, Hud 11:46)

"Nuh (Noah) said: "O my Lord! I seek refuge with You from asking You that of which I have no knowledge. And unless You forgive me and have Mercy on me, I would indeed be one of the losers." (Qur'an, Hud 11:47)

Other Verse: At-Tawbah 9:114.

Abu Hurairah (May Allah have mercy on him) reported: The Apostle of Allah (peace and blessings be upon him) visited the grave of his mother and he wept, and moved others around him to tears, and said: "I sought permission from my Lord to beg forgiveness for her but it was not granted to me, and I sought permission to visit her grave and it was granted to me so visit the graves, for that makes you mindful of death." (Muslim)

The Prophet Ibrahim would not have asked forgiveness for his father but for a promise he made to him.

516. Overburdening Against Others

Allah, the Exalted, says:

"Allah burdens not a person beyond his scope. He gets reward for that (good) which he has earned, and he is punished for that (evil) which he has earned." (Qur'an, Al-Baqarah 2:286)

"The blame is only against those who oppress men and wrongdoing and insolently transgress beyond bounds through the land, defying right and justice: for such there will be a penalty grievous." (Qur'an, Ash-Shuraa 42:42)

"Indeed, Qarun was from the people of Moses, but he tyrannized them. And We gave him of treasures whose keys would burden a band of strong men; thereupon his people said to him, "Do not exult. Indeed, Allah does not like the exultant." (Qur'an, Al-Qasas 28:76)

Anas ibn Malik (May Allah be pleased with him) reported that the Prophet (May Allah's peace and blessings be upon him) said: "Make things easy for the people, and do not make it difficult for them, and make them calm (with glad tidings) and do not repulse (them)." (Bukhari and Muslim)
(https://hadeethenc.com/en/browse/hadith/5866)

Abu Masud al-Ansari (May Allah be pleased with him) reported: A man said: "O Messenger of Allah, I would almost fail to attend the prayer because so-and-so prolongs it when he leads us." I never saw the Prophet (May Allah's peace and blessings be upon him) more angry in giving admonition than he was on that day. He said: "O people, you cause aversion to others. Whoever leads people in prayer should make it brief, for among them are the sick, the weak and those with needs to be fulfilled." (Bukhari)
(https://hadeethenc.com/en/browse/hadith/11295)

Al-Ma'rur ibn Suwaid (May Allah be pleased with him) said, "I saw Abu Dharr wearing a robe and his slave was also wearing a robe. We asked him about that and he said, 'I insulted a man and he complained against me to the Prophet (peace and blessings be upon him) and the Prophet (peace and blessings be upon him) said to me, 'Did you insult him by his mother?' 'Yes,' I replied. He said, 'Your brothers are your property. Allah has put them under your authority. If someone has his brother under his authority, he should feed him from what he eats and clothe him from what he wears and not burden him with anything that will be too much for him. If you burden him with what will be too much for him, then help him.'" (Al-Adab Al-Mufrad, Bukhari)

Abu Hurairah (May Allah be pleased with him) reported Allah's Apostle (peace and blessings be upon him) as saying: "He who emancipates his portion in a slave, full emancipation may be secured for him out of his property (if he has money) if he has enough property to meet (the required expenses), but if he has not enough property, the slave should be put to extra labor (in order to earn money for buying his freedom), but he should not be overburdened." (Muslim)

Abu Hurairah (May Allah be pleased with him) reported that the Prophet (May Allah's peace and blessings be upon him) said: "Anyone who relieves a hardship for a believer in this world, Allah will relieve one of his hardships on the Day of Resurrection. Anyone who makes things easy for a hard-pressed person, Allah will make things easy for him in this world and in the Hereafter. Anyone who covers up the faults and sins of a Muslim, Allah will cover up his faults and sins in this world and in the Hereafter. Allah supports His slave as long as the slave supports his brother. Anyone who travels a path in search of knowledge, Allah will make an easy path for him to Paradise. There are no people who gather in one of the houses of Allah, reciting the Book of Allah, learning it and teaching it, except tranquility descends upon them, mercy covers them, the angels flock and hover around them, and Allah mentions them in the presence of those near Him (in the heavens). And anyone who lags behind in doing good deeds, his noble lineage will not advance him any faster." (Muslim) (https://hadeethenc.com/en/browse/hadith/4801)

517. Prohibition for a Slave to Run Away from his Master

Narrated Jarir bin Abdullah (May Allah be pleased with him): The Messenger of Allah (peace and blessings be upon him) said, "If a slave runs away from his master, his responsibility to him is absolved." (Muslim)

Narrated Jarir bin Abdullah (May Allah be pleased with him): The Prophet (peace and blessings be upon him) said, "When the slave runs away from his master, his Salat (prayer) will not be accepted." (Muslim)

Commentary: The institution of slavery does not exist in the modern world, but if it exists anywhere or a situation arises in which it re-emerges, the principle stated in this Hadith will be applicable. The Hadith also makes it clear that if someone has expressed his commitment to serve somebody, he should not back out. It also urges us to show gratefulness to one's benefactors and to reciprocate the good, one receives. (453)

518. Employer Keeping the Passports of Their Employees

The passport actually does not even belong to the holder of the passport; it belongs to the issuing government (the passport holder's country). No one is entitled to hold this document but the one who has his name on it.

It is illegal for the company to hold the passport of employees. It is not allowed to detain the passport except by the official parties with a judicial order and according to the law. The employer can only hold it for a limited period when they are issuing, renewing or cancelling visa. The employers retain employee's passport because companies want to have control over them. Holding passport also amounts to forcible work in violation of International Labour Organization (ILO) Convention on the Abolition of Forced Labour.

As per UAE law for passport keeping, holding passport of employee is illegal and the employer can be fined up to 20,000 dirham's or three years of jail term.

519. Salary Not Paid or Delayed Without Legal Reason

Allah, the Exalted, says:

"And if someone is in hardship, then (let there be) postponement until (a time of) ease. But if you give (from your right as) charity, then it is better for you, if you only knew." (Qur'an, Al-Baqarah 2:280)

Narrated Abdullah bin 'Umar (May Allah have mercy on him): The Messenger of Allah (peace and blessings be upon him) said: "Pay the worker his dues before his sweat has dried up." (Ibn Majah)

Abu Hurairah (May Allah have mercy on him) reported: The Prophet (peace and blessings of Allah be upon him) said: "Delayed payment by a rich person is an act of injustice." (Bukhari and Muslim)

Wages are an earned right. It addresses the rightful dues of those in employment of others, and emphasizes the prompt disbursement of all dues to the worker upon completion of his or her duties.

It is not permissible to delay payment of salaries to employees beyond the time when they are due, which is when the work is completed or at the end of the agreed-upon period. If the agreement is that the salary be paid monthly, then it must be paid to the worker at the end of each month; delaying it with no excuse is regarded as unfair and unjust. (454)

520. Benefit Fraud

Allah, the Exalted, says:

"Do not wrong (others) and do not be wronged (by others)" (Qur'an, Al-Baqarah 2:279)

"Whosoever does righteous good deed it is for (the benefit of) his ownself, and whosoever does evil, it is against his ownself, and your Lord is not at all unjust to (His) slaves." (Qur'an, Fussilat 41:46)

"Whosoever does a good deed, it is for his ownself, and whosoever does evil, it is against (his ownself). Then to your Lord you will be made to return." (Qur'an, Al-Jathiyah 45:15)

Other Verse: Al-Ma'idah 5:1.

Narrated 'Abdullah bin 'Umar (May Allah be pleased with him): "The Prophet (peace and blessings be upon him) used to give me some money (grant) and I would say (to him), 'Give it to a more needy one than me.' Once he gave me some money and I said, 'Give it to a more needy one than me.' The Prophet (peace and blessings be upon him) said (to me), 'Take it and keep it in your possession and then give it in charity. Take whatever comes to you of this money while you are not keen to have it and not ask for it; take it, but you should not seek to have what you are not given." (Bukhari)

Abu Hurairah (May Allah have mercy on him) narrated that the Prophet (peace and blessings be upon him) said: "A time will come upon the people when one will not care how one gains one's money, legally or illegally." (Bukhari)

Jabir (May Allah have mercy on him) reported God's Messenger (peace and blessings be upon him) as saying, "Flesh which has grown out of what is unlawful will not enter Paradise*, but Hell is more suitable for all flesh which has grown out of what is unlawful." (Ahmad, Darimi and Baihaqi, in *Shu'ab al-Iman*, transmitted it. *The reference here is to people who live on an unlawful source of income.

There is nothing wrong with accepting help from the state if the conditions set out for help apply to you, such as having a certain number of children, or if you have a low income or unemployed, and so on. What is forbidden is using tricks and lies to get this help. (455)

You commit Benefit Fraud by claiming benefits from state you are not entitled to on purpose.

For example, by:

- not reporting a change in your circumstances
- providing false information or falsifying documents

If you have committed Benefit Fraud, one or more of the following may also happen in this life:

- you will be told to pay back the overpaid money
- you may be taken to court or asked to pay a penalty
- your benefits may be reduced or stopped

The following benefits can be reduced or stopped if you commit Benefit Fraud:

- Carer's Allowance
- Employment and Support Allowance
- Housing Benefit
- Incapacity Benefit
- Income Support
- Jobseeker's Allowance
- Severe Disablement Allowance

- Widowed Mother's/Parent's Allowance, etc.

What the Muslim should do is earn his living with his own hands and refrain from taking people's wealth. It is not the characteristic of the Muslim to look for the wealth that is in other people's hands, let alone take it unlawfully. If a Muslim is living in a non-Islamic state, then it is even more necessary for him to refrain from taking their wealth, and he should not humiliate himself by seeking the help that these countries offer to those who are unemployed, as working hard and striving to earn a living is better for him than humiliating himself.

With regard to taking help (benefits) from the government - whether it is Muslim or not - when you are not entitled to it and you do not meet the conditions stipulated, that is haram wealth.

Between you and the state there is a covenant whereby entitlement to this money is subject to conditions, so the conditions must apply to you in order for their wealth to become permissible for you.

If a person is working and has a salary, then he is not entitled to any help (benefits). If he does not work despite the availability of opportunities for permissible work, then the help is also haram for him. (456)

Getting benefits by cheating and making use of deceptive methods by providing the state with false information or falsifying documents includes two forbidden matters:

- The first is telling a lie.
- The second is benefiting and making use of people's money without any right.

521. Withholding Excess Water from Others

Allah, the Exalted, says:

"Have not those who disbelieve known that the heavens and the earth were joined together as one united piece, then We parted them? And We have made from water every living thing. Will they not then believe?" (Qur'an, Al-Anbya 21:30)

"...and the water (rain) which Allah sends down from the sky and makes the earth alive therewith after its death." (Qur'an, Al-Baqarah 2:164)

Narrated Abu Hurairah (May Allah have mercy on him): Allah's Messenger (peace and blessings be upon him) said, "Do not withhold the superfluous water, for that will prevent people from grazing their cattle." (Bukhari)

Narrated Abu Hurairah (May Allah have mercy on him): Allah's Apostle (peace and blessings be upon him) said, "There are three persons whom Allah will not look at on the Day of Resurrection, nor will he purify them and theirs shall be a severe punishment. They are: 1. A man possessed superfluous water on a way and he withheld it from travelers, 2. A man who gave a pledge of allegiance to a ruler and he gave it only for worldly benefits. If the ruler gives him something, he gets satisfied, and if the ruler withholds something from him, he gets dissatisfied, 3. And man displayed his goods for sale after the 'Asr prayer and he said, 'By Allah, except Whom None has the right to be worshipped, I have been given so much for my goods', and somebody believes him (and buys them)." The Prophet then recited: *"Verily! Those who purchase a little gain at the cost of Allah's covenant and their oaths." (Qur'an, Ali 'Imran 3.77)* (Bukhari)

522. Prohibition of the Sale of Excess Water in the Barren Lands and Preventing

People to Use it

Jabir b. 'Abdullah (May Allah be pleased with him) reported that Allah's Messenger (peace and blessings be upon him) forbade the sale of excess water. (Muslim)

Abu Hurairah (May Allah be pleased with him) reported Allah's Messenger (peace and blessings be upon him) as saying: "The excess of water should not be sold in order to enable the sate of herbage." (Muslim)

523. Prohibition of Malpractices in Commerce

Allah, the Exalted, says:

"O you who believe! Eat not up your property among yourselves unjustly except it be a trade amongst you, by mutual consent. And do not kill yourselves (nor kill one another). Surely, Allah is Most Merciful to you." (Qur'an, An-Nisa 4:29)

The Noble Qur'an enunciates the fundamental principles of commerce as follows:

1. To give just measure and weight.
2. Not to withhold from the people the things that are their due.
3. Not to commit evil on the earth with the intent of doing mischief.

4. To be contented with the profit that is left with us by God after we have paid other people their due.

All transactions should be based on the fundamental principle of "Ta'auanu ala birri wa't-taqwa" (mutual cooperation for the cause of goodness or piety).

Unlawful transactions are motivated by lust for money and an ignoble desire to build up prestige.

The Prophet (peace and blessings be upon him) has not only disapproved of certain forms of business transactions, but has also laid down some basic conditions that should be fulfilled in every transaction if it is to be lawful.

The following are some of these basic conditions:

1. **Things sold and money offered as their price to be lawfully acquired.** The things sold and the money to be offered as their price should both be lawfully acquired and clearly specified. This condition demands that the goods sold should have been lawfully obtained. One has no business to sell goods which one has stolen or which one has acquired in a fraudulent manner, nor should one purchase anything with the money which one has accepted as illegal gratification or has acquired in some other deceitful way. This condition holds the buyer and the seller responsible for lawful possession of the goods on the part of one and of the money on the part of other.
2. **Goods not to be sold before obtaining their possession.** The Holy Prophet (peace and blessings be upon him) has warned the Muslims against indulging in forward transactions which means selling goods before obtaining their possession. "Whoever buys cereals shall not tell them until he has obtained their possession", says the Holy Prophet (peace be upon him). According to Ibn Abbas, what applies to cereals also applies to other categories of goods. On another occasion the Holy Prophet (peace be upon him) has said: "Bargain not about that which is not with you."
3. **Goods to be bought in the open market.** Goods and commodities for sale should go into the open market, and the seller or his agents must be aware of the state of the market before proposals are made for the purchase by the buyers. The seller should not be taken unawares lest the buyers should take undue advantage of his ignorance of the conditions and prices prevailing in the market.
4. **No trade and traffic in things, the use of which is prohibited by Islam.** A Muslim can trade in those goods and commodities only the use of which has been declared to be Halal (lawful). There can be no trade and traffic in things the use of which is prohibited by Islam. For example, there can be no trade in wine, swine, dead bodies of animals and idols. A devout Muslim merchant would not even traffic in thin and transparent stuff for ladies because the use of such stuff by ladies is unlawful. One cannot sell the carcass of an animal. He can, however, flay its skin which can be used for making shoes and which can therefore, be sold, but not the

flesh of the dead animal. What is true of the usable skin of animals is also true of the tusks of an elephant.

Prohibited forms of Business

1. Monopoly business.

As monopoly means concentration of supply in one hand, it leads to exploitation of the consumers and the workers, it has, therefore, been declared unlawful by the Holy Prophet (peace and blessings be upon him). Gigantic trusts, cartels and monopolies should not exist in the Islamic society. The monopoly-dominated economic order betrays lack of harmony between private and social good and is, thus, a negation of the principle of maximum social advantage which the Islamic society sets out to achieve.

2. Speculative business based on selfish interest.

Speculation means buying something cheap in bulk at a time and selling it dear at another and, thus, controlling the whole market to achieve personal gains. A close observation will reveal that speculators are primarily interested in private gains regardless of the larger interest of the society. These speculators try to create artificial scarcity of goods and commodities and thereby create an inflationary pressure on the economy. As the poor masses have to pay for this, Islam has condemned such speculative business.

3. Interest transactions.

All transactions involving interest are forbidden in Islam. Some people find it hard to submit to the injunction prohibiting interest, because they think interest and profit earned in trade are similar. Capital invested in trade brings an excess called profit; invested in banking it brings interest. Why should one excess be considered lawful and the other unlawful? They fail to take note of the basic difference between the two. Trade involves risk of loss. Also, in its case, it is not only the capital invested that brings profit which is equally the result of initiative, enterprise and efficiency of the entrepreneur. Hence, its rate cannot be predetermined and fixed. Moreover, trade is productive. A person reaps a benefit after undergoing labour and hardship. It creates conditions of full employment and economic growth. It will also be noted that trade acts as one of the dominant factors in the process of building up civilization through cooperation and mutual exchange of ideas. The spread of Islam and Islamic civilization In the Far East has been mostly due to the efforts of Muslim traders. Interest has no redeeming feature at all. The fixed rate of profit which a person gets from a financial investment without any risk of loss and without augmenting it with human labour creates in man the undesirable weakness of miserliness and Shylockian selfishness and lack of sympathy. In the economic sphere it initiates and aggravates crisis.

Rightly, therefore, has Islam strictly prohibited all transactions based on it or involving it in some form or other.

Advancing money on interest, keeping deposits in a bank for the sake of earning interest or getting concessions in rates of goods or commodities against advance payments of price, mortgaging and utilizing an income-yielding property against a certain sum, to be returned in full when the property is redeemed and investing money in a trade against a predetermined and fixed rate of profit - are all unlawful business transactions because they involve Riba (interest) in some form or the other.

4. Transactions similar (in nature) to gambling.

The Arabic equivalent to gambling is Maisir which literarily means "getting something too easily", "getting a profit without working for it". The literal meaning of the term explains the principle on account of which gambling is prohibited in Islam. Any monetary gain which corns too easily, so much so that one does not have to work for it, is unlawful.

The most familiar form of gambling among the Arabs in the days of the Holy Prophet (May peace be upon him) was gambling by casting of lots by means of arrows drawn from a bag. Some were blank and those who drew them got nothing. Others indicated prizes-big or small ones. Whether one got anything or nothing depended on pure luck, unless there was fraud on the part of someone concerned. The principle on which objection to gambling is based, is that you gain what you have not earned, or lose on a mere chance. Dice, lottery, prize bonds and betting on horse races are to be held within the definition of gambling.

5. Munabadha and Mulamasa.

Islam recognizes barter trade subject to the injunctions of the Qur'an and the Sunnah. In fact, Islam has closed all doors of dishonesty and deceit in business dealings. It has prohibited all forms of transactions which admit of fraud in the least degree. It has impressed on the traders that defective and worthless goods should not be given in exchange for good ones, and if there is a defect in the goods sold it must be pointed out and made manifest to the purchaser. The Messenger of Allah (May peace be upon him) said: "The buyer and the seller have the option of cancelling the contract as long as they have not separated; then, if they both speak the truth and make manifest, their transaction shall be blessed, and it they conceal and tell lies, the blessing of their transaction shall be obliterated." (Muslim, Kitab Al-Buyu' (The Book of Transactions), https://www.iium.edu.my/deed/hadith/muslim/010_smt.html

Anas bin Malik (May Allah be pleased with him) said: "The Messenger of Allah (peace and blessings be upon him) forbade that a person in the city should make a deal on behalf of a villager on commission even if he is his real brother." (Bukhari and Muslim)

Narrated Ibn 'Umar (May Allah be pleased with him): The Messenger of Allah (peace and blessings be upon him) said, "Do not meet the merchandise till they arrive in the market." (Bukhari and Muslim)

Narrated Ibn 'Abbas (May Allah be pleased with him): The Messenger of Allah (peace and blessings be upon him) said, "The caravans carrying merchandise should not be met on the way to purchase from them; a man in the city should not sell for a man of the desert." Tawus asked him (Ibn 'Abbas): "What do these words really imply?" He said: "He should not work as an agent on his behalf." (Bukhari and Muslim)

Narrated Abu Hurairah (May Allah be pleased with him): "The Messenger of Allah (peace and blessings be upon him) forbade that a man in the city should be the commission agent of a man from the desert and prohibited the practice of Najsh (i.e. offering a high price for something in order to allure another customer who is interested in the thing); and that a man should make an offer while the offer of his brother is pending; or that he should make a proposal of marriage while that of his brother is pending; or that a woman should try that a sister of hers might be divorced, so that she might take her place. (Bukhari and Muslim)

Narrated Ibn 'Umar (May Allah be pleased with him): The Messenger of Allah (peace and blessings be upon him) said, "A person should not enter into a transaction when his (Muslim) brother has already negotiated, nor should he make a proposal of marriage when that of his brother is pending, except with the permission of the latter." (Bukhari and Muslim)

Narrated 'Uqbah bin 'Amir (May Allah be pleased with him): The Messenger of Allah (peace and blessings be upon him) said, "A Mu'min is the brother of another Mu'min; and thus, it is not permissible for a Mu'min to make an offer while the offer of his brother is pending, nor should he make a proposal of marriage while that of his brother is pending till he withdraws his proposal." (Muslim)

Commentary:
All the acts prohibited in the Ahadith cited above are such that they can cause or increase ill-will and enmity among people. For this reason, all these things have been forbidden by Islam to obviate all possibilities of dissension and discord and bring about mutual affection, fraternity and accord. (457)

524. Selling the Commodity Before Taking the Possession of it

Ibn Abbas (Allah be pleased with them) reported Allah's Messenger (peace and blessings be upon him) as saying: "He who buys food grain should not sell it until he has taken possession of it." (Muslim)

The Prophet (peace and blessings be upon him) said: "Bargain not about that which is not with you." (Muslim) (https://www.iium.edu.my/deed/hadith/muslim/010_smt.html)

525. Short Weighing or Cheating in Business

Allah, the Exalted, says:

"And observe the weight with equity and do not make the balance deficient." (Qur'an, Ar-Rahman 55:9)

"Woe to Al-Mutaffifin [those who give less in measure and weight (decrease the rights of others)], Those who, when they have to receive by measure from men, demand full measure, And when they have to give by measure or weight to men, give less than due. Think they not that they will be resurrected (for reckoning), On a Great Day, The Day when (all) mankind will stand before the Lord of the 'Alamin (mankind, Jinns and all that exists)?" (Qur'an, Al-Mutaffifin 83:1-6)

"O my people! Serve Allah, you have no god other than He, and do not give short measure and weight. Surely, I see you in prosperity and surely, I fear for you the punishment of an all-encompassing day. And O my people! Give full measure and weight fairly, and defraud not men their things, and do not act corruptly in the land, making mischief." (Qur'an, Hud 11:84-85)

Other Verse: Al-A'raf 7:85.

Narrated Yahya related to me from Malik from Yahya ibn Said that he had heard that Abdullah ibn Abbas said, "Stealing from the spoils does not appear in a people but that terror is cast into their hearts.

Fornication does not spread in a people but that there is much death among them. A people do not lessen the measure and weight but that provision is cut off from them. A people do not judge without right but that blood spreads among them. A people do not betray the pledge but that Allah gives their enemies power over them." (Malik Muwatta)

Narrated Ibn 'Abbas (May Allah be pleased with him): "When the Prophet (peace be upon him) came to Al-Madinah, they were the worst people in weights and measures. Then Allah, Glorious is He, revealed: *"Woe to Al-Mutaffifin [those who give less in measure and weight (decrease the rights of others)]."* (Qur'an, Al-Mutaffifin 83:1) and they were fair in weights and measures after that." (Ibn Majah)

Narrated Isma'il bin 'Ubaid bin Rifa'ah, from his father, that his grandfather Rifa'ah said: "We went out with the Messenger of Allah (peace and blessings be upon him) and the people were trading early in the morning. He called them: 'O merchants!' And when they looked up and craned their necks, he said: 'The merchants will be raised on the Day of Resurrection as immoral people, apart from those who fear Allah and act righteously and speak the truth (i.e. those who are honest).'" (Ibn Majah)

Abu Safwan Suwayd ibn Qays (May Allah be pleased with him) reported: "Makhramah al-'Abdi and I brought some linen garments from Hajar. The Prophet (May Allah's peace and blessings be upon him) came to us and bargained with us for some pants. There was a man present who would weigh merchandise (in scales) for a wage. The Prophet (May Allah's peace and blessings be upon him) said to him: 'Weigh, and add some more.'" (Tirmidhi) (https://hadeethenc.com/en/browse/hadith/3737)

Narrated Abu Hurairah (May Allah be pleased with him): The Messenger of Allah (peace and blessings of Allah be upon him) happened to pass by a heap of eatables (corn). He thrust his hand in that (heap) and his fingers were moistened. He said to the owner of that heap of eatables (corn): "What is this?" He replied: "Messenger of Allah, these have been drenched by rainfall." He (the Holy Prophet) remarked: "Why did you not place this (the drenched part of the heap) over other eatables so that the people could see it? He who deceives is not of me (is not my follower)." (Muslim)

Cheating when weighing or measuring out goods is considered as a type of theft, a breach of faith and consuming other's property through falsehood.

526. Mixing Bad Articles with Good Ones and Selling at the Higher Price

Hakim b. Hazim (May Allah be pleased with him) reported Allah's Messenger (peace and blessings be upon him) as saying: "The buyer and the seller have the option of cancelling the contract as long as they have not separated; then, if they both speak the truth and make manifest, their transaction shall be blessed, and if they conceal and tell lies, the blessing of their transaction shall be obliterated." (Muslim)

Mixing the bad articles with good ones and then selling them all at a high price (of the good merchandise) without clarifying the reality of the truth; it is a Fraud.

527. Falsifying the Origin, Quality or Expiration Date of Goods

Falsifying the origin, quality and expiration date in order to make more profit.

Abdullah b. Dinar (May Allah be pleased with him) narrated that he heard Ibn 'Umar (May Allah be pleased with them) saying: "A man mentioned to the Messenger of Allah (peace and blessings be upon him) that he was deceived in a business transaction, whereupon Allah's Messenger (peace and blessings be upon him) said: "When you enter into a transaction, say: There should be no attempt to deceive." (Muslim)

Narrated Wathilah bin Asqa' (May Allah be pleased with him): "I heard the Messenger of Allah (peace and blessings be upon him) say: 'Whoever sells defective goods without pointing it out, he will remain subject to the Wrath of Allah, and the angels will continue to curse him.'" (Ibn Majah) (https://hadithanswers.com/selling-defective-goods-without-pointing-out-the-defect)

Hakim b. Hazim (May Allah be pleased with him) reported Allah's Messenger (peace and blessings be upon him) as saying: "The buyer and the seller have the option of cancelling the contract as long as they have not separated; then, if they both speak the truth and make manifest, their transaction shall be blessed, and if they conceal and tell lies, the blessing of their transaction shall be obliterated." (Muslim)

528. Lying and Concealing the Defects of Goods

Narrated Uqbah bin Amir (May Allah be pleased with him): "I heard the Messenger of Allah (peace and blessings be upon him) say: 'The Muslim is the brother of another Muslim, and it is not permissible for a Muslim to sell his brother goods in which there is a defect, without pointing that out to him.'" (Ibn Majah)

Hakim b. Hazim (May Allah be pleased with him) reported Allah's Messenger (peace and blessings be upon him) as saying: "The buyer and the seller have the option of cancelling the contract as long as they have not separated; then, if they both speak the truth and make manifest, their transaction shall be blessed, and if they conceal and tell lies, the blessing of their transaction shall be obliterated." (Muslim)

They want to sell, will praise it and swear by Allah that it is good, and they will fabricate reasons why they want to sell it, but Allah knows all secrets and that which is yet more hidden. (458)

529. Misleading Others About Real Price

Narrated Abu Hurairah (May Allah be pleased with him): The Messenger of Allah said: "Do not envy one another, do not inflate prices one to another, do not hate one another, do not turn away from one another, and do not undercut one another, but be you, O servants of Allah, brothers. A Muslim is the brother of a Muslim: he neither oppresses him nor does he fail him, he neither lies to him nor does he hold him in contempt. Piety is right here - and he pointed to his breast three times. It is evil enough for a man to hold his brother Muslim in contempt. The whole of a Muslim for another Muslim is inviolable: his blood, his property and his honor." (Muslim)

Selling at a much higher rate to a person who is ignorant of its actual value, is also a type of Fraud.

530. Ba'i al-Najsh, a type of Impermissible Sale

Narrated Abu Hurairah (May Allah be pleased with him): The Prophet (peace and blessings be upon him) said, "No town dweller should sell for a Bedouin. Do not practice Najsh (i.e. do not offer a high price for a thing which you do not want to buy, in order to deceive the people). No Muslim should offer more for a thing already bought by his Muslim brother, nor should he demand the hand of a girl already engaged to another Muslim. A Muslim woman shall not try to bring about the divorce of her sister (i.e. another Muslim woman) in order to take her place herself." (Bukhari)

Narrated Abu Hurairah (May Allah be pleased with him): "Allah's Apostle (peace and blessings be upon him) forbade:

1) the meeting of the caravan (of goods) on the way,
2) that a residing person sells goods of a Bedouin,
3) that a woman stipulates the divorce of the wife of the would-be husband,
4) that a man tries to cause the cancellation of a bargain concluded by another.

He also forbade An-Najsh (see Hadith 837) and that one withholds the milk in the udder of the animal so that he may deceive people on selling it." (Bukhari)

531. Selling a Product at Different Prices to Different Customers

The vendor should sell the item for the price for which it is sold in the marketplace; if he sells it for a price different from that for which it is sold in the marketplace, one of two scenarios must apply:

1 – He sells it for less than its market value, such as if he wants to do a favor for one of his friends. This is permissible and there is nothing wrong with it, and the seller should not be stopped from doing that unless he intends to cause harm to other merchants, because the Prophet (peace and blessings of Allah be upon him) said: "There should be neither harming no reciprocating harm." (Ibn Majah)

2 – He sells it for more than the market value. If he sells it for slightly more, such as selling something that is worth twenty for twenty-two, then this is permissible because it is something that usually happens and people tolerate it.

But if the price is greatly increased, and the purchaser does not know the usual price – such as if he sells something that is usually worth sixty for ninety, as mentioned in the question – then this is not permissible, and is a kind of cheating and deception. In this case the purchaser has the option, if he is told of the situation, of returning the goods. (See al-Mughni, 4/18)

Sheikh Ibn 'Uthaymeen (May Allah have mercy on him) was asked:

"What is the ruling on merchants who sell things for different prices to different people, even though it is the same product? So, he sells it to one person for ten, to another for twenty, and to a third for five? Is this permissible or not?" He replied:

"If this variation is caused by fluctuations in the market, or the price of this product goes up one day and down the next, then there is nothing wrong with selling it at the market price, and there is nothing haram in that. But if this variation occurs because of the purchaser's skill in bargaining – so if he sees that he is not clever in bargaining, he will increase the price, and if he sees that he is clever in bargaining, then he will give him a lower price – then this is not permissible, because it is a kind of deception and insincerity. It was proven in the Hadith of Tameem al-Daari that the Prophet (peace and blessings of Allah be upon him) said: 'Religion is sincerity.' It was said: 'To whom, O Messenger of Allah?' He said: 'To Allah, to His Book, to His Messenger, to the leaders of the Muslims and to their common folk. (Muslim).'" (459)

532. Hoarding, Black Marketing, Adulteration and Profiteering

Allah, the Exalted, says:

"And those who hoard up gold and silver (Al-Kanz: the money, the Zakah of which has not been paid) and spend them not in the way of Allah, announce unto them a painful torment. On the Day when that (Al-Kanz: money, gold and silver, etc., the Zakat of which has not been paid) will be heated in the Fire of Hell and with it will be branded their foreheads, their flanks, and their backs, (and it will be said unto them): "This is the treasure which you hoarded for yourselves. Now taste of what you used to hoard."
(Qur'an, At-Tawbah 9:34-35)

"The mutual rivalry (for hoarding worldly things) preoccupy you. Until you visit the graves (i.e. till you die). Nay! You shall come to know! Again Nay! You shall come to know! Nay! If you knew with a sure knowledge (the end result of hoarding, you would not have been occupied in worldly things). Verily, you shall see the blazing Fire (Hell)! And again, you shall see it with certainty of sight! Then (on that Day) you shall be asked about the delights (you indulged in, in this world)!" (Qur'an, At-Takathur 102:1-8)

Other Verse: Al-Hashr 59:7, Ali 'Imran 3:185, Al-An'am 6:32.

Ma'mar b. Abdullah (May Allah be pleased with him) reported Allah's Messenger (peace and blessings be upon him) as saying: "No one hoards but the sinner." (Muslim)

Narrated Ibn 'Umar (May Allah be pleased with him): The Messenger of Allah (peace and blessings be upon him) said: "The trustworthy, honest Muslim merchant will be with the martyrs on the Day of Resurrection." (Ibn Majah)

Narrated 'Umar bin Khattab (May Allah be pleased with him): "I heard the Messenger of Allah (peace and blessings be upon him) say: 'Whoever hoards food (and keeps it from) the Muslims, Allah will afflict him with leprosy and bankruptcy.'" (Ibn Majah)

Asma' bint Abu Bakr (May Allah be pleased with her) reported: Messenger of Allah (peace and blessings be upon him) said to me, "Do not hoard; otherwise, Allah will withhold from you." (Bukhari and Muslim)

Asma' reported God's Messenger as saying, "Spend, do not calculate and so have God calculating against you, do not hoard and so have God hoarding from you, but give such small amounts as you can." (Bukhari and Muslim)

'Abdullah bin Ash-Shikhkhir (May Allah be pleased with him) reported: "I came to the Prophet (peace and blessings be upon him) while he was reciting *Surah At-Takathur 102*: *"The mutual rivalry (for hoarding worldly things) preoccupy you. Until you visit the graves (i.e. till you die). Nay! You shall come to know! Again Nay! You shall come to know! Nay! If you knew with a sure knowledge (the end result of hoarding, you would not have been occupied in worldly things). Verily, you shall see the blazing Fire (Hell)! And again, you shall see it with certainty of sight! Then (on that Day) you shall be asked about the delights (you indulged in, in this world)!"* *(102:1-8)* After reciting he (peace and blessings be upon him) said, "Son of Adam says: 'My wealth, my wealth.' Do you own of your wealth other than what you eat and consume, and what you wear and wear out, or what you give in Sadaqah (charity) (to those who deserve it), and that what you will have in stock for yourself." (Muslim)

Hoarding of essential items like wheat, barley, rice, oil, etc. during periods of shortages with the intention of selling them at higher rates to people, who are compelled to purchase them, is prohibited.

Hoarding, indulging in profiteering, adulteration and black marketing of medicines, medical equipments and oxygen cylinders during the pandemic are prohibited.

Buying goods from Black market, if there are stolen, is prohibited.

Narrated Anas ibn Malik (May Allah be pleased with him): The people said: "Messenger of Allah, prices have shot up, so fix prices for us. Thereupon the Messenger of Allah (peace and blessings be upon him) said: "Allah is the One Who fixes prices, withholds, gives lavishly and provides, and I hope that when I meet Allah, none of you will have any claim on me for an injustice regarding blood or property." (Abu Dawud)

With regard to the story of Qaroon, it is a practical, real-life example, and definitive proof, that highlights the message of Verses (*3:185, 6:32*) and others which condemn this world and show how the people whose main focus is this world were distracted by it from the Hereafter, and they were content with it and thus were distracted from obeying and worshipping Allah, and how they were punished in this world.

If people gain all luxuries and all good things in this world, they become insolent and transgress, and they forget to give thanks for Allah's blessings. (460)

533. Trade and Traffic in Haram (Unlawful) and Doubtful Things

Allah, the Exalted, says,

"…Help you one another in Al-Birr and At-Taqwa (virtue, righteousness and piety); but do not help one another in sin and transgression. And fear Allah. Verily, Allah is Severe in punishment." (Qur'an, Al-Ma'idah 5:2)

Narrated Ibn Abbas (May Allah be pleased with him): "I saw the Messenger of Allah (peace and blessings be upon him) sitting near the black stone (or at a corner of the Ka'bah). He (the Prophet) raised his eyes towards the heaven and laughed, and he said: 'May Allah curse the Jews!' He said these three times. Allah declared unlawful for them the fats (of the animals which died a natural death); they sold them and they enjoyed the price they received for them. When Allah declared eating of thing forbidden for the people, He declared it price also forbidden for them. The version of Khalid b. 'Abd Allah al-Tahhan does not have the words "I saw". It has: "May Allah destroy the Jews!" (Abu Dawud)

Jabir b. 'Abdullah (May Allah be pleased with him) reported Allah's Messenger (peace be upon him) as saying in the year of Victory while he was in Makkah: "Verily Allah and His Messenger have forbidden the sale of wine, carcass, swine and idols." It was said: 'Allah's Messenger, you see that the fat of the carcass is used for coating the boats and varnishing the hides, and people use it for lighting purposes.' Whereupon he said: 'No, it is forbidden.' Then Allah's Messenger (peace and blessings be upon him) said: 'May Allah, the Exalted and Majestic, destroy the Jews; when Allah forbade the use of fat of the carcass for them, they melted it and then sold it, and made use of its price (received from it)." (Muslim)

Abdullah ibn Abbas (May Allah be pleased with him) reported: Umar (May Allah be pleased with him) was once informed that so-and-so sold alcohol. Umar said: "May Allah destroy so-and-so! Does he not know that the Messenger (May Allah's peace and blessings be upon him) said: 'May Allah destroy the Jews; the fat of animals was forbidden for them, but they melted it and sold it?'" (Bukhari and Muslim) (https://hadeethenc.com/en/browse/hadith/2976)

Narrated An-Nu'man bin Bashir (May Allah be pleased with him): "I heard Allah's Messenger (peace and blessings be upon him) saying, 'Both legal and illegal things are evident but in between them there are doubtful (suspicious) things and most of the people have no knowledge about them. So, whoever saves himself from these suspicious things saves his religion and his honor. And whoever indulges in these suspicious things is like a shepherd who grazes (his animals) near the Hima (private pasture) of someone else and at any moment he is liable to get in it. (O people!) Beware! Every king has a Hima and the Hima of Allah on the earth is His illegal (forbidden) things. Beware! There is a piece of flesh in the body if it becomes good (reformed), the whole body becomes good but if it gets spoilt, the whole body gets spoilt and that is the heart." (Bukhari)

534. Selling Something that Will Be Used for Sinful Purposes

Allah, the Exalted, says:

"And do not help one another in sin and transgression." (Qur'an, Al-Ma'idah 5:2)

This would include selling juice to someone who uses it to make khamr (intoxicants), selling weapons during periods of fitnah (confusion or instability) or selling a house to someone who will use it for sinful deeds. This prohibition is based upon knowledge of the intention or evidence supporting the suspicion.

If the thing is something which it is haram to use in any way and under any circumstances, then it is not permissible to deal in it or to give it as a gift. (461)

535. Prohibition of Deceiving Others

Allah, the Exalted, says:

"Do not handle the property of the orphans except with a good reason until they become mature and strong. Maintain equality in your dealings by the means of measurement and balance. No soul is responsible for what is beyond its ability. Be just in your words, even if the party involved is one of your relatives and keep your promise with God. Thus, does your Lord guide you so that you may take heed." (Qur'an, Al-An'am 6:152)

"They (think to) deceive Allah and those who believe, while they only deceive themselves, and perceive (it) not!" (Qur'an, Al-Baqarah 2:9)

Abu Hurairah (May Allah be pleased with him) said: The Messenger of Allah (peace and blessings be upon him) said, "He who takes up arms against us is none of us; and he who cheats us is none of us." (Muslim)

Ibn 'Umar (May Allah be pleased with him) said: The Messenger of Allah (peace and blessings be upon him) prohibited the practice of Najsh. (Bukhari and Muslim)

Ibn 'Umar (May Allah be pleased with him) said: A man mentioned to the Messenger of Allah (peace and blessings be upon him) that he was often deceived in dealings. The Messenger of Allah (peace and blessings be upon him) said to him, "When you enter into a transaction you should say: 'There should be no deception.'" (Bukhari and Muslim)

Abu Hurairah (May Allah be pleased with him) said: The Messenger of Allah (peace and blessings be upon him) said, "He who deceives another's wife or his slave is none of us." (Abu Dawud)

Commentary: To incite or provoke someone's wife or slave against her husband or his master, or to create hatred between the two is a great crime, because a Muslim is required to create peace and accord amongst people. It is against his conduct to foment dissension and discord between them. (462)

Narrated Isma'il bin 'Ubaid bin Rifa'ah from his father, from his grandfather, that he went with the Messenger of Allah (peace and blessings be upon him) to the Musalla, and he saw the people doing business, so he said: 'O people of trade!' and they replied to the Messenger of Allah (peace and blessings be upon him) turning their necks and their gazes towards him, and he said: "Indeed the merchants will be resurrected on the Day of Judgment with the wicked, except the one who has Taqwa of Allah, who behaves charitably and is truthful." (Tirmidhi)

536. Taking Things that Do Not Belong to You

Allah, the Exalted, says:

"And eat up not one another's property unjustly (in any illegal way, e.g. stealing, robbing, deceiving)." (Qur'an, Al-Baqarah 2:188)

'Uday ibn 'Umayrah (May Allah be pleased with him) reported that the Messenger (May Allah's peace and blessings be upon him) said: "If any of you is assigned by us to a position but conceals a needle or more from us, it will amount to misappropriation and he will be called upon to restore it on the Day of Judgment." A black man from the Ansar stood up - I can still see him - and said: "O Messenger of Allah, take back your assignment from me." The Prophet (May Allah's peace and blessings be upon him) said: "What has happened to you?" The man replied: "I heard you say such-and-such." The Prophet replied: "I say that even now: Whosoever from you is appointed by us to a position, he should render an account of everything, big or small, and whatever he is given therefrom, he should take, and he should desist from taking what is unlawful.'" (Muslim) (https://hadeethenc.com/en/browse/hadith/5412)

Narrated Abdullah ibn as-Sa'ib ibn Yazid (May Allah be pleased with him): The Messenger of Allah (peace and blessings be upon him) said: "None of you should take the property of his brother in amusement (i.e. jest), nor in earnest." The narrator Sulayman said: 'Out of amusement and out of earnest'. If anyone takes the staff of his brother, he should return it. The transmitter Ibn Bashshar did not say 'Ibn Yazid', and he said: 'The Messenger of Allah (peace and blessings be upon him) said.'" (Abu Dawud)

Narrated Zaid bin Khalid (May Allah have mercy on him): A Bedouin asked the Prophet (peace and blessings of Allah be upon him) about the Luqata. The Prophet (peace and blessings of Allah be upon him) said, "Make public announcement about it for one year and if then somebody comes and describes the container of the Luqata and the string it was tied with (give it to him); otherwise, spend it." He then asked the Prophet (peace and blessings of Allah be upon him) about a lost camel. The face of the Prophet (peace and blessings of Allah be upon him) become red and he said, "You have no concern with it as it has its water reservoir and feet and it will reach water and drink and eat trees. Leave it till its owner finds it." He then asked the Prophet (peace and blessings of Allah be upon him) about a lost sheep. The Prophet (peace and blessings of Allah be upon him) said, "It is for you, for your brother or for the wolf." (Bukhari)

Narrated Ibn Abbas (May Allah be pleased with him): Allah's Messenger (peace and blessings be upon him) also said, "It (i.e. Makkah's) thorny bushes should not be uprooted and its game should not be chased, and picking up its fallen things is illegal except by him who makes public announcement about it, and its grass should not be cut." Abbas said, "O Allah's Messenger! Except Eidhkhir (a kind of grass)." The Prophet (peace and blessings be upon him) said, "Except Eidhkhir." (Bukhari)

Narrated Ubai bin Kab (May Allah be pleased with him): "I found a purse containing one hundred Dinars. So, I went to the Prophet (peace and blessings be upon him) and informed him about it, he said, "Make public announcement about it for one year." I did so, but nobody turned up to claim it, so I again went to the Prophet (peace and blessings be upon him) who said, "Make public announcement for another year." I did, but none turned up to claim it. I went to him for the third time and he said, "Keep the container and the string which is used for its tying and count the money it contains and if its owner comes, give it to him; otherwise, utilize it." The sub-narrator Salama said, "I met him (Suwaid, another sub-narrator) in Makkah and he said, 'I don't know whether Ubai made the announcement for three years or just one year.'" (Bukhari)

Possessing something that belongs to someone else, means intending to deprive the owner of it, including the lost and found things, animals. (463)

537. Internet Fraud

From computer viruses to website hacking and financial fraud, Internet crime became a larger concern. Auction or retail fraud, Investment fraud, non-delivery of merchandise or payment, confidence fraud, etc.

The Internet consumers were invited to view or to access free computer images, when viewers attempted to access the images, their computer modems were surreptitiously disconnected from their local Internet Service Providers (ISPs) and were reconnected to the Internet through the defendants' expensive international modem connections. Exorbitantly priced long-distance telephone charges continued to accrue until the consumer turned off the computer.

Electronic viruses are malicious software programs written to cause harm to unsuspecting computer users. They are designed to spread from computer to computer.

538. Website Redirects

Malicious redirects are typically inserted into a website by attackers with the intent of generating illegal income. You may receive unexpected SMS on your mobile "Thank you for the subscription for… You will be charged weekly, monthly, etc. …"

539. Phishing

Phishing is the fraudulent attempt to obtain the usernames, passwords and credit card details by disguising as a trustworthy entity.

540. Email Fraud

The "request for help" email fraud from someone you do not know or from someone from the dating website you were communicating. Or your email won 1 million dollars or email from a wealthy person, who wants to place his money with mutual benefits into your bank, or business email fraud, where employees with access to company finances, are tricked into making money transfers by an email pretending to be from the CEO or a trusted customer.

"I need your urgent assistance in transferring the sum of $4.5 Million US Dollars. This money has been dormant for years in our bank without claim. I want the bank to release the money to you as the nearest person (next of kin) to our deceased customer; I don't want the money to go into bank treasury as an abandoned fund."

541. Charitable Organization Fraud

Fraudulent charitable organizations solicit people to make donations to various causes that do not actually exist or exist but money never reach the needy people. These fake organizations are very active especially immediately after disaster. They do not believe in the Judgment Day.

Various charity foundations for different diseases researches misappropriate the funds.

There are many reliable government charity organizations in UAE.

542. Pyramid Scheme

Allah, the Exalted, says:

"O you who believe! Intoxicants (all kinds of alcoholic drinks) and gambling, and Al-Ansab (stone altars for sacrifices to idols, etc.), and Al-Azlaam (arrows for seeking luck or decision) are an abomination of Shaytan's (Satan's) handiwork. So, avoid (strictly all) that (abomination) in order that you may be successful." (Qur'an, Al-Ma'idah 5:90)

Pyramid Scheme is based on gambling. Allah has forbidden gambling. Gambling refers to any transaction in which there may be a gain or a loss, and in which a person does not know whether he will be a winner or a loser.

As for not knowing how the money is invested, that is because it is not known where the company puts its money or how it invests it. It is not permissible for anyone to invest his money. Many of these companies do not invest the money at all; rather they cheat people and consume their wealth unlawfully. Hence these kinds of companies are known in some countries as companies that sell dreams, or illusionary pyramids, because no one gains from them except a small number of people, then the company soon folds and ceases operation.

A number of scholars have issued Fatwas stating that it is prohibited to deal with companies that use pyramid schemes, even if they sell some goods or products. (464)

543. Lottery Scam

Allah, the Exalted, says:

"O you who believe! Intoxicants (all kinds of alcoholic drinks) and gambling, and Al-Anaab (stone altars for sacrifices to idols, etc.), and Al-Azlaam (arrows for seeking luck or decision) are an abomination of Shaytan's (Satan's) handiwork. So, avoid (strictly all) that (abomination) in order that you may be successful." (Qur'an, Al-Ma'idah 5:90)

"Shaytan (Satan) wants only to excite enmity and hatred between you with intoxicants (alcoholic drinks) and gambling, and hinder you from the remembrance of Allah, and from As Salah (the prayer). So, will you not then abstain?" (Qur'an, Al-Ma'idah 5:91)

Other Verse: *Al-Baqarah 2:219.*

Sheikh 'Abd al-'Azeez ibn Baaz (May Allah have mercy on him) was asked:

"Are the lotteries or raffles which some charities organize to raise funds for their activities in the educational, medical or social work fields, permissible according to Shariah?" He answered: "Lotteries and raffles are other names for gambling, which is haram according to the Qur'an and Sunnah, and the consensus of the scholars. It is not permissible for the Muslims to engage in any kind of gambling at all, whether the money collected from gambling is to spent on charitable projects or otherwise, because it is evil and forbidden, as indicated by the general meaning of the evidence (daleel), and because the earnings derived from gambling are among the kinds of earnings which we must avoid and beware of. And Allah is the Source of strength. (Fataawa Islamiyyah, 4/442) (465)

544. Bank Fraud

There are different types of Bank Fraud: Accounting fraud, Demand draft fraud, Remotely created check fraud, Uninsured deposits, Bill discounting fraud, Duplication or skimming of card information, Cheque kiting, Forged or fraudulent documents, Forgery and altered cheques, Fraudulent loan applications, Fraudulent loans, Empty ATM envelope deposits, the fictitious 'bank inspector', Identity theft or Impersonation, Money laundering, Payment card fraud, Booster cheques, Stolen cheque, Stolen payment cards, Phishing or Internet fraud, Prime bank fraud, Wire transfer fraud, Rogue traders, etc.

545. Credit Card Fraud

Credit card fraud is an inclusive term for fraud committed using a credit card or debit card. The purpose may be to obtain goods or services, or to make payment to another account, which is controlled by a criminal.

Credit card is a Riba – prohibited by Almighty God.

546. Check Fraud

Check fraud is incredibly widespread. In fact, because there are so many different types of check fraud, no one has the exact numbers on how many people are affected or how much money is lost each year.

Here are examples of some of the most common types of fraud: Paperhanging, Check Kiting, Check Floating, Check Forgery, Check, Identity Check Theft, Chemical Alteration, Counterfeiting, Money Order Fraud, etc.

547. Job Offer Fraud

Fake employment offers have become increasingly common. There are some useful ways on how to spot scams and fraudulent proposals: it seems too good to be true, the email text is unprofessional, the offer was sent from a personal email, you are asked to provide confidential information, it involves money transfers, you are asked to pay for something, it involves working from home, you didn't apply for the job, etc.

548. University Admission Fraud

Parents of high school students conspired with other people to use bribery and other forms of fraud to illegally arrange to have their children admitted to top colleges and universities in USA. Read about Scandal named "Operation Varsity Blues": https://en.wikipedia.org/wiki/Varsity_Blues_scandal.

I received a letter with "Congratulations, you have been (conditionally) accepted to Tilburg University! Now that you have been offered a place…in your envelope you will find the "Welcome to Tilburg University Guide". We would like to inform you that there is small mistake; for statutory fee for the academic year 2019-2020 is 2083 euro and the institutional fee however is correct." The letter was addressed to me, but I had no idea about Tilburg University.

549. Work from Home Scam

Anything that seems too good to be true, to get-rich-quick schemes, should be avoid.

The true purpose of this kind of offer is to extort money from the victim, either by charging a fee to join the scheme or requiring the victim to invest in products, whose resale value is misrepresented.

550. Online Shopping Fraud

The website of Online Shopping can be fake or the items you paid for but they will be fake, other times you will receive nothing at all.

551. Identity Fraud and Identity Theft

Identity fraud is the use by one person of another person's personal information, without authorization, to commit a crime or to deceive or defraud that other person or a third person. Most identity fraud is committed in the context of financial advantages, such as accessing a victim's credit card, bank accounts or loan accounts.

Identity theft is when someone uses your personal information to open and abuse new accounts or services in your name - or possibly to impersonate you in other ways.

552. Passport Fraud

Some organizations offer the second passport or offer their service to obtain, for example, Canadian citizenship, etc. They only try to sell information kits that outline how to apply.

A fake passport is a counterfeit of a passport issued by a nation or authorized agency. Such counterfeits are copies of genuine passports or illicitly modified genuine passports made by unauthorized persons. Its purpose is to be used deceptively. Falsified passports can be used to leave a country from which exit is barred, for identity theft, illegal immigration and organized crime.

Here is one example of documents Fraud online:

"We are the world number one independent group of specialized IT professionals and database technicians base in the USA, we are specialized in the making of genuine passport SSN, ID card, Birth Certificate, Visa, PR, Diplomas and many other documents of very unique quality. We have produced passport, Driver's license, SSN, ID card, Birth Certificate, Diploma and other documents for over 150 countries. We also produce high quality undetectable GBP notes, fake dollar bills, fake euro bills that you can use anywhere." (https://validdocsonline.com)

553. False Advertising

False advertising is the use of false, misleading or unproven information to advertise products. One form of false advertising is to claim that a product has a health benefit that it in fact does not. A false advertisement can further be classified as deceptive if the advertiser deliberately misleads the consumer.

554. Advertising Interrupting Allah's Words, the Qur'an Recitation

Advertising (selling the products) invaded even the Qur'an recitation on youtube. Do you know that your business success and provisions depend only from Allah, the Provider, the Disposer of all affairs?

555. Telecommunication Fraud

Responding to the text message can allow malware to be installed that will silently collect personal information from your phone. You might end up with unwanted charges on your cell phone bill.

The 'Wangiri scam' occurs when people ring back a missed call from an anonymous international number, and are then routed to premium rate numbers. An automated message then plays, which cannot be disconnected unless the user switches off his phone.

As well as recorded messages, victims of the scam have also received other numbers and texts offering contests to win money. When they call back, the pre-recorded response sucks away the user's credit.

The fake callers from Telecom inform the innocent subscribers that they have won lucky draw and ask to follow certain steps to claim the prize money. In the fraudulent call, people are lured to make transactions in order to get hold of their bank details.

556. Prize and Winning Fraud

Be aware of the Unexpected Prize or Winnings. The scammers may notify you that your mobile or your email won 1 million USD. To claim your prize, you will be asked to pay a fee, for example, for taxes, bank fees or courier charges. The scammers may ask for your identity, bank account to steal personal data.

557. Scientific Article Publication Fraud

Pseudo-scientific article publishing platforms accepting any article, based on pay-publish-profit system, without checking the accuracy, without serious Editorial Board. These compagnies want to collect money as much as they can to publish the articles and spread "fake-science".

Some publishing articles companies look US based online to attract people but in reality, they are based in India or somewhere else. Some publishing companies just collect money without publishing.

558. Congress Fraud

The organizer of the Congress may invite you as a valuable speaker at Annual World Congress. These organizing companies do not select the speakers, the quality of the presentations and benefits of attending, with few exceptions, do not bring something useful for the current practice.

The main purpose of these organizing private companies to have financial profits from the registration fees. The Congress has big name like Annual World, in reality, there are only 7-15 attendants and most of them are the speakers.

Some fake Congress organizations collect the registration fees then block the speaker's email.

559. Visa Fraud

Many people are deceived by scamsters who take their money without providing visa or provide them with fake visa.

560. Immigration Fraud

The websites offering immigration or citizenship services are too good to be true. Some promote legitimate representatives' services that you will need to pay for. Others, will offer false guarantees to take your money or steal your private information.

561. Online Travel Agency Fraud

Anyone who travels is always looking for the best available price. Instead of getting the best price, these websites often overcharge on purpose with few avenues of recourse.

Cancelled air ticket with confirmation of the calculated refund but you never receive the refund money. Or payment is done for the air ticket but there is no ticket.

Free airline tickets advertising. Instead, you will reach a third-party "phishing" website unaffiliated with the airline which will access your information.

562. Airline Baggage Lost Coverage Insurance Fraud

Baggage Lost Coverage Insurance can be fake, just collecting money without any action. The passenger can also falsely claim baggage lost with valuable things. Fraud possible from both sides.

563. Property Management Fraud

Property management companies overcharging for the maintenance services or billing for work that has not been completed or that was not needed.

564. Car Repair Fraud

You bring your vehicle for regular service. And you may receive a call that your car needs some job to be fixed or some parts should be replaced, when in reality, your car doesn't need any job.

565. Prohibition of Squandering Wealth

Allah, the Exalted, says:

"O children of Adam, take your adornment at every Masjid, and eat and drink, but be not excessive. Indeed, He likes not those who commit excess." (Qur'an, Al-A'raf 7:31)

"And give the relative his right and (also) the poor, and the traveler, and do not spend wastefully. Indeed, the wasteful are brothers of the Devils, and ever has Satan been to his Lord ungrateful." (Qur'an, Al-Isra 17:26-27)

"...the extravagant are the inmates of the Fire." (Qur'an, Ghafir 40:43)

Narrated Abu Hurairah (May Allah be pleased with him): The Messenger of Allah (peace and blessings be upon him) said, "Verily, Allah likes three things for you and disapproves three things for you. He likes that you should worship Him Alone, not to associate anything with Him (in worship) and to hold fast to the Rope of Allah and not to be divided among yourselves; and He disapproves for you irrelevant talk, persistent questioning and the squandering of the wealth." (Muslim)

Commentary:

Wealth has a great importance in man's life since it is the very source of sustenance and basis of his livelihood, its wastage is akin to cutting the branch of the tree on which one is sitting. (466)

Warrad, the scribe of Al-Mughirah bin Shu'bah (May Allah be pleased with him) said: "Al-Mughirah bin Shu'bah dictated a letter to me addressed to Mu'awiyah (May Allah be pleased with him) that the Prophet (peace and blessings be upon him) used to supplicate at the end of each obligatory salat (prescribed prayer): 'La ilaha illallahu, wahadahu la sharika lahu, lahul-mulku, wa lahul-hamdu, wa Huwa `ala kulli shai'in Qadir. Allahumma la mani`a lima a`taita, wa la mu`tiya lima mana`ta, wa la yanfa`u dhal-jaddi mink-al-jaddu. (There is no true god except Allah, the One, Who has no partner. His is the Sovereignty and His is the Praise, and He is Able to do everything. O Allah! Nobody can withhold what You give; and nobody can give what You withhold; and the high status of a person is of no avail against Your Will).' He also wrote to him that the Prophet (peace and blessings be upon him) used to forbid irrelevant talk, wasteful expenditure, persistent questioning, disobedience of parents (especially mothers), infanticide of daughters by burying them alive, depriving others of their rights and acquisition of property wrongfully." (Bukhari and Muslim)

Abu Umamah (May Allah be pleased with him) reported: The Prophet (peace and blessings be upon him) said, "…My Lord presented me with the valley of Makkah that He might turn it into gold for me." I said: "No, O Lord, rather I will be satiated some days and hungry some days. When I am hungry, I will humble myself to You and remember You. When I am satiated, I will be grateful to You and praise You." (Tirmidhi)

Narrated Abu Hurairah (May Allah be pleased with him): The Prophet (peace and blessings be upon him) said, "Wealth is not in having many possessions, but rather (true) wealth is feeling sufficiency in the soul." (Bukhari)

Extravagance means crossing the limits or spending wastefully. Spending on something useless is haram, even if it is only a single dirham. Throwing away food and drink leftover after drinking and eating, tearing up and throwing away old clothes, having a light on when there is enough sunlight. Spending on the luxury cars, jewelry, dress, vacation, wedding party, fireworks, trip to Mars, etc.

Eating when one is already full is a waste and harmful.

566. Buying Distinct Mobile Phone Numbers and Car Fancy Plate Numbers

Allah, the Exalted, says:

"…and eat and drink but waste not by extravagance, certainly He (Allah) likes not Al-Musrifun (those who waste by extravagance)." (Qur'an, Al-A'raf 7:31)

"And give to the kinsman his due and to the Miskeen (poor), and to the wayfarer. But spend not wastefully (your wealth) in the manner of a spendthrift." (Qur'an, Al-Isra 17:26)

"Verily, the spendthrifts are brothers of the Shayateen (Devils), and the Shaytan (Devil-Satan) is ever ungrateful to his Lord." (Qur'an, Al-Isra 17:27)

Abu Barzah Nadlah ibn 'Ubayd al-Aslami (May Allah be pleased with him) reported that the Prophet (May Allah's peace and blessings be upon him) said: "Man's feet will not move from their place on the Day of Resurrection before he is asked about his life, in what did he let it perish? About his knowledge, what did he do with it? About his wealth, from where did he earn it, and on what did he spend it? About his body, in what did he wear it out?" (Tirmidhi) (https://hadeethenc.com/en/browse/hadith/4950)

Abdullah ibn Umar reported (May Allah be pleased with him): The Messenger of Allah (peace and blessings be upon him) said, "Whoever wears a garment in vanity, Allah will make him wear a garment of humiliation on the Day of Resurrection, then He will set it ablaze with Fire." (Ibn Majah)

Buying distinct mobile phone numbers and car license plates for thousands of riyals is a kind of extravagance and wasteful spending on haram things. Allah will ask everyone about his wealth and what he spent on such things.

Especially since we see the Muslims in most parts of the world suffering misery and hardship in their lives. Some of them cannot find a morsel of food with which to ward off hunger, and others cannot find clothes with which to cover their bodies, or a house in which to shelter themselves, and the houses of some of them have been destroyed.

Yet at such a time of hardship we find some Muslims buying a license plate with the number "1" for the equivalent of 2 million dollars in an auction!

It is similar with mobile phone numbers where a number was sold for the equivalent of 360.000 dollars.

This madness has spread in a number of countries where it would have been better for them to help the Muslims and keep their wealth safe from such foolishness, extravagance and waste.

It is not permissible to buy and sell these custom numbers. Even if it may be permissible in some cases, it is not permissible to sell them for such high prices.

The one whom Allah has blessed with wealth, should be grateful for this blessing and take proper care of it. He should not spend it on things that incur the Wrath of Allah or things which serve no purpose. More questions will be asked for more money on the Day of Resurrection and will be asked from where he acquired it and on what he spent it. (467)

567. Saying "Wealth of People"

Allah, the Exalted, says:

"To Him (Allah) belongs what is in the heavens and what is on the earth, and what is between them, and what is under the soil." (Qur'an, Taha 20:6)

"…give them from the wealth of Allah which He has given you." (Qur'an, An-Nur 24:33)

"Believe in Allah and His Messenger and spend (in charity) out of the (sustenance) whereof He has made you heirs. For those of you who believe and spend (in charity) - for them is a great reward." (Qur'an, Al-Hadid 57:7)

Other Verse: *Al-Hashr 59:8.*

Narrated Anas bin Malik: "…Has Allah ordered you to take Zakat (obligatory charity) from our rich people and distribute it amongst our poor people?" The Prophet (peace be upon him) replied, "By Allah, yes."… (Bukhari)

The wealth belongs to Allah, the Owner of everything. It is not permissible to say "the wealth of people" because that means that the people have the right to dispose of it however they wish. (468)

The rulers do not have the right to distribute the wealth of Allah according to their own whims and desires. Rather they are trustees, deputies and agents; they are not the owners.

The "wealth of Allah" must be spent on the general interests of Muslims, to protect Muslim borders and defend Muslim causes in the east and in the west, above all; to call people to Allah; to strive to defeat the oppressors and those who transgress against Muslims, and to meet the needs of those who are in need.

568. 568. Rulings on Dress for Men

Allah, the Exalted, says:

"Children of Adam! We have sent down clothing to you to conceal your private parts." (Qur'an, Al-A'raf 7:26)

"…and eat and drink but waste not by extravagance, certainly He (Allah) likes not Al-Musrifun (those who waste by extravagance)." (Qur'an, Al-A'raf 7:31)

"Bad statements are for bad people (or bad women for bad men) and bad people for bad statements (or bad men for bad women). Good statements are for good people (or good women for good men) and good people for good statements (or good men for good women), such (good people) are innocent of (each and every) bad statement which they say, for them is Forgiveness and Rizqun Karim (generous provision i.e. Paradise)."
(Qur'an, An-Nur 24:26)

The Rulings on Men's Dress.

1. It should cover the Awrah, the area between navel and knees.
2. It should be loose and not tight on his body.
3. It should not cover his ankles.
4. It should not be decorated or ornate such as to attract onlookers.
5. It should not be considered libaas al-shuhrah (i.e. to show-off or as a status symbol).
6. It should not resemble the dress of women.
7. It should not resemble the dress of the disbelievers.
8. It should not bear crosses or depictions of anything with a soul (humans, animals, birds, etc.).
9. It should not be expensive, extravagant.
10. Should not wear red plain colored garments
11. It should not be from the untanned skin and sinew of dead animals.
12. No silk and gold for men.
13. No bracelet, necklace, earring, piercing for men.
14. Should not wear shoes making noise.

Abdullah ibn 'Umar (May Allah be pleased with him) reported that the Prophet (May Allah's peace and blessings be upon him) said: "Modesty is a part of faith." (Bukhari and Muslim) (https://hadeethenc.com/en/browse/hadith/5478)

Narrated Abu Hurairah (May Allah be pleased with him): The Prophet (peace and blessings of Allah be upon him) said: "The part of an Izar which hangs below the ankles is in the Fire." (Bukhari)

Abdullah ibn Umar (May Allah be pleased with him) reported: The Messenger of Allah (peace and blessings be upon him) said, "Whoever wears a garment in vanity, Allah will make him wear a garment of humiliation on the Day of Resurrection, then He will set it ablaze with Fire." (Ibn Majah)

Ali (May Allah be pleased with him) reported: "I saw the Messenger of Allah (May Allah's peace and blessings be upon him) taking silk in his right hand and gold in his left hand and then he said: "These two are forbidden for the males of my Ummah." Abu Musa al-Ash'ari (May Allah be pleased with him) reported that the Messenger of Allah (May Allah's peace and blessings be upon him) said: "Wearing silk and gold is forbidden for the males of my Ummah and is allowed for their females." (Ibn Majah)

Hudhayfah ibn al-Yaman (May Allah be pleased with him) reported that the Prophet (May Allah's peace and blessings be upon him) said: "Do not wear silk or brocade, and do not drink from gold or silver vessels, nor eat in platters made therefrom, for they are for them in this world and for you in the Hereafter." (Bukhari and Muslim)

Narrated Jarhad (May Allah be pleased with him): The Messenger of Allah (peace be upon him) sat with us and my thigh was uncovered. He said: "Do you not know that thigh is a private part?" (Abu Dawud)

Ibn 'Abbas (May Allah be pleased with him) said: The Messenger of Allah (peace and blessings of Allah be upon him) cursed those men who are effeminate, and women who imitate men." (Bukhari)

Ibn 'Abbas (May Allah be pleased with him) said the Prophet (peace and blessings of Allah be upon him) cursed the mukhannaths among men and the women who imitated men, saying, "Put them out of your houses." (Bukhari)

Anas (May Allah be pleased with him) said: The Prophet (peace and blessings be upon him) prohibited men from wearing saffron-dyed clothes." (Bukhari and Muslim)

Narrated Abdullah bin Ukaym: "There came to us a letter from the Prophet (peace and blessings be upon him) saying: 'Do not make use of the untanned skin and sinew of dead animals.'" (Ibn Majah)

Abu Hurairah (May Allah be pleased with him) reported that the Messenger of Allah (May Allah's peace and blessings be upon him) said: "There are two categories of Hell inmates whom I have not seen: people having whips like the tails of cows with which they will be beating people, and women who will be dressed but appear to be naked, inviting to evil; and they themselves will be inclined to it. Their heads will appear like the humps of the Bactrian camels inclined to one side. They will not enter Paradise, nor will they smell its fragrance, which is smelled from such-and-such a distance." (Muslim)

Mu'adh ibn Anas (May Allah be pleased with him) reported that the Prophet (May Allah's peace and blessings be upon him) said: "Whoever gives up wearing elegant expensive clothes out of humbleness with Allah, while he can afford it, Allah will call him on the Day of Judgment before all people and let him choose whichever of the garments of faith he would like to wear." (Tirmidhi) (https://hadeethenc.com/en/browse/hadith/5432)

569. Rulings on Dress for Women

Allah, the Exalted, says:

"O Prophet! Tell your wives and your daughters and the women of the believers to draw their cloaks (veils) all over their bodies (i.e. screen themselves completely except the eyes or one eye to see the way). That will be better, that they should be known (as free respectable women) so as not to be annoyed. And Allah is Ever Oft-Forgiving, Most Merciful." (Qur'an, Al-Ahzab 33:59)

"And tell the believing women to lower their gaze (from looking at forbidden things), and protect their private parts (from illegal sexual acts) and not to show off their adornment except only that which is apparent (like both eyes for necessity to see the way or outer palms of hands, or one eye, or dress like veil, gloves, headcover, apron), and to draw their veils all over Juyoobihinna (i.e. their bodies, faces, necks and bosoms), and not to reveal their adornment except to their husbands or their fathers, or their husband's fathers, or their sons, or their husband's sons, or their brothers, or their brother's sons, or their sister's sons, or their (Muslim) women (i.e. their sisters in Islam), or the (female) slaves whom their right hands possess, or old male servants who lack vigour, or small children who have no sense of feminine sex. And let them not stamp their feet so as to reveal what they hide of their adornment. And all of you beg Allah to forgive you all, O believers, that you may be successful." (Qur'an, An-Nur 24:31)

"Children of Adam! We have sent down clothing to you to conceal your private parts." (Qur'an, Al-A'raf 7:26)

Other Verses: Al-A'raf 7:27, Al-Ahzab 33:32, An-An'am 6:120, An-Nur 24:26.

Scholars have specified the requirements of the Muslim woman's proper dress from the Glorious Qur'an and Sunnah. (469)

<u>Ruling on Women's Dress:</u>

1. It should cover the whole body.
2. It should be thick enough, i.e. non-transparent or translucent.
3. It should be loose and not tight on her body.
4. It should not be decorated or ornate such as to attract onlookers.
5. It should not be perfumed.
6. It should not be considered libaas al-shuhrah (i.e. to show-off or as a status symbol)
7. It should not resemble the dress of men.
8. It should not resemble the dress of the disbelievers.
9. It should not bear crosses or depictions of anything with a soul (humans, animals, etc.).
10. It should not be expensive, extravagant.
11. It should not be from the untanned skin and sinew of dead animals.
12. It should not be from the skin of the leopard.
13. Should not display the beauty and ornaments to non-Mahram.
14. Should not wear the artificial hair (wig) and make hair extension.
15. Should not wear shoes making noise and high heels.

Abdullah ibn 'Umar (May Allah be pleased with him) reported that the Prophet (May Allah's peace and blessings be upon him) said: "Modesty is a part of faith." (Bukhari and Muslim) (https://hadeethenc.com/en/browse/hadith/5478)

Narrated Ibn 'Abbas (May Allah be pleased with him): The Prophet (peace and blessings be upon him) cursed the *mukhannaths* among men and the women who imitated men, saying, "Put them out of your houses." (Bukhari)

Abu Musa reported: The Prophet (peace and blessings be upon him) said, "Every eye can commit adultery. The woman who adorns herself with fragrances and passes by an assembly of men is as such," meaning an adulteress." (Tirmidhi)

Narrated Amr bin Shu'aib, from his father, that his grandfather said: "The Messenger of Allah (peace be upon him) said: 'Eat and drink, give charity and wear clothes, as long as that does not involve any extravagance or vanity.'" (Ibn Majah)

Abdullah ibn Umar (May Allah be pleased with him) reported: The Messenger of Allah (peace and blessings be upon him) said, "Whoever wears a garment in vanity, Allah will make him wear a garment of humiliation on the Day of Resurrection, then He will set it ablaze with Fire." (Ibn Majah)

Mu'adh ibn Anas (May Allah be pleased with him) reported that the Prophet (May Allah's peace and blessings be upon him) said: "Whoever gives up wearing elegant expensive clothes out of humbleness with Allah, while he can afford it, Allah will call him on the Day of Judgment before all people and let him choose whichever of the garments of faith he would like to wear." (Tirmidhi)

Abu Hurairah (May Allah be pleased with him) reported that the Messenger of Allah (May Allah's peace and blessings be upon him) said: "There are two categories of Hell inmates whom I have not seen: people having whips like the tails of cows with which they will be beating people, and women who will be dressed but appear to be naked, inviting to evil; and they themselves will be inclined to it. Their heads will appear like the humps of the Bactrian camels inclined to one side. They will not enter Paradise, nor will they smell its fragrance, which is smelled from such-and-such a distance." (Muslim)

Narrated 'Abdullah bin 'Ukaym (May Allah be pleased with him): "There came to us a letter from the Prophet (peace and blessings be upon him) saying: 'Do not make use of the untanned skin and sinew of dead animals.'" (Ibn Majah)

570. Prohibition of Wearing Saffron-Colored Dress for Men

Anas (May Allah be pleased with him) said: "The Prophet (peace and blessings be upon him) prohibited men from wearing saffron-dyed clothes." (Bukhari and Muslim)

'Abdullah bin 'Amr bin Al-'As (May Allah be pleased with him) said: "The Prophet (peace and blessings be upon him) saw me dressed in two saffron-coloured garments and asked, "Has your mother commanded you to wear these?" I asked him, "Shall I wash them out?" He replied, "You had better set them to fire."

Commentary: Saffron and safflower are plants with a bright orange-yellow colour. Their use is forbidden because this colour is generally used by women and disbelievers, and men should show no resemblance to women and disbelievers in their dress. (470)

571. Prohibition of Wearing Plain Red Colored Garments for Men

Narrated al-Baraa' ibn 'Aazib (May Allah be pleased with him): "The Prophet (peace and blessings of Allah be upon him) forbade us to use soft red mattresses and qasiy – garments with woven stripes of silk." (Bukhari) (https://www.youtube.com/watch?v=WXGRXxclaCY)

Narrated Ibn Abbas (May Allah be pleased with him): "I was forbidden to wear red garments and gold rings, and to recite Qur'an when bowing," (An-Nasa'i)

Narrated 'Abd-Allah Ibn 'Amr Ibn al-As (May Allah be pleased with him): "A man passed by the Prophet (peace and blessings of Allah be upon him) wearing two red garments and greeted him with salaam, but he (peace and blessings of Allah be upon him) did not return the greeting." (Abu Dawud)

572. Woman Not Covering Whole Body

Allah, the Exalted, says:

"O Prophet! Tell your wives and your daughters, and the believing women, to draw their cloaks (veils) over their bodies. That will be better that they should be known (as respectable woman), so as not to be annoyed. And Allah is Ever Oft-Forgiving, Most Merciful." (Qur'an, Al-Ahzab 33:59)

"O you who believe! Follow not the footsteps of Shaitan (Satan). And whosoever follows the footsteps of Shaitan (Satan), then, verily he commands Al-Fahisha' [i.e. to commit indecency (illegal sexual intercourse, etc.)], and Al-Munkar [disbelief and polytheism (i.e. to do evil and wicked deeds; to speak or to do what is forbidden in Islam, etc.)]. And had it not been for the Grace of Allah and His Mercy on you, not one of you would ever have been pure from sins. But Allah purifies (guides to Islam) whom He wills, and Allah is All-Hearer, All-Knower." (Qur'an, An-Nur 24:21)

"Indeed, Allah orders justice and good conduct, and giving to relatives, and forbids immorality, and bad conduct and oppression. He admonishes you that perhaps you will be reminded." (Qur'an, An-Nahl 16:90)

Usama ibn Zayd (May Allah be pleased with him) reported the Prophet (May Allah's peace and blessings be upon him) said: "I am not leaving a trail behind me that is more harmful to men than women." (Bukhari and Muslim) (https://hadeethenc.com/en/browse/hadith/5830)

Narrated People: The Prophet (peace and blessings be upon him) said, "A single endeavor (of fighting) in Allah's Cause in the afternoon or in the forenoon is better than all the world and whatever is in it. A place in Paradise as small as the bow or lash of one of you is better than all the world and whatever is in it. And if an houri from Paradise appeared to the people of the earth, she would fill the space between heaven and the earth with light and pleasant scent and **her head cover is better than the world and whatever is in it**." (Bukhari) (https://sunnah.com/bukhari:2796)

Abu Hurairah (May Allah be pleased with him) reported that the Messenger of Allah (May Allah's peace and blessings be upon him) said: "There are two categories of Hell inmates whom I have not seen: people having whips like the tails of cows with which they will be beating people, and women who will be dressed but appear to be naked, inviting to evil; and they themselves will be inclined to it. Their heads will appear like the humps of the Bactrian camels inclined to one side. They will not enter Paradise, nor will they smell its fragrance, which is smelled from such-and-such a distance." (Muslim)

Aisha (May Allah be pleased with her) reported that the Prophet (May Allah's peace and blessings be upon him) said: "Allah does not accept the prayer of any woman who has reached the age of menstruation unless (she is) veiled." (Ibn Majah) (https://hadeethenc.com/en/browse/hadith/10637)

Woman must cover whole body including the head (hair, face, neck, feet) because it is not permissible for her to uncover it except before her husband and mahrams. It is also the protection from the destructive Evil Eye.

She should dress in such a manner that strange men do not get an opportunity to glance at those parts of her body which arouse passion, and thus making her an object of desire. If a woman covers herself, then immoral and corrupt men will know that this is not part of their prey, thus Allah will protect her and take care of her.

573. Hijab Ban

The Hijab covers the head and neck but leaves the face clear. The Niqab (or ruband) is a veil for the face that leaves the area around the eyes clear. The Burka is the most concealing of all Islamic veils. It is a one-piece veil that covers the face and body, often leaving just a mesh screen to see through.

The Niqab and Burka are the most appropriate dress to the description in the Qur'an and Sunnah.

I. The Qur'an about Woman's Dress:

Allah, the Exalted, says:

"And tell the believing women to lower their gaze (from looking at forbidden things) and protect their private parts (from illegal sexual acts), and not to show off their adornment except only that which is apparent (like both eyes for necessity to see the way, or outer palms of hands, or one eye, or dress like veil, gloves, headcover, apron), and to draw their veils all over Juyoobihinna (i.e. their bodies, faces, necks and bosoms), and not to reveal their adornment except to their husbands or their fathers, or their husband's fathers, or their sons, or their husband's sons, or their brothers, or their brother's sons, or their sister's sons, or their (Muslim) women (i.e. their sisters in Islam), or the (female) slaves whom their right hands possess, or old male servants who lack vigour, or small children who have no sense of feminine sex. And let them not stamp their feet, so as to reveal what they hide of their adornment. And all of you beg Allah to forgive you all, O believers, that you may be successful." (Qur'an, An-Nur 24:31)

"O Prophet! Tell your wives and your daughters, and the women of the believers to draw their cloaks (veils) all over their bodies (i.e. screen themselves completely except the eyes or one eye to see the way). That will be better, that they should be known (as free respectable women), so as not to be annoyed. And Allah is Ever Oft-Forgiving, Most Merciful." (Qur'an, Al-Ahzab 33:59)

"O you who believe! Enter not the Prophet's houses, unless permission is given to you for a meal, (and then) not (so early as) to wait for its preparation. But when you are invited, enter, and when you have taken your meal, disperse without sitting for a talk. Verily, such (behavior) annoys the Prophet, and he is shy of (asking) you (to go); but Allah is not shy of (telling you) the truth. And when you ask (his wives) for anything you want, ask them from behind a screen, that is purer for your hearts and for their hearts. And it is not (right) for you that you should annoy Allah's Messenger, nor that you should ever marry his wives after him (his death). Verily, with Allah that shall be an enormity." (Qur'an, Al-Ahzab 33:53)

Other Verse: *An-Nur 24:60.*

II. Ahadith about Woman's Dress:

1. Narrated Safiyyah bint Shaybah that Aisha (May Allah be pleased with her) used to say: "When these words were revealed – *"and to draw their veils all over Juyoobihinna (i.e. their bodies, faces, necks and bosoms)"* – they took their izaars (a kind of garment) and tore them from the edges and covered their faces with them." (Bukhari)

2. Narrated Aisha that the wives of the Prophet (peace and blessings of Allah be upon him) used to go out at night to al-Manaasi' (well known places in the direction of al-Baqee') to relieve themselves and 'Umar used to say to the Prophet (peace and blessings of Allah be upon him), "Let your wives be veiled." But the Messenger of Allah (peace and blessings of Allah be upon him) did not do that. Then one-night Sawdah bint Zam'ah, the wife of the Prophet (peace and blessings of Allah be upon him), went out at 'Isha time and she was a tall woman. 'Umar called out to her: "We have recognized you, O Sawdah!" hoping that hijab would be revealed, then Allah revealed the Verse of hijab." (Bukhari and Muslim)

3. Narrated Ibn Shihaab that Anas said: "I am the most knowledgeable of people about hijab. Ubayy ibn Ka'b used to ask me about it. When the Messenger of Allah (peace and blessings of Allah be upon him) married Zaynab bint Jahsh, whom he married in Madinah, he invited the people to a meal after the sun had risen. The Messenger of Allah (peace and blessings of Allah be upon him) sat down and some men sat around him after the people had left, until the Messenger of Allah (peace and blessings of Allah be upon him) stood up and walked a while, and I walked with him, until he reached the door of Aisha's apartment. Then he thought that they had left so he went back and I went back with him, and they were still sitting there. He went back again, and I went with him, until he reached the door of Aisha's apartment, then he came back and I came back with him, and they had left. Then he drew a curtain between me and him, and the Verse of hijab was revealed." (Bukhari and Muslim)

4. Narrated 'Urwah that Aisha said: "The Messenger of Allah (peace and blessings of Allah be upon him) used to pray Fajr and the believing women would attend (the prayer) with him, wrapped in their aprons, then they would go back to their houses and no one would recognize them." (Bukhari and Muslim)

5. Narrated Aisha (May Allah be pleased with her) said: "The riders used to pass by us when we were with the Messenger of Allah (peace and blessings be upon him) in ihram, and when they drew near to us, we would lower our jilbabs from our heads over our faces, then when they had passed, we would uncover them again." (Abu Dawud and Ibn Majah)

6. Narrated Asma' bint Abi Bakr: "We used to cover our faces in front of men." (Ibn Khuzaymah and al-Haakim)

7. Narrated 'Aasim al-Ahwaal: "We used to enter upon Hafsah bint Sireen who had put her jilbab thus and covered her face with it, and we would say to her: 'May Allah have mercy on you. Allah says: *"And as for women past childbearing who do not expect wedlock, it is no sin on them if they discard their (outer) clothing in such a way as not to show their adornment."* (An-Nur

24:60). And she would say to us: 'What comes after that?' We would say: *"But to refrain (i.e. not to discard their outer clothing) is better for them."* And she would say: "That is confirming the idea of hijab." (al-Bayhaqi) (471)

8. Aisha (May Allah be pleased with her) reported that the Prophet (May Allah's peace and blessings be upon him) said: "Allah does not accept the prayer of any woman who has reached the age of menstruation unless (she is) veiled." (Ibn Majah, Tirmidhi, Abu Dawud and Ahmad)

9. Narrated People: The Prophet (peace and blessings be upon him) said, "A single endeavor (of fighting) in Allah's Cause in the afternoon or in the forenoon is better than all the world and whatever is in it. A place in Paradise as small as the bow or lash of one of you is better than all the world and whatever is in it. And if an houri from Paradise appeared to the people of the earth, she would fill the space between heaven and the earth with light and pleasant scent and her head cover is better than the world and whatever is in it." (Bukhari) (https://sunnah.com/bukhari:2796)

574. Women Praying with Uncovered Feet

Narrated Umm Salama (May Allah be pleased with her) that she asked the Prophet (peace and blessings of Allah be upon him): "Can a woman pray wearing a chemise and headcover and no izaar (waist-wrapper)?" He said: "If the chemise is long enough to cover the tops of her feet (then that is fine)." (Abu Dawud)

Narrated Aisha, Ummul Mu'minin: "Asma, daughter of Abu Bakr, entered upon the Messenger of Allah (peace and blessings of Allah be upon him) wearing thin clothes. The Messenger of Allah (peace and blessings of Allah be upon him) turned his attention from her. He said: 'O Asma, when a woman reaches the age of menstruation, it does not suit her that she displays her parts of body except this and this, and he pointed to his face and hands." (Abu Dawud)

The majority of scholars are of the view that it is obligatory for a woman to cover feet. (472-474)

575. Displaying the Beauty and Ornaments

Allah, the Exalted, says:

"And tell the believing women to lower their gaze (from looking at forbidden things) and protect their private parts (from illegal sexual acts), and not to show off their adornment

except only that which is apparent (like both eyes for necessity to see the way, or outer palms of hands, or one eye, or dress like veil, gloves, headcover, apron), and to draw their veils all over Juyoobihinna (i.e. their bodies, faces, necks and bosoms), and not to reveal their adornment except to their husbands or their fathers, or their husband's fathers, or their sons, or their husband's sons, or their brothers, or their brother's sons, or their sister's sons, or their (Muslim) women (i.e. their sisters in Islam), or the (female) slaves whom their right hands possess, or old male servants who lack vigour, or small children who have no sense of feminine sex. And let them not stamp their feet, so as to reveal what they hide of their adornment. And all of you beg Allah to forgive you all, O believers, that you may be successful." (Qur'an, An-Nur 24:31)

Every believing woman is obliged to cover her beauty and adornment before non-Mahram men.

Adornment includes kohl, makeup, jewelry, etc.

The reason why it is haram to show this adornment is so as to protect women's chastity and honor, and to close the door to temptation and prevent her being tempted or tempting others. Those who are sick at heart may have hopes concerning those who show their adornment, but they will leave the one who is modest and covered alone.

Islam closes the doors that lead to men being tempted by women and vice versa. Islam enjoins lowering the gaze and forbids tabarruj (wanton display), free mixing and being alone with woman. This is reflective of the perfection of Islam, for men by nature are affected by women, and if this is not prevented then there will be much fitnah (temptation and tribulation), and corruption will become widespread, as we can see in societies that have neglected the guidelines and rulings of Shariah. (475)

576. Women Doing Da'wah on Television

Allah, the Exalted, says:

"…If you keep your duty (to Allah), then be not soft in speech, lest he in whose heart is a disease (of hypocrisy, or evil desire for adultery, etc.) should be moved with desire, but speak in an honorable manner." (Qur'an, Al-Ahzab 33:53)

"And when you ask (his wives) for anything you want, ask them from behind a screen, that is purer for your hearts and for their hearts." (Qur'an, Al-Ahzab 33:53)

"And tell the believing women to lower their gaze (from looking at forbidden things) and protect their private parts (from illegal sexual acts), and not to show off their adornment except only that which is apparent (like both eyes for necessity to see the way, or outer palms of hands, or one eye, or dress like veil, gloves, headcover, apron), and to draw their

veils all over Juyubihinna (i.e. their bodies, faces, necks and bosoms), and not to reveal their adornment except to their husbands or their fathers, or their husband's fathers, or their sons, or their husband's sons, or their brothers, or their brother's sons, or their sister's sons, or their (Muslim) women (i.e. their sisters in Islam), or the (female) slaves whom their right hands possess, or old male servants who lack vigour, or small children who have no sense of feminine sex. And let them not stamp their feet, so as to reveal what they hide of their adornment. And all of you beg Allah to forgive you all, O believers, that you may be successful."* (Qur'an, An-Nur 24:31)

Narrated Safiyyah bint Shaybah that Aisha (May Allah be pleased with her) used to say: "When these words were revealed – *"and to draw their veils all over Juyubihinna (i.e. their bodies, faces, necks and bosoms)"* – they took their izars (a kind of garment) and tore them from the edges and covered their faces with them." (Bukhari)

In terms of sisters doing Da'wah on social media off camera on platforms, such as Facebook, Instagram, Twitter, etc., then it is permissible according to the scholars provided that the sister who is doing Da'wah is capable and avoids anything haram.

As for sisters going on camera whether on youtube or other social media platforms is something the scholars do not allow.

The sisters must do Da'wah in the manner highlighted in the Qur'an, Sunnah and the practice of the Salaf. The sahabiyyaat and the female scholars of the salaf used to teach the women privately. If they taught both men and women, they would do so from behind a screen.

Abdullah Ibn Masud (May Allah be pleased with him) that the Prophet (peace and blessings be upon him) said, "The woman is 'awrah, so when she goes out, the Shaitan seeks to tempt her." (Tirmidhi)

The Sheikh in that very verdict was asked about recording the sister when she is giving the lecture in front of the mixed audience. The Sheikh said it is not allowed. He said, "However, the act of picture-taking, it is necessary not to do in these affairs. Rather it is necessary to record the voice without the picture because the origin of pictures is that they are haram as the Prophet (peace and blessings be upon him) said, 'The most severe punishment on the Day of Judgement is for the picture-takers." (Bukhari)" (476)

If she makes Da'wah to men she must do so whilst observing hijab and without being alone with any non-Mahram man. She has to keep away from clothing that will distract people, and avoid all kinds of fitnah (temptation) such as displaying her beauty or speaking in a soft manner, for which she may be criticized. She must take care to call people to Allah in a manner which will not harm her religious commitment or her reputation. (477)

577. Shoes Making Noise and High Heels

Allah, the Exalted, says:

"And let them not stamp their feet to make known what they conceal of their adornment. And turn to Allah in repentance, all of you, O believers, that you might succeed." (Qur'an, An-Nur 24:31)

It is prohibited for a woman to wear high heel shoes or any footware that make a sound making woman more attractive and it is a temptation to men.

578. Undesirability of Wearing one Shoe or Sock

Narrated Abu Hurairah (May Allah be pleased with him): The Messenger of Allah (peace and blessings be upon him) said, "None of you should walk wearing one shoe; you should either wear them both or take them off both." (Bukhari and Muslim)

Narrated Abu Hurairah (May Allah be pleased with him): "I heard the Messenger of Allah (peace and blessings be upon him) saying, 'When the lace of one of the shoes of any one of you is cut off, he should not walk with the other until he has got the lace repaired.'" (Muslim)

Narrated Jabir (May Allah be pleased with him): "The Messenger of Allah (peace and blessings be upon him) forbade a person wearing (tying up) his shoe while standing." (Abu Dawud)

Commentary: We learn from this Hadith that it is undesirable to put on one's shoes (or socks, etc.) in the standing position. (478)

579. Prohibition of Using the Skin of the Leopard

Mu'awiyah (May Allah be pleased with him) reported: The Messenger of Allah (peace and blessings be upon him) said, "Do not ride on saddles made from silk or leopard's skin. (Abu Dawud)

Abul-Malih on the authority of his father reported: The Messenger of Allah (peace and blessings be upon him) prohibited the use of the skins of wild animals. (Abu Dawud, Tirmidhi and An-Nasa'i)

Commentary: The Messenger of Allah (peace and blessings be upon him) has forbidden the use of hide of wild beasts. Explaining the ban by Messenger of Allah (peace and blessings be upon him), some say that even the tanning process cannot wipe out hair from a beast's hide. As a result, it retains some impurity. Others think that the prohibitive order is related only to the untanned hides and is inapplicable to the tanned ones. This opinion also goes since such hides are used by extravagant and arrogant people, and its use by Muslims may hold them analogous to the former... (479)

580. Man Wearing the Garment Below the Ankles (Isbaal)

Narrated Abu Hurairah (May Allah be pleased with him): The Prophet (peace and blessings be upon him) said: "The part of an Izar which hangs below the ankles is in the Fire." (Bukhari)

Abu Sa'id al-Khudri (May Allah be pleased with him) reported that the Messenger of Allah (May Allah's peace and blessings be upon him) said: "The Muslim's lower garment should be half way down the leg. There is no harm (if it reaches) between that and the ankles. However, what is below the ankles will be in the Fire. Whoever trails his lower garment out of vanity, Allah will not look at him." (Ibn Majah)
(https://hadeethenc.com/en/browse/hadith/4964)

581. Man who Drags his Clothes Out of Pride

Narrated 'Abdullah bin Umar (May Allah be pleased with him): Allah's Messenger (peace and blessings be upon him) said, "Whoever drags his clothes (on the ground) out of pride and arrogance, Allah will not look at him on the Day of Resurrection." ((Bukhari)

Narrated 'Abdullah bin Umar (May Allah be pleased with him): Allah's Messenger (peace and blessings be upon him) said, "While a man was dragging his Izaar on the ground (behind him), suddenly Allah made him sink into the earth and he will go on sinking into it till the Day of Resurrection." (Bukhari)

582. Men Wearing Silk or Brocade and Gold

Allah, the Exalted, says:

"O Children of Adam! Take your adornment (by wearing your clean clothes), while praying and going round (the Tawaf of) the Ka'bah, and eat and drink but waste not by extravagance, certainly He (Allah) likes not Al-Musrifun (those who waste by extravagance)." (Qur'an, Al-A'raf 7:31)

"Help you one another in Al-Birr and At-Taqwa (virtue, righteousness and piety); but do not help one another in sin and transgression. And fear Allah. Verily, Allah is Severe in punishment." (Qur'an, Al-Ma'idah 5:2)

Hudhayfah ibn al-Yaman (May Allah be pleased with him) reported that the Prophet (May Allah's peace and blessings be upon him) said: "Do not wear silk or brocade, and do not drink from gold or silver vessels, nor eat in platters made therefrom, for they are for them in this world and for you in the Hereafter." (Bukhari and Muslim) (https://hadeethenc.com/en/browse/hadith/2985)

Ali (May Allah be pleased with him) reported: "I saw the Messenger of Allah (May Allah's peace and blessings be upon him) taking silk in his right hand and gold in his left hand and then he said: "These two are forbidden for the males of my Ummah."" (Abu Dawud, An-Nasa'i and Ibn Majah) (https://hadeethenc.com/en/browse/hadith/4292)

'Asim al-Abwal reported on the authority Abu Uthman saying: "Umar wrote to us when we were in Adharba'ijan saying: 'Utba b. Farqad, this wealth is neither the result of your own labour nor the result of the labour of your father, nor the result of the labour of your mother, so feed Muslims at their own places as you feed (members of your family and yourselves at your own residence), and beware of the life of pleasure, and the dress of the polytheists and wearing of silk garments, for Allah's Messenger (peace and blessings be upon him) forbade the wearing of silk garments, but only this much, and Allah's Messenger (peace and blessings be upon him) raised his forefinger and middle finger and he joined them (to indicate that only this much silk can be allowed in the dress of a man).' 'Asim said also: 'This is what is recorded in the letter (sent to us), and Zuhair raised his two fingers (to give an idea of the extent to which silk may be used).'" (Muslim)

583. Prohibition for Men and Women Apeing One Another

Ibn 'Abbas (May Allah be pleased with him) said: "The Messenger of Allah (peace and blessings be upon him) cursed those men who ape women. He also cursed the hermaphrodite of men."

Another narration is: "The Messenger of Allah (peace and blessings be upon him) cursed men who copy women and cursed women who copy men." (Bukhari)

Ibn 'Abbas (May Allah be pleased with him) reported: The Prophet (May Allah's peace and blessings be upon him) cursed the effeminate men and the masculine women. He said: "Turn them out of your houses." Ibn 'Abbas added: "So the Prophet (May Allah's peace and blessings be upon him) turned so-and-so out, and 'Umar turned so-and-so out." (Bukhari)

Many Muslim women have adopted evils and shameless fashions without fear of punishment in the Hereafter. (480)

584. Men Wearing the Earring, Necklace, Bracelet, Piercing

Narrated Ibn 'Abbas (May Allah be pleased with him): "The Messenger of Allah (peace and blessings be upon him) cursed men who imitate women and women who imitate men." (Bukhari)

Wearing bracelets, whether they are of the type mentioned in the question or other types, and whether they are made of leather, metal or anything else, is haram for men, because they come under the heading of women's clothing and adornments. (481)

Some bracelets, necklaces, anklets are used for Black Magic (Taweez and Amulets) and Shirk (idolatry or to attract good luck or ward off the Evil Eye). (482)

'Uqbah ibn 'Amir (May Allah be pleased with him) reported: The Messenger of Allah (peace and blessings be upon him) received a group of men and he accepted the pledge of nine of them, while he refrained from one. They said, "O Messenger of Allah, you accepted the pledge of nine men and left this one out?" The Prophet said, "Verily, there is an amulet upon him." The man took it in his hand and cut it, then the Prophet accepted his pledge and he said, "Whoever hangs an amulet around his neck has committed an act of idolatry." (Ahmad)

'Imran ibn Husayn (May Allah be pleased with him) reported that the Prophet (May Allah's peace and blessings be upon him) saw a man wearing a brass ring on his hand and said: "What is that?" The man said: "It is for weakening ailment." He said: "Take it off, for it will only increase your weakness. If you die with it on, you will never succeed." (Ibn Majah)

585. Men with Whips Like the Tails of Cattle, Women with the Humps of Camels on their Heads

Abu Hurairah (May Allah be pleased with him) reported that the Messenger of Allah (May Allah's peace and blessings be upon him) said: "There are two categories of Hell inmates whom I have not seen: people having whips like the tails of cows with which they will be beating people, and women who will be dressed but appear to be naked, inviting to evil; and they themselves will be inclined to it. Their heads will appear like the humps of the Bactrian camels inclined to one side. They will not enter Paradise, nor will they smell its fragrance, which is smelled from such-and-such a distance." (Muslim) (https://hadeethenc.com/en/browse/hadith/8903)

586. Hair Extension

Narrated Asma (the daughter of Abu Bakr): "A woman came to Allah's Messenger (peace and blessings of Allah be upon him) and said, "I married my daughter to someone, but she became sick and all her hair fell out, and (because of that) her husband does not like her. May I let her use false hair?" On that the Prophet (peace and blessings of Allah be upon him) cursed such a lady as artificially lengthening (her or someone else's) hair or got her hair lengthened artificially." (Bukhari)

Narrated Aisha (May Allah be pleased with her): An Ansari girl was married and she became sick and all her hair fell out intending to provide her with false hair. They asked the Prophet (peace and blessings of Allah be upon him) who said, "Allah has cursed the lady who artificially lengthens (her or someone else's) hair and also the one who gets her hair lengthened." (Bukhari)

Abdullah ibn 'Amr (May Allah be pleased with him) reported: The Messenger of Allah (May Allah's peace and blessings be upon him) cursed the woman who fixes hair extensions (to another) and the woman who has them fixed for her, and the woman who does tattoos and the woman who has them done for her." (Bukhari and Muslim) (https://hadeethenc.com/en/browse/hadith/58099)

587. Prohibition of Wearing False Hair, Tattooing and Filling of Teeth

Allah, the Exalted, says:

"They (all those who worship others than Allah) invoke nothing but female deities besides Him (Allah), and they invoke nothing but Shaitan (Satan), a persistent rebel! Allah cursed him. And he [Shaitan (Satan)] said: 'I will take an appointed portion of your slaves. Verily, I will mislead them, and surely, I will arouse in them false desires; and certainly, I will order them to slit the ears of cattle, and indeed I will order them to change the nature created by Allah.' And whoever takes Shaitan (Satan) as a Wali

(protector or helper) instead of Allah, has surely suffered a manifest loss." (Qur'an, An-Nisa 4:117-119)

Asma (May Allah be pleased with her) said: "A woman came to the Prophet (peace and blessings be upon him) and said: "O Messenger of Allah! I have a daughter who had an attack of smallpox and her hair fell off. Now I want to celebrate her marriage. Can I get her a wig?" Thereupon, the Prophet (peace and blessings be upon him) said, "Allah has cursed the maker and wearer of a wig." (Bukhari and Muslim)

Humaid bin 'Abdur-Rahman (May Allah be pleased with him) said: "I saw Mu'awiyah (May Allah be pleased with him) during the Hajj (pilgrimage) standing on the pulpit. He took from the guard a bunch of hair and said: "O people of Al-Madinah! Where are your scholars? (Why do they do not prohibit you)." I heard the Prophet (peace and blessings be upon him) prohibiting from using this (false hair) and saying, 'The people of Bani Israel were ruined when their women wore such hair.'" (Bukhari and Muslim)

Ibn 'Umar (May Allah be pleased with him) reported: The Messenger of Allah (May Allah's peace and blessings be upon him) cursed the woman who fixes hair extensions (to another) and the woman who has them fixed for her, and the woman who does tattoos and the woman who has them done for her. (Bukhari and Muslim)

Commentary:
Al-Washimah is a woman who practices Al-Washm Al-Washm was performed (in the past) by piercing needle in some part of the body for drawing blood and then filling the cavity caused by it with antimony, indigo, etc., to make the spot green or black. This is called tattooing. In the Arab society of the Prophet's time, this fashion was very popular among women for enhancing their charms and beauty in the same way as the fashion of patching someone's hair with his own. Al-Mustaushima is a woman who asks some women for tattooing and/or a woman who marks tattoos on the skin of another woman. As this act amounts to changing the natural appearance of a person, both women, that is the one who subjects her body to tattooing and the one who makes this operation, are cursed. Such fashions are in vogue in this age also. **Plucking the Eyelashes** and filling them with colours and other material of makeup, or like Hindu women, making mark between the eyebrows with cinnabar, etc., fall in the category of such fashions. Such means of **Makeup** which are practiced nowadays by women and on which huge amounts of money are wasted are the things which have been cursed. Muslim women should, therefore, avoid such evils as they are ruinous for religion as well as worldly life. Similar is the case of **Nail Polish**. In the opinion of some religious scholars, this act invalidates Wudu. Women are now also in the habit of keeping **Long Nails** on which nail polish is applied to give an effect of beastly claws. All such vile fashions have been borrowed by oriental societies from the class of shameless women of the west, and Muslim women have also adopted them. We must strictly abstain from them because they tend to create resemblance to the non-Muslims, which is unlawful and is rated as a **Major sin**. (483)

Ibn Masud (May Allah be pleased with him) said: "Allah has cursed those women who practice tattooing and those women who have themselves tattooed, and those women who get their hair removed from their eyebrows and faces (except the beard and the mustache), and those who make artificial spaces between their teeth for beauty, whereby they change Allah's creation. A woman started to argue with him, saying: "What is all this?" He replied: "Why should I not curse those whom the Messenger of Allah (peace and blessings be upon him) cursed and who are cursed in Allah's Book? Allah, the Exalted, has said in His Book: *"And whatsoever the Messenger (Muhammad (peace and blessings be upon him) gives you, take it; and whatsoever he forbids you, abstain (from it)." (59:7)* (Bukhari and Muslim)

Narrated Abu Hurairah (May Allah be pleased with him): The Prophet (peace and blessing be upon him) said, ""The influence of the evil eye is true," and forbade tattooing. (It would seem from this tradition that tattooing was used as a protection agains; the evil eye). (Bukhari)

588. Prohibition to Dye Hair Black

Jabir (May Allah be pleased with him) said: "Abu Quhafah, father of Abu Bakr (May Allah be pleased with him) was presented to the Messenger of Allah (peace and blessings be upon him) on the day of the conquest of Makkah and his head and bear were snow white. The Messenger of Allah (peace and blessings be upon him) said, 'Change it (i.e. dye it and avoid black colour).'" (Muslim)

Commentary: Abu Quhafah was the Kunyah (nick-name) of Abu Bakr's father. His real name was Usman bin 'Amir. He had embraced Islam on the day Makkah was conquered by the Muslims. "Saghamah" is a herb which grows in mountains and is completely white. Since Abu Quhafah's hair were gray, the Prophet (peace be upon him) ordered him to dye them but forbade him from turning them black. Thus, we learn that except for inevitable circumstances, dying the hair of head and beard in black is prohibited. (484)

Narrated Ibn 'Abbas (May Allah be pleased with him): The Prophet (peace and blessings be upon him) said: "Some people will dye their hair black like the breasts of pigeons at the end of time, but they will not even smell the fragrance of Paradise." (An-Nasa'i)

Abu Dharr (May Allah be pleased with him) reported God's Messenger (peace and blessings of Allah be upon him) as saying, "The best things with which gray hairs are changed are henna and katam (leaves of the salam tree (mimosa flava). This dye applied with henna to the hair is said to preserve its original colour, is also said to lighten the color of the hair)." (Tirmidhi, Abu Dawud and An-Nasa'i)

589. Prohibition of Shaving a Part of Head

Ibn 'Umar (May Allah be pleased with him) said: "The Messenger of Allah (peace and blessings be upon him) forbade cutting hair of the different lengths, cutting hair on the sides of the head more than the middle (Qaza) and said, explaining Qaza: "Shaving part of a boy's head and leaving part." (Bukhari and Muslim)

'Abdullah bin Ja'far (May Allah be pleased with him) said: "The Prophet (peace and blessings be upon him) gave respite for three days to the family of Ja'far (after his martydom). Then he came and said, "Don't weep for my brother after this day." He said, "Bring all of my nephews to me." We were accordingly brought as if we were chickens. Then he said, "Call for me a barber." He directed him to shave our heads which he did. (Abu Dawud)

Commentary: Ja'far was the cousin of the Prophet (peace and blessings be upon him) and he was martyred in the battle of Mu'tah. Although martyrdom is an honor but even then, the bereaved family does feel the shock of the loss. For this reason, the Prophet (peace and blessings be upon him) permitted them to give vent to their grief for three days. It should not, however, be taken to mean that he allowed them to lament and wail, because that is prohibited. What he actually allowed them was the natural weeping which does occur when people come for condolence and speak of the deceased. Such expression of grief is permissible after a period of three days also. Therefore, what the Prophet (peace and blessings be upon him) had advised them was not in the nature of unlawful but natural. The children of the deceased called themselves "chickens" as they were greatly enervated by the tragedy. This Hadith has been mentioned here to confirm the validity of shaving the hair of the head, especially of children, although keeping bobbed hair is more meritorious because the Prophet (peace and blessings be upon him) himself did so. Bobbed hair is cut short and allowed to hang loosely. (485)

Ali (May Allah be pleased with him) said: "The Messenger of Allah (peace and blessings be upon him) prohibited a woman from shaving her head." (An-Nasa'i)

Shaving hair for women is not permissible, except in the case of sickness. The length of hair for women should be below the shoulders. Cutting of hair for women short, imitating men and imitating the styles of the Kuffar and non-Muslim women, is not permissible.

Letting the hair grow long for men, tying it at the back of the head is an imitation of women and immoral people. (486)

590. Prohibition of Plucking Grey Hairs

Narrated 'Amr bin Shu'aib, on the authority of his father and grandfather that the Prophet (peace and blessings be upon him) said, "Do not pluck out grey hair, for they are the Muslim's light on the Day of Resurrection." (Abu Dawud, Tirmidhi and An-Nasa'i)

Commentary: This Hadith makes it abundantly clear that all heresies and violations of Shariah will not be accepted by Allah. Every Muslim is required to be a faithful follower of Divine orders rather than a heretic and a rebel. (487)

591. Trimming or Plucking Eyebrows

Ibn Masud (May Allah be pleased with him) said: "Allah has cursed those women who practice tattooing and those women who have themselves tattooed, and those women who get their hair removed from their eyebrows and faces (except the beard and the mustache), and those who make artificial spaces between their teeth for beauty, whereby they change Allah's creation. A woman started to argue with him, saying: "What is all this?" He replied: "Why should I not curse those whom the Messenger of Allah (peace and blessings be upon him) cursed and who are cursed in Allah's Book? Allah, the Exalted, has said in His Book: *"And whatsoever the Messenger (Muhammad SAW) gives you, take it; and whatsoever he forbids you, abstain (from it)." (59:7)* (Bukhari and Muslim)

592. Wearing Fake Eyelashes

It is not permissible to wear false eyelashes because this comes under the ruling on wearing Hair Extension. (488)

593. Removing Excess Facial Hair

Ibn Masud (May Allah be pleased with him) said: "Allah has cursed those women who practice tattooing and those women who have themselves tattooed, and those women who get their hair removed from their eyebrows and faces (except the beard and the mustache), and those who make artificial spaces between their teeth for beauty, whereby they change Allah's creation. A woman started to argue with him, saying: "What is all this?" He replied: "Why should I not curse those whom the Messenger of Allah (peace and blessings be upon him) cursed and who are cursed in Allah's Book? Allah, the Exalted, has said in His Book:

"And whatsoever the Messenger (Muhammad SAW) gives you, take it; and whatsoever he forbids you, abstain (from it)." (59:7) (Bukhari and Muslim)

594. Not Removing Pubic and Armpit Hair

Narrated Abu Hurairah (May Allah be pleased with him): "I heard the Prophet (peace and blessings be upon him) saying. "Five practices are characteristics of the Fitrah: circumcision, shaving the pubic hair, cutting the short moustaches, clipping the nails and depilating the hair of the armpits."(Bukhari)

Aisha (May Allah be pleased with her) reported that the Prophet (May Allah's peace and blessings be upon him) said: "Ten practices are part of the Fitrah: Trimming the mustache, letting the beard grow, using the tooth stick, rinsing the nose, trimming the nails, washing the finger joints, plucking the armpit hairs, shaving the pubic hair and washing the private parts with water (after answering the call of nature)." One of the narrators said: "I have forgotten the tenth; except if it was rinsing the mouth." (Muslim) (https://hadeethenc.com/en/browse/hadith/3730)

Narrated 'Atiyyah Al-Qurazi (May Allah be pleased with him): "We were presented to the Messenger of Allah (peace and blessings of Allah be upon him) on the day of (the battle of) Quraizah. Whoever had pubic hair, was killed and whoever did not, was left to his way. I was of those who did not have pubic hair, so I was left to my way." (Tirmidhi)

Narrated Jabir ibn 'Abdullah (May Allah be pleased with him): "We were with the Messenger of Allah (peace and blessings of Allah be upon him) on campaign, and when we approached Madinah, we wanted to enter the city straight away, but the Prophet (peace and blessings of Allah be upon him) said: "Delay it until we enter at night, so that the one who is disheveled may tidy herself up and the one whose husband is absent may shave her pubic hair." (Bukhari and Muslim)

595. Mustache Hair Touching the Upper Lip

Aisha (May Allah be pleased with her) reported that the Prophet (May Allah's peace and blessings be upon him) said: "Ten practices are part of the Fitrah: Trimming the mustache, letting the beard grow, using the tooth stick, rinsing the nose, trimming the nails, washing the finger joints, plucking the armpit hairs, shaving the pubic hair and washing the private parts with water (after answering the call of nature)." One of the narrators said: "I have forgotten the tenth; except if it was rinsing the mouth." (Muslim)

Ibn 'Umar (May Allah be pleased with him) reported God's Messenger (peace and blessings be upon him) as saying, "Do the opposite of what the polytheists do; let the beard grow long and clip the moustache." A version has, "Cut the mustache down and leave the beard." (Bukhari and Muslim)

596. Shaving the Beard

Allah, the Exalted, says:

"The only saying of the faithful believers, when they are called to Allah (His Words, the Qur'an) and His Messenger (peace and blessings be upon him), to judge between them, is that they say: 'We hear and we obey.' And such are the successful (who will live forever in Paradise)." *(Qur'an, An-Nur 24:51)*

Aisha (May Allah be pleased with her) reported that the Prophet (May Allah's peace and blessings be upon him) said: "Ten practices are part of the Fitrah: Trimming the mustache, letting the beard grow, using the tooth stick, rinsing the nose, trimming the nails, washing the finger joints, plucking the armpit hairs, shaving the pubic hair and washing the private parts with water (after answering the call of nature)." One of the narrators said: "I have forgotten the tenth; except if it was rinsing the mouth." (Muslim)

597. Growing Fingernails and Using Nail Polish

In the opinion of some religious scholars, **Nail Polish** invalidates Wudu. Women are now also in the habit of keeping **Long Nails** on which nail polish is applied to give an effect of beastly claws. All such vile fashions have been borrowed by oriental societies from the class of shameless women of the west, and Muslim women have also adopted them. We must strictly abstain from them because they tend to create resemblance to the non-Muslims, which is unlawful and is rated as a **Major sin**. (483)

598. Using any Kind of Perfume Going Out for Women

Abu Hurairah (May Allah be pleased with him) reported: The Messenger of Allah (peace and blessings be upon him) said, "The perfume for men is that whose odor is apparent but whose color is hidden and the perfume for women is that whose color is apparent but whose odor is hidden." (Tirmidhi and An-Nisa'i)

Abu Musa (May Allah be pleased with him) reported: The Prophet (peace and blessings be upon him) said, "Every eye can commit adultery. The woman who adorns herself with fragrances and passes by an assembly of men is as such", meaning an adulteress." (Tirmidhi)

Zainab Thaqafiya (May Allah be pleased with him) reported: The Messenger of Allah (peace and blessings be upon him) said: "When any one of you (women) participates in the 'Isha prayer, she should not perfume herself that night." (Muslim)

599. Wearing Colored Contact Lenses

Allah, the Exalted, says:

"... and waste not by extravagance..." (Qur'an, Al-An'am 6:141)

Wearing colored cosmetic contact lenses is not permissible for several reasons: beautifying, wasting money of Allah the Almighty for extravagancy, deceiving as covering the reality. (489)

Additionally, they may cause eye health problems, then she will spend money to visit doctor and for the medications.

600. Makeup, Henna, Jewelry are Forbidden in front of Non-Mahram Men

Allah, the Exalted, says:

"and not expose their adornment except that which (necessarily) appears thereof and to wrap (a portion of) their headcovers over their chests and not expose their adornment except to their husbands..." (Qur'an, An-Nur 24:31)

Makeup which are practiced nowadays by women and on which huge amounts of money are wasted are the things which have been cursed. Muslim women should, therefore, avoid such evils as they are ruinous for religion as well as worldly life. (483)

This beautification should not be for non-Mahram men.

The one for whom a Muslim woman should beautify herself first and foremost is her husband. If she uses cosmetics so that her husband will see her in the best shape, or she appears thus beautified before other women or her mahrams, that is permissible for her.

The materials used for cosmetic purposes should be permissible, such as henna and kohl. It is not permissible for her to use fat from dead meat (i.e. from animals that have not been slaughtered in accordance with Shariah) or impure (najis) substances, because Islam forbids using impure and haram things.

The materials used for cosmetic purposes should not be harmful to her body. It is not permissible for her to use harmful chemical substances, whether the harmful effect will occur immediately or in the future, because Islam forbids harming oneself, as the Prophet (peace and blessings of Allah be upon him) said: "There should be neither causing harm nor reciprocating harm."

The cosmetic effect on the body should be temporary. It is not permissible for her to use those substances that change the creation of Allah, as some women do by having lip treatments, face peeling and tattoos which change the colour of the skin permanently. (490)

Jewelry and other adornments are only for husband (and mahrams) and are permissible so long as there is no obvious extravagance and Shirk (idolatry, Black Magic or Evil Eye) involved.

601. Sleeping and Lying on the Abdomen

Suhayl (May Allah be pleased with him) reported: "Abu Salih used to order us that if anyone of us wanted to sleep, he should lie on his right side and then say: "O Allah, Lord of the heavens and Lord of the earth and Lord of the Magnificent Throne! Our Lord, and the Lord of everything, the Cleaver of grains and date seeds, the Revealer of the Torah, the Gospel and the Criterion (the Qur'an), I seek refuge with You from the evil of everything that You have grasp of its forelock (You have full control over it). O Allah, You are the First, there is nothing before You, You are the Last and there is nothing after You, You are the Highest and there is nothing above You, and You are the Nearest and there is nothing nearer than You. Remove the burden of debt from us and relieve us of poverty." Abu Salih used to narrate this from Abu Hurairah, who narrated it from the Prophet (May Allah's peace and blessings be upon him)." (Muslim) (https://hadeethenc.com/en/browse/hadith/6335)

Ya'ish bin Tikhfah Al-Ghifari (May Allah be pleased with him) reported: My father said: "I was lying down on my belly in the Mosque when someone shook me with his foot and said, "Lying down this way is disapproved by Allah." I looked up and saw that it was Messenger of Allah (peace and blessings be upon him)." (Abu Dawud)

Narrated Abu Dharr (May Allah be pleased with him): "The Prophet (peace and blessings be upon him) passed by me and I was lying on my stomach. He nudged me with his foot and said: 'O Junaidib! This is how the people of Hellfire.'" (Ibn Majah)

Al-Bara' bin 'Azib (May Allah be pleased with him) reported: The Messenger of Allah (peace and blessings be upon him) directed me thus: "Whenever you go to bed, perform Wudu as you do for Salat then (before sleeping) recite: 'O Allah! I have submitted myself to You, I have turned myself to You, committed my affairs to You and sought Your refuge for protection out of desire for You and fear of You (expecting Your Reward and fearing Your Punishment). There is no refuge and no place of safety from You but with You. I believe in the Book You have revealed and in the Prophet (peace and blessings be upon him) You have sent.'" The Messenger of Allah (peace be upon him) added: "If anyone recites these words and dies during the night, he will die on the true Deen, and if he remains alive till the morning, he will obtain good. And make this supplication your last words (before sleeping)." (Bukhari and Muslim)

602. Christmas Celebration

Allah, the Exalted, says:

"And cooperate in righteousness and piety, but do not cooperate in sin and aggression. And fear Allah; indeed, Allah is severe in penalty." (Qur'an, Al-Ma'idah 5:2)

Abdullah ibn 'Umar (May Allah be pleased with him) reported that the Prophet (May Allah's peace and blessings be upon him) said: "Whoever imitates a people is one of them." (Abu Dawud)

Christmas is the celebration of the birthday of Jesus and englobes many Major sins.

1. Christmas is a Shirk, associating partners with Allah, the Creator. Jesus was a Muslim man and the

Messenger of Allah; not god or son of God.

Allah, the Exalted, says:

"Say (O Prophet), "He is Allah, One (and Indivisible); Allah, the Sustainer (needed by all). He has never had offspring, nor was He born. And there is none comparable to Him." (Qur'an, Al-Ikhlas 112:1-4)

"(Jesus) said, "Indeed, I am the servant of Allah. He has given me the Scripture and made me a Prophet." (Qur'an, Maryam 19:30)

"The Jews say, "Ezra is the son of Allah"; and the Christians say, "The Messiah is the son of Allah." That is their statement from their mouths; they imitate the saying of those who disbelieved (before them). May Allah destroy them; how are they deluded?" (Qur'an, At-Tawbah 9:30)

2. Speaking about Allah without knowledge is another Major sin.

Allah, the Exalted, says:

"O People of the Scripture, do not commit excess in your religion or say about Allah except the truth. The Messiah, Jesus, the son of Mary, was but a Messenger of Allah and His Word which He directed to Mary and a soul (created at a command) from Him. So, believe in Allah and His Messengers. And do not say, "Three"; desist - it is better for you. Indeed, Allah is but One God. Exalted is He above having a son. To Him belongs whatever is in the heavens and whatever is on the earth. And sufficient is Allah as Disposer of affairs." (Qur'an, An-Nisa 4:171)

3. Christmas is an innovation (Bid'ah) and every innovation is misguidance, it removes people from the Straight Path. Christmas became a global celebration, exceeding Christianity as a religion and celebrated all over the world even by non-Christian ignorant people.

Allah, the Exalted, says:

"They have certainly disbelieved who say," "Allah is the Messiah, the son of Mary" while the Messiah has said, "O Children of Israel, worship Allah, my Lord and your Lord." Indeed, he who associates others with Allah - Allah has forbidden him Paradise, and his refuge is the Fire. And there are not for the wrongdoers any helpers." (Qur'an, Al-Ma'idah 5:72)

Sharing happiness and joy on Christmas, Easter, etc., it is like shaking hands with Satan.

4. Celebration of the birthday is another innovation. None of the Prophets celebrated the birthday. The birthday of the Prophet Jesus (May Allah have mercy on him) is not in December; it was during the warm period of the year when palm trees deliver ripe fresh dates. When Jesus' mother was in labor pain, delivering him, Allah said to her:

"And shake toward you the trunk of the palm tree; it will drop upon you ripe fresh dates." (Qur'an, Maryam 19:25)

5. Celebration of Christmas involves many sins like unlawful food, smoking, music, singing, dance, females and males mixing, temptation, unlawful sex, etc. Sins remove Allah's blessings. Sins cause diseases, calamities. It cannot be taken in an ignorant or easy way.

6. Alcohol consumption is a Major sin.

7. Killing the trees, the creations of Allah, disturbing the natural environment, is a Major sin.

"Whatever you have cut down of (their) palm trees or left standing on their trunks - it was by permission of Allah and so He would disgrace the defiantly disobedient." (Qur'an, An-Hashr 59:5)

Narrated Abdullah Ibn Habashi: The Prophet (peace and blessings be upon him) said: If anyone cuts the lote-tree, Allah brings him headlong into Hell. (Abu Dawud)

Abu Dawud was asked about the meaning of this tradition. He said: This is a brief tradition. It means that if anyone cuts uselessly, unjustly and without any right a lote-tree under the shade of which travelers and beasts take shelter, Allah will bring him into Hell headlong.

Narrated Anas bin Malik: Allah's Messenger (peace and blessings be upon him) said, "There is none amongst the Muslims who plants a tree or sows seeds, and then a bird, or a person or an animal eats from it, but is regarded as a charitable gift for him." (Bukhari)

"…Bring no harm to the trees, nor burn them with fire, especially those which are fruitful." (Muslim) (https://www.iium.edu.my/deed/hadith/muslim/019)

Anas ibn Malik reported: The Messenger of Allah (peace and blessings be upon him) said, "Even if the Resurrection were established upon one of you while he has in his hand a sapling, let him plant it." (Ahmad)

Islam prohibits the cutting or destruction of trees and plants.

8. Wasting Allah's money for decoration of the Christmas trees, for renting the place to celebrate, for Christmas dinner, exchange gifts, candles, dress, haram food and drink, etc., wasting Allah's money for the Shirk and extravagance.

9. Christmas season traditions have their roots in pagan festivities celebrated on December 25th.

10. Anything related to Christmas like greeting, selling, buying, offering gifts, decorating, taking pictures under the Christmas tree, purchasing the books on Christmas, children asking Santa Claus to make their wishes come true or for the gift, etc.; all these involve sins.

11. Imitating the disbelievers – Christians – means he is a disbeliever

'Abdullah ibn 'Umar (May Allah be pleased with him) reported that the Prophet (May Allah's peace and blessings be upon him) said: "Whoever imitates a people is one of them." (Abu Dawud)
(https://hadeethenc.com/en/browse/hadith/5353)

12. Those who don't remember the Creator, will suffer loss

Abu Hurairah (May Allah be pleased with him) reported: The Messenger of Allah (peace and blessings of Allah be upon him) said, "Whoever sits in a place where he does not remember Allah, the Exalted, he will suffer loss and incur displeasure of Allah; and whoever lies (to sleep) in a place where he does not remember Allah, he will suffer sorrow and incur displeasure of Allah." (Abu Dawud)

DEVASTATING CHRISTMAS

The 2004 Indian Ocean earthquake and tsunami (also known as the Christmas or Boxing Day Tsunami and the Sumatra–Andaman earthquake) occurred at 07:59 am on 26 December after Christmas night, with an epicenter in Sumatra, Indonesia which killed nearly 300.000 people in 14 countries, making it one of the deadliest natural disasters in history. The earthquake was the third-largest ever recorded, the largest in the 21st century and had the longest duration, it caused the planet to vibrate and also remotely triggered earthquakes as far away as Alaska.

The end of December is the peak of the high tourist season in the region. A lot of westerners escape the cold winter at home to spend the Christmas to New Year on the beaches of Indonesia and other countries around. That was the most sinful Christmas night which caused Allah's Anger.

Allah has chosen for all people only two Celebrations:

1. Eid al-Fitr (Festival of Breaking Fast) celebrating the end of the fasting month of Ramadan, accompanied by many charity actions.
2. Eid al-Adha (Festival of Sacrifice) being the commemoration of Prophet Ibrahim. Allah the Almighty ordered Prophet Ibrahim to sacrifice his son Ismail (peace be upon them), but instead of his son, Allah, the All-Wise, sent the sheep to sacrifice to feed the family, the poor and neighbors.

603. New Year Celebration

New Year celebration involves many Major Sins. It is a pagan festivity, wasting Allah's money, music, dance, songs, unlawful food and drink, fireworks, men and women mixing, temptation, etc.

God didn't create a month of 31 days. Satan, however, has cleverly deceived the world into believing the New Year begins on January first!

Almighty God created a month of 29 or 30 days depending on the visibility of the moon, astronomical positioning of the earth and weather conditions. Each month of the Islamic calendar commences on the birth of the new lunar cycle.

The Islamic New Year (Hijri New Year) is the day that marks the beginning of a new lunar Hijri year. The first day of the Islamic year is observed by most Muslims on the first day of the month of Muharram. A day in the Islamic calendar is defined as beginning at sunset. The Islamic lunar year is eleven to twelve days shorter than the solar year as counted by the Gregorian calendar.

The Islamic New Year was not celebrated by God's Messenger.

Muslims should not celebrate any New Year celebrations. It is not permissible for the Muslims to exchange greetings on the occasion of the Gregorian New Year or any other New Year (Gregorian, Persian, Chinese, etc.) and it is not permissible for them to celebrate it, because it involves imitation of the kuffaar, and we have been forbidden to do that. (491)

604. Birthday Celebration

Allah, the Exalted, says:

"Or have they other deities who have ordained for them a religion to which Allah has not consented? But if not for the decisive word, it would have been concluded between them. And indeed, the wrongdoers will have a painful punishment." (Qur'an, Ash-Shuraa 42:21)

"Say (O Muhammad SAW) to these idolaters (pagan Arabs) of your folk) Follow what has been sent down unto you from your Lord (the Qur'an and Prophet Muhammad's Sunnah), and follow not any Auliya' (protectors and helpers, etc. who order you to associate partners in worship with Allah), besides Him (Allah). Little do you remember!" (Qur'an, Al-A'raf 7:3)

"Then We have put you (O Muhammad SAW) on a plain way of (Our) commandment [like the one which We commanded Our Messengers before you (i.e. legal ways and Laws of the Islamic Monotheism)]. So, follow you that (Islamic Monotheism and its Laws), and follow not the desires of those who know not. [Tafsir At-Tabari, vol.25, p.146]." (Qur'an, Al-Jathiyah 45:18)

Other Verse: Al-Jathiyah 45:19.

Narrated by Abu Sa`id Al-Khudri (May Allah be pleased with him): The Prophet (peace and blessings of Allah be upon him) said, warning us against following their ways and traditions: "You would follow the ways of those nations who were before you, span by span and cubit by cubit (i.e. inch by inch) so much so that even if they entered a hole of a mastigure, you would follow them." We said, "O Messenger of Allah, (do you mean) the Jews and the Christians?" He said, "Who else?" (Bukhari)

The evidence in the Qur'an and Sunnah indicates that celebrating birthdays is a kind of Bid'ah or innovation in religion, which has no basis in the Shariah. It is not permitted to accept invitations to birthday celebrations because this involves supporting and encouraging Bid'ah. Celebrating birthdays, accepting the invitation for the party, congratulating with "Happy Birthday", offering and accepting the gifts, even just mentioning "Birthday" is a kind of Bid'ah (innovation). (492)

605. Ruling on Celebrating Valentine's Day

Allah, the Exalted, says:

"Help you one another in Al-Birr and At-Taqwa (virtue, righteousness and piety); but do not help one another in sin and transgression. And fear Allah. Verily, Allah is Severe in punishment." (Qur'an, Al-Ma'idah 5:2)

Origin of Valentine's Day

Valentine's Day is a jahili Roman festival, which continued to be celebrated until after the Romans became Christians. This festival became connected with the saint known as Valentine who was sentenced to death on 14 February 270 CE. The kuffar still celebrate this festival, during which immorality and evil are practiced widely.

Can Muslims celebrate Valentine Day?

Sheikh Ibn Taymiyah (May Allah have mercy on him) said:

"Festivals are part of Shariah, clear way and rituals of which Allah says:

"To each among you, We have prescribed a Law and a clear way." (Qur'an, Al-Ma'idah 5:48)

"For every nation We have ordained religious ceremonies which they must follow." (Qur'an, Al-Hajj 22:67)

- such as the Qiblah (direction faced in prayer), prayer and fasting. There is no difference between their participating in the festival and their participating in all other rituals. Joining in fully with the festival is joining in with kufr, and joining in with some of its minor issues is joining in with some of the branches of kufr. Indeed, festivals are one of the most unique features that distinguish various religions and among their most prominent symbols, so joining in with them is joining in with the most characteristic and

prominent symbols of kufr. No doubt joining in with this may lead to complete kufr.

Partially joining in, at the very least, is disobedience and sin. This was indicated by the Prophet (peace and blessings of Allah be upon him) when he said: "Every people have its festival and this is our festival." This is worse than joining them in wearing the zinar (a garment that was worn only by ahl al-dhimmah) and other characteristics of theirs, for those characteristics are man-made and are not part of their religion, rather the purpose behind them is simply to distinguish between a Muslim and a kafir. As for the festival and its rituals, this is part of the religion which is cursed along with its followers, so joining in with it is joining in with something that is a cause of incurring the Wrath and Punishment of Allah." (Iqtida al-Sirat al-Mustaqim (1/207)

He (May Allah have mercy on him) also said:

"It is not permissible for the Muslims to imitate them in anything that is uniquely a part of their festivals, whether it be food, clothing, bathing, lighting fires, refraining from a regular habit, doing acts of worship or anything else. It is not permissible to give a feast or to give gifts, or to sell anything that will help them to do that for that purpose, or to allow children and others to play games that are part of the festivals, or to wear one's adornments.

To conclude: the Muslims should not do any of their rituals at the time of their festivals; rather the day of their festival should be like any other day for the Muslims. The Muslims should not do anything specific in imitation of them." (Majmu' al-Fataawa (25/329)

It is also haram for the Muslim to help people to celebrate this or any other haram festival by supplying any kind of food or drink, or buying, or selling, or manufacturing, or giving or advertising, etc., because all of that is cooperating in sin and transgression and is disobedience towards Allah, the Creator, and His Messenger (peace and blessings of Allah be upon him). It results in evils and haram things such as wasting time, singing, music, extravagance, unveiling, wanton display, men mixing with women, women appearing before men other than their mahrams, and other haram things or things that are a means that lead to immorality. (493)

606. Conditions for the Acceptance of Good Deeds by Allah

Allah, the Exalted, says:

"So, call you (O Muhammad and the believers) upon (or invoke) Allah making (your) worship pure for Him (Alone) (by worshipping none but Him and by doing religious deeds sincerely for Allah's sake only and not to show off and not to set up rivals with Him in worship)." (Qur'an, Ghafir 40:14)

"And who has (in mind) no favor from anyone to be paid back, Except to seek the Countenance of his Lord, the Most High." (Qur'an, Al-Layl 92:19)

"(Saying): "We feed you seeking Allah's Countenance only. We wish for no reward, nor thanks from you." (Qur'an, Al-Insan 76:9)

Other Verses: *Ash-Shuraa 42:20, Hud 11:15-16, Nuh 71:10-12, Al-Mulk 67:2.*

Ibn al-Qayyim (May Allah have mercy on him) said:

"Allah has made devotion of worship to Him Alone and following the Sunnah the means of deeds being accepted; if these conditions are not met, then deeds are unacceptable." (al-Rooh, 1/135) (494)

Conditions for Acceptance of Good Deeds:

1) Call upon No One Except Allah

Allah, the Exalted, says:

"And they were commanded not but that they should worship Allah, and worship none but Him Alone (abstaining from ascribing partners to Him." (Qur'an, Al-Bayinah 98:5)

Abu al-Abbas 'Abdullah bin 'Abbas (May Allah have mercy on him) reported: The Prophet (peace and blessings of Allah be upon him) said: "…If you ask, then ask Allah (Alone), and if you seek help, then seek the help from Allah (Alone). And know that if the nation were to gather together to benefit you with anything, they would not benefit you except with what Allah had already prescribed for you." (Tirmidhi) (https://sunnah.com/nawawi 40:19)

2) Deeds should be in accordance with the Qur'an and Sunnah

Aisha (May Allah be pleased with her) reported: The Messenger of Allah (May Allah's peace and blessings be upon him) said: "Whoever introduces into this matter of ours (meaning Islam) something that does not belong to it shall have it rejected." (Bukhari and Muslim) (https://hadeethenc.com/en/browse/hadith/4792)

Yahya bin Abu Muta' said: "One day, the Messenger of Allah (peace and blessings of Allah be upon him) stood up among us and delivered a deeply moving speech to us that melted our hearts and caused our eyes to overflow with tears….'I urge you to adhere to my Sunnah and the path of the Rightly-Guided Caliphs, and cling stubbornly to it. And beware of newly-invented matters, for every innovation is a going astray.'" (Ibn Majah)

3) Reward of Deeds Upon the Intentions

Narrated Umar ibn al-Khattab (May Allah be pleased with him) said: "I heard the Messenger of Allah (peace and blessings be upon him) say, "The reward of deeds depends upon the intentions and every person will get the reward according to what he has intended. So, whoever emigrated for worldly benefits or for a woman to marry, his emigration was for what he emigrated for." (Bukhari)

4) Sincerity in Making Du'a to Allah Alone

Sincerity in Du'a means having the firm belief that the One upon Whom you are calling, Allah, may He be Glorified and Exalted, is Alone Able to meet your need.

3) Repentance to Allah

Allah, the Exalted, says:

"See they not that they are put in trial once or twice every year (with different kinds of calamities, disease, famine)? Yet, they turn not in repentance, nor do they learn a lesson (from it)." (Quran, At-Tawbah 9:126)

"But whosoever repents after his crime and does righteous good deeds (by obeying Allah), then verily, Allah will pardon him (accept his repentance). Verily, Allah is Oft-Forgiving, Most Merciful." (Quran, Al-Ma'idah 5:39)

4) Humbling and avoiding aggression, Hoping for Allah's Reward and Fearing His Punishment

This is the spirit, essence and purpose of Du'a.

Allah, the Exalted, says:

"Invoke your Lord with humility and in secret. He likes not the aggressors." (Qur'an, Al-A'raf 7:55)

5) Repeating the Du'a without Getting Exasperated or Bored

Thauban (May Allah be pleased with him) reported: Whenever the Messenger of Allah (peace and blessings of Allah be upon him) finished his Salat (prayer), he would beg forgiveness three times [by saying, 'Astaghfirullah' (3 times)] and then he would say: "Allahumma Antas-Salamu, wa minkas-Salamu, tabarakta ya Dhal-Jalali wal-Ikram. (O Allah! You are the Bestower of security and security comes from You; Blessed are You. O Possessor of Glory and Honor)." Imam Al-Auza'i (one of the subnarrators) of this Hadith was asked: "How forgiveness should be sought?" He replied: "I say: Astaghfirullah, Astaghfirullah (I seek forgiveness from Allah. I seek forgiveness from Allah)." (Muslim)

6) Making Du'as at times of ease and more at times of adversity

Abdullah ibn 'Abbas (May Allah be pleased with him) reported: "One day I was riding behind the Prophet (peace and blessings of Allah be upon him), and he said: "…Be mindful of Allah, and you will find Him in front of you. Recognize and acknowledge Allah in times of ease and prosperity, and He will remember you in times of adversity…" (Tirmidhi) (https://40hadithnawawi.com/hadith/19-be-mindful-of-allah-and-allah-will-protect-you)

7) Calling Allah by His Most Beautiful Names and Attributes

Allah, the Exalted, says:

"And (all) the Most Beautiful Names belong to Allah, so call on Him by them." (Qur'an, Al-A'raf 7:180)

8) Choosing the Best of Du'as

The best of Du'as are the Du'as of the Prophet (peace and blessings of Allah be upon him), but it is permissible to say other words according to the specific needs of a person.

Ibn al-Qayyim (May Allah have mercy on him) said:

"Dua's and Taawwudhaat (prayers seeking refuge with Allah) are like a weapon, and a weapon is only as good as the person who is using it; it is not merely the matter of how sharp it is. If the weapon is perfect and free of faults, and the arm of the person using it is strong, and there is nothing stopping him, then he can lay waste the enemy. But if any of these three features is lacking, then the effect will be lacking accordingly." (al-Daa wal-Dawaa, p.35)

From this it will be clear that there is an etiquette and rulings which must be fulfilled, in the Du'a and in the person making the Du'a. There are also things that may prevent the Du'a reaching Allah or being answered these things must be removed from the person making the Du'a and from the Du'a. (495)

<u>Things which may prevent Du'a from being answered include:</u>

1) When the Du'a involves something inappropriate, sinful

Abu Sa'id al-Khudri reported the Prophet as saying, "Any Muslim who makes a supplication containing nothing which is sinful or which involves breaking ties of relationship will be given for it by God one of three things: He will give him as speedy answer, or store it up for him in the next world, or turn away from him an equivalent amount of evil." Those who heard it said they would then make many supplications and he replied that God was more ready to answer than they were to ask." (Ahmad)

2) Weak Faith

He is faint-hearted in his turning towards Allah. This may be either because of bad manners towards Allah, may He be Exalted, such as raising his voice in Du'a or making Du'a in the manner of one who thinks he has no need of Allah, or because he pays too much attention to the wording and tries to come up with unnecessarily ornate phrases, without paying attention to the meaning, or because he tries too hard to weep or shout without really feeling it, or he goes to extremes in that.

3) Sins prevent from answering to Du'a

Allah, the Exalted, said:

"Verily, Allah accepts only from those who are Al-Muttaqoon (the pious)." (Qur'an, Al-Ma'idah 5:27)

Narrated Abu Hurairah (May Allah be pleased with him): The Messenger of Allah (peace and blessings of Allah be upon him) said: "Allah, may He be Blessed and Exalted, says: 'I am so Self-Sufficient that I am in no need of having an associate. Thus, he who does an action for someone else's sake as well as Mine will have that action renounced by Me to him whom he associated with Me.'" (Muslim)

Abu Hurairah (May Allah be pleased with him) said: The Messenger of Allah (peace and blessings of Allah be upon him) said, "O people! Allah is Pure and, therefore, accepts only that which is pure. Allah has commanded the believers as He has commanded His Messengers by saying: *'O Messengers! Eat of the good things, and do good deeds.' (23:51)* And He said: *'O you who believe (in the Oneness of Allah - Islamic Monotheism)! Eat of the lawful things that We have provided you...'" (2:172)* Then he (peace and blessings of Allah be upon him) made a mention of the person who travels for a long period of time, his hair is disheveled and covered with dust. He lifts his hand towards the sky and thus makes the supplication: 'My Rubb! My Rubb!' But his food is unlawful, his drink is unlawful, his clothes are unlawful and his nourishment is unlawful, how can, then, his supplication be accepted?" (Muslim)

Abu Najeeh al-'Irbaad ibn Saariyah (May Allah be pleased with him) said: The Messenger of Allah (peace and blessings of Allah be upon him) gave us a sermon by which our hearts were filled with fear and tears came to our eyes. So, we said, "O Messenger of Allah! It is as though this is a farewell sermon, so counsel us." He (peace and blessings of Allah be upon him) said, "I counsel you to have Taqwa (fear) of Allah, and to listen and obey (your leader), even if a slave were to become your ameer. Verily he among you who lives long will see great controversy, so you must keep to my Sunnah and to the Sunnah of the Khulafa ar-Rashideen (the rightly guided Caliphs), those who guide to the right way. Cling to it stubbornly (literally: with your molar teeth). Beware of newly invented matters (in the religion), for verily every Bid'ah (innovation) is misguidance." (Abu Dawud and Tirmidhi)

Abu Hurairah (May Allah be pleased with him) said, "When the following Ayat was revealed *"Warn your near relatives." (26:214)*, the Prophet (peace and blessings be upon him) stood up and called out, saying, 'Banu Ka'b ibn Lu'ayy! Save yourselves from the Fire! Banu 'Abdu

Manaf! Save yourselves from the Fire! Banu Hashim! Save yourselves from the Fire! Banu 'Abdu'l-Muttalib! Save yourselves from the Fire! Fatima, daughter of Muhammad! Save yourselves from the Fire! I do not have anything for you in respect to Allah except for the fact that you have ties of kinship.'" (Al-Adab Al-Mufrad, Bukhari)

Ibn 'Umar (May Allah be pleased with him) said, "If someone fears his Lord and maintains ties of kinship, his term of life will be prolonged, he will have abundant wealth and his people will love him." (Al-Adab Al-Mufrad, Bukhari)

4) For God's Answer - Be patient

Abu Hurairah (May Allah be pleased with him) reported that the Messenger of Allah (peace and blessings be upon him) said, "The supplication of any of you is answered as long as he does not make supplication for something which is a wrong action or cutting off ties of kinship, or become impatient and say, 'I made supplication and was not answered, and so he stops making supplication." (Al-Adab Al-Murad, Bukhari)

5) Making the Du'a conditional: "O Allah, forgive me if You will"

Narrated Abu Hurairah (May Allah be pleased with him): The Prophet (peace and blessings of Allah be upon him) said: "None of you should say, 'O Allah, forgive me if You wish, O Allah, be Merciful to me if You wish, but he should always appeal to Allah with determination, whilst knowing that no one can compel Allah to do anything." (Bukhari and Muslim)

6) Should think positively of Allah

Narrated Abu Hurairah (May Allah be pleased with him): The Prophet (peace and blessings of Allah be upon him) said, "Allah says: 'I am just as My slave thinks…'" (Bukhari) (https://hadeethenc.com/en/browse/hadith/3636)

Thinking positively of Allah, may He be Exalted, is a great act of worship of the heart, but many people have not understood it correctly.

Thinking positively of Allah, may He be Exalted, means: believing in what is appropriate to Allah, may He be Exalted, of Names, Attributes and actions; believing in the great impact that they have on His creation, such as believing that Allah, may He be Exalted, bestows Mercy on those who deserve it, and pardons them if they repent and turn to Him, and He accepts their deeds of obedience and worship; believing that Allah, may He be Exalted, has great Wisdom in all that He wills and decrees.

Thinking positively of Allah cannot be sound when one is not doing obligatory deeds or when one is committing sins. Whoever thinks that is deceived, his hope is blameworthy hope, he is resembling the Murji'ah who were innovators, and he is feeling secure from the Plan of Allah; all of these are serious problems which will lead one to doom. (496)

7) Should be focused and mindful of Allah

Abu Hurairah (May Allah be pleased with him) reported: The Messenger of Allah (peace and blessings be upon him) said, "Call upon Allah with certainty that He will answer you. Know that Allah will not answer the supplication of a heart that is unmindful and distracted." (Tirmidhi)

Abu al-'Abbas 'Abdullah bin 'Abbas (May Allah have mercy on him) reported: The Prophet (peace and blessings be upon him) said, 'Young man, I will teach you some words. Be mindful of God, and He will take care of you. Be mindful of Him, and you shall find Him at your side…" (Tirmidhi)
(https://40hadithnawawi.com/hadith/19-be-mindful-of-allah-and-allah-will-protect-you)

8) Should Not Let Du'a Distract you from an Obligatory Prayer

9) Should Not Neglect Parents' Rights on the Basis of Du'a or Voluntary Prayer

Make priority parents' rights over Du'a or voluntary prayer. This is indicated by the story of Jurayj, when he did not answer his mother's calls and turned instead to his prayer. She prayed against him and Allah tested him sorely. (https://sunnah.com/riyadussalihin:259)

Al-Nawawi (May Allah have mercy on him) said:

"The scholars said: 'This indicates that what he should have done is to answer her, because he was offering a supererogatory (naafil prayer), continuation of which was voluntary, not obligatory, whereas answering his mother and honoring her was obligatory and disobeying her was haram.'" (497)

The response to the Du'a may take different forms

Allah the Almighty may respond and fulfil the desire of the person who made the Du'a, or He may ward off some evil from him because of the Du'a, or He can make something good easy for him to attain because of it, or He may save it with Him for him on the Day of Resurrection when he will be most in need of it. (495)

The Best Times and Places when Du'a is more likely to be accepted by Allah

(1) *At the Adhan*

Sa'd ibn Abi Waqqas (May Allah be pleased with him) reported: The Prophet (May Allah's peace and blessings be upon him) said: "Whoever says when he hears the Muezzin: 'I bear witness that there is no god but Allah Alone without any partner and that Muhammad is His slave and Messenger. I am pleased with Allah as a Lord, with Muhammad as a Messenger and with Islam as a religion', his sins shall be forgiven." (Muslim) (https://hadeethenc.com/en/browse/hadith/6272)

Narrated Sahl ibn Sa'd (May Allah be pleased with him): The Prophet (peace and blessings be upon him) said: "There are two that will not be rejected, or will rarely be rejected: Du'a at the time of the Call for Prayer and at the time of battle when the fighting begins." (Abu Dawud)

(2) *Du'a after Wudu*

'Uqba b. 'Amir (May Allah be pleased with him) reported: "We were entrusted with the task of tending the camels. On my turn when I came back in the evening after grazing them in the pastures, I found Allah's Messenger (peace and blessings be upon him) stand and address the people. I heard these words of his: 'If any Muslim performs ablution well, then stands and prays two Rak'ahs setting about them with his heart as well as his face, Paradise would be guaranteed to him.' I said: 'What a fine thing is this!' And a narrator who was before me said: 'The first was better than even this.' When I cast a glance, I saw that it was 'Umar who said: 'I see that you have just come and observed: 'If anyone amongst you performs the ablution, and then completes the ablution well and then says:' I testify that there is no god but Allah and that Muhammad is the servant of Allah and His Messenger.'" (Muslim)

(3) *Between Adhan and Iqamah*

Allah, the Exalted, says:

"And when My slaves ask you (O Muhammad SAW) concerning Me, then (answer them), I am indeed near (to them by My Knowledge). I respond to the invocations of the supplicant when he calls on Me (without any mediator or intercessor). So, let them obey Me and believe in Me, so that they may be led aright." (Qur'an, Al-Baqarah 2:186)

Narrated Sahl bin Sa'd (May Allah be pleased with him): The Messenger of Allah (peace and blessings be upon him) said, "Supplications at two times are never turned down (or said, "Are seldom turned down"), a supplication after the Adhan has been proclaimed, and a supplication during the battle combating the enemy." (Abu Dawud)

Narrated Anas (May Allah have mercy on him): Allah's Messenger (peace and blessings be upon him) said, "A supplication made between the Adhan and Iqamah is not rejected." (Abu Dawud)

(4) *While Reciting Surah Al-Fatihah*

Narrated Abu Hurairah (May Allah be pleased with him): The Prophet (peace and blessings be upon him) said that Allah, Mighty and Sublime be He, had said: 'I have divided prayer between Myself and My servant into two halves, and My servant shall have what he has asked for. When the servant says: 'Al-hamdu lillahi rabbi l-alamin (3)', Allah, Mighty and Sublime be He, says: 'My servant has praised Me.' And when he says:' Ar-rahmani r-rahim (4)', Allah,

Mighty and Sublime be He, says: 'My servant has extolled Me', and when he says: 'Maliki yawmi d-din (5)', Allah says: 'My servant has glorified Me' - and on one occasion He said: 'My servant has submitted to My Power.' And when he says: 'Iyyaka na budu wa iyyaka nasta in (6)', He says: 'This is between Me and My servant, and My servant shall have what he has asked for.' And when he says:' Ihdina s-sirata l- mustaqim, siratal ladhina an amta alayhim ghayril-maghdubi alayhim wa la d-dallin (7)', He says: 'This is for My servant, and My servant shall have what he has asked for.' (1) Surah Al-Fatihah, the first Surah (Chapter) of the Qur'an. (2) i.e. standing behind the imam (leader) listening to him reciting Al-Fatihah. (3) "Praise be to Allah, Lord of the worlds." (4) "The Merciful, the Compassionate." (5) "Master of the Day of Judgement." (6) "It is You we worship and it is You we ask for help." (7) "Guide us to the Straight Path, the Path of those upon whom You have bestowed favors, not of those against whom You are angry, nor of those who are astray." (Muslim)

(5) *Saying 'Ameen' During Prayer*

Narrated Abu Hurairah (May Allah be pleased with him): Allah's Messenger (peace and blessings be upon him) said, "When the Imam says: 'Ghair-il-Maghdubi 'alaihim Walad-Dallin (i.e. not the path of those who earn Your Anger, nor the path of those who went astray (1:7), then you must say, 'Ameen', for if one's utterance of 'Ameen' coincides with that of the angels, then his past sins will be forgiven."

(6) *Du'a when Prostrating at the End of the Prayer*

Narrated Abu Hurairah (May Allah have mercy on him): The Allah's Messenger (peace and blessings be upon him), said: "The nearest a slave can be to his Lord is when he is prostrating, so increase (your) supplications (while in this state)." (Muslim)

(7) *At the End of the Obligatory Prayers*

Narrated Abu Umamah (May Allah have mercy on him): "Allah's Messenger (peace and blessings be upon him) was asked, "O Messenger of Allah, which supplication is heard by Allah, the Exalted." He said. "At the end of the night and at the end of the obligatory Salat (prayer)." (Tirmidhi)

There was some difference of scholarly opinion concerning the phrase dubur al-salawat al-maktubah ("following the prescribed prayers") – does it mean before the salam or afterwards?

Sheikh Ibn Taymiyah and his student Ibn al-Qayyim were of the view that it is before the salam. Ibn Taymiyah said: "The word dubur refers to something that is part of a thing, like dubur al-hayawan (the hindquarters of an animal)." (Zad Al-Ma'ad, 1.305)

Sheikh Ibn 'Uthaymeen (May Allah have mercy on him) said:

"What has been narrated of Du'a following the prayer is before the salam and what has been narrated of Dhikr following the prayer is after the salam, because Allah says: *"When you have finished As-Salah (the congregational prayer), remember Allah standing, sitting down and (lying down) on your sides." (Qur'an, An-Nisa 4:103)* (See: Kitab al-Du'a by Sheikh Muhammad al-Hamad, p.54)

(8) After the Sun Has Passed its Zenith and before Zhuhr

'Abd-Allah ibn al-Saib (May Allah be pleased with him) narrated that the Messenger of Allah (peace and blessings of Allah be upon him) used to pray four Rak'ahs after the sun had passed its zenith and before Zuhr, and he said: "This is a time when the gates of Heaven are opened and I want a good deed of mine to ascend during this time." (Tirmidhi)

(9) *At Midnight*

Masruq (May Allah be pleased with him) reported on the authority of Aisha that she said that the Messenger of Allah (peace and blessings be upon him) used to observe the Witr prayer every night, maybe in the early part of night, at midnight and in the latter part, finishing his Witr at dawn. (Muslim)

(10) *When Waking Up at Night*

Narrated Ubada Bin As-Samit (May Allah be pleased with him): "Allah's Messenger (peace and blessings be upon him) said: 'Whomever wakes up at night and says La ilaha illallahu wahdahu la shrika lahu lahulmulku, wa lahul hamdu, wa huwa ala kulli shai'in qadir. Alhamdu lillahi, wa subhanallahi wa la ilaha illallahu, wallah akbar, wa la hawla wala quwata illa billah (None has the right to be worshipped but Allah, the Exalted. He is the Only One Who has no partners. His is the kingdom and all the praises are for Allah, the Exalted. All the glories are for Allah, the Exalted. And none has the right to be worshipped but Allah, the Exalted, and Allah, the Exalted, is the Most Great, and there is neither might nor power except with Allah, the Exalted, and then says, Allahumma ighfir li (O Allah! Forgive me) or invokes Allah, the Exalted, he will be responded to and if he makes ablution and performs Salat (prayer), his Salat (prayer) will be accepted." (Bukhari)

(11) *The Last Third of the Night*

Abu Hurairah (May Allah be pleased with him) reported Allah's Messenger (peace and blessings be upon him) as saying: "Our Lord Almighty descends to the lowest heaven in the last third of every night, saying: "Who is calling upon Me that I may answer him? Who is asking from Me that I may give him? Who is seeking My Forgiveness that I may forgive him?" (Bukhari and Muslim)

Jabir (May Allah be pleased with him) reported: "I heard the Messenger of Allah (May Allah's peace and blessings be upon him) saying: "There is an hour at night that no Muslim happens to be asking Allah the Almighty any good of this world or the Hereafter except that He will give it to him, and this occurs every night." (Muslim) (https://hadeethenc.com/en/browse/hadith/3625)

(12) *An Hour on Friday*

Narrated Abu Hurairah (May Allah have mercy on him): "Allah's Messenger (peace and blessings be upon him) talked about Friday and said: 'There is an hour on Friday and if a Muslim gets it while offering Salat (prayer) and asks something from Allah, the Exalted, then Allah will definitely meet his demand.' And he (the Prophet, peace and blessings be upon him) pointed out the shortness of that particular time with his hands." (Bukhari)

Narrated Abu Hurairah (May Allah have mercy on him): "Allah's Messenger (peace and blessings be upon him) talked about Friday and said: "On the day of Friday there is a (short) moment in which a Muslim is granted whatever he asks if he occupies this moment with Du'a/ the remembrance of Allah." (Bukhari and Muslim)

There are numerous views of the Scholars regarding the exact moment on a Friday that is being referred to. The following two are the more popular and well substantiated views.

1) Abu Musa Musa Al-Ash'ari (May Allah have mercy on him) reported that Rasulullah (peace and blessings be upon him) said: "It is between the time when the imam sits on the mimbar till after the [Jumu'ah] salah." (Muslim)

Note: Since we are (1) instructed to remain silent while the Khutbah is in motion, as well as (2) forbidden from reciting anything during this time, the 'Ulama have suggested making a Du'a between the two Khutbahs. This should be done in one's heart and not verbally, as the prohibition of verbal utterances still apply even if the imam is quiet at that time (between the two khutbahs).

2) Abdullah ibn Salam (May Allah have mercy on him) has reported that this moment exists after 'Asr Salah till sunset. (Tirmidhi)

This has been reported by other Sahabah (May Allah have mercy on them) as well.

Hafiz Ibn 'Abdil Barr (May Allah have mercy on him) said that this is the most well-established view on this topic. (Fathul Bari, Hadith: 935)

Imam Muhibbuddin Tabari (May Allah have mercy on him) said: "The most authentic Hadith on this is that of Sayyiduna Abu Musa (May Allah have mercy on him), and the most popular view is that of Sayyiduna 'Abdullah ibn Salam (May Allah have mercy on him)." ('Umdatul Qari, & Fathul Bari, Hadith: 935)

Imam Ahmad (May Allah have mercy on him) said: 'Most of the Hadiths on this state that it is after 'Asr. Although we can also hope for it to be after zawal (which concurs with the first Hadith I cited above). (Tirmidhi) (https://hadithanswers.com/the-moment-of-acceptance-on-friday)

(13) *Du'a when Fasting*

Anas ibn Malik (May Allah be pleased with him) reported: The Messenger of Allah (peace and blessings be upon him) said, "The supplications of three are not turned back: the supplication of a parent, the supplication of a fasting person and the supplication of a traveler." (al-Bayhaqi)

Abu Hurairah (May Allah be pleased with him) narrated that the Messenger of Allah (peace and blessings be upon him) said: "There are three whose supplication is not rejected: The fasting person when he breaks his fast, the just leader and the supplication of the oppressed person; Allah raises it up above the clouds and opens the gates of heaven to it. And the Lord says: 'By My Might, I shall surely aid you, even if it should be after a while.'" (Tirmidhi)

(14) *Du'a During Ramadan*

Aisha (May Allah be pleased with her) said: "With the start of the last ten days of Ramadan, Messenger of Allah (peace and blessings be upon him) would pray all the night, and would keep his family awake for the prayers. He tied his lower garment (i.e. avoided sleeping with his wives) and devoted himself entirely to prayer and supplication." (Bukhari and Muslim)

Abu Hurairah (Allah be pleased with him) reported Allah's Messenger (peace and blessings be upon him) as saying: "Every good deed of the son of Adam would be multiplied, a good deed receiving a tenfold to seven hundredfold reward. Allah, the Exalted and Majestic, has said: 'With the exception of fasting, for it is done for Me and I will give a reward for it, for one abandons his passion and food for My sake. There are two occasions of joy for one who fasts, joy when he breaks it, and joy when he meets his Lord, and the breath (of an observer of fast) is sweeter to Allah than the fragrance of musk.'" (Muslim)

(15) *At the Night of Qadr (Decree)*

Narrated Aisha (May Allah be pleased with her): "O Messenger of Allah, what do you think I should say in my supplication, if I come upon Laylatul-Qadr?" He said: "Say: 'Allahumma innaka 'afuwwun tuhibbul-'afwa, fa'fu 'anni (O Allah, You are Forgiving and love forgiveness, so forgive me).'" (Ibn Majah)

Narrated Abu Hurairah (May Allah be pleased with him): The Prophet (peace and blessings be upon him) said, "Whoever established prayers on the night of Qadr out of sincere faith and hoping for a reward from Allah, then all his previous sins will be forgiven; and whoever fasts in the month of Ramadan out of sincere faith, and hoping for a reward from Allah, then all his previous sins will be forgiven." (Bukhari)

(16) *First Ten Days of Dhu al-Hijjah*

Abdullah ibn Abbas (May Allah be pleased with him) reported: The Prophet (May Allah's peace and blessings be upon him) said: "There are no days on which righteous deeds are more beloved to Allah than on these days." (Meaning: the first ten days of Dhu al-Hijjah). They (the Companions) said: "O Messenger of Allah, not even Jihad in the Cause of Allah?" He said: "Not even Jihad in the Cause of Allah, except that of a man who went to Jihad with himself and his property, but did not return with any of them." (Bukhari) (https://hadeethenc.com/en/browse/hadith/6255)

(17) *Du'a Inside the Ka'bah*

Narrated Ibn 'Abbas (May Allah be pleased with him): When the Prophet (peace and blessings be upon him) entered the Ka'bah, he invoked Allah in each and every side of it and did not pray till he came out of it, and offered a two Rak'ahs prayer facing the Ka'bah and said, "This is the Qiblah." (Bukhari)

(18) *Du'a on the Mount of Safa or Marwah During Umrah or Hajj*

Narrated Jabir ibn 'Abd-Allah (May Allah be pleased with him) said: "... then he (the Prophet, peace and blessings of Allah be upon him) went out through the gate to As-Safa and when he drew near to As-Safa he recited: *"Verily, As-Safa and Al-Marwah (two mountains in Makkah) are of the Symbols of Allah" (Al-Baqarah 2:158)* (and he said:) "I begin with that with which Allah began." He began with As-Safa and climbed it until he could see the House, then he turned to face the Qiblah and proclaimed the Oneness of Allah and magnified Him, and said: "Laa ilaaha ill-Allaah wahdahu laa shareeka lah, lahu'l-mulk wa lahu'l-hamd wa huwa 'ala kulli shay'in qadeer; Laa ilaaha ill-Allaah wahdahu anjaza wa'dah wa nasara 'abdah wa hazama al-ahzaaba wahdah (There is no god but Allah Alone, with no partner or associate, His is the dominion and to Him be praise, and He is able to do all things; there is no god but Allah Alone, He fulfilled His promises and granted victory to His slave and defeated the confederates alone)." Then he made Du'a between that and repeated these three times." (Muslim)

Jabir (May Allah be pleased with him) said: "Then he (peace and blessings be upon him) came down towards Al-Marwah and when his feet reached the bottom of the valley he ran until the ground started to rise, then he walked until he came to Al-Marwah, and he did at Al-Marwah as he had done at As-Safa." (Muslim)

(19) *Du'a after Stoning the Jamarat at Hajj*

Narrated Salim (May Allah be pleased with him): Ibn 'Umar used to do Rami of the Jamrat-ud-Dunya (the Jamra near to the Khaif Mosque) with seven small stones and used to recite Takbir on throwing every pebble. He then would go ahead till he reached the level ground where he would stand facing the Qiblah for a long time to invoke Allah while raising his hands (while invoking). Then he would do Rami of the Jamrat-ul-Wusta (middle Jamra) and then he would go to the left towards the middle ground, where he would stand facing the Qiblah. He would remain standing there for a long period to invoke Allah while raising his hands, and would stand there for a long period. Then he would do Rami of the Jamrat-ul-Aqaba from the middle of the valley, but he would not stay by it, and then he would leave and say, "I saw the Prophet doing like this." (Bukhari)

(20) *Du'a on the Day of Arafat*

'Amr ibn Shu'ayb (May Allah be pleased with him) reported: The Prophet (peace and blessings be upon him) said, "The best supplication is that which is made on the day of Arafat. The best of it is what was said by myself and the Prophets before me: There is no God but Allah Alone, without any partners, unto Him belong the dominion and all praise and He has Power over all things." (Tirmidhi)

(21) *While Drinking Zamzam Water*

Narrated Jabir bin 'Abdullah (May Allah have mercy on him): "I heard the Messenger of Allah (peace and blessings be upon him) say: 'The water of Zamzam is for whatever it is drunk for.'" (Ibn Majah)

(22) *Du'a of the Traveler*

Anas ibn Malik (May Allah be pleased with him) reported: The Messenger of Allah (peace and blessings be upon him) said, "The supplications of three are not turned back: the supplication of a parent, the supplication of a fasting person and the supplication of a traveler." (al-Bayhaqi)

(23) *The Parent's Du'a for or against his Child*

The parent's Du'a for or against his child is answered.

Abu Hurairah (May Allah be pleased with him) reported that the Prophet (peace and blessings be upon him) said, "There are three supplications which are answered: the supplication of the person who is wronged, the supplication of the traveler and the supplication of a parent for his child." (Al-Adab Al- Mufrad, Bukhari)

Jabir ibn Abdullah (May Allah be pleased with him) reported: The Prophet (peace and blessings of Allah be upon him) forbade praying against one's children, one's wealth and one's own self, lest that be at a time when Du'as are answered. He (peace and blessings of Allah be upon him) said: "Do not pray against yourselves, do not pray against your children, do not pray against your wealth, lest that coincides with a time when Allah is asked and He gives, so He answers your prayer." (Muslim)

A mistake that is made by many fathers and mothers is that they pray against their children if the latter do something that makes them angry. What they should do is pray for them to be guided and for Allah to set their affairs straight.

By His Mercy, Allah does not answer the Du'a of parents against their children if it is at a time of anger, because Allah says:

"And were Allah to hasten for mankind the evil (they invoke for themselves and for their children, while in a state of anger) as He hastens for them the good (they invoke) then

they would have been ruined. So, We leave those who expect not their Meeting with Us, in their trespasses, wandering blindly in distraction." (Qur'an, Yunus 10:11)

Ibn Kathir (May Allah have mercy on him) said in his Tafseer (Exegesis) (2/554):

"Here Allah tells us of His Forbearance and Kindness towards His slaves, for He does not answer them when they pray against themselves or their wealth, or their children at moments of anger. He knows that they do not really mean any ill, so He does not answer them out of Kindness and Mercy, as He does when they pray for themselves or their wealth, or their children for goodness, blessing and growth. End quote." (498)

(24) *Du'a of the Righteous Child for his Parents*

Abdullah ibn Umar (May Allah be pleased with him) reported: The Messenger of Allah, peace and blessings be upon him, said, "While three men were walking, they were overcome by rain and took refuge in a cave in a mountain. A boulder fell over the mouth of their cave, blocking them inside. One of them said to the others, 'Look at the good deeds you have done for Allah that you may call upon Allah Almighty by them, for perhaps He will relieve you.' One of them said, 'O Allah, I had two old parents with my wife and young child. I tended to a flock and when evening came, I milked them and served my parents first before my child. One day I went in search of fodder and I did not come back until it was evening. I found them both sleeping, so I milked as I had done before. I brought the milk and stood by their heads, for I hated to disrupt their sleep or to serve my child before both of them. My child was crying at my feet, yet I continued standing over them until the approach of dawn. If You know I had done that seeking Your Countenance, then relieve us of this distress that we might see the sky!' Allah shifted the boulder until they could see the sky. Another man said, 'O Allah, I had a cousin whom I loved more than any man could love women. I presented myself to her and she refused unless I could give her one hundred coins. I worked hard until I gathered one hundred coins and brought them to her. When I prepared myself between her legs, she said: 'O servant of Allah, fear Allah and do not break the hymen without right to do so!' I stood and left her. If You know I had done that seeking your Face, then relieve us of this distress!' The boulder was again shifted for them. The last man said, 'O Allah, I employed a worker for a portion of rice. When he finished his work, he said: 'Give me what I deserve!' I offered his share to him but he did not accept it. I continued planting his share until I had amassed cows and flocks. Then he came to me and he said: 'Fear Allah and do not violate my rights!' I said: 'Go to this cow and its flocks and take them.' He said: 'Fear Allah and do not mock me!' I said: 'I do not mock you, take that cow and its flocks.' So, he took them and he left. If You know I had done that seeking Your Face, then relieve us of what remains!' Then Allah relieved them of what remained." (Bukhari and Muslim)

(25) *Du'a of a Muslim for his Absent Brother or Sister Muslim Stemming from the Heart*

Abu Dharr (May Allah be pleased with him) reported: The Prophet (peace and blessings be upon him) said: "There is no believing servant who supplicates for his brother in his absence where the Angels do not say, 'the same be for you.'" (Muslim)

(26) *Du'a of the One Who Is Suffering Injustice and Oppression*

Mu'adh (May Allah be pleased with him) reported that Messenger of Allah (peace and blessings be upon him) sent me (as a governor of Yemen) and instructed me thus: "…Beware of the supplication of the oppressed, for there is no barrier between it and Allah." (Bukhari and Muslim)
(https://sunnah.com/riyadussalihin:208)

(27) *Du'a During the Battle (Jihad)*

Narrated Sahl bin Sa'd (May Allah be pleased with him): The Messenger of Allah (peace and blessings be upon him) said, "Supplications at two times are never turned down (or said, "Are seldom turned down"), a supplication after the Adhan has been proclaimed, and a supplication during the battle combating the enemy." (Abu Dawud)

(28) *When Muslims Gather for the Purpose of Remembering Allah*

Abu Hurairah (May Allah be pleased with him) reported: The Messenger of Allah (peace and blessings be upon him) said, "No people gather to remember Allah Almighty but that the Angels surround them, cover them with mercy, send tranquility upon them, and mention them to Allah among those near to Him." (Muslim)

(29) *Du'a after the Death of a Person*

Umm Salama (May Allah be pleased with her) reported: The Messenger of Allah (peace and blessings be upon him) visited Abu Salamah (May Allah be pleased with him) when his eyes were open soon after he died. He closed them (the eyes) for him and said, "When the soul is taken away, the sight follows it." Some members of his family began to weep. He (peace and blessings be upon him) said: "Do not supplicate for yourselves anything but good, for the angels say 'Amin' to what you say." Then he said, "O Allah! Forgive Abu Salamah, raise his rank among those who are rightly guided and grant him a successor from his descendants who remain behind. Grant him pardon and us, too. O Rubb of the worlds. Make his grave spacious for him and give him light in it." (Muslim)

(30) *Du'a of a Just Ruler*

Abu Hurairah (May Allah be pleased with him) narrated that the Messenger of Allah (peace and blessings be upon him) said: "There are three whose supplication is not rejected: The fasting person when he breaks his fast, the just leader and the supplication of the oppressed person; Allah raises it up above the clouds and opens the gates of heaven to it. And the Lord says: 'By My Might, I shall surely aid you, even if it should be after a while.'" (Tirmidhi)

(31) *When Raining*

Narrated Sahl Ibn S'ad (May Allah have mercy on him): "The Messenger of Allah (peace and blessings be upon him) said: 'Two will not be rejected, supplication when the Adhan (Call of Prayer) is being called, and at the time of the rain.'" (Al-Hakim)

(32) *At the Crowing of a Rooster*

Narrated Abu Hurairah (May Allah have mercy on him): The Prophet (peace and blessings be upon him) said: "When you hear a rooster crowing, then ask Allah for His Bounties, for it has seen an Angel…" (Bukhari and Muslim)

(33) *Visiting the Sick*

'Ali bin Abu Talib (May Allah be pleased with him) reported: "I heard the Messenger of Allah (peace and blessings be upon him) saying, "When a Muslim visits a sick Muslim at dawn, seventy thousand Angels keep on praying for him till dusk. If he visits him in the evening, seventy thousand Angels keep on praying for him till the morning; and he will have (his share of) reaped fruits in Jannah." (Tirmidhi)

Aisha (May Allah be pleased with her) reported: When the Prophet (peace and lessings be upon him) visited any ailing member of his family, he would touch the sick person with his right hand and would supplicate: "Allahumma Rabban-nasi, adhhibil-ba'sa, washfi, Antash-Shafi, la shifa'a illa shifa'uka, shifaan la yughadiru saqaman (O Allah! the Rubb of mankind! Remove this disease and cure (him or her)! You are the Great Curer. There is no cure but through You, which leaves behind no disease)." (Bukhari and Muslim)

(34) *When saying the Du'a,* "La ilaha illa anta, subhanaka, inni kuntu min al-zalimin

[None has the right to be worshipped but You (O Allah)], Glorified and Exalted be You [above all that (evil) they associate with You]! Truly, I have been of the wrongdoers – cf. Al-Anbya 21:87])." It was narrated in a Saheeh Hadith that the Prophet (peace and blessings of Allah be upon him) said: "The prayer of Dhu'l-Nun (Yunus) which he said when he was in the belly of the whale: 'La ilaha illa anta, subhanaka, inni kuntu min al-zalimin [none has the right to be worshipped but You (O Allah)], Glorified and Exalted be You [above all that (evil) they associate with You]! Truly, I have been of the wrongdoers.' No Muslim recites this Du'a concerning any matter but Allah will answer him." (Tirmidhi)

Allah, the Exalted, says:

"And (remember) Dhun-Nun (Jonah), when he went off in anger, and imagined that We shall not punish him (i.e. the calamities which had befallen him)! But he cried through the darkness (saying): La ilaha illa Anta [none has the right to be worshipped but You (O Allah)], Glorified (and Exalted) be You [above all that (evil) they associate with You]! Truly, I have been of the wrongdoers." So, We answered his call and delivered him from the distress. And thus, We do deliver the believers (who believe in the Oneness of Allah, abstain from evil and work righteousness)." (Qur'an, Al-Anbya 21:87-88)

(35) *If a calamity befalls him and he says,*

"Inna Lillahi wa inna ilayhi raji'un, Allahumma ujurni fi musibati w'ukhluf li khayran minha" (Truly, to Allah we belong and truly, to Him we shall return; O Allah, reward me in this calamity and compensate me with something better than it).

Umm Salamah, the wife of the Messenger of Allah (peace be upon him), reported Allah's Messenger (peace be upon him) as saying: "If any servant of Allah who suffers a calamity says: "We belong to Allah and to Him we shall return; O Allah, reward me for my affliction and give me something better than it in exchange for it," Allah will give reward him for affliction, and would give him something better than it in exchange. She (Umm Salamah) said: 'When Abu Salama died. I uttered (these very words) as I was commanded (to do) by the Messenger of Allah (peace and blessings be upon him).' So, Allah gave me better in exchange than him. i.e. (I was taken as the wife of) the Messenger of Allah (peace be upon him).'" (Muslim)

607. Unlawful Innovations (Bid'ah)

Allah, the Exalted, says:

"This day I have perfected your religion for you, completed my favor upon you, and have chosen for you Islam as your religion." (Qur'an, Al-Ma'idah 5:3)

"For that is Allah, your Lord, the Truth. And what can be beyond Truth except error? So how are you averted?" (Qur'an, Yunus 10:32)

"And hold fast, all of you together, to the Rope of Allah (i.e. this Qur'an), and be not divided among yourselves, and remember Allah's Favor on you, for you were enemies one to another but He joined your hearts together, so that, by His Grace, you became brethren (in Islamic Faith), and you were on the brink of a pit of Fire, and He saved you from it. Thus, Allah makes His Ayat (proofs, evidences, verses, lessons, signs, revelations, etc.) clear to you, that you may be guided." (Qur'an, Ali 'Imran 3:103)

Other Verses: *An-Nisa 4:59, An-Nur 24:54 and 24:63, Adh-Dhariyat 51:56, Al-Ahqaf 46:9, An-Nahl 16:36, Al-An'am 6:116, Al-Isra 17:36, Al-Ma'idah 5:55, Ash-Shuraa 42:21.*

Anas ibn Malik reported: The Prophet (peace and blessings be upon him) said, "Some of my companions will come to me at the fountain in the Hereafter, until I recognize them. They will be taken away from me, then I will say: "My companions!" It will be said: "You do not know what they innovated after you." (Bukhari and Muslim)

1. Definition of Bid'ah

Sheikh Muhammad ibn 'Uthaymeen (May Allah have mercy on him) said:

"According to Shariah, the definition is 'Worshipping Allah in ways that Allah has not prescribed.' If you wish you may say, 'Worshipping Allah in ways that are not those of the Prophet (peace and blessings of Allah be upon him) or his rightly guided successors (al-khulafaa' al-raashidoon).'"

The second definition is taken from the Hadith of the Prophet (peace and blessings of Allah be upon him), who said: "I urge you to adhere to my way (Sunnah) and the way of the rightly guided successors (al-khulafa' al-raashidoon) who come after me. Hold fast to it and bite onto it with your eyeteeth (i.e. cling firmly to it), and beware of newly-invented matters."

He also said: "And there is no such thing in Islam as Bid'ah hasanah (good innovation)." (Majmoo' Fataawa Ibn 'Uthaymeen, vol.2, p.291)

2. Categories of Bid'ah

Bid'ah may be divided into two categories:

i) Bid'ah which constitutes kufr.

ii) Bid'ah which does not constitute kufr. (499)

Ali bin Abi Talib (May Allah be pleased with him) said: "Allah's Messenger (peace and blessing of Allah be upon him) informed me about four Judgments of Allah: 1) Allah's Curse is upon the one who slaughters (devoting his sacrifice) to anything other than Allah; 2) Allah's Curse is upon the one who curses his own parents; 3) Allah's Curse is upon the one who shelters an heretic (who has brought a Bid'ah in religion); 4) Allah's Curse is upon the one who alters the landmarks (who changes boundary lines)." (Muslim)

Ibrahim al-Taimi (May Allah be pleased with him) reported on the authority of his father: 'Ali b. Abu Talib (May Allah be pleased with him) addressed us and said: "He who thinks that we (the members of the Prophet's family) read anything else besides the Book of Allah and this Sahifa (and he said that Sahifa was tied to the scabbard of the sword) tells a lie. (This Sahifa) contains (problems) pertaining to the ages of the camels and (the recompense) of the injuries, and it also records the words of the Prophet (peace and blessings of Allah be upon him): 'Madinah is a sacred territory from 'Ayr to Thaur (it is most probably Uhud). He who innovates (an act or practice) or gives protection to an innovator, there is a Curse of Allah and that of His angels and that of the whole humanity upon him. Allah will not accept from him (as a recompense) any obligatory act or supererogatory act, and the responsibility of the Muslims is a joint responsibility; even the lowest in rank can undertake the responsibility (on behalf of others), and he who claims anyone else as his father besides his own father or makes one his ally other than the one (who freed him), there is a Curse of Allah, that of His angels and that of the whole mankind upon him. Allah will not accept the obligatory act of the supererogatory act (as a recompense) from him." (Muslim)

Abu Hurairah (May Allah be pleased with him) reported that the Messenger of Allah (May Allah's peace and blessings be upon him) said: "Whoever calls to guidance shall receive a reward similar to these obtained by those who follow him without that diminishing anything from their rewards. And whoever calls to misguidance shall incur a sin similar to these incurred by those who follow him without that diminishing anything from their sins." (Muslim) (https://hadeethenc.com/en/browse/hadith/3373)

List of Common Bid'ah

1) Fabricated Ahadith with No proof in the Qur'an and Sunnah.

Narrated Salama (May Allah have mercy on him): "I heard the Prophet (peace and blessings of Allah be upon him) saying, "Whoever (intentionally) ascribes to me what I have not said then (surely) let him occupy his seat in Hellfire." (Bukhari)

"O son of Adam! Do not be afraid of any power or sovereignty as long as My Sovereignty remains, and My sovereignty never ceases! O son of Adam! Don't fear restricted sustenance as long as My storehouses are full, and My storehouse are never empty. O son of Adam! Don't ask for anyone but Me; if you ask for Me you will find Me, and if you miss Me you will miss all the goodness! O son of Adam! I created you to worship Me, so don't play. I have already set your share of substance in this world, so don't make yourselves tired. I swear by My Glory and Might, if you are pleased with what I have allocated for you, I will bring comfort to your heart and body and you will praised by Me; on the other hand, if you are not content with what I have allocated for you, I swear with My Glory and Might that I will set the world loose on you in which you will run just like animals run in the wild and you will still not get more than what I originally allocated for you. O son of Adam! Don't ask me for tomorrow's sustenance, just as I have not asked you for tomorrow's deeds. O son of Adam! I love you, so by My right over you, love Me!" (Moulana Suhail Motala, 'O son of Adam, Do not be afraid of any power or Sovereignty.' (https://hadithanswers.com/o-son-of-adam-do-not-be-afraid-of-any-power-or-sovereignty) The Hadith was narrated by al-Tirmidhi, (Kitaab Sifat al-Qiyaamah wa'l-Wara', 2429), where the wording is, "Whoever shames his brother for a sin will not die until he does it too." Sheikh al-Albaani described this hadeeth in Da'if al-Jaami' (5710) as mawdoo' (fabricated).

Fabricated Ahadith described in "Correcting the fake hadith about "Four things that…"

(https://alibaanahtt.wordpress.com/2018/01/16/correcting-the-fake-hadith-about-four-things)

Beware of the website - https://www.al-islam.org – which contains many fabricated Ahadith.

There are three primary ways to determine the authenticity (*sihha*) of a Hadith:

- by attempting to determine whether there are "other identical reports from other transmitters";

- by determining the reliability of the transmitters of the report; and
- "the continuity of the chain of transmission" of the Hadith.

(https://en.wikipedia.org/wiki/Hadith_studies)

Many scholars have compiled these fabricated and weak ahadith in books devoted solely to these type of reports, so that it is easy to find out about them then one can beware of them and warn others about them. These books include al-Ilal al-Mutanaahiyah by Ibn al-Jawzi, al-Manaar al-Muneef by Ibn al-Qayyim, al-Laaali al-Masnooah fil-Ahaadeeth al-Mawdooah by al-Suyooti, al-Fawaaid al-Majmooah by al-Shawkaani, al-Asraar al-Marfooah fil-Ahaadeeth al-Mawdooah by Ibn Arraaq, and Daeef al-Jaami al-Sagheer and Silsilat al-Ahadith al-Daeefah wal-Mawdooah, both by Sheikh al-Albaani (May Allah have mercy on him).

The useful books and websites with authentic Ahadith: Saheeh Bukhari, Saheeh Muslim, Riyad as-Salihin is a selection of Ahadith by Imam Yahya ibn Sharaf an-Nawawi, https://hadithanswers.com, https://sunnah.com, https://islamqa.info/en/answers, https://sunnahonline.com, https://hadeethenc.com/en/browse/hadith, https://hadithcollection.com, etc.

2) Reciting Verses of the Qur'an a specific number of times and with specific intention.

3) Singling Out Certain Verses of the Quran to Recite at Times of Hardship and Difficulty. (500)

4) Fixing a Certain Time Only for the Recitation of the Qur'an, such as after the Asr prayer, is Bid'ah. (501)

5) Writing Verses of the Qur'an on the paper and putting them in water that is later drunk, thinking that it will ease the Qur'an memorization.

6) Leaving the broadcast of the Holy Qur'an playing at the places of business and at home. (82)

7) Accepting the fees for the Qur'an recitation. No Allah's rewards for paid Qur'an recitation.

8) Saying "Sadaqa Allaahu al-'Azeem" (Allah has spoken the Truth).

9) Bid'ah in Qur'an reading.

10) Kissing the Mushaf, kissing ones fingers and swaying whilst reciting Qur'an.

11) Swearing or taking an oath by placing hand on the Mushaf.

12) Celebrating completing the Qur'an.

13) Hanging Verses of the Qur'an and/or the Name of Allah on walls.

14) Writing the Name of Allah on cakes and chocolate?

15) Writing the Name of Allah on the cars (e.g. Ma shaa Allah).

16) Saying "Ma Shaa Allah" to prevent the Evil Eye is a Bid'ah. (354, 355)

17) Distributing and selling the Verses of the Qur'an for the protection.

18) Rejection the Qur'an as the Words of God.

19) Reading the Qur'an in congregation except for teaching purpose.

20) Reading the Qur'an over Zamzam water.

21) Repeating the Name of Allah on its own or the pronoun Huwa (He) is a Sufi Bid'ah

22) Reciting the Names of Allah in certain combinations.

23) Believing that Allah is without image and is formless and disbelieving in His Attributes.

24) Believing that Allah is everywhere.

25) Comparing the Creator to His creation.

26) Calling Allah by the names which are not in the Qur'an or Sunnah.

27) Believing that there are Prophets or Messengers after Muhammad (peace be upon him).

28) Celebrating the birthday of the Prophet Muhammad (peace and blessings be upon him).

29) Encouraging billions of salawat upon the Prophet on the occasion of his Birthday. (502)

30) Sending blessings upon the Prophet (peace and blessings and be upon him) collectively.

31) Sending Salam on the Prophet (peace be upon him) out loud and as a group after every Prayer, especially after Jumu'ah like done by the Barelvi community.

32) Belief that the Prophet (peace be upon him) was created from the Noor (light) of Allah.

33) Believing that the whole world and everything in it was created for the Prophet Muhammad (peace be upon him).

34) Kissing thumbs upon hearing the name of the Prophet (peace be upon him).

35) Celebrating the night of Ascension, the Isra' and Mi'raj.

36) Fasting on the day of the Mi'raj.

37) Going to visit places and Mosques in which the Prophet prayed (apart from Quba', Uhud…)

38) Believing that the Prophet (peace be upon him) is everywhere and/or that he attends certain gatherings of 'Remembrance'.

39) Believing in the altered concept of Tawassul. For example, making Du'a to Allah that He grants you something by the name of His Prophet (peace be upon him).

40) Believing the book of "Al-Hisn Al-Haseen" and others for protection.

41) Claiming that Ali was given specific knowledge of Khilafah (Caliphate), which was not given to anybody else

42) Uttering the intention (niyyah) in acts of worship.

43) Washing mouth and nose separately during Wudu. (https://www.youtube.com/watch?v=y7o4NcklQMA)

44) Abstaining from drying or wiping the water off after Wudu. (https://www.al-feqh.com/en/not-drying-off-after-finishing-wudu)

45) Wiping the hands on the back of the neck during the ablution.

46) Believing that talking during Wudu or smiling/laughing while with Wudu invalidates the ablution.

47) Washing the limbs more than three times during Wudu.

48) Sending blessings on the Prophet (peace be upon him) out loud before making each Adhan.

49) Du'a after Iqamah.

50) Closing the eyes while praying.

51) Raising one's eyes towards the sky during prayer.

52) Glancing in one direction of the other during prayer.

53) Placing the hands on the sides during prayer.

54) Praying with one's hands on one's waist.

55) Sitting with left hand behind the back and leaning on the fleshy part of it.

56) Putting the forearms on the ground in the prostration like a dog.

57) Reciting the Qur'an when bowing and prostrating.

58) Not settling his spine when bowing and prostrating.

59) Regular recitation of the Qunut during the Fajr prayer.

60) Performing regular voluntary Zuhr prayers on Friday Jumu'ah prayer.

61) Rushing when Reciting Qur'an and Praying.

62) Not Separating the Obligatory and Voluntary Prayers.

63) Using anything to count Adhkar other than the fingers.

64) Wiping the face with the hands after Prayer or after Making Du'a.

65) Prostrating for the sake of Du'a is an Innovation.

66) Balancing, moving rhythmically backwards and forwards the body during the prayer.

67) Making Du'a after the obligatory prayers by Raising Hands. It says in Fatawa al-Lajnah al-Daimah: "Making Du'a after the obligatory prayers is not Sunnah if it is done by Raising the Hands, whether that is done by the imam alone or a member of the congregation alone, or it is done by them both together. Rather that is Bid'ah, because it was not narrated that the Prophet (peace and blessings of Allah be upon him) or any of his Companions (May Allah be pleased with them) did that. With regard to making Du'a without doing that (raising the hands, etc.), there is nothing wrong with it, because there are some Ahadith concerning that." (Fataawa al-Lajnah al-Daimah, 7/103) (503)

68) Congregational Du'as, Adhkar after salat or not.

69) Imam praying on minbar other than Jumu'ah.

70) Doing a Khutbah before Eid prayers. Narrated Ibn 'Abbas: The Messenger of Allah (peace and blessings of Allah be upon him) prayed before the Khutbah on Eid, then he gave the Khutbah." (Ahmad)

71) Saying "Taqabbal Allah (May Allah accept it)" after Prayer.

72) Women praying differently from men.

73) Believing that those who achieve the high level of righteousness through piety (like saints) no longer need to follow the Guidelines of the Shariah.

74) Singling out the first third of Ramadan to pray for mercy, the second third to pray for forgiveness and the last third to pray for ransom from Hell is an innovation.

75) There is no specific Du'a for each day and night of Ramadan.

76) Praying Witr with three Rak'ahs like Maghreb.

77) Reciting specific supplications in each circuit of Tawaaf (circumambulation of the Ka'bah) or lap of Sa'i (going between as-Safa and al-Marwah) during Hajj and 'Umrah.

78) Salatul Tasbeeh (Salat al-Tasbeeh is not Sunnah).

79) Salat al-Fatih (Durood Fatih).

80) Salat al-Naariyah (or Salat al-Tafrijiyya (the Prayer of Relief).

81) Salat al-Hajah.

82) Rajab Month Innovations.

83) Sha'ban Month Innovations.

84) Muharram Month Innovations.

85) Asking someone else to do Istikhara for you. Paying someone to do Istikhara.

86) Shaking hands after the end of obligatory prayer.

87) Shaking hands and making Du'a "Allahumma Salli Ala Muhammad."

88) Shaking hands with both hands.

89) Congratulating "Jumu'ah Mubarak".

90) Learning sacred knowledge for the sake of this world or concealing It.

91) Celebrating the birthday of the Prophet Muhammad.

92) Birthday Celebration (reminding people of your birthday, saying "Happy birthday", offering cakes and gifts, etc.)

93) Going to Birthday Celebration.

94) Celebrating New Year (any New Year).

95) Celebrating the innovated festivals (all except Al-Fitr and Al-Adha).

96) Touching the chest (heart) after exchanging hands with people or when leaving.

97) Looking up and pointing towards the sky while reciting the shahada (testimony of Faith) after completion of Wudu (only reciting the Shahada is from the Sunnah).

98) Bi'dah when sneezing

Narrated Naafi': a man sneezed next to Ibn 'Umar and said "Al-hamdu Lillah wa as-salaam 'ala Rasool Allah (praise be to Allah and peace be upon the Messenger of Allah)." Ibn 'Umar said: "And I say: Praise be to Allah and peace be upon the Messenger of Allah, but this is not how the Messenger of Allah (peace and blessings of Allah be upon him) taught us; rather he taught us to say: 'Al-hamdu Lillah 'ala kulli haal (Praise be to Allah in all circumstances)." (Tirmidhi)

99) Sacrificing a horse is a Bid'ah. Sacrifice is limited to lamb, cattle, sheep and camels.

100) Sacrificing animal for anyone than Allah.

101) Believing that only a black sheep can be given as Sadaqah (charity).

102) Exaggeration in praising of the good people.

103) Reciting Naats (Nasheeds/Praises) of the Prophet (peace be upon him) by using musical instruments or techniques which resemble songs and music.

104) The Concept of Taqleed (choosing an imam and sticking with his rulings alone in all matters of the Deen).

105) Separating religious matters from worldly matters like the Christians did with segregation of State and Church.

106) Indulging in Magic, Soothsayers, Palmists, Astrologists, Numerologists, etc., whether you believe or not.

107) Reciting the Qur'an during the funeral, at the grave for a deceased person, during the condolence days, on the death anniversary or singling out other days by hiring imam (or people) or inviting relatives and sharing food.

108) Crying or weeping in a loud voice; following it with incense (bukhoor), etc.; reciting Dhikr in a loud voice in front of the coffin as it is being carried, because that is Bid'ah - it is an imitation of the Christians.

109) Congregational Du'a right after the funeral prayer.

110) Spending money of the deceased person for the charity on his behalf. After the death, money of the deceased belongs to his legal heirs.

111) Erecting structures, gravestones, domes, shrines over grave.

112) Touching graves and looking for help from the occupants.

113) Praying at the grave, in the graveyard

114) Mourning on the 3rd, 10th, 40th and on the yearly death anniversary of the deceased.

115) Women wearing black clothes at times of calamity and death

116) Sitting or Listening to Innovators in Religion.

117) Not going against Innovation even if the person does not practice it.

118) Using of Bandiri.

The Prophet (peace and blessings be upon him) said: "There will be among my Ummah people who will regard adultery, silk, alcohol and musical instruments as permissible." (Bukhari)

This Hadith indicates that all musical instruments are haram, including the daff.

'Abd-Allah ibn 'Abbas (May Allah be pleased with him) said: "The daff is haram, stringed instruments are haram, drums are haram and flutes are haram." (al-Bayhaqi)

119) Dowry from the bride's family to the groom's family.

120) Marriage necklace (thali) presented by groom's family during wedding celebration (India).

121) Naming Ceremony.

122) Going to Naming Ceremony.

123) Inviting Alfa to come and name the baby on the day of Haqeeqah. (504)

124) Ceremony at 40 days of Baby's Birth.

The ceremony is called "balany kyrkynan shygaru" ("Passing forty days") in Kazakhstan. The events and rituals are held, designed to strengthen the health of the baby, to protect him from evil spirits and diseases. Therefore, during the forty-day period, relatives lit a lamp at night near the baby's cradle, sewed amulets to his clothes in order to prevent the baby from evil spirits. People don't show the child to other people from outside family during the first forty days, they don't take photos of baby, and some put ash ("kuye") on the baby forehead to keep any bad luck (evil spirit) away ("koz timesin" or Evil Eye). When a child is 40 days old, he is officially presented to his relatives and friends. (https://el.kz/en/news/obychai_i_traditsii/kazakh_traditions_associated_with_babies)

The tradition involves Shirk, ascribing partners to Allah, sorcery, superstition, etc.

125) Celebration of baby's first steps.

Tusau kesu — cutting the fetters. The ceremony is held when the baby takes the first steps. His legs are tied with a thin mottled lace, which is to be cut by an honorable person. Songs and wishes accompany the ceremony, so that the child is able to go through life on his own legs. The ceremony continues with a feast. Ceremony is done so that in the future the baby could walk confidently and run fast. (https://weproject.media/en/articles/detail/9-kazakh-traditions-that-are-used-with-the-birth-and-upbringing-of-a-child)

The tradition involves Shirk, songs, music, mixing men and women, wasting Allah's money, etc.

126) Revealing the face of bride – "Betashar" Ceremony.

The Neke Qiyu (Wedding) when the bride is revealed to her groom's family, including non-Mahrams. This festive ceremony is called Betashar or "revealing of the face." (https://en.wikipedia.org/wiki/Kazakh_wedding_ceremony)

The tradition involves many sins: meeting and mixing men and women, adornment display, extravagance, photography, video, wasting Allah's money, music, dance, songs, etc.

127) Stinging to "Jazak Allah".

128) Answering to "Jazak Allah Khayran" by "Wa 'antum fa-jazakumu-llāhu khayran".

129) Women doing Da'wah on television.

130) Celebrations commemorating some of the scholars.

131) The Bid'ah of superstition about getting married in Shawwaal. (505)

132) The Bid'ah of Eid al-Abraar, the festival of the righteous.

133) Saying "Innahu Ala Rajihi la Qaadir" to bring back something that has been lost.

134) Congratulating the pilgrim after he returns and decorating the house for him if extravagance and wasting of money involved.

135) Bowing when greeting.

136) Greeting with a gesture.

137) Standing up for someone to venerate him.

138) Saluting the Flag, Standing up for it and Singing the national anthem.

139) Breaking "Laa ilaha illa Allah" into two parts.

Someone leading a group of people in a call-and-response (i.e. the group repeats what he says), and he says "laa ilaha", and they repeat that, then he says "illa Allah", and they repeat. This sentence must not be divided like that because the first part is an assertion that there is no God. The second part (the exception) must always be connected to it.

140) Saying "Allah knows your intention".

141) Saying "Only God can judge me".

142) Believing that believers will not face punishment in this life and/or on Judgment Day.

143) Believing that humans create their actions.

144) Jinn Catching

Proofs Against Bid'ah

Allah, the Exalted, says:

"This day I have perfected your religion for you, completed my favor upon you, and have chosen for you Islam as your religion."(Qur'an, Al-Ma'idah 5:3)

Narrated Aisha (May Allah be pleased with her): The Messenger of Allah (peace and blessings be upon him) said: "Whosoever introduces into this affair of ours (i.e. into Islam) something that does not belong to it, it is to be rejected." (Bukhari and Muslim)

Abu Najeeh al-'Irbaad ibn Saariyah (May Allah be pleased with him) said: The Messenger of Allah (peace and blessings of Allah be upon him) gave us a sermon by which our hearts were filled with fear and tears came to our eyes. So, we said, "O Messenger of Allah! It is as though this is a farewell sermon, so counsel us." He (peace and blessings of Allah be upon him) said, "I counsel you to have Taqwa (fear) of Allah, and to listen and obey (your leader), even if a slave were to become your ameer. Verily he among you who lives long will see great controversy, so you must keep to my Sunnah and to the Sunnah of the Khulafa ar-Rashideen (the rightly guided caliphs), those who guide to the right way. Cling to it stubbornly (literally: with your molar teeth). Beware of newly invented matters (in the religion), for verily every Bid'ah (innovation) is misguidance." (Abu Dawud)

Yazid ibn Sharīk ibn Tariq (May Allah be pleased with him) reported: "I saw 'Ali (May Allah be pleased with him) delivering a speech from the pulpit, and I heard him say: "By Allah! We have no book to read except the Book of Allah and what is written in this scroll." He unrolled the scroll, and it showed a list of the types of camels to be given as blood-money and contained other legal matters relating to the killing of game in the sanctuary of Makkah and the expiation for it. In it was also written: "The Messenger of Allah (May Allah's peace and blessings be upon him) said: 'Madinah is a sanctuary from 'Ayr to Thawr (mountains). Whoever innovates something new (in religion) or shelters an innovator in it will incur the Curse of Allah, the angels and all the people, and Allah will accept from him neither an obligatory nor a supererogatory prayer on the Day of Resurrection. A pledge of protection granted by any Muslim, even of the lowest status is the same and should be honored by all Muslims. Whoever betrays a Muslim in this respect will incur the Curse of Allah, the angels and all the people, and Allah will accept from him neither an obligatory nor a supererogatory prayer on the Day of Resurrection. Whoever attributes his fatherhood to someone other than his (real) father or takes as his master someone other than his (real) master will incur the Curse of Allah, the angels and all the people, and Allah will accept from him neither an obligatory nor a supererogatory prayer on the Day of Resurrection.'" (Bukhari and Muslim)

(https://hadeethenc.com/en/browse/hadith/6381)

Anas ibn Malik (May Allah be pleased with him) reported: "A group from among the Prophet's Companions asked the Prophet's wives about the acts of worship that he performed in private. Some of them said: "I will not marry women." Others said: "I will not eat meat." Some others said: "I will not lie down on a bed." Their words reached the Prophet (May Allah's peace and blessings be upon him). So, he praised Allah and glorified Him and said: "What is the matter with those people who said such-and-such? Indeed, I pray and I sleep too, I fast sometimes and do not fast other times, and I marry women. Whoever turns away from my Sunnah does not belong to me." (Bukhari and Muslim)

(https://hadeethenc.com/en/browse/hadith/6078)

Narrated Abu Hurairah (May Allah be pleased with him): "One day while the Prophet (peace and blessings be upon him) was sitting in the company of some people, the angel Gabriel came and asked, "What is Faith?" Allah's Messenger (peace and blessings be upon him) replied, 'Faith is to believe in Allah, His angels, the meeting with Him, His Apostles and to believe in Resurrection." Then he further asked, "What is Islam?" Allah's Messenger (peace and blessings be upon him) replied, "To worship Allah Alone and none else, to offer prayers perfectly, to pay the compulsory charity (Zakat) and to observe fasts during the month of Ramadan." Then he further asked, "What is Ihsan (perfection)?" Allah's Messenger (peace and blessings be upon him) replied, "To worship Allah as if you see Him, and if you cannot achieve this state of devotion then you must consider that He is looking at you." Then he further asked, "When will the Hour be established?" Allah's Messenger (peace and blessings be upon him) replied, "The answerer has no better knowledge than the questioner. But I will inform you about its portents.

1. When a slave (lady) gives birth to her master.

2. When the shepherds of black camels start boasting and competing with others in the construction of higher buildings. And the Hour is one of five things which nobody knows except Allah.

The Prophet (peace and blessings be upon him) then recited: *"Verily, with Allah (Alone) is the knowledge of the Hour." (Qur'an, Luqman 31:34)* Then that man (Gabriel) left and the Prophet (peace and blessings be upon him) asked his companions to call him back, but they could not see him. Then the Prophet (peace and blessings be upon him) said, "That was Gabriel who came to teach the people their religion." Abu 'Abdullah said: "He (the Prophet) considered all that as a part of Faith." (Bukhari)

Innovations in Worldly Matters:

1. Good worldly innovations such as using technology to propagate the Faith of Islam.

2. Innovation that is purely evil - these are forbidden under Islamic Law. Examples of this type of Bid'ah

include the discovery and synthesis of new intoxicants.

3. All celebrations (except Al-Fitr and Al-Adha): Christmas, New Year (any), Birthday, Women's Day,

Valentine Day, Mother Day, Father Day, Victory Day, National Day, Independence Day,

Halloween, Carnivals, International Worker's Day, Unity Day, Defender of the Fatherland Day, World

Cancer Day, The Day of Dead, Music Festival, Pride Parade, etc.

In all these celebrations there is no remembrance of Allah and there are many sins.

It is forbidden for the Muslims to imitate the kufar by holding parties on the festive occasions, exchanging gifts, distributing sweets or other foods, etc.

The Devils created multiples celebrations to distract people from the Straight Path.

608. Sitting with the Innovators in Religion or Listening to them

Allah, the Exalted, says:

"And when you (Muhammad SAW) see those who engage in a false conversation about Our Verses (of the Qur'an) by mocking at them, stay away from them till they turn to another topic. And if Shaitan (Satan) causes you to forget, then after the remembrance sit not you in the company of those people who are the Zalimun (polytheists and wrong-doers, etc.)." (Qur'an, Al-An'am 6:68)

609. Prohibition of the Music, Singing and Dancing

Allah, the Exalted, says:

"And Istafziz [literally means: befool them gradually] those whom you can among them with your voice (i.e. songs, music and any other call for Allah's disobedience),

make assaults on them with your cavalry and your infantry, mutually share with them wealth and children (by tempting them to earn money by illegal ways usury, etc., or by committing illegal sexual intercourse, etc.), and make promises to them." But Satan promises them nothing but deceit." *(Qur'an, Al-Isra 17:64)*

"Do you then wonder at this recital (the Qur'an)? And you laugh at it and weep not, Wasting your (precious) lifetime in pastime and amusements (singing, etc.)." (Quran, An-Najm 53:59-61)

"And of mankind is he who purchases idle talks (i.e. music, singing, etc.) to mislead (men) from the Path of Allah without knowledge, and takes it (the Path of Allah, the Verses of the Qur'an) by way of mockery. For such there will be a humiliating torment (in the Hellfire)." (Qur'an, Luqman 31:6)

Abu Hurairah (May Allah be pleased with him) reported that the Prophet (May Allah's peace and blessings be upon him) said: "Hellfire is surrounded by lusts, and Paradise is surrounded by adversities." (Bukhari and Muslim) (https://hadeethenc.com/en/browse/hadith/3702)

Narrated Abu Umamah (May Allah be pleased with him): "The Messenger of Allah forbade selling or buying singing girls and their wages, and consuming their price." Ibn Majah)

Narrated Abu 'Amir or Abu Malik Al-Ash'ari: The Prophet (peace and blessings be upon him) said, "From among my followers there will be some people who will consider illegal sexual intercourse, the wearing of silk, the drinking of alcoholic drinks and the use of musical instruments, as lawful; be some people who will stay near the side of a mountain and in the evening their shepherd will come to them with their sheep and ask them for something, but they will say to him, 'Return to us tomorrow.' Allah will destroy them during the night and will let the mountain fall on them, and He will transform the rest of them into monkeys and pigs and they will remain so till the Day of Resurrection." (Bukhari)

Some dances (e.g. Zar Zar) involve rhythmic drumming and singing, animal sacrifices, dancing and ecstatic states during which the Jinns manifest themselves. The Zar confirms the intimate relationship between the Jinns and humans.

610. Parties and Gathering Without Remembering Allah

Allah, the Exalted, says:

"And whoever is blinded from remembrance of the Most Merciful - We appoint for him a Devil, and he is to him a companion. And indeed, the Devils avert them from the way (of guidance) while they think that they are (rightly) guided." (Qur'an, Az-Zukhruf 43:36-38)

"Then as for one whose scales are heavy (with good deeds), He will be in a pleasant life (in Paradise). But as for one whose scales are light; His refuge will be an abyss (Hell)." (Qur'an, Al-Qari'ah 101:6-9)

"Till, when they reach it (Hellfire), their hearing (ears) and their eyes, and their skins will testify against them as to what they used to do. And they will say to their skins, "Why do you testify against us?" They will say: "Allah has caused us to speak, as He causes all things to speak, and He created you the first time, and to Him you are made to return." (Qur'an, Fussilat 41:20-21)

Other Verses: Al-Muddaththir 74:40-46, Al-Isra 17:36, Al-Baqarah 2:152.

Abu Hurairah (May Allah be pleased with him) reported: The Prophet (peace and blessings be upon him) said, "No people sit in a gathering without remembering Allah or sending blessings upon their Prophet, but that they will earn the displeasure of Allah. If Allah wills, he will punish them. If he wills, he will forgive them." (Tirmidhi)

Abu Hurairah (May Allah be pleased with him) reported that the Messenger of Allah (May Allah's peace and blessings be upon him) said: "No people leave a gathering in which they did not remember Allah the Almighty except that it will be as if they are leaving the carcass of a donkey, and it will be a cause of regret for them." (Abu Dawud) (https://hadeethenc.com/en/browse/hadith/3910)

611. Settling in Non-Muslim Country if he is Unable to Practice his Religion Openly

Allah, the Exalted, says:

"Verily! As for those whom the angels take (in death) while they are wronging themselves (as they stayed among the disbelievers even though emigration was obligatory for them), they (angels) say (to them): "In what (condition) were you?" They reply: "We were weak and oppressed on earth." They (angels) say: "Was not the earth of Allah spacious enough for you to emigrate therein?" Such men will find their abode in Hell - What an evil destination! Except the weak ones among men, women and children who cannot devise a plan, nor are they able to direct their way." (Qur'an, An-Nisa 4:97-98)

Some basic Islamic rules about migration:

1. It is Haram for a Muslim to live in or to migrate to a place where he cannot practice his/her religion, unless one is very weak and has no other way. Almighty Allah says, *"Lo! As for those whom the angels take (in death) while they wrong themselves,*

(the angels) will ask: 'In what were ye engaged?' They will say: 'We were oppressed in the land.' (The angels) will say: 'Was not Allah's earth spacious that ye could have migrated therein?' As for such, their habitation will be Hell, an evil journey's end..." (An-Nisa 4:97)

It is obligatory upon Muslims to live in and to migrate to those lands where they can freely practice their religion.

2. It is not recommended for Muslims to migrate to the lands where their and their next generations' religion might be at risk, unless they make every effort to safeguard their own religion and the religion of their next generations. Without such efforts it will be Makruh (reprehensible) (and in some cases even Haram) to migrate to such lands.
3. It is permissible for Muslims to migrate to the lands where they feel confident that they can practice their religion freely and they can raise their children under the Islamic principles. It is, however, better for Muslims to live in Muslim lands where they can live under Islamic Laws to govern their personal as well as collective lives.
4. It is highly recommended for Muslims to migrate to those lands where they feel they can practice Islam and can spread the message of Islam. The Prophet (peace and blessings be upon him) sent many Sahabah (his Companions) to different areas to spread Islam and to teach Islam. After the death of the Prophet (peace and blessings be upon him) many Sahabah left Madinah and went to different lands to live there and to teach Islam to the people of those lands. It is due to their efforts and the efforts of many Muslims after them that Islam spread in many lands. This is also our duty and we must make every effort to convey the message of Allah to the whole world." (506, 507)

612. Driving or Accompanying People to the Place of Sins

Driving or accompanying people to the places of sins (bar, night club, etc.) and taking money (taxi), there is no barakah on it.

613. Renting or Offering the Place for the Gathering with Sins

Someone renting or offering the place for the gathering, where there is no remembrance of Allah and there are other Sins (like alcohol, music, dance, inappropriate language, unlawful sex, etc.)

614. Television, Internet

Allah, the Exalted, says:

"Tell the believing men to lower their gaze (from looking at forbidden things), and protect their private parts (from illegal sexual acts). That is purer for them. Verily, Allah is All-Aware of what they do. And tell the believing women to lower their gaze (from looking at forbidden things), and protect their private parts (from illegal sexual acts)." (Qur'an, An-Nur 24:30-31)

Abu Hurairah (May Allah be pleased with him) reported that the Prophet (May Allah's peace and blessings be upon him) said: "The son of Adam has been destined his share of fornication, which he will inevitably acquire. The eyes fornicate by looking, the ears fornicate by listening, the tongue fornicates by speaking, the hand fornicates by hitting, the foot fornicates by stepping. The heart loves and wishes. The genitals prove or disapprove that." (Bukhari and Muslim)
(https://hadeethenc.com/en/browse/hadith/8898)

The issue of watching films is not free from numerous reservations from a Shariah point of view, such as uncovering 'awrah, listening to music, spreading corrupt beliefs, violence, crime, unlawful sex and calling for imitation of the kufar.

Sheikh Abdul Aziz Ibn Baaz (May Allah have mercy on him) said in al-Fataawa 3/227:

"With regard to television, it is a dangerous device and its harmful effects are very great, like those of the cinema or even worse. This is because it includes the presentation of bad morals, tempting scenes, immoral pictures, semi-nakedness, destructive speech and Kufr. It encourages imitation of their conduct and ways of dressing, respect for their leaders, neglect of Islamic conduct and ways of dressing, and looking down on the scholars and heroes of Islam. It damages their image by portraying them in an off-putting manner that makes people despise them and ignore them. It shows people how to cheat, steal, hatch plots and commit acts of violence against others. Undoubtedly anything that produces so many bad results should be stopped and shunned, and we have to close all the doors that could lead to it." (508)

Internet is an excellent device if used correctly, for example to study beneficial knowledge, Arabic language to read the Qur'an, the Names and Attributes of Allah, Sunnah.

Otherwise, internet is the tool of Satan that destroys belief.

615. Reading Books about Unlawful Things

The Book which everybody should read is the Noble Qur'an which was sent to all mankind as a Mercy from our Creator. You can only distinguish good from bad, right from wrong, lawful from unlawful in the Glorious Qur'an and Sunnah.

Satan beautifies bad as a good, wrong as a right; creates illusions, we live in the deluded world.

Prohibited the books about astrology, witchcraft, love stories, other religions than Islam, etc.

616. Preserving Books that Lead to Deviation in Religion

Preserving the books that lead to deviation in the Religion is not permissible, destroying them is obligatory.

617. Branding Animals on the Face

Jabir (May Allah be pleased with him) reported: "The Messenger of Allah (peace and blessings be upon him) prohibited beating or cauterizing animals on the face." (Muslim)

Ibn 'Abbas (May Allah be pleased with him) said: An ass with a brand on the face happened to pass before the Prophet (peace and blessings be upon him). Thereupon he said, "May Allah curse the one who has branded it (on the face)." (Muslim)

618. Killing, Torturing Animals, Birds, Not Feeding Them

Allah, the Exalted, says:

"...whoever kills a soul unless for a soul or for corruption (done) in the land – it is as if he had slain mankind entirely. And whoever saves one – it is as if he had saved mankind entirely. And our messengers had certainly come to them with clear proofs." (Qur'an, Al-Ma'idah 5:32)

Satan said:

"And I will mislead them, and I will arouse in them (sinful) desires, and I will command them so they will slit the ears of cattle…" *(Qur'an, An-Nisa 4:119)*

Abu Ja'far 'Abdullah ibn Ja'far (May Allah be pleased with him) reported: "The Messenger of Allah (May Allah's peace and blessings be upon him) made me ride behind him one day and confided something to me which I shall never disclose to anyone. What the Messenger of Allah (May Allah's peace and blessings be upon him) liked most to screen himself from others while answering the call of nature was an elevation or a date-palm orchard. Once he entered an orchard belonging to an Ansari man and found a camel therein. When it saw him, it began to groan and its eyes shed tears. The Prophet (May Allah's peace and blessings be upon him) approached it and patted it on the hump and behind its ears until it calmed down. Then, he asked: "Who is the owner of this camel? To whom does it belong?" An Ansari youth stepped forward and said: "It is mine, O Messenger of Allah," He said: "Do you not fear Allah regarding this animal which Allah has placed in your possession? It is complaining to me that you starve it and put it to toil." (Abu Dawud) (https://hadeethenc.com/en/browse/hadith/8842)

Narrated Abu Hurairah (May Allah be pleased with him): The Messenger of Allah (peace and blessings of Allah be upon him) said: "Allah is Gentle and loves gentleness, and He grants reward for it that He does not grant for harshness." (Ibn Majah)

Narrated Abu Hurairah (May Allah be pleased with him): The Prophet (peace and blessings of Allah be upon him) said, "A man felt very thirsty while he was on the way, there he came across a well. He went down the well, quenched his thirst and came out. Meanwhile he saw a dog panting and licking mud because of excessive thirst. He said to himself, 'This dog is suffering from thirst as I did.' So, he went down the well again and filled his shoe with water and watered it. Allah thanked him for that deed and forgave him. The people said, 'O Allah's Apostle (peace and blessings be upon him)! Is there a reward for us in serving the animals?' He replied: 'Yes, there is a reward for serving any animate (living) being.'" (Bukhari)

Narrated Abdullah bin Umar (May Allah be pleased with him): Allah's Apostle (peace and blessings be upon him) said, "A woman was tortured and was put in Hellfire because of a cat which she had kept locked till it died of hunger." Allah's Apostle (peace and blessings of Allah be upon him) further said, Allah knows better. "Allah said (to the woman), 'You neither fed it nor watered when you locked it up, nor did you set it free to eat the vermin of the earth.'" (Bukhari)

Jabir b. 'Abdullah (May Allah be pleased with him) reported: "Allah's Messenger (peace be upon him) forbade that any beast should be killed after it has been tied." (Muslim)

Narrated Hisham bin Zaid (May Allah be pleased with him): "Anas and I went to Al-Hakam bin Aiyub. Anas saw some boys shooting at a tied hen. Anas said, "The Prophet has forbidden the shooting of tied or confined animals." (Bukhari)

Ibn 'Abbas (May Allah be pleased with him) reported Allah's Messenger (peace and blessings be upon him) having said this: "Do not make anything having life as a target." (Muslim)

Sa'id b. Jubair (May Allah be pleased with him) reported that Ibn 'Umar happened to pass by some young men of the Quraish who had tied a bird (and this made it a target) at which they had been shooting arrows. Every arrow that they missed came into the possession of the owner of the bird. So, no sooner did they see Ibn 'Umar they went away. Thereupon Ibn 'Umar said: "Who has done this? Allah has cursed him who does this. Verily Allah's Messenger (May peace be upon him) invoked curse upon one who made a live thing the target (of one's marksmanship)." (Muslim)

Narrated Abdullah ibn Abbas (May Allah be pleased with him): "The Prophet (peace and blessings be upon him) prohibited to kill four creatures: ants, bees, hoopoes and sparrow-hawks." (Abu Dawud)

Narrated Abu Hurairah ((May Allah be pleased with him): I heard Allah's Messenger (peace and blessings be upon him) saying, "An ant bit a Prophet amongst the Prophets, and he ordered that the place of the ants be burnt. So, Allah inspired to him, 'It is because one ant bit you that you burnt a nation amongst the nations that glorify Allah?" (Bukhari)

Releasing hunting dogs against a gazelle that is tied up is a kind of torment and cruelty.

Do not slit the ears, do not cut the tail of animal, do not beat, do not torture, do not overuse.

619. Prohibition of Keeping a Dog Except as a Watchdog or Hunting Dog

Ibn 'Umar (May Allah be pleased with him) said: The Messenger of Allah (peace and blessings be upon him) said, "He who keeps a dog other than one for guarding the fields or herds, or hunting, will lose two Qirat every day out of his rewards." (Bukhari and Muslim)

Abu Hurairah (May Allah be pleased with him) said: The Messenger of Allah (peace and blessings be upon him) said, "He who keeps a dog, will lose out of his good deeds equal to one Qirat every day, except one who keeps it for guarding the fields or the herd." (Bukhari and Muslim)

In a narration of Muslim, the Messenger of Allah (peace and blessings be upon him) is reported to have said: "He who keeps a dog for any reason other than to guard his property (lands) or his flock of sheep, his good deeds equal to two Qirat will be deducted every day."

Commentary:

What is Qirat? It is differently interpreted. There is a Qirat which is mentioned in the funeral prayer. This is equal to the Uhud mountain. Does it signify the same here? Some scholars answer this question in the affirmative while others hold that in the funeral prayer it occurs with reference to Allah's Mercy and Grace but here it relates to His Wrath. As the former is far greater than the latter, the word cannot have the same significance in both contexts. (509)

A dog is a despicable filthy animal, and that is why Islamic Shariah forbade owning it because of the harms and bad consequences resulting from keeping it. Examples of these harms include the following: The honorable and obedient angels turn away from the house where a dog is kept; dogs frighten and terrify people; dogs are a source of impurity and harm; and owning a dog is a sign of foolishness. Therefore, anyone who keeps a dog their rewards of good deeds will decrease considerably every day. This amount is translated into two Qirats, which only Allah knows how big they are, because such a person insists on disobeying Allah by keeping a dog.

However, if there is a need for keeping a dog, it is allowed to do so in three cases:

1- Guarding livestock against wolves and thieves.

2- Guarding crops.

3- Hunting animals.

Narrated Abu Hurairah (May Allah be pleased with him): The Prophet (peace and blessings be upon him) said, "When a dog laps a vessel wash it seven times, rubbing it with earth the first or the last time. If a cat puts its mouth into a vessel, wash it once." (Bukhari and Muslim)

Narrated Abdullah bin Mughaffal (May Allah be pleased with him): The Messenger of Allah (peace and blessings be upon him) said: "Were it not that dogs form one of the communities (or nations - of creatures), I would have commanded that they be killed. But kill those that are all black. There are no people who keep a dog, except for dogs used for herding livestock, hunting or farming, but two Qirat will be deducted from their reward each day." (Ibn Majah)

Narrated Abu Dharr (May Allah be pleased with him): "I asked the Messenger of Allah (peace be upon him), as you are asking me, and he said: 'The black dog is a Devil.'" (Muslim)

Narrated Ibn Mugghaffal (May Allah be pleased with him): "The Messenger of Allah (peace and blessings be upon him) ordered killing of the dogs, and then said: 'What about them, i.e. about other dogs? and then granted concession (to keep) the dog for hunting and the dog for (the security) of the herd', and said: 'When the dog licks the utensil, wash it seven times, and rub it with earth the eighth time.'" (Muslim)

Narrated Abu Talha (May Allah be pleased with him): The Prophet (peace and blessings be upon him) said, "Angels do not enter a house that has either a dog or a picture in it." (Bukhari)

Narrated Ali ibn Abu Talib (May Allah be pleased with him): The Prophet (peace and blessings be upon him) said: "Angels do not enter the house where there is a picture, or a dog, or a person who is sexually defiled." (Abu Dawud)

620. Undesirability of Hanging Bells Round the Necks of Animals

Abu Hurairah (May Allah be pleased with him) said: The Messenger of Allah (peace and blessings be upon him) said, "Angels do not accompany the travelers who have with them a dog or a bell." (Muslim)

Abu Hurairah (May Allah be pleased with him) said: The Prophet (peace and blessings be upon him) said,

"The bell is one of the musical instruments of Satan." (Muslim)

Commentary: Mazamir is the plural of Mizmar meaning musical instrument. It covers the lute, the plectrum and other musical instruments. All these are used by Satan to lead the people astray. (510)

621. Buying and Selling Dogs and Cats

Narrated Aun bin Abi Juhaifa (May Allah be pleased with him): "I saw my father buying a slave whose profession was cupping, and ordered that his instruments (of cupping) be broken. I asked him the reason for doing so. He replied, "Allah's Apostle (peace and blessings be upon him) prohibited taking money for blood, the price of a dog and the earnings of a slave girl by prostitution; he cursed her who tattoos and her who gets tattooed, the eater of Riba (usury), and the maker of pictures." (Bukhari)

Narrated Abu Masud Al-Ansari (May Allah be pleased with him): Allah's Apostle (peace and blessings be upon him) regarded illegal the price of a dog, the earnings of a prostitute, and the charges taken by a soothsayer." (Bukhari)

Narrated Jabir (May Allah be pleased with him): "The Messenger of Allah (peace and blessings be upon him) forbade eating cats and he forbade their price." (Ibn Majah)

Narrated Jabir ibn 'Abd-Allaah (May Allah be pleased with him): "The Messenger of Allah (peace and blessings of Allah be upon him) forbade the price of dogs and cats." (Abu Dawud and Tirmidhi)

It says in Fataawa al-Lajnah al-Daa'imah, 13/37:

"It is not permissible to sell cats, monkeys or dogs, or any other carnivores that have fangs, because the Prophet (peace and blessings of Allah be upon him) forbade that and discouraged it, and because it is a waste of money, and the Prophet (peace and blessings be upon him) forbade wasting money." (511, 512)

622. Cursing the Beasts

'Imran b. Husain (May Allah be pleased with him) reported: "We were with Allah's Messenger (peace and blessings be upon him) in some of his journeys and there was a woman from the Ansar riding a she-camel that it shied and she invoked curse upon that. Allah's Messenger (peace and blessings be upon him) heard it and said: "Unload that and set it free for it is accursed." 'Imran said: "I still perceive that (dromedary) walking amongst people and none taking any notice of that." (Muslim)

Abu Burza al-Aslami (May Allah be pleased with him) reported that a slave-girl was riding a dromedary and there was also the luggage of people upon it. that she suddenly saw Allah's Apostle (peace and blessings be upon him). The way of the mountain was narrow and she said (to that dromedary): "Go ahead." But that dromedary did not move. She (that slave-girl), out of anger, said: "O Allah, let that (dromedary) be damned." Thereupon Allah's Apostle (peace and blessings be upon him) said: "Let the dromedary on which the curse has been invoked not proceed with us." (Muslim)

623. Disturbance to the Natural Environment

Allah, the Exalted, says:

"There is the type of man whose speech about this world's life may dazzle thee, and he calls the God (Allah) to witness about what is in his heart: yet is he the most contentious of enemies? When he turns his back, his aim everywhere is to spread mischief through the earth and destroy crops and cattle. But Allah loves not mischief." (Qur'an, Al-Baqarah 2:204-205)

"Mischief has appeared on the land and sea, because of (the need) that the hands of man have earned, that (Allah) may give them a taste of some of their deeds: in order that they may turn back (from evil)." (Qur'an, Ar-Rum 30:41)

"We will show them Our Signs in the universe, and in their own selves, until it becomes manifest to them that this (the Quran) is the truth. Is it not sufficient in regard to your Lord that He is a Witness over all things?" (Qur'an, Ar-Rum 41:53)

Other Verse: Al-An'am 6:65.

Narrated Anas bin Malik (May Allah have mercy on him): Allah's Messenger (peace and blessings be upon him) said, "There is none amongst the Muslims who plants a tree or sows seeds, and then a bird, or a person or an animal eats from it, but is regarded as a charitable gift for him." (Bukhari)

"…Bring no harm to the trees, nor burn them with fire, especially those which are fruitful." (Muslim) (https://www.iium.edu.my/deed/hadith/muslim/019)

Mischief on the land and sea is inflicted by man's unwary interference with the natural Allah's Laws and environmental systems that are ultimately against his own interests.

Deforestation including killing the trees for the Christmas decoration, flowers to sell or offer, throwing chemicals in the water or air, constructing artificial islands, disturbing or killing marine and earth creations, fireworks, strikes, carnivals, radiation, smoking, the list is endless.

Allah is Beautiful and loves Beauty in all things. Allah, the Most Merciful, created beautiful nature with high concentration of Negative Ions with the healing power for us to enjoy and to be healthy. While the humans, instead of preserving, exploiting the natural resources for their materialistic gain or desire. Meantime the concentration of the harmful Positive Ions has been increasing with the increase of the diseases due to the environmental destructive human intervention.

Natural disasters, such as a flood, earthquake, hurricane, cyclone, tsunami and sandstorm (that cause great damage or loss of life) are caused because of shirk and sins.

624. Not Preserving the Blessings of Allah on Earth

Allah, the Exalted, says:

"And if you would count the graces of Allah, never could you be able to count them. Truly! Allah is Oft-Forgiving, Most Merciful." (Qur'an, An-Nahl 16:18)

The Earth has been given to us a trust from our Lord, and a religious responsibility that He has commanded us to cultivate and construct and settle upon in a way that is demonstrates our concern for preserving its blessings.

Allah, the Exalted, says:

"He has produced you from the earth and settled you in it." (Qur'an, Hud 11:61)

Our obligations and duty with regards to the earth are to take care of it, protect its resources and further develop its prosperity for ourselves and future generations.

Allah, the Exalted, says:

"And the earth He laid (out) for the creatures. Therein is fruit and palm trees having sheaths (of dates)." (Qur'an, Ar-Rahman 55:10-11)

"And cause not corruption upon the earth after its reformation. That is better for you, if you should be believers." (Qur'an, Al-A'raf 7:85)

Allah has forbidden waste and extravagance when He says:

"But be not excessive. Indeed, He likes not those who commit excess." (Qur'an, Al-A'raf 7:31)

Our Prophet (peace and blessings of Allah be upon him) ordered us to be conservative and economical in the consumption of water and do not waste it even if it appears to be a large amount and readily available such as a running river.

Allah, the Exalted, says:

"And (We) made from water every living thing." (Qur'an, Al-Anbya 21:30)

We should maintain air and its purity, this means we should abstain from everything that pollutes it such as harmful emissions, smoking and other such substances.

The Prophet (peace and blessings of Allah be upon him) tasked us to take care of the animal and plant life on earth, he said: "Never does a Muslim plant trees or cultivate land and birds or a man or an animal eat out of them but that is (recorded) as charity on his behalf." (Bukhari and Muslim)

The earth has been created by Allah as a manifestation of His Omnipotent Power. He has placed within its resources for mankind, such that their livelihoods can be supported and continue.

Allah, the Exalted, says:

"And We have certainly established you upon the earth and made for you therein ways of livelihood." (Qur'an, Al-A'raf 7:10)

"It is He who created for you all of that which is on the earth." (Qur'an, Al-Baqarah 2:29)

Everything on earth has been put in a place of balance, with the proportioning and interconnected relationships established by His Wisdom ensuring that everything has a purpose.

Allah, the Exalred, says:

"And (We) caused to grow therein (something) of every well-balanced thing." (Qur'an, Al-Hijr 15:19)

We should grateful for the countless blessings of Allah. We should strive to ensure that its blessings and goodness remains. It is actually a right the future generations have upon us, and we are accountable.

625. Prohibition of Reviling the Wind

Allah, the Exalted, says:

"And We have sent the fertilizing winds." (Qur'an, Al-Hijr 15:22)

"It is Allah Who sends the winds, and they stir the clouds and spread them in the sky however He wills, and He makes them fragments so you see the rain emerge from within them." (Qur'an, Ar-Rum 30:48)

"So, We sent upon them a screaming wind during days of misfortune to make them taste the punishment of disgrace in the worldly life." (Qur'an, Fussilat 41:16)

Other Verses: Al-A'raf 7:57, Al-Qamar 54:19-20, Al-Ahqaf 46:24.

Aisha (May Allah be pleased with her) said: "Whenever the wind blew strongly, The Prophet (peace be upon him) would say: 'Allahumma inni as'aluka khairaha, wa khaira ma fiha, wa khaira ma ursilat bihi. Wa a' udhu bika min sharriha, wa sharri ma fiha, wa sharri ma ursilat bihi. 'O Allah, I beg of You its good and the good of that which it contains and the good of the purpose for which it has been sent; and I seek Your Refuge from its evil and the evil of that which it contains and the evil of the purpose for which it has been sent).'" (Muslim)

Commentary: Like His innumerable other gifts, the wind is a free gift of Allah, which is essential for man's health and sustenance. But if Allah wills, He can turn it into a means of destruction and ruin. Therefore, one should pray to Allah to enable him to benefit from its good effects and save him from bad ones. (513)

Abu Hurairah (May Allah be pleased with him) reported: "I heard the Messenger of Allah (May Allah's peace and blessings be upon him) say: "The wind is from the blessings of Allah. It brings mercy, and it brings punishment. When you see it, do not swear at it, but ask Allah for its goodness and seek Allah's refuge from its evil." (Abu Dawud) (https://hadeethenc.com/en/browse/hadith/8957)

'Abdullah Ibn Abbas (May Allah be pleased with him) narrated that a man cursed the wind in the presence of the Prophet, so he said: "Do not curse the wind, for it is merely doing as ordered, and whoever curses something undeservingly, then the curse returns upon him." (Tirmidhi and Abu Dawud) (https://hadithanswers.com/do-not-curse-the-wind-for-it-is-merely-doing-as-ordered)

626. Football and Other Sport Games

Allah, the Exalted, says:

"Who took their religion as distraction and amusement and whom the worldly life deluded. So today We will forget them just as they forgot the meeting of this Day of theirs and for having rejected Our Verses." (Qur'an, Al-A'raf 7:51)

Abu Hurairah (May Allah be pleased with him) reported that the Prophet (May Allah's peace and blessings be upon him) said: "Competitions with prizes are allowed only in camel racing, horse racing and shooting arrows." (Ibn Majah) (https://hadeethenc.com/en/browse/hadith/64640)

Football matches which are played for money and prizes are haram, because that is gambling, because it is not permissible to take prizes. (514, 515)

Any games which lead to missing obligatory remembrance of our Creator, involving haram income, fitnah and desires, conflicts, violence, uncovering awrah, statues or images of living beings, mixing men and women, music, alcohol, etc. are prohibited.

As for playing football just to strengthen the body and give it energy without falling into any of these haram things, this is something permissible.

627. Yoga

Allah, the Creator, says:

"If you join others in worship with Allah, (then) surely (all) your deeds will be in vain, and you will certainly be among the losers." (Qur'an, Az-Zumar 39:65)

Muhammad 'Abd al-Fattaah Faheem in the book al-Yoga wa'l-Tanaffus (yoga and breathing) (p.19) said:

"Yoga in the sacred Indian language means union and contact with god, i.e. union between the body, the mind and god which helps man attain knowledge and wisdom and develops his thought by developing his knowledge of life; it protects him from sectarianism, religious fanaticism, narrow-mindedness and shortsightedness when searching; it makes him live a life of contentment both physically and spiritually."

Yoga involves various exercises and rituals, but the most important and most famous of them is an exercise called Surya Namaskar (known in English as the "Sun Salutation"), which means in Sanskrit:

"prostration to the sun on eight parts of the body". And they defined these parts as the two feet, the two knees, the two hands, the chest and the forehead. The origin of the Yoga stems from idolatrous Hindu beliefs, it is a Shirk.

Yoga also involves other sins like nakedness, mixing, encourages vegetarian diet for which Allah has not revealed any authority, etc. (516)

628. Persistence in Minor Sins

Allah, the Exalted, says:

"If you shun the great Sins which you are forbidden, We will do away with your small Sins and cause you to enter an honorable place of entering." (Qur'an, An-Nisa 4:31)

"And those who when they commit an indecency or do injustice to their souls remember Allah and ask forgiveness for their faults and who forgives the faults but Allah, and (who) do not knowingly persist in what they have done." (Qur'an, Ali 'Imran 3:135)

The Believer fears his Sins.

Al-Harith ibn Suwaid (May Allah be pleased with him) reported: Abdullah ibn Masud (May Allah be pleased with him) said, "Verily, the believer views his sins as if he were sitting under a mountain, fearing it will fall upon him. The wicked views his sins as if they were a fly passing over his nose." (Bukhari)

Beware of accumulating many Minor sins

Narrated Sahl ibn Sa'd (May Allah be pleased with him): The Messenger of Allah (peace and blessings be upon him) said: "Beware of Minor sins, like a people who camped in the bottom of a valley, and one man brought a stick, another brought a stick, and so on, until they have fire to cook their bread. Verily, when a person is held accountable for these minor sins, they will destroy him." (Ahmad)

Sheikh Ibn Taymiyah (May Allah have mercy on him) said:

"Adultery is a Major sin, but looking and touching are lamam (Minor sins) which may be forgiven if one avoids Major sin. But if a person persists in looking or touching, that becomes a Major sin, and persisting in that may be worse than a small amount of Major sin, for persisting in looking with desire, along with the connected feelings of mixing and touching, may be much worse than the evil of an isolated act of Zina. Hence the fuqaha' said concerning the witness of good character: he does not commit a Major sin or persist in a Minor sin… Indeed, looking and touching may lead a man to Shirk as Allah says:

"And of mankind are some who take (for worship) others besides Allah as rivals (to Allah). They love them as they love Allah." (Qur'an, Al-Baqarah 2:165)

The one who is in love becomes a slave to the one he loves." (End quote from Majmoo' al-Fataawa (15/293) (21)

Sheikh Ibn 'Uthaymeen (May Allah have mercy on him) said:

"Praying for forgiveness is of no benefit when one persists in sin, because it is closer to making a mockery (of Faith) than to good deeds." (End quote from Thamaraat at-Tadween, p.141) (517)

Where not seeking forgiveness is due to carelessness, heedlessness of Divine commands and feeling safe from Divine Anger, considering the sin small and insignificant, it is already a Major sin.

Minor sins become Major under the conditions:

1) When they are committed due to heedlessness.
2) When they are considered insignificant and not punishable.
3) When the person who commits them is pleased and happy with himself.
4) To commit them again and again without feeling any remorse and repenting for them.
5) Being aware of the fact that doing them again and again makes them a Major sin.
6) When the sinner steals the smallest amount of money which is the last remaining money from poor person, leaving him without anything; it becomes a Major sin.

Warning against sins and faults, and do not to underestimate any sin because when Minor sins increase without expiation or their doer insists on committing them, they shall be his destruction.

Refer also to the Chapter "When Minor Sin becomes Major sin and Shirk".

629. Being Pleased with a Sinful Act

Narrated Ibn 'Umar (May Allah be pleased with him): The Prophet (peace and blessings be upon him) said, "While a man was walking, dragging his dress with pride, he was caused to be swallowed by the earth and will go on sinking in it till the Day of Resurrection." (Bukhari)

Abu Hurairah (May Allah be pleased with him) reported Allah's Messenger (peace and blessings be upon him) as saying: "Allah, the Exalted and Glorious, said: 'I live in the thought of My servant and I am with him as he remembers Me.' The Holy Prophet further said: 'By Allah, Allah is more pleased with the repentance of His servant than what one of you would do on finding the lost camel in the waterless desert… '" (Muslim) (https://sunnah.com/muslim:2675h)

Abu Dharr (May Allah be pleased with him) reported: The Messenger of Allah (peace and blessings be upon him) said, "Fear Allah wherever you are, follow a bad deed with a good deed and it will erase it, and behave with good character towards people." (Tirmidhi)

630. Staying in an Assembly of Sin

Allah, the Exalted, says:

"Therefore, proclaim openly (Allah's Message Islamic Monotheism) that which you are commanded, and turn away from Al-Mushrikun (polytheists, idolaters, disbelievers, etc. - see V.2:105)." (Qur'an, Al-Hijr 15:94)

'Abdullah bin Masud (May Allah be pleased with him) reported: The Messenger of Allah (peace and blessings be upon him) said, "The first defect (in religion) which affected the Children of Israel in the way that man would meet another and say to him: 'Fear Allah and abstain from what you are doing, for this is not lawful for you.' Then he would meet him the next day and find no change in him, but this would not prevent him from eating with him, drinking with him and sitting in his assemblies. When it came to this, Allah led their hearts into evil ways on account of their association with others." Then he (peace and blessings be upon him) recited, *"Those among the Children of Israel who disbelieved were cursed* by the tongue of Dawud (David) and 'Isa (Jesus), son of Maryam (Mary). That was because they disobeyed (Allah and the Messengers) and were ever transgressing beyond bounds. They used not to forbid one another from the Munkar (wrong, evildoing, sins, polytheism, disbelief) which they committed. Vile indeed was what they used to do. You see many of them taking the disbelievers as their Auliya' (protectors and helpers). Evil indeed is that which their own selves have sent forward before them; for that (reason) Allah's Wrath fell upon them and in torment will they abide. And had they believed in Allah and in the Prophet (Muhammad (peace and blessings be upon him)) and in what has been revealed to him, never would they have taken them (the disbelievers) as Auliya' (protectors and helpers); but many of them are the Fasiqun (rebellious, disobedient to Allah)." (5:78-81) Then he (peace and blessings be upon him) continued: "Nay, by Allah, you either enjoin good and forbid evil and catch hold of the hand of the oppressor and persuade him to act justly and stick to the Truth or Allah will involve the hearts of some of you with the hearts of others and will curse you as He had cursed them." (Abu Dawud and Tirmidhi) (https://sunnah.com/riyadussalihin:196)

Narrated 'Ubaidullah bin Jarir (May Allah be pleased with him) that his father said: "The Messenger of Allah (peace and blessings be upon him) said: 'There is no people among whom sins are committed when they are stronger and of a higher status (i.e. they have the power and ability to stop the sinners) and they do not change them, but Allah will send His punishment upon them all." (Ibn Majah)

631. Prohibiting Woman from Traveling Alone

Narrated Abu Hurairah (May Allah be pleased with him): The Messenger of Allah (peace and blessings be upon him) said, "It is not permissible for a woman who believes in Allah and the Last Day to make a journey of one day and night unless she is accompanied by a Mahram (husband or any other relative to whom she is prohibited to marry)." (Bukhari and Muslim)

Narrated Ibn 'Abbas (May Allah be pleased with him): The Prophet (peace and blessings be upon him) said, "No man must not be alone with a woman except in the presence of her (Mahram). No woman should travel except in company of a (Mahram)." A man said: "O Messenger of Allah! I have been enrolled for such and such expedition, and my wife left for Hajj." He (peace and blessings be upon him) said to him, "Go and perform Hajj with your wife." (Bukhari and Muslim)

Commentary: This Hadith proves that under no circumstance woman may travel alone. The Shariah strictly bans a meeting of this kind between two opposite sexes. Even if nothing objectionable happens, a mischievous person may exploit this situation and talk about them slanderously. Families disregardful of Hijab provide instances of illicit relationship between a man and a woman related to each other. (518)

Narrated Qaza'a Maula (freed slave of) Ziyad: "I heard Abu Sa'id Al-khudri narrating four things from the Prophet and I appreciated them very much. He said, conveying the words of the Prophet. 1) "A woman should not go on a two-day journey except with her husband or a Dhi-Mahram, 2) No fasting is permissible on two days: Eid-Al-Fitr and Eid-Al-Adha, 3) No prayer after two prayers, i.e. after the Fajr prayer till the sun rises and after the 'Asr prayer till the sun sets, 4) Do not prepare yourself for a journey except to three Mosques, i.e. Al-Masjid Al-Haram, the Mosque of Aqsa (Jerusalem) and my Mosque." (Bukhari)

632. Prohibition Traveling Alone at Night

Ibn 'Umar (May Allah be pleased with him) reported: The Messenger of Allah (peace and blessings be upon him) said, "Were people to know of what I know about the dangers of traveling alone, no rider would travel alone at night." (Bukhari)

Abdullah ibn 'Amr Ibn al-'As (May Allah be pleased with him) reported that the Prophet (May Allah's peace and blessings be upon him) said: "The lonely rider is a Devil, two riders are two Devils and three are a traveling team." (Tirmidhi) (https://hadeethenc.com/en/browse/hadith/5938)

Shaykh al-Albaani said in his commentary on this Hadith in al-Saheehah (62):

"Perhaps the Hadith refers to travelling in the deserts or wilderness where the traveller rarely sees anyone. It does not include travel nowadays on paved and well travelled roads. And Allah knows best. End quote." (519)

633. Trip to Mars

Allah, the Exalted, says:

"Do not throw yourselves with your own hands into destruction." (Qur'an, Al-Baqarah 2:195)

Abu Dharr (May Allah be pleased with him) reported that the Prophet (May Allah's peace and blessings be upon him) said: "I see what you do not see. The sky has squeaked, and it has every right to do so, for it does not have a space of four fingers where there is no angel prostrating his forehead before Allah the Almighty. By Allah! If you knew what I know, you would laugh little and weep much; you would not enjoy women in bed; and you would go out to the open plains loudly imploring Allah the Almighty."

(Ibn Majah) (https://hadeethenc.com/en/browse/hadith/3265)

Sheikh Mohammed Yusuf (Amena Mosque) said:

"Man's life is not his or her own property; it is God's creation, and therefore, suicide is prohibited in all religions and of course by Law." (520)

Narrated Abu Sa'id Al-Khudri (who fought in twelve Ghazawat in the company of the Prophet): "I heard four things from the Prophet (peace and blessings be upon him) and they won my admiration. He (peace and blessings be upon him) said: 1. No lady should travel on a journey of two days except with her husband or a Dhi-Mahram, 2. No fasting is permissible on the two days of Eid Al-Fitr and Eid Al-Adha,

3. No prayer (may be offered) after the morning compulsory prayer until the sun rises; and no prayer after the 'Asr prayer till the sun sets, 4. One should travel only for visiting three Masajid (Mosques): Masjid Al-Haram (Makkah), Masjid Al-Aqsa (Jerusalem), and this (my) Mosque (at Madinah)." (Bukhari)

634. Commercial Insurance Fraud

Commercial insurances of all types are forbidden by our Creator, whether it is life insurance, health insurance or insurance of one's property.

1. Insurances involve ambiguity.

Narrated Abu Hurairah (May Allah be pleased with him) that the Prophet (peace and blessings be upon him) forbade gharar (ambiguous) transactions." (Muslim)

Gharar transactions (risky) include any transactions in which something is not known such as selling fish in the water or birds in the air, because the purchaser may or may not get it. (Mu'jam Maqaayees al-Lughah (4/380-381); Lisaan al-'Arab (6/317)

Al-Nawawi (May Allah have mercy on him) said:

"With regard to the prohibition on ambiguous transactions, this is a very important principle with regard to commercial transactions and includes many issues, such as selling things that are not present or are unknown and so on. All of these are invalid transactions because there is ambiguity with no reason for that."

2. Insurance contracts are a kind of gambling.

What is meant by gambling is when a person pays something of his own money and takes a risk: either he will gain more than it or he will lose the money that he paid.

3. Insurance involves Riba

Narrated 'Ubaadah ibn al-Saamit (May Allah be pleased with him): The Prophet (peace and blessings be upon him) said: "Gold for gold, silver for silver, wheat for wheat, barley for barley, dates for dates, salt for salt, like for like, same for same, hand to hand. But if these commodities differ, then sell as you like, as long as it is hand to hand." (Muslim)

This Hadith indicates that if a person sells gold for gold, it must be equal amounts.

If a person sells gold for gold with a difference in the amount, then they have fallen into Riba al-fadl. If the exchange is not completed during the same meeting, then they have fallen into Riba al-nasee'ah, i.e. interest charged when hand-to-hand exchange is delayed. Riba is prohibited in the Noble Qur'an.

"Those who eat Riba (usury) will not stand (on the Day of Resurrection) except like the standing of a person beaten by Shaitan (Satan) leading him to insanity." *(Qur'an, Al-Baqarah 2:275)*

Insurance is consuming people's wealth unlawfully and it is forbidden by God.

"O you who believe! Eat not up your property among yourselves unjustly except it be a trade amongst you, by mutual consent." *(Qur'an, An-Nisa 4:29)*

Insurance contracts oblige the insurance company to pay compensation, if the risk against which insurance was taken happens. But, on what basis? The insurance company did not cause the danger or make it happen; it did not commit any acts of aggression or shortcoming, so how can it be forced to pay compensation for something for which it is not liable according to Shariah?

Ibn Taymiyah (May Allah have mercy on him):

"The same applies to ambiguous transactions, which are a kind of gambling, but some types may be permissible in the case of need and where it serves a clear interest. End quote." (Majmoo' al-Fataawa, 14/471) He also said:

"Ambiguous transactions are forbidden because they are a kind of gambling which may lead to consuming people's wealth unlawfully. But if that is countered by a greater harm, that makes it permissible so as to ward off the greater of two evils by putting up with the lesser. And Allah knows best." (End quote from Majmoo' al-Fataawa, 29/483) (521)

Commercial insurance can be permissible in two cases:

1) Health Insurance can be obligatory by the government's or company's rules, so the person is forced to do so. In that case the sin is on the one who forces people to do that.

2) When a person is compelled to take out health insurance or he is in great need as he is not able to cover the cost of treatment. This is a need which makes it permissible to deal with health insurance according to a number of scholars, because the reason for the prohibition on this insurance is the ambiguity and the element of gambling, not Riba.

635. Ruling on Medico-Surgical Treatment

Allah, the Exalted, says:

"And when I am ill, it is He Who cures me." (Qur'an, Ash-Shu'ara 26:80)

"And We send down from the Qur'an that which is a <u>Healing</u> and a Mercy to those who believe (in Islamic Monotheism and act on it), and it increases the Zalimun (polytheists and wrong-doers) nothing but loss." (Qur'an, Al-Isra 17:82)

"O mankind! There has come to you a good advice from your Lord (i.e. the Qur'an, ordering all that is good and forbidding all that is evil), and a <u>Healing</u> for that (disease of ignorance, doubt, hypocrisy and differences, etc.) in your breasts, - a Guidance and a Mercy (explaining lawful and unlawful things, etc.) for the believers." (Qur'an, Yunus 10:57)

Other Verses: Fussilat 41:44, At-Tawbah 9:14, An-Nahl 6:17 and 16:69.

<u>Allah is the Physician. You are only kind man</u>

Allah's Name Ash-Shafi - The One Who cures, the Healer. His Healing is Perfect according to His Wisdom and He is the Source from which all cures come!

Abu Ramthah (May Allah be pleased with him) reported that he said to the Prophet (May Allah's peace and blessings be upon him): "Show me this thing on your back (to treat it), for I am a physician." The Prophet (May Allah's peace and blessings be upon him) replied: "Allah is the Physician. You are only a kind man. The One Who heals, it is the One Who created it." (Abu Dawud)

(https://hadeethenc.com/en/browse/hadith/8303)

Suhayb ibn Sinan Ar-Rumi (May Allah be pleased with him) reported that the Prophet (May Allah's peace and blessings be upon him) said: "…The boy used to treat people suffering from congenital blindness, leprosy and other diseases. One of the king's companions, who had become blind, heard about the boy. He brought many gifts for the boy and said: 'All these gifts are for you on condition that you cure me.' The boy said: 'I do not cure anybody; it is only Allah the Almighty, Who can cure people. If you believe in Allah, the Exalted, I will supplicate Him to cure you and He will cure you…" (Muslim)

https://hadeethenc.com/en/browse/hadith/3303

Aisha (May Allah be pleased with her) reported that when the Prophet (May Allah's peace and blessings be upon him) visited some of his family members who were sick, he would pass his right hand over them and say: "O Allah, Lord of mankind, remove the affliction. Cure, for You are the One Who cures; there is no cure but Yours, a cure that leaves behind no trace of sickness." (Bukhari and Muslim)

(https://hadeethenc.com/en/browse/hadith/5542)

Khawlah bint Hakim (May Allah be pleased with her) reported that the Prophet (May Allah's peace and blessings be upon him) said: "Whoever alights somewhere and then says: 'I seek refuge in the Perfect Words of Allah from the evil of what He has created', nothing will harm him until he leaves that place."

(Muslim) (https://hadeethenc.com/en/browse/hadith/5932)

Ibn Al-Qayyim Al-Jawziyya (May Allah have mercy on him) said:

"The Qur'an is the most complete cure from all physical and psychological illnesses - the illnesses of this World and the illnesses of the Hereafter. Not everyone is capable, nor is everyone given the success from Allah to seek a cure from it. If the sick person uses the proper method of using the Qur'an as a Medicine, with belief complete faith and acceptance, and firm belief in it as a cure, and he fulfills all the conditions [of doing so], no disease will ever overcome him. How can a disease overcome the Speech of the Lord of the Heavens and the Earth, the Speech which if it was sent upon a mountain, would render that mountain to dust. The Speech that if it was sent upon the Earth, would break the Earth into pieces? There is no illness of the heart and the body except that the Qur'an contains the means to guide how to cure it, why it happens, and how to protect from it, for those whom Allah gives the understanding of his Book. As for the diseases of the heart, Allah mentions them in detail along with their causes and the method of curing them. So, the one who is not cured by the Qur'an, may Allah not cure him, and the one who the Qur'an is not sufficient for him, May Allah not suffice him in anything! It is known that certain things that we say have particular special qualities and proven benefits, then what do you think of the Speech of the Lord of the Worlds, the One Who the virtue of his Speech over the speech of others, is like the virtue of Him over his creation. The Qur'an is the perfect cure, and it is a beneficial means of protection, and a guiding light and a general mercy. If it was sent upon a mountain it would render it asunder from its greatness and its glory." (Zad Al-Ma'ad) (7)

Ibn Taymiyah (May Allah have mercy upon him) said:

"Applying this knowledge of Quranic Medicine is compulsory upon whoever learns it. Because it is equivalent to relieving the troubled, helping the oppressed, liberating the distressed and supporting the weak." (10)

Disease is a Test, Expiation of Sins or Punishment

For more details, refer to the Chapter "Allah send down the diseases for three reasons".

Trials and Calamities as Remedy

Refer to the Chapter "Medicine of Calamities and Trials".

Medical treatment and Reliance on Allah

Narrated Abud Darda (May Allah be pleased with him): "The Messenger of Allah (peace and blessings of Allah be upon him) said: 'Allah has sent down both the disease and the cure, and He has appointed a cure for every disease, so treat yourselves medically, but use nothing unlawful.'" (Abu Dawud)

Narrated Abu Hurairah (May Allah be pleased with him): The Prophet (peace and blessings be upon him) said "If a house fly falls in the drink of anyone of you, he should dip it (in the drink) and take it out, for one of its wings has a disease and the other has the cure for the disease." (Bukhari)

Seeking a medical treatment (modern medicine) is not obligatory according to the scholars, unless – according to some – it will definitely be of benefit.

The majority of scholars (Hanafi and Maliki) said that medical treatment is mubaah (permitted). The Shaafi'is, and al-Qaadi, Ibn 'Aqeel and Ibn al-Jawzi among the Hanbalis, said that it is mustahabb (recommended), because of the Hadith "Allah has sent down the disease and the cure, and has made for every disease the cure. So, treat sickness, but do not use anything haram," and other Ahadith which contain instructions to seek cure. They said: 'The fact that the Prophet (peace and blessings of Allah be upon him) used cupping and other kinds of treatment indicates that medical treatment is permitted.' For the Shaafi'is, treatment is mustahabb when there is no certainty that it will be beneficial, but when treatment is certain to be beneficial (such as putting a dressing on a wound), then it is wajib or obligatory (an example would be blood transfusions in certain cases).

(See Haashiyat Ibn 'Aabideen, 5/215, 249; al-Hidaayah Takmilat Fath al-Qadeer, 8/134; al-Fawaakih al-Dawaani, 2/440; Rawdah al-Taalibeen, 2/96; Kashshaaf al-Qinaa', 2/76; al-Insaaf, 2/463; al-Aadaab al-Shar'iyyah, 2/359ff, Haashiyat al-Jumal, 2/134).

Ibn al-Qayyim said concerning the Saheeh Ahadith that speak about medical treatment:

"This does not contradict tawakul (putting one's trust in Allah), just as warding off hunger, thirst, heat and cold does not contradict tawakul. The essence of tawakul is not complete without resorting to the means which Allah has set out in order for us to achieve results both according to His Decree (Qadr) and His Laws (shar'). Not using these means is contrary to tawakul: it goes against and undermines the Command and Wisdom of Allah, although the one who neglects the means may think that this makes his tawakul stronger. Ignoring the means is a sign of helplessness that goes against the true essence of tawakul, which is that the heart relies on Allah to bring the slave whatever will benefit him in this world and the next, and to protect him from whatever may harm him in this world and the next. But along with this reliance, it is essential to take the appropriate means, otherwise he will be going against the Wisdom and Command of Allah. Helplessness should not be taken as a sign of tawakul, nor should tawakul make a person helpless." (Zad Al-Ma'ad, 4/15. See al-Mawsoo'ah al-Fiqhiyyah, 11/116)

Seeking a treatment or cure is not obligatory according to the scholars, unless – according to some – it will definitely be of benefit. Since in the situation described in the question there is no certainty that treatment will be of benefit, and indeed it is likely to cause suffering to the patient, then there is nothing at all wrong with not giving the treatment. The patient should not forget to put his trust in Allah and seek refuge in Him, for the gates of heaven are open to those who call on Allah. He may also seek treatment (Ruqyah) by reciting Qur'an, such as reading Al-Fatihah, Al-Falaq and An-Nas over himself. This will benefit him psychologically and physically, as well as bringing him reward. Allah is the Healer and there is no healer but He. (522)

Narrated Abu Sa'id Al-Khudri: "...One of them (the Prophet's companions) started reciting Surah Al-Fatiha and gathering his saliva and spitting it (at the snake-bite or stung by a scorpion). The patient got cured..." (Bukhari) (https://sunnah.com/bukhari:5736)

Seeking medico-surgical treatment is recommended in case of life-threatening conditions (e.g. heavy bleeding, serious injury, bowel occlusion or perforation, septicemia, pneumonia, etc.), delivery which can lead to emergency C-section at any time, etc.

Prophet Muhammad (peace and blessings be upon him) didn't recommend any medical treatment in the diseases caused by Decreased Oxygen Utilization and by the Evil Jinn including Epidemics.

636. Health Care Fraud and Abuse

Health care fraud can be committed by medical providers, patients and others who intentionally deceive the health care system to receive unlawful benefits or payments. (523)

637. Misdiagnosis of Jinn Diseases

Allah, the Exalted, says:

"And remember Our slave Ayub (Job), when he invoked his Lord (saying): "Verily! Shaitan (Satan) has touched me with distress (by losing my health) and torment (by losing my wealth)! (Allah said to him): "Strike the ground with your foot: This is a spring of water to wash in, cool and a (refreshing) drink." (Qur'an, Sad 38:41-42)

"Shall I inform you (O people!) upon whom the Shayateen (Devils) descend? They descend on every lying (one who tells lies), sinful person." (Qur'an, Ash-Shu'ara 26:221-222)

"We have made the Devils allies to those who do not believe." (Qur'an, Al-A'raf 7:27)

Other Verses: *Ali 'Imran 3:36, Maryam 19:83, Al-Baqarah 2:275, Al-Jinn 72:6, Al-Anfal 8:11.*

95% of diseases are caused by the Evil Jinn - confirmed by my Istikhara prayer and Du'a to Allah.

Refer to the Chapter "Diseases caused by Positive Ions".

Menorrhagia, Polymenorrhea, Metrorrhagia are from Devil

Narrated Hamnah daughter of Jahsh: "Hamnah said, "my menstruation was great in quantity and severe. So, I came to the Apostle of Allah (peace and blessings be upon him) be upon him) for a decision and told him. I found him in the house of my sister, Zaynab, daughter of Jahsh. I said: 'Apostle of Allah, I am a woman who menstruates in great quantity and it is severe, so what do you think about it? It has prevented me from praying and fasting.' He said: 'I suggest that you should use cotton, for it absorbs the blood.' She replied: 'It is too copious for that.' He said: 'Then take a cloth.' She replied: 'It is too copious for that, for my blood keeps flowing.' The Apostle of Allah (peace be upon him) said: 'I shall give you two commands; whichever of them you follow, that will be sufficient for you without the other, but you know best whether you are strong enough to follow both of them.' He added: '**This is a stroke of the Devil**, so observe your menses for six or seven days, Allah Alone knows which it should be; then wash. And when you see that you are purified and quite clean, pray during twenty-three or twenty-four days and nights and fast, for that will be enough for you, and do so every month, just as women menstruate and are purified at the time of their menstruation and their purification. But if you are strong enough to delay the noon (Zuhr) prayer and advance the afternoon ('Asr) prayer, to wash, and then combine the noon and the afternoon prayer; to delay the sunset prayer and advance the night prayer, to wash, and then combine the two prayers, do so: and to wash at dawn, do so: and fast if you are able to do so if possible.' The Apostle of Allah (peace be upon him) said: 'Of the two commands this is more to my liking.'" (Abu Dawud)

Aisha (May Allah have mercy on her) reported: "Fatimah b. Abu Hubaish came to the Apostle (peace and blessings be upon him) and said: 'I am a woman whose blood keeps flowing (even after the menstruation period). I am never purified; should I, therefore, abandon prayer?' He (the Holy Prophet) said: 'Not at all, for that is only a vein, and is not a menstruation, so when menstruation comes, abandon prayer, and when it ends wash the blood from yourself and then pray." (Muslim)

Ahadith on the Skin Diseases

1. Narrated Um Salama: that the Prophet (peace and blessings be upon him) saw in her house a girl whose face had a black spot. He said. "She is under the effect of an Evil Eye; so, treat her with a Ruqyah." (Bukhari)

2. Narrated Ash-Shifa', daughter of Abdullah: "The Messenger of Allah (peace and blessings be upon him) entered when I was with Hafsah, and he said to me: "Why do you not teach this one the spell for skin eruptions as you taught her writing." (Abu Dawud)

Watering Eye is from Satan

"There was an old woman who used to enter upon us and perform Ruqyah from Erysipelas: Contagious

disease which causes fever and leaves a red coloration of the skin. We had a bed with long legs, and

when Abdullah entered, he would clear his throat and make noise. He entered one day and when she heard his voice, she veiled herself from him. He came and sat beside me, and touched me, and he found a sting. He said: 'What is this?' I said: 'An amulet against Erysipelas.' He pulled it, broke it and threw it away, and said: 'The family of Abdullah has no need of polytheism.' I heard the Messenger of Allah

(peace and blessings be upon him) say: "Ruqyah (i.e. which consist of the names of idols and devils etc.), amulets and Tiwalah (charms) are polytheism." "I said: 'I went out one day and so-and-so looked at me, and my eye began to water on the side nearest him. When I recited Ruqyah for it, it stopped, but if I did not recite Ruqyah it watered again.' He said: **'That is Satan**, if you obey him, he leaves you alone but if you disobey him, he pokes you with his finger in your eye. But if you do what the Messenger of Allah (peace and blessings be upon him) used to do, that will be better for you and more effective in healing. Sprinkle water in your eye and say: Adhhibil-bas Rabban-nas, washfi Antash-Shafi, la shifa'a illa shafi'uka, shafi'an la yughadiru saqaman (Take away the pain, O Lord of mankind, and grant healing, for You are the Healer, and there is no healing but Your healing that leaves no trace of sickness).'" (Ibn Majah) (https://sunnah.com/urn/1275750)

Ibn Taymiyah (May Allah have mercy on him) said:

"Those who deny the Jinn's existence do not have evidence to support their denial. They merely have a lack of knowledge because the beliefs and experimental knowledge of their profession contain nothing which confirms the Jinn's existence. Such a case of medical doctor who looks after the health of the body by treating the physical symptoms of its sicknesses from the point of view of changes of its physical make up without considering what may can happen to the body from the spiritual point of view or what may happen to the body because of the effect of the Jinn on it. This is often the case even so though he may have learned through means other than his medicine that the soul has greater effect on the body then his medicinal remedies. The Jinn most certainly do have an effect on humans according to the Prophet's clear statement in the following authentic narration, "Verily Satan flows in the blood stream of Adam's descendants." (Narrated by Safiyah and collected in the six books with the exception of Tirmidhi. Narrated by Anas in Saheeh Muslim (English Trans.), vol.3, Hadith no. 1188, and Sunan Abi Dawud (English Trans.), vol.3, p.1390, Hadith no. 497626) For, in the blood is the ether known to doctors as the "animal soul" which is emitted by the heart and which moves throughout the body giving it life.

(A distinction is being made here by the author between the life of the body which may exist independently of the soul as in the case where bodies are kept "alive" today by machines long after their souls have departed. This is also similar to the life of the fetus prior to the introduction of its soul in the fifth month according to the Prophet Muhammad's statement, "Verily the creation of each one of you is brought together in his mother's womb for forty days as an oily drop, then as a leech-like clot of blood for a similar period, then as a chewed clump of flesh for a similar period. Then an angel is sent to him who blows the breath of life into him." (Narrated by 'Abdullah ibn Masud and collected by Bukhari and Muslim. Saheeh al-Bukhari (Arabic-English), vol.4, p.290-291, Hadith no. 430) (10)

"What Ibn Taymiyah said is well known, for everywhere some humans become overcome by fits and speak in unintelligible languages, they are beaten with blows so severe that if a camel were struck by them it would react violently, yet the one possessed does not feel the blows nor realize that he has spoken what people heard him say. The possessed may lift others much heavier than themselves, move heavy machinery, run at unnaturally fast speeds and other such things which have been witnessed and reported by many things which have been witnessed and reported by many reliable sources. All of this evidence clearly indicates that the entity speaking with the human's voice and moving their bodies is definitely another species of being other than man. None of the leading Muslim scholars deny that the Jinn enters the body of the insane. Therefore, whoever denies that this may happen or claims that the religious laws reject it as false, has himself falsified the religious law, for there is nothing in the Divine Law to contradict its occurrence." (10, Appendix Two)

Ibn al-Qayyim stated the following in his book Zad Al-Ma'ad:

"Fits of madness (or epileptic seizures) are of two types: Fits resulting from evil earthly spirits (the Jinn) and fits resulting from bad humours. The latter is that about whose causes and remedies doctors have spoken. As for spirit-possession, leading scholars and intellectuals acknowledge its occurrence and do not attempt to treat it. They recognize that its treatment requires that noble transcendent spirits counter, neutralize and expel the evil spirits. Hippocrates himself spoke on this matter at length in some of his books wherein he mentioned some remedies for epileptic fits then said, 'These (medicines) are beneficial in the case of fits due to humours and other biological causes. As for fits resulting from the effects of spirits, these remedies are of no use.'" "Only ignorant doctors and those pseudo- intellectuals who consider heresy a virtue deny spirit-possession and their effects on the body of the insane. They have no evidence for their denial except their ignorance of its occurrence, as there is nothing in the field of medicine which rejects it, while the senses and experiences of people world-wide confirm it. Their ascribing it to the preponderance of some humours is correct in some instances but not in all. The intelligent and those knowledgeable about these spirits and their effects are amused by the stupidity of such people who deny spirit possession due to their ignorance." (10, Appendix Two)

Blood clots are caused by Devils

Anas ibn Malik (May Allah be pleased with him) reported: Jibreel came to the Messenger of Allah (May Allah's peace and blessings be upon him) while he was playing with his playmates. He took hold of him, laid him on the ground, split open his chest, took the heart out and then extracted a blood clot out of it and said: "That was the Devil's share in you." Then he washed it with Zamzam water in a golden basin and then joined the wounded parts together after he restored the heart to its place. The boys came running to his mother, i.e. his wet nurse, and said: "Muhammad has been killed." They rushed to him and found his color was changed. Anas said: "I used to see the scar of this stitching on his chest." (Muslim) (https://hadeethenc.com/en/browse/hadith/10862)

The diagnosis of the Jinn Possession is easy by application of Negative Ions, recitation of Ruqyah and by Jinn Possession symptoms. (524)

638. Medico-Surgical Treatment in Jinn Diseases

Allah, the Exalted, says:

"O mankind! There has come to you a good Advice from your Lord (i.e. the Qur'an, ordering all that is good and forbidding all that is evil), and a Healing for that (disease of ignorance, doubt, hypocrisy and differences, etc.) in your breasts, a Guidance and a Mercy (explaining lawful and unlawful things, etc.) for the believers." (Qur'an, Yunus 10:57)

"And if an Evil whisper comes to you from Shaytan (Satan), then seek refuge with Allah. Verily, He is All-Hearer, All-Knower." (Qur'an, Al-A'raf: 200)

"And if Allah touches you with harm, none can remove it but He, and if He touches you with good, then He is Able to do all things." (Qur'an, Al-An'am 16:17)

The Jinn most certainly do have an effect on humans according to the Prophet's clear statement in the following authentic narration, "Verily Satan flows in the blood stream of Adam's descendants." (10)

The Prophet didn't recommend medical treatment in Jinn diseases:

Narrated Ya'la ibn Murah: "…On the way, we passed by a woman sitting at the roadside with a young boy. She called out, 'O Messenger of Allah, this boy is afflicted with a trial, and from him we have also been afflicted with a trial. I don't know how many times per day he is seized by fits.' He (peace be upon him) said: 'Give him to me.' So, she lifted him up to the Prophet.

He (peace be upon him) then placed the boy between himself and the middle of the saddle, opened the boy's mouth and blew in it three times, saying, **'In the Name of Allah, I am the slave of Allah, get out, enemy of Allah!'**…" (Musnad Ahmad, vol. 4, p.170), and al-Haakim who declared it authentic) (https://www.kalamullah.com/Books/The%20Exorcist%20Tradition%20In%20Islam.pdf)

Another Hadith was mentioned above: https://sunnah.com/ibnmajah:3532

Epidemics are the Jinn Possession because of Humanity's Sins.

The Prophet didn't recommend medical treatment In Epidemics.

Ibn al-Qayyim (May Allah have mercy on him) stated,

"In summary, this type of seizure and its treatment is only denied by small-minded, intellectually-deficient persons devoid of real understanding. Evil spirits mostly gain control of those having little religious inclination and those whose heart's and tongue's faith has deserted. Those whose souls are desolate of the remembrance of Allah and formulas for strengthening faith. When evil spirits meet a man who is isolated, weaponless and naked, they are easily able to attack him and overcome him." (Zad Al-Ma'ad)

In fact, to exorcise the Jinn is obligatory according to the principles of repelling oppression, aiding the oppressed, enjoining righteousness and forbidding evil, just as it is with humans. It has already been mentioned in authentic Ahadith that the Prophet (peace and blessings be upon him) choked the Devil until its saliva flowed unto his noble hand and that he said, "Were it not for my brother Sulayman's prayer, it would have been tied up so people could see it." (Ahmad, narrated Abu Sa'id al-Khudri) And in Muslim's narration on the authority of Abu ad-Darda: The Prophet (peace and blessings be upon him) said: "Verily the enemy of Allah, Iblees, came with a flame to put in my face, so I said three times, 'I seek refuge in Allah from thee.' Then I said three times, 'I curse thee with Allah's full Curse.' But he did not retreat (on any one of these) three occasions. Thereafter I meant to seize him. I swear by Allah that, had it not been for the supplication of my brother Sulayman, he would have been bound, and made an object of sport for the children of Madinah. (10, Appendix Two)

Medico-Surgical Treatment in the Jinn Diseases is detrimental as excites the Evil Jinn.

Medico-surgical treatment in the Jinn possessed people is detrimental and life threatening as excites the Evil Jinn and excited Jinn spread more disease, additionally to the new diseases created by the drugs' severe side effects.

Some of the examples of Jinn Possession diseases described by different name and syndromes:

Serotonin Syndrome

Serotonin Syndrome symptoms usually occur within several hours of taking a new drug or increasing the dose of a drug you are already taking.

Serotonin syndrome is a serious drug reaction. It is caused by medications that build up high levels of serotonin in the body.

Serotonin is a chemical that the body produces naturally. It is needed for the nerve cells and brain to function. But too much serotonin causes signs and symptoms that can range from mild (shivering and diarrhea) to severe (muscle rigidity, fever and seizures). Severe serotonin syndrome can cause death if not treated.

Serotonin syndrome can occur when you increase the dose of certain medications or start taking a new drug. It is most often caused by combining medications that contain serotonin, such as a migraine medication and an antidepressant. Some illicit drugs and dietary supplements are associated with serotonin syndrome.

Signs and symptoms include:

- Agitation or restlessness
- Insomnia
- Confusion
- Rapid heart rate and high blood pressure
- Dilated pupils
- Loss of muscle coordination or twitching muscles
- High blood pressure
- Muscle rigidity
- Heavy sweating
- Diarrhea
- Headache
- Shivering
- Goose bumps

Severe serotonin syndrome can be life-threatening. Signs include:

- High fever
- Tremor
- Seizures
- Irregular heartbeat
- Unconsciousness (525)

We see the same but on global level with the mass vaccinations. Vaccines excite the hidden Devils and Devils manifest by spreading or accentuating the existing diseases symptoms and/or creating new diseases, additionally to the toxicity of drugs which can alone create new diseases. The pics of death on the graphics correspond to the immediate post mass vaccination periods.

Postoperative Delirium (POD)

Postoperative Delirium is a form of Delirium that manifests in patients who have undergone surgical procedures and anesthesia, Aulus Cornelius Celsus (25 B.C.- 50 A.C.) used the term "becoming mad". In his work *De Medicina,* he said: "Now it is useless to adopt remedies when the delirium is at its height… there is nothing else to do than to restrain the patient, but when circumstances permit, relief must be given with haste…" (526, 527)

Doctors don't know that Postoperative Delirium is a manifestation of the Jinn (Demonic) Possession. Drugs and surgery excite the Evil Jinn.

Steroid Shots for Painful Joints May It Worse

Amy Norton, Steroid Shots for Painful Joints May Make It Worse, https://www.webmd.com/pain-management/news/20191015/steroid-shots-for-painful-joints-may-make-matters-worse

Pain relief treatments for Arthritis, corticosteroid injections, may actually be associated with faster progression of the disease, according to new research. (528)

Arthritis are caused by the Evil Jinn. Medications and invasive procedure excite them.

Here are some cases of the Jinn diseases in my practice:

1. In the Mosque, a lady said that she had tumors on her ovary (and/or uterus?) and two doctors in different countries recommended her the operation. I said that it was caused by Satan and surgery is detrimental in this case, and she should recite Ruqyah. She asked me to do Ruqyah for her but I advised her to recite Qur'an by herself. Two years later in the same Mosque, she approached me and said: "Do you remember me? You asked me to do Ruqyah for my gynecological tumors." She told me that she followed my advice, recited Ruqyah after each obligatory prayer. When she returned back to see her doctor. The doctor said after

performing ultrasound that tumors disappeared. She couldn't believe. Then she went to see another doctor who also previously recommended her a surgery. The second doctor also said that she doesn't need operation as Allah cured her by Ruqyah.

2. I was walking and repeating the Name of Allah As-Samee' meaning the "All-Hearing" as I have learned that by calling Allah by His Beautiful Name, I can have better hearing in one ear. I walked about 1,5 km and from opposite side, a fisherman approached me and complained of his ears problem, "ringing, buzzing, grinding in the ears" and he couldn't sleep because of the noise in his ears. Surprised, I told him that I was repeating Allah's Name As-Samee', then I advised him to call Allah by His Name. When I returned back to the beach two months later, I met him and asked him about his Tinnitus. He told me that he submitted himself to Allah and Allah cured him immediately. Tinnitus is a Jinn Possession disease.

3. A man from New York Mosque complained that his one eye doesn't see well and doctor has already scheduled operation. He had the same problem on another eye two years ago and had surgery.

I suspected that Satan caused the disease and advised him to make istikhara prayer and Du'a as in Jinn diseases, the surgery and drugs excite the Evil Jinn and excited Jinn spread more disease. When I contacted him the day after his scheduled operation, he told me that he followed my advice, did Istikhara prayer and Du'a. Allah cancelled his surgery and cured him.

4. On my way, on the street there was a dying paralyzed bird, breathing rarely. I started to recite Ruqyah. A man came from the opposite side and put few drops of water on bird's head. Paralysis is caused by Satan. Satan is made from fire and doesn't like water. The bird started to blink his eyes. Allah was showing me how I should act in this situation (water against Satan as he is made from the fire). I recited Surah Al-Ikhlasx3, Surah Al-Falaqx3, Surah An-Nasx3 and when I finished Surah Ayatul Kursi, the bird flew out from my hand as there was nothing happened to him. The Qur'an is a Miracle of miracles!

5. During the night flight, I was praying night prayers in the aircraft. Few minutes after finishing prayer, my neighbor, a woman of 50 y-of old, lost consciousness and her daughter was calling for doctor. A man took a bottle of water, took few sips of water and sprayed on her face. She regained consciousness immediately looking very tired and confused. Almighty God was showing me that I should use the water to spray on unconscious patient as Satan is made from fire and fire is extinguished by water. Satan caused unconsciousness. We put her on the floor in the horizontal position with the legs up, while I was reciting Ruqyah. I advised her to pray and read the Noble Qur'an.

Atiyyah reported: The Messenger of Allah (peace be and blessings be upon him) said, "Verily, anger comes from Satan and Satan was created from fire. Fire is extinguished with water, so if you become angry then perform ablution with water." (Abu Dawud)

6. My patient called me about her babysitter who lost consciousness then was in state of lethargy and had severe headache. Ambulance performed the investigations and didn't find

anything abnormal. Worried by her unusual state, my patient asked me to see her. She arrived to the clinic with another lady working with her who said that it was a Jinn Possession. Patient was having headache from time to time for the last 6 months. In my office suddenly she screamed raising hands and trying to catch me. I started recite Ruqyah and she became so aggressive that we were four people on her trying to immobilize her as she wanted to harm me. When she became calm, I remembered the conversation with Jinni described in Ibn Taymiyah's Essay Jinn (Demons) book and asked the name of the Jinni. She answered by male voice: "Ahmad." I asked from where was Ahmad. Patient answered: "From Pakistan." I asked when he entered into lady patient's body and for what reason. Patient answered (Jinni speaking): "I love her and I want to marry her. 6 months ago." Then patient became again very agitated, aggressive and I continued the recitation of Ruqyah, reminded Jinni the purpose of his creation which is the same as of the human creation – to worship Allah Alone. I reminded him to fear Allah, the Judgment Day, and ordered him to leave body through the left foot. Then patient became very calm and very tired. I asked: "Where are you?" Patient (Jinni speaking) answered: "I left." I asked: "Did you leave her by her left foot?" Patient answered: "No, by her head." Patient said that she was going to sleep dressed but in the morning she was naked. I advised her to pray, to stop sins (she had a boyfriend), learn the Qur'an. After some time, she was Jinn re-possessed as continued with sins.

7. During labor of one of my patients, few minutes after epidural anesthesia, her heart rate went up to 200 bpm. She was healthy before. It was her second delivery. First delivery was quick and normal, and under epidural anesthesia. This time, she was in instance of divorce (divorce is caused by Devils). Few minutes later after tachycardia, her baby heart beat went dramatically down and disappeared. We rushed to the operating theater. Emergency C-section was performed. Baby was extracted blue, atonic and without signs of life. There was a silence in the room. After few minutes of neonatal resuscitation, we heard a very weak cry, baby was admitted to NICU. After finishing the surgery, I went to NICU, baby was pink, breathing spontaneously, recovered very quick by Allah' s Grace. Patient was seen by the cardiologist, the investigations were done, all were normal. Two days after the discharge from the hospital, she called me with the severe pain in her bones, joints, muscle, she couldn't move. She presented Jinn Possession symptoms: sudden tachycardia with normal investigations in previously healthy person, which occurred after epidural anesthesia (Satan's excitation by drugs), sudden bone, joints, muscle pain, presenting the autoimmune disease.

8. Two sisters came to see me: one with the history of infertility, ovarian cyst and miscarriage and another with depression, difficulties to get married. On the recitation of Ruqyah, the first had a headache and the second had inappropriate involuntary movements and frequent yawning which are the Jinn Possession symptoms.

9. Young patient with permanent migraine and all normal investigations – it is a Jinn Possession. She had tattoo and tattoo is from Satan.

10. I was contacted by email from Croatia, man said that his wife was in coma for two months and doctors didn't know the cause and couldn't help. I said that she was a Jinn possessed and doctors cannot help. That he should recite Ruqyah over her. He invited one imam from the

Mosque who after the recitation of the Qur'an confirmed what I said and said that it was by Black Magic. Imam said to him to pray. After some time, he found under the pillow the bracelet made from the threads with the knots, it was a Black Magic.

11. The mother of my colleague stopped speaking and moving. She was admitted in ICU. I met my colleague during Fajr prayer in the Mosque and she asked me to recite Ruqyah over her mother. I was already reciting Ruqyah for cancer patient in the same ICU department in American hospital Dubai. When I was entering the room, my colleague was with her mother and she said: "Look, look, my mother raised her hand for the first time, when you entered…" By the end of one-hour Ruqyah, suddenly her mother moved her head and hand, and said long phrase. By this time, we were three doctors in the room: me, her daughter and ICU doctor. The Qur'an is a Miracle of miracles!

12. On my way to the hospital to do Ruqyah for my colleague, at the entrance of the hospital there was a man about 45 y-old, crying from severe shooting pain like electrical shock in the hands, legs and other parts of body, his legs were purple, almost black, because of severe vascular problem (beginning of gangrene). He said that the same day in the morning he had heart attack. He had three diseases (cardiovascular disease, diabetes and the third I don't remember). I started to recite Du'a for pain, then Ruqyah. After about 30 minutes, the pain started to decrease and disappeared. He got up, walked and even tried to clean after other people. He said that he was a successful businessman, had business with his partners. There was a dispute between partners, they were separated. The business went bankrupt. His wife and children left him. And he is alone, sick and with no money. He looked, even sick and suffering, like someone with high degree education and respectable. He was from Makkah. And I was asking him to repeat after me the Du'a in Arabic! This was a typical case of Black Magic.

13. Then I went to hospital room with the intention to recite Ruqyah for my colleague. When I reached him, he said that he recited whole Baqarah and he felt great. This was his second admission. He, 40 y-old, was previously healthy. Suddenly, he had very stressful angina like he was going to die. He was admitted to the hospital; all investigations were normal. He was discharged but re-admitted for angina again. He had more and expensive investigations: all normal. I said it was from Shaytan. He did his researches, it was corresponding more to the Evil Eye.

14. Two Cancer cases were described in my book "Cancer is a Jinn (Demonic) Possession. The Ultimate Cure". Almighty God guided me in the diagnosis of the Jinn Possession as a cause of Cancer. There were several Jinn. The Evil Jinn manifested quickly to Negative Ions. Under Ruqyah recitation, about four Jinn left body within 2 weeks of Ruqyah recitation.

15. Several Infertility Jinn Possession cases were described in my book "Infertility Caused by Decreased Oxygen utilization and Jinn (Demons)".

16. A lady in the Mosque with infertility problem said that she was compressed from behind by invisible force, causing her stress and fear. I said that it was a Jinn. She said that saw a dream

that one woman from her relatives did a Black Magic on her causing infertility. I advised her to recite the Qur'an. Reading the Qur'an, she felt very relaxed. Then, Allah showed her in the dream that she had a daughter. Allah knows best.

17. Constipation during two weeks with normal habitual eating. Patient had Ruqyah water with honey, lemon, ginger and cloves which I prepared myself for her as I drink only Ruqyah water with honey, lemon, ginger and cloves. She drunk Ruqyah water and went to toilet. Almighty Allah relieved her thrice and she felt very happy. She shared her constipation problem only after she was relieved.

18. I heard that my family member was admitted to the hospital for thrombophlebitis for 10 days. I went to visit her after Asr prayer; she was already at home few days. That day, she was attacked by the Evil Jinn (chest tightening) and didn't pray Asr prayer. I advised her to pray immediately. In the house I found Turkish Blue Eye Beads Charms Pendants (Shirk), many pictures and statues of the animated beings (people, birds, animals, insects - attracting Devils and repugning Angels). She was wearing Taweez (Black Magic) on her neck. Blood clots and angina were caused by the Evil Jinn. I advised her to pray Tawbah prayer and ask Allah's forgiveness, pray on time, break and throw Shirks objects and pictures and statues with animated images. I destroyed the Taweez according Islamic procedure under the recitation of the last 3 Surahs of the Qur'an and Du'a for Protection from all evil:

Bismillahil-lazee la ya-dur-ru ma'as-mihi shai'un fil-ardi wa la fis-sama'i, wa Hu-was-Sami'ul-'Alim

Meaning: In the Name of Allah with Whose Name there is protection against every kind of harm in the earth or in the heaven, and he is the All-Hearing and All-Knowning.

19. Woman afflicted by cancer. Husband contacted me for my book "Cancer is a Jinn (Demonic) Possession. The Ultimate Cure." But his wife died few days later. "A week before she passed, she was vomiting strange objects - pieces of brown rolled up (some knotted) symmetrically shaped papers. The Sihr is also confirmed by an ustaz specialised in Ruqya Shariah."

'Uthman bin 'Affan (May Allah be pleased with him) reported: The Messenger of Allah (peace and blessings be upon him) said, "He who recites three times every morning and evening: 'Bismillahil-ladhi la yadurru ma'as-mihi shai'un fil-ardi wa la fis-sama'i, wa Huwas-Sami'ul-'Alim (In the Name of Allah with Whose Name there is protection against every kind of harm in the earth or in the heaven, and He is the All-Hearing and All- Knowing', nothing will harm him. (Ibn Majah) (https://hadeethenc.com/en/browse/hadith/6093)

19. Removal of the Evil Jinn by Miraculous Negative Ions. (524, 529-538)

Complications after taking medications including vaccines in Jinn diseases

Majority of people are Jinn Possessed because of disbelief and transgressions of our Creator's Laws (the Qur'an and Sunnah). When they take drugs or undergo the surgeries, the Jinn react aggressively to the foreign toxic chemical substances named medications, what about the human body and soul?

Complications are countless, here there are only some examples.

1) Hallucinations visual, auditory, olfactory, tactile, gustatory, and general somatic.
2) Leukopenia, Lymphopenia, thrombocytopenia. Lymphopenia may be considered as a cardinal laboratory finding, with prognostic potential. Neutrophil/lymphocyte ratio and peak platelet/lymphocyte ratio may also have prognostic value in determining severe cases.
3) Angina, Heart attack, Stroke, Myocarditis, Pericarditis, Tachycardia, etc.
4) Respiratory diseases, Tonsilitis, sore throat, etc.
5) Encephalopathy, Meningitis, Myelitis, Guillain-Barre syndrome, Multiples Sclerosis, Paralysis, Parkinson, Spinal muscular atrophy (SMA), Epilepsy, Headache, Anosmia, Ageusia, Dementia, Memory loss, etc.
6) Asthma and Allergies.
7) Autoimmune diseases.
8) Skin Diseases.
9) Musculoskeletal diseases.
10) Priapism
11) Disseminated Intravascular Coagulation (DIC), Thromboembolism, Pulmonary Embolism, etc.
12) Kidney insufficience, Liver insufficience, etc.
13) Anxiety, Stress, Depression, Psyhosis, Compulsive Behaviors, etc.
14) Other diseases. (539)

Stevens-Johnson Syndrome (SJS) is a rare, life-threatening hypersensitivity reaction of the skin and mucous membranes. During SJS, large macules rapidly spread and form together, leading to blistering, necrosis and shedding of the skin. The number one cause is medication-related—common ones including sulfonamides, antiepileptics, allopurinol, and nonsteroidal anti-inflammatory drugs. Lamotrigine (Lamictal) is an antiepileptic drug of the phenyltriazine class that is indicated for the prevention of focal and generalized seizures in epileptic patients as well as monotherapy or adjunctive maintenance treatment for Bipolar disorder. Lamotrigine has a relatively high incidence of SJS, especially when initiated at high doses, which led the FDA to require a black box warning on its package labeling to inform consumers of this risk. Other medications that may cause SJS include allopurinol (Zyloprim), acetaminophen (Tylenol), ibuprofen (Motrin), naproxen (Aleve), sulfa drugs, penicillin, barbiturates and other anticonvulsants. (540, 541)

In the UK, the number of **antipsychotic prescriptions** is rising faster than the number of psychosis diagnoses. About 50% of the prescriptions are for people without a diagnosis of psychosis or bipolar disorder. The side-effects of antipsychotic drugs can be severe. Tremors, muscle stiffness, restlessness and muscle spasms are common side-effects with older, first-generation antipsychotic drugs, which are still widely prescribed. Other side-effects with all generations of antipsychotics include constipation, bed wetting, sexual dysfunction and weight gain. There are also health-related side effects like heart problems, liver disorders, seizures and neuroleptic malignant syndrome (a rare but potentially life-threatening reaction to antipsychotic drugs). (542)

Antiarrhythmic agents that list sudden cardiac death within their package inserts include sotalol (Betapace), amiodarone (Cordarone), and procainamide (Procanbid). Lastly, the labeling for morphine and Adderall includes warnings about increased risk of sudden death due to cardiac abnormalities. (543)

Baboon Syndrome resulting from systemic drugs. The term 'baboon syndrome' (BS) was introduced 20 years ago to classify patients in whom a specific skin eruption resembling the red gluteal area of baboons occurred after systemic exposure to contact allergens. (544, 545)

Cholesterol is a natural component in everyone's blood, and supports functions within the body. It's only when bad cholesterol causes plaque to build up in your arteries that it's considered a major risk factor for heart attack, heart disease and stroke.

Doctor prescribed medicine for high cholesterol. "I took 10 mg of atorvastatin. I noticed I started having very detailed and vivid nightmares. (I would rather be awake than be in these nightmares.)… I am also having memory issues (e.g. could not remember the names of close colleagues from only two years ago). I recently saw an article that suggested there may be a link between dementia and use of statins." (546)

All diseases, nightmares and memory loss mentioned above are caused by the Evil Jinn.

Postoperative Complications in Jinn Diseases.

1) Stroke
2) Blood Clots (Deep Vein Thrombosis (DVT) and Pulmonary Embolism (PE)
3) Reduced kidney function
4) Heart rhythm problems
5) Atrial fibrillation
6) Muffled hearing or thumping sensations in your chest, head or ears
7) Postoperative Delirium
8) Nightmare
9) Urinary retention
10) Post-operative cognitive dysfunction (POCD)
11) Blurred vision
12) Tingling and numbness
13) Sleeping problems
14) Memory Loss
15) Death
16) Other (547)

The correct terminology for Postoperative Dellirium is the Jinn (Demonic) Possession.

Devils cannot be cut, they are invisible, that's way the surgery in the majority of diseases are not indicated and even dangerous. When the surgeon tries to cut, Devils move the lesion to another place or spead over the body (metastasis).

It is important to diagnose diseases caused by the Evil Jinn as they are removed only by Allah: Ruqyah, Negative Ions, both in the Noble Qur'an.

639. Undesirability of Departing from or Coming to a Place Stricken by an Epidemic

Allah, the Exalted, says:

"Wheresoever you may be, death will overtake you even if you are in fortresses built up strong and high!" (Qur'an, An-Nisa 4:78)

"And do not throw yourselves into destruction." (Qur'an, Al-Baqarah 2:195)

Ibn 'Abbas (May Allah be pleased with him) reported: 'Umar bin Al-Khattab (May Allah be pleased with him) set out for Ash-Sham (the region comprising Syria, Palestine, Lebanon and Jordan). As he reached at Sargh (a town by the side of Hijaz) he came across the governor of Al-Ajnad, Abu 'Ubaidah bin Al-Jarrah (May Allah be pleased with him) and his companions. They informed him that an Epidemic had broken out in Syria. Ibn 'Abbas relates: 'Umar (May Allah be pleased with him) said to me: "Call to me the earliest Muhajirun (Emigrants)." So, I called them. He sought their advice and told them that an Epidemic had broken out in Ash-Sham. There was a difference of opinion whether they should proceed further or retreat to their homes in such a situation. Some of them said: 'You have set forth to fight the enemy, and therefore you should not go back;' whereas some of them said: 'As you have along with you many eminent Companions of Messenger of Allah (peace and blessings be upon him), we would not advice you to set forth to the place of the Plague (and thus expose them deliberately to a danger).' 'Umar (May Allah be pleased with him) said: 'You can now go away.' He said: 'Call to me the Ansar (the Helpers)." So, I called them to him, and he consulted them and they differed in their opinions as well. He said: 'Now, you may go." He again said: 'Call the old (wise people) of the Quraish who had emigrated before the conquest of Makkah.' I called them. 'Umar (May Allah be pleased with him) consulted them in this issue and not even two persons among them differed in the opinions. They said: 'We think that you should go back along with the people and do not take them to this scourge. 'Umar (May Allah be pleased with him) made an announcement to the people, saying: 'In the morning I intend to go back, and I want you to do the same." Abu 'Ubaidah bin Al-Jarrah (May Allah be pleased with him) said: 'Are you going to run away from the Divine Decree?" Thereupon 'Umar (May Allah be pleased with him) said: 'O Abu 'Ubaidah! Had it been someone else to say this.' ('Umar (May

Allah be pleased with him) did not like to differ with him). He said: 'Yes, we are running from the Divine Decree to the Divine Decree. What do you think if you have camels and you happen to get down a valley having two sides, one of them covered with foliage and the other being barren, will you not act according to the Divine Decree if you graze them in vegetative land? In case you graze them in the barren land, even then you will be doing so according to the Divine Decree. There happened to come 'Abdur-Rahman bin 'Auf who had been absent for some of his needs. He said: 'I have knowledge about it. I heard the Messenger of Allah (peace and blessings be upon him) saying, 'If you get wind of the outbreak of Plague in a land, you should not enter it; but if it spreads in the land where you are, you should not depart from it.' Thereupon 'Umar bin Khattab (May Allah be pleased with him) praised Allah and went back." (Bukhari and Muslim)

Commentary:
This Hadith highlights the following four important points:

1. The test of validity of any decision is its correspondence with Shariah.
2. The desirability of mutual consultation.
3. The power of the Imam to depart from the advice of the consultative body.
4. The responsibility of the Imam to make every possible effort for the security of his subjects. (548)

Narrated Usama bin Zaid: "Allah's Messenger (peace and blessings be upon him) said: "Plague was a means of torture sent on a group of Israelis (or on some people before you). So. if you hear of its spread in a land, don't approach it, and if a Plague should appear in a land where you are present, then don't leave that land in order to run away from it (i.e. Plague)." (Bukhari)

640. Undesirability of Reviling Fever

Jabir (May Allah be pleased with him) reported: "The Messenger of Allah (May Allah's peace and blessings be upon him) visited Umm As-Sā'ib (or Umm al-Musayyab) and asked her: "What ails you, O Umm As-Sa'ib (or Umm al-Mūsayyab)? You are shivering!" She replied: "It is the fever; may Allah not bless it!" He said to her: "Do not curse the fever, for it removes the sins of the children of Adam the same way the bellows remove the impurities of iron." (Muslim)
(https://hadeethenc.com/en/browse/hadith/8961)

Narrated Nazi': Abdullah bin 'Umar said, "The Prophet said, 'Fever is from the heat of Hell, so put it out (cool it) with water.'" Nafi' added: 'Abdullah used to say, "O Allah! Relieve us from the punishment (when he suffered from fever)." (Bukhari)

Narrated Fatima bint Al-Mundhir: "Whenever a lady suffering from fever was brought to Asma' bint Abu Bakr, she used to invoke Allah for her and then sprinkle some water on her body, at the chest and say, "Allah's Apostle used to order us to abate fever with water." (Bukhari)

Narrated 'Aisha (May Allah be pleased with her): The Prophet (peace and blessings be upon him) said, "Fever is from the heat of Hell, so abate fever with water." (Bukhari)

Narrated Ibn 'Abbas: "Allah's Apostle entered upon sick man to pay him a visit, and said to him,

"Don't worry, Allah willing, your sickness will be an expiation for your sins." The man said, "No, it is but a fever that is boiling within an old man and will send him to his grave." On that, the Prophet said, "Then yes, it is so." (Bukhari)

641. Pharma Fraud

Allah, the Exalted, says:

"And believe in what I have sent down (this Qur'an), confirming that which is with you, [the Taurat (Torah) and the Injeel (Gospel)], and be not the first to disbelieve therein, and buy not with My Verses [the Taurat (Torah) and the Injeel (Gospel)] a small price (i.e. getting a small gain by selling My Verses), and fear Me and Me Alone." (Tafsir At-Tabari, vol.1, p.253) (Qur'an, Al-Baqarah 2:41)

"The disbelievers are in nothing but delusion." (Qur'an, Al-Mulk 67:20)

Anas b. Malik reported that Allah's Messenger (peace be upon him) said: "It would be said to the non-believers on the Day of Resurrection: 'If you were to possess gold, filling the whole earth, would you like to secure your freedom by paying that?' He would say: 'Yes.' Thereupon it would be said to him: 'Something easier (than this) was demanded from you (but you paid no heed to it).'" (Muslim)

The Messenger of Allah (peace and blessings be upon him) didn't recommend the medico-surgical treatment in majority of diseases as the cause of the disease is a sin.

Medical and Pharmaceutical companies' monopoly, FDA, WHO, CDC transgressed Almighty God's Laws, with misinformation, misguidance, lying, fraudulent trial and marketing, forced western inappropriate guidelines and fraudulent practice, exaggerated prices, approving poisonous drugs (silent weapons), etc., with the only purpose is to get bumper financial profit and control humanity. Patients are forced into medical-related debt and bankruptcy because of the expensive cost and longue duration of treatment.

Doctors (except few) have no knowledge of the Qur'an healing, Negative Ions and Prophetic Medicine based on natural treatment as in the whole medical education there is nothing about the miraculous Divine Cure which doesn't leave traces of disease, without spending money, time, energy, being at home and having Allah's rewards for the Qur'an recitation and Du'as.

642. Vaccination Fraud

Allah, the Exalted, says:

"Like those before you, they were mightier than you in power, and more abundant in wealth and children. They had enjoyed their portion awhile, so enjoy your portion awhile as those before you enjoyed their portion awhile; and you indulged in play and pastime (and in telling lies against Allah and His Messenger Muhammad SAW) as they indulged in play and pastime. Such are they whose deeds are in vain in this world and in the Hereafter. Such are they who are the losers." (Qur'an, At-Tawbah 9:69)

"(They took to flight because of their) arrogance in the land and their plotting of evil. But the evil plot encompasses only him who makes it. Then, can they expect anything (else), but the Sunnah (way of dealing) of the peoples of old? So, no change will you find in Allah's Sunnah (way of dealing), and no turning off will you find in Allah's Sunnah (way of dealing)." (Qur'an, Fatir 35:43)

"Know that the life of this world is only play and amusement, pomp and mutual boasting among you, and rivalry in respect of wealth and children, as the likeness of vegetation after rain, thereof the growth is pleasing to the tiller; afterwards it dries up and you see it turning yellow; then it becomes straw. But in the Hereafter (there is) a severe torment (for the disbelievers, evildoers), and (there is) Forgiveness from Allah and (His) Good Pleasure (for the believers, good-doers), whereas the life of this world is only a deceiving enjoyment." (Qur'an, At-Hadid 57:20)

Other Verse: *Al-Anfal 8:30.*

People should believe in Predestination. Everything happens only by Allah's Will and Decree.

When people disobey Allah (cause), Allah sent the diseases and calamities (effect) to remind people the purpose of human creation, to expiate sins or punish the wrongdoers.

Vaccines cannot prevent or cure as cannot remove sins or Devils. They only aggravate existing diseases by exciting the Evil Jinn, create new disease and death.

Our Creator warned:

"Because of that We ordained for the Children of Israel that if anyone killed a person not in retaliation of murder, or (and) to spread mischief in the land - it would be as if he killed all mankind, and if anyone saved a life, it would be as if he saved the life of all mankind. And indeed, there came to them Our Messengers with clear proofs, evidences, and signs, even then after that many of them continued to exceed the limits (e.g. by doing oppression unjustly and exceeding beyond the limits set by Allah by committing the Major sins) in the land!" (Qur'an, Al-Ma'idah 5:32)

The Muslim countries should follow the Glorious Qur'an and Sunnah and do not follow blindly the disbelievers following Satan.

Allah, the Exalted, says:

"O Prophet (Muhammad SAW)! Keep your duty to Allah, and obey not the disbelievers and the hypocrites (i.e. do not follow their advices). Verily! Allah is Ever All-Knower, All-Wise." (Qur'an, Al-Ahzab 33:1)

"So, obey not the disbelievers, but strive against them (by preaching) with the utmost endeavour, with it (the Qur'an)." (Qur'an, Al-Furqan 25:52)

The Prophet (peace and blessings be upon him) didn't recommend medical treatment (Chapter "Diseases caused by Positive Ions").

The Prophet (peace and blessings be upon him) introduced the concept of Quarantine 1400 years ago.

Narrated Saud: The Prophet (peace and blessings be upon him) said, "If you hear of an outbreak of Plague in a land, do not enter it; but if the Plague breaks out in a place while you are in it, do not leave that place." (Bukhari)

On December 14th 2020, when I was praying during Pandemic, Allah Allmighty said to me that with the mass vaccination there will be more death and urged me to write a book about vaccination.

We see the highest pic of death after the first mass Covid-19 vaccination (December 2020 – January 2021), then the pics of death after the following mass vaccinations: https://www.worldometers.info/coronavirus.

My book "Vaccines for Coronavirus and Other Diseases Increase Death" describes the history of epidemics, the events which caused the epidemics (cause and effect or action and reaction), vaccines and death after vaccination. (549)

All fraudulent politics around vaccines, claiming that they reduce mortality while they increase death, introducing fine for vaccination refusal, censuring doctors for anti-vaccine claims, threatening people, restricting the travel for unvaccinated people, etc. – all these only confirm the faudulous plan of criminals.

Narrated Abu Sirmah that the Messenger of Allah (peace and blessings pf Allah be upon him) said: "Whoever harms others, Allah Almighty will harm him; and whoever causes hardship to other Allah will cause hardship to him." (Ibn Majah)

Abu Sa'id al-Khudri (May Allah be pleased with him) reported that the Prophet (May Allah's peace and blessings be upon him) said: ''There should be neither harm nor reciprocating harm.'' (Ibn Majah)
(https://hadeethenc.com/en/browse/hadith/4711)

643. Children Vaccination

Allah, the Exalted, says:

"The mothers shall give suck to their children for two whole years, (that is) for those (parents) who desire to complete the term of suckling . . ." *(Qur'an, Al-Baqarah 2:233)*

When the newborn is born, Allah's Miracle, God prepared for him the breast milk, another Allah's Miracle. Breast milk contains everything that baby needs including the antibodies protecting him from diseases. The Creator recommended the breastfeeding for two years.

Threatening that if baby doesn't have vaccines, he may become sick and even die – it is a disbelief in Allah's Predestination which is a Major sin.

What will happen in the future, only Allah knows the Unseen. Will the child be sick or non, it was already written in his book in Lawh Al-Mahfuz which is with Allah.

Following the CDC obligatory vaccination schedules, the healthy innocent child receives around 30 vaccines between his birth and 3 years of old. The injection of multiples vaccines at one time overload increases the harmful effects and lead to death.

Many articles and books were written by doctors warning about danger of vaccines. (549-548)

644. Coronavirus Vaccination

Allah, the Exalted, says:

"No calamity befalls on the earth or in yourselves but is inscribed in the Book of Decrees before We bring it into existence. Verily, that is easy for Allah." (Qur'an, Al-Hadid 57:22)

The Qur'an has predicted Coronavirus in 7th century:

"Over it are nineteen (angels as guardians and keepers of Hell). (Qur'an, Al-Muddaththir 74:30)

"And We have set none but angels as guardians of the Fire, and We have fixed their number (19) only as a trial for the disbelievers, in order that the people of the Scripture (Jews and Christians) may arrive at a certainty [that this Qur'an is the truth as it agrees with their Books i.e. their number (19) is written in the Taurat (Torah) and the Injeel (Gospel)] and the believers may increase in Faith (as this Qur'an is the Truth) and that no doubts may be left for the people of the Scripture and the believers, and that those in whose hearts is a disease (of hypocrisy) and the disbelievers may say: "What Allah intends by this (curious) example?" Thus, Allah leads astray whom He wills and guides whom He wills. And none can know the hosts of your Lord but He. And this (Hell) is nothing else than a (warning) reminder to mankind." (Qur'an, Al-Muddaththir 74:31)

On December 14th 2020, during my prayer, Almighty God said to me that with the mass vaccination will be more death and urged me to write the book. It was shocking to read online that death rate jumped very high immediately after the first mass vaccination campaign in USA confirming our Creator's Statement and He is All-Knowing, All-Seeing, All-Hearing and All-Aware!

"Indeed, Allah does not wrong the people at all, but it is the people who are wronging themselves." (Qur'an, Yunus 10:44)

Coronavirus is a Jinn (Demonic) Possession disease because of humanity's sins. (557, 558)

The most affected countries are the most sinful countries – USA and India on the top of list!

https://www.worldometers.info/coronavirus/countries-where-coronavirus-has-spreadRapid spread of Rapid spread of Coronavirus around the globe in a blink of eye, reaching even the isolated places with no contact with Coronavirus affected people, the diversity of symptoms, accelerated innumerable mutations at an unprecedented speed and scale - can be only explained by the Jinn involvement.

Additionally, the pandemic has set off a wave of scams around the world, including fake vaccines.

The Prophet Muhammad recommended in Epidemics only quarantine and no medical treatment.

Narrated Usama bin Zaid: Allah's Messenger (peace and blessings be upon him) said, "Plague was a means of torture sent on a group of Israelis (or on some people before you). So, if you hear of its spread in a land, don't approach it, and if a Plague should appear in a land where you are present, then don't leave that land in order to run away from it (i.e. Plague)." (Bukhari)

Narrated Abu Hurairah: Allah's Apostle said, 'There is no 'Adha (no disease is conveyed from the sick to the healthy without Allah's permission), nor Safar, nor Hama." A bedouin stood up and said, "Then what about my camels? They are like deer on the sand, but when a mangy camel comes and mixes with them, they all get infected with mangy." The Prophet said, "Then who conveyed the (mange) disease to the first one?" (Bukhari)

Narrated Sa'd: Allah's Messenger (peace and blessings be upon him) said, "He who eats seven 'Ajwa dates every morning, will not be affected by poison or magic on the day he eats them." (Bukhari)

645. Post-Vaccination Diseases

Coma after Vaccination Covid-19

Sarah, the 46-year-old, in England, developed distressing symptoms after getting vaccinated against COVID-19. These included dizziness, backache and tingling in toes and tongue. Later she suddenly collapsed and remained in a coma for four days. She has also been diagnosed with Guillain-Barré syndrome. (552)

Previously there were only some nations touched by Epidemics but now it is a pandemic spread around the globe to remind the disbelievers to turn back to the Creator. The mischief on the earth, on the sea and in the air reached the culminative point including mass obligatory vaccination (killing silently).

Vaccines cannot prevent or cure as cannot remove sins and Devils.

They are dangerous.

646. Death Following Vaccination

Abdullah ibn Masud reported: The Messenger of Allah (peace and blessings be upon him) said, "Verily, Satan has influence with the son of Adam and the angel has influence. As for the influence of Satan, he promises evil and denies the truth. As for the influence of the angel, he promises goodness and affirms the truth. Whoever finds this goodness, let him know that it is from Allah and let him praise Allah. Whoever finds something else, let him seek refuge in Allah from the accursed Satan." Then, the Prophet recited the Verse, "*Satan threatens you with poverty and commands evil, but Allah promises you forgiveness and grace from Him." (2:268)* (Tirmidhi)

On December 14th 2020, Almighty Allah warned me during my prayer that there will be more death with mass Covid-19 vaccination. After prayer I went to my laptop and it was shocking to read:

"Covid's strange moment: Joy over vaccines coincides with new levels of deaths and hospitalizations in U.S." on Stat news.

"The vaccines — the elixirs that will help drag this pandemic to a close — had finally arrived… And yet, even as the images of trucks, planes and unpacked boxes offered a triumphant respite for a public desperate for hope, the bad news kept knocking. The country crossed 300,000 official deaths from the coronavirus on Monday. It hit a record number of Covid-19 patients hospitalized — more than 110,000, according to the Covid Tracking Project. For the week that ended Monday, the average daily toll included more than 2,300 deaths and more than 210,000 infections, according to STAT's Covid-19 Tracker. It would have been a jarring split screen, if not for the fact that so much of the suffering from Covid-19 has seen people dying or mourning alone. While doctors and nurses administered vaccines in front of cameras as governors kept watch, the 1,300 people who died from the virus Monday largely did so isolated in hospital rooms." (554)

The pics of Coronavirus death on the worldmeter chart (https://www.worldometers.info/coronavirus) correspond to immediate postvaccination periods which reflect exactly God's warning Statement.

The fact that the death pics correspond to immediate postvaccination periods (from few hours to few weeks), aggravation of pre-existing diseases and appearance of new diseases after vaccination, diseases and death in fully vaccinated people prove that vaccines trigger new diseases, aggravate pre-existing diseases and causing death by two ways: 1. by exciting the Evil Jinn in Jinn diseases, 2. by toxicity of vaccines.

As vaccination was made obligatory, the harmful effects are more evident.

An analysis of the VAERS database 1990–2019 and review of the medical literature was performed by Neil Z. Miller: "Of 2605 infant deaths reported to VAERS from 1990 through 2019, 58 % clustered within 3 days post-vaccination and 78.3 % occurred within 7 days post-vaccination, confirming that infant deaths tend to occur in temporal proximity to vaccine administration." (551)

Why Do Vaccinated People Represent Most COVID-19 Deaths Right Now?

The share of COVID-19 deaths among those who are vaccinated has risen. In fall 2021, about 3 in 10 adults dying of COVID-19 were vaccinated or boosted. But by January 2022, as we showed in an analysis posted on the Peterson-KFF Health System Tracker, about 4 in 10 deaths were vaccinated or boosted. (555)

Brain death in a double vaccinated patient with COVID-19 infection.

A 60-year-old woman with medical history for type II diabetes, hypertension, atrial fibrillation on apixaban, and systemic lupus erythematosus, treated with steroids, rituximab, and methotrexate. She had been vaccinated twice. She underwent routine COVID testing and tested positive. The patient was admitted to the ICU due to acute hypoxic respiratory failure. She had antibiotics, high dose steroids for lupus, and remdesivir. She received her home dose of apixaban during the initial 5 days of hospitalization; this was subsequently stopped given development of disseminated intravascular coagulopathy (DIC) with platelet count dropping to a nadir of $20 \times 10^3/\mu L$ (platelet count on presentation $164 \times 10^3/\mu L$) on hospital day 8. On hospital day 13, the patient reported headache, and altered mental status. She was intubated at this time for airway protection. Subsequent head CT demonstrated a new acute to subacute infarct involving the right frontal operculum and insular region, new parenchymal hemorrhages versus hemorrhagic infarcts involving the left parietal lobe and left cerebellar hemisphere, and multifocal acute subarachnoid hemorrhage, etc.

In this unfortunate case, despite double vaccination, this patient who notably was on immunosuppression for systemic lupus erythematosus, succumbed to SARS-CoV-2 infection. Hypoxic respiratory failure, complicated by DIC and acute CVD including ischemic, hemorrhagic and venous thrombotic events were contributory to this patient's death. This case not only is illustrative of classic imaging findings of brain death, but also highlights the vulnerability of immunocompromised patients despite vaccination. (556)

Allah, the Owner of Judgment Day, says:

"And never think that Allah is unaware of what the wrongdoers do. He only delays them (i.e. their account) for a Day when eyes will stare (in horror)." (Qur'an, Ibrahim 14:42)

"So, the evil (consequences) of what they did shall afflict them and that which they mocked shall encompass them." (Qur'an, An-Nahl 16:34)

647. Making Vaccination Obligatory

Allah, the Exalted, says:

"(He Alone) the All-Knower of the Ghaib (Unseen), and He reveals to none His Ghaib (unseen)." (Qur'an, Al-Jinn 72:26)

Narrated Masruq: "I said to 'Aisha, "O Mother! Did Prophet Muhammad see his Lord?" Aisha said, "What you have said makes my hair stand on end! Know that if somebody tells you one of the following three things, he is a liar: Whoever tells you that Muhammad saw his Lord, is a liar." Then Aisha recited the Verse: *'No vision can grasp Him, but His grasp is over all vision. He is the Most Courteous Well-Acquainted with all things.' (6.103)* 'It is not fitting for a human being that Allah should speak to him except by inspiration or from behind a veil.' (42.51) 'Aisha further said, "And whoever tells you that the Prophet knows what is going to happen tomorrow, is a liar." She then recited: *'No soul can know what it will earn tomorrow.' (31.34)* She added: "And whoever tell you that he concealed (some of Allah's orders), is a liar." Then she recited: 'O Apostle! Proclaim (the Message) which has been sent down to you from your Lord.' (5.67) 'Aisha added. "But the Prophet (peace and blessings be upon him) saw Gabriel in his true form twice."

Making vaccine obligatory is unjustified assault on the human rights and freedom. (559)

648. Fine for Vaccination Refusal

This is another way to collect more money.

649. Penalties for Anti-Vaccination Claims

Allah, the Exalted, says:

"Verily, Allah enjoins Al-Adl (i.e. justice and worshipping none but Allah Alone - Islamic Monotheism) and Al-Ihsan [i.e. to be patient in performing your duties to Allah, totally for Allah's sake and in accordance with the Sunnah (legal ways) of the Prophet SAW in a perfect manner], and giving (help) to kith and kin (i.e. all that Allah has ordered you to give them e.g. wealth, visiting, looking after them, or any other kind of help, etc.): and forbids Al-Fahsha' (i.e all evil deeds, e.g. illegal sexual acts, disobedience of parents, polytheism, to tell lies, to give false witness, to kill a life without right, etc.), and Al-Munkar (i.e all that is prohibited by Islamic law: polytheism of every kind, disbelief and every kind of evil deeds, etc.), and Al-Baghy (i.e. all kinds of oppression), He admonishes you, that you may take heed." (Qur'an, An-Nahl 16:90)

Doctors were warned to be censured for anti-vaccine claims. (560)

Hudhayfah ibn Al-Yaman reported: The Prophet (peace and blessings be upon him) said, "By the One in Whose Hand is my soul, you must enjoin good and forbid evil, or else Allah will soon send punishment upon you. Then, you will call upon Allah and it will not be answered for you." (Tirmidhi)

Abu Bakr reported: The Messenger of Allah (peace and blessings be upon him) said, "Verily, if people see an oppressor and they do not seize his hand, Allah will soon send His punishment upon all of them." (Tirmidhi)

It is an obligation on individual and communal level to forbid evil.

650. Repeated Vaccination

Allah, the Exalted, says:

"And never think that Allah is unaware of what the wrongdoers do. He only delays them for a Day when eyes will stare [in horror]." (Qur'an, Ibrahim 14:42)

Repeated vaccination increases harmful effects and death.

651. Multivalent Vaccines

There are more deaths when multiple vaccines administered in one shot. More foreign bodies in the human body, more disruption will happen in all levels.

A three-month-old baby died within two hours of receiving three vaccines under a regular immunization programme, in Maharashtra's Nandurbar on Friday. The baby had received pentavalent vaccine, oral polio drops and rotavirus vaccine. (561)

652. Telling that if you Don't Take this Medicine or Vaccine

Allah, the Exalted, says:

"And if Allah touches you with harm, none can remove it but He, and if He touches you with good, then He is Able to do all things." (Qur'an, An-Nahl 6:17)

"No calamity befalls, but with the Leave [i.e. decision and Qadar (Divine Preordainments)] of Allah, and whosoever believes in Allah, He guides his heart [to the

true Faith with certainty, i.e. what has befallen him was already written for him by Allah from the Qadar (Divine Preordainments)], and Allah is the All-Knower of everything." (Qur'an, At-Taghabun 64:11)

The Prophet (peace and blessings of Allah be upon him) said: "Allah wrote the decrees concerning all created beings fifty thousand years before He created the heavens and the earth." (Muslim)

653. Buying and Selling Expensive Drugs

Allah, the Exalted, says:

"O you who believe! Verily, there are many of the (Jewish) rabbis and the (Christian) monks who devour the wealth of mankind in falsehood, and hinder (them) from the Way of Allah (i.e. Allah's Religion of Islamic Monotheism). And those who hoard up gold and silver [Al-Kanz: the money, the Zakat of which has not been paid], and spend it not in the Way of Allah, - announce unto them a painful torment." (Qur'an, At-Tawbah 9:34)

Anas reported: The Messenger of Allah (peace and blessings be upon him) said, "The son of Adam grows old but remains young in two matters: greed for wealth and greed for long life." (Muslim)

Spinal muscular atrophy (SMA) is rare disease with unknown cause and no cure – means Jinn Possession.

Two new medications for treating a rare and deadly neuromuscular disease have high prices. The scientists argue that they offer only modest benefits with possible health risks, leaving patients with unmet medical needs and possibly with substantial healthcare bills.

In 2019, the FDA approved Zolgensma, a gene therapy that provides a functional copy via viral vector of the gene encoding SMN. The one-time treatment, an intravenous infusion, costs $2,125.000 – one of the most expensive single treatment ever. (562)

FDA approved the first gene therapy for the genetic blood-clotting disorder haemophilia B - a one-time treatment that costs US$3,500.000. The most expensive drug in the world. (563)

Clinical trial data suggest that the single dose of Hemgenix will provide people with moderate to severe haemophilia with adequate protection from uncontrolled bleeding for eight years and longer.

Our Creator says:

"And eat up not one another's property unjustly (in any illegal way e.g. stealing, robbing, deceiving, etc.), nor give bribery to the rulers (judges before presenting your cases) that you may knowingly eat up a part of the property of others sinfully." (Qur'an, Al-Baqarah 2:188)

Narrated Abu Hurairah: Allah's Messenger (peace be upon him) said, "…then on the Day of Resurrection his wealth will be made like a bald-headed poisonous male snake with two black spots over the eyes. The snake will encircle his neck and bite his cheeks and say, 'I am your wealth, I am your treasure.'" (Bukhari) (https://sunnah.com/bukhari/24)

Narrated Anas bin Malik: Allah's Messenger (peace and blessings be upon him) said, "If Adam's son had a valley full of gold, he would like to have two valleys, for nothing fills his mouth except dust. And Allah forgives him who repents to Him." (Bukhari)

654. Gene Therapy

Allah, the Exalted, says:

"(Iblees) said: "Because You have sent me astray, surely I will sit in wait against them (human beings) on Your Straight Path." (Qur'an, Al-A'raf 7:16)

"Then I will come to them from before them and behind them, from their right and from their left, and You will not find most of them as thankful ones (i.e. they will not be dutiful to You)." (Qur'an, Al-A'raf 7:17)

"(Allah) said (to Iblees) "Get out from this (Paradise) disgraced and expelled. Whoever of them (mankind) will follow you, then surely I will fill Hell with you all." (Qur'an, Al-A'raf 7:18)

Other Verse: Al-Baqarah 2:171.

Zolgensma, the one-time treatment, an intravenous infusion of $2,125.000 and Hemgenix of US$3,500.000; the most expensive drugs but the cure remains elusive. (562, 563)

Gene therapy is detrimental as excites Devils caused the disease by toxicity and causes bankruptcy.

Devils can create any chromosomal and genetic mutations.

Gene therapy was tried in many diseases: cancer, cystic fibrosis, heart disease, diabetes, hemophilia, Sickle cell anemia, Severe Combined Immunodeficiency (ADA-SCID / X-SCID or the bubble boy disease), AIDS, Duchenne muscular dystrophy, Huntington's disease, Parkinson's, Neurodegenerative Diseases, Hypercholesterolemia, Alpha-1 antitrypsin, Chronic granulomatous disease (CGD), Fanconi Anemia, Gaucher Disease. Schizophrenia, Alzheimer's disease, Blindness (Leber's congenital amaurosis (LCA), Mesothelioma, Spinal muscular atrophy (SMA), etc.

But all these diseases are caused by Devils, mostly because of sins. Sins and Devils are removed by Allah Only.

655. Cancer Treatment

Cancer is a Jinn (Demonic) Possession because of sins. (524)

"Gut commensal dysbiosis, an unhealthy and inflammatory gut microbiome, systemically changes the mammary tissues of mice that do not have cancer", said researcher Melanie R. Rutkowski, PhD, of UVA Cancer Center." (314)

The Ultimate Cure is a Repentance to Allah, giving up sins, restoring people's rights, following the Divine Guidance (the Glorious Qur'an and Sunnah), doing good deeds, fasting, Ruqyah, Negative Ions and Prophetic Medicine.

Cancer cases:

1. Woman afflicted by Cancer. "A week before she passed, she was vomiting strange objects - pieces of brown rolled up (some knotted) symmetrically shaped papers." Cancer was caused by Sorcery. Husband contacted me by email for this case.
2. Two Cancer cases were cured by Allah through Zamzam water.
    2.1. The story of repentance of Leila Lahlou; she wrote a book in Arabic "Do not forget God" about her miracle cure at Ka'bah from terminal stage of Breast Cancer. Allah cured her after her repentance by Zamzam water. (564)
    2.2. Allah cured terminal stage of Liver cancer by Zamzam water. (565)
3. Cancer cured by Allah through the Du'a. (566)
4. Two Cancer cases were described in my book "Cancer is a Jinn (Demonic) Possession. The Ultimate Cure". The Negative Ions helped to diagnose the presence of the Evil Jinn. Under Ruqyah recitation, several Evil Jinn left the body.

656. Chemotherapy and Nanotherapy

Cancer is a Jinn (Demonic) Possession because of sins. (524)

Chemotherapy by toxicity and expensive price makes people sicker, causes death and bankruptcy.

Chemotherapy is a crime against humanity.

657. Radiotherapy

Cancer is a Jinn (Demonic) Possession because of sins. (524)

Radiotherapy is a dangerous treatment with serious complications.

658. Immunotherapy

Disease is an expiation of sins and caused by the Evil Jinn. Sins and Devils are removed by Allah Only.

Immunotherapy is detrimental treatment as excites the Devils and causes new diseases by toxicity.

One of my infertile patients tried everything: IVF, Intralipid, immunotherapy, etc… She ended up with the consultation online with one of best immunologists in USA to whom she paid 500 USD for 30 min or 1 hour. Then she divorced her husband. Infertility and divorce were caused by Devils.

Infertility is an expiation of sins. (567)

659. Proton-Pump Inhibitors (PPIs) in Cancer Treatment

Cancer is a Jinn (Demonic) Possession because of sins. (524)

Proton-Pump Inhibitors (PPIs) cannot cure or enhance anti-cancer treatment and cannot cause cancer as cancer is caused by the Evil Jinn because of sins.

660. Melatonin in Cancer Treatment

Cancer is a Jinn (Demonic) Possession because of sins. (524)

Melatonin cannot remove sins and the Evil Jinn. Sins and Evil Jinn are removed by Allah Only.

661. Prophylactic Mastectomy

Allah, the Exalted, says:

"And if Allah should afflict you with harm, then there is none to remove it but He..." (Qur'an, Yunus 10-107)

Prophylactic mastectomy is prohibited. It cannot prevent from Cancer as Cancer is a Jinn (Demonic) Possession. (524)

The owner of our bodies and souls is Allah. It is not permissible to amputate a healthy limb due to fear and probability that it may become diseased in the future as this is a form of transgression against that which Allah, the Exalted, has created and is not necessary.

662. Heart Diseases Treatment

Allah the Exalted, says:

"In their hearts is a disease (of doubt and hypocrisy) and Allah has increased their disease. A painful torment is theirs because they used to tell lies." (Qur'an, Al-Baqarah 2:10)

"The Day when there will not benefit (anyone) wealth or children, but only one who comes to Allah with a sound heart." (Qur'an, Ash-Shu'ara 26:88-89)

"And whosoever honors the Symbols of Allah, then it is truly from the piety of the heart." (Qur'an, Al-Hajj 22:32)

Other Verses: Al-Baqarah 2:74, Al-Jathiyah 45:23, Ghafir 40:35, Az-Zumar 39:22, Ali 'Imran 3:8,

Ar-R'ad 13:28, Al-Anfal 8:24, Qaf 50:37.

The Blood clot – the sourse of all evils and sins – from Satan!

Anas ibn Malik (May Allah be pleased with him) reported: Jibreel came to the Messenger of Allah (May Allah's peace and blessings be upon him) while he was playing with his playmates. He took hold of him, laid him on the ground, split open his chest, took the heart out and then extracted a blood clot out of it and said: "That was the Devil's share in you." Then he washed it with Zamzam water in a golden basin and then joined the wounded parts together after he restored the heart to its place. The boys came running to his mother, i.e. his wet nurse, and said: "Muhammad has been killed." They rushed to him and found his color was changed. Anas said: "I used to see the scar of this stitching on his chest." (Muslim) (https://hadeethenc.com/en/browse/hadith/10862)

Abu Hurairah narrated: The Messenger of Allah (peace and blessings be upon him) said: "Verily, when the slave (of Allah) commits a sin, a black spot appears on his heart. When he refrains from it, seeks forgiveness and repents, his heart is polished clean. But if he returns, it increases until it covers his entire heart. And that is the 'Ran' which Allah mentioned: *'Nay, but on their hearts is the Ran which they used to earn.'*" (Tirmidhi)

Narrated An-Nu'man bin Bashir: "I heard Allah's Messenger (peace and blessings be upon him) saying, "… (O people!) Beware! Every king has a Hima and the Hima of Allah on the earth is His illegal (forbidden) things. Beware! There is a piece of flesh in the body if it becomes good (reformed) the whole body becomes good but if it gets spoilt the whole body gets spoilt and that is the heart." (Bukhari)

Zayd ibn Arqam (May Allah be pleased with him) reported that the Messenger of Allah (May Allah's peace and blessings be upon him) used to say: "O Allah, I seek refuge in You from incapacity, laziness, miserliness, decrepitude and the torment of the grave. O Allah, grant me piety and purify my soul as You are the best to purify it. You are its Guardian and Master. O Allah, I seek refuge in You from knowledge that is not beneficial, and from a heart that does not fear (You), and from a soul that does not feel content and from a supplication that is not answered." (Muslim)

(https://hadeethenc.com/en/browse/hadith/5878)

Abu Hurairah (May Allah be pleased with him) reported that the Prophet (May Allah's peace and blessings be upon him) said: ''Allah does not look at your bodies or at your forms, rather He looks at your hearts and deeds." (Muslim) (https://hadeethenc.com/en/browse/hadith/4555)

Ibn 'Umar (May Allah have mercy on him) narrated that the Messenger of Allah (peace and blessings be upon him) said: "Do not talk too much without remembrance of Allah. Indeed, excessive talking without remembrance of Allah hardens the heart. And indeed, the furthest of people from Allah is the harsh-hearted." (Tirmidhi)

Shahr ibn Hawshab (May Allah have mercy on him) reported: "I asked Umm Salama (May Allah be pleased with her): 'O Mother of the Believers, what was the supplication that the Messenger of Allah (May Allah's peace and blessings be upon him) used to say most frequently when he was with you?' She said: "The supplication he said most frequently was: 'O Turner of the hearts, keep my heart firm upon Your religion!'" (Tirmidhi) (https://hadeethenc.com/en/browse/hadith/3142)

Abdullah bin 'Amr bin Al-'As (May Allah be pleased with him) reported: The Messenger of Allah (peace and blessings be upon him) supplicated: "Allahumma musarrifal-qulubi, sarrif qulubana 'ala ta'atika (O Allah! Controller of the hearts, direct our hearts to Your obedience)." (Muslim)

Heart diseases are the Jinn Possession diseases because of sins.

Following conditions associated to Heart diseases are the Jinn Possession diseases too.

> High Cholesterol.
> Diabetes.
> Obesity.
> Autoimmune and inflammatory diseases.
> Chronic kidney disease.
> Metabolic syndrome.

Ibn Taymiyah wrote an excellent book "Diseases of the Hearts and their Cure". (568)

663. Obesity Treatment

Allah, the Exalted, says:

"...and eat and drink but waste not by extravagance, certainly He (Allah) likes not Al-Musrifun (those who waste by extravagance)." *(Qur'an, Al-A'raf 7:31)*

Al-Miqdam ibn Ma'di Karib (May Allah be pleased with him) reported: "I heard the Messenger of Allah (May Allah's peace and blessings be upon him) say: "No man fills a container worse than his stomach. A few morsels that keep his back upright are sufficient for him. If he has to, then he should keep one-third for food, one-third for drink and one-third for his breathing." (Timirdhi)

(https://hadeethenc.com/en/browse/hadith/4723) (552)

Narrated Ibn 'Umar (May Allah have mercy on him): Allah's Messenger (peace and blessings be upon him) said, "A believer eats in one intestine (is satisfied with a little food), and a kafir (unbeliever) or a hypocrite eats in seven intestines (eats too much)." (Bukhari)

Narrated Abu Hurairah (May Allah have mercy on him): Allah's Messenger (peace and blessings be upon him) said, "The food for two persons is sufficient for three, and the food of three persons is sufficient for four persons." (Bukhari)

Abu Hurairah (May Allah be pleased with him) reported that the Messenger of Allah (May Allah's peace and blessings be upon him) said: "Food for two persons suffices for three, and food for three persons suffices for four." In Muslim's narration, Jabir (May Allah be pleased with him) reported that the Prophet (May Allah's peace and blessings be upon him) said: "Food for one person suffices for two, and food for two persons suffices for four, and food for four persons suffices for eight." (Muslim) (https://hadeethenc.com/en/browse/hadith/6057)

'Imran bin Husain (May Allah be pleased with them) reported: The Prophet (peace and blessings be upon him) said, "The best of you, are my contemporaries, then those who follow them, then those who will come after them. ('Imran said, I do not know if he said this twice or thrice). Then, they will be followed by those who will testify but will not be called upon to testify; they will betray the trust, and will not be trusted. They will make vows but will not fulfill them, and obesity will prevail among them." (Bukhari and Muslim)

One of the signs of the Judgment Day: Obesity will be rampant among the people. (569-571)

Obesity is the Jinn Possession disease because of sins.

Obesity is associated with other Jinn Possession diseases and symptoms: Hypertension, Heart diseases, Stroke, Diabetes, Autoimmune diseases, Psychiatric diseases, Cancers, Gout, Kidney Diseases, Laziness, etc. (572-575)

Allah, the Exalted, says:

"Verily, the hypocrites seek to deceive Allah, but it is He Who deceives them. And when they stand up for As-Salat (the prayer), they stand with laziness and to be seen of men, and they do not remember Allah but little." (Qur'an, An-Nisa 4:142)

"And nothing prevents their contributions from being accepted from them except that they disbelieved in Allah and in His Messenger (Muhammad), and that they came not to As-Salat (the prayer) except in a lazy state, and that they offer not contributions but unwillingly." (Qur'an, At-Tawbah 9:54)

Narrated Abu Hurairah: Allah's Apostle (peace and blessings be upon him) said, "Satan puts three knots at the back of the head of any of you if he is asleep. On every knot he reads and exhales the following words, 'The night is long, so stay asleep.' When one wakes up and remembers Allah, one knot is undone; and when one performs ablution, the second knot is undone, and when one prays the third knot is undone and one gets up energetic with a good heart in the morning; otherwise one gets up lazy and with a mischievous heart." (Bukhari)

The Ultimate Cure is a Repentance to Allah, giving up sins, restoring people's rights, following the Divine Guidance (the Glorious Qur'an and Sunnah), doing good deeds, fasting, Ruqyah, Negative Ions and Prophetic Medicine.

664. Diabetes Treatment

Diabetes is the Jinn Possession disease because of sins.

Two patients with Diabetes, one of them a surgeon, received Negative Ions and Ozone therapy by one of my colleagues in our clinic, sugar levels were normalized, they were previously under Insulin therapy.

Recent studies suggested that oral microbiota is an important factor in the development of diabetes, and on the other hand, oral microbiota is also an important avenue for diabetes to cause other oral or systemic complications. (576)

Diabetes is associated to other Jinn Possession diseases:

- Cardiovascular disease.
- Stroke (Brain Attack)
- Atherosclerosis.
- Nerve damage (Diabetic neuropathy).
- Kidney damage (Diabetic nephropathy).
- Eye damage (Diabetic retinopathy).
- Foot damage.
- Skin and Mouth conditions.
- Infections.
- Hearing impairment.
- Autoimmune diseases
- Alzheimer's disease. Dementia.
- Depression.
- Infertility.
- Erectile Dysfunction, Retrograde ejaculation,
- Nausea, vomiting, diarrhea or constipation
- Psychiatric diseases

The data clearly show that diabetes is associated with both **Schizophrenia** itself and with **Antipsychotic drug** treatment. It is important to notice that the increased risk starts from a young age, as early as 15–19 years of age. (577)

Understanding the Risk of Diabetes in Multiples Sclerosis (MS)

Having type 1 diabetes is considered a risk factor for MS. People who have type 1 diabetes have a three-fold higher risk of developing MS than people who do not have type 1 diabetes. On the other hand, type 2 diabetes may be a risk among people who already have MS. (578)

665. Autoimmune Diseases Treatment

There are more than 80 Autoimmune diseases: Diabetes, Psoriasis, Vasculitis, Sarcoidosis, Scleroderma, Multiple sclerosis, Sjogren syndrome, Rheumatoid arthritis, Systemic Lupus Erythematosus, Thyroiditis, etc.

Autoimmune diseases are the Jinn Possession diseases because of sins.

Psychiatric symptoms are common to many autoimmune disorders. Patients often will have mood disorders, anxiety, depression, cognitive deficits, schizophrenia, and psychosis. (579, 580)

Neuropsychiatric symptoms that may be caused by an Autoimmune reaction. Obsessions and Compulsions, Motor and Vocal Tics, Attention Deficits and Hyperactivity, Autism Spectrum Disorders, Seizures and Convulsions, Chronic Fatigue. (581)

Psoriasis is a Jinn Possession by physical contact with sorcery, most of the time the person walked on it. When on the head it can cause loss of hair, in the mouth it can create wounds.

Two patients with Diabetes, one of them a surgeon, received Negative Ions and Ozone therapy, sugar levels were normalized, they were previously under Insulin therapy.

Lupus and Scleroderma patients answered amazingly to Negative Ions treatment. Lupus patient was on the wheel chair and she walked almost normally only after two sessions of Negative Ions (bed) with Dr Ahmed Al Jaziri in Dubai.

666. Psychiatric Diseases Treatment

Allah, the Exalted, says:

> *"And be not like those who forgot Allah (i.e. became disobedient to Allah) and He caused them to forget their own selves, (let them to forget to do righteous deeds). Those are the Fasiqun (rebellious, disobedient to Allah)." (Qur'an, Al-Hashr 59:19)*

"Indeed, the criminals are in error and madness." (Qur'an, Al-Qamar 54:47)

"Shall I inform you (O people!) upon whom the Shayateen (Devils) descend? They descend on every lying (one who tells lies), sinful person." (Qur'an, Ash-Shu'ara 26:221-222)

Other Verse: Al-Baqarah 2:275.

Anas ibn Malik (May Allah be pleased with him) reported that the Prophet (May Allah's peace and blessings be upon him) used to say: "O Allah, I seek refuge in You from leukoderma, insanity, leprosy, and evil diseases." (An-Nasa'i) (https://hadeethenc.com/en/browse/hadith/6047)

Abdullah bin Masud (May Allah have mercy on him) said: *"Whoever recites the following ten Verses of Surah Baqarah*

(1) in the morning, will be saved from Shaytan till the evening, and whoever recites it in the evening will be protected from Shaytan till the morning.

(2) Furthermore, he will not experience unpleasant surprises in his family or wealth.

(3) If these Verses are recited on an insane person, he will be cured."

(Sunan Darimi and Shu'abul Iman)

In another narration Ibn Masud (May Allah have mercy on him) added:

(4) "If it is recited in a home, no Shaytan shall enter it till the morning."

(Sunan Darimi and Al-Mu'jamul Kabir)

Those ten Verses are:

1-4. The first four Verses. (according to some 'Ulama this ends at the word: *'Muflihun'*

(Al-Hirzuth Thamin, vol.1 p.521)

5-7. Ayatul Kursi and the two Verses that follow it.

8-10. The last three Verses.

Abdullah ibn Masud's student; Imam Mughirah ibn Subay' (May Allah have mercy on him) said:

5) *'Whoever recites these ten Verses before sleeping, will not forget the Qur'an.'* (Sunan Darimi and Shu'abul Iman) (582)

"Researching the topic of the Jinn is one of the most difficult of subjects, especially since it has to do with finding out about a hidden world that is not visible and cannot be measured in physical or empirical terms." (583)

Ibn Taymiyah said:

"What he (Imam Ahmad) said is self-evident. The Jinn may possess someone and cause them to speak a language he does not even know. A possessed person may be violently beaten, in a way that even a camel may not endure, yet he neither feels the beating nor is aware of the words he says." (10)

According Imam Abdul-Aziz Ibn Baaz:

"Sihr or Sorcery as defined by Islamic Law consists of charms or incantations that are composed to cause illness, loss of mental stability, death, to separate spouses from each other, or to prevent a man from acts of intimacy with his wife…" (339)

Psychiatric diseases are the Jinn Possession diseases.

Listen the following very informative lectures. (584, 585)

667. Anti-HIV/AIDS Therapy

Allah, the Exalted, says:

"And (remember) Loot (Lot), when he said to his people: 'Do you commit the worst sin such as none preceding you has committed in the 'Aalameen (mankind and jinn)? 'Verily, you practice your lusts on men instead of women. Nay, but you are a people transgressing beyond bounds (by committing great sins).'" (Qur'an, Al-A'raf 7:80-81)

"Verily, by your life (O Muhammad), in their wild intoxication, they were wandering blindly. So As-Saihah (torment - awful cry) overtook them at the time of sunrise. And We turned (the towns of Sodom in Palestine) upside down and rained down on them stones of baked clay. Surely, in this are signs for those who see (or understand or learn the lessons from the Signs of Allah). And verily, they (the cities) were right on the highroad (from Makkah to Syria, i.e. the place where the Dead Sea is now)." (Qur'an, Al-Hijr 15:72-76)

"And come not near to unlawful sex. Verily, it is a Faahishah (i.e. anything that transgresses its limits: a great sin), and an evil way (that leads one to hell unless Allah Forgives him)." (Qur'an, Al-Isra 17:32)

Ibn 'Abbas (May Allah have mercy on him) narrated that the Messenger of Allah (peace and blessings be upon him) said: "Whoever you find doing as the people of Lot did (ie homosexuality), kill the one who does it and the one to whom it is done, and if you find anyone having sexual intercourse with animal, kill him and kill the animal." (Ahmad and the four Imams with a trustworthy chain of narrators)

The crime of Homosexuality is one of the greatest of crimes, the worst of sins and the most abhorrent of deeds, and Allah punished those who did it in a way that He did not punish other nations. It is indicative of violation of the Fitrah, total misguidance, weak intellect and lack of religious commitment, and it is a sign of doom and deprivation of the Mercy of Allah. (586)

HIV/AIDS is a Jinn Possession disease because of sins (Zina, mainly homosexuality).

Anti-HIV treatment including vaccines cannot prevent or cure HIV/AIDS.

668. Epilepsy Treatment

The Prophet Muhammad (peace and blessings be upon him) didn't recommend medical treatment in two causes of Epilepsy: Decreased Oxygen Utilization and Jinn Possession:

1) Epilepsy by Decreased Oxygen Utilization

Abdullah ibn 'Abbas (May Allah be pleased with them said to 'Atā' ibn Abi Rabah: "Shall I show you a woman of the people of Paradise?" 'Atā' said: 'Yes.' He said: "This black woman came to the Messenger of Allah (May Allah's peace and blessings be upon him) and said: 'I suffer from Epilepsy and, as a result, my body becomes uncovered. So, please supplicate to Allah for me.' The Messenger of Allah (May Allah's peace and blessings be upon him) said to her: 'If you wish, be patient and you will enter Paradise; or, if you wish, I will supplicate to Allah to cure you.' She said: 'I will remain patient.' She then said: 'But I become uncovered, so please invoke Allah that I do not become uncovered.' So, he supplicated for her." (Bukhari and Muslim) (https://hadeethenc.com/en/browse/hadith/3160)

2) Epilepsy by Jinn Possession

"Ya'la ibn Murah said: 'I saw Allah's Messenger (peace and blessings be upon him) do three things which no one before or after me saw. I went with him on a trip. On the way, we passed by a woman sitting at the roadside with a young boy. She called out, 'O Messenger of Allah, this boy is afflicted with a trial, and from him we have also been afflicted with a trial. I don't know how many times per day he is seized by fits.' He (peace and blessings be upon him) said: 'Give him to me.' So, she lifted him up to the Prophet. He (peace and blessings be upon him) then placed the boy between himself and the middle of the saddle, opened the boy's mouth and blew in it three times, saying, 'In the Name of Allah, I am the slave of Allah, get out, enemy of Allah!' Then he gave the boy back to her and said: 'Meet us on our return at this same place and inform us how he has managed.' We then went. On our return, we found her in the same place with three sheeps. When he said to her, 'How has your son fared?' She replied: 'By the One Who sent you with the truth, we have not detected anything (unusual) in his behavior up to this time... '" (Musnad Ahmad vol.4, p.170, and al-Haakim, who declared it authentic, in Ibn Kathir's Al bidaya wal nihaya vol.6, p.146) (https://www.kalamullah.com/Books/The%20Exorcist%20Tradition%20In%20Islam.pdf)

Hippocrates in his Treatise on Epilepsy distinguished two causes of Epilepsy and warned against medical treatment of Epilepsy by Jinn Possession.

When Hippocrates explained the cures for Epilepsy, he stated that, "These cures are effective in treating the Epilepsy that results from chemical and material causes. As for the Epilepsy that results from negative forces, these remedies (that he explained and detailed) do not cure it." (https://archive.org/details/HealingWithTheMedicineOfTheProphet_201801/page/n81/mode/2up?view=theater, p.83)

669. Paralysis Treatment

Salamah ibn al-Akwa' (May Allah be pleased with him) reported that a man ate with his left hand in the presence of the Messenger of Allah (May Allah's peace and blessings be upon him), whereupon he said: "Eat with your right hand." The man said: "I cannot do that." Thereupon, he said: "May you not be able to do that." It was only arrogance that prevented the man from doing it, and consequently he could not raise it (his right hand) up to his mouth afterwards." (Muslim) (https://hadeethenc.com/en/browse/hadith/3372)

Aban bin 'Uthman said: "I heard 'Uthman bin 'Affan (May Allah have mercy on him) saying: 'The Messenger of Allah (peace and blessings be upon him) said: "There is no worshiper who says, in the morning of every day, and the evening of every night: 'In the Name of Allah, who with His Name, nothing in the earth or the heavens can cause harm, and He is the Hearing, the Knowing (Bismillāh, alladhi lā yaḍurru ma'a ismihi shai'un fil-arḍi wa lā fis-samā', wa huwas-Samī'ul 'Alīm)' – three times, (except that) nothing shall harm him." And Aban had been stricken with a type of semi-paralysis, so a man began to look at him, so Aban said to him, "What are you looking at? Indeed, the Hadith is as I reported it to you, but I did not say it one day, so Allah brought about His Decree upon me." (Abu Dawud, Tirmidhi and Ibn Majah) (https://hadeethenc.com/en/browse/hadith/6093)

Paralysis is caused by Jinn Possession (except in case of injury).

The miracle cures of two paralytic men in Bethesda and Capernaum by Jesus were in fact performed by Allah through His Messenger, Jesus. Human being cannot cure.

Jesus, visiting Jerusalem for a Jewish feast (John 5:1), encounters one of the disabled people who used to lie here, a man who had been paralyzed for thirty-eight years. Jesus asks the man if he wants to get well. Jesus tells him to pick up his bed or mat and walk; the man is instantly cured and is able to do so.

Later, Jesus finds the man in the Temple, and **tells him not to sin again**, so that nothing worse happens to him. (11)

Jesus, Muslim man, was living in Capernaum and teaching the people there, and on one occasion the people gathered in such large numbers that there was no room left inside the house where he was teaching, not even outside the door. Some men came carrying a paralyzed man but could not get inside, so they made an opening in the roof above Jesus and then lowered the man down. When Jesus saw how faithful they had been, he said to the paralyzed man, "Son, your sins are forgiven..." He says to the man "...get up, take your mat and go home." (12)

Sheikh Wahid Abdussalaam Bali described a case of young lady with total body Paralysis for 2 months by Jinn Possession. Allah Almighty cured her just by recitation of the Surah Al-Falaq and one Du'a! (340)

Paralysis cases in my practice:

1. The mother of my colleague stopped moving and speaking. She was admitted to the hospital. My colleague asked me to recite Ruqyah. When I was entering the room, my colleague was with her mother and she said: "Look, look, my mother raised her hand for the first time when you were entering..." When I finished reciting one-hour Ruqyah, we were three doctors in the room. The mother suddenly said a long phrase. The Qur'an is a Miracle of miracles!

2. The bird was on my road, paralysed, breathing rarely, was going to die. From the opposite side, Allah Almighty sent a man, who observed the bird then went to the supermarket. I took the bird and started to recite Ruqyah, the bird blinked his eyes. The man came back with the bottle of water and sprinkled it on the bird's head. The bird was awakened by water and blinked eyes rapidly but was not moving. I continued reciting Ruqyah, the bird was blinking his eyes rapidly. When I finished reciting short Ruqyah, the bird flew out from my hand. Allah's Miracle! The bird was Jinn Possessed. Satan is made from the fire. The water extinguishes the fire. Satan is afraid of Allah: *"Verily! I fear Allah for Allah is Severe in punishment." (Al-Anfal 8:48)*

670. Treatment of Pain

Narrated Aisha (May Allah be pleased with her), the wife of the Prophet (peace and blessings be upon him): "When the Messenger of Allah (peace and blessings be upon him) suffered from some pain, he recited Mu'awwadhat in his heart and blew (them over him). When the pain became severe, I recited (them) over him and wiped him with his hand in the hope of its blessing." (Abu Dawud)

Abu 'Abdullah 'Uthman ibn Abi al-'As (May Allah be pleased with him) reported that he once complained to the Messenger of Allah (May Allah's peace and blessings be upon him) about a pain that he felt in his body. The Messenger of Allah said: "Place your hand where you feel pain in your body and say: 'Bismillah' three times; and then repeat seven times: 'I seek refuge with Allah's Might and Power from the evil of what I suffer from and what I am wary of)." (Malik) (https://hadeethenc.com/en/browse/hadith/6018) (https://www.youtube.com/watch?v=L6d04SNvot0)

The Evil Jinn can cause persistent pain all over the body. This pain can prevent the person from studying, working, walking, having sexual life with no obvious cause.

Migraine in healthy person with normal investigations, drinking and eating normally is caused by Satan.

Persistent unexplained pelvic pain can lead to diagnostic laparoscopic surgery which in most cases doesn't find anything abnormal.

Upper and low back pains are common in diseases caused by the Evil Jinn.

Bone and joints pains are caused by the Evil Jinn.

Pain Jinn Possession Cases:

1) 60 year of old patient had persistent pain on her vulva. She couldn't sleep. She was seen by many doctors, had different treatments without relief. Two doctors suggested surgery going up to total hysterectomy, adnexectomy…

Clinically, the vulva was absolutely normal, there was only small area around 1 cm very painful. I recommended to apply Anion pantiliners. When I called a week later, her husband was very happy and said that the pain disappeared and she was able to sleep normally.

2) Young woman with Rheumatoid Polyarthritis came to see me for vaginal infection. I recommended her Negative Ions products for the infection and Rheumatoid Polyarthritis. She did her researches on Negative Ions and Rheumatoid Polyarthritis and sent her work to me to help other patients.

3) Young man with severe back pain, walking only few steps and with difficulties, there were skin lesions and behavior changes; all together making Jinn Possession diagnosis. His condition was considerably improved during Ramadan with Tarawih prayers and fastings, with natural Negative Ions (sea), Anion napkins applied on his body with Ruqyah water, and sheep sacrifice with the intention that Allah cure him.

4) Middle aged man couldn't sleep because of foot pain, he was taking painkillers every night. I recommended the Winalite Negative Ions Energy stone. Pain disappeared, he had more energy and good sleep. Then he bought many Energy stones to his family members.

5) The story of Jinn Possession which will shake you.
Every person should read.
Misdiagnosed Jinn Possession with terrible consequences.

2015. Maya, a 10-year-old girl, and her younger brother, were playing with sparklers near their home in Florida, when she had a severe Asthma attack. (587)

My commentary:

Asthma is the Jinn Possession disease
The cure: Ruqyah and Negative Ions only
Jinn Possession by revenge, she accidentally harmed Jinn by sparklers
Jinn sees humans. Humans do not see Jinn.
Parents should learn and teach children the Qur'an and Sunnah and the ways of protection from Satan from the age of 3.

Beata, her mother and nurse, took her to the hospital where she began to complain of a burning sensation in her legs and feet. Within weeks, she could barely walk. Her feet turned inward, she developed lesions, and her legs could no longer support her body. At night, Beata could hear Maya's cries from her bedroom on the other side of the house.

My commentary:
All these are the Jinn Possession manifestations.

Doctors were unable to come up with a diagnosis. Doctors at yet another hospital, Tampa General, thought that Maya's muscle weakness could be explained by an oral steroid she'd been prescribed for her asthma.

My commentary:
Medical treatment is detrimental as excites the Evil Jinn, spreads disease and causes new diseases.

Then one of Beata's patients, whose child suffered from an acute pain condition, recommended that they consult a local anesthesiologist that studied complex regional pain syndrome or CRPS; it is sometimes called "the suicide disease" for its lack of viable treatments.

Anesthesiologist recommended directly Ketamine 1,500 milligrams infusions which is a huge dose. Beata took Maya for ketamine infusions every three to four weeks. Anesthesiologist charged $10,000 per four-day session which was not covered by health insurance.

My commentary:
a) Medical treatment is detrimental as excites the Evil Jinn, spreads disease and causes new diseases.
b) Narcotics should be the last resort after using other possibilities.
c) When indicated, the minimal dose should be prescribed.
d) Exorbitant bills causing bankruptcy.
e) Medicine is a commerce, especially in USA (doctor's and hospital bills).
f) Narcotics side effects, complications, addiction, withdrawal requiring other medications, exorbitant price – dangerous, expensive, have very limited medico-legal indications (e.g. postoperative pain) when pain persists to all other painkillers.

Pain and all symptoms were caused by the Evil Jinn and Jinn is removed only by Allah!

Beata (nurse) worked extra shifts and the family sold a rental property to cover the cost… Maya still required a wheelchair under regular Ketamine infusions.

October 2016. In the middle of the night, Maya woke up complaining of severe abdominal pain. She was acutely sensitive to stimuli of all kinds and that disabling pain radiated through her legs and feet. Maya spent 24 hours in the intensive-care unit at All Children's hospital, screaming and writhing. Maya appeared to shake, squirm and cry out in pain. Light, noise, even showers had become distressing, the droplets of water making her feel like her skin was on fire. All happened while she was already receiving regular Ketamine infusions. So, mother had asked for her daughter Ketamine infusion to be given.

My commentary:
All these are the Jinn Possession manifestations which are aggravated with the medical treatment including Ketamine.
Doctors don't know the causes of diseases and don't know the cure
The Ultimate Cure is from Allah Alone: the Qur'an and Negative Ions Only.

Maya was isolated from her family in the hospital based on the suspicion of child abuse (Munchausen syndrome). But as weeks went by with Maya isolated, she continued to report extreme pain; so, pain was not caused by her mother/parents!

December 2016, a hospital pediatrician had changed Maya's diagnosis from Munchausen by proxy to Factitious disorder.

My commentary:
All doctors missed Jinn Possession diagnosis.
Unjustified separation of Maya from her parents based on the suspicion of child abuse causing additional suffering from both sides.

The strange bumps and lesions that continued to appear on her arms, legs and forehead in isolation - were caused the Evil Jinn.

My commentary:
The Evil Jinn moves around body causing bumps and any kind of lesions.
The pain, bumps, lesions persisted in absence of parents which eliminate the child abuse suspicion.

Persistence of symptoms in isolation did not alter her custody status, and she remained separated from her parents. That was lucrative for the hospital. In the months that Maya was forced to remain there, All Children's billed her insurer more than $650,000 for her treatments, including 174 entries for CRPS, the malady Maya supposedly didn't have.

My commentary:
a) a) Unjustified claim of child abuse, separation of the child from parents,
b) b) Forced hospitalization based on unjustified child abuse suspicion.
c) c) Unjustified exorbitant bill – $650,000.

Hospital attorneys argued that sending Maya home could expose her to harm, and Beata's judge issued a series of continuances that kept her confined to the hospital.

My commentary:
Injustice will bring the darkness on Judgment Day.

Narrated Buraydah ibn al-Hasib: The Prophet (peace be upon him) said: "Judges are of three types, one of whom will go to Paradise and two to Hell. The one who will go to Paradise is a man who knows what is right and gives judgment accordingly; but a man who knows what is right and acts tyrannically in his judgment will go to Hell; and a man who gives judgment for people when he is ignorant will go to Hell." (Abu Dawud)

Beata's behavior changed, sad and desperate, one day she came home drunk. Another day, inside the garage, Beata was found hanging motionless from the ceiling. "I'm sorry," her suicide note read, "but I no longer can take the pain being away from Maya and being treated like a criminal. I cannot watch my daughter suffer in pain and keep getting worse while my hands are tied by the state of FL and the judge!"

My commentary:
Jinn Possession in human's weakness state, extreme sadness.
Allah is Al-Musta'an. This means that not only that Allah is the Helper (An-Naseer), but He is the Only One Whose help first and foremost should be sought. He is the One Who knows, sees, hears and controls all affairs and therefore His help is PERFECT at ALL times. The Ultimate Healer and Ultimate Judge is Allah, the Disposer of all affairs, the Owner of the Universe.
The Glorious Qur'an is the solution for all problems and diseases.

671. Autism Treatment

Autism is a Jinn (Demonic) Possession. Medical treatment is detrimental as excites the Evil Jinn.

Listen to the following informative lectures about Autism. (588-593)

672. Dementia and Alzheimer's Disease Treatment

Allah, the Exalted, says:

"Shaitan (Satan) has overtaken them. So, he has made them forget the remembrance of Allah. They are the party of Shaitan (Satan). Verily, it is the party of Shaitan (Satan) that will be the losers!" (Qur'an, Al-Mujadilah 58:19)

"…none but Shaitan (Satan) made me forget to remember it…" (Qur'an, Al-Kahf 18:63)

Other Verses: Ar-Rum 30:54, Al-Hajj 22:5, Yusuf 12:42, Az-Zukhruf 43:36, Al-Hashr 59:19, At-Tawbah 9:67, Al-An'am 6:68, Al-A'raf 7:201, Ali 'Imran 3:135.

Abdullah bin Masud (May Allah have mercy on him) said: *"Whoever recites the following ten Verses of Surah Baqarah*

1) in the morning, will be saved from Shaytan till the evening, and whoever recites it in the evening will be protected from Shaytan till the morning.
2) Furthermore, he will not experience unpleasant surprises in his family or wealth.
3) If these Verses are recited on an insane person, he will be cured."
(Sunan Darimi and Shu'abul Iman)
In another narration Ibn Masud (May Allah have mercy on him) added:
4) "If it is recited in a home, no Shaytan shall enter it till the morning."
(Sunan Darimi and Al-Mu'jamul Kabir)
Those ten Verses are:
1-4. The first four Verses. (according to some 'Ulama this ends at the word: *'Muflihun'* (Al-Hirzuth Thamin, vol.1 p.521)
5-7. Ayatul Kursi and the two Verses that follow it.
8-10. The last three Verses.
Abdullah ibn Masud's student; Imam Mughirah ibn Subay' (May Allah have mercy on him) said:
5) 'Whoever recites these ten Verses before sleeping, will not forget the Qur'an.' (Sunan Darimi and Shu'abul Iman) (582)

Dementia is a Jinn Possession because of sins. (594-596)

673. Infertility Treatment

Infertility is an Expiation of Sins. (567)

95% of Infertility cases are caused by the Evil Jinn because of sins.

I have published a book and many articles about Infertility. (529-537, 597)

In the case of the Prophet Ibrahim (May Allah have mercy on him), infertility was a test, which turned out in his old age (100 years of old) with amazing Allah's blessings, two Prophets were born.

674. Anti-Allergy Treatment

People living with common allergies such as asthma, hay fever and atopic dermatitis are at greater risk of developing depression, bipolar disorder, anxiety and neuroticism. Researchers report the link was likely not causal. (598)

A new study of data from the UK Biobank confirms the correlation between allergies and mental health. These mental health conditions included depression, major depressive disorder, anxiety, bipolar disorder, schizophrenia, and neuroticism. (599)

Seasonal allergies have been associated with mental health problems. (600)

There is a growing body of research that posits a strong link between allergic conditions such as asthma, allergic rhinitis, and atopic dermatitis, and mental health conditions including depression, anxiety, ADHD, hyperactivity, conduct disorder, bipolar disorder and autism. (601)

Gluten Intolerance Linked to Schizophrenia

From the WEBMD archives, Feb. 20, 2004 — Intriguing early research suggests that people with a genetic intolerance to gluten may also be at increased risk for Schizophrenia. (602)

Celiac Disease is a Risk Factor for Schizophrenia.

People with a history of the digestive disorder celiac disease are three times more likely to develop schizophrenia than those without the disease, according to a report by Danish researchers and a researcher at the Johns Hopkins Bloomberg School of Public Health. The report is published in the February 21, 2004, edition of the British Medical Journal. (603)

There is a Link between Allergies and Mental Health Conditions.

Respiratory allergies, skin allergies (such as eczema) and food allergies or sensitivities have been linked to several emotional, behavioral and developmental issues in children, including: Anxiety, Depression, Bipolar disorder, ADHD, Autism, Hyperactivity, Conduct disorders, etc. (604)

The research has shown connections with psychiatric disorders and other types of chronic inflammatory disease, including multiple sclerosis, rheumatoid arthritis and irritable bowel syndrome.

Ashtma is caused by the Jinn Possession (in case of Maya by vengeance). (587)

Allergies are caused by the Evil Jinn.

675. Ruling on Using Relaxants and Sleeping Pills to Treat Anxiety and Insomnia

Sheikh Ibn 'Uthaymeen (May Allah have mercy on him) was asked:

"What is the ruling on taking sleeping pills or what are called relaxants? Do they come under the heading of narcotics or not? Is that permissible in the case of necessity or if it is advised by a doctor?" He replied: "It is not permissible to use these pills except in the case of necessity, on condition that they be recommended by a knowledgeable doctor, because they are dangerous and have an impact on the function of the brain. If someone uses them, they may bring about relaxation for a short time, but that will be followed by a greater evil. So, it is important to note that it is permissible to use them when there is a need for that, on condition that that be done under the supervision of a doctor and on his advice." (End quote from Fataawa Noor 'ala ad-Darb (tape no. 82, side A) (605)

The basic principle regarding any medicine that contains any kind of narcotic is that it is prohibited, but if they must be used for treatment and there is no permissible alternative, then in that case it is permissible to use them, subject to the following conditions:

1. The patient's need for that medicine has reached the level of necessity or urgent need.

5. The trustworthy Muslim doctor testifies that this narcotic medicine is indeed beneficial for the patient.
6. That use of the medicine is limited to the extent to which it will meet the necessity.
7. That this medicine will not cause any harm greater than or equal to the harm for which it is being used.

Treat your anxiety and insomnia by means of beneficial kinds of treatment that are prescribed in Islamic teachings, such as reading Qur'an, remembering Allah and sending blessings upon His Prophet (blessings and peace of Allah be upon him), for that will bring reassurance to the heart and dispel worries.

Allah, the Exalted, says:

"Those who have believed and whose hearts are assured by the remembrance of Allah."
(Qur'an, Ar-Ra'd 13:28)

Ibn Qayyim (May Allah have mercy on him) wrote the Chapters "Guidance in the Treatment of Worry, Anxiety and Sadnesss" and "Guidance in the Treatment of Fear and Sleeplessness" in his book "Provisions for the Hereafter (Zad Al-Ma'ad) (7)

Anxiety and Insomnia can be caused by the Evil Jinn.

676. Ruling on Stem Cells Therapy

The list of diseases that can be treated with Stem Cells is false as the majority of diseases is caused by the Evil Jinn because of sins. The majority of diseases on the list treated by Stem Cells are cancers, autoimmune diseases, rare diseases, other diseases with unknow cause and no cure – they are all caused by the Evil Jinn.

A number of published papers and case studies support the feasibility of treating spinal cord injury with stem cells. Spinal cord injury (SCI) occurs when the spinal cord becomes damaged, mostly after motor vehicle accidents, falls, acts of violence or sports injuries. (606)

677. Stem Cells from Induced Abortion

In the session of the Islamic Fiqh Council, held during its sixth conference in Jeddah, KSA, 17-23 Sha'baan 1410 AH (14-20 March 1990 CE), after studying the research and recommendations on this subject – which was entitled Using Foetuses as a Source for Organ Transplants – which was also one of the topics of the sixth Medical Fiqh conference held in

Kuwait, 23-26 Rabee' al-Awwal 1410 AH (23-26 October 1990 CE) – in cooperation between this Council and the Islamic Medical Sciences Organization, the following was determined:

1) It is not permissible to use foetuses as a source for organs that are needed for transplant into another individual except in some cases that are subject to conditions that must be met:

1.a) It is not permissible to deliberately induce abortion for the purpose of using the foetus in order to transplant organs into another individual. Rather abortion should be limited to that which is natural and spontaneous (i.e. miscarriage) and not deliberate, or abortion that is carried out for a legitimate Shariah reason. Surgery should not be resorted to in order to extract the foetus except where that is necessary in order to save the mother's life.

1.b) If the foetus is viable (i.e. could survive), then medical treatment should focus on saving and preserving its life, and it should not be used for organ transplants. If the foetus is not viable, it is not permissible to use it except after its death.

2) It is not permissible to use the process of organ transplant for commercial gain under any circumstances.

3) It is essential to delegate responsibility for supervision of organ transplants to a committee of specialist and trustworthy individuals. End quote.

It is permissible to make use of the cells found in the umbilical cord, especially when the cord is usually discarded. And Allah knows best.

The Fiqh Council of the Organization of the Islamic Conference issued a statement concerning this matter during its session that was held on 18 Jumada al-Aakhirah 1408 AH (6 February 1988 CE). The text of this statement follows:

"Firstly: it is permissible to transplant an organ from its place in a person's body to elsewhere in his body, whilst making sure that the expected benefit from this procedure outweighs any potential harm, and on condition that this is done for the purpose of replacing a missing organ or reshaping it, or changing its function, or correcting a defect, or removing a deformity that is causing psychological or physical pain. End quote."

Prohibition of Using Spermatozoids and Oocytes to Obtain Stem Cells

We should point out that it is not permissible for anyone to donate sperm or eggs for the purpose of producing zygotes (fertilized eggs) which will then develop into the foetus with the aim of obtaining the stem cells from it.

Prohibition of Cloning to Obtain Stem Cells

It is also not permissible to use cloning in order to obtain foetal stem cells. Rather permission is limited to obtaining stem cells from umbilical cords. (607)

678. Ruling on Medicines that are Mixed with Alcohol and Intoxicants

Allah, the Exalted, says:

"O you who believe! Intoxicants (all kinds of alcoholic drinks), gambling, Al-Ansab, and Al-Azlam (arrows for seeking luck or decision) are an abomination of Shaitan's (Satan) handiwork. So, avoid (strictly all) that (abomination) in order that you may be successful." (Qur'an, Al-Ma'idah 5:90)

"Shaitan (Satan) wants only to excite enmity and hatred between you with intoxicants (alcoholic drinks) and gambling, and hinder you from the remembrance of Allah and from As-Salat (the prayer). So, will you not then abstain?" (Qur'an, Al-Ma'idah 5:91)

Wa'il al-Hadrami reported: Tariq ibn Suwayd al-Ju'fi asked the Prophet (May Allah's peace and blessings be upon him) about alcohol. he forbade him from preparing it. He (Tariq) said: "I only prepare it for medicinal reasons." Whereupon the Prophet (May Allah's peace and blessings be upon him) said: "It is not medicine, but an ailment." (Muslim) (https://hadeethenc.com/en/browse/hadith/58263)

It is not permissible to mix medicines with alcohol. (608, 609)

Intoxicants means alcohol, alcoholic beverage, over-the-counter medication, prescription medication, controlled substances, if such OTC medication is labeled or has a package insert warning against operating machinery or driving after usage, as defined by state or federal law, marijuana, hashish, cocaine, heroin, dangerous drugs, narcotics, mood-altering substances, or any combination of the above. (610)

679. Ruling on Medicine that Contain Pork

Four Verses of the Qur'an prohibit Pork.

Allah, the Exalted, says:

"He has forbidden you only the Maytatah (dead animals), and blood, and the flesh of swine.." (Qur'an, Al-Baqarah 2:173)

"Forbidden to you (for food) are: Al-Maytatah (the dead animals - cattle-beast not slaughtered), blood, the flesh of swine..." (Qur'an, Al-Ma'idah 5:3)

"He has forbidden you only Al-Maytatah (meat of a dead animal), blood, the flesh of swine..." (Qur'an, Al-Nahl 16:115)

Other Verse: Al-A'nam 6:145.

Pig is impure and immoral animal, causes many diseases, changes man's behavior. (611)

Pork gelatin is used for capsules and pills.

680. Homeopathy

In al-Mawsoo'ah al-'Arabiyyah al-'Aalamiyyah it says:

"Homoeopathy is a kind of medical treatment that is based on the principle of "let like cure like." According to the practitioners of this method, the substance that causes symptoms in a healthy person will cure the same symptoms in a sick person. Some plants, for example, cause rashes on the skin, so homoeopathic doctors treat the rash with the same plants. Onions cause tearing in the eyes and make the nose run, so onion is used to treat nasal secretions caused by the cold...

...Many homeopathic remedies contain substances that may be poisonous or dangerous to human beings if the doses were increased. In addition to that, the medical efficacy of the homoeopathic remedies has not been proven scientifically. For these reasons, homeopathy has been subjected to criticism by many doctors. End quote."

Conclusion:
1. Homoeopathy has not been proven to be beneficial according to medical specialists, and there are those who are strongly opposed to it.
2. Do not use any remedy unless it has been proven to be beneficial, for most patients, on the basis of either certainty or overwhelming likelihood.
3. Beware of medicines that contain poisonous substances or alcohol, unless the amount is small and it is proven that that medicine is beneficial for most patients according to confirmed studies and proven results.
4. We advise you to use Ruqyah as prescribed in Shariah, composed of Qur'an and Adhkar and Du'as that are narrated in Shariah; read them over yourself and seek the help of

Allah, asking Him to ward off sickness from you. And we advise you to use medicines that Islam has stated are beneficial and useful, such as Honey and Black Seed. (612)

681. Ruling on Treating Patients with Music

Allah, the Exalted, says:

"And of mankind is he who purchases idle talks (i.e. music, singing, etc.) to mislead (men) from the Path of Allah without knowledge, and takes it (the Path of Allah, the Verses of the Quran) by way of mockery. For such there will be a humiliating torment (in the Hell-fire)." (Qur'an, Luqman 31:6)

Narrated Abu 'Amir or Abu Malik Al-Ash'ari that he heard the Prophet (peace and blessings be upon him) saying, "From among my followers there will be some people who will consider illegal sexual intercourse, the wearing of silk, the drinking of alcoholic drinks and the use of musical instruments, as lawful." (Bukhari)

Narrated Abu Malik Ash'ari that the Messenger of Allah (peace and blessings be upon him) said: "People among my nation will drink wine, calling it by another name, and musical instruments will be played for them and singing girls (will sing for them). Allah will cause the earth to swallow them up, and will turn them into monkeys and pigs." (Ibn Majah)

It is prohibited to play music or listen to it, whether it is with or without singing, but with singing it is worse and more corrupting to sound human nature and morals. (613)

682. Ruling on Dealing in so-called "Healing Crystals"

Narrated Abu'd-Darda': The Messenger of Allah (peace and blessings be upon him) said: "Allah has created the sickness and the remedy, so treat sickness but do not treat sickness with anything that is haram." (Tabarani)

Sheikh Ibn 'Uthaymeen (May Allah have mercy on him) said, explaining the means that it is permissible to use for treating sickness:

"The means that Allah, may He be exalted, has caused to be means are of two types:

1. Means that are prescribed in Islam, such as the Holy Qur'an and Du'aa' (supplication), as the Prophet (peace and blessings of Allah be upon him) said concerning Surah al-Fatihah: "How did you know it is a Ruqyah?" And the Prophet

(peace and blessings of Allah be upon him) used to perform Ruqyah for the sick by offering Du'a asking Allah, may He be exalted, to heal by means of his Du'a whomever He wanted to heal thereby.

2. Physical means such as regular medicine that is known through Shariah, such as honey, and through trial and experience, such as many other kinds of medicine and remedies. For this category, the effect should be direct, not by way of imagination. If it is proven that something has a direct effect, then it is valid to be used to treat sickness and healing will be achieved thereby, by Allah's leave.

But if it is just something imaginary that the sick person imagines will bring him psychological relief based on that imagination and that it will alleviate the sickness, and perhaps this psychological sense of relief may lead to recovery from sickness, then in this case it is not permissible to rely on it and that does not prove that it is a remedy. That is so that people will not pin their hopes on illusions.

Hence it is forbidden to wear halaqah bracelets, strings and the like to cure or ward off disease, because that is not a means that is prescribed in Shariah, nor is it proven on the basis of trial and experience. So long as there is no proof that it is a means of healing in either Shariah or scientific terms, it is not permissible to take it as a means, because taking it as a means is a kind of contesting the sovereignty of Allah, may He be exalted, and it is associating something else with Him, because He is the Only One Who creates cause and effect (and such actions attribute effects to causes that Allah has not made to be such)." (End quote from Majmoo' Fataawa wa Rasaa'il al-'Uthaymeen, 17/70) (614)

So-called "healing crystals" are various kinds of stones, gems or crystals that some people use to seek wellbeing and healing from psychological and physical sickness, because they believe that they have extraordinary powers to strengthen the body and heart, to bring peace of mind and ward off anxiety, tension, depression and so on from the individual.

Based on that, it is not permissible to use these crystals for treating sickness, and what appears to be the case is that it is not permissible to sell them or give them to those who will use them for this purpose, because there is no proof that they are beneficial in treating sickness, either from Shariah sources or from scientific sources. What connection is there between stones or crystals and healing from sickness, whether physical or psychological? Rather this comes under the heading of wearing amulets and seashells (worn for protection against the Evil Eye).

Narrated 'Uqbah ibn 'Aamir (May Allah be pleased with him): "I heard the Messenger of Allah (peace and blessings of Allah be upon him) say: "Whoever wears an amulet, may Allah never fulfil his wish and whoever wears a seashell, may Allah never protect him from what he fears." (Ahmad)

Based on that, it is not permissible to sell these rocks or crystals, and the like, for the purpose of treating sickness or seeking healing from them. And believing that they are of benefit for such purposes comes under the heading of associating others with Allah, may He be Exalted.

683. Ruling on Believing in Auras and Energy Healing

The word aura is part of the terminology used by energy healers, by which they refer to a subtle body which surrounds the physical body. In their view, the aura is the means that connects the human being to the energy of the universe!

Practitioners of energy healing claim that it is possible for some people who have extraordinary vision to see these auras that surround the body, and that these auras are composed of seven layers, which are called the "seven bodies."

They also claim that it is possible for one who does not have these extraordinary powers to see these auras and their different colours with the naked eye by doing specific exercises, which are mostly based on exhausting the retina.

The evidence which proves scientifically that this so-called seeing is false and it has no medical indication, whether for the purposes of diagnosis or treatment, includes the following:

1. Those who claim to see the aura of the same person see it differently.

2. The colours in some experiments differed from the psychological conditions they were supposed to represent.

And there are other reasons mentioned in the article Aura Photography: a Candid Shot, which was published in Skeptical Inquirer Magazine, vol.24, no.3.

It should be noted that the philosophy of the seven bodies is connected to one of the ancient forms of yogic philosophy, according to which each of these seven bodies is connected to one of the centres of energy, which are known as chakras. These are centres of universal spiritual energy which are found in the auras, and have corresponding centres in the body which are known as the nervous system. The Complete Illustrated Book of Yoga (p.344) by Swami Vishnu Denananda. But most of the research into energy science and its therapeutic applications is based on mere speculation and conjecture, and is connected to idolatrous beliefs that have nothing to do with empirical medicine or Islamic teachings, because there is no way to prove it either on the basis of Shariah evidence or of empirical evidence that is acceptable to scientists. In fact, the matter went further, to the realm of astrology, through the philosophy of the five elements, which have to do with stars and zodiac signs. Hence, you will find blatant astrology in some applications of Reiki and Ayurveda, especially with regard to healing with precious stones and crystals. This is in addition to what these practices involve of going to extremes in sanctifying the self, because the focus of one of them is to bring out his hidden divine essence and become one with the universal energy, in order to liberate himself – or so they claim – from materialistic enslavement, until the seeker reaches an advanced stage of self-awareness and realizes that he and his object of worship are one, at which point there is no longer any point in worship!

This matches precisely the belief of the heretics, those who believe in immanence and union with the divine, and they believe in the oneness of all being or pantheism. This is an ancient idolatrous philosophy that found its way to some misguided Sufis who believe in immanence. (615)

684. Ruling on Using a "Biodisc" and the Ruling on Wearing "Chi Pendants" for Healing

We should point out a number of matters having to do with the wearing of Chi Pendant:

a. It is not permissible to wear it unless it has been proven that it is beneficial to the body or that it can protect against disease.

b. It is not permissible for men to wear it; rather it may be worn by women only, because wearing pendants or necklaces on the chest is something that is only for women, and not for men, especially when it is possible to put the pendant in a pocket and it does not have to be worn on the chest.

c. For women who wear it, it is not permissible for the necklace to have a cross on it, because the cross is a symbol of disbelief and disbelievers. Therefore, it was the practice of the Prophet (peace and blessings of Allah be upon him) to erase crosses.

Narrated Aisha (May Allah be pleased with her): The Prophet (peace and blessings of Allah be upon him) did not leave anything in his house on which there was anything that resembled crosses but he would erase them." (Bukhari)

d. One should avoid wearing pendants on which there is written the Name of Allah, may He be exalted, or Verses of the Qur'an.

However, even if it is proven to be beneficial, we should refrain from using these things, because wearing them resembles what is done by ignorant people of wearing such things to bring good luck or to ward off the Evil Eye, and the like. There are magnetic bracelets and copper bracelets, which are claimed to be beneficial if worn as a remedy for rheumatism (or arthritis), and the scholars have responded to questions about the ruling on wearing them by noting that they should be avoided.

Sheikh 'Abd al-'Azeez ibn Baaz (May Allah have mercy on him) was asked: "What is the ruling on wearing magnetic bracelets?" He replied:

"What I think concerning this matter is that such bracelets should not be used, so as to block the means that may lead to shirk, and so as to avoid something that may be a cause of fitnah whereby people would become inclined towards them and form an attachment to them, and so as to encourage the Muslim to turn with all his heart to Allah, may He be glorified, putting his trust in Him and relying on Him, and being content with the means that are prescribed in Islam and are known to be permissible beyond any doubt. That which Allah has permitted to His slaves and made easily available to them is sufficient and there is no need for that which He has prohibited to them or that which is dubious. It is narrated in a sound report from the Prophet (blessings and peace of Allah be upon him) that he said: "Whoever guards against the doubtful matters will protect his religious commitment from shortcomings and will protect his honor from slander, but whoever falls into that which is doubtful will fall into that which is haram, like a shepherd who grazes his flock around prohibited land; he will soon graze in it." Agreed upon. And he (peace and blessings of Allah be upon him) said: "Leave that which makes you doubt for that which does not make you doubt." (Tirmidhi)

Undoubtedly, wearing the bracelet mentioned is similar to what the ignorant did in the time of Jaahiliyyah; so, it is either something that is prohibited and constitutes Shirk, or it is one of the means that lead to Shirk..." (End quote. Fataawa ash-Sheikh Ibn Baaz (1/207) (616)

If the biodisk contains Negative Ions, then it is permissible. The mother of my patient had Diabetes and Hypertension; with the Biodisk with the Negative Ions, her blood pressure and sugar were normalized.

685. Believing that Doctors or Drugs Cure

The Prophet Ibrahim (May Allah have mercy on him) said:

"And when I am ill, it is He (Allah) Who cures me." (Qur'an, Ash-Shu'ara 26:80)

Allah, the Exalted, says:

"O mankind! There has come to you a good advice from your Lord (i.e. the Qur'an, ordering all that is good and forbidding all that is evil), and a <u>Healing</u> for that (disease of ignorance, doubt, hypocrisy and differences, etc.) in your breasts, - a Guidance and a Mercy (explaining lawful and unlawful things, etc.) for the believers." (Qur'an, Yunus 10:57)

Abu Ramthah (May Allah be pleased with him) reported that he said to the Prophet (May Allah's peace and blessings be upon him): "Show me this thing on your back (to treat it), for I am a physician." The Prophet (May Allah's peace and blessings be upon him) replied: "Allah is the Physician. You are only a kind man. The one who heals it is the One who created it." (Abu Dawud)
(https://hadeethenc.com/en/browse/hadith/8303)

Thinking that doctors or drugs cure is a Shirk. The Ultimate Cure is from Allah Alone.

686. Ordering Unnecessary Medical Tests, Medications

Majority of disease are caused by the Evil Jinn because of sins. It is important to diagnose Jinn diseases as medico-surgical treatment is detrimental and death-dealing, excites the Evil jinn and excited Jinn spread more disease, create new diseases, cause death. We cannot cut Demons. Surgery excites the Evil Jinn, thus is not indicated except in emergency cases (e.g. bowel occlusion or perforation; heavy bleeding, injury).

Modern medicine went stray, instead of healing, it contributes to disease progression. There is no Qur'an, no Negative Ions and no Prophetic Medicine, how to except cure?

Medical fraud in the hospital, clinic chains, individual employees and even patients can be involved - as victims or perpetrators. Misdiagnosis intentionally by the dishonest doctors will involve additional investigations and costly treatments with exaggerated bills, overcharging patients or health insurances.

Reasons for excessive ordering of tests by doctors include defensive behavior and fear or uncertainty, lack of experience, the use of protocols and guidelines, inadequate educational feedback and clinician's unawareness about the cost of examinations, or intentionally overcharging for non-indicated investigations, medications and surgery.

687. Surgical Operations Without Medico-Legal Indication

Some of the common types of unnecessary surgeries:

- Cardiac angioplasty and stents.
- Cardiac pacemakers.
- Back surgery and spinal fusion.
- Hysterectomy.
- Knee and hip replacement.
- Cesarean section.

The dishonest obstetrician diagnoses "cord prolapse" following the midwife's examination who found that the cervix was closed and long and patient was not in labor, but doctor performs unjustified emergency C-section which brings more financial profit.

The abdominal pain not related to appendicitis but intentionally misdiagnosed as appendicitis to perform surgery and consequently, overcharging patient.

When a doctor performs unnecessary surgery, it may be medical malpractice. Medical malpractice claims allow an injury victim to recover damages from a negligent doctor or hospital.

688. Euthanasia, Taking a Patient off a Respirator and the Ruling on Mercy Killing

Allah, the Exalted, says:

"And no person can ever die except by Allah's Leave and at an appointed term. And whoever desires a reward in (this) world, We shall give him of it; and whoever desires a reward in the Hereafter, We shall give him thereof. And We shall reward the grateful."
(Qur'an, Ali 'Imran 3:145)

The Islamic Fiqh Council, belonging to the Muslim World League, issued statement during its 10th session on 24/2/1408 AH:

"In the case of a patient whose body has been hooked up to life support, it is permissible to remove it if all his brain functions have ceased completely, and a committee of three specialists, experienced doctors have determined that this cessation of function is irreversible, even if the heart and breathing are still working mechanically with the help of the machine. But he cannot be ruled dead according to Shariah until his breathing and heart stop completely, after the machine is removed. End quote."

So-called mercy killing is not permissible, whether it is done by withholding treatment from the patient or by any other means. It comes under the heading of haram killing which the Prophet (peace and blessings be upon him) regarded as one of the Major sins. There are no exceptions to that except what has been mentioned above concerning one who comes under the rulings of those who have died. As for withholding treatment on which life depends on the basis of reducing the suffering of the patient and putting an end to his pain and suffering, it is not permissible and this comes under the heading of haram killing. (617)

689. Telling that these Food or Drugs Increase Longevity

Allah, the Exalted, says:

"And no aged person is granted (additional) life nor is his lifespan lessened but that it is in a register. Indeed, that for Allah is easy." (Qur'an, Fatir 35:11)

"And for every nation is a (specified) term. So, when their time has come, they will not remain behind an hour, nor will they precede (it)." (Qur'an, Al-A'raf 7:34)

"And spend (in the way of Allah) from what We have provided you before death approaches one of you and he says, 'My Lord, if only You would delay me for a brief term so I would give charity and be among the righteous.' But never will Allah delay a soul when its time has come. And Allah is Acquainted with what you do." (Qur'an, Al-Munaafiqoon 23:10-11)

Other Verse: *Nooh 71:2-4.*

Narrated Anas ibn Malik (May Allah be pleased with him): "I heard the Messenger of Allah (peace and blessings of Allah be upon him) say: "Whoever would like his rizq (provision) to be increased and his life to be extended, should uphold the ties of kinship." (Bukhari and Muslim)

Narrated Salman (May Allah be pleased with him): The Messenger of Allah (blessings and peace of Allah be upon him) said: "Nothing can ward off the Divine Decree except Du'a (supplication) and nothing can increase lifespan except honoring one's parents." (Tirmidhi)

Narrated Thawban: The Messenger of Allah (peace and blessings be upon him) said: 'Nothing extends one's life span but righteousness, nothing averts the Divine Decree but supplication, and nothing deprives a man of provision but the sin that he commits." (Ibn Majah)

Death and lifespan are part of the Will and Decree of Allah that He wrote in Al-Lawh Al-Mahfuz with Him, fifty thousand years before He created all of creation. That is not subject to change or alteration; He, may He be Glorified, wrote it according to His Knowledge that cannot err, and according to His Will that cannot be changed. That does not mean that death and lifespans are not subject to the Laws of cause and effect that Allah has created in this Universe; rather the issue of death, like anything else that is decreed in this world, is based on tangible causes that were also written in Al-Lawh Al-Mahfuz. (618)

Ibn Taymiyah (May Allah have mercy on him) said:

"Allah commanded the angel to write the lifespan and said: 'If he upholds ties of kinship, I will increase it by such and such, but the angel does not know whether his lifespan will be increased or not; rather Allah knows how things will turn out. Then when the end of his lifespan comes, (his death) cannot be brought forward or put back. End quote." (Majmoo' al-Fataawa (8/517)

Seeking medical treatment is one of the tangible means of preserving life and health, by Allah's leave. If a person neglects that, it may lead to harm or death. That does not contradict in any way what the Verses and Ahadith say about a person's lifespan being already defined on the basis of means and measures. It is defined on the basis of means and measures, and everything with Him is by due measure (cf. 13:8). If a person seeks medical treatment and recovers, and lives longer in this world as a result, that happens by the Decree of Allah. If he is negligent or fails to seek medical treatment until he dies, that also happens by the Decree of Allah.

690. Do Not Applying Ruqyah, Negative Ions and Prophetic Medicine

Allah, the Exalted, says:

"And We send down of the Qur'an that which is Healing and Mercy for the believers, but it does not increase the wrongdoers except in loss." (Qur'an, Al-Isra 17:82)

"And when I am ill it is He Who cures me." (Qur'an, Ash-Shu'ara 26:80)

"O mankind! There has come to you a good advice from your Lord (i.e. the Quran, ordering all that is good and forbidding all that is evil), and a Healing for that (disease of ignorance, doubt, hypocrisy and differences, etc.) in your breasts, - a guidance and a mercy (explaining lawful and unlawful things, etc.) for the believers." (Qur'an, Yunus 10:57)

Other Verses: *Fussilat 41:44, Al-Anbiya 21:90, An-Nahl 16:69, Al-An'am 6:17.*

THE QUR'AN HEALING - RUQYAH

Ibn Al-Qayyim (May Allah have mercy on him) said:

"The Qur'an is the perfect cure, and it is a beneficial means of protection, and a guiding light and a general mercy. If it was sent upon a mountain, it would render it asunder from its Greatness and its Glory." (7)

Abdullah ibn Khubayb (May Allah be pleased with him) reported: The Messenger of Allah (May Allah's peace and blessings be upon him) said to me: "Recite Surah Al-Ikhlas, Surah Al-Falaq and Surah An-Nas thrice every morning and evening, and it will be sufficient for you and will grant you protection from everything." (Tirmidhi) (https://hadeethenc.com/en/browse/hadith/6082)

Aisha (May Allah be pleased with her) said: "In his last illness, the Prophet (peace and blessings be upon him) used to blow breath (into his cupped hands) and recite Al-Mu'awwidhatayn (Surahs Al-Falaq and An-Nas) and then wipe over his body. But when his illness aggravated,

I used to recite them over him and pass his own hand over his body for its blessing." (Bukhari and Muslim)

Narrated Abu Khuzaamah that his father said: "I asked the Messenger of Allah (peace and blessings of Allah be upon him): 'O Messenger of Allah, do you think that the Ruqyah by which we seek healing, the medicines with which we treat ourselves, and the means of protection that we seek change the Decree of Allah at all?' He said: 'They are part of the Decree of Allah.'" (Tirmidhi and Ibn Majah)

Abdullah ibn Masud (May Allah be pleased with him) said: "Whoever recites the following ten Verses of Surah Baqarah 1) in the morning, will be saved from Shaytan till the evening, and whoever recites it in the evening will be protected from Shaytan till the morning. 2) Furthermore, he will not experience unpleasant surprises in his family or wealth. 3) If these Verses are recited on an insane person, he will be cured.'" (Darimi and Shu'abul Iman) (582)

MIRACULOUS NEGATIVE IONS (ANION) TREATMENT

The Negative Ions are the Miracles of Allah Almighty in the Glorious Qur'an: *Al-Anfal 8:11 and Sad 38:42.*

Allah, the Exalted, says referring to Negative Ions in the form of Rain:

"...and He caused water (rain) to descend on you from the sky, to clean you thereby and to remove from you the Rijz (whispering, evil-suggestions, etc.) of Shaitan (Satan), and to strengthen your hearts, and make your feet firm thereby." (Qur'an, Al-Anfal 8:11)

The Prophet Ayub was tested by Devil. Devil was removed by Allah through Negative Ions! (619)

Allah, the Exalted, says:

"And remember Our slave Ayub (Job), when he invoked his Lord (saying): "Verily! Shaitan (Satan) has touched me with distress (by losing my health) and torment (by losing my wealth)! (Allah said to him): "Strike the ground with your foot: This is a spring of water to wash in, cool and a (refreshing) drink." (Qur'an, Sad 38:41-42)

Negative Ions are formed by **gaining electrons** and are called **Anions**. Negative Ions are created in nature as air molecules break apart due to sunlight, radiation and moving air and water. You feel energized and relaxed by the power of Negative Ions when you are on the beach, beneath a waterfall, in the mountains, forest. While tired, having headache or pain in the unhealthy Positive Ions places (home, work, malls, airports, etc.). (620)

What does Fiqh-us-Sunnah say about Water

Fiqh 1. Purification

The Shariah has divided water into four kinds:

1. Mutlaq Water,
2. Used Water (for purification),
3. Water mixed with Pure elements,
4. Water mixed with Impure elements. (621)

Fiqh 1.1. Mutlaq Water

This kind of water is considered pure because of its inherent purity and as such, it can be used by an individual to purify him or herself. It consists of the following categories:

Fiqh 1.1.a: Rain Water, Snow and Hail

These substances are pure because Allah says:

"And sent down water from the sky upon you, that thereby He might purify you thereby and to remove from you the Rijz (whispering, evil-suggestions, etc.) of Shaitan (Satan)..." (Qur'an, Al-Anfal 8:11)

"And it is He Who sends the winds as heralds of glad tidings, going before His Mercy (rain), and We send down pure water from the sky." (Qur'an, Al-Furqan 25:48)

Abu Hurairah (May Allah be pleased with him) reported: "Whenever the Messenger of Allah (May Allah's peace and blessings be upon him) said: "Allah is the Greatest" to start the prayer, he would remain silent before reciting. I said: "O Messenger of Allah, may my father and mother be ransomed for you! I notice that you remain silent between the Takbir (saying 'Allah is the Greatest') and the recitation. What do you say (in between them)?" He said: "I say: 'O Allah, distance me from my sins as You have distanced the east from the west. O Allah, purify me from my sins as a white garment is purified from dirt. O Allah, wash out my sins with water, snow and hail.'" (Muslim) (https://hadeethenc.com/en/browse/hadith/10904)

Fiqh 1.1.b: Sea Water

Abu Hurairah related that a man asked the Messenger of Allah (peace and blessings of Allah be upon him) "O Messenger of Allah, we sail on the ocean and we carry only a little water. If we use it for ablution, we will have to go thirsty. May we use sea water for ablution?" The Messenger of Allah (peace and blessings be upon him) said: "Its (the sea) water is pure and its dead (animals) are lawful (i.e. they can be eaten without any prescribed slaughtering)." (This Hadith is related by "the five." Tirmidhi graded it Hassan Saheeh, and al-Bukhari says it is Saheeh)

Fiqh 1.1.c: Water from the well of Zamzam

Zamzam water cures Cancer and all diseases. (564, 565)

Fiqh 1.1.d: Altered Water

This involves water whose form has been altered because of its being in a place for a long period of time or because of the place in which it is located, or because of its being mixed with a substance that cannot be completely removed from it (i.e. water mixed with algae, tree leaves, and so on). The scholars agree that this type of water falls under the heading of Mutlaq water.

The rationale is simple: everything that falls under the general term of water, without any further qualifications, is considered pure, for the Qur'an says, *"...and if you find not water, then go to clean, high ground..." (Al-Ma'idah 5:6)*

Fiqh 1.2. Used Water (for Purification)

This category refers to water which drips from the person after he performs ablution or Ghusl. It is considered pure because it was pure before its use for ablution, and there is no basis to think that it has lost its purity.

Abu Hurairah reported that the Messenger of Allah (peace and blessings be upon him) met him alone in the streets of Madinah while he was in post-sex impurity. He therefore slipped away, made Ghusl and returned. The Messenger of Allah (peace and blessings be upon him) asked him "Where have you been, Abu Hurairah?" He answered, "I was in post-sex impurity and did not want to sit with you while I was in that condition." The Prophet (peace and blessings be upon him) replied, "Glory be to Allah. The believer does not become impure." This is related by "the group."

The Water used for Wudu or Ghusl neutralizes the Evil Eye

Malik related to me from Ibn Shihab that Abu Umama ibn Sahl ibn Hunayf said, "Amir ibn Rabia saw Sahl ibn Hunayf doing a Ghusl and said, 'I have not seen the like of what I see today, not even the skin of a maiden who has never been out of doors.' Sahl fell to the ground. The Messenger of Allah (peace and blessings be upon him) was approached and it was said, 'Messenger of Allah, can you do anything about Sahl ibn Hunayf? By Allah, he cannot raise his head.' He said, 'Do you suspect anyone of it?' They said, 'We suspect Amir ibn Rabia.'" He continued, "The Messenger of Allah (peace and blessings be upon him) summoned Amir and was furious with him and said, 'Why does one of you kill his brother? Why did you not say, "May Allah bless you?" Do Ghusl for it.' Amir washed his face, hands, elbows, knees, the end of his feet, and inside his lower garment in a vessel. Then he poured it over him, and Sahl went off with the people, and there was nothing wrong with him." (Malik Muwatta)

Ibn Abbas reported: The Prophet (peace and blessings be upon him) said, "The Evil Eye is real. If anything could precede the Divine Decree, it would be preceded by the Evil Eye. When you are asked to perform a ritual bath, then do so." (Muslim)

Negative Ions Create Positive Vibes

Nature, God's gift, has regenerative, healing effects due to high concentration of Negative Ions; it cures Cancer and all other diseases by Allah's Will. (622)

Negative Ions are odorless, tasteless and invisible molecules, abundant during the thunderstorm and rain, around the waterfalls, ocean, sea, spring water, river, forest, mountains, etc. Once they reach our bloodstream, Negative Ions are believed to produce biochemical reactions that increase levels of the mood chemical serotonin, helping to alleviate depression, stress, anxiety, boost energy and immunity. (623)

Major Depressive disorder and Bipolar II disorder

"The action of the pounding surf creates Negative Air Ions and we also see it immediately after spring thunderstorms when people report lightened moods", says Ion researcher Michael Terman, PhD, of Columbia University in New York. In his study, people with the winter seasonal pattern of major Depressive disorder or of Bipolar II disorder had considerable improvement after being exposed to high density Negative Air Ions. (624)

<u>Positive Effects of Negative Ions:</u>

1. **Negative Oxygen Ions** are the most commonly recognized Natural Air Ions (NAIs). NAIs (Anions) are those that gain an electron. Reports showed that **Superoxide $O_2^{\cdot-}$** was a kind of NAIs. Among NAIs generated by natural atmosphere and the Lenard effect (waterfall), **Superoxide $O_2^{\cdot-}$** are the major Negative Ions. (625)

The natural and artificial energy sources include:

1) radiant or cosmic rays in the atmosphere;
2) sunlight including ultraviolet;
3) natural and artificial corona discharge including thunder and lightning;
4) shearing forces of water (Lenard effect);
5) plant-based sources of energy.

Oxygen is the most important food for every cell, organ in our body. Without Oxygen, permanent brain damage begins after 4 minutes and death can occur as soon as 4-6 minutes later. Three processes are essential for the transfer of Oxygen from the outside air to the blood flowing through the lungs: ventilation, diffusion and perfusion. Ventilation is the process by which air moves in and out of the lungs.

Positive Ions (Cautions) are formed by losing an electron. Positive Ions cause diseases, infertility, sick building syndrome, fatigue, headache, lack of energy, poor concentration, low immunity, pain, sleep disorder, etc. Positive Ions are abundant in cities, industrial areas, produced by air conditioning, electrical (artificial lights, signboards, microwave, etc.) and electronic (internet, laptop, television, phone, etc.) devices, building and furniture materials, paint, carpets, upholstery, smoking, unhealthy environment, lifestyle, food and drinks, medications, etc.

2. Negative Ions remove the Evil Jinn by Allah's Will.

Allah removed the Devil, caused the disease of the Prophet Ayub, by Negative Ions (Spring water): *(Qur'an, Sad 38:41-42)*

Jinn is created from the smokeless flame of fire (Positive Ions: Carbon Dioxide and steam). (626-628)

Allah, the Exalted, says:

"And the Jinn, We created aforetime from the smokeless flame of fire." *(Qur'an, Al-Hijr 15:27)*

"And the Jinns did He create from a smokeless flame of fire." *(Qur'an, Ar-Rahman 55:15)*

The life-supporting character of Oxygen and the suffocating power of Carbon Dioxide.

Oxygen typifies the Good, and Carbon Dioxide is regarded as a spirit of Evil.

3. Anions Improve erythrocyte deformability, thereby aerobic metabolism. Restore erythrocyte biconcave discoid shape needed to navigate the cardiovascular system and for an increased surface area to support sufficient gas exchange and permits the cell to carry out its function.

4. Natural blood thinner, have anticlotting effects.

5. Prevent and break the agglutination of red cells.

6. Reduce the body's acidity, increase alkalinity in the body, thus reduce the infections and diseases. Bacteria, viruses, the Evil Jinn cannot tolerate alkaline atmosphere.

7. Antibacterial, antiviral effects.

8. Increase sense of well-being, energy, mental concentration, performance and alertness by counteracting debilitating Positive Ions in the environment. (629)

9. Clear the air of dust, pollen, mold spores and other potential allergens.

10. Improve the function of the cilia in respiratory tract, protect the lungs from irritation and Inflammation.

11. Asthma and Allergies are alleviated and cured in atmosphere rich in Negative Ions.

12. Remove bad odour from room, shoes, etc.

13. Anti-Fatigue, boost energy.

14. Anti-Stress, Anti-Anxiety effect, a relaxing effect, relieves tension.

15. Improves sleep quality.

16. Normalize the body's circadian rhythmicity.

17. Boost Immunity.

18. Reduce free radicals.

19. Treat Seasonal Affective Disorder (SAD).

20. Bring Positive outlook and mood.

21. Natural painkiller.

22. Anions reverse the effects of cations and, in addition, reduced suspicion and excitement to levels below those occurring before cationization. (630)

23. Improve physical performance.

24. Boost concentrations of the antioxidant superoxide dismutase (SOD), one of body's primary defenses against oxidative stress.

25. Treat burns, wounds, other skin lesions. (631, 632)

26. Regulate Menstrual Cycles, decrease bleeding, cramps. (537)

27. Enhance Sexual Capacities.

28. Enhance Male and Female Fertility. (529-536)

One of History's Strangest Natural Disasters

The SUDDEN catastrophic release of CARBON DIOXIDE from Lake Nyos on 21 August 1986 caused the deaths of about 1,700 people and 3,000 cattle near the Lake and along drainages up to 10 km north of the Lake in Cameroon. Lake Nyos is a volcanic crater that was formed by a violent explosion only a few hundred years ago.

On Thursday evening, 21 August 1986, tragic events occurred at this idyllic lake that made it known throughout the world as a "killer lake". The early part of the evening began with heavy rains and thunderstorms typical of the rainy season. By 9:30 pm, however, the weather was calm, the air temperature cool... This tranquil scene was suddenly disturbed by a series of rumbling sounds lasting perhaps 15-20 seconds. Many people in the immediate area of the lake came out of their homes, experienced a warm sensation, smelled rotten eggs or gunpowder, and rapidly lost consciousness. Other individuals either became unconscious without preliminary symptoms, or never awakened from their sleep. One observer, who was on high ground above Lake Nyos, reported hearing a bubbling sound. Walking to a better vantage point, he saw a white cloud rise from the lake, accompanied by a large water wave that washed up onto the southern shore. None of the survivors in the valley saw a visible cloud. Any large input of lava or volcanic gas into the lake would add sulfur and chlorine compounds. Again, an example of this is found in Soufriere crater lake, where large increases in concentrations of sulfur and chlorine compounds accompanied volcanic injection (Sigurdsson, 1977). Lake Nyos, however, shows no such enrichment of sulfur and chlorine compounds in either lake waters or sediments. Hydrogen fluoride is also a common volcanic gas, but its aqueous form was nearly absent from Lake Nyos. Based on our field sampling, we estimate that one liter of hypolimnetic water in Lake Nyos contains one to five liters of dissolved gas. Carbon dioxide comprises 98-99 percent of the dissolved gas. The non-volcanic character of the gas is most apparent in the low concentrations of carbon monoxide, hydrogen, hydrogen sulfide and sulfur dioxide compared to those in volcanic gas. Studies of volcanic emanations from magmas similar in composition to those erupted in Cameroon, notably those from Iceland and Hawaii, show that the relative proportions of C02 and sulfur in near-surface volcanic gases vary within certain limits. The weight ratio of CO2 to sulfur in such volcanic gases is typically less than 100 (Gerlach, 1986; Arnorsson, 1986). In contrast, the ratio CO2 to sulfur for Lake Nyos bottom waters is greater than 10 4. The water temperature, composition of dissolved gases and the low sulfur content of Lake Nyos waters and sediments does not support a hypothesis of recent, direct injection of lava or volcanic gas.

The head of the flowing cloud probably maintained the highest concentrations of C02, because it would have been continually recharged from the faster flowing tail (Simpson, 1982). This means that the head of the cloud would have remained lethal to greater distances than one might expect. Significant seismic activity during or preceding the event was not observed at the Kumba recording station 220 km southwest of Lake Nyos. Anecdotal evidence from survivors also does not support the hypothesis of a seismic shock. A similar catastrophic event occurred at Lake Monoun, about 95 km to the southeast in August 1984. In the Monoun disaster, 37 people died after walking into a visible cloud around the lake. An evaluation, done seven months after the incident, concluded that the causative agent was Carbon Dioxide (CO2) released from the lake. (633)

Explanation of this Sudden Disaster in the Light of the Qur'an and Sunnah

1) The Universal Law of "cause and effect" or "action and reaction" is applicable in all areas of life.

2) Sins (Disobedience to Allah) cause calamities, disasters, diseases, hardship, difficulties.

SUDDEN catastrophic release of CARBON DIOXIDE (Devils) are the result of humanity's sins.

Allah, the Exalted, says:

"Evil (sins and disobedience of Allah, etc.) has appeared on land and sea because of what the hands of men have earned (by oppression and evil deeds, etc.), that Allah may make them taste a part of that which they have done, in order that they may return (by repenting to Allah and begging His Pardon)." (Qur'an, Ar-Rum 30:41)

3) Rain, thunderstorm, lake, mountains are Negative Ions, very beneficial for health, well-being.

Rain (Negative Ions, **Superoxide** $O_2^{\cdot-}$ revives the land, fulfills the water needs of living creatures, cattle are multiplying and growing, vegetation is growing, and it is a pure water which cures diseases, removes Devils.

Allah, the Exalted, says:

"Allah is He Who sends the winds, so they raise clouds, and spread them along the sky as He wills, and then break them into fragments, until you see rain drops come forth from their midst! Then when He has made them fall on whom of His slaves as He will, lo! they rejoice!" (Qur'an, Ar-Rum 30:48)

"and He caused water (rain) to descend on you from the sky, to clean you thereby and to remove from you the Rijz (whispering, evil-suggestions, etc.) of Shaitan (Satan), and to strengthen your hearts, and make your feet firm thereby." (Qur'an, Al-Anfal 8:11)

Rain is one of countless Allah's blessings.

Then this beautiful pleasant scenario suddenly replaced by catastrophic release of deadly Carbon Dioxide (Positive Ions). Lake change suddenly the colour from bleu to red.

Allah sent down the Devils (Carbon Dioxide) because some people in the village committed Major sins, disobeying the Creator, causing Allah's Anger.

4) Then, the **sudden catastrophic release of Carbon Dioxide kills the population and cattle**.

Carbon Dioxide here are the Devils (Positive Ions).

Allah, the Exalted, says:

"Shall I inform you (O people!) upon whom the Shayatin (Devils) descend? They descend on every lying (one who tells lies), sinful person." (Qur'an, Ash-Shu'ara 26:221-222)

5) The **SUDDEN onset** of release of Carbon Dioxide confirms the Devils involvement.

6) The was a white cloud from the lake, accompanied by a large water wave that washed up onto

the southern shore. None of the survivors in the valley saw a visible cloud. Devils formed the cloud.

Allah can show to whomever He wants the Unseen.

7) Allah Almighty and His Messenger (peace and blessings be upon him) commanded to forbid evil.

It is an obligation upon every human being on an individual and communal level. As people didn't forbid evil, they were punished along with the sinners.

Allah, the Exalted, says:

"Those who follow the Messenger, the Prophet who can neither read nor write (i.e. Muhammad SAW) whom they find written with them in the Taurat (Torah) (Deut, xviii, 15) and the Injeel (Gospel) (John xiv, 16), - he commands them for Al-Ma'ruf (i.e. Islamic Monotheism and all that Islam has ordained); and forbids them from Al-Munkar (i.e. disbelief, polytheism of all kinds, and all that Islam has forbidden); he allows them as lawful At-Taiyibat [(i.e. all good and lawful) as regards things, deeds, beliefs, persons, foods, etc.], and prohibits them as unlawful Al-Khaba'ith (i.e. all evil and unlawful as regards things, deeds, beliefs, persons, foods, etc.), he releases them from their heavy burdens (of Allah's Covenant), and from the fetters (bindings) that were upon them. So, those who believe in him (Muhammad SAW), honor him, help him, and follow the Light (the Qur'an) which has been sent down with him, it is they who will be successful." (Qur'an, Al-A'raf 7:157)

Abu Bakr As-Siddiq (May Allah be pleased with him) reported: "O you people! You recite this Verse: 'O you who believe! Take care of your own selves. If you follow the Right Guidance (and enjoin what is right (Islamic Monotheism and all that Islam orders one to do) and forbid what is wrong (polytheism, disbelief and all that Islam has forbidden)] no hurt can come to you from those who are in error.' *(Qur'an, Al-Ma'idah 5:105)* But I have heard the Messenger of Allah (peace and blessings be upon him) saying: "When people see an oppressor but do not prevent him from (doing evil), it is likely that Allah will punish them all." (Abu Dawud and Tirmidhi)

Abu Sa'id al-Khudri reported: The Messenger of Allah (peace and blessings be upon him) said: "Whoever among you sees evil, let him change it with his hand. If he is unable to do so, then with his tongue. If he is unable to do so, then with his heart, and that is the weakest level of faith." (Muslim)

If people fail to do its duty of enjoining what is good and forbidding what is evil, wrongdoing, the corruption will spread throughout the Ummah, and it will deserve the Curse of Allah. Enjoining what is good and forbidding what is evil is one of the basic principles of this religion, and doing this is Jihad for the sake of Allah. Jihad requires putting up with difficulties and bearing insults and harm with patience, as Luqman said to his son:

"O my son! Aqim-is-Salah (perform As-Salah), enjoin (on people) Al-Ma'ruf (Islamic Monotheism and all that is good), and forbid (people) from Al-Munkar (i.e. disbelief in the Oneness of Allah, polytheism of all kinds and all that is evil and bad), and bear with patience whatever befalls you. Verily, these are some of the important commandments (ordered by Allah with no exemption." (Qur'an, Luqman 31:17)

Enjoining what is good and forbidding what is evil is a mission which will never end until the Last Hour.

8) People didn't learn from previous Allah's warning by volcanic eruption caused by people's sins.

Allah send down the diseases (calamities) because of humanity's sins, to remind people the purpose of their creation which is to submit to His commands and prohibitions to attain the bliss in this temporary life and Paradise in the next eternal life.

9) This is a lesson for this and next generations to follow the Glorious Qur'an and Sunnah, to fear Allah, for their own benefits and salvation from the torments of Hellfire.

Allah, the Exalted, says:

"Whatever of good reaches you, is from Allah, but whatever of evil befalls you, is from yourself. And We have sent you (O Muhammad SAW) as a Messenger to mankind, and Allah is Sufficient as a Witness." (Qur'an, An-Nisa 4:79)

10) All people are the sinners but the best of them are those who repent immediately, stop sins, restore people's rights, repair the past, follow Allah's Laws (the Qur'an and Sunnah)

"Evil (sins and disobedience of Allah, etc.) has appeared on land and sea because of what the hands of men have earned (by oppression and evil deeds, etc.), that Allah may make them taste a part of that which they have done, in order that they may return (by repenting to Allah, and begging His Pardon)." (Qur'an, Ar-Rum 30:41)

PROPHETIC MEDICINE IS THE DIVINE MEDICINE

Ibn Al-Qayyim (May Allah have mercy on him) said in his excellent work, *Zad Al-Ma'ad*:

"Prophetic Medicine is not like the medicine of the physicians, for the medicine of the Prophet (peace and blessings be upon him) is certain, definitive, emanating from Divine Revelation, the lantern of Prophethood and Perfection of reason.

As for the medicine of others, most of it is conjecture, presumptions and experimentation.

With regard to physical medicine, that is something that is complementary to Islamic teachings and is not something to sought in and of itself; therefore, it is only to be used in the case of necessity."

Refer to the book of Ibn Qayyim "Healing with the Medicine of the Prophet." (634)

Prayer is a Cure

Allah, the Exalted, says:

"O you who have believed, seek help through patience and prayer. Indeed, Allah is with the patient." (Qur'an, Al-Baqarah 2:153)

"Those who have believed and whose hearts are assured by the remembrance of Allah. Unquestionably, by the remembrance of Allah hearts are assured." (Qur'an, Ar-Ra'd 13:28)

Rabia reported: Abu Darda (May Allah be pleased with him) said, "Verily, everything has a polish and the polish of the heart is the remembrance of Allah Almighty." (Shu'ab al-Iman 503)

Narrated Abu Hurairah: "The Prophet (peace and blessings be upon him) set out in the early morning and I did likewise. I prayed, then I sat. The Prophet (peace and blessings be upon him) turned to me and said: 'Do you have a stomach problem?' I said: 'Yes, O Messenger of Allah.' He said: 'Get up and pray, for in prayer there is healing.'" (Ibn Majah)

Miracle of the Ablution Water on Patient with Aphasia

Narrated Umm Jundub: "I saw the Messenger of Allah (peace and blessings be upon him) stoning the 'Aqabah Pillar from the bottom of the valley on the Day of Sacrifice, then he went away. A woman from Khath'am followed him, and with her was a son of hers who had been afflicted, he could not speak. She said: 'O Messenger of Allah! This is my son, and he is all I have left of my family. He has been afflicted and cannot speak.' The Messenger of Allah (peace and blessings be upon him) said: 'Bring me some water.' So, it was brought, and he (peace and blessings be upon him) washed his hands and rinsed out his mouth. Then he (peace and blessings be upon him) gave it to her and said: 'Give him some to drink, and pour some over him, and seek Allah's healing for him.'" She (Umm Jundub) said: "I met that woman and said: 'Why don't you give me some?' She said: 'It is only for the sick one.' I met that woman one year later and asked her about the boy. She said: 'He recovered and became (very) smart, not like the rest of the people.'" (Ibn Majah)

Miracle of the Ablution Water on Unconscious Patient

Narrated Jabir: "Allah's Apostle (peace and blessings be upon him) came to visit me while I was sick and unconscious. He (peace and blessings be upon him) performed ablution and sprinkled the remaining water on me and I became conscious and said, "O Allah's Apostle! To whom will my inheritance go as I have neither ascendants nor descendants?" Then the Divine Verses regarding Fara'id (inheritance) were revealed." (Bukhari)

Saliva with the Dust of the Earth

Aisha (May Allah be pleased with her) reported: When someone complained of an ailment or had a sore, or a wound, the Prophet (May Allah's peace and blessings be upon him) did this with his index finger – the narrator, Sufyan ibn 'Uyaynah, touched the ground with his index finger and then raised it - and said: "In the Name of Allah, the dust of our earth along with the saliva of some of us will cure our ailing people, with the permission of our Lord." (Bukhari and Muslim)

(https://hadeethenc.com/en/browse/hadith/6113)

DU'AS for CURE – there are many.

Abu Sa'id al-Khudri (May Allah be pleased with him) reported: Jibreel came to the Prophet (May Allah's peace and blessings be upon him) and said: "O Muhammad, have you fallen ill?" He said: 'Yes.' So Jibreel said: "In the Name of Allah I recite over you, (to cleanse you) from everything that troubles you, from the evil of every soul or envious eye, Allah will cure you, in the Name of Allah I recite over you)."

(Muslim) (https://hadeethenc.com/en/browse/hadith/5650)

Du'a is Better than Painkillers

Abu 'Abdullah 'Uthman ibn Abi al-'As (May Allah be pleased with him) reported that he once complained to the Messenger of Allah (May Allah's peace and blessings be upon him) about a pain that he felt in his body. The Messenger of Allah said: "Place your hand where you feel pain in your body and say: 'Bismillah' three times; and then repeat seven times: 'I seek refuge with Allah's Might and Power from the evil of what I suffer from and what I am wary of).'" (Malik)
(https://hadeethenc.com/en/browse/hadith/6018)

Du'a when Visiting Sick

Abdullah ibn Abbas (May Allah be pleased with him) reported that the Prophet (May Allah's peace and blessings be upon him) said: "Whoever visits a sick person whose time of death has not come and says, seven times: 'I ask Allah the Great, the Lord of the Great Throne, to cure you', except that Allah will cure him from that sickness." (Tirmidhi) (https://hadeethenc.com/en/browse/hadith/6270)

Sa'd ibn Abi Waqqas (May Allah be pleased with him) reported: The Messenger of Allah (May Allah's peace and blessings be upon him) visited me when I was ill and said: "O Allah, cure Sa'd; O Allah, cure Sa'd; O Allah, cure Sa'd!" (Bukhari and Muslim. This is the wording of Muslim)
(https://hadeethenc.com/en/browse/hadith/5469)

Hijama - Cupping is the Divine Cure from Paradise

Narrated Anas ibn Malik (May Allah be pleased with him): The Prophet (peace and blessings of Allah be upon him) said: "'On the night on which I was taken on the Night Journey (Isra'), I did not pass by any group (of Angels) but they said to me: "O Muhammad, tell your nation to use cupping." (Ibn Majah)

Narrated Abu Hurairah (May Allah be pleased with him): The Prophet (peace and blessings be upon him) said: "The best medical treatment you apply is Cupping." (Abu Dawud)

Narrated Jabir bin 'Abdullah that he paid Al-Muqanna a visit during his illness and said, "I will not leave till he gets cupped, for I heard Allah's Apostle saying, "There is healing in Cupping." (Bukhari)

Anas (May Allah be pleased with him) reported God's Messenger (peace and blessings be upon him) as saying, "The best medical treatments you apply are Cupping and Sea Costus." (Bukhari and Muslim)

Honey is a Miracle of Allah

There are around 50 plants mentioned in the Holy Quran and Sunnah.

Allah, the Exalted, says:

"And your Lord inspired the bee, saying: "Take you habitations in the mountains and in the trees and in what they erect. "Then, eat of all fruits, and follow the ways of your Lord made easy (for you)." There comes forth from their bellies, a drink of varying colour wherein is healing for men. Verily, in this is indeed a sign for people who think." (Qur'an, An-Nahl 16:68-69)

Abdallah b. Masud reported God's Messenger (peace and blessings be upon him) as saying: "Make use of the two remedies: Honey and the Qur'an." (Ibn Majah and Baihaqi)

Ibn 'Abbas reported God's Messenger as saying: "There is a remedy in three things: the incision of a cupping-glass, a drink of Honey or cauterization by fire, but I forbid my people to cauterize." (Bukhari)

Abu Sa'id al-Khudri (May Allah be pleased with him) reported: A man came to the Prophet (May Allah's peace and blessings be upon him) and said: "My brother has some abdominal trouble." The Prophet (May Allah's peace and blessings be upon him) said to him: "Let him drink honey." The man came for the second time and the Prophet (May Allah's peace and blessings be upon him) said to him: "Let him drink honey." He came for the third time and the Prophet (May Allah's peace and blessings be upon him) said: "Let him drink honey." When he came for the fourth time, he said: "I have done that", and the Prophet (May Allah's peace and blessings be upon him) said: "Allah has spoken the truth, and your brother's abdomen has lied. Let him drink honey." So, he made him drink honey and he was cured." (Bukhari and Muslim) (https://hadeethenc.com/en/browse/hadith/8300)

Camel Milk and Urine as Medicine

Narrated Anas: "The climate of Medina did not suit some people, so the Prophet (peace and blessings be upon him) ordered them to follow his shepherd, i.e. his camels, and drink their milk and urine (as a medicine). So, they followed the shepherd that is the camels and drank their milk and urine till their bodies became healthy…" (Bukhari)

Black Seed is a Cure from all Diseases

Narrated Abu Hurairah: "I heard Allah's Apostle (peace and blessings be upon him) saying,

'There is healing in black cumin for all diseases except death.'" (Bukhari)

Narrated Khalid bin Sa'd (May Allah be pleased with him): "…Aisha has narrated to me that she heard the Prophet (peace and blessings be upon him) saying, 'This Black Cumin is healing for all diseases except As-Sam.' Aisha said, 'What is As-Sam?' He said, 'Death.'" (Bukhari)

Ajwa Dates Against Poison and Black Magic

Narrated Sa'd (May Allah be pleased with him): 'I heard Allah's Messenger (peace and blessings be upon him) saying, "Whoever takes seven 'Ajwa dates in the morning will not be effected by magic or poison on that day." (Bukhari)

Olive Oil

Allah, the Exalted, says:

"By the Fig and the Olive." *(Qur'an, At-Tin 95:1)*

Al-Bara b. 'Azib reported that he said prayer with the Messenger of Allah (peace be upon him) and he recited: *"By the Fig and the Olive."* (Muslim)

Zaid b. Arqam told that God's Messenger (peace and blessings be upon him) ordered them to treat pleurisy with Sea Costus and Olive Oil. (Tirmidhi)

Palm Leaves Stopping Bleeding

Narrated Sahl bin Saud As-Sa'idi: "When the helmet broke on the head of the Prophet and his face became covered with blood and his incisor tooth broke (i.e. during the battle of Uhud), 'Ali used to bring water in his shield while Fatima was washing the blood off his face. When Fatima saw that the bleeding increased because of the water, she took a mat (of palm leaves), burnt it, and stuck it (the burnt ashes) on the wound of Allah's Apostle, whereupon the bleeding stopped." (Bukhari)

Talbina is Good for Heart, Sorrow and Grief

Narrated 'Ursa: "Aisha used to recommend At-Talbina for the sick and for such a person as grieved over a dead person. She used to say, "I heard Allah's Apostle saying, 'At-Talbina gives rest to the heart of the patient and makes it active and relieves some of his sorrow and grief.'" (Bukhari)

Indian Incense against Seven Diseases

Narrated Um Qais bint Mihsan: "I heard the Prophet saying, "Treat with the Indian incense, for it has healing for seven diseases; it is to be sniffed by one having throat trouble, and to be put into one side of the mouth of one suffering from pleurisy…" (Bukhari)

Narrated Um Qais that she took to Allah's Apostle one of her sons whose palate and tonsils she had pressed because he had throat trouble. The Prophet (peace and blessings be upon him) said, "Why do you pain your children by getting the palate pressed like that? Use the Ud Al-Hindi (certain Indian incense) for it cures seven diseases one of which is pleurisy." (Bukhari)

Aloes for Inflamed Eye

Nubaih bin Wahb narrated that the eye of ʿUmar bin Ubaidullah became inflamed when he was in ihram, and he wanted to apply kohl to it, but Aban bin ʿUthman (May Allah be pleased with him) forbade him to do that and told him to apply Aloes to it. He said that ʿUthman (May Allah be pleased with him) narrated from the Messenger of Allah (peace and blessings be upon him) that he had done that." (Ahmad)

Truffles for the Eye Diseases

Saʾid b. Zaid reported Allah's Messenger (peace and blessings be upon him) as saying: "Truffles are 'Manna' which Allah, the Exalted, the Majestic, sent to the people of Israel, and its juice is a medicine for the eyes." (Muslim)

691. Non-Islamic Exorcism

The Glorious Qur'an says:

"And when I am ill, it is He who cures me." (Qur'an, Ash-Shuʾara 26:80)

"And your Lord says, "Call upon Me; I will respond to you." Indeed, those who disdain My worship, will enter Hell (rendered) contemptible." (Qur'an, Ghafir 40:60)

Satan said:

"Verily! I fear Allah for Allah is Severe in punishment." (Qur'an, Al-Anfal 8:48)

When the disciples of Jesus asked him (Jesus) how to cast the evil spirits away, he (Jesus, Allah's Messenger) is reported to have said, *"But this kind never comes out except by prayer and fasting." (Matthew 17:21)*

Allah performed His Miracles through His Messenger, Jesus:

"…and ʿmake himʾ a Messenger to the Children of Israelʿ to proclaim', 'I have come to you with a sign from your Lord: I will make for you a bird from clay, breathe into it, and it will become aʿrealʾ bird—by Allah's Will. I will heal the blind and the leper and raise the dead to life—by Allah's Will. And I will prophesize what you eat and store in your houses. Surely in this is a sign for you if youʿtrulyʾ believe." (Qur'an, Ali ʿImran 3:49)

"Andʿon Judgment Dayʾ Allah will say, "O Jesus, son of Mary! Remember My Favor upon you and your mother: how I supported you with the holy spirit[1] so you spoke to people inʿyourʾ infancy and adulthood. How I taught you writing, wisdom, the Torah and the Gospel. How you moulded a bird from clay—by My Will—and breathed into it and it

became a 'real' bird—by My Will. How you healed the blind and the lepers—by My Will. How you brought the dead to life—by My Will. How I prevented the Children of Israel from harming you when you came to them with clear proofs and the disbelievers among them said, "This is nothing but pure magic." (Qur'an, Al-Ma'idah 5:110)

Yahya related to me from Malik from Yahya ibn Said from Amra bint Abd ar-Rahman that Abu Bakr as-Siddiq visited A'isha while she had a (health) complaint and a Jewish woman was making incantation (Ruqyah) for her. Abu Bakr said, "**Do it (incantation) with the Book of Allah.**" (Malik Muwatta, Engl. Ref., Book 50, Hadith 11)

Aisha (May Allah be pleased with her) reported: Allah's Messenger (peace and blessings be upon him) used to recite (this supplication) as the words of incantation: "Lord of the people, remove the trouble for in Thine Hand is the cure; none is there to relieve him (the burden of disease) but only Thou." (Muslim)

'Abdullah ibn Khubayb (May Allah be pleased with him) reported: The Messenger of Allah (May Allah's peace and blessings be upon him) said to me: "Recite Surah al-Ikhlas, Surah al-Falaq, and Surah An-Nas thrice every morning and evening, and it will be sufficient for you and will grant you protection from everything." (Tirmidhi) (https://hadeethenc.com/en/browse/hadith/6082)

Anas reported that he said to Thabit: "Shall I not perform for you the Ruqyah of the Messenger of Allah (May Allah's peace and blessings be upon him)?" He said: 'Yes.' He (Anas) said: "Oh Allah, Lord of mankind, Remover of harm. Cure, You are the Curer. There is no curer but You. A cure that leaves behind no illness." (Bukhari) (https://hadeethenc.com/en/browse/hadith/5541)

Abu Sa'id al-Khudri (May Allah be pleased with him) reported: Jibreel came to the Prophet (May Allah's peace and blessings be upon him) and said: "O Muhammad, have you fallen ill?" He said: 'Yes.' So Jibreel said: "In the name of Allah I recite over you, (to cleanse you) from everything that troubles you, from the evil of every soul or envious eye, Allah will cure you, in the Name of Allah I recite over you)." (Muslim)

(https://hadeethenc.com/en/browse/hadith/5650)

Jabir (May Allah be pleased with him) reported that when the Messenger of Allah (May Allah's peace and blessings be upon him) was asked about the 'Nushrah' (counteracting Magic with Magic), he said: "It is an act of the Devil." (Abu Dawud) (https://hadeethenc.com/en/browse/hadith/3402)

Zainab the wife of 'Abdallah b. Masud told that 'Abdallah saw a thread on her neck and asked what it was. When she told him that it was a thread over which a spell had been recited for her, he took it, cut it up and said, "You, family of 'Abdallah, are independent of polytheism. I have heard God's messenger say that spells, charms and love-spells are polytheism." She replied, "Why do you speak like this? My eye was discharging and I kept going to so and so, the Jew, and when he applied a spell to it, it calmed down." 'Abdallah said, "That was just the work of the Devil who was pricking it with his hand, and when a spell was uttered, he desisted. All you need to do is to say as God's Messenger (peace and blessings be upon him) did, 'Remove the harm, O Lord of men, and heal. Thou art the Healer. There is no remedy but Thine which leaves no disease behind." (Abu Dawud)

Non-Islamic "exorcists" involve Devils by committing Shirk (associating partner with Allah), consolidate people's kufr (disbelief) and Shirk and make them firm in their path towards Hellfire, which is Shaytan's goal for humanity. The fortune teller or non-Islamic "exorcist" calls upon Jesus or another false deity, or another stronger Jinni/Jinn to kick out the present Jinni/Jinn, or the Jinni (or Jinn) leaves as the Shirk was committed, so the present disease will disappear but later on, there will be many other diseases and problems. And Allah knows the best.

Following is an extract from Ibn Taymiyah's Essay on Jinn (Demon):

"The fundamental principle on the basis of which this subject (Exorcism) should be understood is that it may be permissible, recommended or even compulsory to defend or aid one who is possessed, because helping the oppressed is a duty according to one's ability.

In both Saheeh al-Bukhari and Saheeh Muslim there is a narration in which the Prophet's Companion al- Barra' ibn 'Azib (May Allah have mercy on him) said, "Allah's Messenger (peace and blessings be upon him) commanded us to do seven things and prohibited us from doing seven. He enjoined on us: visiting the sick, following funeral processions, wishing well for one who sneezes, fulfilling oaths, helping the oppressed, responding to invitations, and spreading greetings of peace. He forbade the wearing of gold rings, drinking from silver vessels, using silk brocade saddle blankets, wearing silk blend clothes, silk clothes, velvet and silk brocade."

In the Saheeh collections on the authority of Anas it is reported that Allah's Messenger (peace and blessings be upon him) said: "Help your brother whether he is the oppressor or the oppressed. Anas asked, 'O' Messenger of Allah! I would help him if he is oppressed, but how can I help him when he is the oppressor?' He replied, 'By preventing him from oppression you are helping him.'"

Allah's Messenger (peace and blessings be upon him) is reported by Abu Hurairah in Saheeh Muslim to have said: "Whoever relieves a believer of one of the tragedies of this life, Allah will relieve him of one of the calamities of the Day of Resurrection. And whoever goes easy on one in a state of difficulty, Allah will go easy on him in both this life and the next. Furthermore, whoever conceals (the faults of) a Muslim, Allah will conceal his faults in this life and the next. Allah will help His servant as long as the servant helps his brother."

Jabir is also reported in Saheeh Muslim to have said that when Allah's Messenger (peace and blessings be upon him) was asked about incantations, he replied, "Whoever among you is able to help his brother should do so."

However, help should be justly rendered according to the method prescribed by Allah and His Messenger. For example, Islamically based prayers, words and phrases should only be used in the way they were used by the Prophet (peace and blessings be upon him) and his Companions. When commanding the Jinn to righteousness and prohibiting it from evil, it should be done in the same way that man is ordered and forbidden. Whatever is allowable in the case of humans is also allowable in the case of Jinns. For example, repelling Jinns might require scolding, threatening and even evoking God's Curse. In a narration from Abu ad-Darda in Saheeh Muslim he said: "Allah's Messenger stood up (in prayer) and we heard him say, 'I seek refuge in Allah from you.' Then he said thrice, 'I curse you by Allah's Curse.' And he reached out his hand as if he were catching something. When he finished praying, we asked him, 'O' Messenger of Allah! We heard you say something in your Salah which we have never heard you say before and we saw you stretch your arm out.' He said, 'Verily, Allah's enemy, Iblees brought a fiery torch and tried to thrust it in my face, so I said three times, 'I seek refuge in Allah from you.' Then I said thrice, 'I curse you by Allah's perfect Curse.' But he did not back off, so I caught a hold of him, and — by Allah — if it were not for our brother Sulayman's prayer, he would have been tied up for the children of Madinah to play with.'" This Hadith provides the foundation for the practices of seeking refuge in Allah from the Jinn and cursing them by Allah's Curse.

In both Saheeh al-Bukhah and Saheeh Muslim, Abu Hurairah (May Allah have mercy on him) reported that the Prophet (peace and blessings be upon him) said: "Verily the Devil appeared before me and launched an attack on me in order to break my Salah, but Allah gave me mastery over him and I choked him. I intended to tie him to a post until the morning so you could see him, but I remembered my brother Sulayman's prayer, *"... My Lord forgive me and grant me sovereignty not allowed to anyone after me.."* (Qur'an, 38:35) So, Allah sent him (the Devil) back in vain." The Prophet (peace and blessings be upon him) reached out his hand physically repel the Devil's assault by choking him. This was sufficient to ward off his attack and Allah sent him back disgraced. As for the added information with regard to binding the Devil to the post, such an act would have been the conduct of a sovereign and sovereignty over the Jinn was given only to Prophet Sulayman (May Allah have mercy on him). Our Prophet's conduct with the Jinn was the same as his conduct with humans; that of a servant of God and a Messenger. His ability to command them to worship Allah and order them to obey Him was not due to any special sovereignty which he held over them. He was a slave of God and one of His Messengers who was sent with a Book of Revelation, while Sulayman was a prophet of God and a king. The office of slave-Messenger is more honorable than that of prophet-king, just as the believers foremost in faith and nearest to God (as-Sabiqoon, and al-Muqarraboori) are superior to the righteous Companions of the right hand in general…

…One of the opinions is that it breaks Salah based on the previously mentioned Hadith and the Prophet's explanation of his statement that the passage of a black dog breaks Salah. He is reported to have said, "The black dog is a Devil." The reason that he gave for it breaking the Salah is that it is an Evil Jinn and it is as the Messenger of Allah (peace and blessings be upon him) says, "For the black dog is the Devil among dogs and Jinns take its form often, as well as that of black cats, because black rallies satanic forces more readily than any other colour and it contains the power of heat. If one afflicted gets well as a result of prayer, the mention of God, commanding the Jinn to do good and prohibiting them from evil, scolding them, shaming them, evoking curses on them and other such practices, and in doing so a group of the Jinn get sick or die, they are at fault for having oppressed themselves, as long as the one performing the exorcism does not overstep the Islamically defined limits in dealing with them. Many exorcists who use amulets command the Jinn to execute other Jinns whose lives it is not permissible to take, or they may imprison one who does not need to be detained. Consequently, the Jinn may attack and kill them, or cause them, their wives, their children or their animals to become sick.

As for those who follow the path of justice enjoined by Allah and His Messenger in repelling Jinn assaults, the Jinn will not wrong them because such an exorcist is obedient to Allah and His apostle in helping the oppressed and aiding the distressed. Comforting the troubled in an Islamic way, free from idolatry (Shirk) and evil, does not bring harm from the Jinn, either due to their knowledge that it is just or as a result of their inability to do so. If the possessing Demon is an 'Ifreet among Jinns and the exorcist is weak, it could harm him. Consequently, he should shield himself by the recitation of prayers seeking refuge in Allah, the Mu'awwidhatayn (two means of seeking refuge), Ayatul Kursi; by making Salah (formal prayer) and supplications and other similar things which strengthen faith and put aside sins by which the Evil Jinn may gain control over him. Such a person is a soldier of Allah (Mujahidfee Sabeelillah) and exorcism is among the greatest forms of Jihad, so he should beware not to help his enemy to overcome him by his own sins. If the circumstance is beyond his ability, *"Allah does not burden a soul beyond its capacity..." (Qur'an 2:286)*

— so, he should not expose himself to tribulation by taking on what he is unable to handle.

Among the greatest weapons which may be used to exorcise the Jinn is Ayatul Kursi, as confirmed in Saheeh al-Bukhari in a narration from Abu Hurairah (May Allah have mercy on him) who said: "Allah's Messenger (peace and blessings be upon him) put me in charge of the Zakah (charity) of Ramadan. While I was doing so, someone came and began to rummage around in the food so I caught a hold of him. I said, 'By Allah I am going to take you to Allah's Messenger!' The man implored, 'Verily I am poor and I have dependents. I am in great need.' So, I let him go. The next morning, the Prophet (peace and blessings be upon him) asked, 'O' Abu Hurairah, what did your captive do last night?' I said, 'He complained, of being in great need and of having a family so I let him go.' The Prophet replied, 'Surely he lied to you and he will return.' Since I knew that he was going to return, I laid in wait for him. When he returned and began to dig about in the food, I grabbed him and said, 'I am definitely going to take you to Allah's Messenger.' He pleaded, 'Let me go! Verily I'm poor and I do have a family. I won't return.' So, I had mercy on him and let him go. The next morning Allah's Messenger asked, 'O' Abu Hurairah what did your captive do last night?' I said that he complained of being in great need and of having a family so I let him go. The Prophet replied, 'Surely he lied to you and he will return.' So, I waited for him and grabbed him when he began to scatter the food around. I said, 'By Allah, I will take you to Allah's Messenger. This is the third time, and you promised you would not return. Yet you came back anyway!' He said, 'Let me give you some words by which Allah will benefit you.' I said, 'What are they?' He replied, 'Whenever you go to bed, recite Ayatul Kursi from beginning to end. If you do so, a guardian from Allah will remain with you and Satan will not come near you until the morning.' I then let him go. The next morning Allah's Messenger asked,

'What did your captive do last night?' I said that he claimed that he would teach me some words by which Allah would benefit me, so I let him go. When the Prophet asked what they were, I told him that they were saying Ayatul Kursi before going to bed. I also told him that he said that a guardian from Allah would remain with me and Satan would not come near me until I awoke in the morning. The Prophet said, 'Surely he has told the truth, though he is a compulsive liar. O' Abu Hurairah! Do you know who you have been speaking to these past three nights?' I replied, 'No', and he said, 'That was an Evil Jinn.'" (Bukhari)

Besides that, the countless many who have experience in this field unanimously confirm the incredible effectiveness of this Verse in warding off the Devils and breaking their spells. Indeed, it is greatly effective in repelling the Evil Jinns from human souls and exorcising them from the possessed as well as those prodded by Devils: like tyrants, those easily enraged, the lustful and lecherous, musicians and those who ecstatically whistle and clap enraptured by their music. If this Verse is sincerely recited over them, it will drive away the Devils and neutralize their illusions. It will also disrupt the Satanic visions and Devil-aided supernatural feats performed by humans.

The Evil Jinn reveal to their human allies hidden knowledge which the ignorant masses assume to be among the miracles given only to pious God-fearing saints, when in fact they are only Satanic deceptions manifest in the Devils' helpers, on whom is Allah's displeasure and who have gone astray.

A tyrannical Jinn should be repelled whether it is a Muslim or a disbeliever. For, the Prophet (peace and blessings be upon him) has said: "Whoever is killed defending his wealth is a martyr, whoever is killed defending his life is a martyr and whoever is killed defending his religion is a martyr." (https://hadeethenc.com/en/browse/hadith/58224)

If a man is oppressed, he has the right to protect his wealth even if it means taking the life of the attacker. Why then would he not defend his mind, body and soul which he surely holds more sacred? For, surely Satan corrupts and ruins the mind of one possessed and inflicts punishment on their bodies; it might even rape them. Thus, if they can only be repelled by killing them, it then becomes permissible to do so. As for leaving one's (possessed) companion without treating him, it is the same as abandoning anyone who is oppressed. Aiding the oppressed is Fard Kifdyah (a group obligation) on everyone according to his ability, as the Prophet (peace and blessings be upon him) is reported in Saheeh al-Bukhari and Saheeh Muslim to have said: "A Muslim is a brother to another Muslim, he does not leave him in harm nor does he harm him..." If he is unable to help him, or he is busy with something more obligatory, or someone else has gone to help the possessed individual, it is no longer obligatory on him to do so. If, on the other hand, he is the only one present who is able to help, and he is not busy with something more obligatory, it then becomes a compulsory duty to exorcise the possessed.

As regards the question: "Is (Exorcism) legal in Islam?", it is in fact among the most noble deeds. It is among the deeds performed by the Prophets and the righteous who have continually repelled the Devils from mankind using what has been commanded by Allah and His Messenger. The Messiah did it and so did our Prophet (peace and blessings be upon him). (10)

Read also the book of Dr Bilal Philips, The Exorcism Tradition in Islam. (635)

691a. Superiority of Man over Satan

1. Allah has placed Adam on earth as a Khalifa

"Behold, thy Lord said to the angels: "I will create a vicegerent on earth." (Qur'an, Al-Baqarah 2:30)

2. Allah ordered Satan to bow to Adam

"And surely, We created you (your father Adam) and then gave you shape (the noble shape of a human being), then We told the angels, "Prostrate to Adam", and they prostrated, except Iblis (Satan), he refused to be of those who prostrate." (Qur'an, Al-A'raf 7:11)

3. Allah made Satans subjected to the Prophet Sulayman as servants and workforce

By way of illustration, there is an instance of Prophet Sulayman (Solomon) to whom Satans were subjected as servants and workforce. But there is nothing to the effect that people were ever subjected to Satans or the Jinn in general, even partially.

4. Iblees saw in Adam no more than matter and form, constructing his flawed judgments exclusively around those factors. So blinded by his haughtiness, jealousy, pride and self-regard was he that he could not see - let alone appreciate - the spiritual, cerebral and moral considerations in Adam.

5. Allah taught Adam the names of everything

"And He taught Adam all the names (of everything)…" (Qur'an, Al-Baqarah 2:31)

6. Allah honored the Children of Adam and preferred them above all His creation

"And indeed, We have honored the Children of Adam, and We have carried them on land and sea, and have provided them with At-Taiyibat (lawful good things), and have preferred them above many of those whom We have created with a marked preference." (Qur'an, Al-Isra 17:70)

Accepting man as Allah's vicegerent on earth and as an honorable being preferred over much of what Allah had created was not compatible with Satan's delusions, self-absorption, pride and arrogance.

7. Satan Cannot Tolerate Adhan and Surah Al-Baqarah

Abu Hurairah (May Allah be pleased with him) reported that the Prophet (May Allah's peace and blessings be upon him) said: "When the Call to prayer is announced, the Devil takes to his heels and breaks wind with noise so as not to hear the call. When the Call to prayer is over, he returns. When the Iqamah is announced, he takes to his heels, and after it is over, he returns again to distract the attention of the worshiper and make him remember things which were not on his mind before the prayer, saying: 'Remember such-and-such, and remember such-and-such,' until the worshiper forgets how many units of prayer he performed." (Bukhari and Muslim)

Abu Hurairah (May Allah be pleased with him) reported: "I heard the Messenger of Allah (peace and blessings be upon him) saying: "Do not turn your houses into graveyards. Satan runs away from the house in which Surat Al-Baqarah is recited." (Muslim)

8. Satan has the power only on those who follow him

Satan pledged that he will mislead people and will arouse in them sinful desires to such an extent that they will eventually make recourse to the option of changing the creation of Allah.

"Verily, I will mislead them, and surely, I will arouse in them false desires; and certainly, I will order them to slit the ears of cattle, and indeed I will order them to change the nature created by Allah." And whoever takes Shaitan (Satan) as a Wali (protector or helper) instead of Allah, has surely suffered a manifest loss." (Qur'an, An-Nisa 4:119)

9. Allah had already informed Satan about his final destination - Hellfire

Satan knows that his actions warrant him an eternal punishment in Hellfire, but as long as he fills it with multitudes of people as well, who will share with him his fate. Allah thus reminds man:

"Verily Satan is an enemy to you, so treat him as an enemy. He only invites his adherents (his party) that they may become the dwellers of the blazing Fire." (Qur'an, Fatir 35:6)

10. Satan's few strengths and many weaknesses

As far as people are concerned, Satan is neither weak nor strong. His condition is determined by the people themselves. The stronger one's faith in Allah and piety, the weaker Satan becomes. Everything believers do is the antidote to Satan's trickery. Satan is powerless and desperate. He is a lost cause. Believers are furthermore in control of Satan. They do not worry about him, but about how to keep him at bay by intensifying their devotion and worship. By taking care of themselves, believers know that they take care of Satan and of everything that can be associated with him.

Allah, the Exalted, confirms:

"Feeble indeed is the cunning of Satan" (Qur'an, An-Nisa 4:76)

Allah assured Satan that he will have no authority whatsoever over His believing servants,

"except the erring ones who follow you." (Qur'an, Al-Hijr 15:42)

Satan acknowledged that by saying:

"By Your might, I will surely mislead them all, except, among them, Your chosen (sincere and purified) servants" (Qur'an, Sad 38:82-83)

11. Prophet Muhammad (peace and blessings be upon him) was sent to both mankind and the Jinn

Allah, the Exalted, says:

"And We have sent you (O Muhammad SAW) not but as a Mercy for the 'Alamin (mankind, Jinns and all that exists)." (Qur'an, Al-Anbya 21:107)

12. Satan's greatest nemeses are believers

"Verily! My slaves (i.e. the true believers of Islamic Monotheism), you have no authority over them. And All-Sufficient is your Lord as a Guardian." (Qur'an, Al-Isra 17:65)

The Prophet (peace and blessings be upon him) said to Umar b. al-Khattab: "By Him in Whose Hands my life is, whenever Satan sees you taking a way, he follows a way other than yours" (Bukhari)

Satan only lies in wait, placing traps and snares. He whispers and throws up evil suggestions into the hearts, as well as minds of people. He can influence a person only as much as he allows him and opens the doors of his life to Satan. The more permission Satan gets, and the wider the doors are opened, the more authorized he becomes to ruin a person's life.

13. Disbelief and Sins are the open door for Satans

Anything that is associable with whatever form and degree of non-belief and sin, is an invitation to Satan to act. If he gets full permission to enter and conquer somebody's life, Satan then becomes his owner. A person becomes a slave and Satan his deity. He becomes a Satan himself. There are no barriers between the two anymore. As a "reward," Satan yet can appear to such a person in different discernible forms: in dreams and in real life. That explains the existence of certain hallucinations and nightmares. It additionally explains the root cause of certain mental and spiritual diseases that make people insane.

Satan appeared to the polytheists of Makkah when they were bent on committing two of the most inconceivable deeds: when they plotted to kill Prophet Muhammad (peace and blessings be upon him) just before his migration to Madinah, and during the battle of Badr when they also wanted to kill the Prophet and hence forever extinguish the light of Islam.

14. Truth and Paradise with Allah, and Falsehood and Hellfire with Satan

Satan will tell:

"Indeed, Allah had promised you the promise of truth. And I promised you, but I betrayed you. But I had no authority over you except that I invited you, and you responded to me. So do not blame me, but blame yourselves. I cannot be called to your aid, nor can you be called to my aid. Indeed, I deny your association of me (with Allah) before. Indeed, for the wrongdoers is a painful punishment." (Qur'an, Ibrahim 14:22)

15. The nature of Satan's strategies

Since Satan has no power, nor authority over people, his strategies revolve around seducing, tricking, and misleading people via his endless *waswas* (whispers and incitements).

As to how he hoodwinked Adam and his wife, for example, the Qur'an uses the words *dallahuma bi ghurur*, which is normally translated as "he caused them to fall by deceit (through deception)".

"So, he misled them with deception. Then when they tasted of the tree, that which was hidden from them of their shame (private parts) became manifest to them and they began to stick together the leaves of Paradise over themselves (in order to cover their shame). And their Lord called out to them (saying): "Did I not forbid you that tree and tell you: Verily, Shaitan (Satan) is an open enemy unto you?" (Qur'an, Al-A'raf 7:22)

16. Satan's cowardice and fear

Satan is a coward. He pretends to be somebody and strong only when things go his way. However, when the tables are turned on him, he falters. He cracks under real pressure.

The Prophet (peace and blessings be upon him) said: "When the son of Adam recites a Verse of prostration and he prostrates, Satan withdraws and he weeps and he says: 'Woe to me! The son of Adam was commanded to prostrate and he prostrated, so he will go to Paradise. I was commanded to prostrate and I refused, so I will go to Hellfire'" (Muslim)

On the eve of the battle of Badr, furthermore, Satan was with the polytheists making their actions pleasing to them. He motivated them by insisting that no one could overcome them on that day from among the people. Above all, he guaranteed them that he was with them and was their protector.

"And (remember) when Shaitan (Satan) made their (evil) deeds seem fair to them and said, "No one of mankind can overcome you this Day (of the battle of Badr) and verily, I am your neighbour (for each and every help)." But when the two forces came in sight of each other, he ran away and said "Verily, I have nothing to do with you. Verily! I see what you see not. Verily! I fear Allah for Allah is Severe in punishment." (Qur'an, Al-Anfal 8:48)

Satan could sense that the destruction of either party was imminent. Whichever way and outcome, he was set to win. He wanted to make sure that especially the polytheists did not waver, for if the Muslims were to lose, that would signify his double victory. But if the Muslims were to win, he would have at least one victory: the annihilation of the polytheists.

17. Satan admitted twice that he fears Allah, the Lord of the worlds

According to the Qur'an, in addition, Satan admitted twice that he fears Allah, the Lord of the worlds, even though he incites people to the opposite *(Al-Anfal 8:48 and Al-Hashr 59:16)*.

18. Satan and shooting stars

Satan and his army try to eavesdrop on Allah's commands that are transmitted from one group of Angels to another throughout the seven heavens. They snatch what they manage to overhear and carry it to their friends (non-believers, sorcerers, fortune tellers and astrologers) to con people. And when Angels see the Jinn doing so, they attack them with meteors.

19. Satan and mankind's time and space

When Allah cursed and expelled Satan from Jannah, Satan, now an outcast, asked for a respite until the Day of Resurrection. He wanted to have more than enough time to excel in his ungodly mission. However, there was something else in his request. He asked to be reprieved until the Day people are resurrected, that is after everybody has died and has been brought back to life, after which there will be no more death *(Al-Hijr 15:36)*. In other words, Satan wanted to cheat Allah by deviously seeking His permission not to die. He asked for eternity. He schemed to be at least in that particular regard somehow equal with Allah. He was a mischievous fool. If he was ready yet to trick Allah, one can imagine how far he is ready to go to trick and ruin man. Allah told him that his request was granted, but only until the Day of the time well-known, which is the time appointed for the end of days and for his own death *(Al-Hijr 15:38)*. Having secured time as an existential dimension, Satan then proceeded to attempt and secure the space dimension as well. With that, he thought, his domination over man will be complete.

Satan said, outlining his plans:

"I will surely sit in wait for them on Your Straight Path. Then I will come to them from before them and from behind them and on their right and on their left, and You will not find most of them grateful (to You)." (Qur'an, Al-A'raf 7:16-17)

In a nutshell, Satan swore that he will try every possible course of action, leaving no opportunity unexplored, in his pursuit of people's lives (their souls, bodies and minds). He did not mention that he will come to people from above them. That is so because he has no access to that direction. Allah's Mercy descends from above, and being Most Exalted and Most High are the Attributes of Allah Alone. Satan is not qualified to be in correlation with highness and sublimity. Nor did he say that he will come to people from under them. That is so because it was humiliating for him to say such a thing and to act accordingly. Didn't he refuse to fall to the ground and prostrate before Adam? Why should he later do something like that, even if it be most remotely so? Here, too, Satan was wrong. Certainly, it is by means of humility and obedience – personified by believers' recurring prostration to Allah – that one rises and prospers. As a result of their regular "going down," believers constantly keep rising and keep going up. Their truest lives unfold on a vertical axis that connects the terrestrial bases of theirs with the highest points in Heaven. Owing to this, the Qur'an mentions simultaneously the notion of prostration (*Sajdah*) and the notion of drawing near to Allah (*iqtirab*). Believers are explicitly instructed to firstly embrace the former as the cause, then the latter as the effect *(Al-'Alaq 96:19)*.

The Prophet (peace and blessings be upon him) said that whoever humbles himself for the sake of Allah, Allah will raise him (in status in both worlds). Similarly, whoever is arrogant to Allah, Allah will lower (and humiliate) him (in both worlds). (Ibn Majah)

Trapped in the matter and blinded by sheer worldly concerns, Satan could not see all that. Operating on a plain horizontal axis, he cannot even get close to believers, much less influence or dictate their lives. Satan and believers reside on dissimilar ontological planes. He can mislead and get hold only of such as debase themselves and as such, exchange excellence and sublimity for vice and absurdity.

Allah, the Exalted, says:

"Go, for whoever of them follows you, indeed Hell will be the recompense of you - an ample recompense. And incite (to senselessness) whoever you can among them with your voice and assault them with your horses and foot soldiers and become a partner in their wealth and their children and promise them. But Satan does not promise them except delusion. Indeed, over My (believing) servants there is for you no authority. And sufficient is your Lord as Disposer of affairs." *(Qur'an, Al-Isra 17:63-65)*

The Shaytan is close to man, and indeed he flows through him like blood, so he whispers to him at moments of heedlessness and withdraws from him when he remembers Allah. Through this constant closeness he knows what whims and desires occur to man, so he makes them appear attractive to him and he whispers to him regarding them. (636, 637)

Ibn Taymiyah (May Allah have mercy on him) said:

"They smell a good smell or a bad smell [meaning the angels, who smell a good smell when a person is thinking of a good deed, as was narrated from Sufyan ibn 'Uyaynah]. But the

Devils do not need that (smell) in order to know; rather they even know what is in the heart of the son of Adam, and they see and hear what he says to himself. Moreover, the devil has full control over man's heart, then when man remembers Allah he withdraws, and when he neglects to remember Him, he whispers to him. He knows whether he is remembering Allah or is neglecting to remember Him, and he knows the whims and desires of his heart and makes them appear attractive to him." (638)

Narrated Safiyyah (May Allah be pleased with her): The Prophet (peace and blessings of Allah be upon him) said: "The Shaytan flows through the sons of Adam like blood."

The Shaytan is aware of what a person is thinking to himself, and he knows his inclinations and his whims and desires, both good and bad, so he whispers to him accordingly.

Sheikh Ibn Baaz (May Allah have mercy upon him) was asked - in a lengthy question: "If I intend in my heart to do something good, does the Shaytan know and try to divert me from it?"

He replied: "Every person has a Devil and an angel with him, as the Prophet (peace and blessings of Allah be upon him) said: "There is no one who does not have a companion from among the Jinn and a companion from among the angels." They said: "Even you, O Messenger of Allah?" He said: "Even me, but Allah helped me with him and he became Muslim (or: and I am safe from him), so he only enjoins me to do that which is good." And he (peace and blessing of Allah be upon him) told us that the Shaytan dictates evils to man and calls him to evil, and he has some control over his heart. And he can see, by Allah's will, what a person wants and intends to do of both good and bad deeds. The angel also has some control over his heart that makes him inclined towards good and calls him to good. This control is something that Allah has enabled them to have, i.e. He has given some power to the companions from among the Jinn and from among the angels; even the Prophet (peace and blessings of Allah be upon him) had a Shaytan with him who was the companion from among the Jinn as mentioned in the Hadith quoted above. The point here is that every person has with him a companion from among the Angels and a companion from among the Devils. The believer suppresses his Shaytan by obeying Allah and adhering to His religion, and he humiliates his Shaytan until he becomes weak and is unable to prevent the believer from doing good or to make him fall into evil except that which Allah wills. But the sinner, through his sins and bad deeds helps his Shaytan until he becomes strong enough to help him to follow falsehood and he encourages him to do so and he becomes strong enough to keep him from doing good. The believer has to fear Allah and strive to resist his Shaytan by obeying Allah and His Messenger (peace and blessings of Allah be upon him), and seeking refuge with Allah from the Shaytan. And he should be keen (to accept the) support (of) his angel to obey Allah and His Messenger (peace and blessings of Allah be upon him) and to follow the commands of Allah." (End quote from Fataawa al-Shaykh Ibn Baaz) (638)

20. Satan is afraid of water

Allah, the Exalted, says:

"(Allah said to him): "Strike the ground with your foot: This is a spring of water to wash in, cool and a (refreshing) drink." (Qur'an, Sad 38:42)

"He caused water (rain) to descend on you from the sky, to clean you thereby and to remove from you the Rijz (whispering, evil-suggestions, etc.) of Shaitan (Satan), and to strengthen your hearts, and make your feet firm thereby." (Qur'an, Al-Anfal 8:11)

"And the Jinn, We created aforetime from the smokeless flame of fire." (Qur'an, Al-Hijr 15:27)

'Atiyyah reported: The Messenger of Allah, peace be and blessings be upon him, said, "Verily, anger comes from Satan and Satan was created from fire. Fire is extinguished with water, so if you become angry then perform ablution with water." (Abu Dawud)

Wudu and Ghusl water has a miraculous healing effects – the Ahadith were already mentioned before.

From my practice:

1. During my night flight when I finished praying Tahajjud and Witr prayers, my neighbor, a woman of 50 y-old, became unconscious. Her daughter was calling for doctor. I said: "we should put her in horizontal position." But before changing the position, a man took a bottle of water, had water in his mouth and splashed on her face – and a miracle happened – she regained consciousness but was confused. Then, recited Ruqyah. Allah Almighty cured her. Loss of consciousness was caused by the Evil Jinn.

2. A paralysed dying bird with rare breathing on my road. A man put few drops of water on bird's head, bird reacted by quick eye blinkings. The bird flew out of my hand after the recitation of Ruqyah. Allah's Miracle. Bird was paralysed by the Evil Jinn.

692. Jinn Catching

Allah, the Exalted, says:

"And verily, there were men among mankind who took shelter with the males among the Jinn, but they (Jinn) increased them (mankind) in sin and transgression. And they thought as you thought, that Allah will not send any Messenger (to mankind or Jinns)." (Qur'an, Al-Jinn 72:6-7)

"See you not that We have sent the Shayateen (Devils) against the disbelievers to push them to do evil." (Qur'an, Maryam 19:83)

Other Verses: *Al-Isra 17:62, Saba 34:20, Al-A'raf 7:188, Al-An'am 6:59 and 6:128.*

'Iyad b. Him-ar reported that Allah's Messenger (peace and blessings of Allah be upon him), while delivering a sermon one day, said, telling how Allah taught His slaves: "…I have created My servants as one having a natural inclination to the worship of Allah but it is Satan who turns them away from the right religion and he makes unlawful what has been declared lawful for them and he commands them to ascribe partnership with Me, although he has no justification for that…(Muslim)

(https://sunnah.com/muslim:2865a)

Narrated Aisha (May Allah be pleased with her): Allah's Messenger (peace and blessings of Allah be upon him) was affected by Magic, so much that he used to think that he had done something which in fact, he did not do, and he invoked his Lord (for a remedy). Then (one day) he said, "O Aisha! Do you know that Allah has advised me as to the problem I consulted Him about?" Aisha said, "O Allah's Messenger! What's that?" He said, "Two men came to me and one of them sat at my head and the other at my feet, and one of them asked his companion, 'What is wrong with this man?' The latter replied, 'He is under the effect of magic.' The former asked, 'Who has worked Magic on him?' The latter replied, 'Labid bin Al-A'sam.' The former asked, 'With what did he work the Magic?' The latter replied, 'With a comb and the hair, which are stuck to the comb, and the skin of pollen of a date-palm tree.' The former asked, 'Where is that?' The latter replied, 'It is in Dharwan.' Dharwan was a well in the dwelling place of the (tribe of) Bani Zuraiq. Allah's Messenger (peace and blessings of Allah be upon him) went to that well and returned to Aisha, saying, 'By Allah, the water (of the well) was as red as the infusion of Hinna, and the date-palm trees look like the heads of Devils.' Aisha added, Allah's Messenger (peace and blessings of Allah be upon him) came to me and informed me about the well. I asked the Prophet, 'O Allah's Messenger (peace and blessings of Allah be upon him), why didn't you take out the skin of pollen?' He said, 'As for me, Allah has cured me and I hated to draw the attention of the people to such evil (which they might learn and harm others with).'" Narrated Hisham's father: Aisha said, "Allah's Messenger (peace and blessings of Allah be upon him) was bewitched, so he invoked Allah repeatedly requesting Him to cure him from that Magic)." Hisham then narrated the above narration. (Bukhari)

The Prophet (peace and blessings be upon him) when noticed forgetfulness due to the sorcery, made repeatedly Du'a to Almighty Allah asking for help and cure.

Allah, the Exalted, says:

"True, there were some among men who sought refuge in some among the Jinn, but they (the Jinn) only increased their fears." (Qur'an, Al-Jinn 72:6)

"And on the Day when He will gather them (all) together (and say): "O you assembly of Jinns! Many did you mislead of men," and their Auliya' (friends and helpers, etc.) amongst men will say: "Our Lord! We benefited one from the other, but now we have

reached our appointed term which You did appoint for us." He will say: "The Fire be your dwelling place, you will dwell therein forever, except as Allah may will. Certainly, your Lord is All-Wise, All-Knowing." *(Qur'an, Al-An'am 6:130)*

"O you assembly of jinns and mankind! "Did not there come to you Messengers from amongst you, reciting unto you My Verses and warning you of the meeting of this Day of yours?" They will say: "We bear witness against ourselves." It was the life of this world that deceived them. And they will bear witness against themselves that they were disbelievers." *(Qur'an, Al-An'am 6:130)*

Whoever claims to have knowledge of the Unseen is a kaafir.

Allah, the Exalted, says

"(He Alone is) the All-Knower of the Ghayb (Unseen), and He reveals to none His Ghayb (Unseen). Except to a Messenger (from mankind) whom He has chosen (He informs him of the Unseen as much as He likes)." (Qur'an, Al-Jinn 72:25-26)

Dealing with the Jinn is a serious issue, and is a door that leads to evil and mischief; how often have people are affected by this evil? It is sufficient for you to know that Shirk only came to mankind through them. There are believers and Muslims among the Jinn, and also kaafirs and evildoers. But the fact that they are concealed from man means that we cannot be sure about any one of them, and gives us cause for concern about their tricks and treachery, especially with the spread of ignorance and Bid'ah (innovation), which is the harbinger of Shirk. Usually these creatures make man fall into that which is haram, and bring only a little benefit. Hence the fatwas of the scholars state that it is haram to deal with the Jinn at all – whether with the believers or the kaafirs among them – and it is essential not to take this matter lightly, so as to close the door to fitnah and confusion, and out of concern for those who have faith in Allah. (639-641)

Sheikh al-Albaani said in al-Silsilah al-Saheehah (Hadith no. 2760):

"This also includes some who appear outwardly to be righteous treating people by means of that which they call "spiritual medicine (al-tibb al-roohaani)", whether that is in the ancient manner by contacting his qareen or Jinn companion – as they used to do during the Jahiliyyah – or it is done by means of what they call "summoning the spirits". Similar to that in my opinion is hypnotism. All of these are means that are not acceptable in Shariah, because they all boil down to seeking the help of the Jinn who were the cause of the mushrikeen going astray as it says in the Holy Qur'an. *"And verily, there were men among mankind who took shelter with the males among the Jinn, but they (Jinn) increased them (mankind) in sin and transgression." (Al-Jinn 72:6)* The claims of some of those who seek their help, that they only seek the help of the righteous among them, are false claims, because they usually cannot mix with them and live with them in ways that will show whether they are righteous or not. We know from experience that most of the humans with whom you keep company turn out not to be good friends. Allah, the Exalted, says: *"O you who believe! Verily, among your wives and your children there are enemies for you (who may stop you from the obedience of Allah); therefore, beware of them!" (Qur'an, Al-Taghabun 64:14)* This has to do with people who can be seen, so what do you think about the Jinn, concerning whom Allah says: *"Verily, he (Shaytan) and Qabeeluhu (his soldiers from the Jinn or his tribe) see you from where you cannot see them." (Qur'an, Al-A'raf 7:27)* End quote. (642)

Ibn Taymiyah (May Allah have mercy on him) said:

"It is haram to question either the Jinn or those who conversed with them, or to believe in the truth of all that they say." He also said:

"Similarly, it is permissible for one to listen to what they say and inform others about the Jinn in the same way that it is permissible for a Muslim to listen to a disbeliever and a sinner to know what they are about and take a lesson from them. It is also similar to listening to information from the unrighteous and checking it out, without initially believing or disbelieving it, as the Almighty says: *"O you who believe! If a rebellious evil person comes to you with a news, verify it, lest you harm people in ignorance, and afterwards you become regretful to what you have done." (Qur'an, Al-Hujurat 49:6)* He also said:

"Seeking the help of the Jinn or turning to them to fulfill one's desires to cause harm or bring benefit is ascribing partners in worship with Allah (Shirk), because it is a kind of mutual benefitting whereby the Jinn respond to the human's requests and fulfills his needs in return for the human's fulfillment of the Jinn's evil request."

"The Jinn usually communicate by either visions or voices' with those seeking information among the idol worshippers, Christians, Jews and heretical Muslims driven astray by the Devils. Jinns may take the form of a live picture portraying whatever the sorcerers and fortune tellers wish to know about. When these deviants see the image of what they sought, they then inform other humans about it. Some of them may know that the image is actually an illusion, while others may be deluded into believing that they are actually witnessing the real scene. Jinns may also make humans hear the voice of those whom they call upon who are far away. Such cases are frequent among idolaters, Christians, Jews and ignorant Muslims who seek refuge in those whom they consider holy. When some devotees call on their spiritual masters for help saying, "O my Lord so and so!" The Jinn will address them in the voice of their masters. When the masters answer their request, the Jinn, in turn, answer the devotees in the master's voice.

The Devils will often respond while taking the form of the one besought, whether dead or alive, even if he is unaware of those who call on him. Those committing Shirk in this fashion believe that the person beseeched has actually replied when in fact it is the Jinn replying. This frequently happens to Christians who call on those whom they edify, whether dead or alive, like George or other holy figures. It also occurs to heretical Muslims who call on the dead or those not present, and the Devils take the form of the one called upon even without him realizing it. I know of many cases where this has occurred and the people called upon have told me that they did not know that they were called upon, though those beseeching them for help saw their images and were convinced that it was the actual person. More than one person has mentioned that they called on me in times of distress, each telling a different story about how I responded. When I told them that I never answered any of them nor did I know that they were calling on me, some said that it must have been an angel. I told them that angels do not benefit those committing Shirk and that it was actually a Devil trying to further misguide them. Sometimes the Jinn will take the form of those admired and stand at 'Arafat, and those who believe well of him will think that he actually stood in 'Arafat. Many others have also been actually carried by the Devils to 'Arafat and other sacred places. In such cases, they pass the Miqat (boundaries) without formally entering the state of Ihram (consecration) or performing many of the obligatory rites of Hajj like making the Talbeeyah (chant of response to God's call) or circulating the Ka'bah, and walking between the mounts of Safa and Marwah. Among them are some who do not even pass through Makkah, others who stand at 'Arafat without performing the pre-requisite rite of casting stones at the Jamarat, etc. It is by these and other similar feats that Satan leads seemingly pious people into misguidance. Sincere devotees among heretics are in this way enticed to do acts which are prohibited (Haram) or despised (Makrooh) in the religion. Satan is able to make such misdeeds appealing to them by convincing them that they are among the Karamat (supernatural or quasi-miraculous feats) of the righteous. However, they are, without a doubt, Satanic deceptions because Allah cannot be worshipped by any religious injunction which is neither compulsory (Wajib) nor recommended (Mustahabb). Whoever performs an act of worship which is neither Wajib nor Mustahabb believing that it is so, has been deceived by Satan. Even if it is decreed that such a person will be forgiven due to his good intention and striving, the act itself is still unacceptable to Allah. Such acts are not among the things with which Allah honors His pious servants who are close to Him, as there is no honor in performing prohibited (Haram) or despised (Makrooh) acts. Divine Honor lies in protecting one whom Allah loves from such acts and preventing him from doing them. For, committing misdeeds debases one who does them and does not in any way favor him, even if he is not punished for doing them. Doing despised or Haram acts must decrease the spiritual level of both the one who does them as well as his followers who praise such acts and glorify him. For, heaping praise on prohibited and despised acts, and honoring the one who does them is definitely a form of deviation from the Path of Allah. The more a man innovates in the religion as a result of independent judgement (Ijtihad), the farther he becomes from Allah, because innovation (Bid 'ah) removes him from Allah's Path; the Divine Path of *"Those whom Allah has blessed from among the Prophets, the sincerely truthful, martyrs and the righteous..." (Qur'an, An-Nisa 4:69)* unto the path of *"... those with whom Allah is angry and those who have gone astray!" (Qur'an, Al-Fatihah 1:7)*

Ibn Taymiyah mentioned the following historical incident concerning al-Hallaj and a group of his followers:

"Some of them requested some sweets from al-Hallaj, so he got up and went to a spot a short distance away, then returned with a plateful of sweets. It was later discovered that it had been stolen from a candy shop in Yemen and carried by a Devil to that area."

Ibn Taymiyah went on to say, "Incidents similar to this have happened to others who, like al-Hallaj, also achieved the pinnacle of satanic states, and we know of quite a few such people in our time as well as other times. For instance, there is a person presently residing in Damascus whom the Devil used to carry from the Saliheeyah mountain to villages around Damascus. He would appear out of the air and enter the windows of houses in which people were gathered to witness his 'miraculous entrance.'"

Ibn Taymiyah also quoted another mystic master who admitted that he used to fornicate with women and sodomize young boys. The former mystic master said, "A black dog with two white spots between his eyes would come to me and say, 'Verily such and such a person has made an oath by you and he will come to you tomorrow to inform you about it. I have already fulfilled his need for your sake.' The person would then come to him the next day and the Sufi master would reveal the details of his oath to him and how it was fulfilled. The Sufi master went on to say, 'I used to walk about the city and a black pole with a light on top of it would lead the way.'" He said, "When the Sufi master repented and began to pray, fast and avoid the forbidden, the black dog went away."

He also narrated the following about another mystic master who had the aid of Devils whom he would dispatch to possess people: "When the family of the possessed would come to him seeking a cure, he would send a message to his Demon companion and they would leave the possessed persons, as a result, the Sheikh would be given many dirhams for his services. Sometimes the Jinn would bring him dirhams and food which they stole from people, so much so that the Sheikh would request dates from his Devils and they would take them from beehives in which some people had hidden their dates. When the beehive owners would look of their dates, they would find them gone." About yet another mystic, Ibn Taymiyah relates, "There was a Sheikh knowledgeable in the religious sciences and Qur'anic recitation to whom the Devils came and eventually managed to seduce. They told him that Saldh was no longer required of him and that they would bring him whatever he wished. As soon as he complied with their wishes, they began to bring him a variety of sweets and fruit. This continued until he was advised to repent by some scholars that he visited who were firmly following the Sunnah. He subsequently repented and repaid the owners of the sweets for what he ate while under the influence of the Jinn." He then went on to say, "Many of those who call on Sheikhs in time of need saying, 'O' master so and so, or Sheikh so and so, fulfill my need' have seen an image of the Sheikh saying, 'I will fulfill your need and put your heart at ease,' then it fulfils their needs or repels their enemies. In such cases it is a Devil taking the Sheikh 's form when they committed Shirk by associating partners with Allah and calling on others besides Him."

Ibn Taymiyah then went on to enumerate similar instances involving himself saying, "I know of many such incidences even among a group of my Companions who called on me in times when they were struck by calamities. One was afraid of the Romans and another afraid of the Tartars. Both of them mentioned that when they called out to me, they saw me in the air and I repelled their enemies for them. I informed them that I did not hear their cries nor did I repel their enemies. It was a Devil taking my appearance to seduce them when they associated partners with Allah the Almighty. Similar incidents have also happened to the students of my contemporaries among the scholars, whereby some of their students have sought refuge in them and have seen them fulfill their needs. The scholars have also denied doing so and indicated that it was in fact the world of Devils." (10)

693. Not Performing Circumcision

The Prophet (peace and blessings be upon him) said, "There are five things that are of the nature (i.e. of the natural hygiene): removing the pubic hair, circumcision, trimming the mustache, removing the underarm hair and cutting of the nails." (reported in all the six authentic collections of Hadith).

The health benefits of the circumcision were confirmed scientifically.

694. Ruling on Surgery that Causes Sterility

Narrated Samurah that the Messenger of Allah (peace and blessings of Allah upon him) said: "Whoever kills his slave, we will kill him: whoever mutilates (his slave). We will mutilate him, and whoever castrates (his slave), we will castrate him." (An-Nasa'i)

Sheikh Ibn Jibreen (May Allah have mercy on him) said:

"It is not permissible to have medical treatment to prevent or end pregnancy except in cases of necessity, if doctors have determined that giving birth will cause irjaaq, or will exacerbate sickness, or there is the fear that pregnancy and giving birth will lead to the woman's death." (643)

695. Abortion

Allah, the Exalted, says:

"And when the female (infant) buried alive (as the pagan Arabs used to do) shall be questioned. For what sin she was killed?" (Qur'an, At-Takweer 81:8-9)

"And kill not your children for fear of poverty." (Qur'an, Al-Isra 17:31)

"... if anyone killed a person not in retaliation of murder, or (and) to spread mischief in the land — it would be as if he killed all mankind, and if anyone saved a life, it would be as if he saved the life of all mankind..." (Qur'an, Al-Ma'idah 5:32)

Views allowing abortion before forty days in Islam

The jurists differed concerning the ruling on abortion before forty days .

Ibn al-Humam said in Fath al-Qadir (3/401): "Is it permissible to abort a pregnancy? It is permissible so long as it has not developed human features? Then they said: "But that does not happen until after one hundred and twenty days. This implies that what they meant by developing human features is when the soul is breathed into it, otherwise it is wrong, because development of human features could be seen before that."

Ar-Ramli said in Nihayat al-Muhtaj (8/443): "What is most likely to be correct is that it is prohibited after the soul is breathed into it in all cases, but it is permissible before that."

In Hashiyat Qalyubi (4/160), it says: "It is permissible to abort the pregnancy, even by use of medicine, before the soul is breathed into it, in contrast to the view of al-Ghazali."

Al-Mirdawi said in al-Insaf (1/386): "It is permissible to take medicine to abort a nutfah (lit., sperm-drop; embryo soon after conception). Ibn al-Jawzi said in Ahkam an-Nisa: "It is haram." It says in al-Furu': The apparent meaning of the words of Ibn 'Aqil in al-Funun is that it is permissible to abort it before the soul is breathed into it, and he said: "There is an argument to support that."

Views prohibiting abortion before forty days in Islam

The Malikis are of the view that abortion is not permissible in any case. This is also the view of some of the Hanafis, some of the Shaafi'is and some of the Hanbalis. Ad-Dardir said in ash-Sharh al-Kabir (2/266): "It is not permissible to abort an embryo that has become settled in the womb, even before forty days; once the soul has been breathed into it, it is prohibited according to scholarly consensus."

Abortion before forty days for a reason

However, some of the jurists limited the permissibility of abortion to cases where there is a reason. See: al-Mawsu'ah al-Fiqhiyyah al-Kuwaitiyyah (2/57).

The Council of Senior Scholars stated:

1. It is not permissible to abort a pregnancy at any stage, except when there is a legitimate justification for doing so, within very narrow guidelines.
2. If the pregnancy is in the first stage, which is forty days, and aborting it will serve a legitimate Shariah purpose or will ward off harm, it is permissible to abort it. As for aborting it at this stage for fear of hardship in raising children, or for fear of not being able to afford the costs of raising and educating them, or for fear about their future, or because the couple think that they have enough children, that is not permissible. (al-Fataawa al-Jami'ah, 3/1055)

It says in Fataawa al-Lajnah ad-Daimah (21/450):

"The basic principle regarding a woman's pregnancy is that it is not permissible to abort it at any stage, unless there is a legitimate justification for that. If the pregnancy is still a nutfah ("sperm-drop"; embryo soon after conception), which is forty days or less, and aborting it will serve a legitimate purpose or ward off harm that is expected to befall the mother, then it is permissible to abort it in that case. That does not include fear of difficulty in raising the children or not being able to afford their expenses or education, or thinking that a certain number of children is enough, and other justifications that are unacceptable according to Islamic teachings. But if the pregnancy has passed forty days, it is forbidden to abort it, because after forty days it becomes an 'alaqah, which is when it begins to develop human features, so it is not permissible to abort it after it reaches this stage, unless a trustworthy medical committee determines that continuing the pregnancy will pose a danger to the life of the mother, and there is the fear that she may die if the pregnancy continues."

What appears to be the case is that it is permissible to abort it before forty days, if there is a need for that, including the case of having three consecutive pregnancies within a short time, because having three pregnancies in rapid succession causes immense difficulty to the woman and weakens her physically, which may affect the foetus itself, and the mother may not be able to take care of the three children when they are so small. (644)

Abortion after the soul has been breathed into the foetus

The Maaliki faqeeh Ibn Jizzi narrated in al-Qawaaneen al-Fiqhiyyah that there was scholarly consensus that it is haram to have an abortion after the soul has been breathed into the foetus. He said: "When the womb has accepted the sperm it is haram to interfere with it. It is worse (to do so) when it has been formed; and it is worse when the soul has been breathed into it, for that is considered to be the killing of a soul, according to scholarly consensus." (al-Qawaaneen al-Fiqhiyyah, 141)

Similarly, it says in Nihaayat al-Muhtaaj: "The prohibition becomes stronger the closer the time is for the soul to be breathed into the foetus, because it is a crime. Then if it has taken on a human form and the midwives can palpate it, it must be protected fully." (Nihaayat al-Muhtaaj, 8/442)

The author of al-Bahr al-Raa'iq stated that when some of the features of the foetus become distinct, it is to be considered as a child. The author of al-Binaayah said: "It is not permitted to interfere with the foetus once its features have become distinct. If it can be distinguished from the 'alaqah (clot) and the blood, it should be considered as having become a soul, and there is no doubt that the sanctity of the soul is protected by scholarly consensus and by the texts of the Qur'an."

Thus, it is clear to us that abortion after the soul has been breathed into the foetus is a crime which it is not permitted to commit, except in cases of extreme and certain necessity, not where necessity is merely imagined, i.e., where the necessity is proven. This means cases where preserving the foetus would put the mother's life in danger, noting that with the advances in modern medicine and the scientific possibilities available nowadays, abortions performed to save the mother's life have become very rare. (645)

696. Foeticide

The decision of the Committee was in accordance with the Fatwa of the Standing Committee for Academic Research and Issuing Fatwas in the Kingdom of Saudi Arabia, no. 2484, issued on 16/7/1399 AH.

"But if the soul has been breathed into the foetus and it has completed 120 days, then it is not permissible to abort it, no matter what the deformity, unless continuation of the pregnancy would put the mother's life in danger. This is because after the soul has been breathed into the foetus, it is considered to be a person who must be protected, regardless of whether it is free of disease or not, and regardless of whether there is hope of recovery or not. That is because Allah has a reason for everything that He creates, which many people do not know, and He knows best what is right for His creation, as Allah says:

"Should not He Who has created know? And He is the Most Kind and Courteous (to His slaves), All Aware (of everything)." (Qur'an, Al-Mulk 67:14)

In the birth of these deformed children there is a lesson for those who are of sound health, and it teaches us of the power of Allah Who shows His creation the manifestations of His Might and the wonders that He has created. Killing and aborting them is a purely materialistic view which pays no attention to matters of religion and morals. Perhaps the existence of these deformities will make people more humble and submissive towards their Lord, and make them bear them with patience, seeking a great reward from Him. Physical deformity is something that Allah has decreed for some of His slaves. Whoever bears that with patience, will attain victory. This is something that happens and has always happened throughout history, but unfortunately studies indicate that the rate of physical deformity is increasing, as the result of pollution of the environment and the increase of harmful rays in the atmosphere, which was previously unknown. It is by the Mercy of Allah that many deformed foetuses are miscarried or die before they are born.

697. Prohibition on Selling Blood

Narrated Aun bin Abi Juhaifa: "I saw my father buying a slave whose profession was cupping, and ordered that his instruments (of cupping) be broken. I asked him the reason for doing so. He replied, "Allah's Apostle (peace and blessings be upon him) prohibited taking money for blood, the price of a dog, and the earnings of a slave girl by prostitution; he cursed her who tattoos and her who gets tattooed, the eater of Riba (usury), and the maker of pictures." (Bukhari)

It says in Fataawa al-Lajnah al-'Daa'imah li'l-Buhooth al-'Ilmiyyah wa'l-Ifta' (13/71):

"It is not permissible to sell blood, because of the report in Saheeh al-Bukhari from Abu Juhayfah who said that he bought a cupper (as a slave) and ordered that his equipment be broken. He was asked about that and he said: The Messenger of Allah (peace and blessings of Allah be upon him) forbade the price of blood." (646)

698. Cosmetic Surgical Procedures

The Satan said:

"And I will mislead them, and I will arouse in them (sinful) desires, and I will command them so they will slit the ears of cattle, and I will command them, so they will change the creation of Allah." And whoever takes Satan as an ally instead of Allah has certainly sustained a clear loss." (Qur'an, An-Nisa 4:119)

Prohibited Cosmetic Surgical Procedures

There are cosmetic surgical procedures which are haram and are not considered to be excusable; these are seen as tampering with the creation of Allah for the sake of beauty. Examples include: breast enlargement or reduction, and procedures aimed at reversing the signs of ageing, such as face-lifts etc. The Islamic view is that these are not permitted, because there is no urgent need or necessity for them; rather, the aim is to change and tamper with the creation of Allah for reasons of human vanity. This is haram and the one who does it is cursed because it involves two things mentioned in the Hadith: pursuit of beauty and changing what Allah has created. Added to this is the fact that these operations are aimed at deceit, and may involve the injection of materials extracted from aborted foetuses. These are very serious crimes. Moreover, many of these operations result in ongoing pain and other side effects, as the specialists themselves say. (See Ahkam al-Jirahah (Rulings on surgery) by Dr. Muhammad Muhammad al-Mukhtar al-Shanqiti).

Types of Faults that Necessitate Plastic Surgery

Faults may be of two types: physical or congenital faults and faults which result from illness. Congenital faults include abnormally turned out lips, hare-lips, twisted fingers or toes, etc. Faults which result from illness include the scars left by leprosy or other skin diseases, or scars caused by accidents and burns. There is no doubt that such faults and scars cause physical and psychological pain and harm, therefore Islam allows people afflicted with them to remove or reduce them by surgical means. They cause the kind of mental and psychological pain that allows this surgery as an urgent need, where necessity permits something that is ordinarily forbidden. (647)

699. Ruling on Face-Lift, Botox, Skin Exfoliating

Allah, the Exalted, says,

"Help you one another in righteousness and piety, but help you not one another in sin and rancor." (Qur'an, Al-Ma'idah 5:2)

Exfoliation means removing a layer of skin to expose new skin. The reason for doing that may be to remove a blemish on the skin that resulted from a burn or tear, or it may be for cosmetic purposes, to beautify the face. If it is the former, then it is permissible, because removing blemishes makes this action permissible. But if it is for the latter then it is not permissible, because that is changing the creation of Allah, and is a kind of beautification.

Face-lift operations are usually done for purposes of beautification and to remove wrinkles. This comes under the heading of changing the creation of Allah. (648)

Botox and **Dermal fillers** treat scars, wrinkles, lines and other depressions with the intention of improving one's appearance (the treatment involves injecting the materials into the affected area of the skin), they are not prohibited in of themselves. However, certain concerns still remain: These injections may contain unlawful and impure substances such as those from pigs or human albumin (source: US Food and Drug Administration) making them unlawful. Thus, if this indeed is the case, it will not be permitted to have them injected into the skin merely for cosmetic purposes. One may avail of them to help alleviate a medical condition such as cerebral palsy or face burns, under the dispensation of using impermissible substances as medication, but that too is subject to certain conditions – namely: a) the medicine/injection is reasonably known to be effective, b) it is needed, c) there is no Halal alternative, and d) the medical need is established by a specialist preferably a Muslim doctor who is at least outwardly upright and God-fearing. (See: *Radd al-Muhtar ala al-Durr*, 1/210) Becoming embroiled in the cosmetic and fashion industry has its own negatives, and ethically wrong in of itself. Unfortunately, the current fashion industry expects us to not even have a few wrinkles or lines on our faces and hence things like Botox injections and dermal fillers are being used widely. Islam teaches us to age gracefully and be content with what our Creator has created us with. The standard of one's beauty is not the external appearance; but rather, piety, virtuous actions and good conduct towards others. As such, even if these products were to not contain any unlawful substances, they would be ethically wrong, in normal cases, as they go against the spirit of Islamic teachings. The Shariah ruling for carrying out such procedures on patients follows that of the procedure itself. If they are proven to contain unlawful substances, it will not be permitted to deal with them for purely cosmetic reasons. (649)

Botox is a protein made from Botulinum toxin, which the bacterium *Clostridium botulinum* produces. This is the same toxin that causes botulism. Botox is widely used for cosmetic purposes in small doses. Botox is used also in some medical conditions like psoriasis, eczema, Raynaud's syndrome, etc., but these are the Jinn diseases in which any medical treatment is detrimental as excites the Evil Jinn!

Complications of Botox can be explained by toxicity of Botulinum toxin but also by Jinn manifestations/reactions to Botox. (650)

Some of complications of Dermal Fillers (Hyaluronic acid (HA) fillers): (651, 652)

Some of complications of the Face-Lift. (653)

700. Sex-Change Operation from Male to Female or Vice Versa

It is not possible for anyone, no matter who he is, to change the creation of Allah, may He be Exalted, from male to female or vice versa. Whoever Allah, may He be Exalted, has created as a male can never become a female who menstruates and gives birth! The doctors may tamper with him to satisfy his perversion so that he will think that he has become a woman, but he will never be truly female and will live in a state of anxiety and worry, which may lead him to commit suicide. What a person may feel in his mind and heart, that he is of a gender other than what he appears to be to us does not give him an excuse to change his gender; rather it comes under the heading of following the Shaytan in changing the creation of Allah - outwardly but not truly - and those feelings do not make it permissible for him to undergo surgery or take medicines and hormones to change his outward appearance. Rather he must be content with the Decree of Allah, may He be Exalted, and treat his case on the basis of faith and obedience to Allah. It is not permissible for him to make himself appear outwardly to be of a gender other than his real gender with which Allah created him, otherwise he will be committing a Major sin; if this person is really female then she will be masculinized and if he is really male then he will be effeminate. The surgery that is permissible in such cases is if a person was originally created male or female, but his genital organs are hidden. In that case it is permissible to do surgery in order to make those organs appear, and to give him or her medicine or hormones to strengthen the characteristics with which Allah originally created him or her. But in the case of one who was created with both female and male genitalia - this is what is called ambiguous intersex - it is not permissible to be hasty in removing one and making the other more apparent. Rather we should wait until it is known what Allah, may He be Exalted, will decree for this individual, which may become apparent after some time has passed.

There follows a detailed Fatwa from the scholars of the Standing Committee for Issuing Fatwas, who were asked about a case similar to what is mentioned in the question. They replied:

"Firstly: Allah, may He be Exalted, says:

"To Allah belongs the kingdom of the heavens and the earth. He creates what He wills. He bestows female (offspring) upon whom He wills, and bestows male (offspring) upon whom He wills. Or He bestows both males and females, and He renders barren whom He wills. Verily, He is the All-Knower and is Able to do all things." (Qur'an, Ash-Shu'ara 42:49)

So, the Muslim must accept and be content with whatever Allah creates and decrees.

Secondly: once your masculinity is proven and established, then having surgery to turn into a female – as you think – is changing the creation of Allah, and is an expression of discontent on your part with what Allah has chosen for you, even if we assume that the surgery is going to be successful and lead to what you want of becoming female. But there is no way that it can be successful, for both males and females have their own, distinct faculties and physical makeup, the development and characteristics of which are decreed only by Allah, may He be Exalted, and are not just the penis of the male or the vaginal opening of the female. Rather the man has a complete, integrated system comprising the testicles and other organs, each of which has a special function and characteristics, and produces specific secretions and so on. Likewise, the woman has a uterus and other connected parts that work in harmony with it, and each part has its own function and characteristics, and produces specific secretions and so on. Among all of them there are connections and harmony over which none of His creation have any power of estimation, creation, control, management or preservation. Rather all of that is under the control of Allah, the All-Knowing, Most Wise, Most High, Almighty, Most Kind and All-Aware. Therefore, the surgery that you want to do is a kind of tampering and striving for something in which there is no benefit. In fact it may be dangerous; if it does not lead to death, then at the very least it will lead to taking away that which Allah has given you without you attaining what you want, and you will still be affected by what you have mentioned of psychological problems that you want to get rid of by means of this surgery that is bound to fail.

Thirdly: if your masculinity is not established, and you only think that you are a man because of what you see in your body of outward masculine appearance, in contrast to what you feel in yourself of having feminine characteristics and an inclination towards males and being sexually attracted to them, then you should examine your situation and not go ahead with the surgery that you have mentioned. You should consult experienced specialist doctors. If they determine that you are male in outward appearance but are in fact female, then you may submit yourself to their treatment, so that they can bring out your femininity by doing surgery. But that will not in fact be a sex change from male to female, because this will not be up to them; rather it will be bringing out your true nature and removing what is in your body, and what you feel deep inside you of confusion and ambiguity. But if nothing is clear to the experts, then do not take the risk of undergoing this surgery; be content with the Decree of Allah and be patient with what has befallen you, seeking to please your Lord and protecting yourself against the possible consequences of doing an operation without guidance and insight concerning your condition. Turn to Allah and beseech Him to relieve you of what you are facing, and to heal you from your psychological problems, for control of all things is in His Hand, may He be Glorified, and He is able to do all things." End quote. Sheikh 'Abd al-'Azeez ibn Baaz, Sheikh 'Abd ar-Razzaaq 'Afeefi, Sheikh 'Abdullah ibn Qa'ood, Sheikh 'Abdullah ibn Ghadyaan, Fataawa al-Lajnah ad-Daa'imah (25/45-49) (654)

701. Fertility Fraud

Fertility fraud can be on every steps of Fertility treatment.

1. some doctors are hurry to do IVF treatment when there is a chance of the natural conception
2. physician may use his/her own or other's spermatozoids or oocytes
3. using donated human reproductive material.
4. mixing the human reproductive cells or embryos
5. unhealthy IVF laboratory environment contributing to the death of the human cells or embryo
6. Increased number of IVF treatments for one patient (more than 4-6 IVF)
7. Infertility treatment without consent.

702. Ruling on Sperm Donation

If a third party, other than the spouses, is introduced into the process of fertilization, such as eggs coming from another woman or another woman acting as a surrogate mother, or sperm coming from another man, then fertilization in such cases is unlawful, because it is counted as Zina (Adultery). When a woman uses the sperm of a man, this comes under the same rulings as intercourse in terms of what is halal and what is haram. With regard to the child who is born as the result of such a process, he is to be attributed to the mother who bore him, and not to the man who produced the sperm, as is the ruling in the case of Zina (Fornication or Adultery). If that man claims to be the father and no one disputes that, then the child may be attributed to him, because the Lawgiver is keen that people should be named after their fathers. With regard to the Hadith, "The child belongs to the (marriage) bed and for the adulterer is the stone," it is to be interpreted as referring to cases where there is a dispute, as is clear from the incident which gave rise to this Hadith. (655)

703. Ruling on Egg Donation

It is not permissible for a woman to donate eggs to be fertilized with the sperm of anyone other than her husband, even if the embryo will be implanted after that in the uterus of the sister of the donor. The prohibition on this kind of fertilization was issued in a statement by the Islamic Fiqh Council in its statement no. 16 on Test-Tube Babies. In that statement it says:

"In the session of the International Islamic Fiqh Council that was held during the third conference in Amman, the capital of the Hashemite Kingdom of Jordan, 8-13 Safar 1407 AH/11-16 October 1986 CE,

After presentation of papers on the topic of artificial insemination (test-tube babies), and listening to the explanations of experts and doctors, and after a discussion in which it was explained to the council that the methods of artificial insemination that are known nowadays are seven, the council determined the following: Firstly: the five following methods of artificial insemination are prohibited according to Shariah and are completely disallowed, in and of themselves, and because of what they result in of mixing of lineages, confusion as to who is to be regarded as the mother, and other matters that are contrary to Islamic teaching. The first of these (prohibited) methods is where sperm taken from the husband is used to fertilize an egg taken from a woman who is not his wife, then the embryo is implanted in the uterus of his wife. End quote." (656)

704. Prohibition of Mitochondrial Donation IVF

Allah, the Exalted, says:

"...and it may be that you dislike a thing which is good for you and that you like a thing which is bad for you. Allah knows but you do not know." (Qur'an, Al-Baqarah 2:216)

Baby from 3-parents is prohibited. Mitochondrial replacement technique (MRT) (the mother's mitochondria are removed from her egg and replaced by a donor's) is prohibited due to the change of creation, mixing of lineage and other evaluations. The sperm should come from the father, the egg from the mother and the resulting embryo should grow inside the uterus of the mother.

705. Human Embryo Model Made from Stem Cells

"We should point out that it is not permissible for anyone to donate sperm or eggs for the purpose of producing zygotes (fertilized eggs) which will then develop into the foetus with the aim of obtaining the stem cells from it. It is also not permissible to use cloning in order to obtain foetal stem cells. Rather permission is limited to obtaining stem cells from umbilical cords." (657)

706. Prohibition of Infertility Treatment for the Single, Lesbian and Gay Couples

Infertility treatment for the single, lesbian and gay couples are prohibited.
Lesbianism and Homosexuality are prohibited.
Sperm and Egg Donations are prohibited.
Renting the womb of another woman is prohibited.
Mixing of lineages is prohibited.

707. Prohibition of Surrogacy

Sheikh 'Abd-Allah ibn 'Abd al-Rahmaan al-Jibreen answered this question as follows:

"We say that this is something innovated and reprehensible. The scholars have not spoken of it previously and it is not narrated that any of the scholars or imams of this ummah permitted that, or that it crossed their minds, or that they were asked about any such thing, even though the means and the motive existed that may have called for such a thing. This is something that has come up recently, within the last few years, where the idea of renting wombs been made attractive (by the Shaytan) to some people and they say there is nothing wrong with it and so on. Undoubtedly this is haram, primarily because Allah has commanded us to guard our chastity, as He says:

"And those who guard their chastity (i.e. private parts, from illegal sexual acts)

Except from their wives or (the slaves) that their right hands possess, for then, they are free from blame." (Qur'an, Al-Mu'minun 23:5-6)

So, Allah has forbidden us to engage in sexual activity with anyone except our wives and female slaves, i.e. having intercourse with them (female slaves) on the basis of possession. Allah tells us that man is enjoined to protect his lineage and his children. Undoubtedly this womb-renting will lead to confusion of lineage and not knowing who the father or mother is. This confusion of lineage will lead to disputes between the original wife and the woman whose womb is rented, and it will not be known to whom the child belongs. Even if we say that he belongs to one of them, the matter still will not be certain. Hence, we advise women to keep away from such things. Moreover, this undoubtedly requires looking at 'awrahs and at the private parts which it is forbidden to see, and it also requires collecting sperm and extracting the eggs and placing them in other wombs. All of that is not allowed in Shariah, indeed it comes under prohibition mentioned in the Ayah:

"Tell the believing men to lower their gaze (from looking at forbidden things), and protect their private parts (from illegal sexual acts)." (Qur'an, An-Nur 24:30)

What is meant is to protect them by covering them, so that no one will see the 'awrah of another. This is the way of Islam and we pay no attention to those who deviate and go against that, and permit this borrowing and this renting of wombs, the consequences of which will undoubtedly be disastrous. Renting wombs is one of the innovations of western civilization, which is a purely materialistic civilization which does not give any weight to moral values and principles. The issue is not things that may affect inherited characteristics or confuse lineage; that is not the point of the Shariah ruling. Whether that leads to any effect on inherited characteristics or not, whether that results in confusion of lineage or not, it does not matter, because the Shariah ruling forbidding this innovation is based on something else, which is that the womb is a part of a woman's private parts and the private parts (i.e. sexual relations) are not permissible except through the Shariah contract whose conditions are fully met. So, the womb is exclusively for the husband who is married to that woman according to a valid marriage contract, and no one else has any right to use it for an alien pregnancy. If the woman who rents out her womb is not married to that husband, then she is permitting her private parts and her womb to a man who is a stranger to her; she is not permissible for him and he is not permissible for her. Even if this is not full-scale Zina (adultery), it is still definitely haram because it is enabling a man who is a stranger to her (i.e. not married to her) to put his semen in her womb. (Dr. 'Abd al-'Azeem al-Mat'ani, al-Azhaar University)

The foetus is nourished and is influenced by the womb and the environment that surrounds him. Bad habits on the part of the surrogate mother may lead to deformity of the foetus, such as smoking, drinking alcohol, etc. Then what if the doctors discover some physical deformity in the foetus before birth and try to treat that by means of surgical intervention? Will the surrogate mother allow that? Will she put her life at risk for the sake of a child who does not belong to her? Moreover, there are some women who become sick as a result of pregnancy, suffering such diseases as a sudden rise in the level of blood sugar or a rise in blood pressure, or toxemia, some of which may take the life of the pregnant woman and which require medical intervention to sacrifice the foetus in order to save the life of the pregnant woman. How would the surrogate mother and the original mother work this out? How are we to deal with the ethical, legal, social and psychological problems that result from that? Therefore, we can reach only one conclusion, which is that the mother who carries the pregnancy can only be the original mother, the child should be attributed to the marriage bed, and that she should conceive, nourish her foetus and give birth to it. Saying that renting wombs is like hiring wet-nurses has no basis in truth, for a wet-nurse breastfeeds a child whose lineage is known, and she can stop breastfeeding him when she wants or when the original mother wants, if she feels that there is any danger. Moreover, in the relationship between a husband and wife there is no room for any third party, no matter who he or she is, not for renting a womb, or for donating sperm or donating eggs. Because of such things innumerable problems have arisen in western societies. In Britain an original mother gave twenty thousand pounds to a surrogate mother in return for renting her womb for nine months. When that time was over, the surrogate mother demanded many times that amount from the original mother in exchange for giving up possession of the child. So, if this door is opened it will bring us innumerable legal and social problems. (Prof. Jamaal Abu'l-Suroor – Dean of Medicine, al-Azhaar) (658)

708. Prohibition of Cloning of Human Beings

Cloning means producing one or more living beings by transferring the nucleus of a body cell to an egg whose nucleus has been removed or splitting a fertilized egg at the stage before the tissues and organs become distinct. It is obvious that these and similar procedures do not represent the act of creation, in whole or in part. Allah, the Exalted, says:

"Or do they assign to Allah partners who created the like of His creation, so that the creation (which they made and His creation) seemed alike to them?" Say: 'Allah is the Creator of all things; and He is the One, the Irresistible.'" (Qur'an, Ar-R'ad 13:16)

"Then tell Me (about) the (human) semen that you emit. Is it you who create it (i.e. make this semen into a perfect human being), or are We the Creator? We have decreed death to you all, and We are not outstripped, To transfigure you and create you in (forms) that you know not. And indeed, you have already known the first form of creation (i.e. the creation of Adam), why then do you not remember (or take heed)?" (Qur'an, Al-Waqi'ah 56:58-62)

Other Verse:, Al-Mu'minun 23:12-14, Yasin 36:77-82, Ar-Ra'd 13:3, An-Nahl 6:67, Taha 20:89, Al-Ghashiyah 88:17, Az-Zumar 39:1, Al-'Alaq 96:1.

The Committee has decided the following:

1) That human cloning that leads to reproduction of human beings is prohibited.

2) If there is any transgression of the Shariah ruling, then the consequences of that should be discussed to explain the Shariah rulings concerning such cases.

3) All scenarios in which a third party may be added to the marital relationship are forbidden, whether that involves a womb (surrogacy), eggs, sperm or cells for cloning.

4) It is permissible in Islam to use the technology of cloning and genetic engineering in cases of germs and microscopic creatures, plants and animals, within the limits and guidelines of Shariah, for the purpose of serving interests and warding off harm. (659)

709. Prohibition of Hypnotherapy

Hypnotherapy has something to do with using the help of the Jinn, it is a Shirk.

1 – It is not permissible to seek the help of the Jinn or any other creatures in trying to find out matters of the unseen, whether that is by calling upon them, trying to please them or any other method. Rather that is Shirk because this is a kind of worship, and Allah has taught His slaves to worship Him alone and say, *"You (Alone) we worship, and You (Alone) we ask for help (for each and everything)." (Qur'an, Al-Fatihah 1:5)*

And it was proven that the Prophet (peace and blessings of Allah be upon him) said to Ibn 'Abbas:

"If you ask, then ask Allah (Alone); and if you seek help, then seek help from Allah (Alone). And know that if the nation were to gather together to benefit you with anything, they would not benefit you except with what Allah had already prescribed for you…" (Tirmidhi)

(https://sunnah.com/nawawi40:19)

2 – Hypnotism is a kind of fortune telling or magic whereby the hypnotist uses the Jinn to overpower the subject and then speak through his tongue and give him strength to do things by means of controlling his faculties. This is if the Jinni is sincere towards the hypnotist and obeys him in return for the things by means of which the hypnotist draws close to him. So, the Jinni makes the subject obey the wishes of the hypnotist to do things or tell him things, through the help of the Jinni. Thus, using hypnotism as a means of finding out where stolen goods are hidden, or where a lost item is, or as a means of treating disease, or of doing anything else is not permissible. Rather it is Shirk because it implies turning to someone other than Allah and goes beyond the ordinary means which Allah has created for His creatures and permitted them to use. (660)

710. Ruling on Organ Transplants

The Islamic Fiqh Council (Majma' al-Fiqh al-Islami), which has issued the following Fatwa:

1. It is permitted to transplant or graft an organ from one part of a person's body to another, so long as one is careful to ascertain that the benefits of this operation outweigh any harm that may result from it, and on the condition that this is done to replace something that has been lost, or to restore its appearance or regular function, or to correct some fault or disfigurement which is causing physical or psychological distress.

2. It is permitted to transplant an organ from one person's body to another, if it is an organ that can regenerate itself, like skin or blood, on the condition that the donor is mature and understands what he is doing, and that all other pertinent Shariah conditions are met.

3. It is permitted to use part of an organ that has been removed because of illness to benefit another person, such as using the cornea of an eye removed because of illness.

4. It is haram to take an organ on which life depends, such as taking a heart from a living person to transplant into another person.

5. It is haram to take an organ from a living person when doing so could impair an essential vital function, even though his life itself may not be under threat, such as removing the corneas of both eyes. However, removing organs which will lead to only partial impairment is a matter which is still under scholarly discussion.

6. It is permitted to transplant an organ from a dead person to a living person whose life depends on receiving that organ, or whose vital functions are otherwise impaired, on the condition that permission is given either by the person before his death or by his heirs, or by the leader of the Muslims in cases where the dead person's identity is unknown or he has no heirs.

7. Care should be taken to ensure that there is proper agreement to the transplant of organs in the cases described above, on the condition that no buying or selling of organs is involved. It is not permitted to trade in human organs under any circumstances. But the question of whether the beneficiary may spend money to obtain an organ he needs, or to show his appreciation, is a matter which is still under scholarly debate.

8. Anything other than the scenarios described above is still subject to scholarly debate, and requires further detailed research in the light of medical research and Shariah rulings. (661)

711. Prohibition of Doing that which Allah and His Messenger Have Prohibited

Allah, the Exalted, says:

"And Allah warns you against Himself (His punishment)." (Qur'an, Ali 'Imran 3:30)

"Verily, (O Muhammad (peace be upon him)) the Grip (punishment) of your Rubb is severe." (Qur'an, Al-Buruj 85:12)

"Such is the Seizure of your Rubb when He seizes the (population of) towns while they are doing wrong. Verily, His Seizure is painful and severe." (Qur'an, Hud 11:102)

Other Verses: An-Nur 24:63, Al-Hajj 22:30, Muhammad 47:7.

Abu Hurairah (May Allah be pleased with him) said: The Prophet (peace and blessings be upon him) said,

"Allah, the Exalted, becomes angry, and His Anger is provoked when a person does what Allah has declared unlawful." (Bukhari and Muslim)

Commentary: This Hadith warns us against committing sins and all that Allah has forbidden in order to avoid exciting the Anger of Allah. (662, 663)

712. Undesirability of Intercession in Hudud

Allah, the Exalted, says:

"The woman and the man guilty of illegal sexual intercourse, flog each of them with a hundred stripes. Let not pity withhold you in their case, in a punishment prescribed by Allah, if you believe in Allah and the Last Day." (Qur'an, An-Nur 24:2)

Aisha (May Allah be pleased with her), the wife of Allah's Apostle (peace and blessings be upon him), reported that the Quraish were concerned about the woman who had committed theft during the lifetime of Allah's Apostle (peace be upon him), in the expedition of Victory (of Makkah). They said: 'Who would speak to Allah's Messenger (peace be upon him) about her?' They (again) said: 'Who can dare do this but Usama b Zaid, the loved one of Allah's Messenger (peace be upon him)?' She was brought to Allah's Messenger (peace be upon him) and Usama b. Zaid spoke about her to him (interceded on her behalf). The colour of the face of Allah's Messenger (peace be upon him) changed, and he said: 'Do you intercede in one of the prescribed punishments of Allah?' He (Usama) said: 'Messenger of Allah, seek forgiveness for me.' When it was dusk, Allah's Messenger (peace be upon him) stood up and gave an address. He (first) glorified Allah as He deserves, and then said: 'Now to our topic. This (injustice) destroyed those before you that when any one of (high) rank committed theft among them, they spared him, and when any weak one among them committed theft, they inflicted the prescribed punishment upon him. By Him in Whose Hand is my life, even if Fatima daughter of Muhammad were to commit theft, I would have cut off her hand.'" (Bukhari and Muslim)

Commentary:

1. Hadd is the punishment fixed by Shariah and which no one has the authority to increase or decrease. For instance, theft is punishable by the cutting of the hand; the punishment of fornication/adultery is a hundred stripes or Rajm (stoning to death); the punishment of drinking of intoxicants is forty stripes, etc.

2. Nobody has the right to intercede or make any recommendation in this matter.

3. There is no distinction of male or female in the matter of these punishments (Hudud). Whoever commits a crime which is punishable by Hadd, whether that person is male or female, will be liable for punishment prescribed under Hadd - the punishment, the limits of which have been defined in the Qur'an and Hadith.

4. No one is exempted from Hadd, no matter how great he is, because there is no distinction of great or small in the matter of Hadd.

5. We must learn a lesson from the history of past nations so that we can save ourselves from such misdeeds which caused their ruin.

6. This Hadith brings into prominence the distinction and eminence of Usama and his position in the eyes of the Prophet (peace and blessings be upon him). (664)

713. Disbelief on Judgment Day

Allah, the Exalted, says:

"Those are the ones who rejected the signs of their Lord and (the concept of) meeting with Him, so their deeds have gone to waste, and We shall assign to them no weight at all." (Qur'an, Al-Kahf 18:105)

"O people, worship your Lord who created you and those before you, so that you may become God-fearing." (Qur'an, Al-Baqarah 2:21)

"How can you disbelieve in Allah? Seeing that you were dead and He gave you life. Then He will give you death, then again will bring you to life (on the Day of Resurrection) and then unto Him you will return." (Qur'an, Al-Baqarah 2:28)

Other Verses: *Az-Zumar 39:67, Luqman 31:33)*

Ibn Masud reported: The Prophet (peace and blessings be upon him) said, "The son of Adam will not be dismissed from his Lord on the Day of Resurrection until he is questioned about five issues: his life and how he lived it, his youth and how he used it, his wealth and how he earned it and he spent it, and how he acted on his knowledge." (Tirmidhi)

Abdullah b. 'Umar reported Allah's Messenger (peace and blessings be upon him) saying: "Allah, the Exalted and Glorious, would fold the heavens on the Day of Judgment and then He would place them on His right Hand and say: 'I am the Lord; where are the haughty and where are the proud (today)?' He would fold the earth (placing it) on the left Hand and say: 'I am the Lord; where are the haughty and where are the proud (today)?'" (Muslim)

Abdullah ibn Masud (May Allah be pleased with him) reported that the Prophet (May Allah's peace and blessings be upon him) said: "The first cases to be settled among people on the Day of Judgment will be the cases of blood (homicide)." (Bukhari and Muslim. This is the wording of Muslim)
(https://hadeethenc.com/en/browse/hadith/2962)

Abu Hurairah (May Allah be pleased with him) said: "I heard the Messenger of Allah (peace and blessings be upon him) say: 'The first of people against whom Judgment will be pronounced on the Day of Resurrection will be a man who died a martyr. He will be brought and Allah will make known to him His Favors and he will recognize them. The Almighty will say: And what did you do about them? He will say: 'I fought for you until I diedا martyr.' He will say: 'You have lied - you did but fight that it might be said (of you): 'He is courageous.' And so, it was said. Then he will be ordered to be dragged along on his face until he is cast into Hellfire. Another will be a man who has studied (religious) knowledge and has taught it and who used to recite the Qur'an. He will be brought and Allah will make known to him His Favors and he will recognize them. The Almighty will say: 'And what did you do about them?' He will say: 'I studied (religious) knowledge and I taught it, and I recited the Qur'an for Your sake.' He will say: 'You have lied - you did but study (religious) knowledge that it might be said (of you): 'He is learned.' And you recited the Qur'an that it might be said (of you): 'He is a reciter.' And so, it was said. Then he will be ordered to be dragged along on his face until he is cast into Hellfire. Another will be a man whom Allah had made rich and to whom He had given all kinds of wealth. He will be brought and Allah will make known to him His Favors and he will recognize them. The Almighty will say: 'And what did you do about them?' He will say: 'I left no path [untrodden] in which You like money to be spent without spending in it for Your sake.' He will say: 'You have lied - you did but do so that it might be said (of you): 'He is open-handed.' And so, it was said. Then he will be ordered to be dragged along on his face until he is cast into Hellfire." (Muslim, Tirmidhi and An-Nasa'i)

Narrated Abu Hurairah: The Prophet (peace and blessings of Allah be upon him) said: "...I shall be the leader of mankind on the Day of Resurrection. Do you know why? Allah would gather in one plain the earlier and the later (of the human race) on the Day of Resurrection. Then the voice of the proclaimer would be heard by all of them and the eyesight would penetrate through all of them and the sun would come near. People would then experience a degree of anguish, anxiety and agony which they shall not be able to bear and they shall not be able to stand. Some people would say to the others: 'Don't you see in which trouble you are? Don't you see what (misfortune) has overtaken you? Why don't you find one who should intercede for you with your Lord?' Some would say to the others: 'Go to Adam.'

And they would go to **Adam** and say: 'O Adam, thou art the father of mankind. Allah created thee by His Own Hand and breathed in thee of His spirit and ordered the angels to prostrate before thee. Intercede for us with thy Lord. Don't you see in what (trouble) we are? Don't you see what (misfortune) has overtaken us?' Adam would say: 'Verily, my Lord is angry, to an extent to which He had never been angry before nor would He be angry afterward. Verily, He forbade me (to go near) that tree and I disobeyed Him. I am concerned with my own self. Go to someone else; go to Noah.'

They would come to **Noah** and would say: 'O Noah, thou art the first of the Messengers sent on the earth (after Adam), and Allah named thee as a "Grateful Servant", intercede for us with thy Lord. Don't you see in what (trouble) we are? Don't you see what (misfortune) has overtaken us?' He would say: 'Verily, my Lord is angry today as He had never been angry before, and would never be angry afterwards. There had emanated a curse from me with which I cursed my people. I am concerned with only myself, I am concerned only with myself; you better go to Ibrahim (peace be upon him).'

They would go to **Ibrahim** and say: 'Thou art the Apostle of Allah and His Friend amongst the inhabitants of the earth; intercede for us with thy Lord. Don't you see in which (trouble) we are? Don't you see what (misfortune) has overtaken us?' Ibrahim would say to them: 'Verily, my Lord is today angry as He had never been angry before and would never be angry afterwards.' And (Ibrahim) would mention his lies (and then say): 'I am concerned only with myself, I am concerned only with myself. You better go to someone else: go to Moses.' They would come to **Moses** (peace be upon him) and say: 'O Moses, thou art Allah's Messenger, Allah blessed thee with His Messengership and His conversation amongst people. Intercede for us with thy Lord. Don't you see in what (trouble) we are? Don't you see what (misfortune) has overtaken us?' Moses (peace be upon him) would say to them: 'Verily, my Lord is angry as He had never been angry before and would never be angry afterwards. I, in fact, killed a person whom I had not ordered to kill. I am concerned with myself, I am concerned with myself. You better go to Jesus (peace be upon him).' They would come to **Jesus** and would say: 'O Jesus, thou art the Messenger of Allah and thou conversed with people in the cradle, (thou art) His Word which He sent down upon Mary, and (thou art) the Spirit from Him; so, intercede for us with thy Lord. Don't you see (the trouble) in which we are? Don't you see (the misfortune) that has overtaken us?' Jesus (peace be upon him) would say: 'Verily, my Lord is angry today as He had never been angry before or would ever be angry afterwards.' He mentioned no sin of his. He simply said: 'I am concerned with myself, I am concerned with myself; you go to someone else; better go to Muhammad (peace be upon him).' They would come to me and say: 'O **Muhammad** (peace and blessings be upon him), thou art the Messenger of Allah and the last of the Apostles. Allah has pardoned thee all thy previous and later sins. Intercede for us with thy Lord; don't you see in which (trouble) we are? Don't you see what (misfortune) has overtaken us?'

'I shall then set off and come below the Throne and fall down prostrate before my Lord; then Allah would reveal to me and inspire me with some of His Praises and Glorifications which He had not revealed to anyone before me. He would then say: 'Muhammad (peace and blessings be upon him), raise thy head; ask and it would be granted; intercede and intercession would be accepted.' I would then raise my head and say: 'O my Lord, my people, my people…'" (Muslim)
(https://sunnah.com/muslim:194a)

Narrated Abu Sa'id Al-Khudri: "We said, "O Allah's Messenger! Shall we see our Lord on the Day of Resurrection?" He (peace and blessings be upon him) said, "Do you have any difficulty in seeing the sun and the moon when the sky is clear?" We said, "No." He (peace and blessings be upon him) said, "So you will have no difficulty in seeing your Lord on that Day as you have no difficulty in seeing the sun and the moon (in a clear sky)." The Prophet (peace and blessings be upon him) then said, "Somebody will then announce, 'Let every nation follow what they used to worship.' So, the companions of the cross will go with their cross, and the idolators (will go) with their idols, and the companions of every god (false deities) (will go) with their god, till there remain those who used to worship Allah, both the obedient ones and the mischievous ones, and some of the people of the Scripture. Then Hell will be presented to them as if it were a mirage. Then it will be said to the Jews, "What did you use to worship?' They will reply, 'We used to worship Ezra, the son of Allah.' It will be said to them, 'You are liars, for Allah has neither a wife nor a son. What do you want (now)?' They will reply, 'We want You to provide us with water.' Then it will be said to them 'Drink', and they will fall down in Hell (instead). Then it will be said to the Christians, 'What did you use to worship?' They will reply, 'We used to worship Messiah, the son of Allah.' It will be said, 'You are liars, for Allah has neither a wife nor a son. What do you want (now)?' They will say, 'We want You to provide us with water.' It will be said to them, 'Drink', and they will fall down in Hell (instead). When there remain only those who used to worship Allah (Alone), both the obedient ones and the mischievous ones, it will be said to them, 'What keeps you here when all the people have gone?' They will say, 'We parted with them (in the world) when we were in greater need of them than we are today, we heard the call of one proclaiming, 'Let every nation follow what they used to worship', and now we are waiting for our Lord.' Then the Almighty will come to them in a shape other than the one which they saw the first time, and He will say, 'I am your Lord', and they will say, 'You are not our Lord.' And none will speak to Him then but the Prophets, and then it will be said to them, 'Do you know any sign by which you can recognize Him?' They will say. 'The Shin', and so Allah will then uncover His Shin whereupon every believer will prostrate before Him and there will remain those who used to prostrate before Him just for showing off and for gaining good reputation. These people will try to prostrate but their backs will be rigid like one piece of a wood (and they will not be able to prostrate).

Then the bridge will be laid across Hell. We, the companions of the Prophet said, 'O Allah's Messenger! What is the bridge?' He (peace and blessings be upon him) said, 'It is a slippery (bridge) on which there are clamps and (hooks like) a thorny seed that is wide at one side and narrow at the other and has thorns with bent ends. Such a thorny seed is found in Najd and is called As-Sa'dan. Some of the believers will cross the bridge as quickly as the wink of an eye, some others as quick as lightning, a strong wind, fast horses or she-camels. So, some will be safe without any harm; some will be safe after receiving some scratches, and some will fall down into Hellfire. The last person will cross by being dragged (over the bridge).' The Prophet (peace and blessings be upon him) said, 'You (Muslims) cannot be more pressing in claiming from me a right that has been clearly proved to be yours than the believers in interceding with Almighty for their (Muslim) brothers on that Day, when they see themselves safe.'

They will say, 'O Allah! Save our brothers for they used to pray with us, fast with us and also do good deeds with us.' Allah will say, 'Go and take out (of Hell) anyone in whose heart you find faith equal to the weight of one (gold) Dinar.' Allah will forbid the Fire to burn the faces of those sinners. They will go to them and find some of them in Hellfire up to their feet, and some up to the middle of their legs. So, they will take out those whom they will recognize and then they will return, and Allah will say (to them), 'Go and take out (of Hell) anyone in whose heart you find faith equal to the weight of one-half Dinar.' They will take out whomever they will recognize and return, and then Allah will say, 'Go and take out (of Hell) anyone in whose heart you find faith equal to the weight of an atom (or a smallest ant), and so they will take out all those whom they will recognize." Abu Sa'id said: 'If you do not believe me then read the Holy Verse: *'Surely! Allah wrongs not even of the weight of an atom (or a smallest ant) but if there is any good (done) He doubles it.' (Qur'an, An-Nisa 4:40)* The Prophet (peace and blessings be upon him) added, "Then the Prophets and Angels and the believers will intercede, and (last of all) the Almighty Allah will say, 'Now remains My Intercession.' He will then hold a handful of the Fire from which He will take out some people whose bodies have been burnt, and they will be thrown into a river at the entrance of Paradise, called the water of life. They will grow on its banks, as a seed carried by the torrent grows. You have noticed how it grows beside a rock or beside a tree, and how the side facing the sun is usually green while the side facing the shade is white. Those people will come out (of the River of Life) like pearls, and they will have (golden) necklaces, and then they will enter Paradise whereupon the people of Paradise will say, 'These are the people emancipated by the Beneficent. He has admitted them into Paradise without them having done any good deeds and without sending forth any good (for themselves).' Then it will be said to them, 'For you is what you have seen and its equivalent as well.'" (Bukhari) (https://hadeethenc.com/en/browse/hadith/8301)

714. Disbelief in Paradise

Allah, the Exalted, says:

'Adn (Eden) Paradise (everlasting Gardens) will they enter, therein will they be adorned with bracelets of gold and pearls, and their garments there will be of silk (i.e. in Paradise)." (Qur'an, Fatir 35:33)

"Gardens under which rivers flow to dwell therein forever, and beautiful mansions in Gardens of 'Adn (Eden Paradise). But the greatest bliss is the Good Pleasure of Allah. That is the supreme success." (Qur'an, At-Tawbah 9:72)

"Gardens of perpetual bliss." (Qur'an, Ar-Ra'd 13:23)

Other Verses: Al-Hijr 15:45-48, Al-Hadid 57:21, Al-Mutaffifin 83:22-28, Ali 'Imran 3:15, Al-Ghashiyah 88:11-13 and 88:16, Al-Ma'idah 5:119, Muhammad 47:15, At-Tur 52:20, 52:22 and 52:24, Yasin 36:57, Al-Kahf 18:31, Ar-Rahman 55:56, Al-Waqi'ah 56:35-38, As-Saffat 37:48, Az-Zukhruf 43:68-73, Al-Dukhan 44:51-57, Yunus 10:9-10.

Jabir (May Allah be pleased with him) reported: The Messenger of Allah (peace and blessings be upon him) said, "The inhabitants of Jannah will eat and drink therein, but they will not have to pass excrement, to blow their noses or to urinate. Their food will be digested producing belch which will give out a smell like that of musk. They will be inspired to declare the freedom of Allah from imperfection and proclaim His Greatness as easily as you breathe." (Muslim)

Abu Hurairah (May Allah be pleased with him) said: The Messenger of Allah (peace and blessings be upon him) said, "Allah, the Exalted, has said: 'I have prepared for my righteous slaves what no eye has seen, no ear has heard, and the mind of no man has conceived.' If you wish, recite: *'No person knows what is kept hidden for them of joy as a reward for what they used to do.'" (Qur'an, 32:17)* (Bukhari and Muslim)

Abu Hurairah (May Allah be pleased with him) said: The Messenger of Allah (peace and blessings be upon him) said, "The first group (of people) to enter Jannah will be shining like the moon on a full moon night. Then will come those who follow them who will be like the most shining planet in the sky. They will not stand in need of urinating or relieving of nature, or of spitting, or blowing their noses. Their combs will be of gold and their sweat will smell like musk; in their censers the aloeswood will be used. Their wives will be large eyed maidens. All men will be alike in the form of their father 'Adam, sixty cubits tall."

Al-Mughirah bin Shu'bah (May Allah be pleased with him) said: The Messenger of Allah (peace and blessings be upon him) said, "Musa (Moses) (May Allah have mercy on him) asked his Rubb: 'Who amongst the inhabitants of Jannah will be the lowest in rank?' He said: 'It will be a person who will be admitted into Jannah last of all when all the dwellers of Jannah have entered Jannah. It will be said to him: 'Enter Jannah.' But he will say: 'O my Rubb! How should I enter while the people have settled in their apartments and taken their shares?' It will be said to him: 'Will you be satisfied and pleased if you have a kingdom like that of a monarch of the world?' He will say: 'I will be content, my Rubb.' Allah will say: 'For you is that, and like that, and like that, and like that, and like that. He will say at the fifth time: 'I am well pleased, my Rubb.' Allah will say: 'It is for you and ten times more like it. You will have whatever your soul desires and whatever your eyes could delight in.' He will say: 'I am well pleased, my Rubb.'

Musa (May Allah have mercy on him) said: 'Who will be of the highest rank in Jannah.' Allah said: 'They are those whom I chose and I established their honor with My Own Hand. I attest with My Seal that they will be blessed with such bounties as no eye has seen, no ear has heard and no human mind has perceived.'" (Muslim)

Abu Musa (May Allah be pleased with him) said: The Prophet (peace and blessings be upon him) said, "In Jannah the believer will have a tent made of a single hollowed pearl of which the length will be sixty miles in the sky. The believer will have his wives with him and he will visit them and they will not be able to see one another." (Bukhari and Muslim)

Anas (May Allah be pleased with him) said: The Messenger of Allah (peace and blessings be upon him) said, "In Jannah there is a market to which the people will come every Friday. The northern wind will blow and shower fragrance on their faces and clothes and, consequently, it will enhance their beauty and loveliness. They will then return to their wives who will also have increased in their beauty and loveliness, and their families will say to them: 'We swear by Allah that you have been increased in beauty and loveliness since leaving us.' Thereupon they will reply: 'We swear by Allah that you have also been increased in beauty and loveliness since we left you.'" (Muslim)

Sahl bin Sa'd (May Allah be pleased with him) said: "I was in the company of the Prophet (peace and blessings be upon him). He gave a description of Jannah and concluded with these words, "There will be bounties which no eye has seen, no ear has heard and no human heart has ever perceived." He (peace and blessings be upon him) then recited this Verse: *"Their sides forsake their beds, to invoke their Rubb in fear and hope, and they spend (in charity in Allah's Cause) out of what We have bestowed on them. No person knows what is kept hidden for them of joy..." (Qur'an, 32:16-17)* (Bukhari)

Abu Sa'id and Abu Hurairah (May Allah be pleased with them) reported: The Messenger of Allah (peace and blessings be upon him) said, "When the dwellers of Jannah enter Jannah, an announcer will call: (You have a promise from Allah that) you will live therein and you will never die; you will stay healthy therein and you will never fall ill; you will stay young and you will never become old; you will be under a constant bliss and you will never feel miserable." (Muslim)

Abu Hurairah (May Allah be pleased with him) said: The Messenger of Allah (peace and blessings be upon him) said, "The lowest place of any of you in Jannah will be that Allah will tell him to express his wish. He will wish and wish again. Allah will then ask him: 'Have you expressed your wish?' He will answer: 'Yes, I have.' Allah will say: 'You will have what you have wished for and the like thereof along with it.'" (Muslim)

Abu Sa'id Al-Khudri (May Allah be pleased with him) said: The Messenger of Allah (peace and blessings be upon him) said, "Allah, the Rubb of Honor and Glory, will say to the inhabitants of Jannah: 'O inhabitants of Jannah!' They will respond: 'Here we are! At Your service, O our Rubb. All good is in Your Hand!' He will ask them: 'Are you pleased?' They will reply: 'Why should we not be pleased, O Rubb, when You have given us what You have not given to any of Your creatures?' Allah will say: 'Shall I not give you something better than that?' They will ask: 'O Rubb! What can be better than that?' Allah will say: 'I shall bestow My Pleasure upon you and I shall never be displeased with you.'" (Bukhari and Muslim)

Jarir bin 'Abdullah (May Allah be pleased with him) reported: "We were sitting with the Messenger of Allah (peace and blessings be upon him) when he looked at the full moon and observed, "You shall see your Rubb in the Hereafter as you are seeing this moon; and you will not feel the slightest inconvenience in seeing Him." (Bukhari and Muslim)

Commentary: Just as when we witness the moon there is no problem, no rush or troublesome gathering of people and no pushing of one another, the pious will see Allah without any trouble or difficulty. How shall we see Him, we cannot describe this even by any instance or parable. In Surah Ash-Shuraa, Verse 11, it is said that there is nothing like Him. However, we cannot see Him in this world with these worldly eyes. The reason is that, as Imam Malik says, these eyes are just temporary and they cannot bear the sight of Allah. This is why the research scholars claim that the Prophet (peace and blessings be upon him) did not actually see Allah during his journey to the heavens; he only talked to Allah by way of Revelation. The saying of Aisha (May Allah be pleased with her) also proves this contention. However, it would be possible to see Allah in Jannah as everything there will be eternal and indestructible. Similar will be the case with the sight and eyes which will be provided to us there. Such eyes would have the power to see Allah. (665)

Narrated Abu Hurairah: Allah's Apostle said, "All my followers will enter Paradise except those who refuse." They said, "O Allah's Apostle! Who will refuse?" He said, "Whoever obeys me will enter Paradise, and whoever disobeys me is the one who refuses (to enter it)." (Bukhari)

715. Disbelief in Hellfire

Allah, the Exalted, says:

"This Day, We shall seal up their mouths, and their hands will speak to Us, and their legs will bear witness to what they used to earn." (Qur'an, Yasin 36:65)

"And whoever Allah guides - he is the (rightly) guided; and whoever He sends astray - you will never find for them protectors besides Him, and We will gather them on the Day of Resurrection (fallen) on their faces - blind, dumb and deaf. Their refuge is Hell; every time it subsides, We increase them in blazing Fire." (Qur'an, Al-Isra 17:97)

"Verily, those who belie Our Ayat (proofs, evidences, verses, lessons, signs, revelations, etc.) and treat them with arrogance, for them the gates of heaven will not be opened, and they will not enter Paradise until the camel goes through the eye of the needle (which is impossible). Thus, do We recompense the Mujrimun (criminals, polytheists, sinners, etc.)." (Qur'an, Al-A'raf 7:40)

Other Verses: *An-Naba' 78:21-30, Qaf 50:24-26.*

Scorching the Face

The noblest and most dignified part of a person is the face.

Allah, the Exalted, will humiliate the disbelievers and transgressors:

"If only those who disbelieved knew (the time) when they will not be able to ward off the Fire from their faces, nor from their backs; and they will not be helped." (Qur'an, Al-Anbya 21:39)

"The Fire will burn their faces, and therein they will grin, with displaced lips (disfigured)." (Qur'an, Al-Mu'minun 23:104)

"On the Day when their faces will be turned over in the Fire, they will say: "Oh, would that we had obeyed Allah and obeyed the Messenger (Muhammad SAW)." (Qur'an, Al-Ahzab 33:66)

Other Verse: Al-Isra 17:97.

Darkness of the Face

Allah, the Exalted, says:

"On the Day (i.e. the Day of Resurrection) when some faces will become white and some faces will become black; as for those whose faces will become black (to them will be said): "Did you reject Faith after accepting it? Then taste the torment (in Hell) for rejecting Faith." (Qur'an, Ali 'Imran 3:106)

"And those who have earned evil deeds, the recompense of an evil deed is the like thereof, and humiliating disgrace will cover them (their faces). No defender will they have from Allah. Their faces will be covered, as it were, with pieces from the darkness of night. They are dwellers of the Fire, they will abide therein forever." (Qur'an, Yunus 10:27)

Burning the Skin

The Fire of the Almighty will burn the skin of the infidels. The skin is the site of sensation, where the pain of burning is felt, and for this reason, Allah Almighty will replace the burned skin with a new one, to be burned anew, and this will be endlessly repeated:

"Surely! Those who disbelieved in Our Ayat (proofs, evidences, verses, lessons, signs, revelations, etc.) We shall burn them in Fire. As often as their skins are roasted through, We shall change them for other skins that they may taste the punishment. Truly, Allah is Ever Most Powerful, All-Wise." (Qur'an, An-Nisa 4:56)

"I will drive him into Hellfire. And what can make you know what is Hellfire? It lets nothing remain and leaves nothing (unburned), Burning the skins." (Qur'an, Al-Muddaththir 74:26-29)

Melting

One of the kinds of torment will be the pouring of Al-Hamim over their heads. Al-Hamim is ultra-heated water; because of its extreme heat, it will melt their innards and everything inside:

"... then as for those who disbelieve, garments of fire will be cut out for them, boiling water will be poured down over their heads. With it will melt or vanish away what is within their bellies, as well as skins." (Qur'an, Al-Hajj 22:19-20)

Dragging on their Faces

The disbelievers will be dragged on their faces into Fire:

"Verily, the Mujrimun (polytheists, disbelievers, sinners, criminals, etc.) are in error (in this world) and will burn (in the Hellfire in the Hereafter). The Day they will be dragged in the Fire on their faces (it will be said to them): "Taste you the touch of Hell!" (Qur'an, Al-Qamar 54:47-48)

The pain at dragging will increase by being tied up in chains and fetters:

"When iron collars will be rounded over their necks, and the chains, they shall be dragged along. In the boiling water, then they will be burned in the Fire." (Qur'an, Ghafir 40:71-72)

The Food, Drink and Clothing of the People of Hell

Food in Hellfire is a fierce kind of torture. (666)

"No food will there be for them but a poisonous thorny plant, Which will neither nourish nor avail against hunger." (Qur'an, Al-Ghashiyah 88:6-7)

"Verily, the tree of Zaqqum, Will be the food of the sinners, Like boiling oil, it will boil in the bellies, Like the boiling of scalding water." (Qur'an, Ad-Dukhan 44:43-46)

"those who shall dwell for ever in the Fire, and be given, to drink, boiling water, so that it cuts up their bowels?" (Qur'an, Muhammad 47:15)

Other Verse: As-Safat 37:62-67.

Hellfire choking food (ad-Daree (thorny plants), az-Zaqqum (tree like heads of Devils), pus, wound discharge, dripping of people of Hell, vaginal discharge of adulteresses, boiling water and oil, etc.) will choke because of stuckness in the throat, scald their faces, tear their bodies apart, cut up the bowels, release bodily fluids).

"Verily, with Us are fetters (to bind them), and a raging Fire. And a food that chokes, and a painful torment." (Qur'an, Al-Muzzammil 73:12-13)

"Nor any food except filth from the washing of wounds, None will eat except the Khati'un (sinners, disbelievers, polytheists, etc.)." (Qur'an, Al-Haqqah 69:36-37)

"Then let them taste it, a boiling fluid and dirty wound discharges. And other torments of similar kind, all together!" (Qur'an, Sad 38:57-58)

Other Verses: Al-Kahf 18:29, Ibrahim 14:16-17.

Four kinds of drink that the people of Hell have to endure:

1) **al-Hameem**: an extremely hot water.

"They will go between it (Hell) and the boiling hot water!" (Qur'an, Ibrahim 55:44)

"They will be given to drink from a boiling spring." (Qur'an, Al-Ghashiyah 88:5)

"(They will be) in scorching fire and scalding water, And shadow of black smoke, (That shadow) neither cool, nor (even) good." (Qur'an, Al-Waqi'ah 56:42-44)

2) **al-Ghassaaq** is the festering pus that oozes out of the skin of the people of Hell. It was suggested that it refers to the offensive discharge that flows from the private parts of adulterous women, and the decaying skin and flesh of the kuffaar.

And also, with this chain, from the Prophet (peace and blessings be upon him) that he said: "If a bucket of Ghassaq were poured out in the world, the people of the world would rot." (Tirmidhi)

3) **al-Sadeed (pus)**: what flows from the flesh and skin of the Kaafir.

Narrated Abdullah bin 'Amr that the Messenger of Allah (peace and blessings be upon him) said: "Whoever drinks wine and gets drunk, his prayer will not be accepted for forty days, and if he dies, he will enter Hell, but if he repents, Allah will accept his repentance. If he drinks wine again and gets drunk, his prayer will not be accepted for forty days, and if he dies, he will enter Hell, but if he repents, Allah will accept his repentance. If he drinks wine again and gets drunk, his prayer will not be accepted for forty days, and if he dies, he will enter Hell, but if he repents Allah will accept his repentance. But if he does it again, then Allah will most certainly **make him drink of the mire of the pus or sweat on the Day of Resurrection**." They said:

"O Messenger of Allah, what is the mire of the pus or sweat? He said: **"The drippings of the people of Hell**." (Ibn Majah) (https://sunnah.com/ibnmajah:3377)

4) **al-Muhl** - water like molten copper, like thick burning oil, which scalds faces, because of the intensity

of its heat.

Allah, the Exalted, says:

"Those who unjustly eat up the property of orphans, eat us a Fire into their own bellies, and they will soon be enduring a blazing Fire!" (Qur'an, An-Nisa 4:10)

Abu Sa'id Al-Khudri narrated that about Kal Muhl, the Prophet (peace and blessings be upon him) said: "Like boiling oil, such that whenever it is brought near him the skin of his face falls into it." (Tirmidhi)

Anas b. Malik reported that Allah's Messenger (peace and blessings be upon him) said that one amongst the denizens of Hell who had led a life of ease and plenty amongst the people of the world would be made to dip in Fire only once on the Day of Resurrection and then it would be said to him: "O, son of Adam, did you find any comfort, did you happen to get any material blessing?" He would say: "By Allah, no, my Lord." And then that person from amongst the persons of the world be brought who had led the most miserable life (in the world) from amongst the inmates of Paradise and he would be made to dip once in Paradise and it would be said to him: "0, son of Adam, did you face any hardship? Or had any distress fallen to your lot?" And he would say: "By Allah, no, 0 my Lord, never did I face any hardship or experience any distress." (Muslim) (https://sunnah.com/muslim:2807)

The horror and intensity of the Fire will make a man lose his mind, and he would give up everything he holds dear to escape it, but he will never be able to:

"...the sinner's desire will be: Would that he could redeem himself from the Penalty of that Day by (sacrificing) his children, his wife and his brother, his kindred who sheltered him, and all, all that is on earth, so that it could deliver him. By no means! For it would be the Fire of Hell! Plucking out right to the skull." (Qur'an, Al-Ma'arij 70:11-16)

Narrated Samura bin Jundub: "...One morning the Prophet (peace and blessings be upon him) said, "Last night two persons came to me (in a dream) and woke me up and said to me, 'Proceed!' I set out with them and we came across a man lying down, and behold, another man was standing over his head, holding a big rock. Behold, he was throwing the rock at the man's head, injuring it…" (Bukhari) (https://hadeethenc.com/en/browse/hadith/6604)

EFFECTS AND CONSEQUENCES OF SINS

Allah, the Exalted, says:

"Leave (O mankind, all kinds of) sin, open and secret. Verily, those who commit sin will get due recompense for that which they used to commit." (Qur'an, Al-An'am 6:120)

"(And We said): "If you do good, you do good for your own selves, and if you do evil (you do it) against yourselves." (Qur'an, Al-Isra 17:7)

"And whoever does an atom's weight of evil, will see it." (Qur'an, Az-Zalzalah 99:8)

Other Verses: *An-Nisa 4:14, 4:48 and 4:111, Al-Ma'idah 5:33-34, Al-Ahqaf 46:20, Ali 'Imran 3:91, Al-Baqarah 2:48 and 2:161, Al-Hajj 22:46, Al-A'raf 7:179, Ar-Rahman 55:41, Al-An'am 6:32.*

Refraining from sins is more important than performing good deeds.

Abu Dharr (May Allah be pleased with him) reported that the Prophet (May Allah's peace and blessings be upon him) said: "I see what you do not see. Heaven is groaning and it has a right to be groaning: there is no space the width of four fingers in it but an angel placing his forehead in prostration to Allah the Exalted." (Ibn Majah) (https://hadeethenc.com/en/browse/hadith/3265)

Narrated Anas: The Messenger of Allah (peace and blessings be upon him) said: "Envy consumers good deeds just as fire consumes wood, and charity extinguishes bad deeds just as water extinguishes fire. Prayer is the light of the believer and fasting is a shield against the Fire." (Ibn Majah)

'Adyy ibn Hatim (May Allah be pleased with him) reported: The Prophet (May Allah's peace and blessings be upon him) said: "The Jews are people who incurred Allah's Wrath, and the Christians are astray." (Tirmidhi) (https://hadeethenc.com/en/browse/hadith/65061)

Imam Ibn Al-Qayyim (May Allah have mercy on him) explains the effects of sins in his books:

"One hundred pieces of advice" and "Al-Jawab Al-Kafi".

1) Prevention of Beneficial Knowledge

Imam Shaafi'ee said:

- "I complained to Wakee' about the weakness of my memory
- So, he ordered me to abandon disobedience
- And informed me that the knowledge is light
- And that the light of Allah is not given to the disobedient." (667)

2) Prevention of Sustenance

Just as Taqwaa brings about sustenance, the abandonment of Taqwaa causes poverty. There is nothing which can bring about sustenance like the abandonment of disobedience.

Narrated Thawban: The Messenger of Allah (peace and blessings be upon him) said: 'Nothing extends one's life span but righteousness, nothing averts the Divine Decree but supplication, and nothing deprives a man of provision but the sin that he commits.'" (Ibn Majah)

3) Prevention of Obedience to Allah

If there was no other punishment for sin except that it prevents one from obeying Allah then this would be sufficient.

4) Disobedience Weakens the Heart

Disobedience continues to weaken the heart until its life ceases completely.

Narrated Abu Hurairah that the Messenger of Allah (peace and blessings be upon him) said: "When the believer commits sin, a black spot appears on his heart. If he repents and gives up that sin and seeks forgiveness, his heart will be polished. But if (the sin) increases, (the black spot) increases. That is the Ran that Allah mentions in His Book: *"Nay! But on their hearts is the Ran (covering of sins and evil deeds) which they used to earn." (83:14)* (Ibn Majah)

5) Disobedience Reduces one's Lifespan and Destroys any Blessings

Just as righteousness increases one's lifespan, sinning reduces it.

6) Legacy of the Cursed.

Every type of disobedience is the legacy of a nation from among those which Allah destroyed. Sodomy is a legacy of the people of Lot, taking more than one's due right and giving what is less is a legacy of the people of Shu`aib, spreading mischief and corruption is a legacy of the people of Pharaoh and pride, including arrogance and tyranny, is a legacy of the people of Hud. So, the disobedient one is somehow a part of those nations who were the enemies of Allah.

7) Disobedience is a Cause of the Servant Being Held in Contempt by his Lord

Allah, the Exalted, said:

"And he whom Allah humiliates - for him there is no bestower of honor." (Qur'an, Al-Hajj 22:18)

Al-Hasan Al-Basri said: "They became contemptible in (His sight) so they disobeyed Him. If they were honorable (in His sight) He would have protected them."

8) Effect of Sins on Others

The ill-effects of the sinner fall upon those around him as well as the animals as a result of which they are touched by harm. Sense of alienation that comes between a person and his Lord, and between him and other people. One of the salaf (righteous predecessors) said: "If I disobey Allah, I see that in the attitude of my riding beast and my wife."

9) Living in Sin

The servant continues to commit sins until they become very easy for him and seem insignificant in his heart and this is a sure sign of destruction. Every time a sin becomes insignificant in the sight of the servant it becomes great in the sight of Allah.

Narrated Abu Hurairah: "I heard Allah's Messenger (peace and blessings be upon him) saying. "All the sins of my followers will be forgiven except for those of the Mujahirin (those who commit a sin openly or disclose their sins to the people). An example of such disclosure is that a person commits a sin at night and though Allah screens it from the public, then he comes in the morning, and says, 'O so-and-so, I did such-and-such (evil) deed yesterday,' though he spent his night screened by his Lord (none knowing about his sin) and in the morning he removes Allah's screen from himself." (Bukhari)

10) Disobedience Brings Humiliation and Lowliness

Every aspect of honor lies in the obedience of Allah. Ibn Al-Mubarak said: "I have seen sins kill the hearts. And humiliation is inherited by their continuity. The abandonment of sins gives life to the hearts. And the prevention of your soul is better for it."

11) Disobedience Corrupts the Intellect

The intellect has light and disobedience extinguishes this light. When the light of the intellect is extinguished it becomes weak and deficient.

12) Sealing of the Heart

When disobedience increases, the servant's heart becomes sealed so that he becomes of those who are heedless. The Exalted said: "But no! A stain has been left on their hearts on account of what they used to earn (that is, their actions)." *(Al-Mutaffifin 83:14)*

For obedience is light and disobedience is darkness. The stronger the darkness grows, the greater becomes his confusion, until he falls into innovation, misguidance and other things that lead to doom, without even realizing, like a blind man who goes out in the darkness of the night, walking alone This darkness grows stronger until it covers the eyes, then it grows stronger until it covers the face, which appears dark and is seen by everyone.

Abdullah Ibn Abbas (May Allah be pleased with him) said, "Verily, good deeds bring brightness upon the face, a light in the heart, an expanse of provision, strength in the body, and love in the hearts of the creation. And evil deeds bring blackness upon the face, darkness in the grave and in the heart, weakness in the body, a restriction of provision, and hatred in the hearts of the creation." (al-Jawāb al-Kafī 1/54)

13) Sins Cause Various Types of Corruption in the Land

Corruption of the water, the air, the plants, the fruit, and the dwelling places. The Exalted said: *"Mischief has appeared on the land and the sea on account of what the hands of men have earned; that He may give them a taste of some of (the actions) they have done, in order that they may return." (Ar-Rum 30:41)*

14) Disappearance of Modesty

Modesty is the essence of the life of the heart and is the basis of every good. Its disappearance is the disappearance of all that is good. The Prophet (peace and blessings be upon him) said: "Modesty is goodness, all of it."

15) Sins Weaken and Reduce the Magnification of Allah the Almighty

in the Heart of the Servant

16) Sins are the Cause of Allah Forgetting His Servant

Sinning also causes Allah to abandon him and leave him to fend for himself with his soul and his Satan and in this is destruction from which no deliverance can be hoped for.

17) Being Removed from the Realm of Benevolence

When a person sins, benevolence is removed from his heart. When benevolence fills the heart, it prevents it from disobedience.

18) Disobedience (Sins) Causes the Favors (of Allah) to Cease and Makes His Revenge Lawful

Allah, the Exalted, says:

"(They took to flight because of their) arrogance in the land and their plotting of evil. But the evil plot encompasses only him who makes it…" *(Qur'an, Fatir 35:43)*

When a person plans evil for others, evil befalls him and he himself will face problems.

Whoever digs a pit, will fall into it.

If someone rolls a stone, it will roll back on them.

If you set a trap for others, you will get caught in it yourself.

Following are Some Effects and Consequences for Particular Sin:

1. Punishments for Hiraabah (Agression)

The punishment for Aggression is one of the Hudud or punishments prescribed by Shariah, and the punishment varies according to the severity of the crime. This is explained as follows:

1.1. Whoever kills someone and steals their property, should definitely be killed and crucified, so that everyone will know about him. It is not permitted to forgive him, by the consensus of the scholars, as was reported by Ibn al-Mundhir.
1.2. Whoever kills but does not steal, should definitely be killed, but not crucified.
1.3. Whoever steals property but does not kill, his right hand and left foot should be cut off at the same time, then the bleeding should be stopped and he should be released.
1.4. Whoever merely terrorizes people, but does not kill or steal, should be banished from the land to another country, where he should be detained until he has repented sincerely and is reformed.

The evidence for the above is as follows:

(1) The Words of Allah: *"The recompense of those who wage war against Allah and His Messenger and do mischief in the land is only that they shall be killed or crucified or their hands and their feet be cut off on the opposite sides, or be exiled from the land. That is their disgrace in this world, and a great torment is theirs in the Hereafter."* (Qur'an, Al-Ma'idah 5:33)

(2) The report narrated Ibn Abaas (May Allah be pleased with him): The Messenger of Allah (peace and blessings of Allah be upon him) made a peace treaty with Abu Barzah Hilaal ibn Awaymir al-Aslami. Some people came, wanting to embrace Islam, and they were ambushed by the companions of Abu Barzah. Then Jibreel (peace be upon him) brought to the Messenger of Allah (peace and blessings of Allah be upon him) the Revelation of the punishment for killing and stealing property, which is to be killed and crucified, and the punishment for killing without stealing, which is to be killed. Whoever steals property but does not kill should have his hand and foot from opposite sides cut off. Whoever becomes Muslim, Islam cancels out whatever deeds came before it at the time of Shirk. (Tafseer al-Tabari, 10/260-261)

The Reason for Different Levels of Punishment for Aggression

Allah, the Exalted, says:

"The recompense for an evil is an evil like thereof." (Qur'an, Ash-Shuraa 42:40)

Different punishments for different degrees of hiraabah have been prescribed for a very important reason. Hiraabah may take different forms, as is well known, it might not involve only killing, or only stealing. It might involve both stealing and killing, or it may involve neither, only terrorizing people. These different forms of crime dictate different forms of punishment. (423)

1. **Punishment for Ascribing a Partner or Rival to Allah**

Allah, the Exalted, says:

"Surely, they have disbelieved who say: "Allah is the Messiah ['Iesa (Jesus)], son of Maryam (Mary)." But the Messiah ['Iesa (Jesus)] said: "O Children of Israel! Worship Allah, my Lord and your Lord." Verily, whosoever sets up partners in worship with Allah, then Allah has forbidden Paradise for him, and the Fire will be his abode. And for the Zalimun (polytheists and wrongdoers) there are no helpers." (Qur'an, Al- Ma'idah 5:72)

2. **Punishment for Zina**

Allah, the Exalted, says:

"The woman and the man guilty of illegal sexual intercourse, flog each of them with a hundred stripes. Let not pity withhold you in their case, in a punishment prescribed by Allah, if you believe in Allah and the Last Day. And let a party of the believers witness their punishment. (This punishment is for unmarried persons guilty of the above crime but if married persons commit it, the punishment is to stone them to death, according to Allah's Law)." (Qur'an, An-Nur 24:2)

3. **Punishment in Hellfire for Backbiting**

Anas ibn Malik reported: The Messenger of Allah (peace and blessings be upon him) said, "When I was taken on my night journey, I passed by people who had metal hooks in their hands and they were clawing at their faces and necks. I said: "Who are these, O Gabriel? Gabriel said: *"These are the ones who 'eat the flesh of people' (49:12) and attack their honor."* (Abu Dawud)

4. **Talebearers, Gossip-Mongers will not enter Paradise**

Hudhayfah reported: The Prophet, peace and blessings be upon him, said, "The talebearer will not enter Paradise." (Bukhari and Muslim)

5. **Disbelievers in Allah, Criminals, Sinners, etc. will not enter Paradise**

Allah, the Exalted, says:

"Verily, those who belie Our Ayat (proofs, evidences, verses, lessons, signs, revelations, etc.) and treat them with arrogance, for them the gates of heaven will not be opened, and they will not enter Paradise until the camel goes through the eye of the needle (which is impossible). Thus, do We recompense the Mujrimun (criminals, polytheists, sinners, etc.)." (Qur'an, Al-A'raf 7:40)

6. **Punishment for Severing the Kinship Ties**

Jubayr ibn Mut'im (May Allah be pleased with him) reported that the Prophet (May Allah's peace and blessings be upon him) said: "The one who severs the ties of kinship will not enter Paradise." (Bukhari and Muslim) (https://hadeethenc.com/en/browse/hadith/5367)

7. **Punishment for Not Forbidding Evil**

Abu Bakr (May Allah be pleased with him) said: "O people, you recite this Verse: *"O you who believe, upon you is (responsibility for) yourselves. Those who have gone astray will not harm you when you have been guided." (Al-Ma'idah 5:105)*, but I have heard Messenger of Allah (May Allah's peace and blessings be upon him) say: 'When people see an oppressor but do not prevent him committing sin, it is likely that Allah will punish them all.'" (Ibn Majah) (https://hadeethenc.com/en/browse/hadith/3470)

SINS ARE EXPIATED BY FOLLOWING MEANS

Allah, the Exalted, says:

"As for those who repent, mend their ways, and let the truth be known, they are the ones to whom I will turn ˹in forgiveness˺, for I am the Accepter of Repentance, Most Merciful." (Qur'an, Al-Baqarah 2:160)

"And he who repents and does righteousness does indeed turn to Allah with (accepted) repentance." (Qur'an, Al-Furqan 25:71)

"Seek the forgiveness of your Rubb, and turn to Him in repentance." (Qur'an, Hud 11:3)

Other Verses: *Taha 20:82, Al-Furqan 25:68-70, An-Nisa 4:92, Az-Zumar 39:53, At-Tahrim 66:8,*

At-Tawbah 9:104.

Ali Ibn Abi Talib (May Allah be pleased with him) said: "A trial is not sent down but due to a Sin, and it is not lifted but with Repentance." (al-Jawab al-Kafi 1/74)

I. THINGS WHICH FORGIVE MAJOR SINS

1. Becoming Muslim
2. Hajj
3. Hijrah or migrating for the sake of Allah

'Amr ibn al-'As reported: The Prophet, peace and blessings be upon him, said, "Do you not know that embracing Islam wipes away all sins committed before it, that emigration wipes away what came before it, and the Hajj pilgrimage wipes away what came before it?" (Muslim)

When a non-Muslim becomes a Muslim, Allah turns his bad deeds (sayyiat) into good deeds (hasanat), and forgives him all his previous sins, as He, the Exalted, says:

"Say to those who have disbelieved, if they cease (from disbelief), their past will be forgiven." (Qur'an, Al-Anfal 8:38)

II. SINCERE REPENTANCE

Allah, the Exalted, says:

"But whosoever repents after his crime and does righteous good deeds (by obeying Allah), then verily, Allah will pardon him (accept his repentance). Verily, Allah is Oft-Forgiving, Most Merciful." (Qur'an, Al-Ma'idah 5:39)

"And He it is Who accepts repentance from His slaves, and forgives sins, and He knows what you do." (Qur'an, Ash-Shuraa 42:25)

"Truly, Allah loves those who turn unto Him in repentance and loves those who purify themselves." (Qur'an, Al-Baqarah 2:222)

Other Verses: An-Nisa 4:17-18, Al-An'am 6:54, Muhammad 47:2, Al-Ma'idah 5:6.

Abu Musa 'Abdullah ibn Qays al-Ash'ari (May Allah be pleased with him) reported that the Prophet (May Allah's peace and blessings be upon him) said: "Allah the Almighty stretches His Hand during the night so that the sinners of the day may repent, and stretches His Hand during the day so that the sinners of the night may repent. He keeps doing so until the sun rises from the west." (Muslim)
(https://hadeethenc.com/en/browse/hadith/4318)

Conditions of Repentance

Sincere repentance is not merely the matter of words spoken on the tongue. Rather, the acceptance of repentance is subject to the conditions that:

1. the person gives up the sin straight away,
2. he regrets what has happened in the past,
3. he resolves not to go back to the thing he has repented from,
4. he restores people's rights or property if his sin involved wrongdoing towards others, and
5. he repents before the agony of death is upon him.

Ibn 'Abbas and Anas bin Malik (May Allah be pleased with them) reported: The Messenger of Allah (peace and blessings be upon him) said, "If a son of Adam were to own a valley full of gold, he would desire to have two. Nothing can fill his mouth except the earth (of the grave). Allah turns with mercy to him who turns to Him in repentance." (Bukhari and Muslim)

Abu Hurairah (May Allah be pleased with him) reported: The Messenger of Allah (peace and blessings be upon him) said, "Allah, the Exalted, smiles at two men, one of them killed the other and both will enter Jannah. The first is killed by the other while he is fighting in the Cause of Allah, and thereafter Allah will turn in mercy to the second and guide him to accept Islam and then he dies as a Shaheed (martyr) fighting in the Cause of Allah." (Bukhari and Muslim)

Commentary: Even the greatest sins, including those which one has committed before embracing Islam, are forgiven by repentance.

Smiling is also one of the Attributes of Allah, although we are unaware of the nature of it. (668)

Abu Hurairah (May Allah be pleased with him) reported that the Prophet (May Allah's peace and blessings be upon him) said: "He who has wronged his brother, concerning his honor or anything else, let him ask for his pardon today before there comes a time when there will be neither a dinar nor a dirham. If he has good deeds, an amount equivalent to the wrong he has done will be taken from his good deeds (and given to the one whom he has wronged). If he has no good deeds, then some of that person's bad deeds will be taken and loaded upon him." (Bukhari)
(https://hadeethenc.com/en/browse/hadith/5438)

Ibn Taymiyah (May Allah have mercy on him) said in Majmoo' al-Fataawa:

"According to the Saheeh Hadith (authentic narration): "Whoever has wronged his brother with regard to his blood, his wealth or his honor, let him come and set matters straight before there comes a Day on which there will be no dirhams and no dinars, only good deeds and bad deeds, and if he has good deeds (they will be taken and given to the one whom he wronged), otherwise some of the bad deeds of the one whom he wronged will be taken and added to his burden, then he will be thrown into the Fire." This has to do with cases where the one who was wronged was aware of it; but if he was gossiped about or slandered and he does not know, then it was said that one of the conditions of repentance is telling him, or it was said that this is not essential, which is the view of the majority; both views were narrated from Ahmad, but his view on such matters is that one should do good deeds for the one who was wronged, such as praying for him, praying for forgiveness for him and doing good deeds to be given to him, to take the place of that backbiting and slander. (669)

An-Nawawi (May Allah have mercy on him) said:

"The scholars said: Repentance is obligatory from all sins. If the sin has to do with a matter that is between the individual and Allah, may He be Exalted, and does not have to do with the rights of other people, then three conditions must be met:

1. he must give up sin
2. he must regret what he has done
3. he must resolve never to go back to it.

If one of these three is missing, then his repentance is not valid.

But if the sin has to do with other people, then four conditions must be met: the three mentioned above, and he must also absolve himself of any wrongdoing and pay his dues to the one whom he wronged. If it is the matter of money and the like, then he must return it to him. If it has to do with punishment for slandering him and the like, he should submit to the punishment to be carried out on him or seek that person's forgiveness. If it is the matter of backbiting, he must ask him to forgive him for it." (End quote from Riyadh as-Saaliheen (p.14) (670)

Repentance for Stealing

The scholars of the Standing Committee said, concerning a man who stole money from a slave:

"If he knows the slave or he knows someone who knows him, he can tell him to look for him and give him the money in silver or the equivalent, or whatever he agrees upon with him. If he does not know who he is and he thinks that he will never find him, he should give it or the equivalent in cash to a charity on behalf of its owner. If he finds him after that, he should tell him what he did; if he accepts that, all well and good, but if he objects and demands his money, then he should give it to him, and the money he gave in charity becomes an act of charity on his own behalf. He also has to ask Allah for forgiveness and repent to Him, and pray for the other person." (Fataawa Islamiyyah) (379)

Repentance for Backbiting and Slander

The Messenger of Allah (peace and blessings be upon him) said: "Beware of Backbiting, for it is worse than adultery". They (Companions) asked: "O Allah's Messenger, how backbiting is worse than adultery? He (peace and blessings be upon him) said: "A man may commit adultery then he turns in repentance to Allah, and Allah accepts it. But the backbiter will not attain salvation unless the person against whom he backbites him forgives him." (Ad-Darqutni from Jabir bin Abdullah)

Ibn Taymiyah (May Allah have mercy on him) said:

"Whoever wrongs a person by Slandering him, Backbiting about him or insulting him, then repents, Allah will accept his repentance, but if the one who was wronged finds out about that, he has the right to settle the score. But if he slandered him or backbit about him and the person did not hear of that, then there are two views according to the scholars, both of which were narrated from Ahmad, the more correct of which is that he should not tell him that he spoke against him in his absence. It was said that he should rather speak well of him in his absence just as he spoke badly of him in his absence, as al-Hasan al-Basri said: the expiation for ghiiba is to pray for forgiveness for the person about whom you backbit." (Majmoo' al-Fataawa) (412)

Repentance for Gossip

Regarding Repentance for Gossip, the seriousness of this sin is due to two reasons:

1 - It has to do with people's rights, so it is more serious because it involves wrongdoing against people.

2 - It is an easy sin that most people commit, except those on whom Allah has mercy.

People usually regard easy things as insignificant, although they are serious before Allah.

With regard to expiation for gossiping, it is essential to note a few important points:

Firstly:

The expiation for gossip includes praying for forgiveness for the one you gossiped about, and making Du'a (supplication) for him and praising him in his absence.

Secondly:

Stating that praying for forgiveness is the expiation for Gossip does not mean that it is sufficient. The basic principle is that sins cannot be erased except by sincere repentance which is accompanied by giving up the sin, regretting it, resolving not to go back to it and being sincere at heart in one's dealings with the Creator, may He be Glorified. Then there is the hope if one repents in this manner, that Allah will forgive him his sins and pardon his errors. With regard to people's rights and transgressions against people, they can only be expiated if the people affected pardon him and forgive him. The command is to seek forgiveness for wrongdoing before scores are settled among people on the Day of Reckoning, when scores will be settled with hasanat and sayyiat and true losses will be borne by those who wronged people with regard to their wealth, honor and blood.

Thirdly:

What the one who wants to free himself of the sin of Gossip must do is strive hard to seek forgiveness from the one whom he gossiped about, and ask him to pardon him, and apologize to him with kind and good words, and he should be as humble as he can in this, even if he has to buy an extremely valuable gift or offer financial help. The scholars have stated that all of this is permissible when it comes to restoring people's rights. Because the scholars among the righteous salaf (predecessors) and fuqaha (jurists) thought that seeking people's forgiveness for Gossip might lead – in some cases – to greater evils such as grudges or breaking of ties, and people might feel resentment and grudges to an extent that is known only to Allah, most of the scholars granted concessions allowing one not to seek forgiveness (from the victim), and they hoped that it would be sufficient to pray for forgiveness for the victim of Gossip and make Du'a (supplication) for him and praise him in his absence. Other scholars were of the view that nothing could expiate for Gossip but the forgiveness of the one who was wronged. But the correct view is that if the one who gossiped repents sincerely, he does not have to tell the one about whom he gossiped about it, especially if he fears that this would cause more trouble, as is usually the case. Praying for forgiveness for the one he gossiped about is an exceptional case and is a case of necessity dictated by Shariah (Islamic Law), where warding off harm takes precedence over bringing benefits. From the above it may be understood that the one who regards the sin of Gossip as insignificant on the basis that praying for forgiveness is sufficient to expiate this sin is incorrect. His thinking is wrong for three reasons:

1) He forgets that the basic condition for repentance is regret, giving up the sin and sincerely repenting to Allah. This condition may not be truly met in the case of most people.

2) The basic principle in expiation with regard to people's rights is striving to seek their pardon. If he thinks that telling the person about the Gossip will lead to a greater evil, then he may resort to praying for forgiveness for him in this case, otherwise the basic principle is that he should seek pardon from the one whom he wronged.

3) This shows you that if the person who was gossiped about has heard about what another man has said about him, then – in this case – it is essential to seek forgiveness from him directly, so that the harm suffered by the victim will be undone and his resentment may be dispelled. If he does not pardon or forgive, then there is no option after that but to pray for forgiveness for him and make Du'a (supplication) for him.

Fourthly:

As for praying in general terms, it does not seem to be sufficient to achieve what you are hoping for from Allah. Just as you gossiped about him by mentioning his name or describing him, and you singled him out for harm, so too you should pray specifically for him and ask for forgiveness for him. We say that when we hope that Allah will accept our Du'a and prayers for forgiveness as an expiation for bad deeds, it is essential to be sincere towards Allah, to seek out means of drawing close to Allah, and to repeat it in times and places where Du'as are answered, and pray for all goodness and blessings in this world and in the Hereafter. Undoubtedly such a Du'a requires us to specify the person for whom we are praying, either mentioning him by name or describing him, by saying: "O Allah, forgive me and the one whom I have gossiped about and wronged"; "O Allah, pardon us and him, and whatever else you can say in your Du'a. As for praying in general terms, it does not seem to be sufficient to achieve what you are hoping for from Allah. Just as you gossiped about him by mentioning his name or describing him, and you singled him out for harm, so too you should pray specifically for him and ask for forgiveness for him, so that the bad deeds will be replaced by good.

Fifthly:

The purpose behind praying for forgiveness and making Du'a is to ward off bad deeds with good, and to compensate for misdeeds. Hence it is not limited to prayers for forgiveness in exclusion to other good deeds. Rather you can do a good deed and dedicate its reward to the one about whom you gossiped, such as giving charity on his behalf or offering him some help, or supporting him at times of hardship, and trying to compensate him for the wrong you did as much as you can.

Ibn Taymiyah (May Allah have mercy on him) said in Majmoo' al-Fatawa:

"As for the rights of the one who was wronged, they are not waived just because one repents. This is a right and there is no difference between a killer and other wrongdoer. If a person repents from wrongdoing, the rights of the one whom he wronged are not waived because of his repentance, rather it is part of his repentance to compensate him to a level commensurate with his wrongdoing. If he does not compensate him in this world then he will inevitably compensate him in the Hereafter. So, the wrongdoer who has repented, should do a lot of good deeds, so that when those who have been wronged claim their rights, he will not end up bankrupt. And if Allah wants to compensate the one who was wronged then no one can prevent His bounty, such as if He wants to forgive sins less than shirk for whomever He wills. Hence in the Hadith (narration) about qasas (prescribed punishments), for which Jabir ibn 'Abd-Allah rode for a month to 'Abd-Allah ibn Unays to hear it from his lips – which was narrated by Imam Ahmad and others, and which al-Bukhari quoted as evidence in his Saheeh (authentic compilation) – it says: "When the Day of Resurrection comes, Allah will gather all creatures in a single plain so that the announcer will be able to make them all hear his voice and the watcher will be able to see all of them, then He will call them in a voice that will be heard from afar just as it is heard from nearby: 'I am the Sovereign, I am the Judge. None of the people of Hell shall enter Hell if they have any right due from any of the people of Paradise, until the score is settled, and none of the people of Paradise shall enter Paradise if they have any right due from any of the people of Hell, until the score is settled.'"

And in Saheeh Muslim it is narrated from Abu Sa'eed: "When the people of Paradise cross al-sirat (a bridge) and stand on a bridge between Paradise and Hell, they will settle their scores with one another, and when they are cleansed and purified, permission will be given to them to enter Paradise."

Allah, the Exalted, says:

"...neither backbite one another" – as gossip is a transgression against people's honor – He then said: "Would one of you like to eat the flesh of his dead brother? You would hate it (so hate backbiting). And fear Allah. Verily, Allah is the One Who forgives and accepts repentance, Most Merciful." (Qur'an, Al-Hujurat 49:12)

So, He told them to repent from Gossip, because it is a kind of wrongdoing. This applies if the one who was wronged found out about the gossip. But if he gossiped about him or slandered him and he did not know about it, it was said that one of the conditions of repentance is telling him, and it was said that this is not essential, which is the view of the majority. Both views were narrated from Ahmad. But he should still do good things for the one who was wronged, such as making Du'a for him, praying for forgiveness for him, and doing good deeds and giving him the reward for that, so as to make up for gossiping about him and slandering him. Al-Hasan al-Basri said: The expiation for gossip is praying for forgiveness for the one about whom you gossiped. End quote. (671)

Repentance for Borrowing and Destroying Items

In the case when someone borrows and destroys the borrowed items, he should compensate by the same. If the destruction is so important that caused to the owner the important fees for the renovation and loss of the rent, the borrower should cover the cost of the renovation and lost rent. He must pay the dues (rights) of others, so that when he dies, he meets his Lord Almighty without others' having any claim on him.

Repentance for Disrespect to Someone

If he had shown disrespect to someone, he should beg pardon of him and should try his best to please him.

Diyat or Qasas (blood money or retaliation)

If the matter involves Diyat or Qasas (blood money or retaliation) he should hand over himself to the concerned person, so, that he may either take Qasas or blood money, or pardon him, if he so pleases.

Repentance for Zina

But if he is loaded with crimes for which Allah has fixed punishments, like adultery, he should repent, give up the sin forever and follow Allah's commands and prohibitions.

Repentance of the Aggression (muhaarib)

If the muhaarib repents, it can only be either of the following two scenarios:

1. Either he repents before he is caught

In this case, the punishment for hiraabah no longer applies, and he should be treated like one who is not a muhaarib. The punishment of banishment, amputation or execution etc., no longer applies, except in cases where the victim or his family have the right to demand retribution. The evidence for this is the Words of Allah:

"The recompense of those who wage war against Allah and His Messenger and do mischief in the land is only that they shall be killed or crucified or their hands and feet be cut off on the opposite sides, or be exiled from the land. That is their disgrace in this world, and a great torment is theirs in the Hereafter. Except for those who (having fled away and then) come back (as Muslims) with repentance before they fall into your power; in that case, know that Allah is Oft-Forgiving, Most Merciful." (Qur'an, Al-Ma'idah 5:33)

2. Or he repents after he is caught

In this case the punishment for hiraabah still applies, and indeed the ruler is obliged to carry it out, because the exception mentioned in the Ayah clearly applies only to one who repents before he is caught. It is not too difficult for a person who wants to escape the prescribed punishment to feign repentance. This punishment is part of the Islamic Shariah which Allah has prescribed for every time and place, not just for one particular country or period. The Muslims applied this punishment for hiraabah at the time of the Prophet (peace and blessings of Allah be upon him) and until the present time. The fact that some of the Roman and Pharaonic punishments were similar to those prescribed by Islamic Law is of no particular significance, good or bad. These Islamic punishments cannot be regarded as backward or savage or barbaric at all. Any intelligent person who thinks about the severity of the crime of hiraabah and the resulting lack of security in the cities and on the road, terrorizing of the populace, robbing and killing, will know for sure that this ruling is exactly what these criminals deserve. The one who looks at the way the punishments for hiraabah fit the crime exactly will see that this is the essence of justice. How can it be otherwise when the One Who has prescribed this Law is the Almighty, the All-Wise, the All-Knowing, the All-Seeing, the Judge, the Just, the All-Aware? (423)

When someone repents, Allah, the Most High, takes away his torment.

"Was there any town (community) that believed (after seeing the punishment), and its faith (at that moment) saved it (from the punishment)? (The answer is none,) except the people of Yunus (Jonah); when they believed, We removed from them the torment

of disgrace in the life of the (present) world, and permitted them to enjoy for a while."
(Qur'an, Yunus 10:98)

Narrated Abu 'Ubadah bin 'Abdullah, that his father said: The Messenger of Allah (peace and blessings be upon him) said: 'The one who repents from sin is like one who did not sin." (Ibn Majah)

What the Hadith means is: if a person commits a sin, then repents sincerely from it, gives it up, regrets having done it, prays for forgiveness and does not go back to it, Allah will accept his repentance and treat him like one who did not sin; in fact, He will turn his bad deeds into good deeds, and He will love him and make him one of His pious slaves, because he repented to his Lord, turned to Him because of his love for Allah, his keenness to please Him, and his fear of Him, and these are the characteristics of the pious. (672)

III. <u>SEEK ALLAH'S FORGIVENESS</u>

Allah, the Exalted, says:

"And ask forgiveness for your sin..." (Qur'an, Muhammad 47:19)

"And seek the forgiveness of Allah. Certainly, Allah is Ever Oft-Forgiving, Most Merciful." (Qur'an, An-Nisa 4:106)

"And declare the freedom of your Rubb from imperfection beginning with His praise, and ask His forgiveness. Verily, He is the One Who accepts the repentance and Who forgives." (Qur'an, An-Nasr 110:3)

Other Verses: Ali 'Imran 3:15-17 and 3:135, Al-Anfal 8:33, An-Nur 24:31, Nooh 71:10-12.

Narrated Shaddad bin Aus (May Allah be pleased with him): The Prophet (peace and blessings be upon him) said, "The best supplication for seeking forgiveness (Syed-ul-Istighfar) is to say: 'Allahumma Anta Rabbi, la ilaha illa Anta, khalaqtani wa ana 'abduka, wa ana 'ala 'ahdika wa wa'dika mastata'tu, a'udhu bika min sharri ma sana'tu, abu'u laka bini'matika 'alayya, wa abu'u bidhanbi faghfir li, fa innahu la yaghfirudh-dhunuba illa Anta. (O Allah! You are my Rubb. There is no true god except You. You have created me, and I am Your slave, and I hold to Your Covenant as far as I can. I seek refuge in You from the evil of what I have done. I acknowledge the favors that You have bestowed upon me, and I confess my sins. Pardon me, for none but You has the power to pardon).' He who supplicates in these terms during the day with firm belief in it and dies on the same day (before the evening), he will be one of the dwellers of Jannah; and if anyone supplicates in these terms during the night with firm belief in it and dies before the morning, he will be one of the dwellers of Jannah." (Bukhari)

Narrated Ibn 'Umar (May Allah be pleased with him): The Prophet (peace and blessings be upon him) said, "O women folk! You should give charity and be diligent in seeking Allah's forgiveness because I have seen (i.e. on the Night of the Ascension to the highest heavens) that dwellers of the Hell are women." A woman amongst them said: "Why is it that the majority of the dwellers of Hell are women?" The Prophet (peace and blessings be upon him) replied, "You curse frequently and are ungrateful to your husbands. In spite of your lacking in wisdom and failing in religion, you are depriving the wisest of men of their intelligence." Upon this the woman asked: "What is the deficiency in our wisdom and in our religion?" He (peace and blessings be upon him) replied, "Your lack of wisdom can be well judged from the fact that the evidence of two women is equal to that one man. You do not offer Salat (prayer) for some days and you do not fast (the whole of) Ramadan sometimes, it is a deficiency in religion." (Muslim)

Commentary:

1. In this narration, certain weaknesses of the female sex have been pointed out, which are natural and pertain to the woman's biology, psychology and embryology. According to biologists, during and before menstruation, a female's thought process is affected. Similarly, her pulse and blood pressure are also altered. Females are also more prone to hysteria. For these reasons, the Qur'an has declared that when you have to appoint or choose witnesses among women, you should choose two in place of one man. Modern researches have proved this rule to be correct on the basis of biology, psychology and embryology. Again, we know that physically speaking, the female has been named as the weaker sex. For these reasons, females have been excused from earning their livelihood. For earning livelihood, one may have to go out and work hard. Women have been exempted from this duty because of their biological differences and other considerations of Shariah. Present-day women who are ignorant of Islam and modern researches are not prepared to accept these scientifically and religiously proved facts. The West claims equality between the sexes. But this equality has not been established so far. Today all the important posts are occupied by males and all the international policies are framed by them alone. Even matters pertaining to women are decided by them. They have mostly relegated them to the posts of workers, secretaries and stenographers for their sexual satisfaction and enjoyment. After a struggle for hundred years, their condition today proves that they are the weaker sex. So, it is both beneficial and more respectful for her to limit herself to the sphere of action suggested for her by Islam. If she oversteps her sphere, she will certainly lose her female dignity and prestige, as has happened in the West. Her state and condition, there is an eyeopener for all.

2. Women should request forgiveness from Allah very often and be generous in charity. They should not show ungratefulness to their husbands and should avoid backbiting and cursing others so that they may save themselves from Hell. (673)

IV. ALLAH'S MERCY EMBRACES EVERYTHING

Allah, the Exalted, says:

"... and My Mercy embraces all things." (Qur'an, Al-A'raf 7:156)

"And whoever does evil or wrongs himself but afterwards seeks Allah's forgiveness, he will find Allah Oft-Forgiving, Most Merciful." (Qur'an, An-Nisa 4:110)

"O you who have believed, fear Allah and believe in His Messenger; He will (then) give you a double portion of His Mercy and make for you a light by which you will walk and forgive you; and Allah is Forgiving and Merciful." (Qur'an, Al-Hadid 57:28)

Other Verses: *Ash-Shuraa 42:37, An-Najm 53:32, Al-Hijr 15:49-50, Ash-Sharh 94:5-7, An-Nahl 16:61, Yunus 10:58.*

Abu Hurairah reported: The Messenger of Allah (peace and blessings be upon him) said, "Our Lord Almighty descends to the lowest heaven in the last third of every night, saying: Who is calling upon Me that I may answer him? Who is asking from Me that I may give him? Who is seeking My forgiveness that I may forgive him?" (Bukhari and Muslim)

No One Will Enter Paradise by Virtue of his Deeds, rather by the Mercy of Allah, Exalted Is He

Aisha (May Allah be pleased with her), the wife of Allah's Apostle, reported that Allah's Messenger (peace and blessings be upon him) used to say: "Observe moderation (in doing deeds), and if you fail to observe it perfectly, try to do as much as you can do (to live up to this ideal of moderation) and be happy for none would be able to get into Paradise because of his deeds alone." They (the Companions of the Holy Prophet) said: 'Allah's Messenger, not even you?' Thereupon he said: 'Not even I, but that Allah wraps me in His Mercy, and bears this in mind that the deed loved most by Allah is one which is constantly done even though it is small.'" (Muslim)

Allah, the Exalted, says:

"And never would We punish until We sent a Messenger." (Qur'an, Al-Isra 17:15)

Narrated Ibn Dailami: "…He (peace and blessings be upon him) said: 'If Allah were to punish the inhabitants of His heavens and of His earth, He would do so and He would not be unjust towards them. And if He were to have mercy on them, His Mercy would be better for them than their own deeds. If you had the equivalent of Mount Uhud which you spent in the cause of Allah, that would not be accepted from you until you believed in the Divine Decree and you know that whatever has befallen you, could not have passed you by; and whatever has passed you by, could not have befallen you; and that if you were to die believing anything other than this, you would enter Hell…" (Ibn Majah)

Narrated Abu Sa`id: The Prophet (peace and blessings be upon him) said, "Among the people preceding your age, there was a man whom Allah had given a lot of money. While he was in his death-bed, he called his sons and said, 'What type of father have I have been to you? They replied, 'You have been a good father.' He said, 'I have never done a single good deed; so, when I die, burn me, crush my body, and scatter the resulting ashes on a windy day.' His sons did accordingly, but Allah gathered his particles and asked (him), 'What made you do so?' He replied, "Fear of You.' So, Allah bestowed His Mercy upon him. (forgave him)." (Bukhari)

Conceal Yourself with Allah's Veil and Repent

Abdullah bin Masud (May Allah be pleased with him): "A man kissed a woman and he came to the Prophet (peace and blessings be upon him) and made a mention of that to him. It was (on this occasion) that this Ayah was revealed: *"And perform As-Salat (Iqamat-as-Salat), at the two ends of the day and in some hours of the night [i.e. the five compulsory Salat (prayers)]. Verily, the good deeds remove the evil deeds (i.e. small sins)." (Qur'an, Hud 11:114)* That person said, 'O Messenger of Allah (peace and blessings be upon him), does it concern me only?' He (Messenger of Allah (peace and blessing be upon him) said, 'It concerns the whole of my Ummah.'" (Bukhari and Muslim)

Narrated Anas bin Malik (May Allah be pleased with him): "A man came to the Prophet (peace and blessings be upon him) and said, "O Messenger of Allah, I have committed a sin liable of ordained punishment. So, execute punishment on me". Messenger of Allah (peace and blessings be upon him) did not ask him about it, and then came the (time for) Salat (prayers). So, he performed Salat with Messenger of Allah (peace and blessings be upon him). When Messenger of Allah (peace be upon him) finished Salat, the man stood up and said: 'O Messenger of Allah! I have committed a sin. So, execute the Ordinance of Allah upon me.' He (peace be upon him) asked, 'Have you performed Salat with us?' 'Yes', he replied. The Messenger of Allah (peace and blessings be upon him) said, 'Verily, Allah has forgiven you.'" (Bukhari and Muslim)

Abdullah ibn 'Umar (May Allah be pleased with him) reported that the Prophet (May Allah's peace and blessings be upon him) stood up after stoning Al-Aslami and said: "Avoid these filthy practices which Allah has prohibited. The one who commits any of these deeds should conceal himself with Allah's Veil (he should not speak about them) and repent to Allah, for if anyone exposes his hidden sins (to us), we shall inflict the punishment prescribed by Allah the Almighty on him." (Al-Bayhaqi) (https://hadeethenc.com/en/browse/hadith/58240)

Umm Salamah reported: The Messenger of Allah (peace and blessings be upon him) said, "No Muslim is afflicted with a calamity but that he should say what Allah has commanded him: *"Indeed, to Allah we belong and to Allah we will return." (2:156)* O Allah, reward me in my affliction and replace it with something better than it. If he does so, Allah will replace it with something better." (Muslim)

Abdullah ibn Amr reported: The Messenger of Allah (peace and blessings be upon him) said, "The merciful will be shown Mercy by the Most Merciful. Be merciful to those on the earth and the One in the heavens will have Mercy upon you." (Tirmidhi)

Narrated Ma'bad bin Hilal Al-'Anzi: "…Muhammad talked to us saying, 'On the Day of Resurrection the people will surge with each other like waves, and then they will come to Adam and say, 'Please intercede for us with your Lord.' He will say, 'I am not fit for that but you'd better go to Abraham as he is the Khalil of the Beneficent.' They will go to Abraham and he will say, 'I am not fit for that but you'd better go to Moses as he is the one to whom Allah spoke directly.' So, they will go to Moses and he will say, 'I am not fit for that but you'd better go to Jesus as he is a soul created by Allah and His Word.' (Be: And it was) they will go to Jesus and he will say, 'I am not fit for that but you'd better go to Muhammad.' They would come to me and I would say, 'I am for that.' Then I will ask for my Lord's permission, and it will be given, and then He will inspire me to praise Him with such praises as I do not know now. So, I will praise Him with those praises and will fall down, prostrate before Him. Then it will be said, 'O Muhammad, raise your head and speak, for you will be listened to, and ask, for your will be granted (your request); and intercede, for your intercession will be accepted.' I will say, 'O Lord, My followers! My followers!' And then it will be said, 'Go and take out of Hell (Fire) all those who have faith in their hearts, equal to the weight of a barley grain.' I will go and do so and return to praise Him with the same praises, and fall down (prostrate) before Him. Then it will be said, 'O Muhammad, raise your head and speak, for you will be listened to, and ask, for you will be granted (your request); and intercede, for your intercession will be accepted.' I will say, 'O Lord, My followers! My followers!' It will be said, 'Go and take out of it all those who have faith in their hearts equal to the weight of a small ant or a mustard seed.' I will go and do so and return to praise Him with the same praises, and fall down in prostration before Him. It will be said, 'O, Muhammad, raise your head and speak, for you will be listened to, and ask, for you will be granted (your request); and intercede, for your intercession will be accepted.' I will say, 'O Lord, My followers!' Then He will say, 'Go and take out (all those) in whose hearts there is faith even to the lightest, lightest mustard seed. (Take them) out of the Fire.' I will go and do so.'" When we left Anas, I said to some of my companions, "Let's pass by Al-Hasan who is hiding himself in the house of Abi Khalifa and request him to tell us what Anas bin Malik has told us." So, we went to him and we greeted him and he admitted us. We said to him, "O Abu Sa`id! We came to you from your brother Anas Bin Malik and he related to us a Hadith about the intercession the like of which I have never heard." He said, "What is that?" Then we told him of the Hadith and said, "He stopped at this point (of the Hadith)." He said, "What then?" We said, "He did not add anything to that." He said, Anas related the Hadith to me twenty years ago when he was a young fellow. I don't know whether he forgot or if he did not like to let you depend on what he might have said." We said, "O Abu Sa`id! Let us know that." He smiled and said, "Man was created hasty. I did not mention that, but that I wanted to inform you of it. Anas told me the same as he told you and said that the Prophet (peace and blessings be upon him) added, 'I then return for a fourth time and praise Him similarly and prostrate before Him me the same as he 'O Muhammad, raise your head and speak, for you will be listened to; and ask, for you will be granted (your request): and intercede, for your intercession will be accepted.' I will say, 'O Lord, allow me to intercede for whoever said, 'None has the right to be worshipped except Allah.' Then Allah will say, 'By My Power, and My Majesty, and by My Supremacy, and by My Greatness, I will take out of Hell (Fire) whoever said: 'None has the right to be worshipped except Allah.'" (Bukhari) (https://sunnah.com/bukhari:7510)

V. <u>GOOD DEEDS REMOVE BAD DEEDS</u>

Allah, the Exalted, says:

"Verily, the good deeds remove the evil deeds." (Qur'an, Hud 11:114)

"If you disclose your Sadaqat (almsgiving), it is well; but if you conceal them and give them to the poor, that is better for you. (Allah) will expiate you some of your sins." (Qur'an, Al-Baqarah 2:271)

"Know they not that Allah accepts repentance from His slaves and takes the Sadaqah (alms, charity), and that Allah Alone is the One Who forgives and accepts repentance, Most Merciful?" (Qur'an, At-Tawbah 9:104)

Other Verses: *Ar-Rum 30:39, Al-An'am 6:160, Al-Ma'idah 5:27, Al-Baqarah 2:254.*

Abu Dharr Jundub ibn Junadah and Abu 'Abd-ir-Rahman Mu'adh bin Jabal (May Allah be pleased with them) that the Messenger of Allah (peace and blessings of Allah be upon him) said: "Be conscious of Allah wherever you are. Follow the bad deed with a good one to erase it, and engage others with beautiful character." (Tirmidhi)

Abu Hurairah reported: The Messenger of Allah (peace and blessings be upon him) said: "Charity does not decrease wealth, no one forgives another but that Allah increases his honor, and no one humbles himself for the sake of Allah but that Allah raises his status." (Muslim)

Narrated from the Messenger (peace and blessings of Allah be upon him): "Treat your sick by means of charity." (Abu Dawud in al-Maraaseel, Tabaraani, al-Bayhaqi and others, from a number of the Sahabah. All its isnaads are da'eef (weak) but it was classed as hasan by al-Albaani (May Allah have mercy on him) because of corroborating evidence in Saheeh at-Tirmidhi (744)

'Protect your wealth by (discharging) zakat, treat your ill by giving sadaqah and prepare for calamity in advance by engaging in Du'a." Sheikh 'Abdullah Siddiq Al-Ghumari (May Allah have mercy on him) has collected the different versions in his book entitled: Az-Zawajirul Muqalqalah li Munkirit Tadawy bis Sadaqah.' He has ruled that the words: (Treat your sick ones with sadaqah) is an established Hadith from the Messenger (peace and blessings be upon him) which are reported via several chains. Giving abundant sadaqah (charity) is indeed a tried and tested method for gaining shifa (cure) and should not be overlooked. (https://hadithanswers.com/cure-sickness-by-giving-sadaqah)

Narrated Hudhaifah: "We were sitting with 'Umar and he said: 'Which of you has remembered a Hadith from the Messenger of Allah (peace and blessings be upon him) concerning Fitnah?'" Hudhaifah said: "I said: 'I have.' He said: 'You are very bold.' He said: 'How?' He said: 'I heard him say: "The fitnah of a man with regard to his family, his children and his neigbors are expiated by his prayers, fasts, charity and enjoining what is good and forbidding what is evil…" (Ibn Majah)

Ibn Qayyim (May Allah have mercy on him) said:

'There are types of medicines which can treat illnesses which the minds of the senior doctors cannot comprehend, and that which their sciences, experiences and measurements cannot reach. These are the medicines of the heart and soul, and the strength of the heart, its dependence upon Allah and trust upon Him and seeking refuge in Him. Prostrating and feeling in dire need of Allah and humbling oneself for Allah. Likewise giving Sadaqah (charity), making *Du'a*, Repentance and seeking forgiveness, being good to the creation, aiding the distressed and liberating from grief and unhappiness.

Indeed, these types of medication have been used by various nations, who are upon different religions and communities, and they found that they had an effect in the treatment of illnesses, which even the sciences of the most knowledgeable doctors could not reach, and they have no experience nor measurement of it. We have indeed experienced these matters a great deal and as others have, and we have seen what ordinary medicine can and cannot do." (Zad Al-Ma'ad)

Sheikh Ibn Jibreen (May Allah have mercy on him) said:

"Charity is a useful and beneficial remedy that brings healing from disease and alleviates sickness.

This is supported by the words of the Prophet (peace and blessings be upon him): Perhaps some diseases happen as a punishment for a sin that the sick person committed, but when his family give charity on his behalf, this sin is erased and so, is the cause of the sickness, or hasanat (good deeds) are recorded for him because of the charity, so his heart is revived thereby and the pain of the sickness is reduced as a result. End quote." (Al-Fataawa ash-Shariah fi'l-Masaa'il at-Tibbiyyah (2/question no.15) (674)

"Give charity without delay, for indeed, calamity cannot overcome it." (Al Mu'jamul Awsat) The Muhaddithun explain that this Hadith encourages giving charity to those deserving before one becomes ill or passes away for calamities cannot overcome it. The Hadith portrays sadaqah and calamities as two race horses. Whichever one wins the race, will not be beaten/overcome by the other. Therefore, by hastening charity, a person ensures that he is not overcome by calamity. (Refer: Mirqat, Hadith: 1887) (https://hadithanswers.com/explanation-of-the-narration-regarding-giving-charity-without-delay)

Ibn Abbas reported: The Messenger of Allah, peace and blessings be upon him, said, "Take advantage of five before five: your youth before your old age, your health before your illness, your riches before your poverty, your free time before your work, and your life before your death." (Shu'ab al-Imān 9767)

Abu Hurairah (May Allah be pleased with him) reported that the Prophet (May Allah's peace and blessings be upon him) that he said: ''On each joint of humans there is a charity every day on which the sun rises: doing justice between two persons is a charity; helping someone with his mount, lifting him onto it or hoisting his belongings onto it, is a charity; and a good word is a charity; and every step you take towards the prayer (congregation prayer) is a charity, and removing harmful objects from the way is a charity." (Bukhari and Muslim) (https://hadeethenc.com/en/browse/hadith/4568)

VI. CALAMITIES BY MEANS OF WHICH ALLAH EXPIATE SINS

Allah, the exalted, says:

"...but give glad tidings to As-Saabiroon (the patient). Who, when afflicted with calamity, say: 'Truly, to Allah we belong and truly, to Him we shall return.' They are those on whom are the Salawaat (i.e. who are blessed and will be forgiven) from their Lord, and (they are those who) receive His Mercy, and it is they who are the guided ones." (Qur'an, Al-Baqarah 2:155-157)

Narrated Aisha (the wife of the Prophet): Allah's Messenger (peace and blessings be upon him) said, "No calamity befalls a Muslim but that Allah expiates some of his sins because of it, even though it were the prick he receives from a thorn." (Bukhari)

Narrated 'Abdullah: "I visited the Prophet during his ailments and he was suffering from a high fever. I said, "You have a high fever. Is it because you will have a double reward for it?" He said, "Yes, for no Muslim is afflicted with any harm but that Allah will remove his sins as the leaves of a tree fall down." (Bukhari)

VII. WHEN VISITING SICK

Thawban (May Allah be pleased with him) reported that the Messenger (May Allah's peace and blessings be upon him) said: "If a Muslim visits his sick fellow Muslim, he will remain in the Khurfah of Paradise tills he leaves returns." It was asked: "O Messenger of Allah, what the Khurfah of Paradise." He said: "Its fruit garden." (Muslim) (https://hadeethenc.com/en/browse/hadith/5647)

Abdullah Ibn 'Abbas (May Allah be pleased with him) reported: The Prophet (peace and blessings be upon him) said, "He who visits a sick person who is not on the point of death and supplicates seven times: As'alullahal-'Azima Rabbal-'Arshil-'Azimi, an yashfiyaka (I ask Allah the Great, the Lord of the Great Throne, to cure you), Allah will certainly cure him from that sickness." (Abu Dawud and Tirmidhi) (https://hadeethenc.com/en/browse/hadith/6270)

VIII. WHEN ANGELS SEEK FORGIVENESS FOR YOU

Narrated Abu Hurairah: Allah's Messenger (peace and blessings of Allah be upon him) said, "The angels keep on asking Allah's forgiveness for anyone of you, as long as he is at his Musalla (his prayer-place where he offered his prayer) and he does not pass wind (Hadath). They say, 'O Allah! Forgive him, O Allah! be Merciful to him." (Bukhari)

IX. LAST WORDS WHEN DYING – THERE IS NO GOD BUT ALLAH

Abu Hurairah (May Allah be pleased with him) reported: "We were sitting with Messenger of Allah (peace and blessings be upon him). Abu Bakr and 'Umar (May Allah be pleased with them) were also there among the audience. In the meanwhile, the Messenger of Allah (peace and blessings be upon him) got up and left us. We waited long for his return: When we were worried about his safety, and got scared, we got up. I, therefore, went out to look for the Messenger of Allah and came to a garden which belonged to the Ansar. He (peace and blessings be upon him) said to me: "Go and give glad tidings of Jannah to anyone who testifies 'La ilaha illallah (There is no true god except Allah)', being whole-heartedly certain of it." (Muslim)

X. **WHEN MUSLIMS PRAY FOR THE DEAD**

Narrated Ibn Abbas (May Allah be pleased with him): The Messenger of Allah (peace and blessings be upon him) said, "Any Muslim dies and forty men who do not associate anything with Allah (in worship), perform his funeral prayer, Allah makes them interceded for him." (Muslim)

Aisha (May Allah be pleased with her) reported: The Messenger of Allah (peace and blessings be upon him) said, "If a group of Muslims numbering a hundred perform a funeral prayer over a dead person, and all of them ask Allah's forgiveness for him, their prayer for him will be accepted." (Muslim)

XI. **PRAYER PREVENTS, EXPIATES SINS AND CURES**

Narrated that Abu Hurairah said: "The Prophet (peace and blessings be upon him) set out in the early morning and I did likewise. I prayed, then I sat. The Prophet (peace and blessings be upon him) turned to me and said: 'Do you have a stomach problem?' I said: 'Yes, O Messenger of Allah.' He said: 'Get up and pray, for **in Prayer there is Healing**.' Another chain with similar wording. Abu 'Abdullah said: "A man narrated it to his people, then they were stirred up against him." (Ibn Majah)

Narrated 'Uthman bin Hunaif that a blind man came to the Prophet (peace and blessings be upon him) and said: "Pray to Allah to heal me." He said: "If you wish to store your reward for the Hereafter, that is better, or if you wish, I will supplicate for you." He said: "Supplicate." So, he told him to perform ablution and do it well, and to pray two Rak'ahs, and to say this supplication: "Allahumma inni as'aluka wa atawajjahu ilaika bimuhammadin nabiyyir-rahmah. Ya Muhammadu inni qad tawajjahtu bika ila rabbi fi hajati hadhihi lituqda. Allahumma fashaffi'hu fiya (O Allah, I ask of You and I turn my face towards You by virtue of the intercession of Muhammad the Prophet of mercy. O Muhammad, I have turned to my Lord by virtue of your intercession concerning this need of mine so that it may be met. O Allah, accept his intercession concerning me)." (Ibn Majah)

Zayd ibn Khalid reported: The Prophet (peace and blessings be upon him) said, "Whoever performs ablution in the best manner, then prays two cycles, without being unmindful in either of them, his previous sins will be forgiven." (Abu Dawud)

Abu Hurairah reported: The Messenger of Allah (peace and blessings be upon him) said: "Whoever purifies himself for ablution in his house and he walks to a house among the houses of Allah in order to fulfill an obligation among the obligations of Allah, then one step of his will expiate his sins and another step will elevate his status. (Muslim)

XII. FASTING PREVENTS, EXPIATES SINS AND CURES

Allah, the Exalted, says:

"O you who believe fasting is prescribed to you, as it was prescribed to those before you, so that you can learn self-restraint." (Qur'an, Al-Baqarah 2:183)

1. Fasting is the Best Deed

Allah, the Exalted, says:

"Whoever brings a good deed (Islamic Monotheism and deeds of obedience to Allah and His Messenger SAW) shall have ten times the like thereof to his credit, and whoever brings an evil deed (polytheism, disbelief, hypocrisy, and deeds of disobedience to Allah and His Messenger SAW) shall have only the recompense of the like thereof, and they will not be wronged." (Qur'an, Al-An'am 6:160)

Abu Hurairah (May Allah be pleased with him) reported that the Messenger of Allah (May Allah's peace and blessings be upon him) said: "Allah, Glorified and Exalted, said: 'All the actions of the son of Adam are for him, except for fasting. Indeed, it is for Me, and I give reward for it...'" (Bukhari)

Narrated Abu Hurairah: The Messenger of Allah (peace and blessings be upon him) said: "There are no days in this world during which worship is more beloved to Allah, Glorious is He, than the (first) ten days (of Dhul-Hijjah). Fasting one of these days is equivalent to fasting for one year, and one night of them is equal to Lailatul-Qadr." (Ibn Majah)

Narrated Abu Dharr: The Messenger of Allah (peace and blessings be upon him) said: "Whoever fasts three days in every month, that is fasting for a lifetime." Then, in testimony of that, Allah revealed: *"Whoever brings a good deed shall have ten time the like thereof to his credit."* (Qur'an, Al-An'am 6:160) So one day is equivalent to ten (in reward)." (Ibn Majah)

2. Special Reward for Fasting

Abu Hurairah (May Allah be pleased with him) reported that the Messenger of Allah (May Allah's peace and blessings be upon him) said: "Allah, Glorified and Exalted, said: 'All the actions of the son of Adam are for them, except for fasting. Indeed, it is for Me, and I give reward for it.' Fasting is a shield. So, when one of you is fasting, then let him not say obscene speech or make too much noise, and if someone insults him or fights him, then let him say:

'I am fasting.' (I swear) by the One in Whose hand the soul of Muhammad is! The foul smell that emanates from the mouth of the fasting person is more pleasant in the sight of Allah than the smell of musk. The fasting person has two (moments of) joy: one when he breaks his fast, as he feels happy, and the other when he meets his lord, he is happy with his fast." This is the wording of Al-Bukhari's narration. (https://hadeethenc.com/en/browse/hadith/3546)

3. There is a Gate in Paradise called Ar-Raiyan for those who Observe Fasts

Narrated Sahl: The Prophet (peace and blessings be upon him) said, "There is a gate in Paradise called Ar-Raiyan, and those who observe fasts will enter through it on the Day of Resurrection and none except them will enter through it. It will be said, 'Where are those who used to observe fasts?' "They will get up, and none except them will enter through it. After their entry the gate will be closed and nobody will enter through it." (Bukhari)

4. Fasting is a Means for one's Sins to be Forgiven

Abu Hurairah (May Allah be pleased with him) reported that the Prophet (May Allah's peace and blessings be upon him) said: "He who observes fasting during the month of Ramadan faithfully and expecting its reward from Allah will have his past sins forgiven." (Bukhari and Muslim)

5. Fasting is a Shield from the Fire

Narrated Abu Said: "I heard the Prophet (peace and blessings be upon him) saying, 'Whosoever observes Saum (fasts) for one day for Allah's Cause, Allah will keep his face away from the Hellfire for a distance covered by a journey of seventy years.'" (Bukhari)

6. The Supplication of the Fasting Person is Answered

Abu Hurairah narrated that the Messenger of Allah (peace and blessings be upon him) said: "There are three whose supplication is not rejected: The fasting person when he breaks his fast, the just leader, and the supplication of the oppressed person; Allah raises it up above the clouds and opens the gates of heaven to it. And the Lord says: 'By My Might, I shall surely aid you, even if it should be after a while.'" (Tirmidhi)

7. Fasting One Day during Jihad Keeps Away from Hellfire Seventy Years

Abu Sa'id al-Khudri (May Allah be pleased with him) reported that the Messenger of Allah (May Allah's peace and blessings be upon him) said: "If anyone fasts a day for the sake of Allah, Allah shall keep his face away from Hell (the distance of) seventy years." (Bukhari and Muslim)

8. Fasting is a Shield Against one's Base Desires

Narrated ʿAbdullah: "We were with the Prophet (peace and blessings be upon him) while we were young and had no wealth. So, Allah's Messenger (peace and blessings be upon him) said, "O young people! Whoever among you can marry, should marry, because it helps him lower his gaze and guard his modesty (i.e. his private parts from committing illegal sexual intercourse etc.), and whoever is committing illegal sexual intercourse etc.), not able to marry, should fast, as fasting diminishes his sexual power." (Bukhari)

9. Fasting is Half of Patience

A man from Banu Sulaim narrated: "The Messenger of Allah (peace and blessings be upon him) counted them out in my hand" - or - "in his hand: 'At-Tasbīḥ is half of the Scale, and "All praise is due to Allah (Al-Ḥamdulillāh)" fills it, and At-Takbīr (Allahu Akbar) fills what is between the sky and the earth, and Fasting is Half of Patience, and Purification is Half of Faith." (Tirmidhi)

10. Fasting is Against all Diseases

When the disciples of Jesus asked him how to cast the evil spirits away, he is reported to have said,

"But this kind never comes out except by prayer and fasting." (Matthew 17:21)

Prof. Noboru Mizushima showed that the autophagy serves as a dynamic recycling system that produces new building blocks and energy for cellular renovation and homeostasis against all diseases and with anti-aging effects. (675)

Patients, when fasting according Sunnah, experience the remission of disease, less or no pain. Fasting helps regeneration, detoxification, anti-aging process. Fasting weakens the Devils in Jinn possessed diseases, etc.

11. The Angels Pray for Forgiveness and Send Blessing upon Fasting Person

Anas (May Allah be pleased with him) reported: The Prophet (May Allah's peace and blessings be upon him) came to visit Saʿd ibn ʿUbādah (May Allah be pleased with him) so he brought some bread and oil. The Prophet ate then said: "May the fasting people break their fast in your house, and may the righteous eat your food, and may the angels ask forgiveness and mercy for you." (Ibn Majah)
(https://hadeethenc.com/en/browse/hadith/10110)

12. Reward for Giving Food for a Fasting Person to Break his Fast

Narrated Zaid bin Khalid Al-Juhani: The Messenger of Allah (peace and blessings be upon him) said: "Whoever feeds a person who is breaking their fast, he gets the same reward as him without any subtraction from the reward of the fasting person." (Tirmidhi and Ibn Majah)

(https://hadithanswers.com/the-reward-for-feeding-a-fasting-person)

13. Fasting for Deceased

Aisha (May Allah be pleased with her) reported that the Prophet (May Allah's peace and blessings be upon him) said: "Whoever dies while still having some fasts to make up for, his heir should fast on his behalf." (Bukhari and Muslim) (https://hadeethenc.com/en/browse/hadith/4530)

Allah Will Not Accept Fasting if Sins

Narrated Abu Hurairah: The Prophet (peace and blessings be upon him) said, "Whoever does not give up forged speech and evil actions, Allah is not in need of his leaving his food and drink (i.e. Allah will not accept his fasting)." (Bukhari)

XIII. OTHER MEANS OF EXPIATION OF SINS

Allah, the Exalted, says:

"If you disclose your Sadaqat (almsgiving), it is well; but if you conceal them and give them to the poor, that is better for you. (Allah) will expiate you some of your sins." (Qur'an, Al-Baqarah 2:271)

Expiation of Sins by Du'a after eating

Narrated Sahl bin Muadh bin Anas Al-Juhani from his father: The Prophet (peace and blessings be upon him) said: "Whoever eats food and said: Al-hamdu lillahil-ladhi at'amani hadha wa razaqanihi min ghayri hawlin minni wa la quwwatin. (Praise is to Allah Who has fed me this and provided it for me without any strength or power on my part), - his previous sins will be forgiven." (Ibn Majah)

Expiation of Sins by Shaking Hands

Hudhayfah ibn al-Yaman reported: The Prophet (peace and blessings be upon him) said, "Verily, when the believer meets another believer, greets him with peace, and shakes his hand, the sins of them both will shed like leaves falling from a tree." (al-Mu'jam al-Awsaṭ 253, Saheeh according to Al-Albaani)

Whoever makes the Hereafter a primary concern

Anas ibn Malik reported: The Messenger of Allah (peace and blessings be upon him) said, "Whoever is concerned about the Hereafter, Allah will place richness in his heart, bring his affairs together, and the world will inevitably come to him. Whoever is concerned about the world, Allah will place poverty between his eyes, disorder his affairs, and he will get nothing of the world but what is decreed for him." (Tirmidhi)

HEALTHCARE REFORM BASED ON THE QUR'AN AND SUNNAH

The Glorious Qur'an says:

"And when I am ill, it is He Who cures me." (Qur'an, Ash-Shu'ara 26:80)

The Hadith says:

"Allah has not sent down any disease but He has also sent down the cure; the one who knows it, knows it and the one who does not know it, does not know it." (Ahmad; classed as Hasan by al-Albaani in Ghaayat al-Maraam, no. 292)

Jabir (May Allah be pleased with him) reported God's Messenger (peace and blessings be upon him) as saying: "There is a medicine for every disease, and when the medicine is applied to the disease it is cured by God's permission." (Muslim)

1. Modern Medical Monopoly demonstrates how health care slowly evolved from a social good to a simple market where the main goal is a financial profit.
2. Big Pharma is the biggest defrauder, has been making a bumper financial profit. Big Pharma doesn't want you to be healthy, they don't want to kill you either as they need customers buying drugs.
3. Modern medicine didn't follow the Glorious Qur'an and Prophetic Medicine - Divine Medicine.
4. Doctors are not aware that the cause of disease is the disobedience to Allah (sins). Modern medicine didn't follow Allah's Messengers' teachings (Jesus and Muhammad, peace be upon them) that disease is the result of sins and the majority of diseases are caused by Devils.
5. Demons can be cast out only by giving up sins, prayers, Ruqyah, Negative Ions.
6. There are no lectures about the Qur'an Healing when it is Allah Who cures.
7. There are no lectures about Miraculous Negative Ions Healing effects. *(Qur'an, 8:11, 38:41-42)*
8. There are no lectures about Prophetic Medicine which is Superior to any other medicine.
9. Doctors are ordered to follow the western inappropriate guidelines and protocols, wrongly informed, perform thousands unnecessary surgeries while we cannot cut Demons.
10. Modern medicine is detrimental in the Jinn diseases as excites the Evil Jinn and excited Jinn spread more disease and create new diseases and even kill. (303, 525)
11. Toxicity of the drugs is another serious issue, it creates new diseases and causes death. Patients die mostly because of the adverse side effects of drugs, including the excitement of the hidden Jinn. (529)

12. The "evidence-based science" does not believe in Unseen but it is the Unseen Jinn who are involved in all human affairs, calamities, disasters, diseases.

Allah, the Exalted, said:

"O Prophet (Muhammad SAW)! Keep your duty to Allah, and <u>obey not the disbelievers and the hypocrites (i.e. do not follow their advices)</u>. Verily! Allah is Ever All-Knower, All-Wise." (Qur'an, Al-Ahzab 33:1)

Doctors and patients should know:

1. Sins (disobedience to Allah) cause diseases
2. Diseases are caused by Positive Ions: Decreased Oxygen Utilization and Evil Jinn
3. 95% of diseases are caused by the Evil Jinn.
4. Jinn Diseases should be the obligatory part of medical education
5. Qur'an is a cure from all diseases and the solution to all problems
6. Negative Ions cure all diseases and should be a part of medical education
7. Prophetic Medicine is a Divine Medicine, should be a part of medical education
8. No surgery in the Jinn diseases (except in life-threatening conditions)
9. No Chemotherapy - Nanotherapy
10. No Radiation Therapy
11. No Cancer Hormonal Therapy
12. No Immunotherapy
13. No Antihypertensive, Angina, Heart Attack Treatment
14. No Stroke Treatment
15. No Sickle Cell Anemia Treatment
16. No Idiopathic Puimonary Fibrosis Treatment
17. No Asthma, Allergy Treatment
18. No Diabetes Treatment
19. No Autoimmune Diseases Treatment
20. No Fibromyalgia Treatment
21. No Psychiatric Diseases Treatment
22. No Dementia, Alzheimer's Disease Treatment
23. No Autism Treatment
24. No Attention Deficit Hyperactivity Disorder (ADHD) Treatment
25. No Parkinson Treatment
26. No Epilepsy Treatment
27. No Paralysis Treatment
28. No Huntington Disease Treatment
29. No Restless Legs Syndrome Treatment
30. No Myalgic Encephalomyelitis Treatment
31. No Chronic Fatigue Syndrome Treatment
32. No Insomnia Treatment
33. No Anxiety Treatment
34. No Depression Treatment

35. No HIV Treatment
36. No Tuberculosis Treatment
37. No Hepatitis, Cirrhosis, Liver Failure Treatment
38. No Kidney Failure Treatment
39. No Benign Tumors Treatment
40. No Endometriosis Treatment
41. No Ovarian Cysts Treatment
42. No Infertility Treatment (except few cases)
43. No Miscarriage Treatment
44. No Eczema (Atopic Dermatitis) Treatment
45. No Primary Immune Deficiency Diseases (PIDDs) Treatment
46. No Obesity Treatment
47. No Gene Therapy
48. No Epidemic Disease Treatment
49. No Vaccination
50. No Stem Cells Treatment (except for approved sport injury)
51. No Any Medical treatment in Jinn Diseases
52. No Medications Containing Pork
53. No Medications Containing Alcohol and Intoxicants
54. DISEASE MANAGEMENT:
    Repentance of sins to Allah
    Asking Allah's for forgiveness
    Stop sins
    Restore people's rights. Repair the past
    Follow Allah's Commands and Prohibitions in the Qur'an and Sunnah.
    Charity
    Ruqyah Shariah
    Negative Ions Treatment
    Prophetic Medicine
    Fasting
    Say "Inna lillahi wa inna ilayhi raji'un - "Indeed, to Allah we belong and to Allah we shall return" in case of calamity and death.
55. For Diagnosis of the Jinn Diseases: use Negative Ions, Ruqyah and Jinn Possession Symptoms
56. Exorcism Only by the Qur'an
57. No Prophylactic Mastectomy
58. No Cosmetic Procedures (except for birth defects, injury, burn scar)
59. No Euthanasia
60. No World Cancer, Diabetes, Autism Day, etc.
    Wasting Allah's money and time
    There is no remembrance of Allah
61. No Cancer (Diabetes, or Multiples Sclerosis, or Autism etc.) Foundation Funds
    How Foundation Funds can remove sins and Evil Jinn?
    Non-Islamic Charitable Organizations have no knowledge of the Day of Judgment and do not fear Allah and make profit with the people's wealth which is prohibited by our Creator.

62. Researches on Jinn are beyond science, we should follow the Qur'an and Sunnah
63. No Insurance (except emergency or if he cannot afford treatment)

Allah, the Exalted, says:

"Whatever of good reaches you, is from Allah, but whatever of evil befalls you, is from yourself. And We have sent you (O Muhammad SAW) as a Messenger to mankind, and Allah is Sufficient as a Witness." *(Qur'an, An-Nisa 4:79)*

BIBLIOGRAPHY

1. The thrilling Story of Tubba the First and the Good news received About the Greatest Prophet, https://www.darulfatwa.org.au/en/the-thrilling-story-of-tubba-the-first-and-the-good-news-received-about-the-greatest-prophet
2. Dr. Haitham Al Haddad, Amazing Story: People of Tubba' mentioned in Surah Dukhan (44:37), https://www.youtube.com/watch?v=vDvwGc55LTE
3. Dr. Zakir Naik, Virtues of the Day of Arafat: https://www.youtube.com/watch?v=xLU1neKn4kA
4. Dr. Abu Ameenah Bilal Philips, The Fundamentals of Tawheed (Islamic Monotheism)
5. Dr. Abu Ameenah Bilal Philips, The Purpose of Greation, http://islamicbook.ws/english/english-018.pdf
6. Sheikh Muhammad Saalih al-Munajjid, The wisdom behind calamities, https://islamqa.info/en/answers/35914
7. Ibn Qayyim al-Jawziyya, Provisions for the Hereafter (Zad Al Ma'ad), https://d1.islamhouse.com/data/en/ih books/single/ en Complete Zad al Ma'ad.pdf
8. The Special Rewards and Circumstances for the Convert, http://www.almasjid.com/book/export/html/543
9. Al-Qalam 51-52, https://wp-en.wikideck.com/Al-Qalam_51-52
10. Ibn Taymiyah's Essay on Jinn (Demons), https://kalamullah.com/Books/Ibn Taymiyah Essay Jinn.
11. Healing the paralytic at Bethesda, https://en.wikipedia.org/wiki/Healing_the_paralytic_at_Bethesda
12. Healing the paralytic at Capernaum, https://en.wikipedia.org/wiki/Healing_the_paralytic_at_Capernaum
13. Exorcising a boy possessed by a demon, https://en.wikipedia.org/wiki/Exorcising_a_boy_possessed_by_a_demon)
14. Why do Children Suffer? https://www.masjidtucson.org/submission/faq/suffering_and_misery.html
15. Sheikh Muhammad Saalih al-Munajjid, Why Allah creates mentally disabled people, https://islamqa.info/en/answers/7951
16. Mufti Menk, Who Have A Disabled Child, https://www.youtube.com/watch?v=d7VfEeSq9P8
17. Omar Suleiman, Loving Those with Disabilities, https://www.youtube.com/watch?v=9ZYdl2aRauo
18. Sheikh Muhammad Saalih al-Munajjid, Will children who die young go to Paradise or Hell? https://islamqa.info/en/answers/6496

19. Sheikh Muhammad Saalih al-Munajjid, Why do children suffer in this world, https://islamqa.info/en/answers/20785
20. Sheikh Muhammad Saalih al-Munajjid, Ages of children who die in childhood when they enter Paradise, https://islamqa.info/en/answers/117432
21. Sheikh Muhammad Saalih al-Munajjid, They forgot to remember Allah at the time of intercourse; what should they do to protect the child from the Shaytan? https://islamqa.info/en/answers/153633
22. Jinn according to Quran and Sunnah, https://www.islamawareness.net/Jinn/jinn.html
23. Sheikh Muhammad Saalih al-Munajjid, Protection from the Jinn: Any Du'a? https://islamqa.info/en/answers/10513
24. Sheikh Muhammad Saalih al-Munajjid, What are lamam ("small faults")? And what is the ruling on a disobedient Muslim who repeatedly commits them? https://islamqa.info/en/answers/47748
25. Sheikh Muhammad Saalih al-Munajjid, The difference between major sins and minor sins https://islamqa.info/en/answers/127480
26. Din and Theology in Qur'an and Sunnah, https://www.encyclopedia.com/history/news-wires-white-papers-and-books/din-and-theology-quran-and-sunnah
27. Hamza Yusuf, The Meaning of "Din", https://www.youtube.com/watch?v=ySbzyqQMkiE)
28. Sayyid Naquib al-Attas, Man's Indebtedness to Allah (Exalted be He), https://seekersguidance.org/articles/general-artices/mans-indebtedness-to-allah-exalted-be-he-sayyid-naquib-al-attas
29. Khaled Abou El Fad, What does "Submission to God" mean? Excerpted from Reasoning with God: Reclaiming Shari'ah in the Modern Age, https://www.searchforbeauty.org/islam-101/submission- to-god
30. Sheikh Muhammad Saalih al-Munajjid, Meaning of the word Islam, https://islamqa.info/en/answers/10446
31. Sheikh Muhammad Saalih al-Munajjid, Disciplining Oneself, https://islamqa.info/en/answers/22090
32. Dr. M. Ibrahem Elmasry, Islam is a Code of Life, https://knowingallah.com/en/articles/islam-is-a-code-of-life
33. Sheikh Muhammad Saalih al-Munajjid, Did Islam exist before the Prophet (peace and blessings of Allah be upon him)? https://islamqa.info/en/answers/48987
34. Ibn Taymiyah, Tafsir of Chapter 112: Surah al-Ikhlas (Purity), https://sunnahonline.com/library/the-majestic-quran/311-tasfir-of-chapter-112-surah-al-ikhlas-purity
35. Imam Shamsu ed-Deen Dhahabi, Major Sins, https://islamhouse.com/en/books/386056
36. Sheikh Muhammad Saalih al-Muhajjih, What is the true meaning of shirk and what are its types? https://islamqa.info/en/answers/34817
37. Idol Worship, the Unforgivable Sin (if maintained until death) https://www.masjidtucson.org/submission/monotheism/idolworship.html
38. Sheikh Muhammad Saalih al-Muhajjih The Jews' idea that 'Uzayr is "a son of Allah" https://islamqa.info/en/answers/9459
39. Sheikh Muhammad Saalih al-Munajjid, Ruling on seeking the help of the jinn, https://islamqa.info/en/answers/10518

40. List of people who have been considered deities https://en.wikipedia.org/wiki/List_of_people_who_have_been_considered_deities
41. Human deities, https://forgottenrealms.fandom.com/wiki/Category:Human_deities
42. Idolatry, https://en.wikipedia.org/wiki/Idolatry
43. Sheikh Muhammad Saalih al-Munajjid, He is asking: why are most of the people on earth disbelievers, and why does Allah want them to enter Hell? https://islamqa.info/en/answers/159301
44. Sheikh Muhammad Saalih al-Munajjid, Does prostrating or bowing by way of greeting come under the heading of shirk? https://islamqa.info/en/answers/229780
45. Sheikh Muhammad Saalih al-Munajjid, Obligation to destroy idols https://islamqa.info/en/answers/20894
46. Sheikh Muhammad Saalih al-Munajjid, Atheism is a greater sin than shirk https://islamqa.info/en/answers/113901
47. Abu Muhammad al-Maqdisi, Reflections: Expecting the Best from Allah, https://muqith.files.wordpress.com/2015/12/expecting-the-best-from-allah.pdf
48. Sheikh Muhammad Saalih al-Munajjid, Tafseer of the verse "So on that Day no question will be asked of man or jinn as to his sin" [ar-Rahmaan 55:39], https://islamqa.info/en/answers/145728
49. Imam Abu Zakariya Yahya bin Sharaf An-Nawawi Ad-Dimashqi, Riyad as-Saliheen, Chapter 51: Hope in Allah's Mercy
50. Imam Abu Zakariya Yahya bin Sharaf An-Nawawi Ad-Dimashqi, Riyad as-Saliheen, Chapter 52: Excellence of Good Hopes
51. And the answer is … Al-Musta'an! https://understandquran.com/answer-al-mustaaan
52. Imam Abu Zakariya Yahya bin Sharaf An-Nawawi Ad-Dimashqi, Riyad as-Saliheen, Chapter 332: Abomination of saying- "Forgive me if you wish, O Allah!"
53. Imam Abu Zakariya Yahya bin Sharaf An-Nawawi Ad-Dimashqi, Riyad as-Saliheen, Chapter 50: Fear (of Allah)
54. Mohammad Zahid, Only God can judge me! https://www.aljumuah.com/only-allah-can-judge-me-2
55. Not preventing the oppressors is a cause for collective punishment from Allah, Hadith related to ruling with commentary, https://ahadith.co.uk/sixtysultaniyya.php?tid=41
56. Sheikh Muhammad Saalih al-Munajjid, Should they pray behind someone who says that Allah is everywhere? https://islamqa.info/en/answers/218026
57. Permanent Committee for Scholarly Research and Ifta' consisting of Shaykh Abdul Azeez aal-shaykh, Sheikh Abdullah al-Ghudayyan, Shaykh Saalih al-Fawzaan, Shaykh Bakr Abu Zayd, *Faith:* Allah is not Imageless, He has Hands, Eyes, Face and Other Attributes, https://millichronicle.com/2019/10/faith-allah-is-not-imageless-he-has-hands-eyes-face-and-other-attributes
58. Mateen A. Khan, On the Attributes of Allah, https://enterthesunnah.com/2020/07/11/on-the-attributes-of-allah
59. Sheikh Muhammad Saalih al-Munajjid, Ruling on Reciting the Names of Allah in certain combinations, https://islamqa.info/en/answers/3927
60. Sheikh Muhammad Saalih al-Munajjid, Is Al-Rasheed one of the Names of Allah? https://islamqa.info/en/answers/5457

61. Sheikh Assim Al Hakeem, Is Al Rasheed one of Allah's names? Are some names not found in Qur'an and sunnah? Where to find them? https://www.youtube.com/watch?v=E0dgrv-5omw
62. The Attribute of Al-Wujud, https://www.al-feqh.com/en/the-attribute-of-al-wujud
63. Sheikh Muhammad Saalih al-Munajjid, Al-Dahr is not one of the Names of Allah, https://islamqa.info/en/answers/26977
64. Prophet Yahya (AS), https://hadithoftheday.com/prophet-yahya-as/Supplicating to Allah saying Hannan and Mannan, https://www.al-feqh.com/en/supplicating-to-allah-saying-hannan-and-mannan
65. Sheikh Muhammad Saalih al-Munajjid, Is as-Saboor one of the beautiful Names of Allah? https://islamqa.info/en/answers/191329
66. Sabr, https://en.wikipedia.org/wiki/Sabr
67. Sheikh Muhammad Saalih al-Munajjid, Remembering Allah by repeating a single Name such as "Allah", https://islamqa.info/en/answers/26867
68. Sheikh Muhammad Saalih al-Munajjid, Repeating the Name of Allah on its own, or the pronoun "Huwa" (He), is a Sufi bid'ah, https://islamqa.info/en/answers/9389
69. Writing Allah's Name on the Back of the Car, https://www.al-feqh.com/en/writing-allah-s-name-on-the-back-of-the-car
70. Sheikh Muhammad Saalih al-Munajjid, The Salafi way of interpreting the divine attributes and refuting the pantheistic interpretation of the hadith "I will be his hearing", https://islamqa.info/en/answers/163948
71. Sheikh Muhammad Saalih al-Munajjid, Refutation of those who claim that the story of the Isra' and Mi'raaj is a myth, https://islamqa.info/en/answers/84314
72. Sheikh Muhammad Saalih al-Munajjid, Celebrating the night of the Isra' and Mi'raaj, https://islamqa.info/en/answers/60288
73. Sheikh Muhammad Saalih al-Munajjid, Going to visit places and mosques in which the Prophet Prayed, https://islamqa.info/en/answers/11669
74. Sheikh Muhammad Saalih al-Munajjid, Who are Ahl al-Bayt (the members of the Prophet's family)? https://islamqa.info/en/answers/10055
75. Imam Abu Zakariya Yahya bin Sharaf An-Nawawi Ad-Dimashqi, Riyad as-Saliheen, Chapter 367: Prohibition of attributing wrong Fatherhood
76. Sheikh Muhammad Saalih al-Munajjid, Ruling on a person touching the Qur'aan without wudoo', and the meaning of the hadeeth, "The believer is never impure", https://islamqa.info/en/answers/10672
77. Sheikh Muhammad Saalih al-Munajjid, Singling out verses from some soorahs to recite them at times of hardship and difficulty, https://islamqa.info/en/answers/115841
78. Sheikh Muhammad Saalih al-Munajjid, Ruling on hanging Verses of the Quran on walls, https://islamqa.info/en/answers/254
79. Dr. Muhammad Salah, Hanging Names of Allah and Quranic Verse on wall? https://www.youtube.com/watch?v=QcBvSn8cPgM
80. Sheikh Muhammad Saalih al-Munajjid, Ruling on swearing on the Mushaf and the expiation for breaking such an oath, https://islamqa.info/en/answers/98194
81. Assim al Hakeem, Can we swear or take an oath on Quran by placing our hand or by words? https://www.youtube.com/watch?v=Hp_EvJg3CRU
82. Sheikh Muhammad Saalih al-Munajjid, Leaving a recording of the Qur'an playing without listening to it, https://islamqa.info/en/answers/174743

83. Sheikh Muhammad Saalih al-Munajjid, The Qur'an is the Word of Allah, may He be exalted, and is not created, https://islamqa.info/en/answers/227441
84. Sheikh Muhammad Saalih al-Munajjid, Ruling on reciting Qur'aan for another person, living or dead, https://islamqa.info/en/answers/20996
85. Dr. Muhammad Salah, Reciting the Qur'an for the deceased does he receive the reward https://www.youtube.com/watch?v=_z4-EJali3w
86. Imam Abu Zakariya Yahya bin Sharaf An-Nawawi Ad-Dimashqi, Riyad as-Saliheen, Chapter 363: Prohibition of Carrying the Qur'an into the Land of Enemy
87. Sheikh Muhammad Saalih al-Munajjid, Saying "Sadaqa Allah al-'Azeem" https://islamqa.info/en/answers/10119
88. Islamic Miracle 1.618 the Golden Ratio, https://www.youtube.com/watch?v=T0hOhH69vmA
89. Sheikh Muhammad Saalih al-Munajjid, Comment on the publication "Thirty supplications (Du'as) for the thirty days of Ramadan" https://islamqa.info/en/answers/139822
90. Sheikh Muhammad Saalih al-Munajjid Tawassul: Islamic vs. bid'ah, https://islamqa.info/en/answers/3297
91. Multiplication of good deeds in terms of quantity and degree whereas sins in terms of degree only, https://www.alifta.gov.sa/En/IftaContents/IbnBaz/Pages/default.aspx?cultStr=en&View
92. Sheikh Muhammad Salih al-Munajjid, Meaning of belief in al-Qadar (the divine will and decree), https://islamqa.info/en/answers/34732
93. Sheikh Muhammad Salih al-Munajjid, Is man's fate pre-destined or does he have freedom of will, https://islamqa.info/en/answers/20806
94. Sheikh Muhammad Saalih al-Munajjid, Du'a is a Worship, https://islamqa.info/en/answers/320772
95. Sheikh Muhammad Saalih al-Munajjid, Ruling on citing al-qadar (divine will and decree) as an excuse for committing sin or failing to do obligatory duties, https://islamqa.info/en/answers/49039
96. Muhammad Tim Humble, Using the Decree of Allah as an Excuse, http://35.190.94.206/watch?v=U44x1ANgka4
97. Imam Abu Zakariya Yahya bin Sharaf An-Nawawi Ad-Dimashqi, Riyad as-Saliheen, Chapter 333: Abomination of saying- "What Allah Wills and so-and-so Wills"
98. Sheikh Muhammad Saalih al-Munajjid, Ruling on one who Rejects a Saheeh Hadith, https://islamqa.info/en/answers/115125
99. Imam Abu Zakariya Yahya bin Sharaf An-Nawawi Ad-Dimashqi, Riyad as-Saliheen, Chapter 185: The Merits of Ablutions (Wudu')
100. Imam Abu Zakariya Yahya bin Sharaf An-Nawawi Ad-Dimashqi, Riyad as-Saliheen, Chapter 186: The Excellence of Adhan
101. Imam Abu Zakariya Yahya bin Sharaf An-Nawawi Ad-Dimashqi, Riyad as-Saliheen, Chapter 189: The Excellence of Proceeding towards the Mosque Walking
102. Imam Abu Zakariya Yahya bin Sharaf An-Nawawi Ad-Dimashqi, Riyad as-Saliheen, Chapter 190: The Excellence of waiting for As-Salat (The Prayer)
103. Imam Abu Zakariya Yahya bin Sharaf An-Nawawi Ad-Dimashqi, Riyad as-Saliheen, Chapter 187: The Excellence of As-Salat (The Prayer)

104. Imam Abu Zakariya Yahya bin Sharaf An-Nawawi Ad-Dimashqi, Riyad as-Saliheen, Chapter 188: Excellence of the Morning (Fajr) and 'Asr Prayers
105. Sheikh Muhammad Saalih al-Munajjid, Forgetting Intention, https://islamqa.info/en/answers/95095
106. The Importance of Intentions, 40 An-Nawawi Hadith #1, https://www.khutbah.info/hadith-1-of-the-forty-an-nawawi/
107. Moutasem Al-Hameedy, How to purify your intentions https://www.youtube.com/watch?v=B8XOBUUscuc
108. Sheikh Muhammad Saalih al-Munajjid, Ruling on Uttering the Intention Niyyah in acts of worship, https://islamqa.info/en/answers/13337
109. Sheikh Muhammad Saalih al-Munajjid, Water gets in his nose when he washes his face during wudoo', https://islamqa.info/en/answers/71169
110. Assim Al Hakeem, Closing the eyes while praying! https://www.youtube.com/watch?v=QRC7hYJmEwA
111. Moutasem Al-Hameedi, Can we pray with eyes closed? https://www.youtube.com/watch?v=KOaISv7JYAc
112. Imam Abu Zakariya Yahya bin Sharaf An-Nawawi Ad-Dimashqi, Riyad-as-Saliheen, Chapter 208: Inducement to Perform Tahiyyat-ul-Masjid (Upon Entering the Mosque)
113. Imam Abu Zakariya Yahya bin Sharaf An-Nawawi Ad-Dimashqi, Riyad as-Saliheen, Chapter 191: The Excellence of Performing Salat (Prayers) in Congregation
114. Imam Abu Zakariya Yahya bin Sharaf An-Nawawi Ad-Dimashqi, Riyad as-Saliheen, Chapter 194: The Excellence of Standing in the First Row (In Salat)
115. Dr. Mohammad Najeeb Qasmi, Jumu'ah: Excellence, virtues and rulings, https://backup.najeebqasmi.com/articles/english-articles/99-prayer-namaz/1177-jumu-ah-excellence-virtues-and-rulings
116. Dr. Zaik Nakir, The seven Virtues of the Day of Arafah, https://www.youtube.com/watch?v=x3FII3ByJAk
117. Imam Abu Zakariya Yahya bin Sharaf An-Nawawi Ad-Dimashqi, Riyad as-Saliheen, Chapter 210: The Excellence of Friday Prayer
118. Sheikh Muhammad Saalih al-Munajjid, The virtue of sending a great deal of blessings upon the Prophet (blessings and peace of Allah be upon him), https://islamqa.info/en/answers/128455
119. Sheikh Muhammad Saalih al-Munajjid, Ruling on following the translation of the Friday khutbah on one's cell phone whilst listening to it, https://islamqa.info/en/answers/233591
120. Sheikh Muhammad Saalih al-Munajjid, Sunnah prayer before and after Jumu'ah? https://islamqa.info/en/answers/6653
121. Imam Abu Zakariya Yahya bin Sharaf An-Nawawi Ad-Dimashqi, Riyad as-Saliheen, Chapter 203: Sunnah of Friday Prayer
122. Sheikh Muhammad Saalih al-Munajjid, Ruling on using the masbahah (prayer beads), https://islamqa.info/en/answers/3009
123. Imam Abu Zakariya Yahya bin Sharaf An-Nawawi Ad-Dimashqi, Riyad as-Saliheen, Chapter 312: Undesirability of Sitting with Erected Legs during Friday Sermon
124. Sheikh Muhammad Saalih al-Munajjid, Ruling on sitting with the knees drawn up (ihtiba'). https://islamqa.info/en/answers/129182

125. Sheikh Muhammad Saalih al-Munajjid, Ruling on pointing one's feet towards the qiblah, https://islamqa.info/en/answers/12871
126. Sheikh Muhammad Saalih al-Munajjid, Is it permissible for him to complete the purchase when he can hear the call to prayer? https://islamqa.info/en/answers/140662
127. Sheikh Muhammad Saalih al-Munajjid, What is the ruling on offering congratulations on Friday? https://islamqa.info/en/answers/134741
128. Dr. Zakir Naik, Greeting Jumuah Mubarak is Bid'ah, https://zakirnaikfansofficial.blogspot.com/2016/01/greeting-jummah-mubarak-is-bidah.html?
129. Sheikh Muhammad Saalih al-Munajjid, Ruling on rushing when reciting and praying https://islamqa.info/en/answers/146675
130. Nouman Ali Khan, This is what happens when you rush through Salah, https://www.youtube.com/watch?v=Sr452jGQiRw
131. Sheikh Muhammad Saalih al-Munajjid, It is mustahabb to separate between the obligatory prayer and the naafil prayer, by speaking or moving, https://islamqa.info/en/answers/116064
132. Sheikh Muhammad Saalih al-Munajjid, The difference between joining and shortening prayers, https://islamqa.info/en/answers/105109
133. Sheikh Muhammad Saalih al-Munajjid, How should the traveler pray, https://islamqa.info/en/answers/82658
134. Muhammad Salah, Combining prayers without valid reason, https://www.youtube.com/watch?v=slPfB-I0Xpg
135. Abu Amina Elias, Should women pray in the mosque? https://www.abuaminaelias.com/should-women-pray-in-the-mosque/
136. Imam Abu Zakariya Yahya bin Sharaf An-Nawawi Ad-Dimashqi, Riyad as-Saliheen, Chapter 337: Prohibition of raising one's Head before the Imam
137. Imam Abu Zakariya Yahya bin Sharaf An-Nawawi Ad-Dimashqi, Riyad as-Saliheen, Chapter 340: Prohibition of Raising one's Eyes Towards the Sky During As-Salat (The Prayer)
138. Imam Abu Zakariya Yahya bin Sharaf An-Nawawi Ad-Dimashqi, Riyad as-Saliheen, Chapter 341: Undesirability of Glancing in one Direction of the other during Prayer
139. Imam Abu Zakariya Yahya bin Sharaf An-Nawawi Ad-Dimashqi, Riyad as-Saliheen, Chapter 338: Prohibition of Placing the hands on the sides during As-Salat (The Prayer)
140. Moulana Suhail Motala, A Disliked Sitting Posture, https://hadithanswers.com/a-disliked-sitting-posture
141. Sheikh Muhammad Saalih al-Munajjid, Raising the hands during prayer, https://islamqa.info/en/answers/21439
142. Sheikh Muhammad Saalih al-Munajjid, The manner of raising the hands in the prayer; what should the worshipper do if he makes a mistake? https://islamqa.info/en/answers/298825
143. Sheikh Muhammad Saalih al-Munajjid, Raising the hands in the first tashahhud – before or after standing? https://islamqa.info/en/answers/95798
144. Imam Abu Zakariya Yahya bin Sharaf An-Nawawi Ad-Dimashqi, Riyad as-Saliheen, Chapter 343: Prohibition of passing in front of a Worshipper while he is offering Salat (Prayer)
145. Sheikh Muhammad Saalih al-Munajjid, Ruling on Forgetting a Prostration of Forgetfulness, https://islamqa.info/en/answers/134518

146. Dr. Muhammad Salah, Please, explain how to correctly perform the prostration of forgetfulness, https://www.youtube.com/watch?v=3CedLHRd1vE
147. Sheikh Muhammad Saalih al-Munajjid, It is not prescribed to do a single prostration for the sake of du'aa', https://islamqa.info/en/answers/116874
148. Dr. Zakir Naik, Making dua in sujood in my mother tongue, https://www.youtube.com/watch?v=0CwlHJ4A3CY
149. Assim al Hakeem, Is it permissible to make an independent sajda after salah to make dua? https://www.youtube.com/watch?v=7L-NjigFLzA
150. Sheikh Muhammad Saalih al-Munajjid, Can We Say "Taqabbal Allah" after Prayer? https://islamqa.info/en/answers/148124
151. Sheikh Muhammad Saalih al-Munajjid, Ruling on praying Witr in the same way as Maghrib, https://islamqa.info/en/answers/38230
152. Dr. Zakir Naik, The correct Way to perform Witr Salah, https://www.youtube.com/watch?v=5LxP82Y694I
153. Imam Abu Zakariya Yahya bin Sharaf An-Nawawi Ad-Dimashqi, Riyad as-Saliheen, Chapter 309: Prohibition of Spitting in the Mosque
154. Sheikh Muhammad Saalih al-Munajjid, Ruling on building toilets that face the qiblah, https://islamqa.info/en/answers/69808
155. Imam Abu Zakariya Yahya bin Sharaf An-Nawawi Ad-Dimashqi, Riyad as-Saliheen, Chapter 311: Undesirability of Entering the Mosque after Eating raw Onion or Garlic
156. Sheikh Muhammad Saalih al-Munajjid, Salaat al-tawbah (the prayer of repentance) https://islamqa.info/en/answers/98030
157. Sheikh Muhammad Saalih al-Munajjid, No one can pray istikharah on behalf of another https://islamqa.info/en/answers/134612
158. Sheikh Faraz Rabbani, Can I Pay Someone to Perform Salat al-Istikhara for me? https://hadithoftheday.com/can-i-pay-someone-to-perform-salat-al-istikhara-for-me
159. Imam Abu Zakariya Yahya bin Sharaf An-Nawawi Ad-Dimashqi, Riyad as-Saliheen, Chapter 334: Abomination of Holding Conversation after 'Isha' (Night) Prayer
160. Making up for Years of Missed Prayer, https://fiqh.islamonline.net/en/making-up-for-years-of-missed-prayer
161. Sheikh Muhammad Saalih al-Munajjid, How can he make up for missed prayers? https://islamqa.info/en/answers/111783
162. Sheikh Muhammad Saalih al-Munajjid, The virtues of Ramadan, https://islamqa.info/en/answers/13480
163. Sheikh Muhammad Saalih al-Munajjid, Breaking one's fast in Ramadaan deliberately, with no excuse, https://islamqa.info/en/answers/26866
164. Sheikh Muhammad Saalih al-Munajjid, There is no specific Du'a for each day and night of Ramadan https://islamqa.info/en/answers/220647
165. Sheikh Muhammad Saalih al-Munajjid, Comment on the publication "Thirty supplications (Du'as) for the thirty days of Ramadan", https://islamqa.info/en/answers/139822
166. Sheikh Muhammad Saalih al-Munajjid, Is I'tikaf Compulsory? tps://islamqa.info/en/answers/48999
167. Sheikh Muhammad Saalih al-Munajjid, Rules of Zakat al-Fitr, https://islamqa.info/en/answers/207225

168. Sheikh Muhammad Saalih al-Munajjid, All About Zakat al-Fitr, https://islamqa.info/en/articles/69
169. Sheikh Muhammad Saalih al-Munajjid, Can he give zakaat al-fitr to the poor in the form of cash if they will not accept food? https://islamqa.info/en/answers/145858
170. Sheikh Muhammad Saalih al-Munajjid, Is zakat al-fitr waived with the passage of time? https://islamqa.info/en/answers/145563
171. Sheikh Muhammad Saalih al-Munajjid, Zakaah on wealth earned during the year, https://islamqa.info/en/answers/93414
172. Sheikh Muhammad Saalih al-Munajjid, Ruling on one who does not pay zakaah, https://islamqa.info/en/answers/93701
173. Imam Abu Zakariya Yahya bin Sharaf An-Nawawi Ad-Dimashqi, Riyad as-Saliheen, Chapter 233: The Obligation of Hajj (Pilgrimage) and its Excellence
174. Imam Abu Zakariya Yahya bin Sharaf An-Nawawi Ad-Dimashqi, Riyad as-Salihin, Chapter 313: Prohibition of having a Hair cut or paring one's nail during the first ten days of Dhul-Hijjah for one who intends to Sacrifice an Animal
175. Sheikh Muhammad Saalih al-Munajjid, Rulings of Udhiyah (Sacrifice), https://islamqa.info/en/articles/67
176. Sheikh Muhammad Saalih al-Munajjid, Ruling on congratulating the pilgrim after his return and decorating the house, https://islamqa.info/en/answers/97879
177. Sheikh Muhammad Saalih al-Munajjid, Virtue of the month of Allah Muharram, https://islamqa.info/en/answers/204142
178. Sheikh Muhammad Saalih al-Munajjid, The month of Rajab, https://islamqa.info/en/articles/68
179. Sheikh Muhammad Saalih al-Munajjid, The hadeeth "Whoever says in Rajab 'I ask Allah for forgiveness, there is no god but He'…" is fabricated and is not saheeh, https://islamqa.info/en/answers/171509
180. Bidah alert for 15th of Shaban, https://www.islamicboard.com/worship-in-islam/134285605-bidah-alert-15th-shaban.html
181. Sheikh Muhammad Saalih al-Munajjid, Shab e Barat/ 15th Night of Sha'ban: Bidah? https://islamqa.info/en/answers/154850/shab-e-barat-15th-night-of-shaban-bidah
182. Guidance Series, Part 4, The Month of Shaban – Facts & Innovations, https://weeklykhutbah.wordpress.com/2017/10/31/guidance-series-the-month-of-shaban-facts-innovations
183. Sheikh Muhammad Saalih al-Munajjid, What the Shi'ah do on 'Ashoora' is bid'ah (innovation) and misguidance, https://islamqa.info/en/answers/101268
184. Abu Ameerah, Religious innovation (bidah) and sin during the blessed month of Muharram, https://thesunnah.wordpress.com/2007/01/25
185. Sheikh Muhammed Salih Al-Munajjid, Is Salaat al-Haajah prescribed in Islam? If it is proven to work, will that justify doing it? https://islamqa.info/en/answers/70295
186. Imam Abu Zakariya Yahya bin Sharaf An-Nawawi Ad-Dimashqi, Riyad as-Saliheen, Chapter 18: Prohibition of heresies in religion
187. Imam Abu Zakariya Yahya bin Sharaf An-Nawawi Ad-Dimashqi, Riyad as-Saliheen, Chapter 234: Obligation of Jihad
188. Sheikh Muhammad Saalih al-Munajjid, Treatment of the prisoners of war in Islam, https://islamqa.info/en/answers/13241

189. Imam Abu Zakariya Yahya bin Sharaf An-Nawawi Ad-Dimashqi, Riyad as-Saliheen, Chapter 266: Prohibition of Reviling a Muslim without any cause
190. Imam Abu Zakariya Yahya bin Sharaf An-Nawawi Ad-Dimashqi, Riyad as-Saliheen, Chapter 271: Prohibition of Spying on Muslims and to be Inquisitive about Others
191. Imam Abu Zakariya Yahya bin Sharaf An-Nawawi Ad-Dimashqi, Riyad as-Saliheen, Chapter 273: Prohibition of Despising Muslims
192. Sheikh Muhammad Saalih al-Munajjid, The hadith "Whoever harms [others], Allah will harm him, and whoever causes hardship [to others] Allah will cause hardship to him", https://islamqa.info/en/answers/285915
193. Sheikh Muhammad Saalih al-Munajjid, The rights of one Muslim over another include those that are obligatory and those that are mustahabb, https://islamqa.info/en/answers/178639
194. Sheikh Muhammad Saalih al-Munajjid, Is it Sunnah to shake hands using both hands? https://islamqa.info/en/answers/92806
195. Imam Abu Zakariya Yahya bin Sharaf An-Nawawi Ad-Dimashqi, Riyad as-Saliheen, Chapter 326: Prohibition of Calling a Muslim an Infidel
196. Dr. Zakir Naik, Can Muslims keep Non-Muslims as Friends, https://www.youtube.com/watch?v=KbxpPa4n8YY
197. Imam Abu Zakariya Yahya bin Sharaf An-Nawawi Ad-Dimashqi, Riyad as-Saliheen, Chapter 138: Greeting the non-Muslims and Prohibition of taking an Initiative
198. Sheikh Muhammad Saalih al-Munajjid, Ruling on greeting with a gesture, https://islamqa.info/en/answers/6670
199. Sheikh Muhammad Saalih al-Munajjid, Ruling on Military Salutes and Saluting the Flag, http://www.darussalaam.co.uk/Ruling_on_Military_Salutes_And_Saluting_The_Flag_262
200. Sheikh Muhammad Saalih al-Munajjid, Ruling on standing up to welcome a newcomer, https://islamqa.info/en/answers/13776
201. Imam Abu Zakariya Yahya bin Sharaf An-Nawawi Ad-Dimashqi, Riyad as-Saliheen, Chapter 360: Undesirability of Praising a Person in his Presence
202. Imam Abu Zakariya Yahya bin Sharaf An-Nawawi Ad-Dimashqi, Riyad as-Saliheen, Chapter 259: Condemnation of Double-faced People
203. Imam Abu Zakariya Yahya bin Sharaf An-Nawawi Ad-Dimashqi, Riyad as-Saliheen, Chapter 260: Condemnation and Prohibition of Falsehood
204. Henry Otgaar, Alysha Baker, When lying changes memory for the truth, https://www.tandfonline.com/doi/full/10.1080
205. Imam Abu Zakariya Yahya bin Sharaf An-Nawawi Ad-Dimashqi, Riyad as-Saliheen, Chapter 74: Clemency, Tolerance and Gentleness
206. Imam Abu Zakariya Yahya bin Sharaf An-Nawawi Ad-Dimashqi, Riyad as-Saliheen, Chapter 73: Good Conduct
207. Imam Abu Zakariya Yahya bin Sharaf An-Nawawi Ad-Dimashqi, Riyad as-Saliheen, Chapter 76: Endurance of Afflictions
208. Sheikh Muhammad Saalih al-Munajjid, Etiquette of naming children, https://islamqa.info/en/answers/7180
209. Sheikh Muhammad Saalih al-Munajjid, He has doubts about his Christian wife; can he disown the child in her womb? https://islamqa.info/en/answers/33615

210. Imam Abu Zakariya Yahya bin Sharaf An-Nawawi Ad-Dimashqi, Riyad as-Saliheen, Chapter 353: Prohibition of giving preference to Children over one another in giving Gifts, etc.
211. Dr. Zakir Naik, Is Adoption permitted in islam, https://www.youtube.com/watch?v=FL8A-SCIvEU
212. Sheikh Muhammad Saalih al-Munajjid, A Girl Calling Her Stepfather Daddy or Abi (Father), https://islamqa.info/en/answers/1041
213. Sheikh Muhammad Saalih al-Munajjid, The difference between sponsoring orphans and adopting them, https://islamqa.info/en/answers/5201
214. Sheikh Muhammad Saalih al-Munajjid, Is he regarded as sponsoring an orphan if he simply pays money to a charity that sponsors orphans? https://islamqa.info/en/answers/47190
215. Suhad Daher-Nashif, Suzanne H. Hammad, Tanya Kane, etc., Islam and Mental Disorders of the Older Adults: Religious Text, Belief System and Caregiving Practices, https://www.ncbi.nlm.nih.gov/pmc/articles/PMC8137626
216. Imam Abu Zakariya Yahya bin Sharaf An-Nawawi Ad-Dimashqi, Riyad as-Saliheen, Chapter 280: Prohibition of Breaking Ties and Relationships
217. Imam Abu Zakariya Yahya bin Sharaf An-Nawawi Ad-Dimashqi, Riyad as-Saliheen, Chapter 275: Prohibition of Deriding one's Lineage
218. Imam Abu Zakariya Yahya bin Sharaf An-Nawawi Ad-Dimashqi, Riyad as-Saliheen, Chapter 367: Prohibition of attributing wrong Fatherhood
219. Sheikh Muhammad Saalih al-Munajjid, Why a woman should not take her husband's surname, https://islamqa.info/en/answers/6241
220. Imam Abu Zakariya Yahya bin Sharaf An-Nawawi Ad-Dimashqi, Riyad as-Saliheen, Chapter 140: Seeking Permission to enter (somebody's House) and Manners relating to it
221. Imam Abu Zakariya Yahya bin Sharaf An-Nawawi Ad-Dimashqi, Riyad as-Saliheen, Chapter 39: Rights of Neighbours
222. Islamic inheritance jurisprudence, https://en.wikipedia.org/wiki/Islamic_inheritance_jurisprudence
223. Muslim, Kitab Al-Wasiyya (the Book of Bequests, https://www.iium.edu.my/deed/hadith/muslim/013_smt.html
224. Funerals: According to the Qur'an and Sunnah, https://sunnahonline.com/library/fiqh-and-sunnah/276
225. Sheikh Muhammad Saalih al-Munajjid, Ruling on wills which deprive some of one's children of their inheritance, https://islamqa.info/en/answers/1511
226. Muslim, Kitab Al-Fara'id (The Book pertaining to the Rules of Inheritance) https://www.iium.edu.my/deed/hadith/muslim/011_smt.html
227. Dr. Hassan Elhais, United Arab Emirates: Inheritance Under Muslim Law: Framework of Sharia Law, https://www.mondaq.com/wills-intestacy-estate-planning/786544
228. Sheikh Muhammad Saalih al-Munajjid, Ruling on one who forbids marriage for himself, https://islamqa.info/en/answers/87998
229. Sheikh Muhammad Saalih al-Munajjid, Ruling What is the ruling on someone who causes trouble between an engaged couple so that he will call it off and she can snag him? https://islamqa.info/en/answers/187895

230. Sheikh Muhammad Saalih al-Munajjid, Ruling, Adulthood is a condition of being a witness to marriage, https://islamqa.info/en/answers/113868
231. Forced Marriage, https://www.mwnuk.co.uk/Forced_Marriage
232. Dr. Zakir Naik, Rights of wife in Islam, https://www.youtube.com/watch?v=tXwatho_mIE
233. Dowry in Islamic Marriages, https://www.legalserviceindia.com/legal/article-2908-dowry-in-islamic-marriages.html
234. Imam Abu Zakariya Yahya bin Sharaf An-Nawawi Ad-Dimashqi, Riyad as-Saliheen, Chapter 34: Recommendations with regard to Women
235. Sheikh Muhammad Saalih al-Munajjid, Ruling on marrying cousins, https://islamqa.info/en/answers/105
236. Dr. Muzammil H. Siddiqi, Islamic View on Marrying Cousins, https://fiqh.islamonline.net/en/islamic-view-on-marrying-cousins
237. Sheikh Muhammad Saalih al-Munajjid, Should he marry his cousin in secret? https://islamqa.info/en/answers/222086
238. Sheikh Muhammad Saalih al-Munajjid, Attribution of an illegitimate child and rulings that result from that, https://islamqa.info/en/answers/85043
239. Abu Abdillah, The Different types of Iddah, https://arabicvirtualacademy.com/the-different-types-of-iddah
240. Types of women who observe 'Iddah, https://www.al-feqh.com/en/types-of-women-who-observe-%60iddah
241. Sheikh Muhammad Saalih al-Munajjid, Ruling He is asking about the words of Ibraaheem (peace be upon him) to Ismaa'eel: "Change your doorstep" https://islamqa.info/en/answers/98414
242. Sheikh Muhammad Saalih al-Munajjid, Ruling on plural marriage and conditions thereof, https://islamqa.info/en/answers/49044/ruling-on-plural-marriage-and-conditions-thereof
243. Sheikh Muhammad Saalih al-Munajjid, The punishment for homosexuality, https://islamqa.info/en/answers/38622
244. Zahid Law Associates, What is Paper Marriage? Is it permitted in Islam? https://zahidlaw.com/paper-marriage
245. Dr. Zulkifli Mohamad Al-Bakri, Marriage Between Human and Jinn, https://maktabahalbakri.com/416-marriage-between-human-and-jinn
246. Sheikh Muhammad Saalih al-Munajjid, What is the ruling on intimacy with slave women? https://islamqa.info/en/answers/13737
247. Sheikh Muhammad Saalih al-Munajjid, Ruling on wearing engagement and wedding rings, https://islamqa.info/en/answers/21441
248. Imam Abu Zakariya Yahya bin Sharaf An-Nawawi Ad-Dimashqi, Riyad-as-Saliheen, Chapter 35: Husband's rights concerning his Wife
249. Sheikh Muhammad Saalih al-Munajjid, What are the rights of the husband and what are the rights of the wife? https://islamqa.info/en/answers/10680
250. Sheikh Muhammad, Saalih al-Munajjid, Woman going out to visit her parents and relatives without her husband's permission, https://islamqa.info/en/answers/83360
251. Sheikh Muhammad Saalih al-Munajjid, Ruling on her going out of the house without her husband's permission and travelling without a mahram, https://islamqa.info/en/answers/69937

252. Sheikh Muhammad Saalih al-Munajjid, Hitting one's wife? https://islamqa.info/en/answers/41199/hitting-ones-wife
253. Sheikh Muhammad Saalih al-Munajjid, The attitudes of the Messenger of Allah (blessings and peace of Allah be upon him) towards his wives and his good treatment of them, https://islamqa.info/en/answers/191429
254. Sheikh Muhammad Saalih al-Munajjid, Is it one of the wife's rights to have her own accommodation? https://islamqa.info/en/answers/81933
255. James Berry, Muslim marriages and rights for women whose husbands have multiple wives. https://jamesberrylaw.com/news-details/1187
256. Sheikh Muhammad Saalih al-Munajjid, She wants to work but her husband refuses, https://islamqa.info/en/answers/22397
257. A wife exiting her house without her husband's permission, http://dar-alifta.org/Foreign/ViewFatwa.aspx?ID=460
258. A divorced woman remaining at her husband's house during the 'Iddah, https://www.al-feqh.com/en/a-divorced-woman-remaining-at-her-husband-s-house-during-the-iddah
259. Disobedient Wife, How to Deal with Her? https://fiqh.islamonline.net/en/disobedient-wife-how-to-deal-with-her
260. Imam Abu Zakariya Yahya bin Sharaf An-Nawawi Ad-Dimashqi, Riyad as-Saliheen, Chapter 335: Prohibition of Refusal by a Woman when her Husband calls her to his Bed
261. Imam Abu Zakariya Yahya bin Sharaf An-Nawawi Ad-Dimashqi, Riyad as-Saliheen, Chapter 366: Prohibition of observing silence from Dawn till Night
262. Sheikh Muhammad Saalih al-Muhajjid, Etiquette of intimate relations https://islamqa.info/en/answers/5560
263. Imam Abu Zakariya Yahya bin Sharaf An-Nawawi Ad-Dimashqi, Riyad as-Saliheen, Chapter 336: Prohibition of Observing an Optional Saum (Fast) by a Woman without the Permission of her Husband
264. Imam Abu Zakariya Yahya bin Sharaf An-Nawawi Ad-Dimashqi, Riyad as-Saliheen, Chapter 331: Prohibition of Describing the Charms of a Woman to a man without a valid reason approved by the Shariah
265. Sheikh Muhammad Saalih al-Muhajjid, What are the husband's obligations towards his children and his ex-wife who has custody of them? https://islamqa.info/en/answers/264146
266. Muslim, Kitab Al-Talaq (The Book of Divorce), https://www.iium.edu.my/deed/hadith/muslim/009_smt.html
267. Sheikh Muhammad Saalih al-Munajjid, What should be done when a husband withholds his wife's rights in bed? https://islamqa.info/en/answers/9021
268. Sheikh Muhammad Saalih al-Munajjid, Ruling on divorce at a moment of anger, https://islamqa.info/en/answers/45174
269. Sheikh Muhammad Saalih al-Munajjid, Giving talaaq (divorce) three times at once is Bid'ah https://islamqa.info/en/answers/2373
270. Sheikh Muhammad Saalih al-Munajjid, Threefold divorce counts as one according to the correct scholarly opinion, https://islamqa.info/en/answers/96194
271. Sheikh Muhammad Saalih al-Munajjid, Is it permissible to divorce a woman who is breastfeeding? https://islamqa.info/en/answers/150751

272. Sheikh Muhammad Saalih al-Munajjid, Rights of Revocably and Irrevocably Divorced Women https://islamqa.info/en/answers/82641
273. Sheikh Muhammad Saalih al-Munajjid, Revocably Divorced Woman Staying in her Husband's House Until her 'Iddah is Over, https://islamqa.info/en/answers/14299
274. Sheikh Muhammad Saalih al-Munajjid, The 'iddah of a woman divorced by talaaq, https://islamqa.info/en/answers/12667
275. Sheikh Muhammad Saalih al-Munajjid, What is tahleel marriage? https://islamqa.info/en/answers/222367
276. Hassan Elhais, UAE Family Matters Q&A: Types of Divorce Under Sharia Law
277. Sheikh Muhammad Saalih al-Munajjid, Rate of maintenance for children if they are in their mother's custody, https://islamqa.info/en/answers/89708
278. Sheikh Muhammad Saalih al-Munajjid, Divorcing a woman by talaaq when she is pregnant https://islamqa.info/en/answers/12287
279. Harun Yahia, Fate of Pompeii, https://sunnahonline.com/library/purification-of-the-soul/212-fate-of-pompeii-the
280. Sheikh Muhammad Saalih al-Munajjid, Ruling on the things that lead to Zina – kissing, touching and being alone together, https://islamqa.info/en/answers/27259
281. Sheikh Muhammad Saalih al-Munajjid, Incest is a worse and more serious sin, https://islamqa.info/en/answers/84982
282. Sodomy, https://www.law.cornell.edu/wex/sodomy
283. Is cunnilingus (oral sex) permissible? Is it haram? https://questionsonislam.com/question/cunnilingus-oral-sex-permissible-it-haram
284. Dr. Muhammad Salah, Is oral sex permissible in Islam, https://www.youtube.com/watch?v=Z5j9fS3P2cc
285. Sheikh Assim Al Hakeem, Is Oral Sex Permissible in Islam? https://www.youtube.com/watch?v=ooZgyJw1sU4
286. Sheikh Muhammad Saalih al-Munajjid, Why Does Islam Forbid Lesbianism and Homosexuality? https://islamqa.info/en/answers/10050
287. Sheikh Muhammad Saalih al-Munajjid, Ruling on the crime of rape, https://islamqa.info/en/answers/72338
288. Sheikh Muhammad Saalih al-Munajjid, Is Masturbation Haram in Islam? https://islamqa.info/en/answers/329
289. Dr. Muhammad Salah, How to Stop Masturbating -Techniques That Work https://www.youtube.com/watch?v=BEUN47EliEU
290. Imam Abu Zakariya Yahya bin Sharaf An-Nawawi Ad-Dimashqi, Riyad as-Saliheen, Chapter 290: Prohibition of Gazing at Women and Beardless Handsome Boys except in Exigency
291. Sheikh Muhammad Saalih al-Munajjid, First and second glance at women, https://islamqa.info/en/answers/1774
292. Sheikh Muhammad Saalih al-Munajjid, Lowering the gaze, https://islamqa.info/en/answers/85622
293. Ibn Al-Qayyim al-Jawziyya, The Great Virtue of Lowering Gaze, https://sunnahonline.com/library/purification-of-the-soul/216-great-virtue-of-lowering-the-gaze-the
294. Imam Abu Zakariya Yahya bin Sharaf An-Nawawi Ad-Dimashqi, Riyad as-Saliheen, Chapter 291: Prohibition of Meeting a non-Mahram Woman in Seclusion

295. Sheikh Muhammad Saalih al-Munajjid, Evidence Prohibiting of Mixing of Men and Women https://islamqa.info/en/answers/1200
296. Sheikh Muhammad Saalih al-Munajjid, Correspondence between the sexes and its effect on the fast, https://islamqa.info/en/answers/7837
297. Sheikh Muhammad Saalih al-Munajjid, Love which ends in marriage – is it haraam? https://islamqa.info/en/answers/84102
298. Sheikh Muhammad Saalih al-Munajjid, Hadd punishment for slander, https://islamqa.info/en/answers/108955
299. Sheikh Muhammad Saalih al-Munajjid, Ruling on one who slanders 'Aa'ishah, https://islamqa.info/en/answers/954
300. Sheikh Muhammad Saalih al-Munajjid, Ruling on marrying young women, https://islamqa.info/en/answers/1493
301. Islam's View on Porn and its Effects and Danger, https://thesincereseeker.com/2019/06/effects-of-pornography
302. Imam Abu Zakariya Yahya bin Sharaf An-Nawawi Ad-Dimashqi, Riyad-as-Saliheen, Chapter 57: Contentment and Self-esteem and avoidance of unnecessary begging of People
303. 14 Prohibition of Begging in Islam According to the Law, https://azislam.com/prohibition-of-begging-in-islam-2
304. Imam Abu Zakariya Yahya bin Sharaf An-Nawawi Ad-Dimashqi, Riyad as-Saliheen, Chapter 59: Encouraging Livelihood by (working with) Hands and Abstaining from Begging
305. Imam Abu Zakariya Yahya bin Sharaf An-Nawawi Ad-Dimashqi, Riyad as-Saliheen, Chapter 319: About Begging in the Name of Allah
306. Should We Take Advantage of Leniency in Islam? https://aboutislam.net/counseling/ask-about-islam/take-advantage-leniency-islam
307. Mufti Menk, Taking advantage of a kind heart! Say, NO! https://www.youtube.com/watch?v=i7y_2N2slqY
308. Imam Abu Zakariya Yahya bin Sharaf An-Nawawi Ad-Dimashqi, Riyad as-Saliheen, Chapter 285: Undesirability of Giving a Gift and then Ask Back for it
309. Ahmad H. Sakr, Professor of Biochemistry and Nutrition. Pork: Possible Reasons for its Prohibition, http://web.ipb.ac.id/~erizal/pork_reasons.
310. The Brain-Gut Connection, https://www.hopkinsmedicine.org/health/wellness-and-prevention/the-brain-gut-connection.
311. Arthi Chinna Meyyappan, Evan Forth, Caroline J. K. Wallace, etc., Effect of fecal microbiota transplant on symptoms of psychiatric disorders: a systematic review, https://bmcpsychiatry.biomedcentral.com/articles/10.1186/s12888-020-02654-5
312. Faecal transplants may change your personality, https://thewest.com.au/news/medicine/faecal-transplants-may-change-your-personality-ng-b88472873z
313. Laura J. Craven, Michael Silverman, and Jeremy P. Burton, Transfer of altered behaviour and irritable bowel syndrome with diarrhea (IBS-D) through fecal microbiota transplant in mouse model indicates need for stricter donor screening criteria, https://www.ncbi.nlm.nih.gov/pmc/articles/PMC5750285
314. Melanie Rutkowski, PhD, Unhealthy Gut Helps Breast Cancer Spread, Research Reveals https://newsroom.uvahealth.com/2022/09/22/unhealthy-gut-helps-breast-cancer-spread-research-reveals

315. What to know about acidosis? https://www.medicalnewstoday.com/articles/326975#treatment
316. Alkaline Diets, Sonya Collins, https://www.webmd.com/diet/a-z/alkaline-diets
317. What to Know About Acidic Foods? https://www.webmd.com/diet/what-to-know-about-acidic-foods
318. R A Kreisberg, B C Wood, Drug and chemical-induced metabolic acidosis, https://pubmed.ncbi.nlm.nih.gov/6347452
319. Sheikh Muhammad Saalih al-Munajjid, How old should the sacrificial animal be? https://islamqa.info/en/answers/41899
320. Imam Abu Zakariya Yahya bin Sharaf An-Nawawi Ad-Dimashqi, Riyad as-Saliheen, Chapter 364: Prohibition of using Utensils made of Gold and Silver.
321. Imam Abu Zakariya Yahya bin Sharaf An-Nawawi Ad-Dimashqi, Riyad as-Saliheen, Chapter 109: Excellence of Eating with three Fingers and Licking them
322. Sheikh Muhammad Saalih al-Munajjid, Is it prescribed to praise Allah after burping and to seek refuge with Him after yawning? https://islamqa.info/en/answers/226979
323. Sheikh Muhammad Saalih al-Munajjid, Ahaadeeth of the Prophet (peace and blessings of Allah be upon him) which criticize extravagance with regard to food, https://islamqa.info/en/answers/102374
324. Imam Abu Zakariya Yahya bin Sharaf An-Nawawi Ad-Dimashqi, Riyad as-Saliheen, Chapter 101: Prohibition of Criticizing Food
325. Imam Abu Zakariya Yahya bin Sharaf An-Nawawi Ad-Dimashqi, Riyad as-Saliheen, Chapter 105: Prohibition of Eating two Date-fruits Simultaneously
326. Sheikh Muhammad Saalih al-Munajjid, Ruling on drinking whilst standing, https://islamqa.info/en/answers/21147
327. Sheikh Muhammad Saalih al-Munajjid, Ruling on accepting an invitation, and the conditions for doing so, https://islamqa.info/en/answers/22006
328. Imam Abu Zakariya Yahya bin Sharaf An-Nawawi Ad-Dimashqi, Riyad as-Saliheen, Chapter 94: Honoring the Guest
329. Imam Abu Zakariya Yahya bin Sharaf An-Nawawi Ad-Dimashqi, Riyad as-Saliheen, Chapter 103: What should one say to the Host if an uninvited Person is accompanied with an invited person.
330. Imam Abu Zakariya Yahya bin Sharaf An-Nawawi Ad-Dimashqi, Riyad as-Saliheen, Chapter 345: Abomination of Selecting Friday for Fasting
331. Sheikh Muhammad Saalih al-Munajjid, Ruling on fasting on Saturdays, https://islamqa.info/en/answers/81621
332. Imam Abu Zakariya Yahyaa Ibn Sharaf An-Nawawi Ad-Dimashqi, Riyad as-Saliheen, Chapter 346: Prohibition of Extending Fast beyond one Day
333. Imam Abu Zakariya Yahyaa Ibn Sharaf An-Nawawi Ad-Dimashqi, Riyad as-Saliheen, Chapter 351: Prohibition of Relieving Nature on the Paths
334. Sheikh Muhammad Saalih al-Munajjid, Ruling on eating and drinking in the bathroom, https://islamqa.info/en/answers/161383
335. Imam Abu Zakariya Yahya bin Sharaf An-Nawawi Ad-Dimashqi, Riyad as-Saliheen, Chapter 99: Excellence of using the right Hand for Performing various good Acts
336. Imam Abu Zakariya Yahya bin Sharaf An-Nawawi Ad-Dimashqi, Riyad as-Saliheen, Chapter 298: Prohibition of using the right hand for cleaning after toilet without a valid reason

337. Imam Abu Zakariya Yahya bin Sharaf An-Nawawi Ad-Dimashqi, Riyad as-Saliheen, Chapter 352: Prohibition of Urinating into Stagnant Water
338. Imam Abu Zakariya Yahya bin Sharaf An-Nawawi Ad-Dimashqi, Riyad as-Saliheen, Chapter 362: Prohibition of Magic
339. 'Abdul-'Azeez Ibn Baaz, The Ruling on Magic and Fortunetelling https://d1.islamhouse.com/data/en/ih_books/single/en_The_Ruling_on_Magic.pdf
340. Wahid Ibn Abdessalam Bali, Sword against Black Magic&Evil Magicians, https://d1.islamhouse.com/data/en/ih_books/single2/en_black_magic_evil_magicians.pdf
341. Muhammad Tim Humble, Abracadabra: The Sinister World of Magic, https://www.youtube.com/watch?v=an0BUey2eKM
342. Fortune-telling, https://en.wikipedia.org/wiki/Fortune-telling
343. Imam Abu Zakariya Yahya bin Sharaf An-Nawawi Ad-Dimashqi, Riyad as-Saliheen, Chapter 303: Prohibition of Consultation with Soothsayers
344. Imam Abu Zakariya Yahya Ibn Sharaf An-NawawI Ad-Dimashqi, Riyad Us-Saliheen, Chapter 304: Forbiddance of Believing in Ill Omens
345. Sheikh Muhammad Saalih al-Munajjid, Ruling on horoscopes, https://islamqa.info/en/answers/2538
346. Imam Abu Zakariya Yahya bin Sharaf An-Nawawi Ad-Dimashqi, Riyad as-Saliheen, Chapter 325: Prohibition of Attributing Rain to the Stars
347. Sheikh Muhammad Saalih al-Munajjid, Ruling on popular bracelets that are made out of threads, https://islamqa.info/en/answers/88485
348. Abu Ameenah Bilaal Philips, The Fundamentals of Tawheed (Islamic Monotheism), p.75, https://books.google.ae/books?id=8BxlVBPmGlcC&pg=PA75&lpg=PA75&dq
349. Dr. Muhammad Salah, Ruling on wearing amulets against jinn and evil eye, https://www.youtube.com/watch?v=GxBJ0M-yGMQ
350. Sheikh Muhammad Saalih al-Munajjid, Protection from the Evil Eye: How? https://islamqa.info/en/answers/20954
351. Sheikh Muhammad Saalih al-Munajjid, Does Ludo come under the heading of dice games which are prohibited? https://islamqa.info/en/answers/181642
352. Imam Abu Zakariya Yahya bin Sharaf An-Nawawi Ad-Dimashqi, Riyad as-Saliheen, Chapter 270: Prohibition of Envy
353. Sheikh Muhammad Saalih al-Munajjid, Ruling on amulets and hanging them up; do amulets ward off the Evil Eye and hasad (Envy)? https://islamqa.info/en/answers/10543
354. Assim al-Hakeem, Does Saying "Ma sha Allah" Prevent the Evil Eye? https://www.youtube.com/watch?v=87HBOEh0d0g
355. Sheikh Muhammad Saalih al-Munajjid, Barak Allahu Laka or 'Alayk: Ward off the Evil Eye by It, https://islamqa.info/en/answers/130786
356. Alfahim AR. Chapter of the day of judgement and inhabitants of paradise and inhabitants of Hell. *The 200 Hadith (200 sayings and doings of the Prophet Mohammed)*: 76–9)
357. Anil Kumar Mysore Nagaraj, Raveesh Bevinahalli Nanjegowda and S. M. Purushothama, The mystery of reincarnation, https://www.ncbi.nlm.nih.gov/pmc/articles/PMC3705678
358. Sheikh Muhammad Saalih al-Munajjid, Reincarnation in Islam, https://islamqa.info/en/answers/14379/reincarnation-in-islam

359. Dr. Zakir Naik, Reincarnation Tanāsukh According to Islam, https://www.youtube.com/watch?v=rWnnBnST6I8
360. Imam Abu Zakariya Yahya bin Sharaf An-Nawawi Ad-Dimashqi, Riyad-as-Saliheen, Chapter 271: Prohibition of Spying on Muslims and to be Inquisitive about Others
361. Dr. Khalid Al Mosleh, The ruling on spying on the mobile phone of the wife or children, https://www.youtube.com/watch?v=-KuEPj7wsSM
362. Dr. Hassan Elhais, What are the punishments for spying on an individual regardless of the relation?
363. Imam Abu Zakariya Yahya bin Sharaf An-Nawawi Ad-Dimashqi, Riyad as-Saliheen, Chapter 327: Prohibition of Obscenity
364. Imam Abu Zakariya Yahya bin Sharaf An-Nawawi Ad-Dimashqi, Riyad as-Saliheen, Chapter 329: Abomination of Self-Condemnation
365. Imam Abu Zakariya Yahya bin Sharaf An-Nawawi Ad-Dimashqi, Riyad as-Saliheen, Chapter 268: Prohibition of Maligning
366. Imam Abu Zakariya Yahya bin Sharaf An-Nawawi Ad-Dimashqi, Riyad as-Saliheen, Chapter 269: Prohibition of Nursing Rancor and Enmity
367. Imam Abu Zakariya Yahya bin Sharaf An-Nawawi Ad-Dimashqi, Riyad as-Saliheen, Chapter 281: Prohibition of two Holding Secret Counsel to the Exclusion of Conversing together a Third
368. Imam Abu Zakariya Yahya bin Sharaf An-Nawawi Ad-Dimashqi, Riyad as-Saliheen, Chapter 274: Prohibition of Rejoicing over another's Trouble
369. Imam Abu Zakariya Yahya bin Sharaf An-Nawawi Ad-Dimashqi, Riyad as-Saliheen, Chapter 282: Prohibition of Cruelty
370. Sheikh Muhammad Saalih al-Munajjid, Is it permissible to rebel against the ruler? https://islamqa.info/en/answers/9911
371. Sheikh Muhammad Saalih al-Munajjid, Is he sinning if he sees an evil action and does not denounce it? https://islamqa.info/en/answers/96662
372. Muhammad Alshareef, When the Night Equals a Thousand, http://www.unm.edu/~msa/main/night_of_power, https://hadithanswers.com/the-repenter- during-drought-in-the-era-of-nabi-musa-alayhisalam
373. Dua of Musa For Rain, Story of Repentance, https://www.youtube.com/watch?v=19klk2llx5Y
374. Sheikh Muhammad Saalih al-Munajjid, Attitude towards sinners who commit sin openly, https://islamqa.info/en/answers/239089
375. Aisha, https://en.wikipedia.org/wiki/Aisha
376. Sheikh Muhammad Saalih al-Munajjid, The meaning of the hadeeth, "Whoever taunts his brother with a sin" and how sound it is, https://islamqa.info/en/answers/13731
377. Imam Abu Zakariya Yahya bin Sharaf An-Nawawi Ad-Dimashqi, Riyad-as-Saliheen, Chapter 287: Prohibition of taking Ar-Riba (The Usury)
378. Sheikh Muhammad Saalih al-Munajjid, Ruling on dealing with mortgages in a non-Muslim country, https://islamqa.info/en/answers/159213
379. Sheikh Muhammad Saalih al-Munajjid, Credit cards, https://islamqa.info/en/answers/13735
380. Sheikh Muhammad Saalih al-Munajjid, The difference between shares and stocks https://islamqa.info/en/answers/69941

381. Sheikh Muhammad Saalih al-Munajjid, Ruling on currency exchange when it is not possible to make the exchange hand-to-hand because of the war situation, https://islamqa.info/en/answers/268658
382. Sheikh Muhammad Saalih al-Munajjid, Dealing with a company that buys and sells currencies, https://islamqa.info/en/answers/93334
383. Sheikh Assim Al Hakeem, Islamic ruling on Bitcoin and Cryptocurrency, https://www.youtube.com/watch?v=O80kKW_k3bg
384. Dr. Muhammad Salah, Islamic ruling on cryptocurrency, https://www.youtube.com/watch?v=XGwzmPyJ1VA
385. Imam Abu Zakariya Yahya bin Sharaf An-Nawawi Ad-Dimashqi, Riyad as-Saliheen, Chapter 286: Prohibition of devouring the Property of an Orphan
386. Sheikh Muhammad Saalih al-Munajjid, Rulings on seizing things wrongfully, https://islamqa.info/en/answers/10323
387. Sheikh Assim Al Hakeem, Punishment of taking someone's Land or Property unjustly, https://www.youtube.com/watch?v=sLRA_ZI9wSc
388. Sheikh Muhammad Saalih al-Munajjid, What should he do with a tenant who does not want to leave the house? https://islamqa.info/en/answers/45653
389. Sheikh Muhammad Saalih al-Munajjid, Trust (amaanah) in Islam, https://islamqa.info/en/answers/232749
390. Imam Abu Zakariya Yahya bin Sharaf An-Nawawi Ad-Dimashqi, Riyad as-Saliheen, Chapter 79: The Just Ruler
391. Imam Abu Zakariya Yahya bin Sharaf An-Nawawi Ad-Dimashqi, Riyad as-Saliheen, Chapter 80: Obligation of Obedience to the Ruler in what is Lawful and Prohibition of Obeying them in what is Unlawful
392. Sheikh Muhammad Saalih al-Munajjid, Is it permissible to rebel against the ruler? https://islamqa.info/en/answers/9911
393. Sheikh Muhammad Saalih al-Munajjid, Ruling on going on strike, https://islamqa.info/en/answers/5230
394. Atique Tahir, Atiq uz Zafar Khan and Ataullah Khan, Right to Basic Necessities of Life in Islam: Meaning and Concept, https://www.qurtuba.edu.pk/thedialogue/The%20Dialogue/11_2/Dialogue_April_June2016_202-212.pdf
395. Sheikh Muhammad Saalih al-Munajjid, Enjoining what is good and forbidding what is evil, https://islamqa.info/en/answers/11403
396. Imam Abu Zakariya Yahya bin Sharaf An-Nawawi Ad-Dimashqi, Riyad-as-Saliheen, Chapter 293: Prohibition of following the Manners of Satan and Disbelievers
397. Imam Abu Zakariya Yahya bin Sharaf An-Nawawi Ad-Dimashqi, Riyad as-Saliheen, Chapter 72: Condemnation of Pride and Self-Conceit
398. Imam Abu Zakariya Yahya bin Sharaf An-Nawawi Ad-Dimashqi, Riyad as-Saliheen, Chapter 279: Prohibition of Arrogance and Oppression
399. Imam Abu Zakariya Yahya bin Sharaf An-Nawawi Ad-Dimashqi, Riyad as-Saliheen, Chapter 26: Unlawfulness of Oppression and Restoring Others Rights
400. Imam Abu Zakariya Yahya bin Sharaf An-Nawawi Ad-Dimashqi, Riyad as-Saliheen, Chapter 321: Prohibition of Conferring a Title of Honor upon a Sinner, a Hypocrite, and the Like
401. Imam Abu Zakariya Yahya bin Sharaf An-Nawawi Ad-Dimashqi, Riyad as-Saliheen, Chapter 357: Prohibition of Pointing with a Weapon at another Brother in Faith

402. Imam Abu Zakariya Yahya bin Sharaf An-Nawawi Ad-Dimashqi, Riyad as-Saliheen, Chapter 283: Prohibition of Chastisement with Fire
403. Imam Abu Zakariya Yahya bin Sharaf An-Nawawi Ad-Dimashqi, Riyad as-Saliheen, Chapter 300: Prohibition of Leaving the Fire Burning
404. Imam Abu Zakariya Yahya bin Sharaf An-Nawawi Ad-Dimashqi, Riyad as-Saliheen, Chapter 301: Prohibition of putting oneself to Undue Hardship
405. Sheikh Muhammad Saalih al-Munajjid, Concept of democracy in Islam, https://islamqa.info/en/answers/98134
406. Sheikh Muhammad Saalih al-Munajjid, Can we do what we want? https://islamqa.info/en/answers/21521
407. Paul L. Heck, Skepticism in Classical Islam, Moments of Confusion, https://www.routledge.com/Skepticism-in-Classical-Islam-Moments-of-confusion/Heck/p/book/9780367868574
408. Dr. Nazir Khan, Atheism and Radical Skepticism: Ibn Taymiyah's Epistemic Critique, https://yaqeeninstitute.org/read/paper/atheism-and-radical-skepticism-ibn-taymiyyahs-epistemic-critique
409. Imam Abu Zakariya Yahya bin Sharaf An-Nawawi Ad-Dimashqi, Riyad as-Saliheen, Chapter 257: Prohibition of Calumny
410. Imam Abu Zakariya Yahya bin Sharaf An-Nawawi Ad-Dimashqi, Riyad as-Saliheen, Chapter 258: Prohibition of Carrying tales of the Officers
411. Imam Abu Zakariya Yahya bin Sharaf An-Nawawi Ad-Dimashqi, Riyad as-Saliheen, Chapter 254: The Prohibition of Backbiting and the Commandment of Guarding one's Tongue
412. Sheikh Muhammad Saalih al-Munajjid, Backbiting in Islam and Its Expiation, https://islamqa.info/en/answers/23328/backbiting-in-islam-and-its-expiation
413. Imam Abu Zakariya Yahya bin Sharaf An-Nawawi Ad-Dimashqi, Riyad as-Saliheen, Chapter 255: Prohibition of Listening to Backbiting
414. Imam Abu Zakariya Yahya bin Sharaf An-Nawawi Ad-Dimashqi, Riyad as-Saliheen, Chapter 256: Some cases where it is permissible to Backbite
415. Imam Abu Zakariya Yahya bin Sharaf An-Nawawi Ad-Dimashqi, Riyad as-Saliheen, Chapter 262: Ascertainment of what one Hears and Narrates
416. Imam Abu Zakariya Yahya bin Sharaf An-Nawawi Ad-Dimashqi, Riyad as-Saliheen, Chapter 264: Prohibition of Cursing one Particular Man or Animal
417. Imam Abu Zakariya Yahya bin Sharaf An-Nawawi Ad-Dimashqi, Riyad as-Saliheen, Chapter 265: Justification of Cursing the Wrongdoers without Specifying one of them
418. Sheikh Ahmed Fareed, Censure of Ignorance, https://www.kalamullah.com/ilm08.html
419. Sheikh Muhammad Saalih al-Munajjid, If the ignorant person is excused, can he be left in his ignorance? https://islamqa.info/en/answers/118144
420. Imam Abu Zakariya Yahya bin Sharaf An-Nawawi Ad-Dimashqi, Riyad-as-Saliheen, Chapter 284: Prohibition of Procrastinating by a Rich Person to Fulfill his Obligation
421. Imam Abu Zakariya Yahya bin Sharaf An-Nawawi Ad-Dimashqi, Riyad-as-Saliheen, Chapter 314: Prohibition of Swearing in the name of anything besides Allah
422. Sheikh Muhammad Saalih al-Munajjid, It is not permissible to cheat in exams no matter what the motives, https://islamqa.info/en/answers/175744
423. Sheikh Muhammad Saalih al-Munajjid, Questions about the punishment for hiraabah (aggression), https://islamqa.info/en/answers/2936

424. Imam Abu Zakariya Yahya bin Sharaf An-Nawawi Ad-Dimashqi, Riyad as-Saliheen, Chapter 277: Prohibition of the Treachery and Breaking one's Covenant
425. Imam Abu Zakariya Yahya bin Sharaf An-Nawawi Ad-Dimashqi, Riyad as-Saliheen, Chapter 316: Desirability of Expiating the Oath taken by a Person who afterwards Breaks it for a better Alternative
426. Imam Abu Zakariya Yahya bin Sharaf An-Nawawi Ad-Dimashqi, Riyad as-Saliheen, Chapter 317: Expiation of Oaths
427. Imam Abu Zakariya Yahya bin Sharaf An-Nawawi Ad-Dimashqi, Riyadas-Saliheen, Chapter 318: Abomination of Swearing in Transaction
428. Sheikh Muhammad Saalih al-Munajjid, Ruling on working as a tax adviser, https://islamqa.info/en/answers/243867
429. Sheikh Muhammad Saalih al-Munajjid, Ruling on financial penalties in Islam, https://islamqa.info/en/answers/21900
430. Sheikh Muhammad Saalih al-Munajjid, Should he pay money in order to get a job? https://islamqa.info/en/answers/60183
431. Sheikh Muhammad Saalih al-Munajjid, Paying a bribe in order to get one's rights, https://islamqa.info/en/answers/72268
432. Imam Abu Zakariya Yahya bin Sharaf An-Nawawi Ad-Dimashqi, Riyad-as-Saliheen, Chapter 288: Prohibition of Show-off
433. Imam Abu Zakariya Yahya bin Sharaf An-Nawawi Ad-Dimashqi, Riyad-as-Saliheen, Chapter 289: Things not to be Considered as Showing off
434. Imam Abu Zakariya Yahya bin Sharaf An-Nawawi Ad-Dimashqi, Riyad-as-Saliheen, Chapter 278: Prohibition of Recounting of Favors
435. Sheikh Muhammad Saalih al-Munajjid, Praying for the one who treats you kindly by saying "Jazak Allaahu khayran", https://islamqa.info/en/answers/84976
436. Imam Abu Zakariya Yahya bin Sharaf An-Nawawi Ad-Dimashqi, Riyad as-Saliheen, Chapter 242: The Obligation of Gratitude
437. Sheikh Muhammad Saalih al-Munajjid, How to Thank Allah for His Blessings, https://islamqa.info/en/answers/125984
438. Imam Abu Zakariya Yahya bin Sharaf An-Nawawi Ad-Dimashqi, Riyad-as-Saliheen, Chapter 305: Prohibition of Drawing Portraits
439. Sheikh Muhammad Saalih al-Munajjid, Ruling on photographs https://islamqa.info/en/answers/365
440. Imam Abu Zakariya Yahya bin Sharaf An-Nawawi Ad-Dimashqi, Riyad-as-Saliheen, Chapter 302: Prohibition of Bewailing the Deceased
441. Sheikh Muhammad Saalih al-Munajjid, Praying at graves and the conditions of intercession, https://islamqa.info/en/answers/13490
442. Imam Abu Zakariya Yahya bin Sharaf An-Nawawi Ad-Dimashqi, Riyad-as-Saliheen, Chapter 342: Prohibition of facing the Graves during Salat (Prayer)
443. Sheikh Muhammad Saalih al-Munajjid, Ruling on congregational du'aa' for the deceased and paying the imam for reciting the du'aa', https://islamqa.info/en/answers/174715
444. Imam Abu Zakariya Yahya bin Sharaf An-Nawawi Ad-Dimashqi, Riyad-as-Saliheen, Chapter 354: Prohibition of Mourning beyond Three Days (for Women)
445. Imam Abu Zakariya Yahya Ibn Sharaf An-Nawawi Ad-Dimashqi, Riyad Us-Saliheen, Chapter 347: Prohibition of Sitting on the Graves

446. Imam Abu Zakariya Yahya Ibn Sharaf An-Nawawi Ad-Dimashqi, Riyad Us-Saliheen, Chapter 348: Prohibition of Plastering and Building over the Graves
447. Sheikh Muhammad Saalih al-Munajjid, Visiting graves and attending occasions on which they say that the souls of the awliyaa' are present, https://islamqa.info/en/answers/6744
448. Imam Abu Zakariya Yahya Ibn Sharaf An-Nawawi Ad-Dimashqi, Riyad Us-Saliheen, Chapter 267: Prohibition of Abusing the Deceased without a valid legal reason approved by Shari'ah
449. Imam Abu Zakariya Yahya Ibn Sharaf An-Nawawi Ad-Dimashqi, Riyad Us-Saliheen, Chapter 154: Prohibition of Disclosing the Physical defects of the Deceased
450. Sheikh Muhammad Saalih al-Munajjid, Stages of trials for the deceased in his grave and du'aa' for him at that time, https://islamqa.info/en/answers/197749
451. Sheikh Muhammad Saalih al-Munajjid, Ruling on wearing black in mourning for the dead https://islamqa.info/en/answers/47488
452. Imam Abu Zakariya Yahya bin Sharaf An-Nawawi Ad-Dimashqi, Riyad as-Saliheen, Chapter 67: Abomination of longing for Death
453. Imam Abu Zakariya Yahya Ibn Sharaf An-Nawawi Ad-Dimashqi, Riyad as-Saliheen, Chapter 349: Prohibition for a Slave to run away from his Master
454. Sheikh Muhammad Saalih al-Munajjid, His company is late in giving him his salary; what should he do? https://islamqa.info/en/answers/95294
455. Sheikh Muhammad Saalih al-Munajjid, Can he accept help from the state? https://islamqa.info/en/answers/127193
456. Sheikh Muhammad Saalih al-Munajjid, He works in a mixed environment in a non-Muslim country; should he leave it and take unemployment benefit or carry on working there? https://islamqa.info/en/answers/125118
457. Imam Abu Zakariya Yahya bin Sharaf An-Nawawi Ad-Dimashqi, Riyad as-Saliheen, Chapter 355: Prohibition of Malpractices in Commerce
458. Sheikh Muhammad Saalih al-Munajjid, The phenomenon of cheating, https://islamqa.info/en/answers/22845
459. Sheikh Muhammad Saalih al-Munajjid, Selling a product at different prices to different customers, https://islamqa.info/en/answers/13641
460. Sheikh Muhammad Saalih al-Munajjid, Meaning of the verse "And were it not that all mankind would have become of one community…" [az-Zukhruf 43:33], https://islamqa.info/en/answers/225941
461. Sheikh Muhammad Saalih al-Munajjid, It is not permissible to sell something that will be used for sinful purposes, https://islamqa.info/en/answers/34587
462. Imam Abu Zakariya Yahya bin Sharaf An-Nawawi Ad-Dimashqi, Riyad as-Saliheen, Chapter 276: Prohibition of Deceiving others
463. Sheikh Muhammad Saalih al-Munajjid, Can she use things that her father takes from work unlawfully? https://islamqa.info/en/answers/31217
464. Sheikh Muhammad Saalih al-Munajjid, Dealing with companies that use pyramid marketing, https://islamqa.info/en/answers/96708
465. Sheikh Muhammad Saalih al-Munajjid, Buying lottery tickets, https://islamqa.info/en/answers/6476
466. Imam Abu Zakariya Yahya bin Sharaf An-Nawawi Ad-Dimashqi, Riyad as-Saliheen, Chapter 356: Prohibition of Squandering Wealth

467. Sheikh Muhammad Saalih al-Munajjid, Ruling on selling exorbitantly expensive telephone numbers and "custom" license plates, https://islamqa.info/en/answers/40752
468. Sheikh Muhammad Saalih al-Munajjid, It is not permissible to say that rule belongs to the people or that wealth is the wealth of the people, https://islamqa.info/en/answers/14061
469. Sheikh Muhammad Saalih al-Munajjid, Requirements for proper Islamic dress for a woman, https://islamqa.info/en/answers/235
470. Imam Abu Zakariya Yahya bin Sharaf An-Nawawi Ad-Dimashqi, Riyad as-Saliheen, Chapter 365: Prohibition of Wearing Saffron-Colored Dress
471. Sheikh Muhammad Saalih al-Munajjid, Verses and Ahadeeth about hijab, https://islamqa.info/en/answers/13998
472. Sheikh Muhammad Saalih al-Munajjid, Ruling concerning women covering their feet in prayer, https://islamqa.info/en/answers/1046
473. Sheikh Muhammad Saalih al-Munajjid, If a woman did not cover her feet when praying, out of ignorance, does she have to repeat her prayer? https://islamqa.info/en/answers/193034
474. Muhammad Salah, Can Women Pray Without Socks, https://www.youtube.com/watch?v=Qc_7EvzHW3U
475. Sheikh Muhammad Saalih al-Munajjid, Is it permissible for her to wear kohl when going out of the house? https://islamqa.info/en/answers/67897
476. Faisal Ibn Abdul Qaadir Ibn Hassan and Abu Sulaymaan, Ruling on Sisters Giving Dawah Online and Off Camera, https://torontodawah.com/ruling-on-sisters-giving-dawah-online-and-off-camera
477. Sheikh Muhammad Saalih al-Munajjid, Women and da'wah, https://islamqa.info/en/answers/21730
478. Imam Abu Zakariya Yahya bin Sharaf An-Nawawi Ad-Dimashqi, Riyad as-Saliheen, Chapter 299: Undesirability of Wearing one Shoe or Sock
479. Imam Abu Zakariya Yahya bin Sharaf An-Nawawi Ad-Dimashqi, Riyad as-Saliheen, Chapter 124: Prohibition of using the skin of the Leopard
480. Imam Abu Zakariya Yahya bin Sharaf An-Nawawi Ad-Dimashqi, Riyad as-Saliheen, Chapter 292: Prohibition for Men and Women Apeing One Another
481. Sheikh Muhammad Saalih al-Munajjid, Are Muslim Men Allowed to Wear Bracelets? https://islamqa.info/en/answers/148059
482. Muhammad Salah, Wearing Wristbands for Men, https://www.youtube.com/watch?v=9AEkgtkQMbo
483. Imam Abu Zakariya Yahya bin Sharaf An-Nawawi Ad-Dimashqi, Riyad as-Saliheen, Chapter 296: Prohibition of Wearing False Hair, Tattooing and Filling of Teeth
484. Imam Abu Zakariya Yahya bin Sharaf An-Nawawi Ad-Dimashqi, Riyad as-Saliheen, Chapter 294: Forbidding to Dye Hair Black
485. Imam Abu Zakariya Yahya bin Sharaf An-Nawawi Ad-Dimashqi, Riyad-as-Saliheen, Chapter 295: On Prohibition of Shaving a part of Head
486. Sheikh Muhammad Saalih al-Munajjid, Ruling on a man tying up his long hair, https://islamqa.info/en/answers/128184
487. Imam Abu Zakariya Yahya bin Sharaf An-Nawawi Ad-Dimashqi, Riyad as-Saliheen, Chapter 297: Prohibition of Plucking Grey Hairs

488. Sheikh Muhammad Saalih al-Munajjid, Are Fake Eyelashes Haram? https://islamqa.info/en/answers/39301
489. Sheikh Muhammad Saalih al-Munajjid, Wearing coloured contact lenses, https://islamqa.info/en/answers/926
490. Sheikh Muhammad Saalih al-Munajjid, Is Makeup Haram? https://islamqa.info/en/answers/119359
491. Sheikh Muhammad Saalih al-Munajjid, Ruling on Muslims congratulating one another on the occasion of the Gregorian New Year, https://islamqa.info/en/answers/177460
492. Sheikh Muhammad Saalih al-Munajjid, Celebrating birthdays is not allowed, https://islamqa.info/en/answers/1027
493. Sheikh Muhammad Saalih al-Munajjid, Ruling on Celebrating Valentine's Day, https://islamqa.info/en/answers/73007
494. Sheikh Muhammad Saalih al-Munajjid, Conditions Acceptability of Deeds by Allah, https://islamqa.info/en/answers/14258
495. Sheikh Muhammad Saalih al-Munajjid, Why doesnt Allah answer our duaas? https://islamqa.info/en/answers/5113
496. Sheikh Muhammad Saalih al-Munajjid, What is meant by thinking positively of Allah, and practical examples thereof, https://islamqa.info/en/answers/150516
497. Sheikh Muhammad Saalih al-Munajjid, Conditions of du'aa' being accepted by Allah, https://islamqa.info/en/answers/13506
498. Sheikh Muhammad Saalih al-Munajjid, Parents' Du'a Against Children, https://islamqa.info/en/answers/90178
499. Sheikh Muhammad Saalih al-Munajjid, Detailed discussion of Bid'ah and Shirk, https://islamqa.info/en/answers/10543
500. Sheikh Muhammad Saalih al-Munajjid, Singling Out Ayat to Recite at Times of Hardship and Difficulty, https://islamqa.info/en/answers/115841
501. What do the scholars say about reading the Quran after the Asr prayer? https://www.majesticquran.co.uk/what-do-the-scholars-say-about-reading-the-quran-after-the-asr-prayer
502. Sheikh Muhammad Saalih al-Munajjid, The Bid'ah (innovation) of encouraging billions of salawaat upon the Messenger of Allah on the occasion of the Mawlid (Prophet's Birthday), https://islamqa.info/en/answers/126367
503. Sheikh Muhammad Saalih al-Munajjid, Making Du'a After Obligatory Salah: Bid'ah? https://islamqa.info/en/answers/21976
504. Ustaadh Abu Ubaydah, Bid'ah (Innovation) and it's examples, https://trulysalafiyyah.wordpress.com/2014/03/05/bidah-innovation-and-its-examples-by-abu-ubaydah
505. Sheikh Muhammad Saalih al-Munajjid, The Bid'ah of superstition about getting married in Shawwaal, https://islamqa.info/en/answers/12364
506. Immigration to a Majority Non-Muslim Country, https://fiqh.islamonline.net/en/immigration-to-a-majority-non-muslim-country
507. Sheikh Muhammad Saalih al-Munajjid, Can Muslims settle in kaafir countries for the sake of a better life? https://islamqa.info/en/answers/13363
508. Sheikh Muhammad Saalih al-Munajjid, Ruling on watching TV, https://islamqa.info/en/answers/3633
509. Imam Abu Zakariya Yahya bin Sharaf An-Nawawi Ad-Dimashqi, Riyad as-Saliheen, Chapter 306: Prohibition of Keeping a Dog except as a Watchdog or Hunting Dog

510. Imam Abu Zakariya Yahya bin Sharaf An-Nawawi Ad-Dimashqi, Riyad as-Saliheen, Chapter 307: Undesirability of Hanging Bells round the Necks of Animals
511. Sheikh Muhammad Saalih al-Munajjid, Ruling on selling cats, https://islamqa.info/en/answers/69770
512. Assim al Hakeem, Can we sell cats, dogs, snakes & other exotic animals & Can we keep them as pets? https://www.youtube.com/watch?v=r1MNsmg9HFc
513. Imam Abu Zakariya Yahya bin Sharaf An-Nawawi Ad-Dimashqi, Riyad as-Saliheen, Chapter 323: Prohibition of Reviling the Wind
514. Sheikh Muhammad Saalih al-Munajjid, What is the ruling on professional pursuit of football (soccer)? https://islamqa.info/en/answers/75644
515. Sheikh Muhammad Saalih al-Munajjid, Is it permissible to watch football (soccer) games on television? https://islamqa.info/en/answers/146844
516. Sheikh Muhammad Saalih al-Munajjid, What Is the Ruling on Yoga? https://islamqa.info/en/answers/101591
517. Sheikh Muhammad Saalih al-Munajjid, If a person is persisting in Minor sins, will praying for forgiveness be of any benefit so that they do not become Major sins? https://islamqa.info/en/answers/184515
518. Imam Abu Zakariya Yahya bin Sharaf An-Nawawi Ad-Dimashqi, Riyad as-Saliheen, Chapter 179: Prohibiting Woman from Traveling Alone
519. Sheikh Muhammad Saalih al-Munajjid, Ruling on travelling alone, https://islamqa.info/en/answers/105280
520. Islam Prohibits Mars Trips: UAE Fatwa, https://islamstory.com/en/artical/17017, http://onislam.net/english/news/middle-east/469405
521. Sheikh Muhammad Saalih al-Munajjid, Evidence for the prohibition on commercial insurance, https://islamqa.info/en/answers/130761
522. Sheikh Muhammad Saalih al-Munajjid, Ruling on medical treatment, https://islamqa.info/en/answers/2438
523. Health Care Fraud, https://www.fbi.gov/scams-and-safety/common-scams-and-crimes/health-care-fraud
524. Dr Mira Bajirova, Cancer is a Jinn (Demonic) Possession. The Ultimate Cure.
525. Serotonin Syndrome, https://www.mayoclinic.org/diseases-conditions/serotonin-syndrome/symptoms-causes/syc-20354758
526. Elizabeth L. Whitlock, Andrea Vannucci and Michael S. Avidan, Postoperative Delirium, https://www.ncbi.nlm.nih.gov/pmc/articles/PMC3615670
527. Muhammad Salman Janjua, Benjamin C. Spurlin, Mary E. Arthur, Postoperative Delirium, https://www.ncbi.nlm.nih.gov/books/NBK534831
528. Angela Yang, Common treatment for joint pain may be linked to faster arthritis progression, research suggests, https://www.nbcnews.com/health/health-news/common-pain-treatment-arthritis-faster-progression-rcna58975
529. Dr. Mira Bajirova, Miraculous Effects of Negative Ions on Male Infertility, https://www.researchgate.net/publication/324030908
530. Dr Mira Bajirova, Infertility Caused by Decreased Oxygen Utilization and Jinn (Demon)
531. Dr. Mira Bajirova, Natural Pregnancy by Negative Ions in Young Woman with Premature Menopause, https://www.researchgate.net/publication/324031250

532. Dr. Mira Bajirova, Natural Pregnancy by Negative Ions in Young Woman with Ovarian Poor Reserve after Four Failed IVF, https://www.ecronicon.com/ecgy/pdf/ECGY-SPI-0S103....
533. Dr. Mira Bajirova, Ovarian Dermoid Cyst: Ruqya and Negative Ions Treatment, https://www.researchgate.net/publication/327551384
534. Dr. Mira Bajirova, Negative Ions and Ovarian Cancer, https://www.researchgate.net/publication/324031376
535. Dr. Mira Bajirova, Urological Diseases: Ruqya and Negative Ions Treatment, https://lupinepublishers.com/reproductive-medicine-journal/fulltext/urological-diseases-ruqya-and-negative-ions-treatment.ID.000123.php
536. Dr. Mira Bajirova, Miraculous effects of Negative Ions on Urogenital Infections, https://medcraveonline.com/OGIJ/miraculous-effects-of-negative-ions-on-urogenital-infections.html
537. Dr. Mira Bajirova, Negative Ions (Anion) Sanitary Napkins and Women Health, https://www.researchgate.net/publication/324031377
538. Dr Mira Bajirova, Ruqya and Negative Ions Treatment, https://opastpublishers.com/wp-content/uploads/2018/11/ruqya-and-negative-ions-treatment-jcrc-18.pdf
539. All about side effects, https://www.medicalnewstoday.com/articles/196135
540. Amber N. Edinoff, Long H. Nguyen, Mary Jo Fitz-Gerald, etc., Lamotrigine and Stevens-Johnson Syndrome Prevention, https://www.ncbi.nlm.nih.gov/pmc/articles/PMC8146560
541. Amanda M. Oakley, Karthik Krishnamurthy, Stevens Johnson Syndrome, https://www.ncbi.nlm.nih.gov/books/NBK459323
542. Laura Lindsey, Lecturer, Pharmacy Practice, Newcastle University, Antipsychotic withdrawal – an unrecognised and misdiagnosed problem, January 2023, https://theconversation.com/antipsychotic-withdrawal-an-unrecognised-and-misdiagnosed-problem-196989
543. 10 Scariest Prescription Drug Side Effects https://www.pharmacytimes.com/view/10-scariest-prescription-drug-side-effects
544. P. Häusermann, Th. Harr, A. J. Bircher, Baboon syndrome resulting from systemic drugs: is there strife between SDRIFE and allergic contact dermatitis syndrome? https://onlinelibrary.wiley.com/doi/abs/10.1111/j.0105-1873.2004.00445.x
545. James Peter Blackmur, Simon Lammy, David E C Baring, Baboon syndrome: an unusual complication arising from antibiotic treatment of tonsillitis and review of the literature, https://casereports.bmj.com/content/2013/bcr-2013-201977
546. Dr. Keith Roach: Cholesterol medications produce rare side effect, https://www.detroitnews.com/story/life/advice/2022/11/29/dr-roach-cholesterol-medications-produce-rare-side-effect/69683307007
547. Side-effects and complications of heart surgery, https://www.ctsnet.org/sites/default/files/images/Side-effects.pdf
548. Imam Abu Zakariya Yahya bin Sharaf An-Nawawi Ad-Dimashqi, Riyad as-Saliheen, Chapter 361: Undesirability of departing from or coming to a Place stricken by an Epidemic
549. Dr. Mira Bajirova, Vaccines for Coronavirus and Other Diseases Increase Death

550. Osawa, Motoki MD, PhD; Nagao, Ryoko MD and others, Sudden Infant Death After Vaccination Survey of Forensic Autopsy Files, https://journals.lww.com/amjforensicmedicine/fulltext/2019/09000
551. Neil Z.Miller, Vaccines and sudden infant death: An analysis of the VAERS database 1990–2019 and review of the medical literature, https://www.sciencedirect.com/science/article/pii/S2214750021001268
552. Coronavirus: Woman left in coma after COVID jab, diagnosed with a serious condition and is in constant pain, https://timesofindia.indiatimes.com/life-style/health-fitness/health-news/coronavirus-woman-left-in-coma-after-covid-jab-diagnosed-with-a-serious-condition-and-is-in-constant-pain/photostory/95943254.cms?picid=95943317
553. Yue Chen, Zhiwei Xu, Peng Wang and others, New-onset autoimmune phenomena post-COVID-19 vaccination, https://pubmed.ncbi.nlm.nih.gov/34957554
554. Andrew Joseph, Covid's strange moment: Joy over vaccines coincides with new levels of deaths and hospitalizations in U.S., Dec. 15, 2020, https://www.statnews.com/2020/12/15/even-as-vaccines-raise-hope-record-hospitalizations-covid-19
555. Cynthia Cox, Krutika Amin, Jennifer Kates, etc., Why Do Vaccinated People Represent Most COVID-19 Deaths Right Now? https://www.kff.org/policy-watch/why-do-vaccinated-people-represent-most-covid-19-deaths-right-now
556. Jennifer M. Watchmaker, Puneet B. Belani, Brain death in a vaccinated patient with COVID-19 Infection, https://www.ncbi.nlm.nih.gov/pmc/articles/PMC8502685
557. Dr. Mira Bajirova, Coronavirus is the Result of Humanity's Sins
558. Dr. Mira Bajirova, The Divine Cure of Coronavirus and Widespread Diseases
559. Vaccine Mandates: an unjustified assault on our human rights and freedoms https://humanrights.gov.au/sites/default/files/2020-09/sub_148_-_australian_vaccination-risks_network_inc.pdf
560. Casey Ross, Cleveland Clinic to censure doctor who promoted anti-vaccine claims, https://www.statnews.com/2017/01/08/cleveland-clinic-vaccines-response
561. Baby dies 2 hrs after being vaccinated under regular immunization programme in Nandurbar https://indianexpress.com/article/cities/mumbai/baby-dies-2-hrs-after-being-vaccinated-under-regular-immunisation-programme-in-nandurbar-7216054
562. Concerns over Efficacy and Cost of Muscle Wasting Treatments, https://www.the-scientist.com/news-opinion/concerns-over-efficacy-and-cost-of-muscle-wasting-treatments-68144
563. Miryam Naddaf, $3.5-Million Hemophilia Gene Therapy Is World's Most Expensive Drug, https://www.scientificamerican.com/article/3-5-million-hemophilia-gene-therapy-is-worlds-most-expensive-drug
564. Ibrahim Abdullah Al Hazemy, Those who repented to Allah (Cancer led me to My Creator...A Story of Repentance), https://www.islamicboard.com/general/17990-cancer-led-creator-story-repentance.html
565. Nedium Botic, A Bosnian Man Was Cured of a Tumor After He Went to Hajj and Drank Only, https://ilmfeed.com/bosnian-man-cured-tumor-went-hajj-drank-zamzam-water
566. Nouman Ali Khan, Dua Cured My Cancer, https://www.youtube.com/watch?v=RrzKJeftwqc
567. Sheikh bin Baaz, Infertility is an Expiation of Sins, https://www.youtube.com/watch?v=VAGWshVE-Kk

568. Ibn Taymiyah, Diseases of the Hearts and their Cures, https://www.kalamullah.com/Books/Diseases
569. Samer Elkassem, Islam and Obesity, https://www.virtualmosque.com/society/health-and-fitness/islam-and-obesity
570. Yasir Qadhi, Obesity in the Final days (Prophecy of the end times), https://www.youtube.com/watch?v=9rT9gJ0jptg
571. Dr. Bilal Philips, The Worst Container, Obesity, https://www.youtube.com/watch?v=0w4Y6hpK6Eg
572. Melinda Ratini, DO, MS, Health Risks Linked to Obesity, https://www.webmd.com/diet/obesity/obesity-health-risks
573. Obesity plays major role in triggering autoimmune diseases, https://www.sciencedaily.com/releases/2014/11/141110110722.htm
574. Jensen P. and Skov L., Psoriasis and Obesity, https://www.karger.com/Article/Fulltext/455840
575. Aniyizhai Annamalai, Urska Kosir, and Cenk Tek, Prevalence of obesity and diabetes in patients with schizophrenia, https://www.ncbi.nlm.nih.gov/pmc/articles/PMC5561038
576. Wei-Zheng Li, Kyle Stirling, Jun-Jie Yang, and Lei Zhang, Gut microbiota and diabetes: From correlation to causality and mechanism, https://www.ncbi.nlm.nih.gov/pmc/articles/PMC7415231
577. Ole A. Andreassen, M.D., Ph.D. Diabetes and Schizophrenia - New Findings for an Old Puzzle, https://ajp.psychiatryonline.org/doi/10.1176/appi.ajp.2017.17040409
578. Anastasia Climan, How Are MS and Diabetes Related? Risks and Management, https://www.mymsteam.com/resources/how-are-ms-and-diabetes-related-risks-and-management
579. Magdalena Celińska-Löwenhoff, Jacek Musiał Psychiatric manifestations of autoimmune diseases – diagnostic and therapeutic problems, http://Psychiatriapolska.pl/uploads/images/pp 62012/engvercelinkska-lowenhoff2012v4616.pdf
580. David B Weiss, Jarl Dyrud, Robert M House, Thomas P Beresford, Psychiatric manifestations of autoimmune disorders, https://pubmed.ncbi.nlm.nih.gov/16079045
581. Neuropsychiatric symptoms that may be caused by an Autoimmune reaction. https://www.moleculeralabs.com/neuropsychiatric-symptoms)
582. 10 Verses of Surah al Baqarah: a key to treasures, https://muslimvillage.com/2018/12/07/118398/last-10-verses-sura-al-baqarah
583. Abul Mundhir Khaleel, The Jinn and Human Sickness.
584. Sheikh Abu Mujahid, Can schizophrenia be from Jinn Possession? https://www.youtube.com/watch?v=oMqM4ZH57T0
585. Mufti Menk, Mental Health Issues & How to Solve Them, https://www.youtube.com/watch?v=u1DTdmaSY9o
586. Sheikh Muhammad Saalih al-Munajjid, The punishment for homosexuality, https://islamqa.info/en/answers/38622/the-punishment-for-homosexuality
587. Dyan Neary, What Happened to Maya When a 10-year-old girl complained of mysterious pain, a doctor suspected child abuse. How far would she go to prove it? https://www.thecut.com/2022/10/child-abuse-munchausen-syndrome-by-proxy.html
588. Dr. Karim AbuZaid, Children with Autism: A Possible Jinni possession, https://www.youtube.com/watch?v=_spl0R8OG6Q

589. Autism documentary: Somalis have no word for it - and some doubt it exists, https://www.youtube.com/watch?v=IIrG5KgzW-U
590. M. Farhan, Autism Awareness in Islam, https://www.youtube.com/watch?v=tgZ5KPsQXuY
591. AbdulRahman Hassan, Islam and Autism, https://www.youtube.com/watch?v=8CeAQnQcE6g
592. Mufti Menk, You have disabled autistic child must listen, https://www.youtube.com/watch?v=R46Wu_ZjsBI
593. Sheikh Yasir Fazaga, Friday khutbah. Autism Islamic Perspective, https://www.youtube.com/watch?v=sHLPyn37eeE
594. Mufti Menk, Memory loss because of Sin, https://www.youtube.com/watch?v=A1vsvfHOC0Q
595. Wife of Alzheimer's patient recalls violent behavior in latter stage, https://www.youtube.com/watch?v=QVhGKnRZLBA
596. 5 Most common Alzheimer's behaviors / Knowledge is Power, https://www.youtube.com/watch?v=O4PsmwWeuio
597. Dr. Mira Bajirova, Infertility caused by Jinn, https://www.lupinepublishers.com/oajrsd/pdf/OAJRSD...
598. Study Uncovers Link Between Allergies and Mental Health Conditions, https://neurosciencenews.com/mental-health-allergies-19421
599. What's the link between mental health and allergies? https://www.medicalnewstoday.com/articles/whats-the-link-between-mental-health-and-allergies
600. Hans Oh, Ai Koyanagi, Jordan E. De Vylder and Andrew Stickley, Seasonal Allergies and Psychiatric Disorders in the United States, https://www.ncbi.nlm.nih.gov/pmc/articles/PMC6164754
601. Allergic conditions and Mental Illness, https://allergyexperts.com/allergic-conditions-mental-illness-is-there-a-link
602. Salynn Boyles, Gluten Intolerance Linked to Schizophrenia, https://www.webmd.com/schizophrenia/news/20040219/gluten-intolerance-linked-to-schizophrenia
603. Celiac Disease is a Risk Factor for Schizophrenia, https://publichealth.jhu.edu/2004/celiac-schizophrenia
604. Nicole Beurkens, There is a Link Between Allergies And Mental Health Conditions, http://www.drbeurkens.com/there-is-a-link-between-allergies-and-mental-health-conditions)
605. Ruling on Using Relaxants and Sleeping Pills to Treat Anxiety and Insomnia, https://islamqa.info/en/answers/297773
606. Stem Cell Therapy for Spinal Cord Injury, https://www.cellmedicine.com/stem-cell-therapy-for-spinal-cord-injury.
607. Sheikh Muhammad Saalih al-Munajjid, Stem cells: definition, ruling on setting up stem cell banks and using them for medical purposes, https://islamqa.info/en/answers/108125
608. Sheikh Muhammad Saalih al-Munajjid, Ruling on medicines that are mixed with alcohol, https://islamqa.info/en/answers/40530
609. Sheikh Muhammad Saalih al-Munajjid, The doctor prescribed medicine that contains narcotics; is it permissible for him to take it? https://islamqa.info/en/answers/192321
610. Intoxicants definition, https://www.lawinsider.com/dictionary/intoxicants

611. Ahmad H. Sakr, Professor of Biochemistry and Nutrition. Pork: Possible Reasons for its Prohibition, http://web.ipb.ac.id/~erizal/pork_reasons.
612. Sheikh Muhammad Saalih al-Munajjid, Ruling on homoeopathy, https://islamqa.info/en/answers/111004
613. Sheikh Muhammad Saalih al-Munajjid, Ruling on Treating Patients with Music https://islamqa.info/en/answers/106605
614. Sheikh Muhammad Saalih al-Munajjid, Ruling on dealing in so-called "healing crystals" https://islamqa.info/en/answers/192206
615. Sheikh Muhammad Saalih al-Munajjid, What is the ruling on believing in auras and energy healing? https://islamqa.info/en/answers/276254
616. Sheikh Muhammad Saalih al-Munajjid, Ruling on using a "Biodisc" and the ruling on wearing "Chi pendants" for benefit or healing, https://islamqa.info/en/answers/138578
617. Sheikh Muhammad Saalih al-Munajjid, Taking a patient off a respirator and the ruling on mercy Killing, https://islamqa.info/en/answers/129041
618. Sheikh Muhammad Saalih al-Munajjid, Lengthening and shortening lifespans, https://islamqa.info/en/answers/110439
619. Ibn Kathir, The Story of Ayub (Job), https://sunnahonline.com/library/stories-of-the-prophets/820-the-story-of-prophet-ayyub-job
620. Joan Arehart-Treichel, Negative Ions May Offer Unexpected MH Benefit, https://psychnews.psychiatryonline.org/doi/full/10.1176/pn.42.1.0025
621. Fiqh-us-Sunnah, vol.1. https://www.iium.edu.my/deed/lawbase/fiqh_us_sunnah/vol1/fsn_vol1a.html
622. Dr. Noburu Horiguchi, Science: Power of Negative Ions - Restorative Medicine of Nature, https://www.youtube.com/watch?v=PTRtKby8P80
623. Denise Mann, Negative Ions Create Positive Vibes, https://www.webmd.com/balance/features/negative-ions-create-positive-vibes
624. Michael Terman, Treatment of Seasonal Affective Disorder with a High-Output Negative Ionizer, https://www.researchgate.net/publication/13833748
625. Shu-Ye Jiang, Ali Ma, and Srinivasan Ramachandran, Negative Air Ions and Their Effects on Human Health and Air Quality Improvement, https://www.ncbi.nlm.nih.gov/pmc/articles/PMC6213340
626. Dr. Ibrahim B. Syed, The Jinn- A Scientific Analysis, https://www.irfi.org/articles/articles_1_50/jinn_a_scientific_analysis.htm
627. Ali Shahzad, A Jinn-A Scientific Outlook, http://qolumnist.com/ en/author/ali-shahzad
628. Mahmood Jawaid, The Nature of the Jinns. An Explanation based on the Quran and Science, https://www.academia.edu/9642981
629. Dr. Pierce Howard, The Owner's Manual for the Brain (4th Edition): The Ultimate Guide to Peak Mental Performance at All Ages
630. A J Giannini, B T Jones, R H Loiselle, Reversibility of serotonin irritation syndrome with atmospheric anions, https://pubmed.ncbi.nlm.nih.gov/3949723
631. Jean-Yves Cote, The Ion Miracle: The effects of Negative Ions on physical and mental well-being
632. Baby Rupert Scalded Skin Syndrome Anion pads helping to heal, https://www.youtube.com/watch?v=CuiB9bXsuK4
633. Michele L. Tuttle U.S Geological Survey Michael A. Clark, M.D. Armed Forces Institute of Pathology, Harry R. Compton U.S. Department of the interior U.S.

633. Geological Survey 21 August 1986 Lake Nyos Gas Disaster, Cameroon Final Report of the United States Scientific Team to the Office of U.S. Foreign Disaster Assistance of the Agency for International Development Environmental Protection Agency, https://pubs.usgs.gov/of/1987/0097/report.pdf
634. Ibn Al-Qayyim, Healing with the Medicine of the Prophet, https://kalamullah.com/Books/Medicine.pdf
635. Dr Bilal Philips, The Exorcism Tradition in Islam
636. 9 Facts About Satan You Should Know https://www.islamicity.org/77304/9-amazing-facts-about-satan-to-defeat-him
637. Sheikh Muhammad Saalih al-Munajjid, Shaytaan's Enmity Towards Man, https://islamqa.info/en/answers/13308
638. Sheikh Muhammad Saalih al-Munajjid, Does the Devil Know the Thoughts and Intentions of Man? https://islamqa.info/en/answers/118151
639. Sheikh Muhammad Saalih al-Munajjid, He found out that his Shaykh deals with jinn, https://islamqa.info/en/answers/102843/he-found-out-that-his-shaykh-deals-with-jinn
640. Assim al Hakeem, Is it permissible to watch videos of people who have been possessed by jinn? https://www.youtube.com/watch?v=8n3rDRQMdlM
641. Assim al Hakeem, Is it permissible to interact with Jinn? https://www.youtube.com/watch?v=898Yo0IILxY
642. Dr. Muhammad Salah, Can we interact with Jinn? Is it shirk to ask them favours? https://www.youtube.com/watch?v=KjClnrhxJYw
643. Sheikh Muhammad Saalih al-Munajjid, Ruling on surgery that causes sterility. https://islamqa.info/en/answers/2160
644. Sheikh Muhammad Saalih al-Munajjid, Ruling on aborting a foetus before Forty days, https://islamqa.info/en/answers/171943
645. Sheikh Muhammad Saalih al-Munajjid, Abortion after the soul has been breathed into the foetus, https://islamqa.info/en/answers/13319
646. Sheikh Muhammad Saalih al-Munajjid, Prohibition on Selling Blood, https://islamqa.info/en/answers/38605
647. Sheikh Muhammad Saalih al-Munajjid, Is Plastic Surgery Haram? https://islamqa.info/en/answers/1006
648. Sheikh Muhammad Saalih al-Munajjid, Ruling on exfoliation of the face and face-lifts, https://islamqa.info/en/answers/83565
649. Mufti Muhammad ibn Adam, Is It Permissible to Get Botox Injections? https://daruliftaa.com/miscellaneous/is-it-permissible-to-get-botox-injections
650. Botox injections, https://www.mayoclinic.org/tests-procedures/botox/about/pac-20384658
651. Anne Barmettler, MD, Complications of Hyaluronic Acid Fillers, https://eyewiki.aao.org/Complications_of_Hyaluronic_Acid_Fillers
652. Martin Kassir MD, Mrinal Gupta MD, DNB, Hassan Galadari MD, Complications of botulinum toxin and fillers: A narrative review, https://onlinelibrary.wiley.com/doi/full/10.1111/jocd.13266
653. Face-Lift, https://www.mayoclinic.org/tests-procedures/face-lift/about/pac-20394059
654. Sheikh Muhammad Saalih al-Munajjid, When is it permissible to do a sex-change operation from male to female or vice versa? https://islamqa.info/en/answers/138451

655. Sheikh Muhammad Saalih al-Munajjid, Ruling on using eggs or sperm from someone other than the spouses in artificial insemination, https://islamqa.info/en/answers/21871
656. Sheikh Muhammad Saalih al-Munajjid, Ruling on donating eggs for artificial insemination, https://islamqa.info/en/answers/101970
657. Sheikh Muhammad Saalih al-Munajjid, Stem cells: definition, ruling on setting up stem cell banks and using them for medical purposes, https://islamqa.info/en/answers/108125
658. Sheikh Muhammad Saalih al-Munajjid, Renting wombs is haram, https://islamqa.info/en/answers/22126
659. Sheikh Muhammad Saalih al-Munajjid, Ruling on cloning of human beings, https://islamqa.info/en/answers/21582
660. Sheikh Muhammad Saalih al-Munajjid, Ruling on hypnotherapy, https://islamqa.info/en/answers/12631
661. Sheikh Muhammad Saalih al-Munajjid, Ruling on organ transplants. https://islamqa.info/en/answers/2117
662. Imam Abu Zakariya Yahya bin Sharaf An-Nawawi Ad-Dimashqi, Riyad as-Saliheen, Chapter 368: Prohibition of doing that which Allah and His Messenger have Prohibited
663. Imam Abu Zakariya Yahya bin Sharaf An-Nawawi Ad-Dimashqi, Riyad as-Saliheen, Chapter 77: Indignation against the Transgression of Divine Laws
664. Imam Abu Zakariya Yahya bin Sharaf An-Nawawi Ad-Dimashqi, Riyad as-Saliheen, Chapter 350: Undesirability of Intercession in Hudud
665. Imam Abu Zakariya Yahya bin Sharaf An-Nawawi Ad-Dimashqi, Riyad as-Saliheen, Chapter 372: Some of the Bounties which Allah has prepared for the Believers in Paradise
666. The Food, Drink and Clothing of the People of Hell, https://www.arabnews.com/news/488191
667. Ibn Al-Qayyim Al-Jawziyah, The Impact of Sins, https://islam2011.tumblr.com/post/35482404806
668. Imam Abu Zakariya Yahya bin Sharaf An-Nawawi Ad-Dimashqi, Riyad as-Saliheen, Chapter 2: Repentance
669. Sheikh Muhammad Saalih al-Munajjid, Expiation for Transgression Against Rights of Others, https://islamqa.info/en/answers/65649
670. Sheikh Muhammad Saalih al-Munajjid, Acceptance of repentance, https://islamqa.info/en/answers/46683
671. Sheikh Muhammad Saalih al-Munajjid, Expiation for Gossip, https://islamqa.info/en/answers/99554/expiation-for-gossip
672. Sheikh Muhammad Saalih al-Munajjid, Discussion of the hadeeth, "The one who repents from sin is like one who did not sin." https://islamqa.info/en/answers/182767
673. Imam Abu Zakariya Yahya bin Sharaf An-Nawawi Ad-Dimashqi, Riyad as-Saliheen, Chapter 371: Seeking Forgiveness
674. Sheikh Muhammad Saalih al-Munajjid, Offering the udhiyah with the intention of seeking healing, https://islamqa.info/en/answers/107549
675. Dr Noboru Mizushima, Autophagy: Renovation of Cells and Tissues, 2011. Cell 147(4): 728-741), https://www.sciencedirect.com/science/article/pii/S0092867411012761

www.ingramcontent.com/pod-product-compliance
Lightning Source LLC
Chambersburg PA
CBHW020717180526
45163CB00001B/1